Women's Primary Health Care

PROTOCOLS FOR PRACTICE

Women's Primary Health Care

PROTOCOLS FOR PRACTICE

Library of Congress Cataloging-in-Publication Data
Women's primary health care : protocols for practice / [edited by]
  Winifred L. Star, Lisa L. Lommel, Maureen T. Shannon.
        p.   cm.
     Includes bibliographical references and index.
     ISBN 1-55810-094-6
     1. Women's health services.   2. Primary health care.   3. Women-
—Health and hygiene.   I. Star, Winifred L.   II. Lommel, Lisa L.
III. Shannon, Maureen T.
     [DNLM: 1. Primary Health Care.   2. Women's Health.   WA 300 W87298
1995]
     RA564.85.W688   1993
     362.1′082—dc20
ISBN 1-55810-094-6

Published by American Nurses Publishing
600 Maryland Avenue, SW
Suite 100 West
Washington, DC 20024-2571

MS-20   7.5M   2/95

CONTENTS

DEDICATION

To Mom, whose lifetime love and generosity have been an enabler of all things good and great; and to Paul, whose music keeps my heart alive.
—WLS

To Michael, for his constant love and support, and to Liam and Tess for sharing their first years.
—LLL

To Matthew, Gregory, and Megan, for helping me keep life's priorities in order; and to Bob, for his patience, encouragement, and sense of humor.
—MTS

CONTRIBUTORS

*Editors and
Principal Authors*

Winifred L. Star, R.N., C., N.P., M.S.
Women's Health Nurse Practitioner
Coordinator, Young Mother's Clinic
Department of Obstetrics and Gynecology
Kaiser Permanente Medical Center
San Francisco, California

Assistant Clinical Professor
Department of Family Health Care Nursing
University of California, San Francisco
San Francisco, California

Lisa L. Lommel, R.N., C., F.N.P., M.P.H.
Associate Clinical Professor
Associate Director
Women's Primary Care Program
Department of Family Health Care Nursing
University of California, San Francisco
San Francisco, California

Director, Young Women's Clinic
Department of Obstetrics
University of California, San Francisco
San Francisco, California

Maureen T. Shannon, C.N.M., F.N.P., M.S.
Research Nurse Practitioner
Coordinator, Women's Services
Bay Area Perinatal AIDS Center
Department of Obstetrics, Gynecology, and Reproductive
  Immunology and Infectious Disease
San Francisco General Hospital
University of California, San Francisco
San Francisco, California

Contributing Authors

Susan Adams, R.N., N.P., M.S.
Women's Health Nurse Practitioner
Obstetrics Practice
Ambulatory Care Center
University of California, San Francisco
San Francisco, California

Assistant Clinical Professor
Department of Family Health Care Nursing
University of California, San Francisco
San Francisco, California

Toni Ayres, Ed.D., R.N., M.F.C.C.
Lecturer
Department of Counseling
San Francisco State University
San Francisco, California

Lecturer
Departments of Holistic Health Education
    and Transpersonal Counseling
John F. Kennedy University
Orinda, California

Marriage, Family, and Child Counselor
(Private practice)
Berkeley, California

Wendy L. Berk, C.A.N.P.
Headache/Facial Pain Clinic
Internal Medicine Clinic
Kaiser Permanente Medical Center
Hayward, California

Pilar Bernal de Pheils, R.N., M.S., F.N.P.
Assistant Clinical Professor
Women's Primary Care Program
Department of Family Health Care Nursing
University of California, San Francisco
San Francisco, California

Jeanette M. Broering, R.N., M.S., C.P.N.P.
Associate Clinical Professor
Departments of Family Health Care Nursing
    and Pediatrics
Division of Adolescent Medicine
University of California, San Francisco
San Francisco, California
(During the preparation of this work the author was supported in
part by a grant from the California Bureau of Maternal and Child
Health and Resources Development [MCJ 000978A]).

Barbara J. Burgel, R.N., M.S., A.N.P., C.O.H.N.
Associate Clinical Professor
Occupational Health Nursing Program
Department of Mental Health, Community, and
    Administrative Nursing
University of California, San Francisco
San Francisco, California

Carole Deitrich, R.N., C., M.S., G.N.P.
Associate Clinical Professor
Director, Gerontological Nurse Practitioner Program
Department of Physiological Nursing
University of California, San Francisco
San Francisco, California

Director, Health Corner, A Nurse-Managed Health
    Center
Menorah Park Senior Health Center
San Francisco, California

Rozane Moon Gee, R.D., M.S.
Clinical Nutritionist
Assistant Clinical Professor
Department of Family Health Care Nursing
University of California, San Francisco
San Francisco, California

Lynn N. Hanson, N.P., M.S.
Women's Health Nurse Practitioner
Gynecology Practice
Ambulatory Care Center
University of California, San Francisco
San Francisco, California

Assistant Clinical Professor
Department of Family Health Care Nursing
University of California, San Francisco
San Francisco, California

Marty Jessup, R.N., M.S.
Associate Clinical Professor
Department of Family Health Care Nursing
University of California, San Francisco
San Francisco, California

Catherine M. Kelber, R.N., C., M.S., A.N.P.
Assistant Clinical Professor
Adult and Occupational Health Nurse Practitioner
    Programs
Department of Mental Health, Community, and
    Administrative Nursing
University of California, San Francisco
San Francisco, California

Michelle M. Marin, R.N., M.S., A.N.P.
General Medicine Practice
Ambulatory Care Center
University of California, San Francisco
San Francisco, California

Carolyn Muir, R.N., C., N.P., M.S.
Women's Health Nurse Practitioner
Obstetrics Practice
Ambulatory Care Center
University of California, San Francisco
San Francisco, California

Assistant Clinical Professor
Department of Family Health Care Nursing
University of California, San Francisco
San Francisco, California

Joan R. Murphy, R.N., C., M.S., N.P., C.N.S.
Women's Health Nurse Practitioner
Perinatal Clinical Specialist
Department of Obstetrics and Gynecology
Kaiser Permanente Medical Center
San Francisco, California

Sandra L. Norman, R.N., N.P., M.S.
Women's Health Nurse Practitioner
Department of Obstetrics and Gynecology and
    Department of Urology
Kaiser Permanente Medical Center
Walnut Creek and Park Shadelands Facilities
Walnut Creek, California

Elisabeth O. O'Mara, R.N., M.S., A.N.P., C.D.E.
Department of Internal Medicine
Kaiser Permanente Medical Center
Walnut Creek, California

Assistant Clinical Professor
Adult Health Nurse Practitioner Program
Department of Mental Health, Community, and
    Administrative Nursing
University of California, San Francisco
San Francisco, California

Diane C. Putney, R.N., C., M.N., N.P.
Orthopedic Nurse Practitioner
Orthopedic Department
Kaiser Permanente Medical Center
South San Francisco, California

Jan Reddick, M.S., F.N.P.
Family Nurse Practitioner
Lyon-Martin Women's Health Services
San Francisco, California

Julie Richards, R.N., C., M.S., M.S.N.
Assistant Clinical Professor
Women's Primary Care Program
Department of Family Health Care Nursing
University of California, San Francisco
San Francisco, California

JoAnne M. Saxe, R.N., A.N.P., C.S.
Associate Clinical Professor
Adult and Occupational Health Nurse Practitioner
    Programs
Department of Mental Health, Community, and
    Administrative Nursing
University of California, San Francisco
San Francisco, California

Ellen Scarr, M.S.N., F.N.P.
Screening and Acute Care Clinic
Ambulatory Care Center
University of California, San Francisco
San Francisco, California

Kellie Sheehan, R.N., C., M.S.N., F.N.P.
General Medicine Practice
Ambulatory Care Center
University of California, San Francisco
San Francisco, California

Diana Taylor, Ph.D., R.N., F.A.A.N.
Associate Professor
Director, Women's Primary Care Program
Department of Family Health Care Nursing
University of California, San Francisco
San Francisco, California

Jacqueline W. Wasserman, R.N., C., M.S., F.N.P.
San Francisco Public Health Department
Chinatown, Visitacion Valley, and Tenderloin
    Neighborhoods
San Francisco, California

Lori M. Weseman, R.N., M.S., N.P.
Women's Health Nurse Practitioner
Del Mar, California

Medical Editors

Susan Bertolli, M.D.
Staff Physician
Department of Obstetrics and Gynecology
Kaiser Permanente Medical Center
San Francisco, California

Ellen Hughes, M.D., Ph.D.
Assistant Clinical Professor of Medicine
University of California, San Francisco
San Francisco, California

DISCLAIMER

The American Nurses Foundation, as publisher of *Women's Primary Health Care: Protocols for Practice,* wishes the readers of this publication to understand that the American Nurses Foundation does not hold itself out as a provider of medical advice. Clinicians must consult the *Physicians' Desk Reference,* drug package inserts, and/or a clinical pharmacist for information concerning drug therapy. Clinicians remain fully responsible for the outcome of the general evaluation and treatment/management of the clinicians' patients to whom any protocols in this publication are applied, including instances in which specific drug therapy has been delineated in this publication.

The authors of this publication disavow any responsibility for the outcomes of the patients to whom any protocols in this publication are applied. It is the individual practicing clinician who shall remain fully responsible for the outcome of the evaluation and treatment/management of the patients to whom any protocols in this publication are applied, including instances in which specific drug therapy has been delineated herein. Clinicians should consult the *Physicians' Desk Reference,* drug package inserts, and/or a clinical pharmacist for information concerning drug therapy.

PREFACE

Women's Primary Health Care: Protocols for Practice was written collaboratively by advanced-practice nurse (APN) clinicians, clinical nursing faculty, and a registered dietitian. It is intended primarily for nurse practitioners (NPs) working in primary care or specialty care settings. Nurse-midwives, physicians' assistants, and resident physicians may also find this book quite useful. The popularity of this publication's already released "sister book," *Ambulatory Obstetrics: Protocols for Nurse Practitioners/Nurse-Midwives* (Star et al. 1990),* necessitated a more comprehensive volume concerning women's primary health care.

The practice of women's primary care by NPs is legally sanctioned by standardized procedures and protocols as defined by individual states' nurse practice acts. These acts vary from state to state as do standards of care in the community.

In many health care settings the NP has primary responsibility for formulating and maintaining practice protocols. This book provides guidelines and a framework from which to develop standards that meet the needs of individual practice settings. As times and technologies change, so will the protocols which guide practice. Thus, a regular protocol review process at the workplace is necessary to reflect these changes and the ever-growing practice of nursing.

The book is divided into several unique parts. The first section presents an overview of primary care and women's primary health care, followed by a review of standards of practice and medicolegal issues, and, finally, a discussion of health care of women across the life span. In the main body of the book are disease-specific protocols, each following a "S-O-A-P" ("Subjective-Objective-Assessment-Plan") format for quick referencing. Lastly, a general nutrition section complements information contained in specific protocols. For more in-depth information on selected conditions the reader is directed to the "Bibliography" or each section of protocol or a current textbook.

---

*Star, W.L., Shannon, M.T., Sammons, L.N., Lommel, L.L., Gutierrez, Y., 1990. *Ambulatory obstetrics: Protocols for nurse practitioners/nurse-midwives*, 2nd ed. San Francisco: University of California, San Francisco.

It is our hope that this publication will provide a guide for the process of protocol development as well as contribute to the practice bases of our readers. The authors welcome comments and suggestions. Address all correspondence to: Publications Editor, the American Nurses Association, 600 Maryland Avenue SW, Suite 100 West, Washington, DC   20024-2571.

ACKNOWLEDGMENTS

The publication of *Women's Primary Health Care: Protocols for Practice* was facilitated by the work and support of a number of people. The editors offer thanks to the medical editors of the book, Susan Bertolli, M.D., and Ellen Hughes, M.D., Ph.D.

A special thank you goes to Roxanne Stiles-Donnelly, research assistant, for her good-natured support and the numerous hours spent in the library assembling a multitude of journal articles. Thanks also to Seth Feigenbaum, M.D., for his contributions to the **Hirsutism** and **Infertility** protocols, and to Darlene Peck, N.P., for her contributions to the **Perimenopausal Symptoms and Hormone Therapy** protocol.

The contributing authors thank a number of people for their support and assistance. Wendy Berk would like to acknowledge Wayne Barger, M.D., F.A.C.S.; Allan Bernstein, M.D.; Gregory Hong, D.D.S.; and Felice O'Ryan, D.D.S., for their contributions to the **Face Pain**, **Bell's Palsy**, and **Temporomandibular Disorder** protocols. Sandra Norman would like to acknowledge Hernan C. Alvarado, M.D., for his contributions to the **Urinary Tract Disorders** Protocols. Pilar Bernal de Pheils thanks Caren Cascio for her assistance in reviewing the **Anxiety Disorders, Depression**, and **Eating Disorders** procotols. Toni Ayres wishes to thank Susan Burnett, N.P., for her clinical insight, experience, and helpful suggestions in reading several drafts of the **Sexual Dysfunction** Protocol. Rozane Gee would like to thank Roger Gee for his assistance in the preparation of the **General Nutrition Guidelines** chapter.

And, finally, we thank Beth Gyorgy, Publications Editor at American Nurses Publishing, and the typesetters who assisted her in the preparation of the manuscript and the book's final production.

SECTION 1
Lisa L. Lommel, R.N., C., F.N.P., M.P.H.

Women's Primary Health Care

In the United States, the history of the concept of primary care can be traced back to an early attempt in the 1940s to conceptualize health care delivery (McGivern 1986).

Primary Care

Early definitions of primary care were associated with medical practice where direct patient-care services for illness management were provided.

By the 1960s, this definition was expanded to include the ambulatory client, using a family-centered and interdisciplinary approach to care. At this point, the concept of primary care became the impetus for the development of special medical programs for the education of "primary care" practitioners. Along with the expansion of primary care in medical practice, the role of the nurse practitioner (NP) in such care was introduced. The NP role was a natural one because nursing had traditionally combined the concepts of collaboration and comprehensive care with an orientation toward psychosocial and physical well-being (McGivern, Mezey, and Glynn 1990).

In the 1970s, the concept of primary care grew even broader to include first-contact care, contact with longitudinal responsibility, and integration of all aspects of care. Simultaneously, health—as opposed to disease and illness—began to be emphasized. Aspects of health included health promotion, health maintenance, self-care, and health teaching (McGivern 1986).

The definitions of primary care and NP practice had merged by the 1980s. Primary care was inherent in the development of the NP role (Fagin 1976). As the scope of primary care widened, so did the role of the NP.

Today, primary care focuses on organizing care for the individual and his or her family over time. The contemporary definition involves the concept of *primary health care*, of which primary care is a component. Primary health care consists of primary care services as well as other systems of care:

→ *disease prevention* (primary, secondary, tertiary);
→ *health promotion* (maintenance and enhancement of health);
→ *care coordination* (outreach, advocacy, referral, service coordination);
→ *community health development* (consumer involvement, public health functions); and,
→ *managed care* (cost containment, outcome evaluation) (Taylor 1993).

Primary health care services are provided to clients as individuals, families, and groups within specific communities, cultures, and environments.

Within the primary health care model, the NP provides specific primary care services including assessment, diagnosis, treatment, referral, and follow-up, along with prevention, health promotion, and case management for acute and chronic physical and mental health problems that adversely affect health. It is within the primary health care model that health providers can respond to society's demand for accountable, accessible, and affordable health care. Primary health care ensures optimal and individualized care.

Women's Health

Approximately 52 percent of the population of the United States is female and the majority of health-care services consumers are women. Traditionally, health care for women has been defined by their reproductive status. A more comprehensive and individualized definition of women's health includes primary health care services and: 1) women's health experiences across the life span, 2) women's health in relation to environment, and, 3) the process of attaining, maintaining, and regarding health as women experience it (Woods 1988).

This expanded definition of women's health attempts to include major health risks that have not been included by traditional medical services. It is these health risks that result in significant morbidity and mortality among women. The lack of health norms for these risks means health professionals often do not adequately understand or address the needs of women who deviate from them (Oiler 1982). It is therefore critically important that the women's health care provider define these norms in order to respond appropriately.

Following are examples of how the expanded definition of women's health can be used in practice:

Primary Health Care

→ Primary care to include services for eating disorders and effects of violence and physical or sexual abuse.
→ Disease prevention to include smoking, alcohol, and drug cessation activities.
→ Health promotion to include nutrition, safer sex, and stress management activities.
→ Care coordination to include development of culturally sensitive primary care for new immigrants or refugees.
→ Community health development to include organizing a neighborhood community advisory group on health.
→ Managed care to include the evaluation of cost containment, access, and early disease identification components of disease prevention programs.

Women's Health Experience across the Life Span

→ Tailoring care to women's biological/social/behavioral experience (i.e., women at adolescence, reproductive age, midlife, and older women).

Women's Health Experience

→ Women's definition of health and illness as it relates to their interactions with their social, physical, community, political, and cultural environments.

In providing an expanded scope of women's health care services, the health care provider must recognize how health risks and concerns affect certain subgroups of women—i.e., women of color, women living in poverty, substance abusers, lesbians, and immigrants. It is within the context of individual experience that health care should be assessed and managed. In these contexts, the value of the health norm should be evaluated and individualized. The focus of change may be on the environment as opposed to the individual—e.g., an emphasis on social support networks, time and role management, or stress in the workplace.

Expanding the definition of women's health to include primary health care is critical to meeting the needs of women. By understanding primary care and women's health, the health care provider will be better able to provide optimal and appropriate care to this population. While it is impossible to include all the criteria for primary health care for every condition and every woman, the authors of this book hope to have started the process by providing selected aspects and conditions of women's health.

Bibliography

Fagin, C. 1976. Nature and scope of nursing practice in meeting primary care needs. In *Primary care by nurses: Sphere of responsibility and accountability*. Kansas City, MO: American Nurses Association.

McGivern, D.O. 1986. The evolution of primary care nursing. In *Nurses, nurse practitioners: The evolution of primary care*, eds. M. D. Mezey and D. O. McGivern. Boston: Little, Brown & Co.

McGivern, D. O., Mezey, M. D., and Glynn, P. M. 1990. Evolution of primary care roles. *Nurse Practitioner Forum* 1(3): 163–168.

Oiler, C. 1992. The phenomenological approach in nursing research. *Nursing Research* 31(3): 178–181.

Taylor, D. 1993. Primary care and primary health care in the United States. *Primary care medicine, principles and practice*. San Francisco: University of California, San Francisco.

Woods, N. F. 1988. Women's health. In *Annual review of nursing research*, eds. J. J. Fitzpatrick, R. L. Tauton, and J. Q. Benoliel, vol. 6. New York: Springer.

SECTION 1
Winifred L. Star, R.N., C., N.P., M.S.

Scope of Practice and Medicolegal Issues

The boundaries of nursing practice are delineated in statutes passed by the legislatures in individual states (Hogue 1989).

Standardized Procedures

These nursing practice acts, designed to safeguard the public interest, legally sanction the practice of nursing. In some states, there is legislative intent to realize the existence of overlapping functions between nurses and physicians, implemented via the development of standardized procedures and protocols. Through these procedures and protocols nurses are within legal bounds to amplify their practices into areas originally considered within the realm of medicine (California Nurses Association 1989). In other words, written protocols provide the means for expanding the practice of nursing beyond what is commonly perceived as traditional to the role (Kauffroath 1990).

Nurse practitioners (NPs) should be knowledgeable regarding their respective nursing practice acts and guidelines for development of standardized procedures, copies of which may be obtained from their state's board of registered nursing (BRN). California requires that standardized procedures be developed through collaborative efforts among administrators, physicians, and nurses, and that these procedures must specify the scope of supervision required for their performance (e.g., physician supervision). Standardized procedures are not subject to prior approval by the BRN or board of medical quality assurance (BMQA). However, they must be developed according to guidelines jointly promulgated by these boards (California Board of Registered Nursing 1987).

In California, standardized procedures have two components: 1) the policy component—i.e., the general intent to allow registered nurses to perform a specific clinical function or service in a particular setting; and, 2) the protocols—i.e., the rules or procedures to be followed in performing the clinical function or service authorized by the policy (CNA 1989, 22).

There are two types of protocols—*disease-specific* or *procedure-specific protocols* and *process protocols*. Disease-specific/procedure-specific protocols delineate steps for the treatment and management of a specific disease or carrying out a specific procedure. Process protocols are function-based and describe the steps to be taken in performing a given function, such as evaluation of chronic illness. Process protocols specify requirements for care but do not mandate medical content (CNA 1989).

The protocols contained in *Women's Primary Health Care: Protocols for Practice* represent disease-specific protocols. They are intended as guidelines for practice and should be adapted for use in different practice settings based on limitations and variations unique to the institution or type of practice and the needs/resources of the patient. In addition, these protocols should not be considered as *the* standard of care; everyday practice has no one standard of care for every situation encountered (Gillstrap 1992). Rather, the protocols herein should be viewed with the same intent as the American College of Obstetricians and Gynecologists (ACOG) regards its "Technical Bulletins":

"[These protocols do] not define a standard of care, nor [are they] intended to dictate an exclusive course of management. [They present] recognized methods and techniques of clinical practice for consideration by [primary care providers] for incorporation into their practices . . ." (ACOG *Technical Bulletin* 201, 1995, 6).

Prescriptive Authority and Reimbursement

Individual states' laws concerning the furnishing of drugs and devices must be adhered to for nursing practice to be within legal bounds. Forty-eight states and the District of Columbia grant advanced practice nurses (APNs) some form of prescriptive authority; however there is wide disparity in the degree of prescriptive autonomy and no national consensus or policy on the issue (Mahoney 1992; Pearson 1995, 16). Ten states have specific plans to seek independent prescriptive authority for APNs in the upcoming year (Pearson 1995, 13, 16).

With regard to reimbursement, all states except Ohio (and the District of Columbia), directly reimburse APNs for Medicaid clients; however, of the 49 states, 37 have specified that NPs are paid 80 percent to 100 percent of the amount paid a physician billing for the same service (Pearson 1995, 16). Thirty-five states now allow third-party reimbursement for APNs; some of these states, however, within narrowly specified situations only (Pearson 1995, 16).

Restrictive barriers to nursing practice must be removed. For advanced practice nursing to fulfill its mission to provide primary health care to all individuals, legislative reforms are needed nationwide. Lobbying by APNs is critical to changing laws governing prescriptive authority and third-party reimbursement.

Malpractice and Professional Liability Insurance

All health care providers are affected by the medical malpractice crisis in this country. With the expansion of the role of the APN comes increased responsibility and liability. Despite surveys which show there have been few malpractice cases against NPs, nurses today are being held personally accountable for their actions and malpractice claims against nurses are increasing (Feutz-Harter 1989; Nettles-Carlson and Wolfe 1988).

Though medicolegal issues of health care are not routinely taught in nursing schools, nurses are responsible for knowing the law and how to comply with it (Feutz-Harter 1989). Ignorance is not defensible in a malpractice action!

Lawsuits occur when legal limits of practice allegedly have been breached and may occur despite legitimate practice. It is reported that of all medical malpractice claims filed, less than 50 percent result in any type of payment; less than 10 percent proceed to trial; and, of those that do, around 80 percent result in verdicts for the defendant (Feutz-Harter 1989).

Legal liability for malpractice means an individual is accountable for acts of negligence which he or she committed. However, liability can expand to include that individual's site manager, supervisory person, or employer (Feutz-Harter 1989). Areas of practice of particular importance with respect to liability include: charting and documentation, informed consent and treatment decisions, and confidentiality and privacy issues. APNs must be aware of the implications of all these areas.

The level of conduct for which a nurse is held accountable is referred to as the *standard of care* (Feutz-Harter 1989, 15). As discussed previously, standards of care should be flexible and individualized according to the particular situation. NPs must keep abreast of advances in health care as they apply to clinical practice, both regionally and nationally. Competency mandates a continual process of updating knowledge and skills (Feutz-Harter 1989).

Unfortunately, protocols of care or practice standards can be used against the health care provider in a lawsuit. Failure to comply precisely with the written standard may constitute a breach of conduct and thus increase liability. Moniz (1992) suggests that to minimize malpractice risk, protocols should be realistic, represent the minimum requirements for safe care instead of the maximum for ideal care, and should be updated regularly as knowledge develops. Once adopted, Moniz warns, protocols must be *followed*: deviation can have legal implications.

Professional liability insurance offers protection for nurses in the event of patient harm, when the acceptable standard of care allegedly has been breached (Feutz-Harter 1989). Nurses must be knowledgeable about which professional services are covered under their professional liability insurance policy. In securing an individual policy, the nurse should consider his or her security needs; advanced practice and professional activities in and outside the work site; personal assets; amount of coverage provided by the employer; and the individual's area of nursing practice, its potential for lawsuits, and the amount of past awards (Feutz-Harter 1989).

There are many misconceptions regarding the extent to which a nurse is afforded protection under the employer's liability insurance policy. Coverage is provided for actions performed within the scope of employment and the job description. In the event of a malpractice suit, the employer may, however, seek compensation for damages awarded against the institution for acts of commission or omission by the nurse (Feutz-Harter 1989). According to Feutz-Harter (1989), this "going after" the nurse occurs rarely (if at all), as it sets up too adversarial a relationship between nurse and employer.

Actions performed outside the scope of employment may also result in malpractice claims and the "Good Samaritan" law cannot be relied upon to provide absolute immunity. Even the offering of well-intentioned advice may expose a nurse to malpractice action.

For additional information on legal issues in nursing, please refer to *Nursing and the Law*, by Sheryl Feutz-Harter, listed in the bibliography.

Bibliography

American College of Obstetricians and Gynecologists. January 1995. *Technical Bulletin* 201. Washington, DC: the Author.

California Board of Registered Nursing. 1987. *An explanation of the scope of RN practice including standardized procedures.* Sacramento: the Author.

California Nurses Association. 1989. *Nursing practice in California: Rights, responsibilities, and regulations.* San Francisco: the Author.

Feutz-Harter, S. 1989. *Nursing and the law.* Eau Claire, WI: Professional Education Systems, Inc.

Gillstrap, L. C. III. July 1992. *Legal issues in obstetrics.* Lecture presented at the Tenth National Kaiser Permanente Obstetrics and Gynecology Conference, Kamuela, Hawaii.

Hogue, E. 1989. The importance of supporting nursing colleagues on scope of practice issues. *Pediatric Nursing* 15(1): 82–83.

Kauffroath, K. A. 1990. *California statutes affecting nursing practice.* Eau Claire, WI: Professional Education Systems, Inc.

Mahoney, D. F. 1992. Nurse practitioners as prescribers: Past research trends and future study needs. *Nurse Practitioner* 17(1): 44–51.

Moniz, D. M. 1992. The danger of written protocols and standards of practice. *Nurse Practitioner* 17(9): 58–60.

Nettles-Carlson, B., and Wolfe, J. 1988. Survey shows few malpractice claims against NPs. *Tar Heel Nurse* 50(1): 1–11.

Pearson, L. J. 1993. 1992–93 update: How each state stands on legislative issues affecting advanced nursing practice. *Nurse Practitioner* 18(1): 23–38.

———. 1994. Annual update: How each state stands on legislative issues affecting advanced nursing practice. *Nurse Practitioner* 19(1): 11–53.

———. 1995. Annual update: How each state stands on legislative issues affecting advanced nursing practice. *Nurse Practitioner* 20(1):13–51.

SECTION 1

Maureen T. Shannon, C.N.M., F.N.P., M.S.
Jeanette M. Broering, R.N., M.S., C.P.N.P.
Carole Deitrich, R.N., C., M.S., G.N.P.
Diana Taylor, Ph.D., R.N., F.A.A.N.

Women's Health across the Life Span: An Overview

Introduction

The purpose of this section of *Women's Primary Health Care: Protocols for Practice* is to present strategies for screening and illness prevention based on the age of a woman. It is designed to help practitioners incorporate health maintenance and illness prevention concepts into clinical practice. These strategies will eventually change as a result of the development of better methods to improve health within our society.

Overview of Women's Health Care Issues
Maureen T. Shannon, C.N.M., F.N.P., M.S.

As the concept of primary care underwent significant changes during the past two decades, it became evident that health care for women needed to change as well. Aside from reproductive health care, the majority of health care recommendations for women are based on studies done primarily on male research subjects. Furthermore, much of medical education and research has demonstrated a gender bias regarding health maintenance, disease prevention, and treatment of conditions for women (National Institutes of Health [NIH] 1992).

In response to this discrepancy in health care and research, NIH established the Office of Research on Women's Health (ORWH) in 1990. ORWH was established to promote women's health and to ensure that clinical research trials supported by NIH include an adequate number of women cohorts so that results extrapolated from studies would be applicable to both sexes.

During its first year of existence, ORWH convened a public hearing and a workshop to develop a research agenda on women's health. Data analyzed by ORWH during these meetings revealed the following facts about women's health in the United States (NIH 1992, 7):

→ "Women will constitute the larger population and will be the most *susceptible* to disease in the future.
→ "Overall, women have *worse* health than men.
→ "Certain health problems are more *prevalent* in women than in men.
→ "Certain health problems are *unique* to women or affect women *differently* than they do men."

Although these findings apply to all women, ethnic and racial differences among women do appear to have an effect on morbidity and mortality rates associated with various diseases (NIH 1992).

Women generally live longer than men but face greater morbidity during their lifetimes. Except for injuries, categories of self-reported chronic illnesses and acute conditions are more common for women than men (Wingard 1984). Several chronic diseases have a higher reported incidence in women. These include obesity, diabetes, anemia, respiratory diseases, autoimmune diseases, gastrointestinal problems, osteoporosis, and Alzheimer's disease (NIH 1992; Strickland 1988).

Reproductive-age women report or seek care for acute conditions and short-term disabilities more frequently than men; and more women than men report and seek care for chronic conditions and associated disabilities during mid- to late life (NIH 1992).

Certain health problems affect women exclusively or differently than they do men. The morbidity and mortality associated with complications of pregnancy (e.g., ectopic pregnancies, gestational diabetes, pregnancy-induced hypertension) and reproductive system cancers (e.g., ovarian, cervical, uterine) are particular to women. Breast cancer, although occurring rarely in men, is a leading cause of death of women. The incidence of this disease has increased from one in 20 women in the 1960s to one in nine women today (NIH 1992).

Each year, six million women acquire a sexually transmitted disease (STD), with 50 percent of these women between the ages of 13 years and 19 years (NIH 1992). STD-associated morbidity (e.g., infertility, ectopic pregnancy, chronic herpes simplex virus [HSV] infection, human papillomavirus [HPV] infection, human immunodeficiency virus [HIV] infection) and mortality will also increase as a result of these infections.

Behavioral factors contribute directly and indirectly to both health promotion and the development of disease. Of particular concern is the increased and sustained incidence of cigarette smoking among women compared to men. During the years between 1935 and 1965, the rate of smoking by women increased from 18 percent to 34 percent. Currently, 29 percent of adolescent girls report smoking (NIH 1992). As a result, an increased incidence of adverse health consequences associated with smoking is reported among women smokers and includes lung and other types of cancer, heart disease, respiratory diseases, hypertension, osteoporosis, increased pregnancy complications (e.g., pre-term births), and increased perinatal and neonatal morbidity and mortality (e.g, low birth-weight infants) (NIH 1992).

Behavioral factors associated with the development of adverse health conditions in women include high dietary fat consumption (which may contribute to heart disease and cancers), delay in accessing medical or prenatal care; use of oral contraceptives in women over the age of 35 years who smoke (which places them at an increased risk for cardiovascular disease), and unprotected sexual activity in women at risk for STDs.

Psychosocial issues faced by women are also different from those faced by men. Role expectations, role burdens (e.g., traditionally the care giver), and abilities to cope with and adapt to stressful situations have a direct impact on a woman's health (Woods 1988). Imbalances in role relationships (e.g., power, control) can also affect women's health adversely. For example, women are at greater risk of physical and sexual assault than are men (Council on Scientific Affairs, American Medical Association [AMA]

1992), and are more likely to be subjected to sexual harassment and sexual discrimination. It has been estimated that during a one-year period, two million women are assaulted by their male partners (Council on Scientific Affairs, AMA 1992).

The psychological stressors women face often require therapeutic interventions. Data indicate that approximately three percent of women in midlife have a major depressive episode while seven percent have experienced an affective disorder of some type (NIH 1992). However, some studies indicate that the diagnosis of psychological problems in women is often the result of gender bias on the part of the clinician, a bias resulting from a lack of knowledge about women's health care. Such a perspective is cited as being the reason physicians more frequently prescribe psychotropic medications for women compared to men (Bernstein and Kane 1981).

Socioeconomic status, ethnicity, and age play significant roles in women's access to health and health services. Recent data show that diabetes is two to three times more common in African American, Hispanic, and Native American women compared to white women. African American women experience the highest rate of coronary heart disease of all ethnic groups—three times higher than white women. While breast cancer has a reportedly higher incidence in white women, African American women have a higher mortality rate associated with breast cancer (National Center for Health Statistics 1992; NIH 1992). Lung and colon cancer rates are higher for African American women than white women. Disability—the inability to carry on one or more major activities of daily life—is higher among African American women compared to white women (U.S. Department of Commerce 1991).

As a group, women are economically disadvantaged compared to men, regardless of age, race, ethnicity, education, or employment status. Although women provide a substantial contribution to the labor force, they consistently receive less pay than men for similar jobs (U.S. Department of Commerce 1991). Most low-income women of all races perceive that their health is poor, with 75 percent of poor minority women and 60 percent of poor white women reporting poor health (National Center for Health Statistics 1992; NIH 1992).

African American, Hispanic, and Native American women—particularly those who are single and heads of households—have long had high rates of poverty. They are now being joined by white, middle-class women rearing children alone and older women subsisting on small fixed incomes. Almost 78 percent of the poor in the United States are women and children (U.S. Department of Commerce 1991). In 1988, 54 percent of all households with children and headed by a female had an income below the poverty level (U.S. Department of Commerce 1991). Twenty-eight percent of families maintained by white women are below the poverty level, compared to 56 percent of those maintained by African American women (U.S. Department of Commerce 1991).

The financial constraints women face are compounded by the lack of affordable medical insurance available to individuals today. In 1988, 31 million Americans had no health insurance coverage. From 1985 to 1987, a total of 36 million Americans had no insurance for a substantial period of time (U.S. Department of Commerce 1991). And insurance companies use data demonstrating sex differentials in longevity to reduce women's benefits on the grounds that women live longer than men (Ramey 1982). Because women are the major recipients of Medicare/Medicaid they are vulnerable to changes in health and social services provided by the federal government.

Improvements in women's health status are no longer likely to come solely from technological breakthroughs. Instead, they must incorporate environmental and social changes, behavioral (i.e., lifestyle) changes, and allow individuals to participate directly in their own health promotion/disease prevention.

Reform at the level of health delivery systems is critical to improving women's health. The present system of health care for women often results in overlapping services for women (e.g., obstetrical care, gynecological care) with duplication of some services (e.g., Pap smears) and lack of attention to issues that can have major health consequences (e.g., substance abuse, eating disorders, domestic violence) (Clancy and Massion 1992).

A plan for health care reform that targets the unique aspects of women's health has been recommended by national nursing organizations. This plan shifts the focus of health care from sophisticated technological interventions and institutional care to community-based primary health care services (Joel 1992). While the structure of the plan will be the same for both men and women, the focus of primary care, prevention, and health promotion will include recommendations specific to women's health care needs. Furthermore, attending to the personal health of women is not possible without altering the environmental factors that affect health and illness (e.g., improved access to primary health care, adequate child-care facilities, reduction of violent behavior, and reproductive options).

Adolescent Health Care Issues (Women 13 Years to 19 Years of Age)
Jeanette M. Broering, R.N., M.S., C.P.N.P.

In the 1990s, demographic trends for adolescents reveal changes in population and racial composition (Brindis, Irwin, and Millstein 1992). It is estimated that although the absolute number of adolescents will increase, the relative proportion of adolescents in the population will decline slightly from 14.8 percent to 14.3 percent. By the year 2000, the age composition of this population will shift, with an increase among the youngest adolescents (10-year- to 15-year-olds) and decrease among the oldest adolescents (15-year- to 19-year-olds).

Racial and ethnic minority shifts are also occurring. By 2000, 31.2 percent of adolescents will represent a racial or ethnic group compared to 25.6 percent among the general population. The most rapid growth will occur among Hispanic youth (41 percent increase), with an increase in the number of Asian American youth also anticipated. However, African Americans will continue to comprise the largest group of minority youth.

Although adolescence is thought to be a time of optimal wellness and developmental and physical growth, morbidity and mortality do occur. Cause-specific mortality by age is attributable to behavioral etiologies which include unintentional injuries such as motor vehicle accidents (MVAs) and intentional injuries such as homicide or suicide (Gans and Blyth 1990). Likewise, the majority of morbidity during adolescence results from risk behaviors with outcomes such as unintentional pregnancy, STDs, substance abuse, injuries, and mental health problems. Some of these behaviors occur together—e.g., alcohol consumption has been highly correlated with adverse outcomes such as MVAs, suicides, and homicides; poor contraceptive and safer-sex practices can result in pregnancy and STDs. Clinicians need to be mindful of the clustering of these behaviors and during interviews of adolescents ask appropriate questions regarding their social behaviors.

Health risks associated with the early onset of sexual activity have a significant effect on adolescents, and can generate long-term health and social problems. The percentage of sexually experienced teenage females increased from 47 percent in 1982 to 55 percent in 1990. The percentage of sexually active teenage females increases as age increases. In 1990, 41 percent of 15-year- to 17-year-olds were sexually experienced compared with 74 percent of 18-year- to 19-year-olds.

As a result, STDs are the most common and potentially destructive infectious diseases occurring among adolescents. It is estimated that 33 percent to 50 percent of all STD cases reported annually will occur in adolescents (Chacko and Taber 1993; Irwin and Shafer 1992; NIH 1992). In adolescent females, negative sequelae associated with STDs include pelvic inflammatory disease (PID) with resultant tubal scarring, ectopic pregnancy, infertility, chronic pelvic pain, exposure to viruses with oncogenic potential (e.g., HPV), and HIV infection.

In 1988, there were 1,033,730 adolescent pregnancies, and, of these, 28,000 involved girls younger than 15 years of age. Pregnancy outcomes included 488,941 live births, 406,370 induced abortions, and an estimated 138,420 miscarriages and stillbirths (U.S. Department of Health and Human Services [HHS] 1993). The majority of these pregnancies are reported to be unintentional.

Furthermore, adolescents are less likely to receive early prenatal care, thus increasing the possibility of adverse maternal and fetal outcomes. Factors that increase the risk a mother will not seek out prenatal care include her being less than 18 years of age, unmarried, with low educational attainment, and a member of a minority group (HHS 1993).

Confidentiality is a major concern of adolescents when they are seeking medical services. One survey of middle-class suburban adolescents reported that if parental knowledge were required, only 45 percent would seek care for severe depression, 19 percent for contraception, 15 percent for STDs, and 17 percent for drug abuse. If assured that medical care would be confidential, an additional 12 percent would seek care for depression, 45 percent for contraception, 50 percent for STDs, and 49 percent would seek care for drug abuse (Marks et al. 1983).

The provisions of the law regarding minors' consent for health care are not always clear. For the practicing clinician, the interpretation and implementation of existing law concerning the reproductive health care of adolescent females can be confusing, particularly since the age of majority varies from ages 18 years to 21 years according to individual states' laws (Gans 1993). Generally, when obtaining consent for routine medical or surgical procedures for an adolescent, it is advisable for the clinician to obtain written consent from both the adolescent and his or her parent or guardian.

There are situations in which a minor can give consent for her own care. Legally emancipated minors can give consent for all forms of health care and their parents do not share fiduciary responsibility for the cost of care. The three categories of emancipated minors include: married minors, minors serving in the armed forces, and those emancipated through court declaration (English 1988). Conditions for which minors may give consent independently include prescription and non-prescription contraceptive devices, pregnancy diagnosis, prenatal and postpartum care, testing for contagious diseases such as STDs and HIV, rape and sexual assault, and, to a limited extent, drug, alcohol, and outpatient mental health counseling. State guidelines regarding an unemancipated, unmarried minor's right to seek medical care, abortion, and other important health care services are available for the practicing clinician (Gans 1993).

Another legal issue pertaining to adolescents is the responsibility for payment, which may constitute a significant barrier to accessing medical services. Adolescents who are 18 years old or emancipated minors are financially responsible for their own care. Federally funded programs such as Title X of the Family Planning Act provide reproductive health services for adolescents in addition to other state-based programs such as Medicaid.

Essential to the assessment of an adolescent female's health is the evaluation of her physical and psychosocial maturation. Although the pubertal process in adolescent females is sequential and predictable, great variations in the intensity and duration of this event have been described (Tanner 1982). Chronological age is a poor prognosticator of pubertal status. However, classification of an adolescent female's pubertal status can be achieved through clinical assessment utilizing **Tanner Staging or Sexual Maturity Rating (SMR) of Females, Table 1.1** (Tanner 1982; Slap 1986).

Table 1.1. TANNER STAGING OR SEXUAL MATURITY RATING (SMR) OF FEMALES

Breast

Breast Stage 1
  Breast-prepubertal; no glandular tissue.
  Areola and papilla-areola conform to general chest line.

Breast Stage 2
  Breast-breast bud; small amount of glandular tissue.
  Areola and papilla-areola widen.

Breast Stage 3
  Breast-larger and more elevation; extends beyond areolar parameters.
  Areola and papilla-areola continue to enlarge but remain in contour with the breast.

Breast Stage 4
  Breast-larger and more elevation.
  Areola and papilla-areola and papilla form a mound projecting from the breast contour.

Breast Stage 5
  Breast-adult (size is variable).
  Areola and papilla-areola and breast in same plane, with papilla projecting above areola.

Pubic Hair

Pubic Hair Stage 1
  None

Pubic Hair Stage 2
  Small amount of long, slightly pigmented, downy hair on the labia majora.

Pubic Hair Stage 3
  Moderate amount of pubic hair, more curly, coarse, and pigmented; the hair also extends more laterally.

Pubic Hair Stage 4
  Hair that resembles adult hair in coarseness and curliness but does not extend down the medial aspects of the thigh.

Pubic Hair Stage 5
  Adult type and quantity of hair extending down the medial aspects of the thighs.

Source: Reprinted with permission from Tanner, J.M. 1982. *Growth at adolescence*, 2nd ed. Oxford: Blackwell Scientific Publications; Slap, G.B. 1986. Normal physiological and psychological growth in the adolescent. *Journal of Adolescent Health Care* 7:139.

Similarly, adolescents vary in their psychological development. The major psychosocial outcomes of adolescence include cognitive and affective identity formation, emancipation from parents and family with the establishment of personal intimacy outside the primary family unit, and educational or vocational achievement as part of beginning some type of life's work. Generally, this process occurs in three stages: early (11 years to 13 years), middle (14 years to 15 years), and late (17 years to 21 years). Major areas for assessment include growth, body image concerns, and sexuality; cognitive development; and relationships with family, peers, and school (see **Table 1.2, Characteristics of Female Adolescent Psychosocial Development**).

Table 1.2. CHARACTERISTICS OF FEMALE ADOLESCENT PSYCHOSOCIAL DEVELOPMENT

Early Adolescence (11 Years to 13 Years)	Mid-Adolescence (14 Years to 17 Years)
Cognition 1. Concrete thought dominant. 2. Cannot perceive long-range implications of current decisions and acts. **Psychosocial** 1. Preoccupation with rapid body change. "Am I normal?" Concerns about appearance and attractiveness. **Family** 1. Defining independence/dependence boundaries. 2. No major conflicts over parental control. **Peer Group** 1. Peer affiliation emerging in relative importance. 2. Compares own normality and acceptance with same-sex age mates. **Sexuality** 1. Self-exploration and evaluation. 2. Limited dating. 3. Limited intimacy.	**Cognition** 1. Rapidly gaining competence in abstract thought. 2. Capable of perceiving future implications of current acts and decisions, though capability variably applied. **Psychosocial** 1. Re-establishes body image as growth decelerates and stabilizes. 2. Preoccupations with fantasy and idealism in exploring expanded cognition and future options. **Family** 1. Potential conflicts over control. 2. Struggle for emancipation. **Peer Group** 1. Strong need for identification to affirm self-image. 2. Looks to peer group to define behavioral code during emancipation process. **Sexuality** 1. Heightened sexual activity. 2. Testing abilities to attract and parameters of femininity. 3. Preoccupation with romantic fantasy.

Late Adolescence (17 Years to 21 Years)	
Cognition 1. Established abstract thought processes. 2. Future-oriented. 3. Capable of perceiving and acting on long-range options. **Psychosocial** 1. Emancipation completed. 2. Intellectual and functional identity established. 3. May experience crisis at age 21 years when facing societal demands for autonomy. **Family** 1. Transition of child/parent dependency relationship to the adult/adult model.	**Peer Group** 1. Recedes in importance in favor of individual friendships. **Sexuality** 1. Forms stable relationships. 2. Capable of mutuality and reciprocity in caring for another rather than former narcissistic orientation. 3. Plans for future in thinking of marriage, family. 4. Intimacy involves commitment rather than exploration and romanticism.

Source: Reprinted with permission from Slap, G.B. 1986. Normal physiological and psychological growth in the adolescent. *Journal of Adolescent Health Care* 7:139.

Because changes in adolescent mortality and morbidity are linked primarily to behavioral etiologies such as unintentional pregnancy, STDs, and alcohol- and drug-related consequences, current health promotion for adolescents emphasizes health guidance and prevention of behavioral and emotional disorders in addition to traditional biomedical conditions (see **Table 1.3, Leading Causes of Death for Women by Age Group; Table 1.4, Health Assessment for Women 13 Years to 19 Years of Age;** and **Table 1.5, Risk Assessment, Prevention Measures, and Counseling for Women 13 Years to 19 Years of Age**).

Table 1.3. LEADING CAUSES OF DEATH FOR WOMEN BY AGE GROUP

Women 13 Years to 19 Years of Age
Motor vehicle accidents
Malignant neoplasms
Homicide
Suicide
Heart disease

Women 20 Years to 39 Years of Age
Motor vehicle accidents
Malignant neoplasms
Homicide
Suicide
Heart disease

Women 40 Years to 64 Years of Age
Malignant neoplasms
Heart disease
Cerebrovascular disease
Chronic obstructive pulmonary disease
Motor vehicle accidents/Diabetes mellitus

Women 65 Years of Age and Older
Heart disease
Cerebrovascular disease
Malignant neoplasms
Chronic obstructive pulmonary disease
Diabetes mellitus

Source: Reprinted from U.S. Department of Commerce. 1991. *Statistical abstract of the United States 1991*, 111th ed. Washington, DC: the Author.

Guidelines for Adolescent Preventive Services (GAPS) (AMA 1993) is a comprehensive set of recommendations providing a framework for the organization and content of preventive health services, with recommendations in three areas—health guidance, screening, and immunizations. *GAPS* can direct clinicians regarding appropriate health maintenance and preventive aspects of the care of adolescents. Copies of *Guidelines for Adolescent Preventive Services* are available at no charge from:

Department of Adolescent Health
American Medical Association
515 North State Street
Chicago, Illinois 60610
(312) 464-5570

**Table 1.4. HEALTH ASSESSMENT FOR WOMEN
13 YEARS TO 19 YEARS OF AGE**

	Health Assessment **(Every One to Three Years)**
History	■ Medical history—including childhood illnesses, immunizations ■ Obstetrical/gynecological history (as indicated)—including age at the time of menarche, menstrual history, age at time of first coitus (consensual, non-consensual), sexual and safer sex practices, contraception, sexually transmitted diseases (STDs), number of partners, sexual orientation ■ Surgical history ■ Family history ■ Current medications—prescription and over-the-counter (OTC) ■ Dietary intake ■ Regular exercise practices ■ Tobacco/alcohol/drug use ■ Psychosocial history—including history of child abuse/neglect, domestic violence, emotional/physical abuse by parents or dating partner(s)
Physical Examination	■ Height, weight, and vital signs ■ Complete physical examination including: • visual acuity • oral cavity examination • palpation of thyroid • cardiovascular assessment • skin examination • lymph node assessment • breast examination • pelvic examination as indicated* • rectal examination as indicated* • scoliosis screening • Tanner staging or sexual maturity rating (SMR)
Laboratory Tests	■ Tuberculin skin tests in high-risk individuals* ■ STD screening as indicated*—including *Gonorrhea* and *Chlamydia* cultures, VDRL or RPR, HIV counseling and testing ■ Pap smear as indicated* ■ Vision screening as indicated* ■ Pregnancy test as indicated*

*See specific protocols for indications/guidelines.

Sources: Adapted from: American Academy of Pediatrics. 1988. *Guidelines for health supervision II.* Elk Grove, IL: the Author; American College of Obstetricians and Gynecologists. 1993. Routine cancer screening. ACOG Committee Opinion 128:1-5. Washington, DC: the Author; U.S. Department of Health and Human Services. 1994. *Clinician's handbook of preventive services.* Washington, DC: U.S. Government Printing Office; and U.S. Preventive Services Task Force. 1989. *Guide to clinical preventive services. An assessment of the effectiveness of 169 interventions.* Baltimore: Williams & Wilkins.

Table 1.5.   RISK ASSESSMENT, PREVENTION MEASURES, AND COUNSELING FOR WOMEN 13 YEARS TO 19 YEARS OF AGE

Risk Assessment

Behaviors
- Tobacco/alcohol/drug use
- Symptoms of physical and/or emotional abuse
- Symptoms of depression, suicide
- Evidence of social isolation, increased stress at home or school
- Risk factors associated with STDs, unintended pregnancy
- Driving motor vehicles: use of seat belts, driving under the influence of alcohol/drugs
- Lack of regular physical exercise
- Excessive dietary intake of fat, cholesterol; inadequate intake of iron, calcium; bingeing and/or purging behaviors for weight control
- Sun/ultraviolet light exposure
- Evidence of social isolation, increased stress at home or school

Prevention Measures and Counseling

Prevention Strategies
- Use of motor vehicle seat belts; use of helmet when bicycling, skateboarding
- Prevention/cessation of tobacco/alcohol/drug use
- Avoidance of driving/being a passenger in a vehicle driven by a person under the influence of alcohol/drugs
- Dietary restriction of fat, cholesterol; adequate intake of iron, calcium; iron supplementation (as indicated); maintenance of balanced diet; avoidance of bingeing and purging for weight control
- Regular exercise program
- Teach/review breast self-examination (when appropriate)
- Discussion of contraceptive options (when appropriate)
- Discussion of behaviors to reduce STD exposure (when appropriate)
- Discussion of violent behavior and strategies to reduce exposure to violence; available resources
- Sun/ultraviolet-light skin protection
- Discussion of stress reduction in home and at school

Immunizations
- Tetanus/diphtheria booster once during adolescence
- Measles/Mumps/Rubella once during adolescence
- Hepatitis B vaccine
- Influenza vaccine annually in high-risk individuals*
- Pneumococcal vaccine as indicated in high-risk individuals*

Referrals (as indicated)
- Primary care clinician
- Dentist
- Obstetrician/gynecologist
- Psychologist/psychiatrist
- Alcohol/drug treatment programs
- STD clinic for partner testing/treatment when indicated*
- Community groups/resources (specific to the needs of the woman)

*See specific protocols for indications/guidelines.

Sources: Adapted from: American Academy of Pediatrics. 1988. *Guidelines for health supervision II.* Elk Grove, IL: the Author; American Academy of Pediatrics. 1994. Report of the Committee on Infectious Diseases, 23rd ed., pp. 232-233. Elk Grove, IL: the Author; American College of Obstetricians and Gynecologists. 1993. Routine cancer screening. ACOG Committee Opinion 128:1-5. Washington, DC: the Author; U.S. Department of Health and Human Services. 1994. *Clinician's handbook of preventive services.* Washington, DC: U.S. Government Printing Office; and U.S. Preventive Services Task Force. 1989. *Guide to clinical preventive services. An assessment of the effectiveness of 169 interventions.* Baltimore: Williams & Wilkins.

Health Care Issues for Reproductive-Age Women (20 Years to 39 Years of Age)

Maureen T. Shannon, C.N.M., F.N.P., M.S.

In 1989, women between the ages of 20 years and 39 years constituted 32.2 percent of the total United States population, with the median age for American women being 34 years (U.S. Department of Commerce 1992). Currently, 40 percent of the U.S. labor force is made up of women in this age group, a percentage equal to that of employed males in the same age category. Although 58 percent of working women have children who are less than six years old, less than six percent of employers provide either on-site child-care (2.1 percent) or assist employees with child-care expenses (3.1 percent) (U.S. Department of Commerce 1991).

Demographic and employment data regarding reproductive-age women can be misleading because one could infer from it that women in this age category are a healthy group of individuals. In reality, personal lifestyle patterns of women between 20 years and 39 years of age reveal risk behaviors that contribute considerably to the mortality and morbidity observed in this population (see **Table 1.3**).

Many of the leading causes of death for women in this age group— e.g., MVAs, and homicide and suicide—involve personal and social factors that could be altered to prevent injuries and death. The incidences of heart disease and malignant neoplasms could also be influenced by preventive measures. Of the deaths attributed to cancer in adult women, 33 percent are related to diet (e.g., high fat consumption) and 30 percent are related to smoking (HHS 1990). Improved nutrition, cessation of smoking and substance abuse (i.e., alcohol, prescription medications, illicit drugs), regular exercise, consistent use of seat belts, personal screening for evidence of cancer (e.g., self breast examination), and early access to appropriate medical evaluation and treatment (see **Table 1.6, Health Assessment for Women 20 Years to 39 Years of Age** and **Table 1.7, Risk Assessment, Prevention Measures, and Counseling for Women 20 Years to 39 Years of Age**) are measures that can significantly reduce mortality rates observed in women of this and older age groups.

Reproductive health is usually the reason women in this age group seek medical care. When they do, the clinician is provided with an opportunity to educate, screen, and intervene to prevent adverse outcomes associated with unintended pregnancies, improper contraceptive method use, and STDs. It is essential that appropriate and adequate screening, testing, and treatment of STDs occur since these infectious diseases are associated with significant morbidity (e.g., PID, infertility, ectopic pregnancy, cancer) and mortality (e.g., HIV infection).

Counseling women about safer sex methods should be an integral component of their reproductive and primary health care. However, recommendations about contraception and safer sex must be made within the context of the individual woman's social and cultural milieu. Determination of obstacles to negotiating safer sex and the use of certain contraceptive methods are essential if successful incorporation of these practices is to be attained.

The majority of pregnant women are between 20 years and 39 years of age. Their health is of particular importance, since inadequate or delayed prenatal care can have an adverse impact on the health of the woman and her

Table 1.6. HEALTH ASSESSMENT FOR WOMEN 20 YEARS TO 39 YEARS OF AGE

	Health Assessment (Every One to Three Years)
History	■ Medical history ■ Review of systems—including signs/symptoms of cancer, heart disease ■ Obstetrical/gynecological history—including menstrual history, sexual and safer sex practices, contraception, STDs, number of partners, sexual orientation ■ Surgical history ■ Family history—including history of breast/ovarian cancer, cardiovascular disease, diabetes ■ Current medications—prescription and OTC ■ Dietary intake ■ Regular exercise practices ■ Tobacco/alcohol/drug use ■ Psychosocial history—including history of domestic violence

Physical Examination	■ Height, weight, and vital signs
	■ Complete physical examination including:
	  • visual acuity as indicated*
	  • oral cavity examination
	  • palpation of thyroid
	  • breast examination
	  • cardiovascular assessment
	  • skin examination
	  • lymph node assessment
	  • pelvic examination
	  • rectal examination

Laboratory Tests	■ Pap smear as indicated* ■ Mammogram as indicated* ■ STD screening as indicated*—including *Gonorrhea* and *Chlamydia* cultures, VDRL or RPR, and HIV counseling and testing ■ Tuberculin skin tests in high-risk individuals* ■ Rubella antibody titer as indicated* ■ Non-fasting total blood cholesterol every 5 years, more frequently as indicated* ■ Fasting plasma glucose as indicated* ■ Urinalysis for bacteriuria as indicated* ■ Pregnancy test as indicated*

*See specific protocols for indications/guidelines.

Sources: Adapted from American Cancer Society. 1992. Update January 1992. The American Cancer Society guidelines for the cancer-related check-up. *CA-A Cancer Journal for Clinicians* 42(1):44-45; American College of Obstetricians and Gynecologists. 1993. Routine cancer screening. ACOG Committee Opinion No. 128:1-5. Washington, DC: the Author; National Heart, Lung, and Blood Institute. 1988. *Report of the Expert Panel on Detection, Evaluation, and Treatment of High Blood Cholesterol in Adults.* National Cholesterol Education Program. Bethesda, MD: National Institutes of Health; U.S. Department of Health and Human Services. 1994. *Clinician's handbook of preventive services.* Washington, DC: U.S. Government Printing Office; and U.S. Preventive Services Task Force. 1989. *Guide to clinical preventive services. An assessment of the effectiveness of 169 interventions.* Baltimore: Williams & Wilkins.

fetus. Infant mortality rates are a barometer of the overall health of a nation, and reflect not only infant outcomes but maternal antenatal health as well.

In the United States, where only 76 percent of women receive any prenatal care (National Center for Health Statistics 1992), inequity exists among infant mortality rates for various ethnic groups, with infant mortality rates for African American infants twice that of white infants (National Center for Health Statistics 1992). The greatest single hazard to infant health is low birth weight, which results from lack of prenatal care, poor maternal

Table 1.7. RISK ASSESSMENT, PREVENTION MEASURES, AND COUNSELING FOR WOMEN 20 YEARS TO 39 YEARS OF AGE

Risk Assessment

Behaviors	▪ Tobacco/alcohol/drug use ▪ Symptoms of depression, suicide, abnormal bereavement ▪ Symptoms of physical and/or emotional abuse ▪ Risk factors associated with STDs, unintended pregnancy, high-risk pregnancy ▪ Driving motor vehicles: use of seat belts, driving under the influence of alcohol/drugs ▪ Lack of regular physical exercise ▪ Excessive dietary intake of fat, cholesterol; inadequate intake of iron, calcium ▪ Sun/ultraviolet light exposure

Prevention Measures and Counseling

Prevention Strategies	▪ Use of smoke detector in home ▪ Use of motor vehicle seat belts ▪ Cessation of tobacco/alcohol/drug use ▪ Limiting alcohol consumption ▪ Avoidance of driving/being a passenger in a vehicle driven by a person under the influence of alcohol/drugs ▪ Dietary restriction of fat, cholesterol; adequate dietary intake of iron, calcium; iron, calcium supplementation (as indicated) ▪ Exercise program (appropriate to physical capabilities) ▪ Review/teach self breast examination ▪ Review/teach signs and symptoms of cancer, cardiovascular disease ▪ Discussion of contraceptive options (when appropriate) ▪ Discussion of behaviors to reduce STD exposure (when appropriate) ▪ Discussion of osteoporosis prevention ▪ Discussion of domestic violence and available resources ▪ Sun/ultraviolet-light skin protection ▪ Discussion of stress reduction in home and employment settings
Immunizations	▪ Tetanus/diphtheria every 10 years ▪ Rubella vaccine as indicated* ▪ Hepatitis B vaccine as indicated in high-risk individuals* ▪ Pneumococcal vaccine as indicated in high-risk individuals* ▪ Influenza vaccine annually in high-risk individuals*
Referrals (as indicated)	▪ Primary care clinician ▪ Dentist ▪ Obstetrician/gynecologist ▪ Psychologist/psychiatrist ▪ Alcohol/drug treatment programs ▪ STD clinic for partner testing/treatment when indicated* ▪ Community groups/resources (specific to particular needs of the woman)

*See specific protocols for indications/guidelines.

Sources: Adapted from U.S. Department of Health and Human Services. 1994. *Clinician's handbook of preventive services.* Washington, DC: U.S. Government Printing Office; and U.S. Preventive Services Task Force. 1989. *Guide to clinical preventive services. An assessment of the effectiveness of 169 interventions.* Baltimore: Williams & Wilkins.

nutrition, maternal smoking, maternal alcohol/drug use, and maternal age (increases observed in women less than 18 years and more than 40 years old) (National Center for Health Statistics 1992; HHS 1990). Early and comprehensive prenatal care reduces the rates of infant mortality and number of low birth-weight infants.

The socioeconomic status of a woman will have an impact on her ability to access needed medical services. Currently, 14 million women of childbearing age (i.e., 20 years to 39 years) do not have medical coverage (either medical insurance or Medicaid) (U.S. Department of Commerce 1991). Furthermore, five million of these women with medical insurance have policies that will not cover prenatal care and delivery expenses (Harvey 1990). Such lack of financial coverage for medical and preventive services will often delay a woman's seeking medical or prenatal care and may contribute to adverse medical, obstetrical, and neonatal outcomes. Ultimately, the need for more costly interventions is often the result of health care services delayed because of such financial barriers.

Psychosocial and cultural aspects of a woman's life can have an impact on her health and her perception of illness. Conflicts regarding family, employment, and personal time commitments have been cited as major sources of stress for women between 25 years and 34 years of age (Woods 1988). In one survey, those under 35 years of age reported an increased incidence of physical and emotional symptoms compared to women over 35 years of age, possibly as a result of attempting to meet high expectations set by themselves or others during these years of anticipated professional success (Griffith 1983). Other studies have demonstrated increased levels of family-related (not employment-related) stress in women compared to male managers, executives, and professionals (Staats and Staats 1983).

Personal relationships within the family, particularly those between the woman and her partner, also contribute to a woman's overall sense of well-being. Studies have indicated that a partner's emotional and psychological support of a woman has a protective effect on her health (Woods 1988). On the other hand, a woman can suffer emotional and physical injuries as a consequence of her partner's violent behavior.

For women of reproductive age, pregnancy can be a stimulus for the emergence of violent tendencies in their partners. In one report, up to 37 percent of women surveyed reported having been assaulted by their partners during pregnancy (Helton, McFarlane, and Anderson 1987). This situation emphasizes the need for clinicians to carefully screen and adequately educate women about domestic violence, and to be particularly vigilant in their assessment of women for partner abuse during pregnancy.

Health Care Issues for Women during Midlife (40 Years to 64 Years of Age)
Diana Taylor, Ph.D., R.N., F.A.A.N.

At the start of the next century, more than 50 million American women will be older than 50 years, compared with only five million women in 1900. Midlife and older women are the fastest growing segment of American society and, when combined with males of the same ages, will represent over 34 percent of the United States population in the first decade of the 21st century (U.S. Department of Commerce 1992).

Midlife for women in the United States is considered to encompass the years between the ages of 40 years and 64 years, and midlife represents a crisis or an opportunity, depending, in part, on the woman's perception of midlife, on how she copes with the transition, on her resources and demands on her, and the support she receives (Frank 1992). How a woman adjusts to midlife is likely to have an impact on her general health, reproductive status, and psychosocial well-being.

Historically, little attention has been given to midlife women's health beyond reproductive biology. The end of reproductivity for a woman signals merely a transition from childbearing to non-childbearing capability, a physiological process that is anticipated in much the same way as puberty is for adolescents. A woman's life, rather than being linear, progresses with overlapping events involving various roles, positions, and biopsychosocial states that occur in a variety of sequences.

Women in their middle years are at varying points in their own life cycles. One woman at age 40 years may be a grandmother, another may be having her first child. Multiple markers such as age, reproductive events, life events, parenting, work, menstruation, and retirement have been used to describe a woman's experiences in midlife. Too often, only one of these experiences of life has been singled out for investigation at the expense of others (e.g., menopause). During this phase of a woman's life, the impact of the "empty nest," entering or re-entering the job market, caring for elderly parents, perimenopausal symptoms, and daily stressors cannot be isolated from one another as separate and distinct events.

Many women in midlife have limited incomes. Compounding the stress associated with financial limitations is the lack of either private or government health coverage for 20 percent of American women between the ages of 44 years and 64 years (U.S. Department of Commerce 1991). With cutbacks in federal programs for "medically needy" individuals, women in this age group may postpone seeking and obtaining essential medical services because of their financial limitations.

Economic disadvantage is a recognized contributing factor for increased morbidity and mortality in any age group. This is in part a result of poor access to necessary health screening and assessment. For example, in 1987, only 22 percent of low-income women 40 years of age or older had ever received a clinical breast examination and a mammogram compared to 36 percent of women in the total population (HHS 1990).

Because diseases that are the leading causes of death for women in this age group can be prevented in many instances (see **Table 1.3**), healthy behaviors and close monitoring for the emergence of diseases is especially important during midlife. Malignant neoplasms—particularly lung and breast cancer, followed by heart disease—account for the majority of deaths of women between ages 40 years and 64 years. Cerebrovascular events, cirrhosis, accidents, and suicide are also significant causes of death observed in this population. Such causes of mortality are preventable only if early, comprehensive health education, health assessments, and medical interventions are integrated into the primary care of women during their midlife (see **Table 1.8, Health Assessment for Women 40 Years to 64 Years of Age**, and **Table 1.9, Risk Assessment, Prevention Measures, and Counseling for Women 40 Years to 64 Years of Age**).

**Table 1.8.   HEALTH ASSESSMENT FOR WOMEN
40 YEARS TO 64 YEARS OF AGE**

	Health Assessment (Every One to Three Years)
History	■ Medical history ■ Review of systems—including signs/symptoms of cardiovascular disease, cancer ■ Obstetrical/gynecological history—including menstrual history (when appropriate), sexual and safer sex practices, contraception, STDs ■ Surgical history ■ Family history—including history of breast/ovarian cancer, cardiovascular disease, diabetes ■ Current medications—prescription and OTC ■ Dietary intake ■ Regular exercise practices ■ Tobacco/alcohol/drug use ■ Psychosocial history—including history of domestic violence

Physical Examination	■ Height, weight, and vital signs
	■ Complete physical examination including:
	  • visual acuity (as indicated)
	  • oral cavity examination
	  • palpation of thyroid
	  • breast examination
	  • cardiovascular assessment
	  • skin examination
	  • lymph node assessment
	  • pelvic examination
	  • rectal examination

Laboratory Tests	■ Non-fasting total blood cholesterol every five years, more frequently as indicated ■ Pap smear as indicated* ■ Mammogram every two years ages 40 years to 49 years, annually starting at age 50 years ■ Fecal occult blood testing annually after age 50 years, earlier as indicated* ■ Sigmoidoscopy every three to five years after age 50 years, earlier as indicated* ■ Tuberculin skin tests in high-risk individuals* ■ STD screening as indicated—including *Gonorrhea* and *Chlamydia* cultures, VDRL or RPR, and HIV counseling and testing in high-risk individuals* ■ Glaucoma testing as indicated* ■ Fasting plasma glucose as indicated*

*See specific protocols for indications/guidelines.

Sources: Adapted from American Cancer Society. 1992. Update January 1992. The American Cancer Society guidelines for the cancer related check-up. *CA-A Cancer Journal for Clinicians* 42(1):44-45; American College of Obstetricians and Gynecologists. 1993. Routine cancer screening. ACOG Committee Opinion 128:1-5. Washington, DC: the Author; National Heart, Lung, and Blood Institute. 1988. *Report of the Expert Panel on Detection, Evaluation, and Treatment of High Blood Cholesterol in Adults.* National Cholesterol Education Program. Bethesda, MD: National Institutes of Health; U.S. Department of Health and Human Services. 1994. *Clinician's handbook of preventive services.* Washington, DC: U.S. Government Printing Office; and U.S. Preventive Services Task Force. 1989. *Guide to clinical preventive services. An assessment of the effectiveness of 169 interventions.* Baltimore: Williams & Wilkins.

Table 1.9.   RISK ASSESSMENT, PREVENTION MEASURES, AND COUNSELING FOR WOMEN 40 YEARS TO 64 YEARS OF AGE

Risk Assessment

Behaviors
- Tobacco/alcohol/drug use
- Symptoms of depression, suicide, abnormal bereavement
- Symptoms of physical and/or emotional abuse
- Risk factors associated with STDs, unintended pregnancy
- Driving motor vehicles: use of seat belts, driving under the influence of alcohol/drugs
- Lack of regular physical exercise
- Excessive dietary intake of fat, cholesterol
- Sun/ultraviolet light exposure
- Evidence of social isolation, increased stress at home or work

Prevention Measures and Counseling

Prevention Strategies
- Use of smoke detector in home
- Use of motor vehicle seat belts
- Cessation of tobacco/alcohol/drug use
- Limiting alcohol consumption
- Avoidance of driving/being a passenger in a vehicle driven by a person while under the influence of alcohol/drugs
- Dietary reduction of fat, cholesterol; adequate dietary intake of calcium
- Exercise program (appropriate to physical capabilities)
- Review/teach self breast examination
- Review/teach signs and symptoms of cardiovascular disease, cancer
- Discussion of contraceptive options (as appropriate)
- Discussion of behaviors to reduce STD exposure
- Discussion of hormone therapy
- Discussion of domestic violence and available resources
- Sun/ultraviolet-light skin protection
- Discussion of stress reduction in home and employment settings

Immunizations
- Tetanus/diphtheria (every 10 years)
- Hepatitis B vaccine as indicated in high-risk individuals*
- Pneumococcal vaccine as indicated in high-risk individuals*
- Influenza vaccine annually in high-risk individuals*

Referrals (as indicated)
- Primary care clinician
- Dentist
- Ophthalmologist (for glaucoma testing)
- Obstetrician/gynecologist
- Psychologist/psychiatrist
- Alcohol/drug treatment programs
- STD clinic for partner testing/treatment (when indicated)*
- Community groups/resources (specific to particular needs of the woman)

*See specific protocols for indications/guidelines.

Sources: Adapted from U.S. Department of Health and Human Services. 1994. *Clinician's handbook of preventive services.* Washington, DC: U.S. Government Printing Office; and U.S. Preventive Services Task Force. 1989. *Guide to clinical preventive services. An assessment of the effectiveness of 169 interventions.* Baltimore: Williams & Wilkins.

Health Care Issues of Older Women (Aged 65 Years and Older)
Carole Deitrich, R.N., C., M.S., G.N.P.

By the year 2030, 22 percent of the United States population will be age 65 years or older, with 45 percent of this group over age 75 years. Women have a longer life expectancy than men. A 65-year-old woman can expect to live an additional 18 years, and, for those women who reach age 75 years, life expectancy is 88 years (Institute of Medicine 1990). Services for long-term chronic illness and disability will also need to increase as our country's elderly population (particularly individuals age 85 years and older) increases.

The quality of life that a woman can anticipate during her older years is important. In addition to physical well-being concerns, there are economic ones. Among the elderly poor, 74 percent are women. The level of poverty observed in women in this age group is attributable to low-paying jobs, the lack of retirement benefits in jobs often held by women, widowhood, and divorce (U.S. Public Health Service 1985).

Among older women, physiological changes that accompany the aging process can contribute to psychological and functional decline. Visual impairment occurs in five percent of older individuals, and 25 percent to 50 percent of this population experiences impaired hearing. Physical inactivity is a major factor in the loss of quality of life for women in this age group (HHS 1990).

Problems such as loss of cognitive function, falling, and incontinence are not normal consequences of aging. The presence of such symptoms indicates a need to assess an individual for an underlying pathology that could require treatment. Under-treatment of older women can result if physiological or psychological symptoms are too quickly attributed to old age.

Psychosocial aspects of older women's lives can be especially stressful. In the United States, 50 percent of women are widows by the age of 60 years (Rowe, Grossman, and Bond 1987). The loss of close family members and friends, compounded by physical limitations or disabilities, can result in social isolation and depression. Depression is often undetected and untreated in geriatric clients. Although depression occurs more frequently in midlife women than in women over 65 years of age, an increased incidence of depression is observed in older women who have medical illnesses associated with disabilities (McIntosh 1992).

Abuse of alcohol and non-prescription drugs is expected to increase among this age group (Glantz and Backenheimer 1988). However, most substance abuse observed in geriatric clients is a result of improper use, including overuse, of prescription medications. Medical providers may be contributing to this problem because they often prescribe incorrect dosages of medications for older clients. A reduction in the doses of certain medications is recommended in older clients because of the physiological changes associated with aging.

In addition, polypharmacy can be a significant problem, since geriatric clients often have several clinicians prescribing medications for them. Coordination of care by a designated primary-care clinician can help reduce occurrences of this problem.

In older age individuals, health promotion is often overlooked because of negative, erroneous assumptions about aging. The aging process is not a disease, and age alone is not an indicator of health or functional capacity. Variation in health status is more likely a function of lifelong habits (e.g., smoking, dietary patterns, exercise, chronic illnesses, coping skills) than chronological age. Assessment of functional capacity is frequently more informative than medical diagnoses alone, and often provides information more useful to the clinician than elaborate diagnostic studies.

Primary health care goals for older women are preventing disability and supporting function. Maintaining normal levels of weight, activity, and exercise, and stopping smoking bring health benefits that cannot be over-emphasized. Annual physical assessment, risk behavior screening, and preventive measures will promote the health of older women so that their quality of life is maintained (see **Table 1.10, Health Assessment for Women 65 Years of Age and Older,** and **Table 1.11, Risk Assessment, Prevention Measures, and Counseling for Women 65 Years of Age and Older**).

Table 1.10. HEALTH ASSESSMENT FOR WOMEN 65 YEARS OF AGE AND OLDER

	Annual Health Assessment
History	■ Medical history ■ Review of systems—including signs/symptoms associated with cardiovascular disease and cancer ■ Obstetrical/gynecological history ■ Surgical history ■ Family history ■ Current medications—prescription and OTC ■ Dietary intake ■ Level of physical activity ■ Functional status ■ Tobacco/alcohol/drug use ■ Psychosocial history

Physical Examination	■ Height, weight, and vital signs
	■ Complete physical examination including:
	  • visual acuity
	  • hearing assessment
	  • oral cavity examination
	  • palpation of thyroid
	  • cardiovascular assessment
	  • breast examination
	  • skin examination
	  • lymph node assessment
	  • neurological examination
	  • pelvic examination
	  • rectal examination

Laboratory Tests	■ Non-fasting total blood cholesterol every five years, more frequently as indicated* ■ Fasting plasma glucose as indicated* ■ Dipstick urinalysis ■ Fecal occult blood testing ■ Sigmoidoscopy every three to five years, more frequently as indicated ■ Glaucoma testing ■ Pap smear as indicated* ■ Mammogram ■ Thyroid function tests as indicated* ■ Tuberculin skin tests in high-risk individuals*

*See specific protocols for indications/guidelines.

Sources: Adapted from American Cancer Society. 1992. Update January 1992: The American Cancer Society guidelines for the cancer-related check-up. *CA-A Cancer Journal for Clinicians* 42(1):44-45; American College of Obstetricians and Gynecologists. 1993. Routine cancer screening. ACOG Committee Opinion No. 128:1-5. Washington, DC: the Author; National Heart, Lung, and Blood Institute. 1988. *Report of the Expert Panel on Detection, Evaluation, and Treatment of High Blood Cholesterol in Adults.* National Cholesterol Education Program. Bethesda, MD: National Institutes of Health; U.S. Department of Health and Human Services. 1994. *Clinician's handbook of preventive services.* Washington, DC: U.S. Government Printing Office; and U.S. Preventive Services Task Force. 1989. *Guide to clinical preventive services. An assessment of the effectiveness of 169 interventions.* Baltimore: Williams & Wilkins.

Table 1.11. RISK ASSESSMENT, PREVENTION MEASURES, AND COUNSELING FOR WOMEN 65 YEARS OF AGE AND OLDER

Risk Assessment

Behaviors
- Changes in cognitive function
- Symptoms of depression, suicide, abnormal bereavement
- Tobacco/alcohol/drug use
- Driving motor vehicles: use of seat belts, driving under the influence of alcohol/drugs
- Symptoms/signs of physical abuse
- Lack of physical exercise
- Excessive dietary intake of fat, cholesterol; unbalanced nutrient intake
- Evidence of social isolation
- Sun/ultraviolet light exposure

Prevention Measures and Counseling

Prevention Strategies
- Prevention of falls/trauma
- Use of smoke detector in home
- Use of motor vehicle seat belts
- Hot water heater temperature reduction to <130°F/54°C
- Cessation of tobacco/alcohol/drug use
- Limiting alcohol consumption
- Avoid driving/being a passenger in a vehicle driven by a person under the influence of alcohol/drugs
- Dietary reduction of fat (specifically saturated fats), cholesterol
- Exercise program (appropriate to physical capabilities)
- Review/teach self breast examination
- Review/teach signs and symptoms of cardiovascular disease, cancer
- Sun/ultraviolet-light skin protection
- Discussion of hormone therapy

Immunizations
- Influenza vaccine annually
- Pneumococcal vaccine
- Tetanus/diphtheria every 10 years
- Hepatitis B vaccine as indicated in high-risk individuals*

Referrals (as indicated)
- Primary care clinician
- Ophthalmologist (for glaucoma testing)
- Dentist
- Geriatrician
- Gynecologist
- Psychologist/psychiatrist
- Physical therapist
- Alcohol/drug treatment programs
- Community groups/resources (specific to particular needs of individual)

*See specific protocols for indications/guidelines.

Sources: Adapted from U.S. Department of Health and Human Services. 1994. *Clinician's handbook of preventive services*. Washington, DC: U.S. Government Printing Office; and U.S. Preventive Services Task Force. 1989. *Guide to clinical preventive services. An assessment of the effectiveness of 169 interventions*. Baltimore: Williams & Wilkins.

Bibliography

American Academy of Pediatrics. 1988. *Guidelines for health supervision II.* Elk Grove, IL: the Author.

———. 1994. Report of the Committee on Infectious Diseases, 23rd ed., pp. 232–233. Elk Grove Village, IL: the Author.

American Cancer Society. 1992. Update January 1992: The American Cancer Society guidelines for the cancer-related checkup. *CA-A Cancer Journal for Clinicians* 42(1):44–45.

American College of Obstetricians and Gynecologists. 1993. Routine cancer screening. *ACOG Committee Opinion* 128:1–5. Washington, DC: the Author.

American Medical Association. 1993. *Guidelines for adolescent preventive services.* Chicago: the Author.

Bernstein, B., and Kane, R. 1981. Physicians' attitudes toward female patients. *Medical Care* 19:600–608.

Brindis, C.D., Irwin, C.E., and Millstein, C.A. 1992. United States profile. In *Textbook of adolescent medicine*, eds. E.R. McAnarney, R.E. Kreipe, D.P. Orr, and G.D. Comerci. Philadelphia: W.B. Saunders.

Chacko, R.R., and Taber, L.H. 1993. Epidemiology of sexually transmitted diseases in children and adolescents in the United States. *Seminars in Pediatric Infectious Diseases* 14(2):71–76.

Clancy, C.M., and Massion, C.T. 1992. American women's health care. A patchwork quilt with gaps. *Journal of the American Medical Association* 268(14):1918–1920.

Council on Scientific Affairs, American Medical Association. 1992. Violence against women. Relevance for medical practitioners. *Journal of the American Medical Association* 267(23):3184–3189.

Davis K., and Rowland, D. 1990. Uninsured and underinsured: Inequalities in health care in the United States. In *The nation's health*, 3rd ed., eds. P.R. Lee and C.L. Estes. Boston: Jones and Bartlett.

English, A. 1988. *Adolescent health care: A manual of California law,* 3rd ed. San Francisco: National Center for Youth Law.

Frank, M.V. 1992. Transition into midlife. *Clinical Issues in Perinatal and Women's Health Nursing* 2(4):421–428.

Gans, J.E. 1993. *Policy compendium on confidential health services for adolescents.* Chicago: American Medical Association.

Gans, J.E., and Blyth, D.A. 1990. *American Medical Association profiles of adolescent health: America's adolescents: How healthy are they?* Chicago: AMA Department of Adolescent Health.

Glantz, M.D., and Backenheimer, M.S. 1988. Substance abuse among elderly women. *Clinical Gerontologist* 8(1):3–26.

Griffith, J. 1983. Women's stressors according to age groups. *Issues in the Health Care of Women* 6:311–326.

Harvey, B. 1990. A proposal to provide health insurance to all children and all pregnant women. *New England Journal of Medicine* 323:1216–1220.

Helton, A., McFarlane, J., and Anderson, E. 1987. Battered and pregnant: A prevalence study. *American Journal of Public Health* 77:1337–1339.

Institute of Medicine. 1990. *The second 50 years.* Washington, DC: National Academy of Sciences.

Irwin, C.E., and Shafer, M.A. 1992. Adolescent sexuality: The problem of negative outcomes of a normative behavior. In *Adolescents at risk: Medical and social perspectives*, eds. E.E. Rogers and E. Ginzberg. Boulder, CO: Westview Press.

Joel, L.A. 1992. Nursing's proposal for health care reform. *Scholarly Inquiry for Nursing Practice* 6:221–223.

Marks, A., Malizio, J., Hoch, J., Brody, R., and Fischer, M. 1983. Assessment of health needs and willingness to utilize health care resources of adolescents in a suburban population. *The Journal of Pediatrics* 102(3):456–460.

McIntosh, J.L. 1992. Epidemiology of suicide in the elderly. *Suicide and Life Threatening Behavior* 22(1):15–35.

National Center for Health Statistics. 1992. *Health United States 1991.* Hyattsville, MD: U.S. Public Health Service.

National Heart, Lung, and Blood Institute. 1988. *Report of the expert panel on detection, evaluation, and treatment of high blood cholesterol in adults.* National Cholesterol Education Program. Bethesda, MD: National Institutes of Health.

National Institutes of Health. 1992. *Report of the National Institutes of Health: Opportunities for research on women's health.* Bethesda, MD: the Author.

Ramey, E.R. 1982. The national capacity for health in women. In *Women: A developmental perspective* (NIH Publication No. 82–2290), eds. P.W. Berman and E.R. Ramey. Washington, DC: U.S. Government Printing Office.

Rowe, J.W., Grossman, E., and Bond, E. 1987. Academic geriatrics for the year 2000: An Institute of Medicine report. *New England Journal of Medicine* 316:1425–1428.

Slap, G.B. 1986. Normal physiological and psychological growth in the adolescent. *Journal of Adolescent Health Care* 7:139.

Staats, M., and Staats, T. 1983. Differences in stress levels, stressors, and stress responses between managerial and professional males and females on the Stress Vector Analysis—research edition. *Issues in the Health Care of Women* 5:165–176.

Strickland, B.R. 1988. Sex-related differences in health and illness. *Psychology of Women Quarterly* 12:381–399.

Tanner, J. M. 1982. *Growth at adolescence*, 2nd ed. Oxford: Blackwell Scientific Publications.

U.S. Department of Commerce. 1991. *Statistical abstract of the United States 1991*, 111th ed. Washington, DC: the Author.

———. 1992. *1990 Census of population. General population characteristics United States.* Washington, DC: U.S. Government Printing Office.

U.S. Department of Health and Human Services. 1990. *Healthy people 2000. National health promotion and disease prevention objectives.* Washington, DC: the Author.

———. Maternal and Child Health Bureau. 1993. *Child health USA '92.* Washington, DC: U.S. Government Printing Office.

———. *Clinician's handbook of preventive services.* Washington, DC: U.S. Government Printing Office.

U.S. Preventive Services Task Force. 1989. *Guide to clinical preventive services. An assessment of the effectiveness of 169 interventions.* Baltimore: Williams & Wilkins.

U.S. Public Health Service. 1985. Report of the Public Health Service task force on women's health issues. *Public Health Reports* 100:73.

Wingard, D.L. 1984. The sex differential in morbidity, mortality, and lifestyle. *Annual Review of Public Health* 5:433–458.

Woods, N.F. 1988. Women's health. *Annual Review of Nursing Research* 6:210–235.

SECTION 2

Ophthalmological Disorders

Lisa L. Lommel, R.N., C., F.N.P., M.P.H.

2-A

Blepharitis

Blepharitis is a chronic bilateral inflammation of the eye-lid margins. *Anterior blepharitis* is more common and involves the eyelid skin, eyelashes, and associated glands. There are two major types of anterior blepharitis—*staphylococci blepharitis*, which may become ulcerative, and *seborrheic blepharitis*, which usually involves the scalp, brows, and ears (Riordan-Eva and Vaughan 1993).

Posterior blepharitis is inflammation of the eyelid secondary to dysfunction of the meibomian glands. There may be an associated staphylococci infection. Posterior blepharitis caused by a primary glandular dysfunction is strongly associated with acne rosacea (Riordan-Eva and Vaughan 1993).

DATABASE

SUBJECTIVE

→ Symptoms may include:
- irritation, burning, and itching of the eyes.
- anterior blepharitis:
  - staphylococci—scaling, lesions, red lid margins, loss of lashes, crusting of lid margins.
  - seborrheic—less lid margin redness and scaling and no lesions or crusting of lid margins.
  - mixed type—red lid margin, crusting, scaling, lesions.
- posterior blepharitis:
  - red lid margins, tearing, lid margin rolled in.

OBJECTIVE

→ Patient may present with:
- anterior blepharitis:

- staphylococci—red lid margins, dry scales, broken or missing lashes, ulcerations, inflamed conjunctiva.
- seborrheic—greasy scales, less lid redness, no ulcerations, inflamed conjunctiva.
- mixed type—dry and greasy scales, red lid margins and ulcerations, inflamed conjunctiva.
- posterior blepharitis:
  - lid margins hyperemic with telangiectasias.
  - inflamed meibomian gland orifice.
  - entropion.
  - frothy or greasy tears.

→ Both anterior and posterior blepharitis may present with signs of hordeolum, chalazion, abnormal lid protrusion, conjunctivitis, keratitis, and increased vascularization and thinning of inferior cornea (more common with posterior) (see **Hordeolum and Chalazion, Conjunctivitis, Keratitis** protocols).

ASSESSMENT

→ Blepharitis

→ R/O hordeolum

→ R/O chalazion

→ R/O conjunctivitis

→ R/O acne rosacea

PLAN

DIAGNOSTIC TESTS

→ Usually not required for diagnosis and treatment.

TREATMENT/MANAGEMENT

Anterior Blepharitis

→ Responds well to lid hygiene and topical antibiotics.

- Dilute Johnson's Baby Shampoo® 1:1 with water, stabilize eyelid by gently pulling laterally, and scrub eyelids with cotton-tipped applicator or clean washcloth. Rinse well with water.
- Follow with application of warm compress for 5 to 10 minutes to each eye.
- Lastly, apply antibiotic ophthalmic ointment to lid margin with clean fingers or cotton-tipped applicator and rub it in for 5 to 10 strokes.
- Bacitracin 500-1000 units/gram ointment (Zun and Mathews 1988)

OR

- Erythromycin 0.5 percent ointment (Zun and Mathews 1988)

OR

- Sulfacetamide sodium (Sodium Sulamyd®) 10 percent ointment (Zun and Mathews 1988).

→ Co-existing seborrheic dermatitis is treated with selenium sulfide shampoo for the scalp and eyebrows (Howes 1988) or low-potency topical steroid. Consider consultation with ophthalmologist before prescribing steroids.

- Prednisolone 0.125 percent solution BID.

→ Repeat above regime 3 to 4 times a day.

Posterior Blepharitis

→ Mild cases may be controlled with regular meibomian gland expression (Riordan-Eva and Vaughan 1993).

→ Inflammation of the conjunctiva and cornea requires treatment with (Riordan-Eva and Vaughan 1993):

- tetracycline (Achromycin®, Sumycin®) 250 mg p.o. BID

OR

- erythromycin (Ilotycin®) 250 mg p.o. TID

AND

- prednisolone 0.125 percent solution BID.
- only short-term course of topical steroids should be used.

→ Dry eye symptoms may be relieved with artificial tears (see **Dry Eye** Protocol).

CONSULTATION

→ Referral is indicated when there is poor response to treatment or if corneal disease is present.

→ As needed for prescription(s).

PATIENT EDUCATION

→ See "Treatment/Management" section.

→ Explain pathophysiology, chronicity, and treatment plan.

→ Advise patient to avoid rubbing eyes at all times.

→ Advise patient to wash hands well before and after eye treatment.

→ Advise patient to keep eye ointment clean and not to share it with others.

→ Maintenance therapy for normal lid margins includes daily lid shampoo and warm compresses.

FOLLOW-UP

→ Document in progress notes and problem list.

2-B

Ceratacts

A *cataract* is an opacification of the crystalline lens of the eye. The majority of cataracts occur with aging. Sixty-five percent of people aged 50 to 59 years and all of those over age 80 years have opacities (Elkington and Khaw 1988).

The exact cause of cataract formation is unclear. Near-ultraviolet radiation, present in sunlight and commonly used in artificial light, recently has been found to be a contributory influence (Bienfang et al. 1990). Smoking also is thought to increase the risk of cataract formation, with risk rising with the number of cigarettes smoked (Hankinson et al. 1992; Christen et al. 1992).

Other conditions associated with cataracts include diabetes, myotonic dystrophy, atopic dermatitis, uveitis, persistent retinal detachment, trauma, prolonged steroid therapy, and congenitally acquired conditions (e.g., intrauterine infections with rubella or cytomegalovirus, galactosemia, and Down syndrome) (Riordan-Eva and Vaughan 1993; Jackson and Finlay 1991).

DATABASE

SUBJECTIVE

→ Symptoms may include:
- blurred vision, usually worse when viewing distant objects, progressive over months or years.
- monocular diplopia (double vision out of one eye).
- decreased visual acuity with extraneous light source (glare from sunlight). Commonly disturbs ability to drive.
- no pain or redness.

OBJECTIVE

→ Reduced visual acuity may be present depending on density and position of opacity on lens.

→ Early-stage cataracts can be seen through the ophthalmoscope at 50 cm. Opacities are seen as black spokes against the red reflex.

→ Senile cataracts are wedge-shaped, pointing toward the center of the pupil.

→ Ability to visualize fundus on close examination depends on density and location of opacity.

→ Slit-lamp examination can reveal the morphology of the cataract—e.g., cataracts due to uveitis or drug use may first appear in the posterior subcapsular region.

ASSESSMENT

→ Cataract

→ R/O concomitant condition contributing to cataract formation

PLAN

DIAGNOSTIC TESTS

→ A complete eye examination should be performed.

→ Examination of the eye for measurement of best eyeglass correction should be completed before a decision is made regarding surgery.

→ Additional diagnostic tests may be appropriate to rule out conditions contributing to cataract formation.

MANAGEMENT/TREATMENT

→ There is no medical treatment for cataracts.

→ Eyeglasses and/or contact lenses may provide satisfactory correction for some patients.

→ Surgery is the treatment of choice for individuals with functional visual impairment.
  - Includes removal of the opacity and implanting an intraocular lens which eliminates the need for heavy cataract glasses or contact lenses.

→ Management of condition contributing to formation of cataract as indicated.

CONSULTATION

→ Referral to an ophthalmologist is indicated for comprehensive work-up and management decision.

PATIENT EDUCATION

→ Explain pathophysiology and treatment options.

→ Specifics of patient education will depend on treatment option.

→ For patients with surgical correction, advise adherence to post-surgical care.

→ Advise all individuals to protect their eyes from ultraviolet radiation with protective sunglasses and wide-brimmed hats.

→ Advise patients who smoke to stop. Referral to a smoking-cessation support group may be indicated.

→ Advise patients that a diet rich in vitamins C and E and beta carotene has been shown to lower the risk of cataract formation (*University of California at Berkeley Wellness Letter* 1993).

FOLLOW-UP

→ Document in progress notes and problem list.

Lisa L. Lommel, R.N., C., F.N.P., M.P.H.

2-C
Conjunctivitis

Conjunctivitis is an inflammation of the conjunctiva, caused most commonly by bacteria, chlamydia, viruses, or allergies. The most common bacteria causing conjunctivitis include staphylococci, streptococci (including *S. pneumoniae*), *Hemophilus* sp., *Pseudomonas* sp., *Moraxella* sp., and *Neisseria gonorrhoeae*. The most common viral pathogen is adenovirus 3, often occurring in epidemics ("pink eye"). Other causes of conjunctivitis include fungus, parasites (see **Keratitis** Protocol), and keratoconjunctivitis (see **Dry Eye** Protocol) (Riordan-Eva and Vaughan 1993).

DATABASE

SUBJECTIVE

Bacterial

→ Precipitating factors include a history of contact with a person with similar symptoms.

→ Symptoms begin in one eye, spreading to the other.

→ Symptoms include:
- copious mucopurulent discharge.
- crusting of eyelids in morning.
- mild discomfort and grittiness.
- no pain, blurred vision, or photophobia.

Gonococcal

→ Precipitating factors include contact with infected genital secretions.

→ Symptoms include:
- copious purulent discharge.
- associated symptoms of genital infection.

Chlamydial

→ Precipitating factors include:
- contact with infected genital secretions.
- young, sexually active women.

→ Symptoms include:
- acute redness and irritation.
- watery to mucopurulent discharge.
- associated symptoms of genital infection.

Viral

→ Symptoms usually involve one eye at onset with less severe involvement of second eye after one week.

→ Symptoms include:
- copious watery discharge.
- eye gritty and irritated.
- photophobia.
- associated symptoms of cough, malaise, fever, and sore throat.

Seasonal and perennial allergy

→ Symptoms include:
- itching, irritation, burning, photophobia.

→ History includes:
- associated allergic problems including rhinitis, eczema, food allergies.
- seasonal allergy (hay fever conjunctivitis):
  - most common in spring and summer.
  - related to appearance of specific allergens or pollens.
- perennial allergy:
  - chronic and usually year-round.

- symptoms usually less severe than seasonal allergy.
- may experience seasonal exacerbation of symptoms.
  - watery discharge.
  - red conjunctiva.
  - mild to moderate discomfort.
  - commonly associated symptoms of nasal and/or pharyngeal complaints.
→ Symptoms usually bilateral.

Contact allergy

→ Wide variety of substances—most commonly including medications, cosmetics, and contact lens solutions—may cause contact allergy.

→ Symptoms include:
  - itching, burning, and watery discharge.
  - photophobia.

OBJECTIVE

→ Patient may present with:

Bacterial
  - copious purulent discharge.
  - no keratitis or preauricular lymph nodes.

Gonococcal
  - copious purulent discharge.
  - red conjunctiva with edema.
  - possible corneal involvement.
  - preauricular lymph node.

Chlamydial
  - watery to mucopurulent discharge.
  - diffuse conjunctival redness.
  - conjunctival follicles.
  - possible corneal involvement.
  - non-tender preauricular lymph node.

Viral
  - pharyngitis.
  - fever.
  - red palpebral conjunctiva.
  - watery eye discharge.
  - stringy exudate.
  - palpebral conjunctival follicles and central keratitis as hallmark clinical signs seen with slit-lamp examination.
  - preauricular lymph node.

Seasonal and perennial allergy
  - red conjunctiva with edema.
  - tarsal conjunctival follicles.
  - clear, stringy discharge.

- signs of perennial allergy that are less severe than seasonal allergy or may be absent.

Contact allergy
  - red conjunctiva with edema.
  - skin of eyelids reddened, edematous, scaling, and papular.
  - inferior fornix presenting with a follicular response.
  - severe cases that may involve cornea with infiltrates and opacities.

ASSESSMENT

→ Conjunctivitis
  - R/O bacterial
  - R/O gonococcal
  - R/O chlamydial
  - R/O viral
  - R/O seasonal and perennial allergy
  - R/O contact allergy
→ R/O trauma
→ R/O uveitus
→ R/O narrow angle closure glaucoma
→ R/O concomitant sexually transmitted disease (STD)

PLAN

DIAGNOSTIC TESTS

→ Eye acuity should be measured before instillation of flourescein.
→ Slit-lamp examination may be helpful.
→ Fluorescein staining may be indicated to rule out corneal involvement (see **Eye Injury**, **Keratitis** protocols).

Bacterial
→ Severe inflammation and purulent discharge should be cultured to guide appropriate treatment.

Gonococcal
→ Suspected cases should be confirmed by culture of discharge.
→ Test for concomitant STDs—syphilis, trichomonas, chlamydia, HIV.

Chlamydial
→ Suspected cases should be confirmed by culture with cytologic examination of discharge.
→ Test for concomitant STDs—syphilis, gonorrhea, trichomonas, HIV.

Viral

→ No specific diagnostic tests.

Seasonal and perennial allergy

→ In severe cases, allergy testing may be recommended to identify specific allergens.

Contact allergy

→ No specific diagnostic tests.

→ Skin testing can be useful in identifying specific allergens.

TREATMENT/MANAGEMENT

Bacterial

→ Usually self-limiting, lasting 10 to 14 days if left untreated.

→ For mild cases:
- sodium sulfacetamide (Sodium Sulamyd®) 30 percent ophthalmic solution, instill 1 drop to 2 drops every 2 to 3 hours, or 10 percent ointment, instill QID and at bedtime, in affected eye(s) for 1 week (Riordan-Eva and Vaughan 1993). Alert patient to stinging on instillation. See *Physicians' Desk Reference* (*PDR*) for side effects.

→ The following are broad-spectrum antibiotics for moderate to severe cases (Benson and Lanier 1992):
- polymycin B sulfate, bacitracin, and neomycin ophthalmic ointments (Neosporin®), instill every 3 to 4 hours for 7 to 10 days
    OR
- polymycin B, bacitracin ophthalmic ointments (Polysporin®), instill every 3 to 4 hours for 7 to 10 days.
- ciprofloxacin hydrochloride (Ciloxan®) 0.3 percent ophthalmic solution, instill 1 drop to 2 drops every 2 hours while awake for the first 2 days, and then 1 drop to 2 drops every 4 hours while awake for the next 5 days.

→ The following antibiotics may be used alone or in combination for a broader spectrum of coverage (Benson and Lanier 1992):
- erythromycin (Ilotycin®) 0.5 percent ophthalmic ointment, instill in affected eye(s) QID for 1 week
    OR
- bacitracin 500 units/gram ophthalmic ointment, instill in affected eye(s) QID for 1 week
    AND/OR
- gentamycin (Garamycin®) 0.3 percent ophthalmic solution, 1 drop to 2 drops every 3

to 4 hours or ophthalmic ointment, instill in affected eye(s) QID for 1 week
    OR
- tobramycin (Tobrex®) 0.3 percent ophthalmic solution, 1 drop to 2 drops QID or ophthalmic ointment, instill in affected eye(s) QID for 1 week.

Gonococcal

→ If cornea is involved, immediate referral to an ophthalmologist is indicated, since corneal involvement may lead to perforation.

→ If cornea not involved (Riordan-Eva and Vaughan 1993):
- ceftriaxone (Rocephin®) 1 gram I.M. for 1 dose
    AND
- erythromycin (Ilotycin®) 0.5 percent ophthalmic ointment, instill in affected eye(s) QID for 7 to 10 days
    OR
- bacitracin 500 units/gram ophthalmic ointment, instill in affected eye(s) QID for 7 to 10 days.

→ Normal saline conjunctival irrigation for 15 minutes, QID.

→ Treat associated STDs.

Chlamydial (Riordan-Eva and Vaughan 1993)

→ Doxycycline (Vibramycin®) 300 mg initially p.o. followed by 100 mg BID for 2 weeks
    OR

→ Tetracycline (Achromycin®, Sumycin®) 250 mg-500 mg p.o. QID for 2 weeks
    OR

→ Erythromycin (Ilotycin®) 250 mg-500 mg p.o. QID for 2 weeks

→ Treat associated STDs.

Viral

→ Usually self-limiting, lasting approximately two weeks.

→ Corticosteroids not recommended as they might prolong course.

→ Warm compresses may relieve discomfort.

→ Often difficult to distinguish clinically from bacterial infection. Topical antibiotic often is prescribed (Riordan-Eva and Vaughan 1993):
- sodium sulfacetamide (Sodium Sulamyd®) 30 percent ophthalmic solution, instill 1 drop to 2 drops every 2 to 3 hours, or 10 percent ointment, instill QID and at bedtime, in affected eye(s) for 1 week (Riordan-Eva and

Vaughan 1993). Alert patient to stinging on instillation.

Seasonal and perennial allergy

→ Initial management is focused on identifying causative antigen(s) and eliminating them from environment.

→ Desensitization is less effective in ocular disease than in allergic rhinitis (Ehlers and Donshik 1992).

→ Mild cases of allergic conjunctivitis may be relieved with topical vasoconstrictors and topical decongestants. However, the overall effectiveness of these products has been challenged in the literature (Riordan-Eva and Vaughan 1993). Long-term use of these medications is not recommended due to the risk of rebound vasodilatation (Riordan-Eva and Vaughan 1993).

  ■ The following is a list of commonly used ophthalmic decongestants that are usually combined with an astringent and/or antihistamine (Roy and Tindall 1991):

  • naphazoline hydrochloride (Ak-Con®, Alabon®, Clear Eyes®, Degest 2®, Naphcon®, Vasoclear®) 1 to 2 drops in each eye up to 5 times a day

OR

  • phenylephrine hydrochloride (Ak-Nefrin®, Efricel®, Eye Cool®, Isopto Frin®, Prefrin Liquifilm®, Relief®) 1 to 2 drops in each eye up to 5 times a day

OR

  • tetrahydrozoline hydrochloride (Collyrium®, Murine Plus®, Soothe®, Visine®, Tetracon®) 1 to 2 drops in each eye up to 5 times a day

OR

  • decongestant/astringent combinations:
  –phenylephrine hydrochloride plus zinc sulfate (Prefrin-Z®, Zincfrin®) 1 to 2 drops in each eye up to 5 times a day

OR

  –tetrahydrozoline plus zinc sulfate (Visine A.C.®) 1 to 2 drops in each eye up to 5 times a day.

→ Systemic antihistamines may be effective against more severe ocular symptoms and associated nasal and pharyngeal symptoms (see **Rhinitis Protocol**).

Contact allergy

→ Eliminate contact with offending substance.

→ Self-limiting, should subside after contact discontinued.

→ Cool compresses may provide relief from discomfort.

→ If cornea is involved, immediate referral to an ophthalmologist is indicated.

CONSULTATION

→ May be indicated for chlamydial or gonococcal conjunctivitis.

→ May be indicated with severe cases of conjunctivitis.

→ Physician consultation is recommended if symptoms are not improved in one week or if condition worsens after beginning treatment.

→ Referral to an ophthalmologist is indicated if symptoms of bacterial conjunctivitis are not improved in one week.

→ Immediate referral to an ophthalmologist is indicated with corneal involvement.

→ As needed for prescription(s).

PATIENT EDUCATION

→ Instruct patient regarding pathophysiology, risk factors, and treatment plan.

→ Advise patient to maintain good hygiene practices:
  ■ avoid contact with towels, or other fomites from infected individual.
  ■ wash hands well before and after touching eyes or instilling ocular medications.
  ■ avoid touching ocular medication container with infected eye.

→ Teach patient proper instillation of ocular medications:
  ■ tilt head back.
  ■ place a finger on the cheek and gently pull downward, forming a pocket.
  ■ instill drops or approximately ½-inch ribbon of ointment into pocket without touching tip of tube to the eye.
  ■ look downward before closing eye.

→ For patients with gonococcal or chlamydial conjunctivitis:
  ■ instruct patient regarding transmission of STDs, including using condoms to avoid contracting them.
  ■ advise patient to avoid contact with infected genital lesions.

- advise patient to have sexual partners treated for infection (see **Gonorrhea** and *Chlamydia Trachomatis* protocols).
- advise patient regarding the need for additional STD testing and treatment as indicated.

→ For patient with seasonal and perennial allergic conjunctivitis:
- instruct patient to avoid allergens precipitating symptoms.

FOLLOW-UP

→ See "Consultation" section.

→ Document in progress notes and problem list.

Lisa L. Lommel, R.N., C., F.N.P., M.P.H.

2-D

Dacryocystitis

Dacryocystitis, an infection of the lacrimal sac, usually develops when the lacrimal system becomes partially or totally blocked. *Staphylococcus aureus* and B-hemolytic streptococci are the most common infecting organisms.

This infection may be acute or chronic and is most common in females over 40 years of age. It can be complicated by cellulitis of the surrounding skin.

DATABASE

SUBJECTIVE
→ Patients with acute cases present with:
  ▪ pain.
  ▪ swelling.
  ▪ redness around inner canthus of eye.
  ▪ increased tearing.
→ Patients with advanced cases may present with generalized skin swelling and tenderness.
→ Patients with chronic cases may present with only tearing and discharge.

OBJECTIVE
→ Patients may present with:
  ▪ tenderness.
  ▪ swelling.
  ▪ redness around inner canthus of eye.
  ▪ pressure over the lacrimal sac possibly producing mucopurulent drainage through the lacrimal puncta.
→ Advanced cases may present with:
  ▪ generalized swelling and tenderness.
  ▪ enlarged cervical lymph nodes.

ASSESSMENT

→ Dacryocystitis
→ R/O orbital cellulitis
→ R/O acute conjunctivitis

PLAN

DIAGNOSTIC TESTS
→ Usually none needed for diagnosis.
→ Culture of duct drainage may assist in choice of antibiotic treatment if first-line therapy is not improving symptoms.

TREATMENT/MANAGEMENT
→ Warm compresses and massage over the lacrimal duct area 3 times a day.
→ Oral antibiotics:
  ▪ ampicillin (Polycillin®, Omnipen®) 500 mg p.o. QID (Wilhelmus 1988)
            OR
  ▪ dicloxicillin (Dynapen®, Pattiocil®) 250 mg-500 mg QID (Yanosfky 1988).

CONSULTATION
→ Referral to an ophthalmologist is indicated when above measures are not helping resolve infection, or with recurrent infections/abscess formation.
→ Immediate emergency referral is warranted when orbital cellulitis is present.
→ As needed for prescription(s).

PATIENT EDUCATION
→ Instruct patient regarding pathophysiology, chronicity, and treatment plan.
→ See ''Treatment/Management'' section.
→ Advise patient to avoid rubbing eyes.
→ Advise patient to wash hands well before and after treatment.

FOLLOW-UP
→ Document in progress notes and problem list.

2-E

Dry Eye

Dry eye may result from a deficiency in one or more of the three components of tear film: aqueous fluid, mucin, or lipid. Aqueous fluid, secreted by the main and accessory lacrimal glands, makes up 90 percent of tear film.

A deficiency in aqueous production is called *keratoconjunctivitis sicca* and occurs most often as a result of aging, most commonly in the aging female. Aqueous deficiency may also occur as a result of systemic disease (Sjögren's syndrome, rheumatoid arthritis, sarcoidosis, Hodgkin's disease, lupus erythematosus, scleroderma), acne rosacea, drug use (e.g., phenothiazines, atropinic agents, antihistamines), or as a result of neurological disease (Greenberg 1995).

Mucin secretion occurs primarily by conjunctival goblet cells. A deficiency in mucin production may occur with Vitamin A deficiency, benign ocular pemphigoid, trachoma, Accutane® use, and following chemical burns (Greenberg 1995).

Lipid secretion occurs from the meibomian glands. Chronic blepharitis and meibomitis will alter the amount of lipid in tear film (Greenberg 1995).

Eyelid defects causing inadequate wetting may lead to dry eye. These conditions include incomplete blinking, 5th or 7th cranial nerve palsy, exophthalmos, and exposure during sleep as a result of deficient lid closure (Greenberg 1995).

DATABASE

SUBJECTIVE

→ Symptoms may include:
- burning, itching, soreness, sandy, gritty, foreign-body sensation in eye.
- increased mucus; patient able to remove strands from inner canthus in morning.
- difficulty in closing eye when eyelid defects are present.

→ Symptoms:
- are worse at end of day.
- are precipitated by dry environment, tobacco smoke, indoor environment with heating and low humidity, forced air in car.
- may begin with excessive tearing.

→ If contact lenses are used, patient may present with soreness, and difficulty removing lenses.

→ A variety of symptoms may present with systemic diseases causing dry eyes (see **Blepharitis, Rheumatoid Arthritis** protocols).

OBJECTIVE

→ Patient may present with:
- minimal eye wetness.
- increased eye debris and mucus.
- hyperemic, edematous bulbar conjunctiva.
- corneal dullness.
- inadequate lid closure.

→ A variety of signs may present with systemic diseases causing dry eyes (see **Blepharitis, Rheumatoid Arthritis** protocols).

ASSESSMENT

→ Dry eyes (keratoconjunctivitis sicca)
→ R/O systemic disease
→ R/O neurological disorder

→ R/O drug use

→ R/O mucin deficiency

→ R/O lipid deficiency

→ R/O eyelid disorder

PLAN

DIAGNOSTIC TESTS

→ Aqueous deficiency can be measured by performing the Schirmer Test:
  - using Whatman No. 41 filter paper, 5 mm by 35 mm.
  - folded end is hooked over lower lid nasally.
  - instruct patient to keep eyes lightly closed during test.
  - wetting is measured after 5 minutes.
  - less than 5 mm is abnormal.

→ A variety of diagnostic tests may be indicated with systemic diseases causing dry eyes (see **Blepharitis, Rheumatoid Arthritis** protocols).

TREATMENT/MANAGEMENT

→ Systemic, neurological, and ocular disease should be ruled out before treatment is begun. Refer to appropriate protocols for management of specific conditions causing dry eye (see **Blepharitis, Rheumatoid Arthritis** protocols).

→ In cases of dry eye due to aging, environmental dryness, and/or drug use, symptomatic relief may be attempted with artificial tears (Greenberg 1995; Roy and Tindall 1991).
  - Polyvinyl alcohol (Liquifilm Tears®, 1.4 percent; Liquifilm Forte® 3 percent; Hypo Tears®, Aqua Tears®, Tears Plus®)

    OR
  - Methylcellulose (Visulose®, 0.5 percent or 1 percent; Isopto Plain®, Methopto®, Methulose®, Murocel®)

    OR
  - Hydroxypropyl methycellulose 1 percent (Ultra Tears®, Tears Naturale®, Absorbotear®, Isopto Alkaline®, Lacril®, Tearisol®).

→ Ophthalmic ointment may be used at night when tear production is minimal.
  - Petroleum ointment (Lacri-Lube®, Akwa-Tears®, Duolube®, Duratears®, Hypotears®, Refresh P.M.®):
    • 1 drop to 2 drops in each eye QID can be used in mild cases, increasing up to hourly to relieve symptoms.
    • risk factors include topical sensitivity and corneal damage.

→ Reduce environmental drying by using a room humidifier and avoiding tobacco smoke and forced air.

CONSULTATION

→ Referral is indicated for management of systemic, neurological, or ocular disease.

→ Referral to an ophthalmologist is indicated if artificial tears do not provide relief.

→ As needed for prescription(s).

PATIENT EDUCATION

→ Explain pathophysiology and treatment plan.

→ See "Treatment/Management" section.

→ Teach patient how to instill eye drops properly:
  - tilt head back or lie on back.
  - rest the hand with medicine bottle on forehead.
  - instill one drop into lower fornix.
  - apply digital pressure in punctal inner region of lower lid to reduce drainage.
  - avoid dropper contact with eye.
  - instill one drop at a time and wait for absorption.

→ Advise patient to wash hands well before and after treatment.

→ Advise patient to avoid sharing eye medications with others.

FOLLOW-UP

→ Document in progress notes and problem list.

2-F

Eye Injury

Eye injuries run the gamut from serious emergencies requiring immediate referral to an ophthalmologist, to minor trauma—e.g., a foreign body lodged in an eye and extracted in an outpatient setting. The primary care provider's responsibility to a patient who presents with a serious emergency is to provide diagnosis and immediate management and transport to an ophthalmologist and/or emergency setting. Non-emergency conditions can be managed in consultation with a physician.

This protocol presents common eye injuries and their management plans.

DATABASE

SUBJECTIVE

Chemical, thermal, or radiation burn; penetrating injury; blunt trauma

→ History should include:
  ▪ how, when, and where injury occurred.
  ▪ protective eye wear, contact lens, or glasses usually worn.
  ▪ loss of vision, and presence of pain or associated manifestations.
  ▪ presence of foreign-body sensation.

→ Identify injuring object.

→ With radiation burns (from sunlight, sunlamp, welding arc), symptoms are usually delayed six to 12 hours, then manifest as severe pain and photophobia.

→ Tetanus immunization status should be obtained in cases of penetrating injury.

Corneal abrasion

→ Symptoms include:
  ▪ pain, tearing, photosensitivity, blurring of vision, sensation of foreign body.

→ History includes object contact with eye (e.g., contact lens, particulates).

→ Tetanus immunization status should be obtained.

Foreign body

→ Symptoms include:
  ▪ pain, burning, and foreign-body sensation increasing with lid movement.

→ Tetanus immunization status should be obtained.

Retinal detachment

→ Symptoms include:
  ▪ sudden onset of floaters, flashing lights, pain on moving eye, headache, or peripheral field defect.

→ Patient has history of "curtain coming down over eye."

OBJECTIVE

→ Signs will be influenced by nature of injury.

→ Physical examination may include some or all of the following, depending on nature of injury (Silverman, Nunez, and Feller 1992):
  ▪ measurement of visual acuity and visual fields.
  ▪ inspection and palpation of eyelids, orbit, and facial structure. (Do not press on eye with penetrating or blunt trauma.)
  ▪ assessment of facial and corneal sensation.
  ▪ assessment of pupils for size, shape, symmetry, and reaction to light and accommodation.

- assessment of extraocular muscle function.
- assessment of ocular motility.
- inspection for subconjunctival injection or hemorrhage and chemosis.
- inspection of cornea, anterior chamber, and lens for clarity.
- eversion of eyelids to assess for foreign body.
- ophthalmoscopy to evaluate red reflex, lens opacities, vitreous and retinal abnormalities, papilledema, and vessel occlusion.

→ Instillation of fluorescein will reveal abnormal staining (i.e., darker green) if corneal abrasion is present. May also highlight foreign body. Linear abrasion in a vertical pattern may indicate foreign body under eyelid.

ASSESSMENT

→ Eye injury
- R/O chemical burn
- R/O thermal burn
- R/O radiation burn
- R/O penetrating eye injury
- R/O blunt trauma
- R/O corneal abrasion
- R/O foreign body
- R/O retinal detachment

PLAN

DIAGNOSTIC TESTS

→ A slit lamp facilitates examination through magnification.

→ Fluorescein staining and ultraviolet light may be used for assessing for corneal epithelial defects and foreign bodies.
- May first anesthetize eye with: Proparacaine 0.5 percent, 1 drop to 2 drops.
- Pull down lower lid and place edge of fluorescein paper against conjunctiva until a small amount of dye is taken up.
- Remove paper and rinse eye with normal saline to remove excess dye.
- Examine with penlight or ultraviolet light.

→ Orbital x-rays (including Waters' and Caldwell projections) may be indicated to rule out fracture with penetrating or blunt trauma injury.

→ Further diagnostic testing may be indicated as per ophthalmologist.

TREATMENT/MANAGEMENT

Chemical burn (e.g., flares, sparklers, acid, or alkali [lye, lime, liquid ammonia]) (Silverman, Nunez, and Feller 1992)

→ Constitutes true emergency.

→ Topical anesthetic may be instilled before irrigation and every 20 minutes. Proparacaine 0.5 percent, 1 drop to 2 drops.

→ Immediate eye irrigation—with any clean, non-toxic liquid (preferably water or normal saline, if available)—using a hose, tap, or shower for at least 15 minutes before transport to an ophthalmologist or emergency setting.

→ Alkali burns are more serious and may require prolonged irrigation.

→ Remove small particles from conjunctival sac with wet cotton-tip applicator.

→ Consultation with a physician may be sought before transport.

Thermal burn (e.g., hot grease, molten metal, tobacco ash) (Silverman, Nunez, and Feller 1992)

→ For small abrasion of conjunctiva, sclera, or cornea, see "Corneal abrasion," "Treatment/ Management" section, p. 2-18.

→ For large burns or burn over pupil, cover eye with non-pressure patch and refer immediately to ophthalmologist or emergency setting.

Radiation burn (e.g., ultraviolet light sources; sunlamp, sunlight, welding arcs) (Riordan-Eva and Vaughan 1993)

→ To relieve discomfort of ciliary spasm instill cyclopentolate 1 percent, 1 drop to 2 drops.
- Do not prescribe local anesthetics.
- Patch both eyes.

→ Most patients will recover in 24 to 48 hours.

→ With severe burns, refer to ophthalmologist.

Perforating eye injury (e.g., bullet, glass, knife, fishing hook, blade) (Silverman, Nunez, and Feller 1992)

→ Apply non-pressure protective eye shield and provide immediate referral to ophthalmologist or emergency setting.

→ Administer tetanus immunization as indicated.

Blunt trauma (Silverman, Nunez, and Feller 1992)

→ For mild trauma with subconjunctival hemorrhage:

- apply cold compresses.
- provide pain relief, avoiding platelet-inhibiting analgesic products (e.g., aspirin).
→ For moderate to severe trauma, refer immediately to ophthalmologist or emergency setting.

Corneal abrasion (Silverman, Nunez, and Feller 1992)

→ For small abrasion of cornea, conjunctiva, or sclera:
- apply sodium sulfacetamide, gentamycin, or tetracycline ophthalmic ointment.
- tape lid closed.
- apply pressure patch, using two patches.
→ For large abrasion or abrasion over the pupil, refer promptly to ophthalmologist.
→ If the patient has a contact-lens-associated injury, refer promptly to ophthalmologist to rule out corneal ulcer.

Foreign body (Silverman, Nunez, and Feller 1992)

→ Topical anesthetic agent may be used before attempting foreign body removal. With prolonged usage, topical anesthetics are toxic to the cornea and should never be dispensed to the patient for relief of ocular discomfort (Bensin and Lanier 1992).
- Proparacaine 0.5 percent, 1 drop to 2 drops.
→ Mobile foreign body may be removed with normal saline irrigation.
→ Foreign body on conjunctiva may be removed by everting the lid and gently wiping with wet cotton-tip applicator.
→ After removal of foreign body, instill polymycin-bacitracin ophthalmic ointment.
→ If foreign body is imbedded in cornea or conjunctiva, patch eye and refer immediately to ophthalmologist.
→ For small abrasion of the conjunctiva, sclera, or cornea, see "Corneal abrasion," "Treatment/Management" section, above.
→ Administer tetanus immunization as indicated.

Retinal detachment (Silverman, Nunez, and Feller 1992)

→ Refer immediately to an ophthalmologist.

→ See "Treatment/Management" section for consultation and referral.
→ As needed for prescription(s).

→ Advise all patients to wear safety glasses when using hazardous materials and during sporting activities.
→ Teach patient how to instill eye medications properly:
- lie down, both eyes open and looking up.
- slightly retract lower eyelid.
- instill medication into lower eyelid cul-de-sac without touching eye. Look down with eyelid still retracted so eyes do not squeeze shut.
→ Teach patient to apply eye patch properly:
- pressure patches should be applied firmly enough to hold lid against cornea.
- non-pressure patches are laid lightly across eye and secured at forehead and cheek.

Corneal abrasion

→ Instruct patient to call provider in case of sudden redness, pain, or tearing.

Blunt trauma

→ Instruct patient with mild trauma to call provider in case of increased pain or decrease in vision.
→ Advise patients to avoid platelet-inhibiting analgesic products for pain relief (e.g., aspirin).

Corneal abrasion

→ For small abrasions, remove eye patch after 24 to 48 hours. If healing, re-patch and check in 24 hours. If not healing, refer to ophthalmologist.
→ Patient who had a foreign body removed should be examined 24 hours later to assess for secondary infection. Early infection presents with white necrotic area around crater and gray exudate. If infection is present, immediate referral to an ophthalmologist is indicated (Riordan-Eva and Vaughan 1993).
→ Document in progress notes and problem list.

Lisa L. Lommel, R.N., C., F.N.P., M.P.H.

2-G

Glaucoma

Glaucoma is defined as any condition in which intraocular pressure is raised with subsequent damage to the optic nerve and vision loss. The pressure in the eye is maintained by the equilibrium of aqueous humor production and outflow. Elevated intraocular pressure is caused by an increase in production or obstruction to outflow of the aqueous. Elevated intraocular pressure is defined as a pressure greater than 21 mm Hg. This number, however, is not diagnostic for glaucoma as many individuals have elevated pressures and do not develop glaucoma.

The two most common types of *primary glaucoma* are *acute angle-closure glaucoma* and *chronic open-angle glaucoma*. Acute angle-closure glaucoma is uncommon and usually presents as an acute, painful condition. It occurs in individuals who have a narrow anterior chamber usually resulting from an enlarging lens associated with aging. Elevated intraocular pressure is precipitated by the closure of the narrow anterior chamber, causing the iris to obstruct the trabecular mesh work which is necessary to aqueous outflow. Angle closure also is associated with pupillary dilatation secondary to being in a darkened room, stress, or mydriatic or cycloplegic drugs.

An uncontrolled, acute attack of open-angle glaucoma can lead to permanent loss of vision or chronic angle closure. Approximately one-half of patients with acute angle-closure glaucoma will develop the condition in the other eye if prophylactic surgery is not performed.

Chronic open-angle glaucoma is common, accounting for 90 percent of all glaucoma cases. It occurs in one to two percent of the population over age 40 years (Riordan-Eva and Vaughan 1993). Elevated intraocular pressure is thought to be caused by an obstruction in aqueous outflow at the microscopic level of the trabecular

mesh work. The intraocular pressure is consistently elevated and over months or years causes optic nerve atrophy and vision loss. This condition is insidious and often silent, causing extensive damage before the patient is aware of vision loss. Approximately 25 percent of cases are undetected (Riordan-Eva and Vaughan 1993).

Primary glaucoma also may be due to congenital glaucoma which is extremely rare. Secondary glaucoma may develop due to uveitis, neoplasm, lens-induced glaucoma, post-trauma, retinal vein thrombosis, diabetes, or prolonged ophthalmic steroid use (Galloway 1985).

DATABASE

SUBJECTIVE

Acute angle-closure glaucoma

→ Risk groups include:
  ▪ individuals who are *hypermetropic* (farsighted).
  ▪ older individuals who have larger lenses.
  ▪ Asian Americans.

→ Symptoms may include:
  ▪ sudden onset of reddening, pain in eye.
  ▪ headache, usually unilateral.
  ▪ nausea and vomiting.
  ▪ blurred vision, with halos around lights (looking through frosted glass).
  ▪ those often precipitated by pupil dilatation at night, darkened rooms, stress, or mydriatic or cycloplegic drugs.
  ▪ history of similar attacks in the past that subsided after going to sleep (causing pupil constriction).

→ Degree of vision loss depends on extent of corneal edema.

→ If acute episode has resolved, no signs and symptoms may be present: thus, the importance of history. Before an acute attack presents, there may be a long history of sub-acute attacks that resolve spontaneously.

Chronic open-angle glaucoma

→ Risk groups and factors include:
  ▪ males.
  ▪ older individuals.
  ▪ African Americans.
  ▪ diabetics.
  ▪ extreme myopia (shortsightedness).
  ▪ arterial disease, including vascular hypertension, atherosclerotic heart disease, and cerebrovascular disease.
  ▪ family history of glaucoma.
  ▪ history of ocular trauma.

→ Patient is usually asymptomatic until severe damage has occurred.

→ Gradual loss of peripheral vision over years.

→ Halos around lights if intraocular pressure is markedly elevated.

→ Severity of symptoms is related to level of intraocular pressure.

OBJECTIVE

Acute angle-closure glaucoma

→ Patient presents with:
  ▪ reddened eye, hazy cornea.
  ▪ semi-dilated, fixed, unreactive pupil.
  ▪ ciliary injection.
  ▪ affected eye harder and tender to touch.
  ▪ decreased visual acuity.

→ Narrow anterior angle can be identified by shining light parallel to iris plane from temporal side of globe. Eyes with narrow angle will have a shadow fall on nasal iris (may be more effectively done on unaffected eye) (Richter 1995).

Chronic open-angle glaucoma

→ Peripheral visual field and visual acuity loss may be present, but only with severe damage.

→ In early glaucoma, optic disc becomes notched on the supertemporal or inferotemporal rim.

→ Later optic disc changes include:
  ▪ increase in depth and width of physiologic cup.
  ▪ nasal displacement of central retinal vessel.
  ▪ progressive pallor of optic disc head.

→ Asymmetrical disc cupping and hemorrhages are associated signs.

→ Almost always bilateral.

→ Severity of signs are related to level of intraocular pressure.

ASSESSMENT

→ Acute angle-closure glaucoma

→ Chronic open-angle glaucoma

→ R/O conjunctivitis

→ R/O acute uveitis

→ R/O corneal disorders

PLAN

DIAGNOSTIC TESTS

→ The Schiotz Tonometer, used for measuring intraocular pressure, should not be used in the outpatient setting when there is suspicion of acute closed-angle glaucoma. Measurement of pressure should only be attempted by the ophthalmologist.

→ Ophthalmoscopy should be performed on all patients when there is suspicion of glaucoma.

→ The Schiotz Tonometer is the most feasible method of measuring intraocular pressure for the primary care provider when there is no suspicion of acute closed-angle glaucoma. Though mass screening with this method has been found to be inefficient and insensitive (Sommer 1990), other tonometers are available but can be very expensive and require considerable skill to use accurately.

→ Visual field testing with the more sensitive perimetry devices should be completed by the ophthalmologist.

TREATMENT/MANAGEMENT

Acute angle-closure glaucoma

→ Requires urgent referral to an ophthalmologist.

→ Immediate consultation with an ophthalmologist is indicated for treatment before urgent referral. It is usually recommended that pupillary constriction be attempted with (Richter 1995):
  ▪ pilocarpine: 1 drop of 4 percent ophthalmic solution into affected eye every 20 minutes
                    AND
  ▪ acetazolamide (Diamox®) 250 mg by mouth or 500 mg I.V.

→ Treatment of choice is laser iridotomy or surgical peripheral iridotomy. Prophylactic laser iridotomy is indicated in the unaffected eye (Richter 1995).

Chronic open-angle glaucoma

→ Referral to an ophthalmologist is indicated for patients with suspected elevated intraocular pressure (> 21 mm Hg).

→ All primary care providers should be familiar with medications that increase intraocular pressure and use them cautiously (e.g., systemic and topical steroids, drugs with anticholinergic effects).

→ All primary care providers should be familiar with their patient's ocular medications, specifically, their side effects and interactions with other drugs. See *PDR*.

Screening

→ Mass screening efforts have been shown ineffective in detecting glaucoma. Current recommendations include comprehensive eye examinations (by an ophthalmologist) for the asymptomatic individual, based on risk factors of age and race (Sommer 1990):
- Caucasian patients:
  - 20 years to 39 years: once.
  - 40 years to 64 years: every 2 to 4 years.
  - older than 65 years: every 1 to 2 years.
- African American patients:
  - 20 years to 39 years: every 3 to 5 years.
  - 40 years to 64 years: every 2 to 4 years.
  - older than 65 years: every 1 to 2 years.

→ Following are special situations in which referral to an ophthalmologist for complete eye examination or follow-up to control glaucoma is recommended (Sommer 1990):
- any patient aged 40 years to 64 years with:
  - no comprehensive eye examination in the past 2 to 4 years (African American patients should be every 2 years).
  - use of glaucoma medications at any time in the past.

- visual acuity: best eye worse than 20/40, or a difference of greater than two Snellen chart lines between eyes.
- any patient aged 65 years and older:
  - recommendations same as above.
- patients who have additional risk factors (e.g., family history, diabetes, myopia, history of ocular trauma or history of arterial disease) should be referred to an ophthalmologist on a more frequent basis.
- patients with symptoms of glaucoma should be referred immediately to an ophthalmologist.

CONSULTATION

→ See "Treatment/Management" section.

→ As needed for prescription(s).

PATIENT EDUCATION

→ Explain pathophysiology, risk factors, management plan for glaucoma.

→ Explain to asymptomatic patients importance of comprehensive eye examinations (Sommer 1990). See "Screening" in "Treatment/Management" section for recommendations.

→ See "Treatment/Management" section for special situations necessitating referral.

→ Emphasize importance of using ocular medications as prescribed, even if the patient is asymptomatic.

FOLLOW-UP

→ Emphasize importance of follow-up examinations with ophthalmologist.

→ Document in progress notes and problem list.

Lisa L. Lommel, R.N., C., F.N.P., M.P.H.

2-H

Hordeolum and Chalazion

A *hordeolum* is a common staphylococcal abscess of the upper or lower lid margin secondary to inflammation of an eyelash follicle. An internal hordeolum points into the conjunctival surface of the lid. An external abscess (*sty*) is an infection of the glans of Moll or Zeis on the lid margin. Cellulitis is a complication of this condition.

A *chalazion* is a common sterile granulomatous inflammation of a meibomian gland that may follow an internal hordeolum (Riordan-Eva and Vaughan 1993). Characteristically, it is centered away from the lid margin, distinguishing it from a hordeolum.

DATABASE

SUBJECTIVE

Hordeolum

→ Symptoms may include:
- swelling and redness surrounding abscess.
- possible abscess on upper or lower conjunctival surface.
- possible abscess on upper or lower lid margin.
- pain related to amount of swelling.
- increased tearing.

Chalazion

→ Symptoms may include:
- non-tender, hard lump on upper or lower lid.
- conjunctiva possibly red and swollen.
- lesion, which, if large enough, may distort vision.
- increased tearing.

→ Symptoms are commonly multiple and recurrent.

OBJECTIVE

Hordeolum

→ Patient presents with:
- red, swollen, acutely tender abscess on upper or lower lid of conjunctival surface or lid margin.
- external abscesses usually smaller than internal.
- swelling and redness surrounding abscess.
- usually a head of pus present at point of follicle.

Chalazion

→ Patient presents with:
- hard, non-tender swelling of upper or lower lid.
  - May be tender with abscess formation.
  - Conjunctiva may be red and swollen.

ASSESSMENT

→ Hordeolum

→ Chalazion

→ R/O sebaceous cyst

→ R/O molluscum contagiosum

→ R/O basal cell carcinoma

PLAN

DIAGNOSTIC TESTS

→ None

TREATMENT/MANAGEMENT

Hordeolum

→ Clean, warm compresses to affected eye for 15 minutes QID.

→ Bacitracin ophthalmic ointment 500-1000 units/ gram into conjunctival sac every 3 hours for 1 week (Riordan-Eva and Vaughan 1993)

OR

→ Erythromycin (Ilotycin®) ophthalmic ointment 0.5 percent into conjunctival sac every 3 hours for 1 week (Riordan-Eva and Vaughan 1993)

OR

→ Sodium Sulfacetamide 10 percent (10 percent-30 percent ophthalmic solution) (Sodium Sulamyd®) ophthalmic ointment into conjunctival sac TID for 1 week (Zun and Mathews 1988).

→ Referral to physician is indicated for incision if resolution does not begin within 48 hours.

Chalazion

→ Warm compresses for 15 minutes QID may reduce swelling and tenderness if present with small lesion.

→ Referral to an ophthalmologist is indicated for incision and curettage for large lesion causing vision impairment or for cosmetic reasons.

CONSULTATION

→ Referral to a physician is indicated for a hordeolum that has not resolved after 48 hours.

→ Referral to an ophthalmologist is indicated for a chalazion.

→ As needed for prescription(s).

PATIENT EDUCATION

→ Explain pathophysiology, transmission, and treatment plan.

→ Advise patient not to rub, scratch, or touch eye.

→ Advise patient to wash hands well before and after instilling eye ointment.

→ Advise patient not to re-use or share eye ointment.

→ Advise patient to apply clean, warm compresses to affected eye QID.

FOLLOW-UP

→ If hordeolum has not improved after 48 hours of treatment, consider referral to a physician.

→ Recurrent lesions should be referred for biopsy to rule out basal cell carcinoma.

→ Document in progress notes and problem list.

2-1

Keratitis

Keratitis is an inflammation of the corneal stroma caused by bacteria, viruses, fungi, or amoebas. The most common bacterial pathogens invading the cornea are *Pseudomonas aeruginosa*, pneumococcus, *Moraxella* sp., and staphylococcus (Riordan-Eva and Vaughan 1993). Herpes simplex and Herpes zoster are major causes of viral keratitis. *Acanthamoeba* is a common cause of amebic keratitis, especially among contact lens wearers.

Corneal ulcers may occur as a result of corneal infection, though there are several non-infectious causes. Because ineffective treatment of corneal ulcers and corneal infections may lead to corneal scarring and permanent vision loss, immediate referral of patients with these conditions to an ophthalmologist is essential.

DATABASE

SUBJECTIVE

→ Symptoms include pain, photophobia, red eye, tearing, reduced vision, conjunctival discharge.

→ If corneal ulcer is present, patient may have sensation of something in the eye as a result of lid moving over corneal defect.

Bacterial

→ Precipitating factors may include:
- contact lens wear, especially extended wear.
- corneal trauma.
- contaminated medications or fluorescein solution.
- adjacent ocular infection—chronic bacterial conjunctivitis, dacryocystitis.
- disorders reducing natural antimicrobial barrier—severe dry eye, inadequate eyelid closure, severe allergic eye disease, loss of corneal sensation.

Viral

→ Herpes simplex characterized by:
- recurrences precipitated by stress, fever, sunlight exposure, menstruation (see **Genital Herpes Simplex Virus** Protocol).

→ Herpes zoster characterized by:
- malaise, fever, headache, burning, itching in periorbital region.
- vesicular rash becoming pustular then crusting.
- rash involving tip of nose or lid margin indicates high likelihood of intraocular involvement (Riordan-Eva and Vaughan 1993)
- ocular symptoms include those of conjunctivitis, anterior uveitis, episcleritis (see **Conjunctivitis, Uveitis, Varicella Zoster Virus** protocols).

Fungal

→ Precipitating factors may include:
- corneal injury from plant material or in agricultural setting.
- immunocompromised individuals.

Amebic

→ Precipitating factors may include:
- contact lens wear.
- homemade saline solutions (for cleaning contact lenses).

→ Eye pain may be severe.

OBJECTIVE

→ Patient may present with:
- red eye with circumcorneal injection.
- purulent or watery discharge.

→ Corneal ulcer may present as gray, necrotic area.

→ With history of trauma, eye should be examined for presence of foreign body.

Bacterial

→ Patient may present with:
- cornea hazy with central ulcer and adjacent stromal abscess.
- pus seen in anterior chamber in front of iris and behind cornea (*hypopyon*).

Viral

→ Patient may present with:
- herpes simplex characterized by:
  - *dendritic* (branching) ulcer.
  - "geographic" ulcers if topical steroid is used.
- herpes zoster characterized by:
  - ocular signs include those of conjunctivitis, anterior uveitis, episcleritis (see **Conjunctivitis, Uveitis, Varicella Zoster Virus** protocols).

Fungal

→ Patient may present with multiple stromal abscesses.

Amebic

→ Patient may present with perineural and ring infiltrates in the corneal stroma.

→ Earlier changes confined to the corneal epithelium may be present.

ASSESSMENT

→ Keratitis
- R/O bacterial
- R/O viral
- R/O fungal
- R/O amebic
- R/O corneal ulcer

PLAN

DIAGNOSTIC TESTS

→ Visual acuity should be measured.

→ Slit-lamp examination may be performed with fluorescein staining, though this test is usually reserved for the ophthalmologist.

→ Further testing and cultures should be completed by an ophthalmologist.

TREATMENT/MANAGEMENT

→ Immediate referral to an ophthalmologist is indicated.

CONSULTATION

→ Immediate referral to an ophthalmologist is indicated in all cases of corneal infection or ulcer.

→ As needed for prescription(s).

PATIENT EDUCATION

→ Teach patient regarding pathophysiology, risk factors, and management plan for keratitis.

→ Advise patient that a delay in or inadequate treatment of keratitis could lead to permanent vision loss.

→ Advise patient to follow treatment plan from the ophthalmologist carefully.

→ Advise patients with herpes simplex:
- to avoid steroid medication which may increase viral activity.
- that recurrences are common and to avoid activities that may precipitate a herpes outbreak.

→ See **Genital Herpes Simplex Virus** and **Varicella Zoster Virus** protocols.

FOLLOW-UP

→ Document in progress notes and problem list.

Lisa L. Lommel, R.N., C., F.N.P., M.P.H.

2-J

Pinguecula and Pterygium

Pinguecula is an elevated nodule on either side of the cornea at the limbus. Caused by hyperplasia of yellow elastic tissue, it is more common on the nasal side and in persons over 35 years of age.

Pterygium is a triangular, vascularized, hyperplastic process occurring medially where the bulbar conjunctiva encroaches on the cornea. Predisposing factors to pterygium include genetic predisposition and chronic exposure to ultraviolet radiation, wind, and dust (Hill and Maske 1989).

DATABASE

SUBJECTIVE

Pinguecula

→ Patient is usually asymptomatic.
  ▪ Though may present with signs of inflammation, redness, tearing, and tenderness.
→ Nodule rarely increases in size.

Pterygium

→ Patient is usually asymptomatic.
  ▪ Though may notice visual disturbance if nodule is encroaching on pupillary area.

OBJECTIVE

Pinguecula

→ Patient presents with:
  ▪ yellow, elevated nodule on either side of cornea.
  ▪ redness and tenderness.

Pterygium

→ Patient presents with pale yellow, pink, or white triangular, thin nodule on nasal side of cornea.

→ Recent or progressive lesion may be thick and vascular.
→ Opaque zone preceding tip of lesion indicates activity.

ASSESSMENT

→ Pinguecula
→ Pterygium
→ R/O corneal ulceration

PLAN

DIAGNOSTIC TESTS

→ Corneal staining to exclude ulceration may be indicated (Jackson and Finlay 1991).

TREATMENT/MANAGEMENT

Pinguecula

→ Benign, not requiring treatment.
→ Excision may be desired for cosmetic purposes.

Pterygium

→ Usually requires no treatment.
→ Excision may be indicated if it is interfering with vision.

CONSULTATION

→ Referral to an ophthalmologist for excision of a pinguecula or pterygium.

PATIENT EDUCATION

→ Explain pathophysiology and treatment plan.

→ Explain that discomfort usually follows excision of a pterygium.

→ Advise individuals who spend a large amount of time outdoors to wear protective glasses.

FOLLOW-UP

→ Advise patient that recurrence is common after pterygium excision.

→ Document in progress notes and problem list.

2-K

Uveitis

Uveitis is inflammation of the uveal tract which includes the iris, ciliary body, and choroid. Uveitis occurs as *anterior, intermediate*, and *posterior uveitis*. The patient may also experience *panuveitis*, which includes inflammation in all three areas.

Anterior uveitis involves inflammation of the iris and ciliary body (*iridocyclitis*). This condition is divided into *granulomatous* or *nongranulomatous uveitis* depending on the type of keratotic precipitate seen on examination. Anterior uveitis due to a traumatic etiology commonly acute can be caused by direct penetrating trauma to the eye, including operative procedures or spread of adjacent or systemic infection (Yanofsky 1988). Non-traumatic anterior uveitis can be acute, subacute, or chronic. In the majority of patients with anterior uveitis, there is no identifiable cause.

Anterior uveitis is associated with a variety of systemic diseases including ankylosing spondylitis, psoriatic arthritis, Reiter's syndrome, Behçet's syndrome, inflammatory bowel disease, sarcoidosis, and a variety of chronic infections including herpes simplex, herpes zoster, syphilis, tuberculosis, toxoplasmosis, histoplasmosis, and gonorrhea (Yanofsky 1988).

Intermediate uveitis indicates that the most intense inflammation is in the vitreous. *Posterior uveitis* involves inflammation of the choroid. Like anterior uveitis, there is often no identifiable cause. There are several systemic conditions that have been associated with posterior uveitis. These include toxoplasmosis, tuberculosis, sarcoidosis, histoplasmosis, syphilis, Behçet's syndrome, Vogt-Koyanagi-Harada syndrome, autoimmune retinal vasculitis, and pars planitis (Galloway 1985; Riordan-Eva and Vaughan 1993).

Complications of uveitis include corneal decompensation, glaucoma, cataracts, vitreous opacities, vitreous hemorrhages, optic atrophy, and cystoid macular edema—all of which are sight-threatening (Bienfang et al. 1990).

DATABASE

SUBJECTIVE

→ Patients may have signs and symptoms of uveitis either as the presenting manifestation of a systemic disease as outlined above or as a part of a constellation of symptoms.
  ▪ If a patient presents with uveitis, consultation should be sought for evaluation of systemic disease.

→ See specific protocols as they relate to associated systemic diseases as outlined above.

→ Anterior uveitis due to trauma presents with:
  ▪ history of trauma.
  ▪ acute onset of pain localized to periorbital area.
  ▪ decreased vision.

→ Non-traumatic anterior uveitis may present with (Yanofsky 1988):
  ▪ superficial burning or stinging pain progressing to deep-seated ache.
  ▪ pain when focusing on near objects.
  ▪ photophobia.
  ▪ decreased vision.

→ Posterior uveitis most often presents with blurring and/or loss of vision.

OBJECTIVE

→ Patients may have signs and symptoms of uveitis either as the presenting manifestation of a systemic disease as outlined above or as a part of a constellation of symptoms. It is recommended:
  ▪ if a patient presents with uveitis, consultation should be sought for evaluation of systemic disease.

→ See specific protocols as they relate to associated systemic diseases as outlined above.

→ Traumatic anterior uveitis presents with tenderness and redness of the conjunctivae, perilimbal area, and surrounding tissues.

→ Non-traumatic anterior uveitis may present with (Yanofsky 1988):
  ▪ small, irregular, poorly reactive pupil.
  ▪ red eye.
  ▪ inflammation into the peripheral cornea (pink flush) due to limbal circulation.
  ▪ cloudy anterior chamber upon slit-lamp examination.
  ▪ inflammatory cells suspended in aqueous humor, visible with magnification.
  ▪ cells on corneal endothelium (i.e., keratic precipitates) with smaller iris nodules (nongranulomatous disease).
  ▪ larger keratic precipitates known as "mutton fat" keratic precipitates with larger iris nodules (granulomatous disease).

→ Posterior uveitis may present with:
  ▪ usually a white eye (not red).
  ▪ grey or yellowish raised area, single or multiple on fundus.
  ▪ extensive inflammation causing vitreous humor to be cloudy, preventing visualization of fundus.
  ▪ inflammatory cells in the vitreous seen on slit-lamp examination.

ASSESSMENT

→ Uveitis, anterior and/or posterior
→ R/O trauma
→ R/O conjunctivitis
→ R/O episcleritis
→ R/O systemic disease

PLAN

DIAGNOSTIC TESTS

→ Diagnosis is usually made on clinical grounds by an ophthalmologist.

→ Slit-lamp examination may be helpful to evaluate extent of disease.

→ Chest, skull, and sinus x-rays, and erythrocyte sedimentation rate (ESR), VDRL, and FTA-ABS tests may be considered with the initial work-up.

→ A variety of diagnostic tests may be indicated to rule out concomitant systemic disease.

TREATMENT/MANAGEMENT

→ Immediate referral to an ophthalmologist is warranted in all cases of uveitis.

CONSULTATION

→ Consultation is warranted to rule out concomitant systemic disease. See this protocol's introductory discussion of specific diseases, p. 2-28.

→ Immediate referral to an ophthalmologist is warranted in all cases of uveitis.

PATIENT EDUCATION

→ Explain pathophysiology and treatment of uveitis.

→ Explain pathophysiology of concomitant systemic disease as indicated.

FOLLOW-UP

→ Document in progess notes and problem list.

2-L
Bibliography

Benson, W.H., and Lanier, J.D. 1992. The red eye: Avoiding pitfalls from topical ocular therapy. *The West Virginia Medical Journal* 88:6–8.

Bienfang, D.C., Kelly, L.D., Nicholson, D.H., and Nussenblatt, R.B. 1990. Ophthalmology. *The New England Journal of Medicine* 323(14):956–967.

Christen, W.G., Manson, J.E., Seddon, J.M., Glynn, R.J., Buring, J.E., Rosner, B., and Hennekens, C.H. 1992. A prospective study of cigarette smoking and risk of cataract in men. *Journal of the American Medical Association* 268(8):989–993.

Ehlers, W.H., and Donshik, P.C. 1992. Allergic ocular disorders: A spectrum of diseases. *The Contact Lens Associations of Ophthalmologists Journal* 18(2):117–124.

Elkington, A.R., and Khaw, P.T. 1988. *ABC of eyes.* London: British Medical Association.

Galloway, N.R. 1985. *Common eye diseases and their management.* Berlin: Springer-Verlag.

Greenberg, D.A. 1995. Evaluation of dry eyes. In *Primary care medicine*, eds. A.H. Goroll, L.A. May, and A.G. Gulley, pp. 845–847. Philadelphia: J.B. Lippincott.

Hankinson, S.E., Willett, W.C., Colditz, G.A., Seddon, J.M., Rosner, B., Speizer, F.E., and Stampfer, M.J. 1992. A prospective study of cigarette smoking and risk of cataract surgery in women. *Journal of the American Medical Association* 268(8):994–998.

Hill, J.C., and Maske, R. 1989. Pathogenesis of pterygium. *Eye* 3:218–226.

Howes, D.S. 1988. The red eye. *Emergency Medicine Clinics of North America* 6(1):43–56.

Jackson, C.R.S., and Finlay, R.D. 1991. *The eye in general practice.* Edinburgh: Churchill Livingstone, Inc.

Richter, C.U. 1995. Management of glaucoma. In *Primary care medicine*, eds. A.H. Goroll, L.A. May, and A.G. Gulley, pp. 852–854. Philadelphia: J.B. Lippincott.

Riordan-Eva, P., and Vaughan, D.G. 1993. Eye. In *Current medical diagnosis and treatment*, eds. L.M. Tierney, S.J. McPhee, M.A. Papadakis, and S.A. Schroeder. East Norwalk, CT: Appleton & Lange.

Roy, H., and Tindall, R. 1991. An update in the use of drugs for common eye problems in older patients. *Geriatrics* 46(11):51–60.

Silverman, H., Nunez, L., and Feller, D.B. 1992. Treatment of common eye emergencies. *American Family Physician* 45(5):2279–2287.

Sommer, A. 1990, September/October Glaucoma screening: Too little, too late? *Journal of General Internal Medicine.* 5(Suppl.):S33–S37.

University of California at Berkeley Wellness Letter. 1993. 9(4):1–8.

Wilhelmus, K.R. 1988. The red eye. *Infectious Disease Clinics of North America* 2(1):99–116.

Yanofsky, N.N. 1988. The acute painful eye. *Emergency Medicine Clinics of North America* 6(1):21–42.

Zun, L.S., and Mathews, J. 1988. Formulary of commonly used ophthalmologic medication. *Emergency Medicine Clinics of North America* 6(1):121–126.

SECTION 3

Dermatological Disorders

Jan M. Reddick, M.S., F.N.P.
Maureen Shannon, C.N.M., F.N.P., M.S.

3-A

Acne Vulgaris

Acne is an inflammation of the sebaceous hair follicles *(pilosebaceous units)*. Acne, the most common skin condition, usually begins at puberty, but the onset may not occur until the third or fourth decade of a person's life (Goldstein and Odom 1994). The actual etiology of acne is unknown, but a genetic predisposition to the effects of androgens is a proposed theory.

The inflammatory process occurs with the presence and interaction of several different factors. Under the stimulation of androgens, the sebaceous glands produce sebum, which—together with fatty acids and bacteria—cause a sterile inflammatory response in the pilosebaceous unit. The collection of this material within the sebaceous glands eventually obstructs the follicular duct and results in hyperkeratinization and plugging. The resultant visible skin lesion is known as a *closed comedone* or *whitehead*.

When whiteheads mature and expand so as to provide a portal of entry at the skin, the keratin, sebum, and bacteria mixture forms a plug, which oxidizes, turns black, and then becomes a *blackhead*. If the distended follicular duct wall ruptures into the surrounding dermis, there is an inflammatory foreign body response to the irritating sebum mixture. The resulting lesions are *papules, pustules, nodules,* and suppurative nodules known, mistakenly, as *cystic acne* (Fitzpatrick et al. 1992; Orkin, Maibach, and Dahl 1991).

Certain factors can aggravate acne—medications (e.g., corticosteroids, oral contraceptives, antibiotics), oil-based skin products, emotional stress, and mechanical irritation (e.g., pressure on skin). Although acne is commonly associated with adolescence, if left untreated it may persist for several decades. Eventually, most untreated acne will resolve, but it may lead to scarring, cyst

formation, pigment changes, and psychological problems (Goldstein and Odom 1994).

Classifying acne according to its various clinical manifestations helps determine effective therapeutic interventions. The presence of comedones constitutes noninflammatory acne. Papules, pustules, and pitted or keloid scarring are classified as inflammatory acne.

Further delineation of acne based upon the severity of the condition provides additional guidelines for management using the following criteria: 1) *mild acne*—presence of <10 lesions without scarring; 2) *moderate acne*—presence of 10 to 25 lesions with possible scarring; and 3) *severe acne*—presence of >25 lesions with possible scarring (Berger, Elias, and Wintroub 1990; Orkin, Maibach, and Dahl 1991).

DATABASE

SUBJECTIVE

→ Acne vulgaris:
- primarily affects adolescents.
- is more severe in men (Fitzpatrick et al. 1992; Orkin, Maibach, and Dahl 1991).
- may persist in women to age 35 years (Fitzpatrick et al. 1992).
- may involve:
  - exposure to medications that exacerbate acne including: lithium, bromides, iodides, hydantoin, corticosteroids, and oral contraceptives with high androgenic activity (Fitzpatrick et al. 1992; Orkin, Maibach, and Dahl 1991).
  - history of use of oily skin products.

- history of emotional stress.
- compulsive face washing.
  - may involve chronic antibiotic treatment (causing superimposed gram-negative infection) (Fitzpatrick et al. 1992).
→ Pressure on skin (e.g., leaning on face with hands, chin straps) may aggravate lesions.
→ Lesions may be worse in fall and winter.
→ Lesions may be mildly painful and pruritic.

OBJECTIVE

→ Lesions observed primarily on face and trunk.
→ Lesions may be isolated, scattered discrete, or coalescent (Berger, Elias, and Wintroub 1990).
→ Acne caused by corticosteroids usually presents as papulopustular lesions with absence of comedones (Orkin, Maibach, and Dahl 1991).

Noninflammatory acne

→ Comedones are:
  - open = blackheads.
  - closed = whiteheads.

Inflammatory acne

→ Papules are:
  - < 0.5 cm diameter.
  - with or without inflammation.
→ Nodules are:
  - 0.5-2 cm diameter.
  - deep.
→ Pustules are:
  - filled with pus.
  - superficial.
→ Scars are:
  - atrophic depressed (pitted).
  - hypertrophic (keloid).

ASSESSMENT

→ Acne (inflammatory, noninflammatory; mild, moderate, or severe)
→ R/O chronic folliculitis
→ R/O acne rosacea
→ R/O drug eruption
→ R/O contact dermatitis
→ R/O perioral dermatitis
→ R/O adenoma sebaceum (rare)
→ R/O acne fulminans (systemic signs and symptoms, fever, arthralgia, and leukocytosis (Orkin, Maibach, and Dahl 1991).

PLAN

DIAGNOSTIC TESTS

→ No specific diagnostic tests are recommended to confirm this condition. However, the following tests may be ordered in severe pustular forms of acne:
  - gram stain to identify a possible pathogen.
  - culture and sensitivity of pustular lesion drainage to confirm presence of a pathogen and any resistant strains of organisms.

TREATMENT/MANAGEMENT

→ The treatment of acne spans several months. Once a good response occurs, treatment should be continued for (at least) another 3 months.
→ Tapering of medications can begin by decreasing both the dose and strength of agents used.
   NOTE: Variations of drug strengths and dosages appear throughout this protocol. If tapering is to begin, the clinician can refer to the specific therapeutic agents listed within each part of the "Treatment/Management" section.

Noninflammatory acne

→ Topical retinoic acid (tretinoin, Retin-A®). Begin with low-strength 0.025 percent gel or 0.025 percent cream every other day at bedtime. After 1 month, increase to every day. Advance to higher concentrations as tolerated (0.01 percent gel or 0.05-0.1 percent cream). Use gels for oily skin and creams for dry skin (creams are less irritating).
  - Improvement may not be noticed for 2 to 5 months.
  - Warn client of local irritation and potential photosensitivity. Recommend sunscreen (noncomedogenic, non-oily).
  - Acne may flare after 2 to 3 weeks of tretinoin therapy. Resolution should occur within 6 to 8 weeks (Berger, Elias, and Wintroub 1990; Fitzpatrick et al. 1992; Orkin, Maibach, and Dahl 1991).
→ Topical therapy with antibacterial agents can have an anti-inflammatory as well as an antimicrobial effect.
  - Clindamycin 1 percent (Cleocin®) lotion or gel applied to lesions every day to BID for several weeks to months (to years).
  - Erythromycin 2 percent (Erycette®) topical solution applied to lesions every day to BID for several weeks to months (to years).

→ Benzoyl peroxide 2 percent-10 percent gels or solutions (Acne Dome®, Brevoxyl®, Xerac BP®), applied to lesions every day to BID for several weeks to months (to years), may be helpful in reducing inflammation but should be discontinued if irritation develops (Orkin, Maibach, and Dahl 1991).

Moderate inflammatory acne

→ Treatment measures combine the above therapeutic interventions with systemic antibiotic therapy, including one of the following:
- tetracycline (Achromycin®) 500 mg p.o. BID for several weeks to months.
- erythromycin (E-Mycin®, Ery-Tab®) 500 mg p.o. BID for several weeks to months.
- minocycline (Minocin®) 50 mg-100 mg p.o. BID for several weeks to months.
  NOTE: Warn patient about possible side effects of medications (e.g., vertigo with minocycline; vaginal candidiasis when systemic antibiotics are used) and contraindication for use of tetracycline during pregnancy.

→ Oral contraceptives with low androgenic activity (e.g., Demulen® 1/35, Ovcon® 1/35) can be used in women, provided there are no contraindications to their use (Berger, Elias, and Wintroub 1990).

Severe inflammatory acne

→ Refer to dermatologist for treatment. Isotretinoin (Accutane®) may be prescribed by the physician for treatment of severe, recalcitrant cystic acne. **NOTE:** Accutane is teratogenic; a woman should not become pregnant while taking this drug.

→ Intralesional injections of corticosteroids and dermabrasion may also be employed by the physician for the treatment of severe acne.

CONSULTATION

→ Physician referral for evaluation and treatment of severe acne.

→ Physician consultation is indicated in any patient with adverse reactions to medications or with acne unresponsive to appropriate therapeutic interventions.

→ As needed for prescription(s).

PATIENT EDUCATION

→ Educate the patient about acne, including its cause, clinical course, treatment (especially length of treatment), possible side effects of treatment, and follow-up.

→ Advise patients that at least four to six weeks of therapy will be required to notice improvement. Encourage them not to abandon any new treatment regimen sooner than after one month (Berger, Elias, and Wintroub 1990; Fitzpatrick et al. 1992).

→ Educate patient to wash the affected area(s) twice a day with a washcloth and non-creamy soap (e.g., Dial®, Neutrogena®) (Sauer 1991).

→ Advise patient to wait ten to thirty minutes after washing to apply tretinoin (less irritation develops if tretinoin is applied to *dry* skin) (Goldstein and Odom 1994; Orkin, Maibach, and Dahl 1991).

→ Advise patient to avoid moisturizers—e.g., Vaseline®, baby oil, and Oil of Olay®—since these products can aggravate acne. Nutraderm® and Moisturel® lotions can be used for dryness.

→ Advise patient that makeup should be oil-free and water-based.

→ Advise that picking of comedones and pustules should be avoided. Healing is facilitated and scarring minimized only if these are properly removed by the health care provider (Sauer 1991).

→ Because tetracycline may increase skin's sensitivity to sunlight, dosage may be lowered or drug discontinued four days prior to travel to sunny area (Sauer 1991). In addition, tetracycline should not be taken if a woman is pregnant because it stains fetal teeth after 20 weeks gestation.

→ Some antibiotics (e.g., tetracycline) may decrease efficacy of oral contraceptives, so an additional form of birth control (e.g., condoms) may be advised (Berger, Elias, and Wintroub 1990).

→ Advise patient to watch for black macules at sites of acne lesions since this may indicate gram-negative folliculitis.

→ There is controversy regarding the role of diet in acne. Explain that foods may or may not be acne precipitants. Some authorities feel that chocolate, nuts, whole milk products, fatty meats, and spicy foods aggravate acne (Sauer 1991).

FOLLOW-UP

→ Individualized according to case presentation.

→ See "Treatment/Management" and "Consultation" sections.

→ Document in progress notes and problem list.

Jan M. Reddick, M.S., F.N.P.

Maureen Shannon, C.N.M., F.N.P., M.S.

3-B

Atopic Dermatitis (Atopic Eczema)

Atopic dermatitis is a chronic or chronically relapsing pruritic inflammation of the epidermis and dermis, usually occurring in patients who have a hereditary predisposition to atopic disease (Fitzpatrick et al. 1992; Orkin, Maibach, and Dahl 1991). Although the role of IgE antibodies is not clear, there exists in atopic dermatitis an IgE-mediated hypersensitivity reaction from vasoactive substances released by mast cells and basophils. These substances have been sensitized by the interaction of an antigen with IgE (Fitzpatrick et al. 1992).

One of the major symptoms of atopic dermatitis is pruritus. The associated scratching is the cause of the characteristic lichenification of the skin, which is pathognomonic of atopic dermatitis (Fitzpatrick et al. 1992; Orkin, Maibach, and Dahl 1991). Additional criteria indicating atopic dermatitis rather than other types of dermatitis include: xerosis-ichthyosis-hyperlineal palms, facial pallor, intraorbital darkening, Dennie Morgan intraorbital fold, *keratosis pilaris* (chronic inflammation of the skin surrounding hair follicles), *pityriasis alba* (scaling and atrophy of skin), elevated serum IgE, a tendency toward recurrent skin infections, and nonspecific hand dermatitis (Goldstein and Odom 1994).

DATABASE

SUBJECTIVE

→ Patient may report rough, red patches of skin on face, neck, upper trunk, and at bends of elbows and knees.

→ Black individuals may report a decreased pigmentation associated with chronic irritation around the wrists and ankles (Goldstein and Odom 1993).

→ Severe pruritus may be precipitated by wool, detergents, soaps, a change in room temperature, or stress.

→ Affected individuals will report history of condition from early childhood (60 percent incidence of onset is by age one year).

→ Family history of atopy (e.g., asthma, allergic rhinitis, atopic dermatitis) (Fitzpatrick et al. 1992).

→ May report a tendency toward cutaneous infections (especially *Staphylococcus aureus* and herpes simplex) (Orkin, Maibach, and Dahl 1991). These infections may trigger fresh exacerbations of the dermatitis (Berger, Elias, and Wintroub 1990).

OBJECTIVE

→ Facial pallor common.

→ Infraorbital folds often present.

→ White *dermatographism* (i.e., with firm stroking of the skin, the area stroked turns white) in 80 percent of patients.

→ Orbital darkening ("allergic shiner") may be present.

→ *Keratoconus* (i.e., cone-shaped cornea) (Orkin, Maibach, and Dahl 1991) may be present.

→ Decreased pigment in areas of lichenification may be evident in black individuals.

→ Lesions may be present:
  - erythema, papules, pustules, erosions, dry and wet crusts, fissures, excoriations, lichenified plaques.

- usually confluent and ill-defined.
- distribution may be generalized on flexor areas, neck, eyelids, lips, forehead, nipples, and dorsa of feet and hands (Fitzpatrick et al. 1992).

ASSESSMENT

- → Atopic dermatitis
- → R/O contact dermatitis
- → R/O superimposed bacterial infection
- → R/O gluten-sensitive enteropathy
- → R/O hyper IgE syndrome
- → R/O selective IgA deficiency
- → R/O herpes simplex virus infection

PLAN

DIAGNOSTIC TESTS

→ Laboratory tests are not routinely ordered but may be indicated in some cases (e.g., significant bacterial infection). The following tests may be ordered as indicated:
  - serum IgE (may be increased).
  - culture and sensitivity for bacteria and culture for herpes.
  - complete blood count (CBC) (may reveal eosinophilia).

TREATMENT/MANAGEMENT

→ General measures include reducing irritation by:
  - bathing, with the use of soap, only once a day and only in the axillary region, groin, and feet. Brushes and washcloths should not be used.
  - use of nondrying soap (e.g., Dove®, Aveeno®, Alpha Keri®, Basis®).
  - after bathing, patting dry (do not rub) using a soft towel. Application of a thin emollient film of Eucerin®, mineral oil, Nivea®, or Vaseline® on body (except for face) is recommended.
  - wearing clothing made of nonirritating fabrics (i.e., avoid wool, acrylics) and fabrics that can breathe (e.g., cotton).
→ Initial treatment (for acute inflammation):
  - weeping lesions should be treated by applying astringent compresses of Burow's solution (Domeboro®, Bluboro®) or colloidal oatmeal (Aveeno®) to the lesions for 10 to 30 minutes 2 to 4 times/day.
  - high-potency topical steroid lotion or cream (not ointment) should be applied to the lesions after the astringent compress/bath treatment.

Recommended fluorinated steroid preparations include:
  - fluocinonide 0.05 percent (Lidex®) cream—thin coating applied to lesion(s) BID until acute inflammation resolves.
  - halcinonide 0.1 percent (Halog®) cream—thin coating applied to lesion(s) BID until acute inflammation resolves.
  - see also **Table 12TB.1, Potency Ranking of Topical Corticosteroids,** p. 12-228.
    NOTE: Avoid use of fluorinated topical steroids on the face.
- systemic antihistamines will reduce associated pruritus:
  - hydroxyzine (Atarax®) 10 mg-50 mg p.o. every 6 hours prn.
  - diphenhydramine (Benadryl®) 25 mg-50 mg p.o. every 6 hours prn.
    NOTE: Advise patient about associated drowsiness and the need to avoid activities requiring concentration (e.g., driving).
- secondary bacterial infection can be treated with either local or systemic antimicrobials, depending upon extent and severity of symptoms.
  - topical treatment:
    –mupirocin 2 percent (Bactroban®) ointment applied to infected lesions TID for 10 days.
  - systemic treatment:
    –dicloxacillin (Dynapen®) 250 mg-500 mg p.o. QID for 10 days.
    –erythromycin (E-Mycin®) 250 mg-500 mg p.o. QID for 10 days.
→ subsequent therapy (subacute or chronic stages):
  - continue systemic antihistamines as needed.
  - compresses are no longer needed but daily colloidal oatmeal baths may promote hydration.
  - reduce topical corticosteroid agent from high-potency to mid-potency agents in ointment form, such as:
    - triamcinolone acetonide 0.1 percent (Aristocort®, Kenalog®) applied BID to affected area(s).
    - betamethasone dipropionate 0.05 percent (Diprosone®) applied BID to affected areas.
    - See **Table 12TB.1,** p. 12-228.
  - therapy should continue until pruritus, scaling, and elevated skin lesions resolve. Patients should then begin to taper from BID to daily, then to alternate day use over the next 2 to 4 weeks to avoid tachyphylaxis.

CONSULTATION

→ Physician consultation is indicated for any patient with extensive involvement (since systemic corticosteroids may be needed), resistant episodes, or with severe secondary bacterial infection.

→ As needed for prescription(s).

PATIENT EDUCATION

→ Educate the patient about atopic dermatitis including the cause, clinical course, treatment, possible complications, side effects of medications, and indicated follow-up.

→ Warn patient about sedating effects of antihistamines and need to avoid activities requiring concentration (e.g., driving).

→ Advise patient to avoid known irritants (e.g., wool and acrylic clothing).

→ Advise patient to avoid rubbing and scratching affected areas.

→ Advise patient to trim nails to avoid excoriation.

→ Advise patient to use soaps that are nondrying (e.g., Dove®, Aveeno®, Eucerin®). The patient should only use soap on axilla, groin, and feet.

→ Advise patient to avoid frequent baths because of their drying effect on skin.

→ Advise patient to avoid lotions and creams that can exacerbate underlying dry skin conditions.

→ Recommend a cool-air humidifier, which can be especially helpful during the winter.

→ Suggest evening primrose oil (contains γ-linolenic acid) which may help severe atopic dermatitis (Berger, Elias, and Wintroub 1990).

→ Discuss methods to reduce stress.

→ See "Treatment/Management" section.

FOLLOW-UP

→ Individualized according to case presentation.

→ See "Consultation" section.

→ Document in progress notes and problem list.

Jan M. Reddick, M.S., F.N.P.
Maureen Shannon, C.N.M., F.N.P., M.S.

3-C

Burns—Minor

Thermal burns are classified according to the depth of tissue damage. First- and second-degree burns will be covered in this section.

First-degree burns are the result of damage to the epidermis. The release of histamines, kinins, prostaglandins, and other mediators leading to vasodilation and edema are responsible for the clinical manifestations associated with first-degree burns. Recovery is usually quick and there is no blistering.

Second-degree burns result from damage to the epidermis and variable levels of the dermis. Blistering is common. Recovery usually takes one to three weeks (Orkin, Maibach, and Dahl 1991). Reepithelization is dependent upon vascularization of the damaged area(s); rapid healing and minimal or no scarring occurs in areas with good circulation (Goldstein and Odom 1993). Secondary bacterial infections may convert a partial-thickness second-degree burn to a full-thickness burn (Goldstein and Odom 1993).

When assessing burns, it is essential to determine the amount of body surface affected by the burn as well as the level of skin traumatized. For adults, the *rule of nines* can be used to assess the extent of the burn rapidly, dividing the surface area of the body as follows: head, neck, and each upper extremity is 90 percent; anterior torso, posterior torso, and each lower extremity is 90 percent; and the perineum is 1 percent (Littler and Momany 1990).

DATABASE

SUBJECTIVE

→ Pain is present (**NOTE**: absence of pain is more indicative of third-degree burn).

→ There is erythema of exposed area. Blistering may be reported in second-degree burn.

→ Patient has history of exposure to sun or heat.

OBJECTIVE

First-Degree burn

→ Blanches with pressure.

→ Erythematous, smooth skin.

→ No blisters.

Second-Degree burn

→ Red, pink, or white thickened skin.

→ Blisters common.

ASSESSMENT

→ First-degree burn

→ Second-degree burn

→ R/O third-degree burn

→ Evaluate percentage of body affected

→ R/O secondary bacterial infection

PLAN

DIAGNOSTIC TESTS

→ No specific diagnostic tests are indicated for the diagnosis or management of uncomplicated minor burns covering ≤ 5 percent of the body.

TREATMENT/MANAGEMENT

First- and Second-Degree burn

→ Immediate management:
- immerse burned area in cool or room-temperature water or saline solution—immediately after the burn has occurred—for up to 20 minutes to reduce further damage. Avoid prolonged application of cold water or ice packs to large surfaces (possible causes of hypothermia or arrhythmias).
- remove clothing in contact with the area.
- if melted synthetics, tar, or molten metal are in contact with the area, cool this/these substance(s) as rapidly as possible and do not remove immediately after the injury because of possibility of increasing tissue damage and depth of injury.

First-Degree burn

→ Will usually resolve within a few days and require minimal treatment.

→ Topical corticosteroid therapy with low-potency agents can be initiated, with one of the following:
- hydrocortisone 1 percent (Hytone®) cream or ointment applied to affected area BID for 1 to 2 days.
- dexamethasone 0.1 percent (Decaderm®) gel applied to affected area BID for 1 to 2 days.

→ Aspirin or acetaminophen can be used for analgesia.

Second-Degree burn

→ Apply a topical antibacterial cream (e.g., 1 percent silver sulfadiazine [Silvadene®], mafenide [Sulfamylon®]) to area and cover with a sterile dressing TID–QID.

NOTE: Sulfa preparations are contraindicated in patients who are pregnant, have G6PD deficiency, or a history of hypersensitivity to the particular drug (Littler and Momany 1990). Mafenide use should be limited to no more than 10 percent of total body surface because of its metabolic effects (Cohen 1994).

→ Prophylactic systemic antibiotics usually are not recommended, regardless of the severity of the burn (Cohen 1994).

→ Administer tetanus/diphtheria (Td) booster to patients who have completed the initial immunization series and whose last Td injection was more than 5 years ago.

→ In patients with unknown tetanus immunization status or incomplete initial immunization series, human tetanus immune globulin (TIG) is indicated for passive immunization. These patients should also receive Td to initiate the active immunization series (CDC 1991). Consultation with a physician is indicated in such situations (Orkin, Maibach, and Dahl 1991).

→ Aspirin or acetaminophen can be used for analgesia.

→ Deep second-degree burns which do not heal in 7 to 10 days with local measures usually require excision and autograft (Cohen 1994). Refer to physician.

CONSULTATION

→ Physician consultation is warranted in any patient with more than five percent of her body affected, with unknown Td immunization status, with evidence of infection, or with burns(s) that do not heal.

→ As needed for prescription(s).

PATIENT EDUCATION

→ Instruct patient in care of the burn.

→ Discuss signs of infection and instruct patient to return for follow-up if infection occurs.

→ Educate patient with history of sunburn about risks associated with overexposure (e.g., skin cancer, melanoma) and ways to decrease exposure with use of sunblock.

→ If patient experienced thermal burn because of accidental exposure (e.g., cooking accident, accidental spill), educate about ways to prevent similar accidents, especially when small children are around.

FOLLOW-UP

→ See "Consultation" section.

→ For individuals with second-degree burns, follow-up evaluation in 24 to 48 hours.

→ Document in progress notes and problem list.

Jan M. Reddick, M.S., F.N.P.
Maureen Shannon, C.N.M., F.N.P., M.S.

3-D

Cellulitis

Cellulitis is a diffuse, spreading infection of the dermis and subcutaneous tissue (Fitzpatrick et al. 1992; Orkin, Maibach, and Dahl 1991). It can occur either as a primary condition or as a complication to a preexisting dermatosis (e.g., tinea pedis, stasis ulcer) (Berger, Elias, and Wintroub 1990).

An increased risk of cellulitis is seen among injection drug users and persons with diabetes mellitus, hematologic malignancies, chronic lymphedema, and immunosuppression. (Fitzpatrick et al. 1992). Group A beta-hemolytic *Streptococci* and *Staphylococcus aureus* are the most common etiologic agents. However, other organisms, including gram-negative rods, may be responsible for cellulitis in diabetics or immunocompromised individuals (Fitzpatrick et al. 1992; Orkin, Maibach, and Dahl 1991).

Lymphangitis and lymphadenitis may arise as common manifestations of cellulitis at the site of an infected wound. Lymphatic involvement may progress rapidly and can lead to septicemia and death (Tierney 1993).

DATABASE

SUBJECTIVE

→ Symptoms may include:
  ▪ fever.
  ▪ chills.
  ▪ malaise.
  ▪ anorexia.
  ▪ tenderness at site of infection.

→ History may include:
  ▪ recent break in the skin (e.g., puncture wound, laceration, abrasion, or surgical incision).

OBJECTIVE

→ Vital signs may include:
  ▪ elevated temperature.

→ Patient may present with:
  ▪ diffuse, sharply defined, hot erythema of variable size.
  ▪ brawny edema.
  ▪ vesicles, bullae, erosions, abscesses, hemorrhage, and necrosis (Fitzpatrick et al. 1992).
  ▪ red streaks from area of cellulitis toward regional lymph node with tender, enlarged lymph node if lymphangitis/lymphadenitis exists.

ASSESSMENT

→ Cellulitis

→ R/O lymphangitis/lymphadenitis.

→ R/O superficial/deep-vein thrombophlebitis

→ R/O soft-tissue infection

→ R/O necrotizing fasciitis

→ R/O gangrene

→ R/O contact dermatitis

→ R/O giant urticaria

→ R/O fixed drug eruptions

→ R/O erythema migrans

→ R/O prevesicular herpes zoster

→ R/O erysipelas

→ R/O cat scratch fever

PLAN

DIAGNOSTIC TESTS

→ Cultures and gram stain may identify a specific pathogen but often specimens for these tests cannot be obtained (Berger, Elias, and Wintroub 1990).

→ Erythrocyte sedimentation rate (ESR) is increased.

→ CBC evidences increased leukocytes; left shift.

TREATMENT/MANAGEMENT

→ During the febrile stage of illness, the patient should rest, increase fluid intake, and take antipyretic medications (e.g., acetaminophen).

→ Immobilization of affected area(s).

→ Elevation of affected extremity or extremities.

→ Moist heat applied to area(s) for 20 to 30 minutes BID-TID.

→ For mild early cellulitis (Fitzpatrick et al. 1992):
  ▪ dicloxacillin (Dynapen®) 0.5 gm-1.0 gm p.o. every 6 hours for 10 days.
  ▪ erythromycin (E-Mycin®) 500 mg p.o. every 6 hours for 10 days for penicillin-allergic individuals.

→ If underlying dermatosis, institute appropriate therapy. See appropriate protocols.

→ Patients with severe systemic symptoms or associated complications should be referred to physician immediately.
  ▪ Hospitalization may be required.

CONSULTATION

→ Physician consultation is warranted in any patient with systemic symptoms, lymphangitis/lymphadenitis, cellulitis of the face, suspected necrotizing cellulitis, history of immune suppression (e.g., HIV infection) or other immune-suppressive medical condition (e.g., diabetes mellitus, hematologic malignancies), or patients not demonstrating significant improvement after 48 hours of antibiotic therapy.
  ▪ Hospitalization may be indicated in some of these circumstances.

→ As needed for prescription(s).

PATIENT EDUCATION

→ Educate patient regarding cause of cellulitis, signs/symptoms of complications, and indicated follow-up.

→ If patient has history of injection drug use, provide information about available treatment programs. Educate regarding adverse effects of drug use and need to consider HIV testing.

FOLLOW-UP

→ Have patient return for follow-up evaluation in 24 to 48 hours. If no improvement, consult with/refer patient to physician.

→ Refer patient with injection drug use to appropriate treatment programs and social services.

→ See "Consultation" section.

→ Document in progress notes and problem list.

Jan M. Reddick, M.S., F.N.P.
Maureen Shannon, C.N.M., F.N.P., M.S.

3-E

Contact Dermatitis (Contact Eczema): Irritant and Allergic

Contact dermatitis is an acute, subacute, or chronic inflammation of the epidermis and dermis caused by direct skin contact with chemicals or allergens. It is characterized by itching, burning, and erythema (Fitzpatrick et al. 1992; Orkin, Maibach, and Dahl 1991). The skin manifestations from exposure to irritating chemicals are a result of toxic reactions and are concentration-dependent. Those from exposure to allergens are the results of an immunologic response (Berger, Elias, and Wintroub 1990; Orkin, Maibach, and Dahl 1991).

Common irritants and allergens responsible for contact dermatitis include soaps, detergents, organic solvents, hair dye, topical medications (e.g., antibiotics [especially neomycin], antihistamines, anesthetics [e.g., benzocaine]), perfumes, certain metals (especially nickel), rubber products, and poison ivy or poison oak. Most episodes of contact dermatitis are self-limited and resolve in two to three weeks unless the individual is reexposed or if a superimposed bacterial infection occurs.

DATABASE

SUBJECTIVE

→ Symptoms may include:
- pruritus or burning sensation (or pain) at site of contact with irritant or allergen.
- fever in severe cases.

→ History may include work involving exposure to
- water (e.g., cleaning, dishwashing)
- nickel products (e.g., costume jewelry).
  - Individuals at high risk for development of nickel allergy include:
    - hairdressers, restaurant workers, nurses, cashiers, workers in metal industries.
- chromates (e.g., cement, leather products tanned with chromates).
- rubber products.
- topical drugs or cosmetics (e.g., lanolin, neomycin, local anesthetics, formaldehyde, and preservatives such as the parabens and benzoisothiozides).
- perfumes and fragrances.
- epoxy resin.
- plants (e.g., poison oak and poison ivy).

→ History may include a prior similar dermatitis (Orkin, Maibach, and Dahl 1991).

OBJECTIVE

→ Lesions vary in appearance depending on stage of response, with a distribution pattern that may be localized (to the site of contact) or generalized. **NOTE:** The site of reaction will often suggest the cause (e.g., facial involvement may be due to soap, cosmetics; scalp involvement may be due to hair products).

→ Acute inflammation:
- irregular, poorly demarcated patches of erythema, edema, and oozing; vesicles, bullae, and crusting (Fitzpatrick et al. 1992; Orkin, Maibach, and Dahl 1991).

→ Subacute inflammation:
- patches of mild erythema with small, dry scales or superficial desquamation.

→ Chronic inflammation:
- mild erythema with patches of lichenification; satellite papules and excoriations (Fitzpatrick et al. 1992).

ASSESSMENT

→ Contact dermatitis

→ R/O secondary infection of lesions

→ R/O atopic dermatitis

→ R/O seborrheic dermatitis

→ R/O psoriasis

→ R/O dermatophytosis (fungal infections)

→ R/O nummular eczema

→ R/O dyshidrotic eruptions

→ R/O lichen planus

→ R/O drug eruptions

→ R/O scabies

PLAN

DIAGNOSTIC TESTS

→ Patch testing to identify a specific allergen cannot be done during the acute episode if the individual's back is involved, because a false-positive reaction can result. Patch testing can be done after the contact dermatitis has resolved, though not all potential allergens are available for testing (Goldstein and Odom 1994).

TREATMENT/MANAGEMENT

→ Identify and avoid contact with etiological agent. **NOTE:** Animals and clothing can cause re-exposure to some types of allergens (e.g., poison oak) (Orkin, Maibach, and Dahl 1991).

→ Topical therapy usually is effective for most individuals with mild, uncomplicated dermatitis and involves:

  ▪ compresses of Burow's solution (Domeboro®) can be applied to weeping areas for 15 to 20 minutes BID–TID. The astringent effect of the solution will help dry the lesion(s).

  ▪ potent topical corticosteroids in a drying vehicle can be used as follows:

    • fluocinomide (Lidex®) gel 0.5 percent applied to affected areas BID.

  ▪ nonfluorinated topical corticosteroid agents should be used for lesions of the face or intertriginous areas.

    • Hydrocortisone 2.5 percent (Hytone®) cream applied to affected area BID.

    • Dexamethasone 0.1 percent (Decaderm®) gel applied to affected area BID.

→ Systemic corticosteroid therapy is indicated for severe episodes (e.g., significant skin involvement, swelling of the face or genitalia, large areas of bullae). The course of treatment should be 14 days; otherwise a rebound flaring of symptoms can occur. The following regimen is one example of recommended dosing (Kaiser Permanente, San Francisco, Dermatology Department 1993):

  ▪ prednisone (Deltasone®) 20 mg #30:

    • 3 tablets every morning, all at once for 5 days.

    • 2 tablets every morning, all at once for 5 days.

    • 1 tablet every morning for 5 days.

→ Oral antihistamine therapy may be helpful in relieving pruritus:

  ▪ diphenhydramine (Benadryl®) 25 mg-50 mg p.o. every 6 hours prn.

  ▪ hydroxyzine (Atarax®) 10 mg-25 mg p.o. every 6 hours prn.
  NOTE: Warn patient about drowsiness associated with these agents and the need to avoid activities requiring concentration (e.g., driving).

CONSULTATION

→ Physician consultation is warranted in any patient with severe manifestations (e.g., generalized distribution) or evidence of secondary bacterial infection and/or in cases where systemic corticosteroid therapy is being considered.

→ As needed for prescription(s).

PATIENT EDUCATION

→ Educate the patient about contact dermatitis—the probable cause, clinical course, diagnostic tests, treatment options, possible complications, adverse effects of medications, and indicated follow-up.

→ Advise patient to avoid additional exposure to known allergens or irritants.

→ Advise patient that if she is a cement worker, ferrous sulfate added to cement can prevent occupational chromate allergy (Orkin, Maibach, and Dahl 1991).

→ Patients using systemic corticosteroids should be educated about the possible side effects, including emotional lability. See *Physicians' Desk Reference (PDR)*.

FOLLOW-UP

→ Individualized according to case presentation.

→ See "Consultation" section.

→ Document in progress notes and problem list.

Jan M. Reddick, M.S., F.N.P.
Maureen Shannon, C.N.M., F.N.P., M.S.

3-F

Dyshidrotic Eczema

Dyshidrotic eczema is an acute, chronic, or recurrent self-limited dermatosis of the hands and feet characterized by vesicles (Fitzpatrick et al. 1992). Usually, the condition does not occur until a patient's second or third decade of life (Goldstein and Odom 1994). Fifty percent of individuals report an atopic history and note increased incidence when experiencing stressful events. It has been postulated that this condition may be an allergic or hypersensitive condition (Fitzpatrick et al. 1992; Goldstein and Odom 1994).

DATABASE

SUBJECTIVE

→ Patient may report an atopic history.

→ Patient may report an allergy to nickel.

→ Patient may deny symptoms occuring prior to second decade of life.

→ Symptoms may include:
  ▪ pruritus.
  ▪ blister-like eruptions on sides of fingers, the palms, and soles of feet.
  ▪ pain if fissures develop.

OBJECTIVE

→ Vesicles are:
  ▪ usually about 1.0 mm in diameter.
  ▪ deep-seated.
  ▪ "like tapioca pudding" when appearing in clusters.

→ Scaling, lichenification, fissures, and erosions may be present.

→ Lesions usually observed on sides of fingers, and palms and soles of feet.

→ Nails may be ridged, pitted, or thickened.

ASSESSMENT

→ Dyshidrotic eczema

→ R/O acute contact dermatitis

→ R/O vesicular tinea

→ R/O herpes simplex viral infection

PLAN

DIAGNOSTIC TESTS

→ No specific diagnostic tests are required since the clinical presentation and history are characteristic of the condition. However, if the patient has a vesicular eruption, the following tests may be ordered:
  ▪ potassium hydroxide (KOH) 10 percent preparation of scraping from a vesicle to rule out the presence of tinea (i.e., evidence of hyphae would indicate a fungal infection).
  ▪ if the patient is immunocompromised, a viral culture may be sent to rule out herpes simplex infection.

TREATMENT/MANAGEMENT

→ Lesions often spontaneously resolve within 2 to 3 weeks.

→ Vesicular stage (early) treatment may include:

- ■ Burow's solution (Domeboro®) compresses applied to affected areas for 15 to 20 minutes BID–TID to help dry the vesicles.
- ■ so-called "black cat" ointment (10 percent crude coal tar in equal parts acetone and flexible collodion) applied daily to help dry the vesicles (Fitzpatrick et al. 1992).
- → Eczematous stage treatment may include:
  - ■ high-potency topical steroids which are beneficial in treating the scaling and fissuring that occurs after the vesicular stage.
    - • Fluocinomide 0.05 percent (Lidex®) ointment or cream applied to affected areas BID until resolution.
    - • Betamethasone dipropionate 0.05 percent (Diprosone®) ointment applied to affected areas BID until resolution.
- → Systemic steroid therapy is not indicated because this is a chronic condition.
- → After acute episode, the patient should avoid contact with any irritating substance(s), use gloves when exposure to water is necessary, and apply hand cream to prevent a recurrence.

- → In patients with a history of nickel allergy along with several recurrences, a nickel-free diet may be necessary. Referral to a nutritionist for proper instruction is indicated.

CONSULTATION

- → Referral to a nutritionist for proper evaluation and instruction regarding a nickel-free diet.
- → As needed for prescription(s).

PATIENT EDUCATION

- → Educate the patient about dyshidrotic eczema—the possible cause(s), clinical course, treatment, prevention, and indicated follow-up.
- → Reassure the patient that symptoms will usually resolve in two to three weeks.

FOLLOW-UP

- → Individualized according to case presentation.
- → See "Consultation" section.
- → Document in progress notes and problem list.

Jan M. Reddick, M.S., F.N.P.

Maureen Shannon, C.N.M., F.N.P., M.S.

3-G

Folliculitis

Folliculitis is a superficial inflammation or infection of hair follicles without involvement of the surrounding skin (Orkin, Maibach, and Dahl 1991). Bacterial and nonbacterial (irritant) forms of folliculitis can occur.

Bacterial folliculitis is usually caused by penicillin-resistant strains of *Staphylococcus aureus* (Berger, Elias, and Wintroub 1990), although *Pseudomonas aeruginosa* (responsible for "hot-tub" folliculitis) and a range of gram-negative organisms (noted in individuals taking antibiotics) have also been implicated (Goldstein and Odom 1994).

Nonbacterial folliculitis can result from follicle occlusion by oils or oil-based cosmetics, or by friction (e.g., shaving skin) and sweating that occurs with tight clothing (Goldstein and Odom 1994). Folliculitis associated with systemic steroid use (*steroid acne*) usually occurs during the first week of steroid therapy and often resolves as the dose is tapered.

Abscess formation is the major complication associated with folliculitis. Cavernous sinus thrombosis, although rare, is a serious, life-threatening complication that can occur if folliculitis involves the upper lip, nose, or eyes. Usually, bacterial folliculitis will respond to therapy without complications, but the condition can persist for weeks or months. *Irritant folliculitis* will respond if exposure to the irritant is avoided (Goldstein and Odom 1994).

DATABASE

SUBJECTIVE

→ Symptoms may:
- include itching and/or burning, usually mild.
- be aggravated by shaving and other sorts of friction against skin.

→ Patient may report recent use of systemic antibiotics or steroids.

→ Patient may report history of:
- exposure to tar, mineral oil, oil-based cosmetics, adhesive tape, or plastic occlusive dressing.
- recent hot tub use (one to four days prior to symptoms).
- diabetes mellitus.

OBJECTIVE

→ Patient may present with small, erythematous pustules at hair follicle.

→ Lesions may be isolated, scattered, discrete, or grouped (Fitzpatrick et al. 1992).

→ Scalp and extremities affected most often (Orkin, Maibach, and Dahl 1991).

ASSESSMENT

→ Folliculitis

→ R/O acne vulgaris

→ R/O warts

→ R/O molluscum contagiosum

→ R/O tinea corporis

→ R/O impetigo

→ R/O staphyloccal carriage (if frequent recurrences of bacterial folliculitis)

→ R/O diabetes mellitus (if frequent recurrences of bacterial folliculitis)

PLAN

DIAGNOSTIC TESTS

→ Though diagnostic tests usually are not necessary in uncomplicated, localized episodes of folliculitis, the following tests may be ordered as indicated by history and physical findings:
  ▪ gram stain to identify infecting organism.
  ▪ culture and sensitivity on specimen from inflamed follicle for confirmation of infecting organism and any resistant strains.

TREATMENT/MANAGEMENT

→ General measures:
  ▪ avoid friction, irritation of affected area(s).
  ▪ cleanse affected area(s) with chlorhexidine (Hibiclens®) daily.
  ▪ if extensive involvement (e.g., thighs, legs) bathe daily with chlorhexidine (Berger, Elias, and Wintroub 1990).

→ Bacterial folliculitis:
  ▪ localized, uncomplicated folliculitis can be treated with topical antimicrobials:
    • mupirpocin (Bactroban®) ointment applied to affected area(s) TID for 10 days.
  ▪ if folliculitis is resistant to topical therapy or there is evidence of severe, extensive involvement, systemic antibiotic therapy should be prescribed, using:
    • dicloxacillin (Dynapen®) 250 mg-500 mg p.o. QID for 10 days.
    • erythromycin (E-Mycin®) 250 mg-500 mg p.o. QID for 10 days.
  ▪ most hot-tub folliculitis resolves without the need for antibiotic therapy. However, in patients with persistent symptoms, consider systemic antibiotic therapy with:
    • ciprofloxacin (Cipro®) 500 mg p.o. BID for 10 days.

→ Irritant folliculitis:
  ▪ in addition to the general measures listed above, the application to the affected area(s) of anhydrous ethyl chloride containing 6.25 percent aluminum chloride (Xerac Ac®) every day to BID will aid in drying the lesions.

→ Steroid folliculitis:
  ▪ usually resolves as steroid dose is tapered. The use of isotretinoin (Accutane®) is recommended. See **Acne Vulgaris** Protocol and *PDR*. **NOTE:** Use with caution. Teratogenic.

CONSULTATION

→ Physician consultation is indicated for any patient with recurring episodes of folliculitis for work-up of persistent nasal carriage of *S. aureus*, for complications associated with folliculitis, or if there is an underlying medical condition such as diabetes mellitus (Berger, Elias, and Wintroub 1990).

→ As needed for prescription(s).

PATIENT EDUCATION

→ Educate the patient about folliculitis—causes, treatment options, possible complications of condition, possible side effects of medication, prevention, and indicated follow-up.

→ Instruct the patient to avoid tight-fitting clothing and potential irritants that may aggravate the condition. Wearing cotton underwear should be recommended (Berger, Elias, and Wintroub 1990).

→ Patients with hot-tub folliculitis should be instructed in the proper treatment of water (i.e., with chlorine) used in hot tubs and spas.

→ Instruct the patient to return if complications develop or if symptoms persist despite therapy.

FOLLOW-UP

→ Individualized according to case presentation.

→ See "Consultation" and "Patient Education" sections.

→ Document in progress notes and problem list.

Jan M. Reddick, M.S., F.N.P.
Maureen Shannon, C.N.M., F.N.P., M.S.

3-H

Fungal Infections

Dermatophytes, or parasitic skin fungi, have an affinity for keratin and therefore affect the keratinized tissues of the body: nails, hair, and stratum corneum of the skin (Aly and Maibach 1987). This protocol covers the common dermatomycoses, or superficial, noninvasive dermatophytosis.

Tinea refers to all noninvasive cutaneous mycoses, except those caused by *Candida,* which are called *candidiasis* or *moniliasis* (Orkin, Maibach, and Dahl 1991). The following discussion of fungal infections includes: *Tinea versicolor* (Pityriasis versicolor), *Tinea capitis, Tinea pedis, Tinea cruris* (Eczema marginatum), and *Candidiasis* (Moniliasis).

Tinea Versicolor

Versicolor means variegated or changing color. Caused by a lipophilic yeast, *Pityrosporon orbiculare,* tinea versicolor infection usually results in hypopigmentation, but can cause hyperpigmentation as well. *P. orbiculare* can be isolated from the skin of 90 percent of the nonaffected population and is not considered contagious. Rather, the organism grows when the skin's micro-environment is suitable (Orkin, Maibach, and Dahl 1991). Infected individuals usually become symptomatic during hot, humid weather. The recurrence rate associated with this infection is probably a result of asymptomatic human colonization of the organism (Goldstein and Odom 1994).

DATABASE

SUBJECTIVE

→ Symptoms may include:
- changes in skin pigmentation, especially hypopigmentation; may also include tan, pink, whitish, or brown macules varying in size.
- mild itching aggravated by bathing or sweating.

OBJECTIVE

→ Lesions are:
- chamois-colored (but may be hypo- or hyperpigmented).
- fine scaling, maculopapular.

→ Involvement may be anywhere from small area (a few millimeters) to a large, confluent distribution.

→ Trunk, neck, and upper extremities most often affected. However, lesions may appear on the face and groin.

→ Palms, soles, and mucous membranes never affected.

ASSESSMENT

→ Tinea versicolor

→ R/O vitiligo (no scaling)

→ R/O cafe-au-lait spots (no scaling)

→ R/O seborrheic dermatitis

→ R/O pityriasis rosea

→ R/O allergic contact dermatitis

→ R/O erythrasma

→ R/O psoriasis

PLAN

DIAGNOSTIC TESTS

→ Potassium hydroxide (KOH) 10 percent microscopic exam of skin scrapings reveals "spaghetti and meatballs" pattern, i.e., large blunt hyphae with clusters of budding spores (Orkin, Maibach, and Dahl 1991).

→ Lesions will fluoresce bright yellow with Wood's light (Aly and Maibach 1987).

→ Mycologic cultures not necessary since the causative organisms are common colonizers of unaffected individuals.

TREATMENT/MANAGEMENT

→ Topical therapy includes application of one of the following solutions:

■ selenium sulfide shampoo (Selsun®, Exsel® most economical).

■ zinc parathion, sulfur, and salicylic acid shampoos (e.g., Sebulex®) are equally effective topical agents (Berger, Elias, and Wintroub 1990).

• Before bedtime, wet skin and apply shampoo to the neck, trunk, arms (wrists), and legs (knees). In the morning, shampoo scalp for 5 minutes, then rinse off shampoo completely from scalp and body.

• A less irritating regimen involves applying the shampoo to the areas described above for 10 to 20 minutes a day, followed by a scalp shampoo every day for 2 weeks (Berger, Elias, and Wintroub 1990).

• Shampooing the same areas described above once a month as maintenance therapy is recommended (Goldstein and Odom 1994).

→ Systemic therapy may be necessary for the treatment of widespread or recalcitrant infections. Current recommendations include:

■ ketoconazole (Nizoral®) 400 mg-800 mg p.o. once

OR

■ ketoconazole (Nizoral®) 200 mg p.o. every day for 7 days.

After ingesting ketoconazole, the patient should be encouraged to exercise to the point of sweating. She should allow the sweat to dry and wait several hours before washing (Berger, Elias, and Wintroub 1990; Orkin, Maibach, and Dahl 1991).

NOTE: Ketoconazole therapy has been associated with hepatotoxicity and drug reactions. Refer to *PDR*.

CONSULTATION

→ Physician consultation is indicated in widespread or recalcitrant infection.

→ As needed for prescription(s).

PATIENT EDUCATION

→ Educate the patient about tinea versicolor—the cause, clinical course, treatment options, recurrence, possible complications, side effects of medications, and indicated follow-up.

→ Inform the patient that return of pigmentation may lag behind completion of therapy by several months and is influenced by skin color and exposure to the sun.

FOLLOW-UP

→ As indicated by case presentation.

→ See "Consultation" section.

→ Document in progress notes and problem list.

Tinea Corporis (Body Ringworm)

Tinea corporis affects the smooth, non-hairy portions of skin, i.e., *glabrous* skin (Aly and Maibach 1987). Typically, it manifests as erythematous, scaling lesions with central clearing, but it also can appear as vesicles, pustules, and psoriatic-like lesions as well (Aly and Maibach 1987; Orkin, Maibach, and Dahl 1991). *Trichophyton rubrum* is the most common dermatophyte causing tinea corporis (Orkin, Maibach, and Dahl 1987).

Tinea corporis is more frequently reported among adults and is more common in hot, humid climates. Occasionally, individuals report exposure to an infected cat. Complications are rare, but include extension of infection to scalp, hair, or nails, secondary bacterial infection, and *dermatophytid* (i.e, an allergy or sensitivity to a fungus) (Goldstein and Odom 1994).

DATABASE

SUBJECTIVE

→ Pruritus is commonly reported.

→ Symptoms may include pain/tenderness at site of lesion(s).

→ Patient may report exposure to an infected cat.

→ Patient may report annular, erythematous skin eruption(s) on exposed areas of body (e.g., face, arms).

OBJECTIVE

→ Erythematous, papulosquamous, circumscribed, raised, and scaling lesion(s) with central clearing are those most commonly observed.

→ Lesions may appear as papulosquamous plaques covering a large area.

→ Concentric, red, scaly rings may be observed.

→ Vesicles and/or pustules may be present with secondary bacterial infection.

ASSESSMENT

→ Tinea corporis

→ R/O annular lesions of psoriasis

→ R/O seborrheic dermatitis

→ R/O contact dermatitis

→ R/O pityriasis rosea

→ R/O erythema multiform

→ R/O furunculosis

→ R/O erythema chronica migrans

PLAN

DIAGNOSTIC TESTS

→ Potassium hydroxide (KOH) 10 percent microscopic exam of scraping of scaly lesion will reveal hyphae.

→ Fungal cultures can be helpful in confirming diagnosis (Berger, Elias, and Wintroub 1991).

TREATMENT/MANAGEMENT

→ Skin should be kept dry and clean.

→ Topical antifungal agents are effective when applied twice a day to lesion(s) until 1 to 2 weeks after the lesions disappear. Commonly used agents include:

  ▪ miconazole 2 percent (Monistat®, Micatin®) cream or lotion.

  ▪ clotrimazole 1 percent (Lotrimin®, Mycelex®) cream or lotion.

  ▪ ketoconazole 2 percent (Nizoral®) cream.

  ▪ sulconazole 1 percent (Exelderm®) cream.

→ If the lesions appear acutely inflamed, consider therapy with:

  ▪ betamethasone dipropionate with clotrimazole (Lotrisone®) applied BID to affected areas for 3 to 5 days.

When inflammation has subsided, or after 5 days of therapy, the patient should continue therapy with a topical antifungal preparation *without* a steroid component (e.g., miconazole 1 percent cream or lotion, clotrimazole 1 percent cream or lotion) (Goldstein and Odom 1994).

→ Use of systemic agents for the treatment of cutaneous dermatophyte infections requires consultation with a physician prior to treatment.

CONSULTATION

→ Seek dermatology consultation for chronic, scaly ringworm as it may require a long-term oral antifungal agent and may sometimes be associated with severe underlying medical problems such as lymphoma and immunological deficiencies (Orkin, Maibach, and Dahl 1991).

→ As needed for prescription(s).

PATIENT EDUCATION

→ Educate patient about cause and indicated treatment, emphasizing need to continue therapy for one to two weeks after lesions have disappeared.

→ Advise the patient to avoid contact with infected animals.

→ Discuss proper laundering of clothing to prevent re-exposure.

FOLLOW-UP

→ Individualized according to case presentation.

→ See "Consultation" section.

→ Document in progress notes and problem list.

Tinea Capitis (Scalp Ringworm)

Tinea capitis, or ringworm of the scalp and hair, is the most common fungal infection in children and is rarely reported in adults (Orkin, Maibach, and Dahl 1991). Two dermatophyte species are responsible for this infection: *Microsporum*, which accounts for a minimal number of cases, and *Trichopyton tonsurans*, the most common etiological pathogen and the organism that is responsible for resistant infections which may persist into adulthood (Goldstein and Odom 1994).

Noninflammatory tinea capitis is usually characterized by annular, gray, scaly patches of alopecia on the scalp with or without pruritus. However, acutely inflamed, localized lesions with indurated pustular areas can occur and are called *kerion celsi* (Goldstein and Odom 1994). Although tinea capitis can persist into adulthood, it usually resolves by puberty. The only potential complications associated with this condition include scarring secondary to kerion celsi and superimposed bacterial infection of exudative lesions.

DATABASE

SUBJECTIVE

→ Symptoms may include pruritus of affected areas, mild to moderate in intensity.

→ Patient may complain of persistent dandruff, unrelieved by proper use of dandruff shampoos.

→ Patient may report:
  ▪ exposure to infected farm animals or pets (Aly and Maibach 1987; Fitzpatrick et al. 1992).
  ▪ a history of tinea capitis prior to or during adolescence.

OBJECTIVE

→ Patient may present with:
  ▪ dry, round scaly lesions with patches of alopecia.
  ▪ acutely inflamed exudative lesions, with or without pustules (Orkin, Maibach, and Dahl 1991).
  ▪ hair looking dry, lusterless.
  ▪ broken hairs at or just above the scalp (Orkin, Maibach, and Dahl 1991). Because broken hairs may be seen as black dots on the scalp, this variety is known as "black dot" tinea capitis (Aly and Maibach 1987).
  ▪ regional lymphadenopathy (especially if chronic infection) (Fitzpatrick et al. 1992).

ASSESSMENT

→ Tinea capitis
→ R/O seborrheic dermatitis
→ R/O psoriasis
→ R/O pyoderma
→ R/O alopecia from other causes
→ R/O lupus erythematosus

PLAN

DIAGNOSTIC TESTS

→ Potassium hydroxide (KOH) 10 percent microscopic examination of the scalp scales and black dystrophic hairs should be done. Evidence of spores indicates tinea capitis infection (Goldstein and Odom 1994).

→ Hair shaft may be pulled from its follicle and sent for fungal culture to identify species (Orkin, Maibach, and Dahl 1991).

→ Wood's light not helpful since *T. tonsurans* does not fluoresce (Orkin, Maibach, and Dahl 1991).

TREATMENT/MANAGEMENT

→ Selenium sulfide shampoo (Selsun®, Exsel®) can be used to reduce the shedding of spores.

→ Topical antifungal agents are not effective in the treatment of adult tinea capitis.

→ Systemic therapy is indicated in adults and includes the following agents:
  ▪ microcrystalline griseofulvin (Fulvicin®, Gris-Peg®) 500 mg p.o. every day for 6 to 8 weeks or until culture is negative.
  ▪ ketoconazole (Nizoral®) 200 mg p.o. every day for 6 to 8 weeks or until culture is negative.

NOTE: Significant side effects, toxicities (e.g., hepatotoxicities, neutropenia) and drug interactions can occur with these agents. Consult *PDR*.

CONSULTATION

→ Physician consultation is indicated in patients undergoing systemic therapy with long-term use of griseofulvin or ketoconazole.

→ Consultation with dermatologist is indicated for patients with kerion celsi. Oral steroids may be indicated to prevent scarring and resultant permanent hair loss (Orkin, Maibach, and Dahl 1991).

→ As needed for prescription(s).

PATIENT EDUCATION

→ Educate the patient about tinea capitis—cause, treatment options, and indicated follow-up.

→ Educate the patient about possible side effects associated with systemic treatments.

→ Advise the patient against sharing her hats, combs, or brushes with others (Berger, Elias, and Wintroub 1990).

FOLLOW-UP

→ As indicated by case presentation.
→ See "Consultation" section.
→ Document in progress notes and problem list.

Tinea Pedis

Tinea pedis, commonly known as *athlete's foot*, is the most prevalent acute or chronic fungal infection (Orkin, Maibach, and Dahl 1991). Several different dermatophytes colonize the skin then penetrate the stratum corneum, the outermost layer of the epidermis. Variable and complex host/parasite reactions follow, resulting in three basic forms of tinea pedis that occur in various locations on the foot: *interdigital, vesicular,* and *dry, scaly moccasin* (Aly and Maibach 1987; Orkin, Maibach, and Dahl 1991).

DATABASE

SUBJECTIVE

→ Symptoms may include:
- pruritus which may be intense.
- burning, stinging at site of infection.
- pain associated with blisters, cracks, or fissures (Orkin, Maibach, and Dahl 1991).
- erythema, edema, purulent drainage if secondary bacterial infection.
- enlarged, tender regional lymph nodes if concomitant lymphadenitis.

OBJECTIVE

→ Interdigital:
- typically does not spread beyond intertriginous areas.
- patient presents with:
  - scaling, maceration, fissuring (Orkin, Maibach, and Dahl 1991).
  - fourth interspace most commonly affected (Aly and Maibach 1987).

→ Vesicular:
- patient presents with:
  - intense inflammation.
  - lesions occurring anywhere on foot, usually in clusters (Orkin, Maibach, and Dahl 1991).

→ Dry, scaly moccasin:
- patient presents with:
  - minimal inflammation.
  - dull erythema, powdery white to pinkish red hue of plantar surface, dryness, scaling, and hyperkeratosis (Orkin, Maibach, and Dahl 1991).
  - involvement of entire plantar skin in moccasin distribution.
- this form may be chronic (Aly and Maibach 1987; Orkin, Maibach, and Dahl 1991).

ASSESSMENT

→ Tinea pedis
→ R/O interdigital intertrigo
→ R/O candidiasis
→ R/O psoriasis
→ R/O contact dermatitis
→ R/O atopic dermatitis
→ R/O cellulitis
→ R/O lichen planus
→ R/O ichthyosis

PLAN

DIAGNOSTIC TESTS

→ Potassium hydroxide (KOH) 10 percent microscopic exam of affected skin scrapings may reveal hyphae (Orkin, Maibach, and Dahl 1991).
→ Fungal cultures may be positive and confirm the diagnosis (Goldstein and Odom 1993).

TREATMENT/MANAGEMENT

→ Topical therapeutic interventions are divided into remedies for the treatment of macerated lesions and for dry, scaly lesions.
  Macerated lesions:
  - apply aluminum subacetate (Domeboro®) solution soaks for 20 minutes BID–TID to help dry lesions.
  - apply topical antifungal agents after completely washing and drying affected area(s). The following antifungal preparations can be used:
    - miconazole 2 percent (Monistat®, Micatin®) cream or lotion applied BID for 2 weeks after lesions resolve.
    - tolnaftate (Tinactin®) preparations can be used BID but are less effective than miconazole or clotrimazole preparations.

  Dry, scaly lesions:
  - can be treated with the topical antifungal agents listed above.

→ Systemic therapy may be necessary in patients with recurrent, severe, or persistent symptoms, and includes (Berger, Elias, and Wintroub 1990):
  - microcrystalline griseofulvin (Fulvin®, Gris-Peg®) 500 mg p.o. every day for 3 to 6 weeks.
  - ketoconazole (Nizoral®) 200 mg p.o. every day for 3 to 6 weeks.
NOTE: Significant side effects, toxicities (e.g., hepatotoxicities, neutropenia) and drug interactions can occur with these agents. Consult *PDR*.

CONSULTATION

→ Physician consultation is indicated for severe secondary bacterial infections because cellulitis, ascending lymphangitis, and lymphadenitis are potential complications of tinea pedis (Orkin, Maibach, and Dahl 1991).

→ As needed for prescription(s).

PATIENT EDUCATION

→ Educate patient about tinea pedis—the cause, treatment options, possible complications, preventive measures, and indicated follow-up.

→ Teach patient that moisture will promote fungal infections. Whenever possible, shoes should be removed to reduce moisture. Encourage use of cotton socks. Advise complete drying of toes and feet after bathing/swimming.

→ Educate patient about the need for twice daily application of antifungals since improvement is unlikely if the medication is used less frequently.

FOLLOW-UP

→ As indicated by case presentation.

→ See "Consultation" section.

→ Document in progress notes and problem list.

Tinea Cruris (Eczema marginatum)

Tinea cruris is an infection caused by various dermatophytes and affecting the groin, perineum, and perianal regions. (Aly and Maibach 1987). The pathology of tinea cruris is similar to that of tinea pedis with moisture, maceration, carbon dioxide tension, and friction thought to be promoting factors (Orkin, Maibach, and Dahl 1991). Tinea cruris is more common in hot, humid climates (Goldstein and Odom 1994) and in males, obese individuals, athletes, and individuals who report increased perspiring tendencies.

DATABASE

SUBJECTIVE

→ Patient may be asymptomatic.

→ Patient may report:
  ▪ history of increased perspiring.
  ▪ moderate to severe itching in intertriginous areas.
  ▪ erythema and/or macular lesions in affected areas.
  ▪ concomitant fungal infection of feet (Fitzpatrick et al. 1992).

OBJECTIVE

→ Lesions are confined to the groin and gluteal fold. Characteristics include (Orkin, Maibach, and Dahl 1991):

  ▪ sharply marginated borders with thin scales, erythema, and central clearing.
  ▪ vesicles and pustules at borders of lesion (rare).
  ▪ usually dry.

ASSESSMENT

→ Tinea cruris

→ R/O candidiasis

→ R/O erythrasma (less inflamed, fluoresces red with Wood's light)

→ R/O seborrheic dermatitis

→ R/O intertrigo

→ R/O psoriasis

→ R/O contact dermatitis

→ R/O neurodermatitis (indistinct borders)

→ R/O Bowen's disease (asymmetrical)

→ R/O extramammary Paget's disease (asymmetrical distribution)

PLAN

DIAGNOSTIC TESTS

→ Potassium hydroxide (KOH) 10 percent microscopic exam of skin scrapings from the lesions' borders will reveal hyphae (Orkin, Maibach, and Dahl 1991).

→ Fungi culture will differentiate tinea cruris from *Candida albicans*.

TREATMENT/MANAGEMENT

→ The affected area should be kept clean and dry, and excessive bathing avoided.

→ Clothing should be loose-fitting and made of absorbent material (e.g., cotton). Avoid irritating and rough materials (Goldstein and Odom 1994).

→ Topical antifungal therapy is effective when recommended regimens are followed. Initiation of any of the following agents in solution or lotion form (for increased penetration of skin folds) is acceptable, but therapy must continue for up to 2 weeks after resolution of the lesion(s):
  ▪ miconazole 2 percent (Monistat®, Micatin®) applied to affected area BID.
  ▪ clotrimazole 1 percent (Lotrimin®, Mycelex®) applied to affected area BID.
  ▪ ketoconazole 2 percent (Nizoral®) applied to affected area every day.
  ▪ sulconazole 1 percent (Exelderm®) applied to affected area every day.

→ Systemic antifungal therapy is not routinely indicated unless the patient is experiencing severe symptoms. If systemic therapy is being considered, consultation with a physician is indicated.

CONSULTATION

→ Physician consultation is warranted with severe or recurrent tinea cruris, or if secondary bacterial infection is suspected (because lymphangitis can occur) (Orkin, Maibach, and Dahl 1991)

→ As needed for prescription(s).

PATIENT EDUCATION

→ Educate patient about tinea cruris—the cause, treatment options, possible complications, preventive measures, and indicated follow-up.

→ Advise patient to avoid tight clothing, thereby decreasing moisture and friction.

→ Advise patient to keep affected areas dry.

→ Advise patient to apply medication as instructed to promote resolution of infection.

FOLLOW-UP

→ Individualized according to case presentation.

→ See "Consultation" section.

→ Document in progress notes and problem list.

Candidiasis (Moniliasis)

Cutaneous candidiasis is most often caused by *Candida albicans*, although other candida species can cause the classic beefy-red, intertriginous fungal infection (Orkin, Maibach, and Dahl 1991). A complex complement reaction of the host is activated by the invading candida organism, resulting in pustule formation (Orkin, Maibach, and Dahl 1991). Precipitating factors which include moisture, obesity, diabetes mellitus, antibiotic therapy, immune deficiency, oral contraceptive use, and pendulous breasts contribute to infection (Aly and Maibach 1987; Fitzpatrick et al. 1992; Orkin, Maibach, and Dahl 1991). Cutaneous candidiasis can be prolonged, especially in patients with depressed immune function.

DATABASE

SUBJECTIVE

→ Symptoms may include burning, stinging, and itching of affected areas (Orkin, Maibach, and Dahl 1991).

→ Patient may report:

- a history of diabetes, obesity, and immunological deficiency.
- episodes of vulvar/vaginal burning, itching, discharge (see **Vaginitis** Protocols).

OBJECTIVE

→ Lesions are:
- beefy-red, with scalded-looking skin.
- irregular, with sharp margins.
- occasionally scaly.

→ Lesions have satellite pustules.

→ Paronychia may be evident.

→ Lesions usually occur in intertriginous areas of groin, axilla, inframammary areas, and between third and fourth fingers (Fitzpatrick et al. 1992; Orkin, Maibach, and Dahl 1991).

ASSESSMENT

→ Candidiasis (cutaneous)

→ R/O intertrigo (nonspecific and psoriatic)

→ R/O contact dermatitis

→ R/O tinea cruris (usually less red)

→ R/O pityriasis rosea

→ R/O underlying medical condition (e.g., diabetes mellitus, HIV infection)

PLAN

DIAGNOSTIC TESTS

→ Potassium hydroxide (KOH) 10 percent microscopic exam of the contents of a vesicle or pustule reveals budding cells or short hyphae (scraping of the beefy-red area will not demonstrate hyphae) (Orkin, Maibach, and Dahl 1991).

→ Fungal culture of scales or curd-like lesions will be positive (Orkin, Maibach, and Dahl 1991).

TREATMENT/MANAGEMENT

→ Affected areas should be kept dry. Whenever possible, expose affected areas to air.

→ Topical antifungal therapy for cutaneous lesions includes:
- nystatin (Mycostatin®, Nilstat®) cream 100,000 u/g applied TID to affected area(s) until complete resolution.
- miconazole 2 percent (Monistat®, Micatin®) cream or lotion applied TID–QID to affected area(s) until complete resolution.

■ clotrimazole 1 percent (Lotrimin®, Mycelex®) applied TID–QID to affected area(s) until complete resolution.
■ ketoconazole 2 percent (Nizoral®) applied TID to affected area(s) until complete resolution.
→ Topical anti-inflammatory therapy may help reduce severe symptoms:
■ hydrocortisone (Hytone®) 1 percent cream applied BID to affected area(s) for a limited time (3 to 5 days).

CONSULTATION

→ Physician consultation is indicated in patients with recurrent, persistent, or severe cutaneous candidiasis infections.
→ As needed for prescription(s).

PATIENT EDUCATION

→ Educate patient about cutaneous candidiasis infection—the cause, treatment options, possible side effects of medications, and indicated follow-up.
→ Advise patient to minimize moisture, occlusion, and maceration to promote resolution and diminish chance of recurrence.
→ For individuals with diabetes, stricter surveillance and control of blood sugar levels to be considered (Orkin, Maibach, and Dahl 1991).

FOLLOW-UP

→ Individualized according to case presentation.
→ See "Consultation" section.
→ Document in progress notes and problem list.

Jan M. Reddick, M.S., F.N.P.

Maureen Shannon, C.N.M., F.N.P., M.S.

3-1

Furuncles and Carbuncles

A *furuncle (abscess* or *boil)* is a deep-seated acute infection of a hair follicle involving the surrounding subcutaneous tissue (Aly and Maibach 1987; Orkin, Maibach, and Dahl 1991). A *carbuncle* is a group of multiple, coalescing furuncles with multiple drainage points. The usual infecting organism is coagulase-positive *Staphylococcus aureus* (Fitzpatrick et al. 1992; Goldstein and Odom 1994; Orkin , Maibach, and Dahl 1991).

The most frequent sites on the body for furuncle/carbuncle formation are hairy portions exposed to friction, irritation, moisture, or the obstructive effect of petrolatum products (Goldstein and Odom 1994). The development of furuncles/carbuncles occurs more commonly in obese individuals with oily skin, and in staphylococcal carrier states (Aly and Maibach 1987; Fitzpatrick et al. 1992). Rare complications associated with manipulation of furuncles include osteomyelitis, perinephric abscess, endocarditis, and cavernous sinus thrombosis (secondary to manipulation of a nasolabial fold or central upper-lip furuncles) (Goldstein and Odom 1994).

DATABASE

SUBJECTIVE

→ Symptoms may include:
- redness and swelling at site of affected follicle.
- usually extremely painful.
- fever and/or malaise.

OBJECTIVE

→ Vital signs include possible low-grade temperature.

→ Lesions start as hard, indurated nodules with a surrounding erythematous flame.

→ The nodule develops into a pustule or becomes a fluctuant abscess.

→ Usually spontaneous rupture with discharge of pus occurs after a few days to one to two weeks.

→ Most frequent sites are face, neck, upper back, axillae, buttocks, and groin.

ASSESSMENT

→ Furuncle

→ Carbuncle

→ R/O inflamed epidermal inclusion cyst

→ R/O pustular acne

→ R/O erysipelas

→ R/O cellulitis

→ R/O necrotic herpes simplex virus infection

→ R/O hidradenitis suppurativa

→ R/O ecthyma (deep form of impetigo)

→ R/O anthrax

→ R/O staphylococcal carrier state

→ R/O diabetes mellitus (if recurrent, severe furuncle/carbuncle)

PLAN

DIAGNOSTIC TESTS

→ Culture and sensitivity after incision and drainage (I & D) is recommended since 80 percent of hospital stains of *S. aureus* are resistant to penicillin (Orkin, Maibach, and Dahl 1991).

→ CBC is rarely indicated but, if done, may reveal a slight leukocytosis.

TREATMENT/MANAGEMENT

→ Immobilization of the affected part is indicated to prevent over-manipulation (Goldstein and Odom 1994).

→ Apply moist heat for 20 to 30 minutes TID to help localize the lesion (Orkin, Maibach, and Dahl 1991).

→ Systemic antibiotics are indicated and should provide antimicrobial activity against coagulase-positive *S. aureus*. The following antibiotics may be used:
 ▪ dicloxacillin (Dynapen®) 250 mg-500 mg p.o. QID for 10 to 14 days.
 ▪ cephalexin (Keflex®) 250 mg-500 mg p.o. QID for 10 to 14 days.
 ▪ ciprofloxacin (Cipro®) 250 mg-500 mg p.o. QID for 10 to 14 days.
 ▪ erythromycin (E-Mycin®) 250 mg-500 mg p.o. QID for 10 to 14 days can be used in penicillin-allergic patients if isolate is sensitive to it.

→ After lesions are "mature," I & D may be performed.

→ Recurrent furunculosis may require combination antimicrobial therapy. Consultation with a physician is indicated in such instances.

→ In patients with recurrent furunculosis, evaluation and possible concomitant antimicrobial therapy for family members/intimate contacts who are determined to be chronic staphylococcal carriers may be indicated. Topical therapy with mupirocin (Bactroban®) applied to the individual's nares, axillae, and anogenital area TID for 5 to 7 days usually resolves the carrier state. **NOTE:** Mupirocin may be irritating when applied intranasally (Goldstein and Odom 1994).

CONSULTATION

→ Consultation with a physician is indicated in a patient with a nasolabial fold or central upper-lip furuncles, who has recurrent furunculosis, who has carbuncles, or who does not respond to therapy.

→ As needed for prescription(s).

PATIENT EDUCATION

→ Educate the patient regarding furuncles/carbuncles—the cause, clinical course, treatment, possible complications, possible side effects of medications, and indicated follow-up.

→ Advise patients to wear loose-fitting clothing and cotton underwear and to avoid using oil-based body lotions and make-up (Berger, Elias, and Wintroub 1990).

→ After I & D, advise the patient to apply an antibacterial ointment and keep the area loosely bandaged (Goldstein and Odom 1994).

FOLLOW-UP

→ Patients should return for evaluation and I & D of a mature furuncle. If packing is inserted into wound site, advise patient to return for advancement/removal of packing material.

→ If the patient develops signs or symptoms of complications, she should return for immediate evaluation.

→ See "Consultation" section.

→ Document in progress notes and problem list.

Jan M. Reddick, M.S., F.N.P.
Maureen Shannon, C.N.M., F.N.P., M.S.

3-J

Molluscum Contagiosum

Molluscum contagiosum is a contagious and relatively common skin disorder (especially in children and sexually active adults) caused by *Molluscipoxvirus*, a member of the poxvirus family (Orkin, Maibach, and Dahl 1991). Infection usually results in the development of flesh-colored, smooth, spherical, centrally umbilicated lesions ranging in size from 2 mm to 6 mm in diameter, though giant molluscum papules larger than 15 mm in diameter have occurred.

In adults, lesions are usually found on the lower abdomen, pubic region, and inner thighs. Facial or neck lesions or a general distribution often are seen in immunocompromised individuals (e.g., HIV-infected).

Molluscum contagiosum is transmitted through close physical contact, including sexual contact. Autoinoculation is another means. The incubation period is between one week to six months. The period of communicability is unknown but probably lasts as long as lesions are present. If left untreated in immune-competent hosts, lesions may persist for six months to two years and then resolve spontaneously (Berenson 1990; Goldstein and Odom 1993).

Complications of molluscum contagiosum include bacterial superinfection (seen in up to 40 percent of cases) and molluscum dermatitis (appearing 1 to 15 months after onset of lesions in 10 percent of cases) (Douglas, Jr. 1990).

DATABASE

SUBJECTIVE

→ Men are affected more often than women.

→ Lesions are asymptomatic.

→ For individuals with multiple lesions—especially on the face or in a disseminated pattern—ask about HIV status (Berger, Elias, and Wintroub 1990; Fitzpatrick et al. 1992; Orkin, Maibach, and Dahl 1991).

→ Patient may report symptoms of other sexually transmitted diseases (STDs).

OBJECTIVE

→ Patient presents with discrete, umbilicated, pearly white, smooth papules.
  - Usually 2.0 mm to 6.0 mm, but lesions may be as large as 1.5 cm to 2.0 cm in diameter.

→ Pubic and genital areas are those most commonly affected. Lesions also may appear on the neck, trunk, and face (Orkin, Maibach, and Dahl 1991; Fitzpatrick et al. 1992).

→ Eyelid lesions may be associated with a unilateral conjunctivitis.

→ Molluscum dermatitis presents with a sharply bordered eczematoid reaction 3 cm to 10 cm in diameter; may involve only a portion of a molluscum lesion; usually disappears as lesion resolves (Douglas, Jr. 1990).

ASSESSMENT

→ Molluscum contagiosum

→ R/O warts (especially condyloma acuminata)

→ R/O keratoacanthoma

→ R/O syringoma

→ R/O lichen planus

→ R/O epithelial/intradermal nevi

→ R/O seborrheic dermatitis

→ R/O papillomas

→ R/O basal cell epithelioma

→ R/O atopic dermatitis

→ R/O herpes simplex virus infection

→ R/O varicella virus infection

→ R/O pyoderma

→ R/O coexistent STDs

→ R/O HIV infection (if evidence of disseminated and/or persistent infection)

PLAN

DIAGNOSTIC TESTS

→ The diagnosis is usually made on the basis of physical findings. However, in patients where confirmation of diagnosis is desired, the following tests may be performed:

- Wright's or Geimsa's stain of the lesion's central core. Will demonstrate large cytoplasmic inclusion bodies.
- biopsy for confirmation of diagnosis (Orkin, Maibach, and Dahl 1991).

→ Screen for other STDs as indicated.

TREATMENT/MANAGEMENT

→ Treatment of lesions will reduce transmission and includes:

- removal of lesion and its core through curettage or use of a #11 blade. This may be followed by cauterization of the lesion base with electrodesiccation or a chemical agent (e.g., silver nitrate, trichloroacetic acid) (Douglas, Jr. 1990).
- application of liquid nitrogen (for shorter period than required for warts: See **Human Papillomavirus** Protocol).
- for tiny lesions difficult to curette—podophyllin, trichloroacetic acid, or silver nitrate. This often requires multiple treatments (Douglas, Jr. 1990).

→ If bacterial superinfection or molluscum dermatitis exists, patient may require systemic antibiotics or topical corticosteroids. See **Furuncles/Carbuncles** and **Atopic Dermatitis** protocols.

→ Treatment of coexisting STDs as indicated.

→ In patients with disseminated or persistent molluscum, testing and counseling for HIV should be offered.

CONSULTATION

→ Physician consultation is indicated in a patient with disseminated or persistent molluscum, and/or in cases of significant bacterial superinfection or molluscum dermatitis.

→ Curettage and liquid nitrogen treatments may be performed only by physicians in certain settings. Refer as indicated.

PATIENT EDUCATION

→ Educate patient about molluscum contagiosum—the cause, communicability, clinical course, treatment options, length of treatment, possible complications, and indicated follow-up.

→ Advise patient that as long as lesions are present, they are probably infectious and to avoid close, intimate contact with others.

→ Discuss the need for additional STD testing (including HIV, especially if patient has disseminated infection) and treatment as indicated.

→ Inform patient that intimate contacts should be evaluated for molluscum contagiosum or other STDs as indicated.

FOLLOW-UP

→ Patients should return every two weeks for retreatment until no lesions are present.

→ See "Consultation" section.

→ Document in progress notes and problem list.

Jan M. Reddick, M.S., F.N.P.
Maureen Shannon, C.N.M., F.N.P., M.S.

3-K

Paronychia

Paronychia is an inflammation of the tissue fold surrounding the nail. The usual causative organism of acute paronychia is *staphylococci,* while *candida* is the usual cause of chronic infection (Berger, Elias, and Wintroub 1990; Fitzpatrick et al. 1992). Fingernail folds are more commonly affected than toenail folds.

DATABASE

SUBJECTIVE

→ Symptoms include pain and tenderness of affected finger.

→ Patient has history of frequent water exposure (e.g., in dishwashers) (Fitzpatrick et al. 1992).

OBJECTIVE

→ Patient presents with:
  ▪ edema surrounding nail fold.
  ▪ erythema of nail fold.
  ▪ affected area warm to touch.

ASSESSMENT

→ Paronychia (bacterial or candidal)

→ R/O cellulitis

PLAN

DIAGNOSTIC TESTS

→ Potassium hydroxide (KOH) 10 percent preparation and microscopic evaluation of purulent material will reveal hyphae if *candida* present.

→ Culture and sensitivity of purulent material may be ordered if there is evidence of significant infection or when there is a history of recurrence (Berger, Elias, and Wintroub 1990).

TREATMENT/MANAGEMENT

Bacterial Paronychia

→ Incision and drainage is indicated when there is pustule formation.

→ For deep pustular lesions, systemic antibiotic therapy should be initiated with:
  ▪ dicloxacillin (Dynapen®) 250 mg p.o. QID for 10 days

OR

  ▪ erythromycin (E-Mycin®) 250 mg-500 mg p.o. QID for 10 days in penicillin-allergic patients (Fitzpatrick et al. 1992).

Candida Paronychia

→ Incise and drain the lesion if fluctuant.

→ Topical antifungal therapy includes:
  ▪ miconazole 2 percent (Monistat®, Micatin®) cream applied TID for 1 to 2 weeks after resolution of lesion.
  ▪ clotrimazole 1 percent (Lotrimin®, Mycelex®) cream applied TID for 1 to 2 weeks after resolution of lesion.

→ If evidence of superimposed bacterial infection, initiation of systemic antibiotics is indicated. See "Bacterial Paronychia" section above, and **Furuncle/Carbuncle** Protocol.

→ With chronic paronychia in absence of water exposure, consider an evaluation for diabetes mellitus (Berger, Elias, and Wintroub 1990).

CONSULTATION

→ Refer patient to dermatologist if paronychia is progressing or if it is associated with cellulitis, severe pain, fever, or significantly elevated white blood-cell (WBC) count (Berger, Elias, and Wintroub 1990).

→ As needed for prescription(s).

PATIENT EDUCATION

→ Educate the patient about paronychia—the causes, treatment, possible complications, and any indicated follow-up.

→ Advise patient to keep hands dry and warm. If rubber gloves are worn to keep hands dry, they should be placed over cotton gloves (Fitzpatrick et al. 1992).

FOLLOW-UP

→ Individualized according to case presentation.

→ See "Consultation" section.

→ Document in progress notes and problem list.

Jan M. Reddick, M.S., F.N.P.
Maureen Shannon, C.N.M., F.N.P., M.S.

3-L

Pediculosis

Pediculosis is a parasitic infestation caused by three species of lice: *Pediculus humanus capitis* (the head louse, infesting the scalp), *Pediculus humanus corporis* (the body or clothing louse, infesting the trunk), and *Pthirus pubis* (the crab louse, infesting pubic areas).

Transmission of *pediculosis capitis* usually occurs through the use of contaminated hats and/or hair grooming articles; *pediculosis corporis* as a result of overcrowded living conditions or poor hygiene; and *pediculosis pubis* through sexual contact (Goldstein and Odom 1994). Head and body lice are highly mobile (i.e., can migrate 23 cm/minute), while pubic lice are very slow (10 cm/day). Head lice are able to survive off the human host 6 to 20 hours, body lice 1 to 7 days, and pubic lice 12 to 48 hours (Orkin, Maibach, and Dahl 1991).

The manifestations of pediculosis are a result of the host's reaction to saliva or anticoagulant injected by the louse into the dermis while feeding (Orkin, Maibach, and Dahl 1991).

DATABASE

SUBJECTIVE

→ Symptoms include mild to intense pruritus, worsening at night.

Pediculosis capitis

→ More common in children, but also occurs in adults.

Pediculosis corporis

→ Patient has history of poor hygiene.

→ More common among homeless populations. (Orkin, Maibach, and Dahl 1991).

Pediculosis pubis

→ More common among females ages 15 years to 19 years and in males over age 20 years.

→ May coexist with other STDs (Orkin, Maibach, and Dahl 1991).

OBJECTIVE

Pediculosis capitis

→ Typically confined to the occipital region.

→ Patient may present with:
  - erythema and scaling.
  - linear excoriations at hairline, from scratching.
  - urticarial eruption over neck and shoulders.
  - variable macular papular rash on trunk.
  - excoriations, crusts, and secondary impetiginized lesions involving the neck, forehead, face, and ears. In extreme secondary infections, the scalp becomes a confluent mass of matted hair, lice, mites, crusts, and purulent discharge called plica polonica (Fitzpatrick et al. 1992).
  - cervical lymphadenopathy, especially if secondary bacterial infection.

→ Unlike dandruff, the egg casings cannot be pulled from the hairs (Orkin, Maibach, and Dahl 1991).

Pediculosis corporis

→ Patient may present with:
- hemorrhagic macules.
- numerous excoriations caused by intense itching.
- postinflammatory pigmentation of lesions.
- few or no adult organisms evident.
- nits found in seams of clothing (Orkin, Maibach, and Dahl 1991).

Pediculosis pubis

→ Usually affects pubic area, but can affect any hairy area (e.g., eyelashes).

→ Often evidences characteristic maculae cerulae (sky-blue spots) on the trunk and thighs (Orkin, Maibach, and Dahl 1991). The blue color is thought to be a breakdown product of heme. (Fitzpatrick et al. 1992).

→ Adult organisms can be seen with the naked eye or with the aid of a magnifying lens.

ASSESSMENT

→ Pediculosis capitis (Fitzpatrick et al. 1992)
- R/O hair casts, hair gels
- R/O seborrheic dermatitis
- R/O contact dermatitis
- R/O eczema
- R/O impetigo
- R/O psoriasis
- R/O lichen simplex chronicus

→ Pediculosis corporis (Orkin, Maibach, and Dahl 1991)
- R/O atopic blepharitis
- R/O seborrheic dermatitis
- R/O infectious eczematous blepharitis
- R/O pyoderma
- R/O impetigo
- R/O psoriasis
- R/O pruritus vulvae
- R/O folliculitis
- R/O contact dermatitis

→ Pediculosis pubis
- R/O pruritus vulvae
- R/O folliculitis
- R/O concomitant STDs

PLAN

DIAGNOSTIC TESTS

→ On microscopic examination in patients with pediculosis capitis and pubis, a plucked hair will show oval nits (eggs) cemented to it (Orkin, Maibach, and Dahl 1991).

TREATMENT/MANAGEMENT

Pediculosis capitis

→ Permethrin (1 percent) (Elimite®, NIX®) cream rinse applied to the head and scalp and washed off after 10 minutes.

Pediculosis corporis

→ Lindane lotion 1 percent (Kwell®) applied to the entire skin surface from the patient's neck down, and washed off after 8 to 12 hours. Retreatment 7 to 10 days after initial application is necessary to destroy eggs (Berenson 1990). Not recommended for pregnant or lactating women.

→ Proper hygiene practices are essential.

Pediculosis pubis

→ Lindane 1 percent shampoo (Kwell®) applied for 4 minutes and then thoroughly washed off. Not recommended for pregnant or lactating women.

→ Permethrin 1 percent cream (Elimite®, NIX®) applied to the pubic area, then completely washed off after 10 minutes. **NOTE:** Lindane is least expensive. Permethrin has less potential for toxicity in the event of inappropriate use (CDC 1993).

→ Shaving the affected area also may be effective (Fitzpatrick et al. 1992).

→ Patients with this condition need counseling and possible testing for other STDs as indicated.

→ Additional considerations
- Systemic treatment for secondary bacterial infection may be necessary, including:
  - dicloxacillin (Dynapen®) 250 mg-500 mg p.o. QID for 10 days

    OR
  - erythromycin (E-Mycin®) 250 mg-500 mg p.o. QID for 10 days.
- If bacterial infection is minimal and confined to a small area, consider topical antibiotic therapy with mupirocin 2 percent (Bactroban®) applied to affected area(s) TID for 10 days. The recommended regimens should not be applied to the eyes.
- Infestation of eyelashes can be treated with thick application of petrolatum BID for 8 days or an occlusive ophthalmic ointment to the eyelid margin BID for 10 days (CDC 1993) with

removal of nits after therapy (Goldstein and Odom 1993).

CONSULTATION

→ Physician consultation is indicated in persistent or recurrent infestations, or if there is evidence of significant superimposed bacterial infection.

→ As needed for prescription(s).

PATIENT EDUCATION

→ To prevent future infestations, advise patient not to share her towels, combs, clothing, or bedding with others and to avoid exposing herself to known contaminated persons/areas.

→ Advise patient to treat combs/brushes by soaking them in peducilocidal solution (e.g., Kwell®, Elimite®) for 15 minutes, and then rinsing them completely (Orkin, Maibach, and Dahl 1991).

→ Advise patient to comb out nits after treatment.

→ Bedding and clothing should be machine washed and dried using the heat cycle or removed from body contact for at least 72 hours.

→ Advise patient to vacuum floors and furniture completely.

→ Household and close contacts of the infested individual should be examined and treated accordingly.

→ See "Patient Education" section of **Scabies** Protocol for management of clothing and bed linens.

FOLLOW-UP

→ Retreatment may be necessary if lice or eggs are seen. **NOTE:** New viable eggs are a creamy-yellow color; empty egg casings are white (Fitzpatrick et al. 1992).

→ Alternative treatment regimens may be tried if patient is not responding to the primary regimen(s).

→ See "Consultation" section.

→ Document in progress notes and problem list.

Jan M. Reddick, M.S., F.N.P.
Maureen Shannon, C.N.M., F.N.P., M.S.

3-M

Pityriasis Rosea

Pityriasis rosea is a common, mild, self-limited inflammatory skin eruption that is believed to be caused by a picornavirus (Fitzpatrick et al. 1992; Goldstein and Odom 1994; Orkin, Maibach, and Dahl 1991). The lesions that develop with this condition will spontaneously resolve within six to eight weeks (Goldstein and Odom 1994). It most often affects young adults, especially women, with an increased incidence during spring and fall. Although infections may be reported in household members (e.g., two percent of married couples have concurrent episodes), pityriasis rosea is not highly infectious (Goldstein and Odom 1994).

DATABASE

SUBJECTIVE

→ A "herald patch," a single plaque, precedes the generalized rash by one to two weeks.

→ Pruritus is absent to severe (Fitzpatrick et al. 1992).

→ Patient may report an oval, pale brown macular eruption on trunk, back, and extremities, preceded by a bright red, scaly patch.

OBJECTIVE

→ Patient presents with:
  ▪ herald patch (80 percent of patients), 2 cm to 5 cm in diameter, bright red, fine scaly lesion (Fitzpatrick et al. 1992; Orkin, Maibach, and Dahl 1991).
    • resembles tinea corporis.
  ▪ generalized maculopapular oval lesions 4 mm to 5 mm in diameter with fine scaling, typically distributed symmetrically over the trunk, along cleavage lines, and over the back in a "Christmas tree" pattern.
  • Central portion of lesions may have a crinkled appearance.
  • Lesions usually limited to trunk and proximal parts of arms and legs; absent from the face, hands, and feet (Fitzpatrick et al. 1992; Orkin, Maibach, and Dahl 1991).

ASSESSMENT

→ Pityriasis rosea

→ R/O secondary syphilis (feet and hands usually affected)

→ R/O drug eruption

→ R/O tinea corporis

→ R/O tinea versicolor

→ R/O seborrheic dermatitis

→ R/O psoriasis (especially guttate psoriasis)

→ R/O erythema migrans

PLAN

DIAGNOSTIC TESTS

→ Though specific diagnostic tests to confirm diagnosis are not necessary, the following tests may be done:
  ▪ VDRL or RPR to rule out syphilis (Orkin, Maibach, and Dahl 1991).
  ▪ a scraping of the eruption can be examined microscopically using potassium hydroxide (KOH) 10 percent to rule out a fungal infection (Goldstein and Odom 1994).

TREATMENT/MANAGEMENT

→ In patients with pruritus, the following antipruritic solutions can be applied to the affected areas as needed (varying results reported):
- camphor 5 percent, menthol 5 percent, phenol 5 percent (Sarna®) lotion (an over-the-counter [OTC] product)
- pramoxine hydrochloride (Prax®) 1 percent cream or lotion.

→ Medium-strength topical corticosteroids may be prescribed if moderate to severe pruritus persists. These include:
- triamcinolone acetonide (Aristocort®, Kenalog®) 0.1 percent cream or lotion applied to affected areas BID–TID.
- alclometasone dipropionate (Aclovate®) 0.5 percent cream or ointment applied to affected areas BID–TID.
- See also **Table 12TB.1,** p. 12-228.

→ Antihistamines may be prescribed if the patient is experiencing severe pruritus:
- hydroxyzine (Atarax®) 25 mg every 6 hours as needed. **NOTE:** Warn patient regarding associated drowsiness. It may be beneficial for the patient to take 50 mg at bedtime.

CONSULTATION

→ Refer to dermatologist patients whose lesions do not clear up after eight weeks.

→ As necessary for prescription(s).

PATIENT EDUCATION

→ Reassure patient that spontaneous clearing will occur, usually within six to eight weeks.

→ Although pityriasis rosea is infectious, it is not highly contagious, so affected individuals do not need to isolate themselves from others.

→ Educate the patient regarding possible side effects associated with recommended medications.

FOLLOW-UP

→ Individualized according to case presentation.

→ See "Consultation" section.

→ Document in progress notes and problem list.

Jan M. Reddick, M.S., F.N.P.
Maureen Shannon, C.N.M., F.N.P., M.S.

3-N

Psoriasis

Psoriasis is a common acute or chronic skin condition characterized by scaling papules or plaques appearing, typically, on elbows, knees, or scalp (Fitzpatrick et al. 1992; Orkin, Maibach, and Dahl 1991). The cause of psoriasis is not known, but a genetic predisposition exists. An abnormality in the growth-control mechanism of the epidermis has been postulated (the epidermis renews itself 10 to 18 times faster in individuals with psoriasis.) (Orkin, Maibach, and Dahl 1991). There are various types of psoriasis, including the plaque-like form, guttate psoriasis (which often follows streptococcal pharyngitis), and a generalized erythrodermic pustule form which is rare but may be life-threatening (Fitzpatrick et al. 1992; Goldstein and Odom 1994).

DATABASE

SUBJECTIVE

→ Symptoms include:
  - pruritus (common).
  - obesity.
  - arthritis.
  - fever.

→ History may include:
  - minor trauma of affected area *(Koebner phenomenon)* in 45 percent of patients.
  - use of systemic corticosteroids, lithium, alcohol, or chloroquine.
  - exposure to sunlight.
  - stress.
  - family history of psoriasis.

OBJECTIVE

→ Patient may present with sharply marginated erythematous papules and plaques, covered with silver-white scales, usually on the extensor surfaces of the elbows and knees. The scalp, sacrum, perineum, genitalia, and nails may be involved.

→ *Auspitz's sign/phenomenon* (pinpoint bleeding) may occur if scale(s) removed.

→ Lesions:
  - may be round, oval, polycyclic, or annular.
  - usually bilateral, often symmetric (Fitzpatrick et al. 1992; Orkin, Maibach, and Dahl 1991).
  - on hands are usually less erythematous than other sites (Orkin, Maibach, and Dahl 1991).

→ Facial eruption can occur but is rare.

→ Nails may be stippled or pitted, yellow, thick, or distorted; with swelling, redness, and scaling of the paronychial margin and arthritis of the distal interphalangeal joint (Orkin, Maibach, and Dahl 1991). "Oil spots" (yellowish-brown spots under the nail bed) are pathognomonic.

→ Psoriasis of the vulva is rarely seen in isolation (Friedrich 1983).

→ Guttate psoriasis (rare) presents as 2.0 mm to 1.0 cm, salmon-pink, "drop-like" lesions, distributed diffusely over trunk, face, and scalp. Palms and soles are unaffected (Orkin, Maibach, and Dahl 1991).

ASSESSMENT

→ Psoriasis

→ R/O seborrheic dermatitis

→ R/O lichen simplex chronicus

→ R/O candidiasis (confused with intertriginous psoriasis)

→ R/O psoriasiform drug eruptions (especially beta-blockers, gold, and methyldopa)

→ R/O glucogonoma syndrome (malignant tumor of pancreatic islet cells)

→ R/O pityriasis rosea

→ R/O secondary syphilis

→ R/O tinea

→ R/O onychomycosis

PLAN

DIAGNOSTIC TESTS

→ Usually, the skin eruption and distribution is diagnostic. However, the following tests may be ordered as indicated:

- VDRL or RPR to rule out syphilis.
- skin scrapings of lesions to rule out fungal infections.
- throat culture—may be positive for group A beta-hemolytic streptococcus in guttate psoriasis (Fitzpatrick et al. 1992).

TREATMENT/MANAGEMENT

→ The type of therapy depends upon the severity of the condition.

→ Mild, limited disease can be managed with the following therapeutic interventions:

- after soaking the lesion and removing the scaling skin, application of a mid- to high-potency topical corticosteroid such as:
  - fluocinonide (Lidex®) 0.05 percent cream or gel applied BID for 14 to 21 days.
  - fluocinolone (Synalar®) 0.2 percent cream or 0.025 percent ointment applied BID for 14 to 21 days.
  - see also **Table 12TB.1,** p. 12-228.
    NOTE: It often is beneficial to apply an occlusive plastic-wrap covering over the area after using the topical steroid, especially if the covering can be left in place overnight (Fitzpatrick et al. 1992; Goldstein and Odom 1994; Orkin, Maibach, and Dahl 1991). Avoid use of mid- to high-potency topical

corticosteroids on the face, breasts, genitalia, or body folds.

- in patients with mild, isolated lesions, occlusive dressings using Duoderm® (applied to lesion and left in place for 5 to 7 days) may be beneficial without topical corticosteroids (Goldstein and Odom 1994).
- scalp involvement can be treated initially with a tar shampoo (Neutrogena T/Gel®, Ionil T Plus®) used daily. If thick scales are present, the application of salicylic acid gel 6 percent (Keralyt®, Compound W®) to the scalp, then covering the scalp with a shower cap, may be beneficial (Goldstein and Odom 1994).

→ If moderate to severe pruritus is reported by the patient, consider prescribing an antihistamine such as:

- hydroxyzine (Atarax®) 10 mg-50 mg p.o. at bedtime prn. **NOTE:** Advise patient regarding drowsiness associated with this medication and to avoid driving or other potentially dangerous activities while taking it.

→ Psoriasis that covers more than 30 percent of the body surface is difficult to treat with topical corticosteroids and usually requires outpatient UVB-light exposure three times a week for several weeks. Refer to physician.

CONSULTATION

→ Consultation is indicated if guttate psoriasis is suspected.

→ Consult with physician as needed for prescription(s) and when using high-potency topical corticosteroids (see **Table 12TB.1,** p. 12-228).

→ Refer patient with psoriasis which covers more than 30 percent of the body to dermatologist for tar or phototherapy.

PATIENT EDUCATION

→ Educate patient regarding psoriasis—the cause(s), possible therapeutic interventions, length of treatment, possible complications/side effects of medications, and indicated follow-up.

→ Advise patient to avoid factors which can aggravate psoriasis (e.g., sunlight exposure, stress, trauma to area).

→ Review hygiene and advise patient to avoid rubbing or scratching lesions to prevent the *Koebner phenomenon* and the possibility of a secondary bacterial infection.

FOLLOW-UP

→ Individualized according to case presentation.

→ See "Consultation" section.

→ Document in progress notes and problem list.

Jan M. Reddick, M.S., F.N.P.
Maureen Shannon, C.N.M., F.N.P., M.S.

3-0

Scabies

Scabies, a skin infestation caused by a mite, *Sarcoptes scabiei*, is often described as a sexually transmitted disease. However, since the mite can remain alive off the host for over two days, transmission is likely through close personal contact or shared clothing or bedding (Fitzpatrick et al. 1992; Orkin, Maibach, and Dahl 1991). In a primary scabies infection, there is an incubation period of two to six weeks between the time of infection and the onset of itching. In subsequent infestation, because the person is sensitized to the mite, symptoms will begin one to four days after reinfestation (Fitzpatrick et al. 1992).

In immunocompromised individuals and debilitated or senile patients, scabies infection may present with a generalized dermatitis that is widely distributed and characterized by scaling, vesicles, and crusting of the eruption. Pruritus may be absent or minimal. These clinical manifestations are associated with a type of scabies called *Norwegian scabies* which is highly transmissible because of the high concentration of mites in the exfoliating scales (Berenson 1990).

DATABASE

SUBJECTIVE

→ Patient may report exposure to a close contact with scabies.

→ Symptoms may include:
- moderate to severe generalized itching, worsening at night.
- papulovesicular lesions.

OBJECTIVE

→ Patient may present with:
- evidence of "burrows" or "runs" that are 0.5 cm to 1.0 cm long, linear or wavy; usually found in/on digital webs, palms, wrists, vulva, nipples, gluteal folds, buttock, axillae, or toes, with a minute vesicle or papule at end (Fitzpatrick et al. 1992). Infestation of the face and neck is rare (Goldstein and Odom 1994).
- vesicles in isolation, often on sides of fingers.
- nodules that are indurated, brownish-red, 0.5 cm to 2.0 cm in diameter, often on axillary folds, upper back, groin, buttocks.
- papules on abdomen, buttocks, thighs.
- eczematous plaques and/or excoriations; if on the breasts, may resemble Paget's disease.
- crusting of lesions, indicating secondary bacterial infection.
- Norwegian or "crusted" scabies present as psoriasiform lesions of palms and soles (Fitzpatrick et al. 1992).

→ Atypical crusted or "exaggerated" scabies may occur in HIV-infected patients (Orkin and Maibach 1990).

ASSESSMENT

→ Scabies

→ R/O atopic dermatitis

→ R/O papular urticaria

→ R/O pyoderma

→ R/O insect bites

→ R/O dermatitis herpetiformis

PLAN

DIAGNOSTIC TESTS

→ For microscopic detection of mites:
  - locate a burrow in typical sites for burrows (as described above) and isolate a "dark point" (the mite) at the end of burrow (magnifying lens may aid this process).
  - slowly open burrow at the dark point, using a needle or thin surgical blade. The mite will stick to the point of the needle/blade.
  - it can then be transferred to a slide containing immersion oil or mineral oil and viewed microscopically (Berenson 1990; Fitzpatrick et al. 1992).

TREATMENT/MANAGEMENT

→ Permethrin 5 percent cream (Elimite®) is the drug of choice, because many scabies infestations are resistant to other antiscabies medications. The cream is applied to the entire skin surface from the neck down (with special attention to hands, feet, intertriginous areas), left on for 8 to 14 hours, then washed off (shower or bath). Generally, one application is curative.

→ Other agents which have been used include lindane (Kwell®) and crotamiton (Eurax®). See *PDR* for details on use and contraindications.

→ Because scabicidal therapy is antibacterial, most patients with secondary bacterial infection do not require antibiotic therapy. However, in certain cases, antibiotic therapy may be indicated.
  - Topical therapy—if a few small areas are involved—using:
    - mupirocin 2 percent (Bactroban®) ointment applied to affected area(s) TID for 10 days.
  - Systemic therapy should be instituted in cases of extensive secondary bacterial infection, with one of the following:
    - dicloxacillin (Dynapen®) 500 mg p.o. every 6 hours for 10 days.
    - erythromycin (E-Mycin®) 500 mg p.o. every 6 hours for 10 days.

→ Systemic antipruritic therapy may include the use of an antihistamine such as hydroxyzine (Atarax®) 25 mg p.o. every 6 hours prn.
  NOTE: Advise patient regarding drowsiness associated with this medication and to avoid activities requiring concentration (e.g., driving).

CONSULTATION

→ Refer patient with recalcitrant nodules to a dermatologist. These lesions may require intralesional corticosteroids (Fitzpatrick et al. 1992).

→ For cases in which there is severe secondary bacterial infection.

→ As necessary for prescription(s).

PATIENT EDUCATION

→ Educate the patient about scabies—the cause, infectivity, clinical course, treatment, and prevention.

→ Advise patient:
  - not to wash hands after applying medication because of the need to treat any infestation involving hands (Berger, Elias, and Wintroub 1990).
  - not to overtreat the condition, as this may lead to irritant dermatitis.
  - that 24 hours after completing therapy, she is no longer able to transmit the disease. However, symptoms may persist for weeks as a result of a hypersensitivity reaction to the mite (Orkin and Maibach 1990).

→ Sexual and close personal or household contacts of the patient should be treated prophylactically (Orkin and Maibach 1990).

→ Clothing and bed linen should be changed before treatment to avoid reinfestation. Bedding and recently worn clothing should be machine washed in hot, soapy water and dried on hot cycle or removed from body contact for at least 72 hours. Nonwashable clothing or bedding should be stored in plastic for two weeks or dry cleaned (Berger, Elias, and Wintroub 1990).

→ Infested individuals should stay away from work or school until 24 hours after completing recommended treatment (Berenson 1990).

FOLLOW-UP

→ If itching or lesions persist, or new lesions appear more than one week after treatment, a second application of antiscabies medication may be indicated (Fitzpatrick et al. 1992).

→ See "Consultation" section.

→ Document in progress notes and problem list.

Jan M. Reddick, M.S., F.N.P.
Maureen Shannon, C.N.M., F.N.P., M.S.

3-P

Seborrheic Dermatitis

Seborrheic dermatitis is an acute or chronic inflammatory condition of the skin characterized by erythema, dry, scaling skin; and yellow, crusted patches; usually occurring on the scalp, central face, body folds, umbilicus, and presternal and interscapular areas of the body (Goldstein and Odom 1993).

Though the etiology is unknown, causal relationships have been postulated. These include a genetic predisposition to the condition and an inflammatory response to *Pityrosporum ovale*, a yeast organism that is found on the scalp of all humans (Berger, Elias, and Wintroub 1990; Fitzpatrick et al. 1992; Goldstein and Odom 1993; Orkin, Maibach, and Dahl 1991). Additional factors that may aggravate seborrheic dermatitis include certain medications (e.g., methyldopa [Aldomet®]), emotional stress, alcohol intake, hormones, and other types of infections (Fitzpatrick et al. 1992; Orkin, Maibach, and Dahl 1991).

Seborrheic dermatitis often exists with other dermatologic conditions such as psoriasis, acne rosacea, and acne vulgaris (Berger, Elias, and Wintroub 1990). The majority of individuals affected are adults between 20 years to 50 years of age. Exacerbations are frequently noted during winter months or when the individual is exposed to high temperatures or increased humidity. Patients with HIV infection and Parkinson's disease frequently develop this condition (Goldstein and Odom 1994; Orkin, Maibach, and Dahl 1991).

DATABASE

SUBJECTIVE

→ Symptoms may include:
  ▪ pruritus.
  ▪ dry scaling and erythema of eyelid margins.
  ▪ erythematous, dry scaling of skin of scalp, face, chest, back, skin folds.
→ Patient may report:
  ▪ a family history of seborrheic dermatitis.
  ▪ coexisting dermatological conditions.
  ▪ medical conditions associated with increased incidence of seborrheic dermatitis (e.g., HIV infection, Parkinson's disease).

OBJECTIVE

→ Characteristics of lesions include:
  ▪ erythema.
  ▪ may have a yellow or orange hue.
  ▪ vary in size from 5 mm to 20 mm.
  ▪ sharp margins.
  ▪ may be psoriasiform and plaque-like.
  ▪ dry, moist, or greasy scaling may be evident (Orkin, Maibach, and Dahl 1991).
  ▪ sticky or weeping crusts may be observed (Fitzpatrick et al. 1992).

→ Lesions are most often located in/on:
  ▪ perinasal areas.
  ▪ ears.
  ▪ scalp.
  ▪ supraorbital areas.
  ▪ eyelids.
  ▪ genitalia.
  ▪ perianal area and gluteal folds.
  ▪ chest, submammary areas.
  ▪ umbilicus.
  ▪ back.
  ▪ axillae.

ASSESSMENT

→ Seborrheic dermatitis

→ R/O pityriasis rosea

→ R/O tinea versicolor

→ R/O tinea faciale

→ R/O psoriasis

→ R/O dermatophytosis

→ R/O candidiasis

→ R/O zinc deficiency

→ R/O lupus erythematosus

→ R/O pemphigus foliaceous

PLAN

DIAGNOSTIC TESTS

→ Usually, no specific diagnostic tests are required to confirm the diagnosis in the majority of patients. However, the following tests may be ordered as indicated to eliminate the possibility of other conditions:

- scraping of lesion for microscopic examination with potassium hydroxide (KOH) 10 percent to evaluate for presence of fungal organisms.
- fungal culture if a particular fungal organism is suspected and a definitive diagnosis is desired.

TREATMENT/MANAGEMENT

→ Underlying conditions (e.g., Parkinson's disease, emotional stress) that may aggravate seborrheic dermatitis should be treated.

→ Seborrhea of scalp (mild to moderate):

- may be treated with OTC shampoos that contain tar, zinc, pyrithione, or selenium (e.g., Neutrogena T/Gel®, Selsun®). The patient should shampoo daily with one of these products.
- ketoconazole (Nizoral®) 2 percent shampoo can be used twice a week (Goldstein and Odom 1993).
- topical corticosteroid solutions or lotions can be added if symptoms persist. To prevent tachyphylaxis, use these agents intermittently and only when the symptoms persist. The patient should apply a small amount of one of the following agents to the affected areas at bedtime:
  - triamcinolone acetonide (Aristocort®) 0.1 percent.

- betamethasone dipropionate (Diprosone®, Maxivate®) 0.05 percent.
- fluocinonide (Lidex®) 0.05 percent.

→ Seborrhea of face:

- use mild soaps to cleanse the face as a means of avoiding further irritation.
- scalp treatment usually reduces facial involvement.
- use of fluorinated topical corticosteroids on the face is not recommended because of the possibility of atrophy, telangiectasia, or steroid rosacea.
- if symptoms persist after scalp therapy and use of mild soaps, ketoconazole (Nizoral®) 2 percent cream can be applied to the affected areas BID for 4 weeks.

→ Seborrhea of body:

- use of mild soaps in axillary and groin areas only with daily bathing.
- low-potency topical steroids can be effective in non-hairy areas, including:
  - hydrocortisone (Hytone®) 1.0 percent-2.5 percent cream BID–TID to affected areas until resolution.
  - desonide (Tridesilon®) 0.05 percent cream BID–TID to affected areas until resolution.
  - alclometasone dipropionate (Aclovate®) 0.5 percent cream BID–TID until resolution.
  - See also **Table 12TB.1,** p. 12-228.
- ketoconazole (Nizoral®) 2 percent cream BID to affected areas can be used as an alternate therapy to topical steroids but is reportedly less effective (Fitzpatrick et al. 1992).

→ Seborrhea of intertriginous areas:

- application of low-potency topical steroids (see "Treatment" section, "Seborrhea of body") BID for 5 to 7 days, and then once or twice a week. See also **Table 12TB.1,** p. 12-228.
- avoid the use of oil-based or greasy ointments in these areas.

→ Seborrhea of eyelids:

- gentle cleansing of the eyelid margins with undiluted Johnson & Johnson Baby Shampoo® using a soft cotton-tipped swab at bedtime is usually effective (Goldstein and Odom 1994).

CONSULTATION

→ Refer severe or resistant cases to dermatologist for further evaluation and treatment.

→ As needed for prescription(s).

PATIENT EDUCATION

→ Educate the patient about seborrheic dermatitis, including the cause(s), aggravating factors, treatment options and length of treatment, possible side effects of medications, and indicated follow-up.

→ Advise patient to avoid prolonged use of fluorinated corticosteroids to prevent telangiectasia and erythema.

→ If tar shampoos dry hair, advise patient on use of hair conditioners.

FOLLOW-UP

→ Individualized according to case presentation.

→ See "Consultation" section.

→ Document in progress notes and problem list.

Jan M. Reddick, M.S., F.N.P.
Maureen Shannon, C.N.M., F.N.P., M.S.

3-Q

Warts

Warts are caused by *human papillomaviruses* (HPVs), each papovavirus manifesting as a different form of wart (Fitzpatrick et al. 1992). There are four types of warts: *flat warts* (*verruca plana*), *common warts* (*verruca vulgaris*), *plantar warts* (*verruca plantaris*), and *genital warts* (*condyloma acuminata*) (Berger, Elias, and Wintroub 1990). There is an increased incidence of warts in younger individuals, with a reduction in common warts noted after the age of 25 years. Flat warts and plantar warts are more common in women. (Genital warts will be discussed in the **Sexually Transmitted Diseases** Protocols.)

Warts may be spread by personal contact or by fomites and autoinoculation from one part of the body to another. The average incubation period is approximately three months, with a range of 2 to 18 months (Goldstein and Odom 1994; Orkin, Maibach, and Dahl 1991). In 50 percent of individuals, warts spontaneously resolve, though they also can be unresponsive to any form of treatment (Goldstein and Odom 1994). Twenty-one of over 60 HPV subtypes are associated with malignant neoplasms—types 5, 8, and 14 are associated with squamous cell carcinoma (American College of Obstetricians and Gynecologists 1994; Goldstein and Odom 1994).

DATABASE

SUBJECTIVE

→ The majority of patients are asymptomatic.

→ Symptoms may include:
- occasional pain with pressure in plantar warts.
- mechanical obstruction, which may be reported if wart is located in nostril or ear canal.

→ Plantar warts may appear at sites of trauma or pressure (Fitzpatrick et al. 1992).

OBJECTIVE

Verruca vulgaris (common wart) (Fitzpatrick et al. 1992):

→ firm papules 1 mm to 10 mm.

→ hyperkeratotic, cleft, with multiple conical projections (vegetations).

→ skin-colored, "reddish-brown dots" (thrombosed capillary loops) may be seen.

→ isolated or scattered discrete lesions.

→ usually occur on hands, fingers, and knees.

Verruca plantaris (plantar wart) (Fitzpatrick et al. 1992):

→ shiny, sharply marginated papule or plaque with hyperkeratotic surface.

→ skin-colored; may need to pierce wart with a scalpel to see reddish-brown dots diagnostic of warts.

→ usually appear as isolated lesion but more may be present.

Verruca plana ("flat wart") (Fitzpatrick et al. 1992):

→ mesa-like, flat-topped, round, oval, polygonal, or linear papules, usually 1 mm to 2 mm thick.

→ skin-colored or light brown.

→ numerous, discrete, and closely set.

→ favor face, dorsa of hands, and shins.

ASSESSMENT

→ Verruca vulgaris

→ Verruca plantaris

→ Verruca plana

→ R/O basal cell carcinoma

→ R/O squamous cell carcinoma

→ R/O seborrheic keratosis

→ R/O actinic keratosis

→ R/O molluscum contagiosum

→ R/O condyloma acuminata

→ R/O inflammatory dermatoses

→ R/O callus

→ R/O foreign body

PLAN

DIAGNOSTIC TESTS

→ Though the physical findings usually are adequate to make the diagnosis of warts, a biopsy of a wart-like lesion may be indicated in the following situations to rule out squamous cell carcinoma:
- large, chronic warts in an older individual.
- wart-like lesions in sun-damaged skin areas.

TREATMENT/MANAGEMENT

Verruca vulgaris

→ Keratolytic agents are safe and effective, with minimal or no side effects when used properly (Goldstein and Odom 1994).

→ Small lesions: salicylic acid-lactic acid collodion (Compound W®, Keralyt®, Occusal®, Occusal-HP®, Dufilm®) gel or liquid applied to affected area under occlusion at bedtime, then washed off in the morning.
NOTE: Patient should hydrate the area prior to application to enhance the effects of the preparation (Ellsworth et al. 1991).

→ Large lesions: 40 percent salicylic-acid plaster for one week, followed by salicylic acid-lactic acid collodion or liquid nitrogen for 10 to 30 seconds to flat lesions. The area of freezing should extend 1 mm to 2 mm beyond the lesion and thaw time should be 30 to 45 seconds. A second freezing is done as above. A blister will appear in 12 to 24 hours. This should be left intact. The client should be seen again in 2 to 3 weeks and assessed for retreatment (Berger, Elias, and Wintroub 1990).

Verruca plana

→ Usually involute spontaneously over months to years without scarring, so avoid destructive treatments (Berger, Elias, and Wintroub 1990; Fitzpatrick et al. 1992).

→ Retinoic acid 0.1 percent cream or 0.25 percent gel applied BID for 4 to 6 weeks (will clear warts in 50 percent of clients) (Berger, Elias, and Wintroub 1990).

Verruca plantaris

→ If asymptomatic, do not treat because 50 percent will involute in 6 months.

→ Do not excise, or the wart will recur with painful scars (Fitzpatrick et al. 1992).

→ Salicylic-acid 40 percent plaster applied every day under adhesive tape, after soaking the warts in warm water and scraping off dead tissue. This is continued until normal skin lines return (Berger, Elias, and Wintroub 1990).

→ Soaking the warts in hot water for ½ to ¾ hour 2 or 3 times a week for 16 treatments can be effective because warts are thermolabile (Fitzpatrick et al. 1992).

CONSULTATION

→ Refer to dermatologist patient with periungal warts, facial warts, unresponsive warts, suspicious, wart-like lesions; and individuals with peripheral vascular diseases or diabetes mellitus who have warts on their extremities (Berger, Elias, and Wintroub 1990).

PATIENT EDUCATION

→ Educate the patient regarding warts—the cause, clinical course, treatment options, possible side effects or complications associated with treatment(s), and indicated follow-up.

→ Teach patients to avoid shaving flat warts since this may spread lesions (Berger, Elias, and Wintroub 1990).

FOLLOW-UP

→ See "Treatment/Management" and "Consultation" sections.

→ Document in progress notes and problem list.

3-R
Bibliography

Aly, R., and Maibach, H.I. 1987. *Skin infections—fungal and bacterial*. Somerville, NJ: Hoechst-Roussel Pharmaceuticals.

American College of Obstetricians and Gynecologists. 1994. Genital human papillomavirus infections. *ACOG Technical Bulletin* No. 193. Washington, DC: the Author.

Berenson, A. S. 1990. *Control of communicable diseases in man*, 15th ed. Washington, DC: American Public Health Association.

Berger, T., Elias, P.M., and Wintroub, B.U. 1990. *Manual of therapy for skin diseases*. New York: Churchill Livingstone.

Centers for Disease Control. 1991. Update on adult immunization. Recommendations of the Immunization Practices Advisory Committee (ACIP). *Morbidity and Mortality Weekly Report* 15(RR-12):17–19.

————. 1993. Sexually transmitted disease treatment guidelines. *Morbidity and Mortality Weekly Report* 42 (RR-14):94–96.

Cohen, R. 1994. Disorders due to physical agents. In *Current medical diagnosis and treatment*, 32d ed., eds. L.M. Tierney, Jr., S.M. McPhee, and Papadakis, M.A., pp. 1302–1307. Norwalk, CT: Appleton & Lange.

Douglas, Jr., J.M. 1990. Molluscum contagiosum. In *Sexually transmitted diseases*, 2nd ed., eds. K.K. Holmes, P-A Mardh, P.F. Sparling, P.K. Wiesner, W. Cates, Jr., S.M. Lemon, and W.E. Stamm, pp. 443–447. New York: McGraw-Hill.

Ellsworth, A.J., Bray, R.F., Bray, B.S., and Geyman, J.P. 1991. *The family practice drug handbook*. St. Louis: Mosby Year Book.

Fitzpatrick, T.B., Johnson, R.A., Polano, M.K., Suurmond, D., and Wolff, K. 1992. *Color atlas and synopsis of clinical dermatology*, 2nd ed. New York: McGraw-Hill.

Friedrich, E.G. 1983. *Vulvar disease*, 2nd ed. Philadelphia: W.B. Saunders.

Goldstein, S.M., and Odom, R.B. 1993. Skin and appendages. In *Current medical diagnosis and treatment*, 32d ed., eds. L.M. Tierney, Jr., S.M. McPhee, M.A. Papadakis, and S.A. Schroeder, pp. 64–124. Norwalk, CT: Appleton & Lange.

————. 1994. Skin and appendages. In *Current medical diagnosis and treatment*, 33d ed., eds. L.M. Tierney, Jr., S.M. McPhee, and M.A. Papadakis, pp. 89–149. Norwalk, CT: Appleton & Lange.

Kaiser Permanente Medical Center. 1993. *Suggested treatments for common skin diseases*. Internal document.

Littler, J.E., and Momany, T. 1990. *University of Iowa. The family practice handbook*. Chicago: Year Book Medical Publishers.

Orkin, M., and Maibach, H. 1990. Scabies. In *Sexually transmitted diseases*, 2nd ed., eds. K.K. Holmes, P-A Mardh, P.F. Sparling, P.K. Wiesner, W. Cates, Jr., S.M. Lemon, and W.E. Stamm, pp. 473–479. New York: McGraw-Hill.

Orkin, M., Maibach, H.I., and Dahl, M.V. 1991. *Dermatology*. Norwalk, CT: Appleton & Lange.

Sauer, G.C. 1991. Manual of skin diseases, 6th ed. Philadelphia: J.B. Lippincott.

Tierney, L.M. 1993. Blood vessels and lymphatics. In *Current medical diagnosis and treatment*, 32d ed., eds. L.M. Tierney, Jr., S.M. McPhee, M.A. Papadakis, and S.A. Schroeder, pp. 393–394. Norwalk, CT: Appleton & Lange.

SECTION 4

Breast Disorders

Lisa L. Lommel, R.N., C., F.N.P., M.P.H.

4-A

Breast Pain and Nodularity

Breast pain (*mastalgia*) is the most common breast complaint for women. Three discrete patterns of breast pain have been recognized: *cyclical mastalgia, noncyclical mastalgia,* and *non-breast pain* (Maddox and Mansel 1989).

Cyclical breast pain is pain occurring the week preceding menses and relieved with menstruation, though pain of varying degrees may persist throughout the menstrual cycle. It is most common in women 30 years to 50 years of age and resolution perimenopausally is common. Though the exact etiology of cyclical breast pain is unclear, it is thought to be related to hormonal fluctuations of the menstrual cycle. Cyclical mastalgia often coexists with cyclical nodularity, but each may occur independently.

Cyclical swelling and nodularity is also secondary to the variation in concentration of gonadotrophic and ovarian hormones. Prior to menses, breast lobules, stroma, and ducts become engorged, causing swelling and nodularity. With the onset of menses, the ducts regress and epithelial cells desquamate and are maintained until the second week of the cycle, when proliferation begins again.

Occuring in pre- and post-menopausal women, non-cyclical mastalgia does not coincide with events in the menstrual cycle. Pain may begin and resolve at any time, often without a defined pattern. While the etiology of non-cyclical pain is poorly understood, radiological abnormalities consistent with coarse calcification and ductal dilatation are commonly seen. There is no histological evidence, however, that noncyclical pain results from the pathological changes of duct ectasia (Souba 1991). Nodularity is much less prominent than in the cyclical pain pattern.

Post-biopsy mastalgia (trauma-related), fat necrosis, and sclerosing adenosis, although less common, may be the cause of breast pain. Breast pain associated with cancer is uncommon (see **Breast Cancer Screening Protocol**) (Souba 1991).

Non-breast pain may be felt as breast pain, but may be caused by a painful costochondral junction syndrome (*Tietze's syndrome*). This pain is a chronic condition, often unilateral, and can occur at any age. The pain emanates from the area of the breast that overlies the tender costocartilage (Souba 1991).

DATABASE

SUBJECTIVE

→ Symptoms include:
- cyclical pain—heaviness, achiness, tenderness, unilaterally or bilaterally, beginning approximately one week—but may be as long as four weeks—prior to menses and resolving with onset of menses.
  - Usually is not well-localized, occurring most typically in upper outer quadrants.
  - May radiate to axilla, and down medial aspect of upper arm.
  - Some women report mastalgia for the first time with estrogen-replacement therapy or oral contraceptive use.
- diffuse lumpiness or nodularity without a dominant mass.
  - Nodularity more common in upper outer quadrants.
  - More commonly, a cyclical pattern beginning mid-cycle and progressing in intensity prior to

menses. Symptoms usually subside after menses begins.

- possible breast swelling, causing change in breast contour and size and bra feeling tighter.
  - Symptom severity may fluctuate from cycle to cycle.
- non-cyclical pain of duct ectasia:
  - burning pain, exacerbated by cold.
  - site precisely located most often subareolar or upper inner quadrant, tender to touch (see **Duct Ectasia/Periductal Mastitis** Protocol).
- non-cyclical pain of sclerosing adenosis:
  - spontaneous onset of well-localized pain.
- non-cyclical pain of fat necrosis:
  - history of trauma by injury, compression by an abscess, or incision for biopsy, localized to area of trauma. Pain may occur months to years after trauma (see **Fat Necrosis** Protocol).
- Tietze's syndrome:
  - unilateral chronic, sharp, or aching pain in the medial quadrants of the breast over the costocartilages. Pain occurs on pressure over affected cartilage.

OBJECTIVE

→ Carefully document findings using descriptive terms.
  - Mass(es) should be described by using a clock position, locating the mass in distance from the base of the nipple, the dimensions measured with a centimeter ruler or tape.
  - The consistency, shape, presence of tenderness, mobility, and associated skin changes should be described. Diagrams are helpful.

Cyclical pain

→ Inspection and palpation of the breasts—supraclavicular, and axillary regions (supine and sitting)—may not reveal a definite mass. If premenstrual, breasts may feel fuller and tense and demonstrate a prominent venous pattern.
  - Finely granular to grossly lumpy nodularity may be palpated particularly in upper outer quadrants.

Non-cyclical pain

→ No discrete palpable masses may be felt at the site of pain. Nodularity less prominent. Scar tissue may be felt over site of pain with post-biopsy trauma. A small, firm, fixed, mass may be felt in fat necrosis.

Tietze's syndrome

→ No discrete palpable mass at the site of pain but the involved costal cartilage may be enlarged. Palpation may elicit pain.

ASSESSMENT

→ Mastalgia—cyclical
→ Mastalgia—non-cyclical
  - R/O duct ectasia
  - R/O fat necrosis
  - R/O sclerosing adenosis
  - R/O post-biopsy trauma
  - R/O breast cancer
→ Non-breast mastalgia
  - R/O Tietze's syndrome
  - R/O degenerative disorders
  - R/O hiatal hernia
  - R/O angina
  - R/O cholelithiasis
  - R/O pulmonary disorders
→ Cyclical nodularity

PLAN

DIAGNOSTIC TESTS

→ In absence of a dominant mass, no specific diagnostic test is recommended.

→ Mammography may be recommended in women over 30 years of age for reassurance or because of suspicion of mass.

TREATMENT/MANAGEMENT

→ Ask a second examiner to corroborate findings.

→ Refer to breast specialist if a dominant mass is present.

→ Pain chart (kept for a minimum of 3 months) is helpful to define the pain pattern severity and to give a baseline measurement of the number of days of pain per cycle. This alone may provide reassurance if the pain is hormonally related.
  - Emphasize to the patient that her symptoms are normal and hormonally related. This should be first-line therapy.

→ For those patients who request treatment despite reassurance that their symptoms are due to a benign condition, and/or when mastalgia continues to severely affect their lives, pharmacological therapy should be offered.

→ Generalized nodularity, alone, usually does not require treatment. Reassurance that the condition is benign and normal should be offered. If pain and nodularity coexist, some reduction in nodularity is seen with danazol (Danocrine®) and bromocriptine (Parlodel®).

Cyclical pain

→ Combined oral contraceptives may be of benefit to women with a history of mild to moderate cyclical mastalgia. Breast pain usually ceases with the first pill cycle and clinical improvement is evident after 6 months.
  ▪ Routine cycling of a low-dose pill containing 30μg-35μg of estrogen and a low-dose/potency progestin is recommended (American College of Obstetricians and Gynecologists 1991; Reifsnider 1990).

→ For women who experience mastalgia or nodularity after starting oral contraceptives, withdrawal of the pill may decrease symptoms.
  ▪ If the patient wants to continue use, a change to a higher progestin pill may be of benefit.

→ For women on estrogen replacement therapy, complete withdrawal or substitution to a low-dose combined preparation may be of benefit (Gateley and Mansel 1991). (See also **Perimenopausal Symptoms and Hormone Therapy** Protocol).

→ In patients with severe symptoms, danazol or bromocriptine may be recommended (see following discussion).
  ▪ Tamoxifen and Gonadotropin-releasing hormone (GnRH) analogs are reserved for cases resistant to the other drugs (Gateley and Mansel 1991).

→ Danazol is effective in relieving breast mastalgia and nodularity in approximately 70 percent to 80 percent of treated patients, although nodularity decreases more slowly. It is also the best agent for severe mastalgia and nodularity (Hughes, Mansel, and Webster 1989).
  ▪ Symptoms recur in 30 percent to 65 percent of patients following discontinuation.
  ▪ Nipple discharge of duct ectasia decreases in 60 percent of patients (Jones and Hendler 1990).
  ▪ Dosage recommendations: 100 mg-300 mg daily then reduce to low maintenance doses of 25 mg-50 mg/day.
    • Adjustment in accordance with symptoms and side effects (Hughes, Mansel, and Webster 1989).
  ▪ Common side effects include amenorrhea, irregular menses, mild androgenic effects such as weight gain, acne and hirsutism, voice change, reduction in breast size. These are

generally dose-dependent. See *Physicians' Desk Reference (PDR)*.
  ▪ Contraindications: Pregnancy, lactation, abnormal vaginal bleeding, markedly impaired renal and/or cardiac function, or liver dysfunction.

→ Bromocriptine, a dopamine antagonist, is effective in lowering prolactin levels, thereby reducing mastalgia and nodularity in 70 percent of patients (Maddox and Mansel 1989).
  ▪ Usually reserved for moderate to severe mastalgia, its severe side effects may reduce its utility.
  ▪ Dosing recommendations (Hughes, Mansel, and Webster 1989):

Day of Menstrual Cycle	Dose
1-3	1.25 mg at night with food
4-7	2.5 mg at night with food
8-11	1.25 mg in morning with food and 2.5 mg at night with food
12 onward	2.5 mg in morning with food and 2.5 mg at night with food

  ▪ Common side effects can be severe and include nausea, vomiting, dizziness, and headache. See *PDR*. Should not be used in patients on a diuretic or hypotensive drug therapy.

→ Tamoxifen binds to estrogen receptors and has both agonistic and antagonistic actions. It has a response rate of approximately 70 percent in the treatment of mastalgia (Maddox and Mansel 1989).
  ▪ It has been demonstrated to be more effective than danazol in treating mastalgia (Speroff 1992).
  ▪ Response rates for nodularity are not available.
  ▪ It completely inhibits the action of estradiol on the breast and is therefore used to treat some estrogen-receptor-positive breast cancers. Studies are underway looking at tamoxifen use in the prevention of breast cancer.
  ▪ Dosage recommendations (Belieu 1994): 20 mg/day p.o. on cycle days 5 to 25 or 15 to 25, or daily for 1 to 4 cycles.
  ▪ Side effects: menstrual irregularity, bleeding secondary to endometrial hyperplasia, vaginal

atrophy, menopausal symptoms (hot flashes), and leukorrhea. See *PDR*.
- Contraindications: pregnancy.

→ GnRH agonists have had some success in treating mastalgia, and to a lesser extent, nodularity.
- GnRH agonists work by increasing the body's secretion of *luteinizing hormone* (LH) and *follicle-stimulating hormone* (FSH). Eventually, there is a depletion of stores of these hormones which decreases the amount of estrogen. The decreased amounts of estrogen then limit the breast symptoms.
- Although case studies have demonstrated the effectiveness of this drug, randomized controlled studies are pending (Preece 1990; Richardson and Njemanze 1990).
- Side effects include those of the perimenopause: menstrual irregularity, vasomotor symptoms, vaginal dryness, theoretical loss of bone density begining after 6 months of therapy, and effects on lipoprotein chemistry. See *PDR*.
- Contraindications: pregnancy.

→ Evening primrose oil is a rich source of *essential fatty acids* (EFAs). A hypothesis of mastalgia proposes an abnormality of prostaglandin production secondary to deficient EFA intake. A deficiency in EFAs increases the prolactin effects on the breast because of deficient production of prostaglandin.
- Studies suggest a 44 percent response rate in mild to moderate cases of mastalgia with no evidence showing reduction in nodularity (Hughes et al. 1989; Belieu 1994).
- Dosage recommendations: 3 grams daily (Maddox and Mansel 1989).
- Side effects: Mild nausea.
- Younger patients who are likely to need treatment of long duration, women who want to continue on oral contraceptives, or women with less severe symptoms may initially have evening primrose oil recommended to them (Gateley and Mansel 1991).

→ A pregnancy test should be done before initiating treatment with danazol, tamoxifen, bromocriptine, or GnRH agonists.

→ Clients at risk for pregnancy who are taking bromocriptine, danazol, or tamoxifen should use a barrier contraceptive method because these agents are potentially teratogenic and may reduce effectiveness of oral contraceptives. Women using oral contraception may take evening primrose oil.

→ An association between methylxanthine (caffeine, theophylline, theobromine) consumption or Vitamin E supplements and mastalgia/nodularity has not been substantiated (Hughes, Mansel, and Webster 1989; Simpson 1992). However, empiric use of Vitamin E (400-600 international units/day) has been effective for some women.

Non-Cyclical pain

→ Danazol appears to be effective with 31 percent of patients responding to treatment (Gateley and Mansel 1991). Recommended dosages for non-cyclical mastalgia are similar to the cyclical mastalgia treatment.

→ Evidence from controlled studies shows bromocriptine, tamoxifen, and evening primrose oil are equivalent to placebo (Hughes, Mansel, and Webster 1989).

→ Non-breast pain from Tietze's syndrome may be treated with lidocaine/steroid injection for intense, localized, persistent pain. For less severe pain, a trial of non-steroidal anti-inflammatory drugs (NSAIDs) is warranted.

CONSULTATION

→ For suspicion of a mass.

→ Advised for management of non-cyclical and non-breast pain.

→ Consultation and/or referral to physician for management with danazol, bromocriptine, tamoxifen, or GnRH agonists.

→ Physician management is warranted for injection treatment of chest wall pain.

→ As needed for prescription(s).

PATIENT EDUCATION

→ Non-pharmaceutical modalities which might help some women include:
- lower salt intake, especially prior to and during mastalgia symptoms.
- heat to breasts; wearing a well-fitting, supportive bra, especially with exercise.
- wearing a bra at night.
- analgesics.

→ Teach/review breast self-examination (BSE).

→ Allay patient's concerns regarding breast findings.

→ Teach/review use of pain chart.

→ Advise correct use of oral contraceptive, danazol, bromocriptine, or evening-primrose oil therapy including dose, regimen, side effects, and treatment plan.

→ Although an association between methylxanthine and mastalgia/nodularity has not been substantiated, a reduction in caffeine intake is safe.

FOLLOW-UP

→ In two to three months, re-examine breasts during the first half of the menstrual cycle, when pain and nodularity are minimal, to re-evaluate for discrete masses.

→ Continue danazol, bromocriptine, and evening primrose oil treatment for three months. Women who have some therapeutic response but ongoing severe pain should continue with an additional three-month treatment of original drug. If there is no response, consider an alternative therapy (Hughes, Mansel, and Webster 1989).

→ Continue breast pain chart throughout treatment to provide a quantitative means of measuring response to treatment.

→ Teach American Cancer Society's recommendation for routine breast screening (American Cancer Society 1992):
- BSE monthly starting at age 20 years.

- clinical breast examination every three years ages 20 years to 40 years and every year after age 40 years.
- mammography: every 2 years ages 40 years to 49 years. Every year starting at age 50 years.

NOTE: The National Cancer Institute's (NCI) summary of evidence for breast cancer screening with mammography concludes (National Cancer Institute 1994):
- ages 40 years to 49 years—there is no evidence to make an informed decision regarding efficacy of screening.
- ages 50 years and over—routine screening every one to two years with mammography and clinical breast examination can reduce breast cancer mortality by about one-third.

→ Women with a personal or family history of breast cancer may need more frequent clinical breast examinations and/or mammograms. Physician consultation should be sought.

→ Document in progress notes and problem list.

4-B

Breast Cancer Screening

One out of every nine American women will develop breast cancer during her lifetime. Breast cancer is the second leading cause of cancer death in women (lung cancer ranks first), and it accounts for 28 percent of all female cancers. Approximately two-thirds of all women with breast cancer are over age 50 years (American Cancer Society 1992).

Despite advances in diagnostic and surgical techniques, breast cancer remains very lethal. No more than twenty-five percent of breast cancer patients are "cured" (Speroff, Glass, and Kase 1989).

Cancer of the breast is of great concern to many women, especially those who have significant risk factors. Since only 25 percent of cancers of the breast occur in defined risk groups, screening for breast cancer should be applied to all asymptomatic women (American Cancer Society 1992). It should be emphasized that screening guidelines apply only to asymptomatic women. Women who have a suspicious breast mass warrant immediate evaluation.

DATABASE

SUBJECTIVE

→ Risk factors include:
- increasing age.
  - Progressive rise in incidence with age.
  - Rare in women under 30 years (Luce 1992).
- family history.
  - First-degree relative (mother or sister) with breast cancer confers a two to three times higher risk. If mother and sister are both affected the reported risk is as high as 50

percent by age 65 years (Kelsey and Gammon 1991).
  - Relatives of women with bilateral disease have even higher risk (Mulley 1995).
  - Families with ataxia-telangiectasia, an autosomal recessive syndrome, have an increased risk (Luce 1992; Kelsey and Gammon 1991).
- previous breast cancer.
  - Women with a history of primary breast cancer have a threefold to fourfold increase in risk for primary cancer in the contralateral breast (Kelsey and Gammon 1991).
  - History of endometrial cancer will slightly increase risk of breast cancer (Mulley 1995).
- menarche.
  - Increased risk of breast cancer in women who had early menarche (Luce 1992).
- menopause.
  - Late menopause increases risk twofold.
  - Early menopause, either natural or artificial, decreases the risk (Luce 1992).
- pregnancy.
  - Risk is higher in women who have never had a child or whose first full-term pregnancy occurred after age 30 years (Luce 1992).
  - Aborted pregnancy does not affect breast cancer risk (Mulley 1995).
- socioeconomic.
  - There is more breast cancer in upper-class women in more affluent countries. It is unknown to what extent this is due to better detection, diet, or environmental pollution factors (Luce 1992).

Table 4B.1. PATHOLOGICAL CLASSIFICATION OF BENIGN BREAST DISORDERS

I. Nonproliferative lesions of the breast
  A. cysts and apocrine metaplasia
  B. duct ectasia
  C. mild ductal epithelial hyperplasia
  D. calcifications
  E. fibroadenoma and related lesions
II. Proliferative breast disorders without atypia
  A. sclerosing adenosis
  B. radial and complexing sclerosing lesions
  C. moderate and florid ductal epithelial hyperplasia
  D. ductal involvement by cells of atypical lobular hyperplasia
  E. intraductal papillomas
III. Atypical proliferative lesions
  A. atypical lobular hyperplasia (ALH)
  B. atypical ductal hyperplasia (ADH)

Source: Reprinted with permission from Souba, W.W. 1991. In *The breast*, eds. K.I. Bland and E.M. Copeland. Philadelphia: W.B. Saunders.

Table 4B.2. RISK FOR DEVELOPMENT OF INVASIVE CARCINOMA AFTER BREAST BIOPSY

Lesion	Approximate Relative Risk
Nonproliferative lesions	no increased risk
Sclerosing adenosis	no increased risk
Intraductal papilloma	no increased risk
Moderate and florid hyperplasia (of usual type)	1.5-fold to twofold
Atypical lobular hyperplasia	fourfold
Atypical ductal hyperplasia	fourfold
Ductal involvement of cells of atypical ductal hyperplasia	sevenfold
Lobular carcinoma *in situ*	tenfold
Ductal carcinoma *in situ*	tenfold

Source: Reprinted with permission from Souba, W.W. 1991. In *The breast*, eds. K.I. Bland and E.M. Copeland. Philadelphia: W.B. Saunders.

- alcohol.
  - There is a positive dose-dependent association between alcohol consumption and risk for breast cancer.
  - Study results (as to degree of dose-dependent association) vary according to type of beverage, and pattern of consumption (Kelsey and Gammon 1991; Luce 1992; Stampfer, Bechtel, and Hunter 1992).
- irradiation.
  - A dose-response relationship has been found between radiation exposure and risk for breast cancer.
  - Peak effects appear to be in adolescents and young adults.
  - No complete data exists for risk associated with very low levels of exposure (Kelsey and Gammon 1991; Luce 1992).
- biopsy-proven breast changes.
  - Risk for breast cancer is increased in women with certain types of breast tissue changes. The **Pathological Classification of Benign Breast Disorders** is outlined in **Table 4B.1** (Souba 1991). The relative risk of developing breast cancer, based on pathological evaluation of breast tissue, is outlined in **Table 4B.2, Risk for Development of Invasive Carcinoma after Breast Biopsy** (Souba 1991).
→ Unsubstantiated risk factors include:
  - ethnicity.
    - About half as common in Asians as in Caucasians and African Americans.
    - Unknown to what extent environment, diet, or other socioeconomic factors influence risk.
    - Asian Americans have higher rates than their native Asian counterparts, though the rates of

breast cancer in China and Japan are rising sharply (Luce 1992).
- oral contraceptives.
  - No association has been confirmed between the risk for breast cancer and oral contraceptive use.
  - Controversy exists regarding long-term use of oral contraceptives at an early age, increasing the risk of breast cancer in women up to 45 years (Kelsey and Gammon 1991; McGonigle 1992).
- estrogen replacement.
  - No firm conclusions can be drawn about the risk for breast cancer associated with use of estrogen replacement therapy.
  - Studies suggest that estrogen use for 15 to 20 years or more may be associated with a modest elevated risk (Gibbons 1992).
- diet.
  - Dietary fat—specifically, saturated and animal fat—thought to be involved in breast cancer etiology.
  - However, recent literature reports weak or no association between fat intake and breast cancer risk.
  - Further studies are needed (Kelsey and Gammon 1991; Stampfer, Bechtel, and Hunter 1992).

DATABASE

SUBJECTIVE

→ Patient may have one or more risk factor(s) for breast cancer.

→ Breast mass almost always painless.

→ Symptoms may include:

- spontaneous, unilateral, serous, or bloody nipple discharge in non-lactating breast.
- itching, burning, dimpling, swelling, or redness of the skin.
- change in contour of the breast.
- nipple retraction.
- axillary swelling.

OBJECTIVE

→ Inspection and palpation of the breasts—supraclavicular and axillary regions (supine and sitting)—may reveal a breast mass, nipple retraction, skin dimpling (*peau d'orange*), erythema, edema, induration, and/or change in breast contour.

→ Patient may present with:
- unilateral, serous, or bloody discharge or crusting on nipple.
- supra/infraclavicular or axillary adenopathy.
- screening mammogram suspicious for breast cancer.

→ Carefully document findings using descriptive terms.
- Mass(es) should be described assuming a clock position, locating the mass in distance from the base of the nipple, the dimensions measured with a centimeter tape or ruler.
- Consistency, shape, presence of tenderness, mobility, and associated skin changes should be described. Diagrams are helpful.

ASSESSMENT

→ Breast mass (with or without adenopathy, nipple discharge, or skin changes)

→ R/O breast cancer

→ R/O benign breast disease

→ R/O cervical/dorsal radiculitis

→ R/O Tietze's syndrome (costochondritis)

PLAN

DIAGNOSTIC TESTS

→ Technologies for evaluating breast masses include:
- mammography—effective in diagnosing early-stage cancers.
  - Most effective in women over 30 years old, whose breasts are less dense.
  - Not recommended in pregnancy.
- sonography—primary use is for differentiating between a solid versus cystic palpable mass.

- Cannot reliably detect microcalcifications or lesions smaller than 1 cm.
- More effective diagnostic tool for fibrous tissue in women less than 30 years old.
- diaphanography (transillumination)—currently under investigation as a screening tool.
- ductography—used to evaluate nipple discharge in non-lactating breast. Involves cannulating involved duct, injecting radiopaque dye, and evaluating by x-ray.
- fine-needle aspiration (FNA)—utilizing a needle to aspirate fluid or tissue from a mass.
  - Solid masses can be aspirated for cytological study. If negative, cannot assume benign mass.
    - If suspicion persists, an excisional biopsy is recommended.
  - Needle aspiration can be useful for assessing palpable lymph nodes.

→ Biopsy for histological evaluation is the only definitive diagnostic procedure for breast cancer.

TREATMENT/MANAGEMENT

→ Second examiner to corroborate breast findings.

→ Refer to breast specialist if a dominant mass or any suspicious findings are present.

→ Discussion of treatment of breast cancer is beyond the scope of this protocol. Refer to current publication on breast cancer management.

CONSULTATION

→ For suspicious mass or findings.

→ Patients with diagnosed breast cancer are managed by a surgeon and oncologist.

PATIENT EDUCATION

→ Teach/review BSE.

→ Allay patient's concerns regarding breast findings.

→ Advise risk modification: decrease fat and alcohol intake, avoid excessive radiation exposure (mammography not included).

FOLLOW-UP

→ Follow-up appointment with breast specialist as indicated.

→ Teach American Cancer Society's recommendations for routine breast screening (American Cancer Society 1992):
- BSE: monthly starting at age 20 years.

■ clinical breast examination every three years ages 20 years to 40 years, every year after age 40 years.

■ mammography: every two years ages 40 years to 49 years, every year starting at age 50 years.

NOTE: NCI's summary of evidence for breast cancer screening with mammography concludes (National Cancer Institute 1994):

■ ages 40 years to 49 years—there is no evidence to make an informed decision regarding efficacy of screening.

■ ages 50 years and over—routine screening every one to two years with mammography and clinical breast examination can reduce breast cancer mortality by about one-third.

→ Patients with a personal or family history of breast cancer may need more frequent clinical breast examinations and/or mammograms. Physician consultation should be sought.

→ Document in progress notes and problem list.

Lisa L. Lommel, R.N., C., F.N.P., M.P.H.

4-C

Duct Ectasia/Periductal Mastitis

Mammary *duct ectasia/periductal mastitis* is the result of inflammation and enlargement of the ducts behind the nipple. The sequence and pathogenesis of events is not clear, although certain histological changes have been found to predominate with age.

Severe inflammation with lack of duct dilitation is seen more often in younger women. "Scanty" inflammatory changes but more mutiple duct dilitation was seen in older women. From these findings, Dixon et al. (1983) concluded that duct ectasia begins as periductal inflammation. As the inflammation resolves, the involved ducts become fibrotic and dilated (Ellerhorst-Ryan, Turba, and Stahl 1988).

Other authors postulate that duct ectasia/periductal mastitis is probably not a single entity and that additional research is needed to explain this complex condition (Hughes, Mansel, and Webster 1989).

Duct ectasia does not increase a women's risk for breast cancer. However, this condition can be complicated by severe inflammation which can cause significant morbidity.

DATABASE

SUBJECTIVE

→ Duct ectasia/periductal mastitis is more common in women ages 45 years to 55 years.

→ Periareolar or subareolar mass may be palpable incidentally or during BSE.

→ Pain of varying intensity may be felt depending on the degree of inflammation.
  ▪ Burning in nature.
  ▪ Exacerbated by cold.

  ▪ Located in subareolar area or in the upper inner quadrant.
  ▪ Usually non-cyclical.
  ▪ Tends to affect younger patients.

→ Duct ectasia is considered a primary cause of non-cyclical breast mastalgia (see **Breast Pain and Nodularity** Protocol).

→ Symptoms include spontaneous, intermittent, unilateral, or bilateral nipple discharge.
  ▪ More commonly thin and watery in the younger patient, and thick, sticky, or toothpaste-like in the older patient.
  ▪ May be off-white, cream-colored, brown, gray, green, greenish-brown, or bloodstained.

OBJECTIVE

→ Inspection and palpation of the breasts—supraclavicular and axillary regions (supine and sitting)—may reveal a 1- to 2-cm worm-like or tubular firm and tender mass in the subareolar region, not attached to surrounding tissue.
  ▪ Mass may appear rapidly and subside spontaneously within a week.
  ▪ May recur at the same site, at intervals of a few months to ten years or more.
    • With each recurrence, the condition tends to be more severe than the last.
  ▪ Bilateral masses may develop or the original mass may subside and a new mass begin in the opposite breast.
  ▪ Mass may also persist and become chronic in nature.
  ▪ Any of these masses may form abscesses.

→ Depending on the extent of inflammation, the nipple and areola may be red and swollen and the nipple flat or inverted.

→ Mild degrees of nipple retraction may occur in early inflammation. Retraction is present in 75 percent of patients with periareolar inflammation.
  ▪ Mean age is 53 years (Dixon 1989).

→ Young patients commonly present with pain and/ or an inflammatory mass. Older patients more likely have nipple retraction or a non-tender mass. This correlates with the suggested pathogenesis of this condition (Dixon 1989).

→ Findings should be carefully documented using descriptive terms.
  ▪ Mass(es) should be described assuming a clock position, locating the mass in distance from the base of the nipple, the dimensions measured with a centimeter ruler or tape.
  ▪ Consistency, shape, presence of tenderness, mobility, and associated changes should be described. Diagrams are helpful.

→ Attempt to elicit nipple discharge.
  ▪ Apply mild pressure over each quadrant of the periareolar region.
  ▪ Note the location of pressure and discharge, and the consistency and color of the discharge.

ASSESSMENT

→ Duct ectasia/periductal mastitis

→ R/O breast cancer

PLAN

DIAGNOSTIC TESTS

→ Mammography is recommended in women over 30 years of age to evaluate for breast cancer.

TREATMENT/MANAGEMENT

→ Ask a second examiner to corroborate findings.

→ Refer to a breast specialist if mass is present.

→ In early stages of inflammation, no intervention may be necessary. Advise patient to keep nipples clean.

→ When nipple discharge resembles galactorrhea, serum prolactin should be done to rule out prolactinemia (see **Galactorrhea** Protocol).

→ Development of moderate to severe inflammation and/or periareolar mass or abscess warrants antibiotic therapy and incision and drainage by a physician.

→ Local excision of involved ducts may be effective in controlling symptoms (Ellerhorst-Ryan, Turba, and Stahl 1988).

CONSULTATION

→ For confirmation of diagnosis.

→ Physician management for dominant mass, or moderate to severe inflammation or abscess is warranted.

→ As needed for prescription(s).

PATIENT EDUCATION

→ Teach/review BSE.

→ Allay patient's concerns regarding breast findings.

→ Advise patient to keep nipples clean with mild soap and water and to refrain from nipple manipulation.

FOLLOW-UP

→ For patients with only mild inflammation, re-examine at routine visits.

→ Follow-up appointment with breast specialist for patients with moderate to severe inflammation or abscess.

→ Teach American Cancer Society's recommendation for routine breast screening (American Cancer Society 1992):
  ▪ BSE—monthly starting at age 20 years.
  ▪ clinical breast examination: every three years ages 20 years to 40 years, every year after age 40 years.
  ▪ mammography—every two years ages 40 years to 49 years, every year starting at age 50 years.

NOTE: NCI's summary of evidence for breast cancer screening with mammography concludes (National Cancer Institute 1994):
  ▪ ages 40 years to 49 years—there is no evidence to make an informed decision regarding efficacy of screening.
  ▪ ages 50 years and over—routine screening every one to two years with mammography and clinical breast examination can reduce breast cancer mortality by about one-third.

→ Women with a personal or family history of breast cancer may need more frequent clinical breast examinations and/or mammograms. Physician consultation should be sought.

→ Document in progress notes and problem list.

Lisa L. Lommel, R.N., C., F.N.P., M.P.H.

4-D
Fat Necrosis

Necrosis of adipose tissue within the breast is a benign condition that is clinically uncommon. It can be linked to direct trauma of the breast in approximately 50 percent of patients (Osuch 1987). Fat necrosis also is reported secondary to breast biopsy, reduction mammoplasty, infection, duct ectasia, lumpectomy, radiotherapy, and malignant neoplasms (Morrow 1991; Ramzy 1990). Actual ecchymosis on physical examination is found in 20 percent to 30 percent of patients (Osuch 1987).

   Since this condition may simulate cancer (on physical examination and mammography), which is more common than fat necrosis, a history of trauma should not rule out the possibility of carcinoma. Fat necrosis does not increase a woman's risk for breast cancer.

DATABASE

SUBJECTIVE

→ Fat necrosis is more common in overweight, perimenopausal, large-breasted women.

→ Patient has history of:
  ▪ trauma to the breasts (50 percent of patients).
  ▪ breast biopsy, reduction mammoplasty, infection, duct ectasia, lumpectomy, radiotherapy, or malignant neoplasm.
  ▪ ecchymosis (20 percent to 30 percent of patients).
  ▪ non-cyclical breast pain, though more commonly painless.

→ Breast mass may be felt, more commonly subareolar.

→ Retraction of the skin may be present.

OBJECTIVE

→ Inspection and palpation of the breasts—supraclavicular and axillary regions (supine and sitting)—may reveal a small, firm, rounded, and smooth or irregular mass fixed to surrounding breast tissue and sometimes associated with skin retraction.

→ Ecchymosis may be present, or there may be evidence—in the form of pigmentation—of recent hemorrhage.

→ Mammography appearance may mimic carcinoma; cannot reliably distinguish between the two.

→ Carefully document findings using descriptive terms.
  ▪ Mass(es) should be described assuming a clock position, locating the mass in distance from the base of the nipple, the dimensions measured with a centimeter ruler.
  ▪ Consistency, shape, presence of tenderness, mobility, and associated skin changes should be described. Diagrams are helpful.

ASSESSMENT

→ Fat necrosis

→ R/O breast cancer

→ R/O benign breast disease

PLAN

DIAGNOSTIC TESTS

→ FNA for cytology is warranted in the presence of a mass.

→ Biopsy may be indicated.

TREATMENT/MANAGEMENT

→ Second examiner to corroborate breast findings.

→ Refer to a breast specialist if dominant mass or any suspicious findings are present.

→ When major trauma to the breast has occurred, accompanied by ecchymosis and a palpable mass, expectant management may be employed.

→ In the absence of clear evidence of trauma and presence of mass, biopsy is warranted.

CONSULTATION

→ Consultation is recommended with history and evidence of trauma and palpable mass.

→ Referral is warranted in absence of clear history and absence of evidence of trauma and a palpable mass.

PATIENT EDUCATION

→ Teach/review BSE.

→ Allay patient's concerns regarding breast findings.

→ Advise ways to avoid trauma to the breasts—e.g., wearing supportive bra, placing seat belt strap below breast, avoiding sports-related injuries.

FOLLOW-UP

→ A mass associated with trauma and ecchymosis may exhibit an initial increase in size followed by regression, or the mass may remain unchanged for years.

→ Follow-up appointment with breast specialist as indicated.

→ Teach American Cancer Society's recommendations for routine breast screening (American Cancer Society 1992):
- BSE—monthly starting at age 20 years.
- clinical breast examination: every three years ages 20 years to 40 years, every year after age 40 years.
- mammography—every two years ages 40 years to 49 years, every year starting at age 50 years.

NOTE: NCI's summary of evidence for breast cancer screening with mammography concludes (National Cancer Institute 1994):
- ages 40 to 49 years—there is no evidence to make an informed decision regarding efficacy of screening.
- ages 50 years and over—routine screening every one to two years with mammography and clinical breast examination can reduce breast cancer mortality by about one-third.

→ Patients with a family or personal history of breast cancer may need more frequent clinical breast examinations and/or mammograms. Physician consultation should be sought.

→ Document in progress notes and problem list.

4-E

Fibroadenoma

Fibroadenomas are the most common benign solid tumor of the female breast. A fibroadenoma is considered an abnormal growth of two types of normal breast tissue—*fibrous tissue* and *ductal tissue*. Under hormonal influence, these two tissues proliferate and grow in size, becoming large enough to be palpable.

A fibroadenoma may grow progressively, remain the same size, or regress. Most fibroadenomas grow to 1 cm to 2 cm in size (Dixon 1991). Fibroadenomas may grow rapidly, reaching a size larger than 4 cm, though this is uncommon. Such tumors are called giant fibroadenomas and occur most commonly in adolescent and menopausal age groups.

Like normal breast lobules, fibroadenomas will develop hyperplastic changes during pregnancy, secrete milk during lactation, and involute at menopause (Hughes, Mansel, and Webster 1989).

Fibroadenomas are most common in African American women in their 20s and early 30s. Twelve percent to 16 percent of all women will have bilateral lesions. Fibroadenomas are not considered a risk factor for breast cancer (Dent and Cant 1989).

DATABASE

SUBJECTIVE

→ Breast mass may be palpable during BSE.
- Unless very large, almost always painless.
- More commonly singular but may be multiple.
- No evidence of change during the menstrual cycle, either in size or consistency.

OBJECTIVE

→ Inspection and palpation of breasts—supraclavicular and axillary regions (supine and sitting)—may reveal a mass that is firm, rubbery, smooth, discrete, mobile, and non-tender.
- After menopause, mass may regress—becoming stony, hard, discrete, and moderately mobile—but it usually will not disappear totally.
- Single mass more common, though there may be multiple and/or bilateral masses.
  - Multiple masses occur in 10 percent to 20 percent of women (Ellerhorst-Ryan, Turba, and Stahl 1988).
- Majority of masses located in upper outer quadrants, more commonly in the left breast.
- Mass may be found incidentally on mammography.
- Masses may grow rapidly during pregnancy.
→ Findings should be carefully documented using descriptive terms.
- Masses should be described assuming a clock position, locating the mass in distance from the base of the nipple, the dimensions measured with a centimeter tape or ruler.
- Consistency, shape, presence of tenderness, mobility, and associated skin changes should be described. Diagrams are helpful.

ASSESSMENT

→ Fibroadenoma
→ R/O fluid cyst

→ R/O benign mass

→ R/O breast cancer

→ R/O cervical/dorsal radiculitis

→ R/O Tietze's syndrome (costochondritis)

PLAN

DIAGNOSTIC TESTS

→ Sonography may be employed to differentiate a solid from a cystic mass.

- Not effective in differentiating a benign from a malignant mass.
- For women under 25 years of age (when the risk for cancer is rare), sonography, together with clinical examination, can aid in the differentiation of a cystic or solid mass and may obviate the need for aspiration cytology.
- In women ages 25 to 30 years, sonography can be used in conjunction with clinical examination and aspiration cytology to improve diagnostic accuracy.
- Not effective assessment tool for women older than 30 years whose breasts are less dense, and because of the increasing risk of breast cancer (Bassett and Kimme-Smith 1991).
- Other limitations to sonography include:
  - cannot detect microcalcifications.
  - difficulty in imaging fatty breast.
  - unreliably depicts solid masses smaller than 1 cm (Bassett Kimme-Smith 1991).

→ Mammography is recommended in women older than 30 years who have a breast mass.

→ FNA is indicated for palpable masses in women older than 25 years (Dent and Cant 1989).

- Cytological testing should be completed on all solid tumor aspirates for specific diagnosis.

TREATMENT/MANAGEMENT

→ Ask second reviewer to corroborate breast findings.

→ Refer to breast specialist if dominant mass is present.

→ Since the risk of cancer is low in women younger than 25 years, the younger woman with a fibroadenoma smaller than 3 cm can be given a choice regarding excision. Excision is recommended for women older than 25 years or those with larger fibroadenomas (Simpson 1992).

CONSULTATION

→ For suspicion of a mass.

→ Physician management is warranted with presence of a dominant mass.

PATIENT EDUCATION

→ Teach/review BSE.

→ Allay patient's concerns regarding breast findings.

FOLLOW-UP

→ Follow-up appointment with breast specialist as indicated.

→ Teach American Cancer Society's recommendation for routine breast screening (American Cancer Society 1992):

- BSE: monthly starting at age 20 years.
- clinical breast examination: every three years ages 20 years to 40 years, every year after age 40 years.
- mammography: every two years ages 40 years to 49 years, every year starting at age 50 years.

NOTE: NCI's summary of evidence for breast cancer screening with mammography concludes (National Cancer Institute 1994):

- ages 40 years to 49 years—there is no evidence to make an informed decision regarding efficacy of screening.
- ages 50 years and over—routine screening every one to two years with mammography and clinical breast examination can reduce breast cancer mortality by about one-third.

→ Women with a personal or family history of breast cancer may need more frequent clinical breast examinations and/or mammograms. Physician consultation should be sought.

→ Document in progress notes and problem list.

Lisa L. Lommel, R.N., C., F.N.P., M.P.H.

4-F

Fluid Cysts

A simple, gross, fluid-filled cyst can exist alone or in conjunction with breast nodularity. A simple cyst is defined sonographically as one with smooth margins, a well-defined posterior wall, enhanced sound transmission distally, and an echo-free interior (Bassett and Kimme-Smith 1991). It is the most common dominant mass in the female breast, found most often in women ages 35 years to 50 years.

Fluid-filled cysts usually cease with menopause except for women on hormone replacement therapy. There is no evidence that simple cysts increase a woman's risk for breast cancer (Haagensen 1991).

DATABASE

SUBJECTIVE

→ Symptoms include:
- single or multiple masses palpable during BSE, more commonly in the left breast.
  - Mass may have developed as rapidly as overnight.
  - Mass may be visible when patient is lying down.
- possible nipple discharge, evident when a duct is involved.

→ Pain:
- is not associated with the menstrual cycle.
- may be associated with a mass that develops rapidly, a large mass, or with rapid disappearance of a mass (due to rupture or discharge of contents into a duct).

OBJECTIVE

→ Inspection and palpation of breasts—supraclavicular areas and axillary regions (supine and sitting)—may reveal a single or multiple mass that is firm, mobile, partially attached to the breast tissue, well delineated, and tense and tender if fully filled, or soft, fluctuant, and tender, if partially filled.
- Two-thirds occur in upper outer quadrant.

→ A cyst may be found incidentally on mammography for breast cancer screening.

→ Carefully document findings using descriptive terms.
- Mass(es) should be described assuming a clock position, locating the mass in distance from the base of the nipple, the dimensions measured with a centimeter ruler.
- Consistency, shape, presence of tenderness, mobility, and associated skin changes should be described. Diagrams are helpful.

ASSESSMENT

→ Fluid cyst

→ R/O fibroadenoma

→ R/O fat necrosis

→ R/O other benign mass

→ R/O breast cancer

PLAN

DIAGNOSTIC TESTS

→ Sonography is recommended as the primary imaging technique for women under 30 years of age to differentiate between a cystic and a solid mass.

- If needle aspiration is done, sonography may be excluded or used to aid in directed aspiration.

→ Mammography is recommended for women over 30 years of age to assist in the diagnosis of a cyst and to exclude an incidental cancer.

→ FNA is both diagnostic and therapeutic for simple cysts and is recommended for a palpable mass in women older than 25 years.

- Cytological testing should be completed on aspirates that are bloodstained. Normal cyst fluid ranges in color from pale yellow to dark green to brown.

TREATMENT/MANAGEMENT

→ Ask a second examiner to corroborate breast findings.

→ Refer to breast specialist if a dominant mass is present.

→ FNA is therapeutic. Re-aspiration may be necessary if cyst recurs.

→ Further evaluation in consultation with a breast specialist is necessary if (Hughes, Mansel, and Webster 1989):

- the cyst does not disappear with aspiration.
- the fluid in cyst is bloody.

→ If the mass is not seen by ultrasound, mammography may be indicated, primarily to look for microcalcifications.

- Single-view mammogram may be used for young women (Jackson 1990).

→ Multiple cyst formation can be treated with Danazol (Danocrine®) 200 mg-400 mg/day. See *PDR*.

→ Physician consultation is warranted (Dixon 1990).

CONSULTATION

→ For suspicion of a mass.

→ Physician management is warranted with presence of a dominant mass.

→ For drug management of multiple cysts.

PATIENT EDUCATION

→ Teach/review BSE.

→ Allay patient's concern regarding breast finding.

FOLLOW-UP

→ Follow-up appointment with breast specialist as indicated.

→ Re-examine in three to four weeks to confirm that cyst has not refilled.

→ Teach American Cancer Society's recommendations for routine breast screening (American Cancer Society 1992):

- BSE—monthly starting at age 20 years.
- clinical breast examination—every three years ages 20 years to 40 years, every year after age 40 years.
- mammography—every two years ages 40 years to 49 years, every year starting at age 50 years.

NOTE: NCI's summary of evidence for breast cancer screening with mammography concludes (National Cancer Institute 1994):

- ages 40 years to 49 years—there is no evidence to make an informed decision regarding efficacy of screening.
- ages 50 years and over—routine screening every one to two years with mammography and clinical breast examination can reduce breast cancer mortality by about one-third.

→ Women with a personal or family history of breast cancer may need more frequent clinical breast examinations and/or mammograms. Physician consultation should be sought.

→ Document in progress notes and problem list.

4-G

Galactocele

A *galactocele* is an uncommon, milk-filled mass caused by over-distention and/or obstruction of a lactiferous duct. Most galactoceles develop after cessation of lactation. Infrequently, they are associated with galactorrhea or contraceptive use (Ramzy 1990). Galactoceles are not risk factors for breast cancer.

DATABASE

SUBJECTIVE

→ Symptoms may include:
  - milky-white nipple discharge may occur, and in later stages the discharge may be green or yellow.
  - painless mass that is commonly subareolar or periareolar.

→ Typical history includes:
  - abrupt cessation of lactation.
  - possible gradual cessation of lactation or galactorrhea.
  - oral contraceptive use.

OBJECTIVE

→ Inspection and palpation of breasts—supra-clavicular and axillary regions (supine and sitting)—may reveal a mass that is smooth, mobile, well delineated, and firm or soft and fluctuant.

→ Patient may present with:
  - single or multiple masses.
  - milky-white, green, or yellow discharge.

→ Findings should be carefully documented using descriptive terms.

- Mass(es) should be described assuming a clock position, locating the mass in distance from the base of the nipple, the dimensions measured with a centimeter tape or ruler.
- Consistency, shape, presence of tenderness, mobility, and associated skin changes should be described. Diagrams are helpful.

ASSESSMENT

→ Galactocele

→ R/O fluid-filled cyst

→ R/O fibroadenoma

→ R/O other benign mass

→ R/O breast cancer

PLAN

DIAGNOSTIC TESTS

→ FNA is advised in any woman older than 25 years who has a breast mass. FNA is recommended in women younger than 25 years if there is suspicion of a cyst and with history of recent lactation.
  - Withdrawal of milky discharge is diagnostic for galactocele.
  - Evidence of fat lobules can be identified with microscopy.

TREATMENT/MANAGEMENT

→ Ask a second examiner to corroborate breast findings.

→ Refer to breast specialist if a dominant mass is present.

→ FNA often is curative, although multiple aspirations may be needed.

→ Galactocele may be self-limiting and may subside in a few weeks.

→ Galactocele may recur after aspiration.

CONSULTATION

→ For suspicion of a mass.

→ Physician management is warranted with presence of a dominant mass.

PATIENT EDUCATION

→ Teach/review BSE.

→ Allay patient's concerns regarding breast findings.

→ Advise patient to taper weaning and not abruptly discontinue breast-feeding to decrease risk of recurrence.

FOLLOW-UP

→ Re-examine in three to four weeks to confirm that cyst has not refilled.

→ Follow-up appointment with breast specialist as indicated.

→ Teach American Cancer Society's recommendation for routine breast screening (American Cancer Society 1992):

- BSE—monthly starting at age 20 years.
- clinical breast examination—every three years ages 20 years to 40 years, every year after age 40 years.
- mammography—every two years ages 40 years to 49 years, every year starting at age 50 years.

NOTE: NCI's summary of evidence for breast cancer screening with mammography concludes (National Cancer Institute 1994):

- ages 40 years to 49 years—there is no evidence to make an informed decision regarding efficacy of screening.
- ages 50 years and over—routine screening every one to two years with mammography and clinical breast examination can reduce breast cancer mortality by about one-third.

→ Women with a personal or family history of breast cancer may need more frequent clinical breast examinations and/or mammograms. Physician consultation should be sought.

→ Document in progress notes and problem list.

Lisa L. Lommel, R.N., C., F.N.P., M.P.H.

4-H

Galactorrhea

Galactorrhea is a multiple-duct, milky nipple discharge most commonly seen in the non-lactating woman during childbearing years. It is most often caused by an increase in production of prolactin (*hyperprolactinemia*), either by direct pituitary gland action or indirectly by an inadequate hypothalamic inhibition of the pituitary gland (Leis 1989).

Chronic hyperprolactinemia can result from physiological, pharmacological, pathological, or functional causes. See **Table 4H.1,** for **Causes of Chronic Hyperprolactinemia in the Non-Pregnant Female.**

Although galactorrhea is a classic symptom of hyperprolactinemia, 30 percent of patients with galactorrhea will not have elevated prolactin levels. The cause of this is unclear. Also, hyperprolactinemia is not always associated with galactorrhea (Katz and Adashi 1990).

DATABASE

SUBJECTIVE

→ Symptoms may include:
  ▪ milky discharge—spontaneous and intermittent or persistent, unilateral or bilateral.
  ▪ in patients with moderate to severe hyperprolactinemia, *hypoestrogenic symptoms* (menopausal symptoms)—e.g., vasomotor symptoms, decreased breast size, vaginal atrophy.
→ Elicited discharge may be physiological (see **Nipple Discharge—Physiological** Protocol) but should be evaluated per **Galactorrhea** Protocol.
→ Patient may experience menstrual irregularities varying from polymenorrhea to amenorrhea.

▪ Oligomenorrhea and amenorrhea are the most common.
▪ Approximately one-third of women with galactorrhea will have normal menses (Speroff, Glass, and Kase 1989) (see **Amenorrhea—Secondary** Protocol).
→ Mild hirsutism may accompany ovulatory dysfunction (see **Hirsutism** Protocol).
→ Patient may have history or signs and symptoms of:
  ▪ any of the causes of hyperprolactinemia (see **Table 4H.1**).
    • For example, neoplastic lesions may produce headaches and visual changes (Katz and Adashi 1990).
  ▪ infertility.

OBJECTIVE

→ Inspection and palpation of the breasts—supraclavicular and axillary regions (supine and sitting) and compression of the breast, areola, or nipple—may reveal a milky nipple discharge. A mass usually is not present.
→ Patients with a history or symptoms of any of the causes of hyperprolactinemia may elicit manifestations of the condition (See **Table 4H.1**).
→ Clinical symptoms of galactorrhea or menstrual irregularities do not always correlate with prolactin levels.
→ Confrontation testing of the visual fields and a fundoscopic examination should be done.
→ See **Amenorrhea—Secondary** Protocol.

Table 4H.1. CAUSES OF CHRONIC HYPERPROLACTINEMIA IN THE NON-PREGNANT FEMALE

Physiological	Excessive breast manipulation
	Stress, surgery, venipuncture, etc.
Pharmacological	Depletion of tuberoinfundibular dopamine stores (by extrusion from intracellular granule to cytosol)
	Reserpine
	Blockade of dopamine receptor binding
	Phenothiazines (Thorazine®, Mellaril®, Compazine®, Trilafon®, Stelazine®)
	Thioxanthenes (Taractan®)
	Butyrophenones (Haldol®)
	Benzamines (Metoclopramide [Reglan®], Sulpiride)
	Dibenzoxapine antidepressants (amoxapine [Asendin®])
	Inhibition of dopamine release
	Chronic opiate use (methadone, morphine)
	Blockade of histamine (H_2) receptor binding
	Cimetidine (Tagamet®)
	Estrogen-containing oral contraceptives
	Interference with the synthesis of dopamine
	α-Methyldopa
	Calcium channel blockers (Verapamil®)
	Mechanism unknown
	Tricyclic antidepressants (imipramine [Tofranil®], amitryptiline [Elavil®], etc.)
	Papaverine derivatives
Pathological	Primary hypothyroidism
	Hypothalamic disorders
	Neoplastic, infectious, vascular, degenerative, or granulomatous hypothalamic lesions
	Pituitary stalk section
	Pituitary disorders
	Prolactin-secreting adenoma
	Acromegaly, Cushing's disease, Nelson syndrome
	Ectopic production of prolactin
	Bronchogenic carcinoma, hypernephroma
	Chronic renal failure
	Chest wall lesions
	Surgical scars, herpes zoster
Functional	Idiopathic (no demonstrable tumor)

Source: Reprinted with permission from Katz, E. and Adashi, E.Y. 1990. Hyperprolactinemic disorders. *Clinical Obstetrics and Gynecology* 33(3):622-639.

ASSESSMENT

→ Galactorrhea

→ R/O hyperprolactinemia

→ R/O any of the possible causes of hyperprolactinemia (See **Table 4H.1**)

PLAN

DIAGNOSTIC TESTS

→ A serum prolactin level should be obtained in all cases of spontaneous discharge and in cases of elicited discharge when physiological causes cannot be ruled out (see **Nipple Discharge—Physiological** Protocol).

- Optimal sampling time is between 8:00 a.m. and 12:00 noon.
- Avoid sampling during and after events that may result in transient physiological hyperprolactinemia: excessive breast stimulation, stress, pelvic examination, coitus, surgical procedures, during mid-cycle, after an extended sleep, and following a protein-rich meal (Katz and Adashi 1990).

NOTE: The half-life for prolactin is 50 to 60 minutes.

→ Computerized axial (assisted) tomographic (CAT, CT) scanning or magnetic resonance imaging (MRI) is indicated with a prolactin greater than or equal to 50 ng/ml, or for lesser values, in consultation with a physician.

- CT scan more useful in the diagnosis of small pituitary tumors that do not distort or alter the size of the gland.
- MRI, although more expensive and not as widely available, is an improvement over CT scanning for the visualization of structures adjacent to the pituitary, which may be affected by tumoral growth, and to diagnose empty-sella syndrome (Katz and Adashi 1990).

→ Thyroid-stimulating hormone (TSH) should be obtained to rule out thyroid disease.

→ A variety of diagnostic tests to rule out underlying disorders may be obtained, depending on the history and physical examination.

→ See **Amenorrhea—Secondary** Protocol.

TREATMENT/MANAGEMENT

→ Hyperprolactinemia due to physiological causes should be managed by discontinuing or reducing the precipitating events (e.g., a decrease in breast manipulation).

→ Hyperprolactinemia of pharmacological origin is managed by eliminating the causative drug.

- In cases where the drug is necessary or when an alternative drug is not available, the presence of galactorrhea and associated symptoms should be weighed against the consequences of discontinuing the drug.

→ Management of hyperprolactinemia—due to pathology other than pituitary tumors or idiopathic hyperprolactinemia—should include treatment of the underlying condition—e.g., treatment of hypothyroidism.

→ Hyperprolactinemia due to prolactin-secreting pituitary tumors should be managed by a physician with dopaminergic agents (e.g., bromocriptine [Parlodel®]) or, rarely, surgery.

→ Hyperprolactinemia due to idiopathic causes should be managed by a physician.
  ▪ Expectant management and/or bromocriptine have/has been employed.

→ Women with a normal prolactin and regular menses have a low risk of pituitary tumor and can be managed expectantly.
  ▪ Periodic prolactin levels should be done to confirm the stability of the underlying process.
  ▪ If the presence or amount of galactorrhea is unsatisfactory to the patient, bromocriptine may be used to reduce the occurrence (Speroff, Glass, and Kase 1989).

→ See **Amenorrhea—Secondary** Protocol.

CONSULTATION

→ Physician management is necessary for management with bromocriptine or when surgery is indicated.

PATIENT EDUCATION

→ Teach/review BSE.

→ Allay patient's concerns regarding breast findings.

→ Patient should be advised before withdrawal of pharmacological agents that may be causing hyperprolactinemia.

→ For women with physiological causes of hyperprolactinemia, advise ways of omitting the offending event.
  ▪ For example, to reduce breast stimulation, if sexually related, teach alternative means of stimulation.
  ▪ For example, if stress-induced, provide suggestions for stress reduction.

→ Advise women using bromocriptine to use an effective form of contraception because of its teratogenic potential.

▪ Review common side effects of this drug:
  • nausea.
  • vomiting.
  • headaches.
  • faintness.
  • dizziness.
  • nasal congestion.
  • fatigue.
  • abdominal cramps.
  • (rarely) neuropsychiatric symptoms (Speroff, Glass, and Kase 1989). See *PDR*.

→ See **Amenorrhea—Secondary** Protocol.

FOLLOW-UP

→ Women with galactorrhea, normal prolactin levels, and normal menses can be followed with periodic prolactin levels every year.
  ▪ If prolactin levels increase, CT scan or MRI can be ordered.

→ Teach/encourage American Cancer Society's recommendation for routine breast screening (American Cancer Society 1992):
  ▪ BSE—monthly starting at age 20 years.
  ▪ clinical breast examination—every three years, ages 20 years to 40 years, every year after age 40 years.
  ▪ mammography—every two years, ages 40 years to 49 years, every year starting at age 50 years.

NOTE: NCI's summary of evidence for breast cancer screening with mammography concludes (National Cancer Institute 1994):
  ▪ ages 40 years to 49 years—there is no evidence to make an informed decision regarding efficacy of screening.
  ▪ ages 50 years and over—routine screening every one to two years with mammography and clinical breast examination can reduce breast cancer mortality by about one-third.

→ Women with a personal or family history of breast cancer may need more frequent clinical breast examinations and/or mammograms. Physician consultation should be sought.

→ Document in progress notes and problem list.

Lisa L. Lommel, R.N., C., F.N.P., M.P.H.

4-1

Intraductal Papilloma

Intraductal papillomas are finger-like projections that invade the lumen of the duct. They are caused by proliferation of the ductal epithelium. Trauma to the ducts that contain papillomas will cause bleeding into the duct lumen and subsequent spontaneous serous or bloody discharge.

Intraductal papillomas are the most common cause of nipple discharge in women who are not pregnant or lactating. Papillomas are more common in the perimenopausal and menopausal woman. Solitary forms of intraductal papilloma (i.e., only one duct involved) do not increase a women's risk for breast cancer, though multiple forms of this condition (i.e., involving multiple ducts) have been shown to be linked with malignant transformation (Ellerhorst-Ryan, Turba, and Stahl 1988; Hughes, Mansel, and Webster 1989). Multiple forms of intraductal papilloma usually affect younger women and are more likely to present with a mass than with nipple discharge.

DATABASE

SUBJECTIVE

→ Symptoms may include:
- bloody (approximately 50 percent of patients) or serous (another 50 percent of patients), spontaneous, intermittent nipple discharge noticed on undergarments or nightclothes (Hughes, Mansel, and Webster 1989).
  - More commonly unilateral, though may be bilateral.
- mass felt but evident in only approximately 50 percent of patients (Osuch 1987).
- tenderness felt with pressure over the involved duct.

OBJECTIVE

→ Inspection and palpation of the breasts—supraclavicular and axillary regions (supine and sitting)—may reveal a subareolar mass, though these are uncommon.
- With multiple forms of intraductal papilloma, mass more commonly in the periphery of the breast.

→ For women with a history of nipple discharge, involved duct can be located by exerting gentle pressure at areolar margin in a circular path around nipple.
- When discharge seen, document location, whether it emanates from a single duct or multiple ducts, and its consistency and color.

→ Carefully document findings using descriptive terms.
- Mass(es) should be described assuming a clock position, locating the mass in distance from the base of the nipple, the dimensions measured with a centimeter ruler or tape.
- Consistency, shape, presence of tenderness, mobility, and associated skin changes should be described. Diagrams are helpful.

ASSESSMENT

→ Solitary intraductal papilloma
→ R/O multiple intraductal papilloma
→ R/O duct ectasia
→ R/O physiological nipple discharge
→ R/O breast cancer

PLAN

DIAGNOSTIC TESTS

→ Mammography is recommended in women over age 30 years to rule out breast cancer.

→ Cytological analysis of the discharge may be recommended, though it is not reliable in evaluating abnormal cells.

  ▪ If a mass is present, aspiration cytology more appropriate.

→ A ductogram can aid in the diagnosis of a papilloma.

TREATMENT/MANAGEMENT

→ Ask a second examiner to corroborate breast finding.

→ Referral to a breast specialist for management.

→ Surgical excision of the involved duct is the usual treatment.

→ If mammogram is normal, expectant management may be chosen. Nipple discharge may cease with time, probably as a result of necrosis of the papilloma.

CONSULTATION

→ For suspicion of a mass.

→ Physician referral is recommended for diagnosis.

PATIENT EDUCATION

→ Teach/review BSE.

→ Allay patient's concerns regarding breast finding.

FOLLOW-UP

→ Encourage follow-up appointment with breast specialist.

→ Teach American Cancer Society's recommendations for routine breast screening (American Cancer Society 1992):

  ▪ BSE—monthly starting at age 20 years.
  ▪ clinical breast examination—every three years ages 20 years to 40 years, every year after age 40 years.
  ▪ mammography—every two years ages 40 years to 49 years, every year starting at age 50 years.

NOTE: NCI's summary of evidence for breast cancer screening with mammography concludes (National Cancer Institute 1994):

  ▪ ages 40 years to 49 years—there is no evidence to make an informed decision regarding efficacy of screening.
  ▪ ages 50 years and over—routine screening every one to two years with mammography and clinical breast examination can reduce breast cancer mortality by about one-third.

→ Women with a personal or family history of breast cancer may need more frequent clinical breast examinations or mammograms. Physician consultation should be sought.

→ Document in progress notes and problem list.

Lisa L. Lommel, R.N., C., F.N.P., M.P.H.

4-J

Mastitis—Non-Lactational

Non-lactational mastitis, an inflammatory condition of the breast, is not associated with lactation. Non-lactational breast infections can present as peripheral or subareolar abscesses. Although they are distinct conditions, their management is similar. When cultured, non-lactational abscesses usually yield multiple organisms including anaerobes (Smith 1991).

Rarely, non-lactational mastitis can be the result of diseases such as tuberculosis, actinomycosis, typhoid, syphilis, or carcinoma.

DATABASE

SUBJECTIVE

Peripheral mastitis

→ More common in younger, premenopausal women:
- who may have a history of diabetes, rheumatoid arthritis, steroid treatment, trauma to the breasts, or silicone implants, but, commonly, have no predisposing factor.

Subareolar mastitis

→ More common in older, premenopausal women.
- Fifty percent will have nipple abnormality— partial nipple inversion or nipple retraction.
  - Symptoms may include:
    - a small palpable mass.
    - tenderness to intense subareolar pain.
    - erythema and/or induration.
- May have a history of squamous epithelial metaplasia or duct ectasia (see **Duct Ectasia/ Periductal Mastitis** Protocol).

→ Unlike lactational mastitis, malaise and fever usually are not present.

OBJECTIVE

→ Inspection and palpation of the breasts— supraclavicular and axillary regions (supine and sitting)—may reveal a tender peripheral mass and axillary lymphadenopathy.

→ Inflammatory changes of the breasts—i.e., edema, erythema, and/or induration—may be present.

→ Findings should be carefully documented using descriptive terms.
- Mass(es) should be described assuming a clock position, locating the mass in distance from the base of the nipple, the dimensions measured with a centimeter ruler or tape.
- Consistency, shape, presence of tenderness, mobility, and associated skin changes should be described. Diagrams are helpful.

ASSESSMENT

→ Non-lactational mastitis

→ R/O duct ectasia

→ R/O concomitant condition—e.g., diabetes, rheumatoid arthritis, steroid treatment, trauma to the breasts.

PLAN

DIAGNOSTIC TESTS

→ FNA for diagnostic culture may be indicated, though it usually does not alter the management plan.

TREATMENT/MANAGEMENT

→ Ask second examiner to corroborate breast findings.

→ Peripheral abscesses are most effectively treated by incision and drainage with appropriate antibiotic coverage (Smith 1991).

→ Subareolar abscesses have a very high recurrence rate with standard incision and drainage.
  ■ Antibiotic therapy does not improve course.
  ■ Recommendation is to incise and drain and provide appropriate antibiotics during acute phase.
    • When major inflammatory process has resolved, duct excision may be indicated (see **Duct Ectasia/Periductal Mastitis** Protocol) (Smith 1991).

CONSULTATION

→ For suspicious mass or finding.

→ Referral to a physician is indicated for diagnosis and treatment.

→ Referral to a physician is warranted if an abscess is present.

→ As needed for prescription(s).

PATIENT EDUCATION

→ Teach/review BSE.

→ Allay patient's concerns regarding breast findings.

→ Advise patient to complete course of antibiotics.

FOLLOW-UP

→ Reexamine patient in 24 to 48 hours after antibiotics started.

→ Follow-up appointment with breast specialist as indicated.

→ Teach American Cancer Society's recommendations for routine breast screening (American Cancer Society 1992):
  ■ BSE—monthly starting at age 20 years.
  ■ clinical breast examination—every three years ages 20 years to 40 years, every year after age 40 years.
  ■ mammography—every two years ages 40 years to 49 years, every year starting at age 50 years.

NOTE: NCI's summary of evidence for breast cancer screening with mammography concludes (National Cancer Institute 1994):
  ■ ages 40 years to 49 years—there is no evidence to make an informed decision regarding efficacy of screening.
  ■ ages 50 years and over—routine screening every one to two years with mammography and clinical breast examination can reduce breast cancer mortality by about one-third.

→ Patients with a personal or family history of breast cancer may need more frequent clinical breast examinations/mammograms. Physician consultation should be sought.

→ Document in progress notes and problem list.

4-K

Nipple Discharge—Physiological

Nipple discharge can be elicited manually from the breasts of the majority of non-pregnant, non-lactating women. This discharge is most always benign. The volume will increase with additional stimulation to the breasts. Spontaneous nipple discharge, although most often benign, should be evaluated (see **Galactorrhea** Protocol).

DATABASE

SUBJECTIVE

→ Patient may notice nipple discharge either unilaterally or, frequently, bilaterally during compression of the breast, areola, or nipple during BSE or sexual stimulation.
  ▪ Discharge may be milky, multicolored and opalescent, serous, or bloody (Hughes, Mansel, and Weber 1989).

OBJECTIVE

→ Inspection and palpation of the breasts—supraclavicular and axillary regions (supine and sitting)—may reveal a few drops of nipple discharge that is sticky, milky-gray or greenish, multicolored and opalescent, or serous.
→ With physiological nipple discharge, usually no mass is found.

ASSESSMENT

→ Physiological nipple discharge
→ R/O galactorrhea
→ R/O mastitis
→ R/O duct ectasia
→ R/O intraductal papilloma
→ R/O breast cancer

PLAN

DIAGNOSTIC TESTS

→ Occult blood testing of the nipple discharge is recommended to rule out presence of blood.
→ Mammography is recommended for women over 30 years of age.

TREATMENT/MANAGEMENT

→ Ask a second examiner to corroborate breast findings.
→ With milky discharge, see **Galactorrhea** Protocol.
→ With serous or bloody discharge, refer to a breast specialist.
→ For women with physiological nipple discharge, no treatment is necessary.

CONSULTATION

→ As appropriate for milky discharge (see **Galactorrhea** Protocol).
→ For serous discharge.
→ For abnormal mammogram.
→ For suspicion of a mass.

PATIENT EDUCATION

→ Teach/review BSE.
→ Allay patient's concerns regarding breast findings.

→ For women with milky discharge, see **Galactorrhea** Protocol.

→ Encourage proper nipple hygiene—i.e., washing with mild soap and water and keeping nipples dry.

→ Patient may use breast pads (commercially bought, or clean cotton pads) if she finds discharge embarrassing.

→ Discourage manual or oral breast stimulation to decrease amount of discharge.

FOLLOW-UP

→ Encourage follow-up appointment with breast specialist.

→ Teach American Cancer Society's recommendations for routine breast screening (American Cancer Society 1992):
- BSE—monthly starting at age 20 years.
- clinical breast examination—every three years ages 20 years to 40 years, every year after age 40 years.
- mammography—every two years ages 40 years to 49 years, every year starting age 50 years.

NOTE: NCI's summary of evidence for breast cancer screening with mammography concludes (National Cancer Institute 1994):
- ages 40 years to 49 years—there is no evidence to make an informed decision regarding efficacy of screening.
- ages 50 years and over—routine screening every one to two years with mammography and clinical breast examination can reduce breast cancer mortality by about one-third.

→ Women with a personal or family history of breast cancer may need more frequent clinical breast examinations and/or mammograms. Physician consultation should be sought.

→ Document in progress notes and problem list.

4-L

Paget's Disease

Paget's disease of the breast is characterized by infiltration of breast carcinoma cells into the epidermis of the nipple, along the mammary ducts, without direct invasion. The associated infiltration can be microscopic or present with erosion, scaling, or ulceration of the areola and/or nipple. When a palpable tumor is also present, it is easier to identify the nipple lesion as Paget's disease. If no palpable tumor is present, nipple lesions may be diagnosed as dermatitis, delaying correct diagnosis and treatment (Aktan, Gokoz, and Goksel 1990). Paget's disease of the breast is rare, constituting only one to three percent of all breast cancers (Bulens et al. 1990).

DATABASE

SUBJECTIVE

→ Symptoms include:
- nipple and/or areolar itching, burning, or pain.
- nipple and/or areolar scaling, erythema, erosion, or ulceration.
- subareolar mass; may be palpable.

OBJECTIVE

→ Patient may present with:
- inspection and palpation of the breasts, supraclavicular, and axillary regions (supine and sitting) may reveal nipple and/or areolar scaling, erythema, erosion, or ulceration.
- subareolar mass; may be palpable.
- axillary or clavicular lymph nodes possibly enlarged.

ASSESSMENT

→ Paget's disease
→ R/O dermatitis
→ R/O fluid cyst
→ R/O fibroadenoma

PLAN

DIAGNOSTIC TESTS

→ Mammography is indicated in cases of discrete mass. Mammography is also recommended in patients with nipple/areolar involvement without a palpable mass (Aktan, Gokoz, and Goksel 1990).
→ Physician referral is indicated for biopsy.

TREATMENT/MANAGEMENT

→ Referral to a physician is indicated for mammography follow-up.
→ Physician management is indicated with diagnosis of Paget's disease.

CONSULTATION

→ Referral is indicated for mammography follow-up and management if diagnosis of Paget's disease is made.

PATIENT EDUCATION

→ Explain need for diagnostic mammography and biopsy.
→ When providing BSE education, stress importance of patient consulting provider when evidence of nipple/areolar skin changes.

FOLLOW-UP

→ Teach American Cancer Society's recommendations for routine breast screening (American Cancer Society 1992).
- BSE—monthly starting at age 20 years.
- clinical breast examination—every three years ages 20 years to 40 years, every year after age 40 years.
- mammography—every two years ages 40 years to 49 years, every year starting at age 50 years.

NOTE: NCI's summary of evidence for breast cancer screening with mammography concludes (National Cancer Institute 1994):

- ages 40 years to 49 years—there is no evidence to make an informed decision regarding efficacy of screening.
- ages 50 years and over—routine screening every one to two years with mammography and clinical breast examination can reduce breast cancer mortality by about one-third.

→ Women with personal/family history of breast cancer may need more frequent clinical breast examinations and/or mammograms. Physician consultation should be sought.

→ Document in progress notes and problem list.

Lisa L. Lommel, R.N., C., F.N.P, M.P.H.

4-M

Superficial Phlebitis (Mondor's Disease)

Superficial phlebitis of the breast (*Mondor's disease*) is an inflammation of a subcutaneous vein most commonly located in the breast and the chest wall, beneath and beside the breast. Although any vein may be involved, the vein usually affected is the thoraco-epigastric vein, which runs from the hypochondrium up across the lateral aspect of the breast to the anterior axillary fold. Mondor's disease is a rare condition and is benign. Etiology is unknown, but it may be observed after biopsy for benign conditions; with unusual exercise involving arms above the head; secondary to tight bandages; with heavy, poorly supported, pendulous breasts; or after traumatic injury (Camiel 1986).

DATABASE

SUBJECTIVE

→ Symptoms may include:
- dull aching or acute pain and tenderness in the breast.
- slight elevation in temperature over the affected area.
- an elongated mass in area of tenderness.

OBJECTIVE

→ Inspection and palpation of the breasts—supraclavicular and axillary regions (supine and sitting)—may reveal acute, tender, thickened cord typical of a thrombosed vein.
- With arm and breast elevated, the cord-like or tubular vein may be taut and raised above the level of the skin.
- Dimpling of the skin may occur over the affected area.

- The affected vein may be v-shaped and if there is branching, vein may have an inverted v-shape.

→ No mass should be palpable.

→ Rarely both breasts involved.

→ Findings should be carefully documented using descriptive terms.
- Mass(es) should be described assuming a clock position, locating the mass in distance from the base of the nipple, the dimensions measured with a centimeter tape or ruler.
- Consistency, shape, presence of tenderness, mobility, and associated skin changes should be described. Diagrams are helpful.

ASSESSMENT

→ Superficial thrombophlebitis (Mondor's disease)

→ R/O breast cancer

PLAN

DIAGNOSTIC TESTS

→ Mammography is not recommended for diagnosis but may be indicated to exclude other pathology.

→ Biopsy is not indicated unless there is suspicion of malignancy.

TREATMENT/MANAGEMENT

→ Ask a second examiner to corroborate breast findings.

→ Acetaminophen, application of heat will ease discomfort.

→ Rest to the arm and support for the breast are recommended (Hughes, Mansel, and Webster 1989).

→ Refer to breast specialist if dominant breast mass is present.

→ This condition is self-limiting and usually lasts 2 to 4 weeks.

CONSULTATION

→ Recommended for diagnosis.

→ With breast specialist if a dominant mass is present.

PATIENT EDUCATION

→ Teach/review BSE.

→ Allay patient's concern regarding breast findings.

FOLLOW-UP

→ Teach American Cancer Society's recommendations for routine breast screening (American Cancer Society 1992).

- BSE—monthly starting at age 20 years.
- clinical breast examination: every three years ages 20 years to 40 years, every year after age 40 years.
- mammography—every two years ages 40 years to 49 years, every year starting at age 50 years.

NOTE: NCI's summary of evidence for breast cancer screening with mammography concludes (National Cancer Institute 1994):

- ages 40 years to 49 years—there is no evidence to make an informed decision regarding efficacy of screening.
- ages 50 years and over—routine screening every one to two years with mammography and clinical breast examination can reduce breast cancer mortality by about one-third.

→ Women with personal or family history of breast cancer may need more frequent clinical breast examinations and/or mammograms. Physician consultation should be sought.

→ Document in progress notes and problem list.

4-N
Bibliography

Aktan, A.O., Gokoz, A., and Goksel, H. 1990. Paget's disease without a palpable mass in the breast. *British Journal of Surgery* 77:226–227.

American College of Obstetricians and Gynecologists 1991. *Nonmalignant conditions of the breast* Technical Bulletin No. 156. Washington, DC: the Author.

American Cancer Society. 1992. Update January 1992: The American Cancer Society guidelines for the cancer related checkup. *CA-A Cancer Journal for Clinicians* 42(1):44–45.

Bassett, L., and Kimme-Smith, C. 1991. Breast sonography. *American Journal of Radiology* 156:449–455.

Belieu, R.M. 1994. Mastalgia: Differential diagnosis, evaluation and treatment. *Primary Care Update for OB/GYNs* 1(3):117–121.

Brucker, M.C., and Scharbo-DeHaan, M. 1991. Breast disease: The role of the nurse-midwife. *Journal of Nurse-Midwifery* 36(1):63–73.

Bulens, P., Vanuystel, L., Rijnders A., and van der Schueren, E. 1990. Breast conserving treatment of Paget's disease. *Radiotherapy and Oncology* 17:305–309.

Camiel, M.R. 1986. Mondor's disease in the breast. *Contemporary OB/GYN* 28(6):38–39.

Chetty, U. 1990. Nipple discharge. In *Benign breast disease*, eds. J.A. Smallwood and I. Taylor. Baltimore: Urban & Schwarzenberg.

Consensus Meeting, Cancer Committee of the College of American Pathologists. 1986. Is fibrocystic disease of the breast precancerous? *Archives in Pathological and Laboratory Medicine* 110:171–173.

Dent, D.M., and Cant, P.J. 1989. Fibroadenoma. *World Journal of Surgery* 13(6):706–710.

Dixon, J.M. 1989. Periductal mastitis/duct ectasia. *World Journal of Surgery* 13:715–720.

———. 1990. Cystic disease of the breast. In *Benign breast disease*, eds. J.A. Smallwood and I. Taylor. Baltimore: Urban & Schwarzenberg.

———. 1991. Cystic disease and fibroadenomas of the breast: Natural history and relation to breast cancer risk. *British Medical Journal* 47(2):258–271.

Dixon, J.M., Anderson, T.J., Lumsden, A.B., Elton, R.A., Roberts, M.M., and Forrest, A.P.M. 1983. Mammary duct ectasia. *British Journal of Surgery* 70(10):601–603.

Ellerhorst-Ryan, J.M., Turba, E., and Stahl, D. 1988. Evaluating benign breast disease. *Nurse Practitioner* 13(9):13–28.

Farber, M., Chhibber, G., and Hewlett, G. 1990. Medical management of benign breast disease. In *The female breast and its disorders*, eds. G.W. Mitchell and L.W. Bassett. Baltimore: Williams & Wilkins.

Gateley, C.A., and Mansel, R.E. 1991. Management of the painful and nodular breast. *British Medical Bulletin* 47(2):284–294.

Gibbons, W.E. 1992. Evaluating studies linking HRT and breast cancer. *Contemporary OB/GYN* 37(6):127–136.

Haagensen, D.E., Jr. 1991. Is cystic disease related to breast cancer? *The American Journal of Surgical Pathology* 15(7):687–694.

Hindle, W.H., and Alonzo, L. 1991. Conservative management of breast fibroadenomas. *American Journal of Obstetrics and Gynecology* 164(6, part 1):1647–1650.

Hughes, L.E., Mansel, R.E., and Webster, D.J.T. 1989. *Benign disorders and diseases of the breast: Concepts and clinical management*. London: W.B. Saunders.

Jackson, V.P. 1990. The role of ultrasound in breast imaging. *Radiology* 177(2):305–311.

Jones, R.C., and Hendler, F.J. 1990. Fibrocystic changes of the breast. In *Breast disease for gynecologists*, ed. W.H. Hindle, East Norwalk, CT: Appleton & Lange.

Katz, E., and Adashi, E.Y. 1990. Hyperprolactinemic disorders. *Clinical Obstetrics and Gynecology* 33(3):622–639.

Kelsey, J.L., and Gammon, M.D. 1991. The epidemiology of breast cancer. *CA-A Cancer Journal for Clinicians* 41(3):146–165.

Leis, H.P. 1989. Management of nipple discharge. *World Journal of Surgery* 13(6):736–742.

Lichtman, R., and Papera, S. 1990. *Gynecology*. East Norwalk, CT: Appleton & Lange.

Luce, J. 1992 (March). *Advances in the management of breast cancer.* Lecture presented at the meeting of the Annual Review in Family Medicine, San Francisco, CA.

Maddox, P.R., and Mansel, R.E. 1989. Management of breast pain and nodularity. *World Journal of Surgery* 13(6):699–705.

McGonigle, K.F. 1992. How OCs affect breast disease. *Contemporary OB/GYN* 37(5):156–180.

Morrow, M. 1991. Breast trauma, hematoma, and fat necrosis. In *Breast diseases*, eds. J.R. Harris, S. Hellman, I.C. Henderson, and D.W. Kinne. Philadelphia: J.B. Lippincott.

Mulley, A.G. 1995. Screening for breast cancer. In *Primary care medicine*, eds. A.H. Goroll, L.A. May, and A.G. Mulley. Philadelphia: J.B. Lippincott.

National Cancer Institute. 1994 (May 1). *Physician data query cancer screening/prevention summary on breast cancer screening. Summary of evidence.* 208/04723. Washington, DC: the Author.

Osuch, J.R. 1987. Nonfibrocystic benign lesions of the breast. *Obstetrics and Gynecology Clinics of North America* 14(3):703–710.

Preece, P.E. 1990. Mastalgia. In *Benign breast disease*, eds. J.A. Smallwood and I. Taylor. Baltimore: Urban & Schwarzenberg.

Ramzy, I. 1990. Pathology of benign breast disease. In *The female breast and its disorders*, eds. G.W. Mitchell and L.W. Bassett. Baltimore: Williams & Wilkins.

Reifsnider, E. 1990. Educating women about benign breast disease. *American Association of Occupational Health Nurses Journal* 38(3):121–126.

Richardson, M.R., and Njemanze, J. 1990. Management of severe fibrocystic disease of the breast with leuprolide acetate. *Fertility and Sterility* 54(5):942–943.

Rogers, K. 1990. Breast abscesses and problems with lactation. In *Benign breast disease,* eds. J.A. Smallwood and I. Taylor. Baltimore: Urban & Schwarzenberg.

Simpson, J.F. 1992. Benign conditions affecting the breast. *Contemporary OB/GYN* 37:11–20.

Smith, B.L. 1991. Duct ectasis, periductal mastitis, and breast infections. In *Breast diseases*, eds J.R. Harris, S. Hellman, I.C. Henderson, and D.W. Kinne. Philadelphia: J.B. Lippincott.

Souba, W.W. 1991. In *The breast*, eds. K.I. Bland and E.M. Copeland. Philadelphia: W.B. Saunders.

Speroff, L. 1992. Tamoxifen: Special considerations for gynecologists. *Contemporary OB/GYN* 37:50–61.

Speroff, L., Glass, R.H., and Kase, N.G. 1989. *Clinical gynecologic endocrinology and infertility*, 4th ed. Baltimore: Williams & Wilkins.

Stampfer, M.J., Bechtel, S.D., and Hunter, D.J. 1992. Fat, alcohol, selenium and breast cancer risk. *Contemporary OB/GYN* 37:42–47.

Stehman, F.B. 1990. Benign neoplasms of the breast. In *Breast disease for gynecologists*, ed. W.H. Hindle. East Norwalk, CT: Appleton & Lange.

SECTION 5

Respiratory/ Otorhinolaryngological Disorders

Maureen Shannon, C.N.M., F.N.P., M.S.

5-A

Asthma

Asthma is a lung disease resulting from airway hyper-responsiveness and inflammation characterized by intermittent reversible airway obstruction (National Institutes of Health [NIH] 1991). The airways of patients with asthma are hyper-responsive to a variety of inhaled irritants including allergens, pollens, dust mites, chemical irritants, viruses, or cold air. Some individuals experience symptoms principally following exercise (i.e., *exercise induced bronchospasm*). Asthma occurs in individuals genetically predisposed to it. Many individuals have family members with asthma or other atopic disorders such as allergic rhinitis or eczema.

When the individual's airway is exposed to a triggering agent or *antigen*, there is immediate bronchoconstriction of smooth muscle and degeneration of mast cells that leads to release of inflammatory mediators. These, in turn, cause an inflammatory response involving a variety of cells and other mediators.

The physiological response to this inflammatory sequence is smooth muscle contraction (i.e., *bronchospasm*), edema, and excess mucus production and plugging. The narrowing of small airways can lead to air trapping, hypoxemia, carbon dioxide (CO_2) retention, increasing pulmonary vascular resistance, and negative pleural pressure. These physiological processes are responsible for the common clinical symptoms of wheezing, shortness of breath, and cough, and can lead to progressive use of accessory muscles, pulsus paradoxicus, and respiratory failure.

Asthma is classified on a continuum from mild to moderate to severe. Clinical characteristics and lung function measurement are used to determine an individual's classification which, in turn, determines a specific level of therapy. The current classification system is described in **Figures 5A.1, 5A.2, 5A.3,** and **5A.4**. Additionally, some patients will have the majority of their symptoms during sleep (i.e., *nocturnal asthma*) while others experience exercise-induced bronchospasm (see **Figure 5A.1, Exercise-Induced Asthma**).

In 1991, with over 8.8 million physicians' office visits, asthma was the tenth-ranking medical diagnosis in the United States (Schappert 1993). Although mortality and hospitalization rates for asthma increased in the 1980s, both these events are uncommon (Weiss and Wagener 1990).

Because asthma is such a widespread chronic disease, with acute exacerbations causing considerable patient dysfunction and extensive use of health care services, the National Heart, Lung, and Blood Institute of NIH created a National Asthma Education Program (NAEP) that has developed *Guidelines for the Diagnosis and Management of Asthma* (NIH 1991). The guidelines still have to be tested to document their effectiveness, but they should nevertheless be considered for incorporation into clinical practice.

Many have been incorporated into this protocol which presents the care plan for individuals with mild to moderate asthma. The care of an individual with severe asthma or asthma that is unresponsive to appropriate therapy is beyond the scope of this protocol. An individual with these conditions should be referred to a physician for evaluation and treatment.

Figure 5A.1. EXERCISE-INDUCED ASTHMA

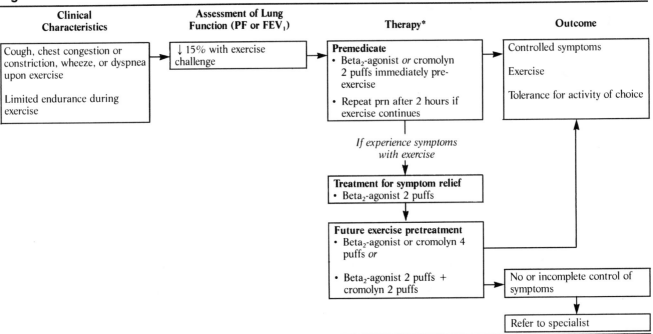

*All therapy must include patient education about prevention (including environmental control where appropriate) as well as control of symptoms.

Source: Reprinted with permission from *Guidelines for the diagnosis and management of asthma, executive summary.* June 1991. Bethesda, MD: National Asthma Education Program, National Institutes of Health. Publication No. 91-3042A.

DATABASE

SUBJECTIVE

→ History may include:
- other allergic disorders (e.g., allergic rhinitis, sinusitis, eczema, nasal polyps).
- lower respiratory infections in childhood (e.g., bronchitis, pneumonia).
- passive exposure to smoke.
- smoking.
- environmental/occupational exposure to allergens, pets.
- environmental/occupational exposure to chemicals/pollutants/irritants (e.g., aerosols, perfumes, detergents, construction materials, fumigants).
- medications (especially aspirin, other nonsteroidal anti-inflammatories, beta-blockers).
- exposure to weather (temperature) change.
- exacerbation of symptoms with exercise.
- endocrine factors (e.g., pregnancy, menses, thyroid disease).
- family history of asthma, allergic rhinitis, eczema.

→ Note early age of initial diagnosis of asthma.

→ Patient may report one or more of the following symptoms:

- wheezing.
- chest tightness.
- shortness of breath.
- daytime cough.
- nighttime cough.
- sputum production (adults).
- activity limitation.
- fever.
- chest pain.
- lethargy.
- anxiety.
- confusion.
- palpitations.

NOTE: When assessing the patient's symptoms, it is important to determine the following: onset, duration, pattern (e.g., episodic, continuous symptoms with intermittent exacerbations), course of disease, treatment(s) that relieved symptoms, aggravating factors or seasonal variations, and any use of medical services (e.g., hospital, emergency room, or urgent-care clinic).

OBJECTIVE

→ Physical examination may reveal the following:
- vital signs:
  - elevation in temperature, along with increased pulse and respirations. Blood pressure may

Figure 5A.2. MANAGEMENT OF ASTHMA IN ADULTS—CHRONIC MILD ASTHMA

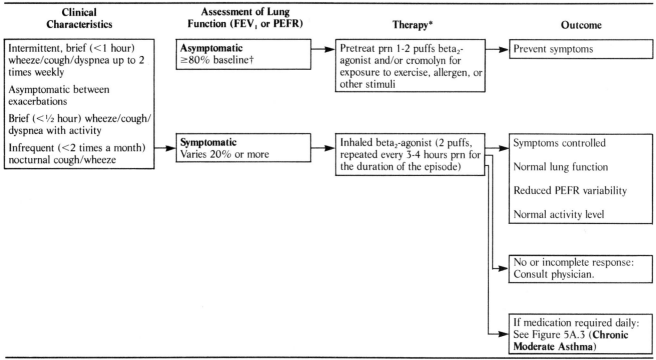

*All therapy must include patient education about prevention (including environmental control where appropriate) as well as control of symptoms.

†PEFR % baseline refers to the norm for the individual, established by the clinician. This may be % predicted of standardized norms *or* % patient's personal best.

Source: Reprinted with permission from *Guidelines for the diagnosis and management of asthma, Executive summary.* June 1991. Bethesda, MD: National Asthma Education Program, National Institutes of Health. Publication No. 91-3042A.

reveal pulsus paradoxicus. These measurements, in part, determine therapeutic interventions.
- patient appearing fatigued, lethargic, disoriented, or too breathless when attempting to talk.
- cyanosis.
- evidence of eczema.
- rhinitis.
- nasal flaring.
- nasal polyps.
- neck vein distention.
- use of accessory muscles of respiration—i.e., neck, chest, abdomen.
- stridor.
- hunched posture while breathing.
- pigeon chest.
- hollow sound upon chest wall percussion.

→ Auscultation of chest may reveal:
- decreased intensity of breath sounds.
- prolonged expiration.
- wheezing.
- crackles.
- rhonchi.

→ Auscultation of the heart may reveal a cardiac gallop or increased P_2.

ASSESSMENT

→ Asthma

→ R/O chronic bronchitis (chronic obstructive pulmonary disease [COPD] Type B)

→ R/O emphysema (COPD Type A)

→ R/O congestive heart failure

→ R/O drug reaction (e.g., to beta-blockers, aspirin, angiotensin-converting enzyme inhibitors)

→ R/O acute inhalation of irritating substance

→ R/O mechanical obstruction

→ R/O pulmonary embolism

→ R/O pulmonary infiltration with eosinophilia

PLAN

DIAGNOSTIC TESTS

→ It is recommended that all patients have objective measures of lung function performed to establish a diagnosis, monitor progress, and judge severity

Figure 5A.3. MANAGEMENT OF ASTHMA IN ADULTS—CHRONIC MODERATE ASTHMA

*All therapy must include patient education about prevention (including environmental control where appropriate) as well as control of symptoms.

†PEFR % baseline refers to the norm for the individual, established by the clinician. This may be % predicted based on standardized norms *or* % patient's personal best.

††If exceed 3-4 doses a day, consider additional therapy other than inhaled beta$_2$-agonist.

Source: Reprinted with permission from *Guidelines for the diagnosis and management of asthma, executive summary.* June 1991. Bethesda, MD: National Asthma Education Program, National Institutes of Health. Publication No. 91-3042A.

during acute exacerbations of asthma. It is important to use objective measures of lung function since a patient's history and physical examination findings may not correlate with the severity of air flow obstruction (Rivo and Malveaux 1992).

→ The following tests are usually ordered (see **Table 5D.2, Pulmonary Function Tests**, p. 5-21 in **Chronic Obstructive Pulmonary Disease** Protocol.
  ▪ Spirometry.
    • Airway obstruction will impact flow rates and produce changes in the *forced vital capacity* (FVC), *forced expiratory volume in one second* (FEV$_1$), and the *maximum midexpiratory flow*

rate (MMEF). An obstructive pattern will be demonstrated.
    • Spirometry equipment is not frequently found in most primary care offices.
  ▪ *Peak Expiratory Flow Rate* (PEFR).
    • These meters measure PEFR which correlates well with FEV$_1$. Asthma reduces PEFR and FEV$_1$.
    • Peak expiratory flow rate meters are widely available as small office equipment or inexpensive plastic portable models.

→ Depending on clinical history and physical examination, the following additional tests may be ordered after consultation with a physician:

Figure 5A.4. MANAGEMENT OF ASTHMA IN ADULTS—CHRONIC SEVERE ASTHMA

Clinical Characteristics	Assessment of Lung Function (FEV$_1$ or PEFR)	Therapy*	Outcome
Continuous symptoms Limited activity level Frequent exacerbations Frequent nocturnal symptoms Occasional hospitalization and emergency treatment	<60% baseline† Highly variable: 20%-30% changes with routine medicine Varies more than 50% during worst exacerbations	• Inhaled beta$_2$-agonist prn-QID†† *and* • Anti-inflammatory agents —Inhaled corticosteroid 2-6 puffs BID–QID *with or without* —Cromolyn 2 puffs QID *with or without* (especially for nocturnal symptoms) • Oral sustained released theophylline, *and/or* • Oral beta$_2$-agonist ------ *with* • Episodic extra beta$_2$-agonist (2–4 puffs MDI or nebulized treatment) for exacerbations *and* **Oral corticosteroids** • Burst for active symptoms (40 mg a day, single or divided dose, for 1 week, then tapered for 1 week) *Consider* • Daily or alternate day use (single dose a.m.)	Improved pulmonary function Reduced peak flow variability Almost normal activity Infrequent awakening at night Reduced frequency of exacerbations Reduced frequency of prn inhaled beta$_2$-agonist Reduced need for corticosteroid burst Reduced need for emergency department treatment

Note: Individuals with severe asthma should be evaluated by an asthma specialist.

*All therapy must include patient education about prevention (including environmental control where appropriate) as well as control of symptoms.

†PEFR % baseline refers to the norm for the individual, established by the clinician. This may be % predicted based on standardized norms *or* % patient's personal best.

††If exceed 3-4 doses a day, consider additional therapy other than inhaled beta$_2$-agonist.

Source: Reprinted with permission from *Guidelines for the diagnosis and management of asthma, executive summary*. June 1991. Bethesda, MD: National Asthma Education Program, National Institutes of Health. Publication No. 91-3042A.

- chest x-ray.
  - To rule out pneumonia in febrile patients, to assess other cardiopulmonary disease, if other obstructive phenomena are suspected, and to assess pneumothorax or atelectasis in acutely ill patients.
- sputum for gram stain and/or culture-and-sensitivity.
  - To rule out a coexisting pulmonary infection.
- complete blood count (CBC).
  - May reveal eosinophilia.
- skin testing.
  - To determine hypersensitivity to specific allergens.
- nasal secretions smear.
  - For eosinophilia.

- serum theophylline level (as a baseline or to evaluate therapeutic levels in patients using theophylline for symptom relief).
→ In *acute* exacerbations of asthma with moderate to severe symptoms, the following tests can be ordered after consultation with a physician:
- oxygen saturation.
- blood gases:
  - pO$_2$—will be decreased.
  - pCO$_2$—will be increased in severe asthma episodes; normal or low in mild to moderate asthma (because of hyperventilation).
  - pH—will be reduced.

NOTE: Although some sources recommend arterial blood gas measurement (NIH 1991), this test is technically difficult and potentially has more complications than other sampling methods. Oxygenation is adequately assessed by measuring transcutaneous oxygen saturation with a digital pulse oximeter (Elborn, Finch, and Stanford 1991; Holmgren and Sixt 1992), and elevations in pCO_2 and reductions in pH are obtainable with capillary or venous blood. The NAEP guidelines use pCO_2 values that are based on arterial blood; pCO_2 measured on capillary or venous blood or transcutaneously will be slightly higher. Transcutaneous pO_2 also will be lower than corresponding arterial values (Holmgren and Sixt 1992).

TREATMENT/MANAGEMENT

→ A wide variety of treatment strategies are available to control asthma.

■ There are a number of different symptom patterns that can be classified as mild, moderate, or severe. The more severe or frequent the symptoms, the greater the dosages of medications.

■ Tailoring the medication regimen to allow maximum patient functioning with the minimum of symptoms and medication side effects is the goal of individualized management.

→ The following are *general* guidelines for environmental control and medication management for asthma therapy:

■ environmental control should be based on the patient's history of allergic/irritant exposure.

• Among outdoor measures:
  –patients do not have to avoid the outdoors, but should avoid activities that may increase symptoms (e.g., mowing the lawn) or involve unnecessarily heavy exposure to outdoor allergens (e.g., pollens, ragweed, molds).

• Among indoor measures:
  –keeping the house as clean as possible, especially the patient's bedroom.
  –the patient wearing a mask when vacuuming and using special vacuums with HEPA filters.
  –having pets sleep outdoors, or, if not possible, in areas where there is limited exposure for the patient to animal hair, fur, and dander.
  –maintaining low humidity to discourage mold growth.
  –encasing mattresses and pillows in plastic covers.

–washing bedding every week in water with a temperature of at least 54°C/130°F.
  –having a minimum of rugs, upholstered furniture, and stuffed animals, and not keeping any in the bedroom if possible.
  –remove carpets on concrete slabs, etc. if possible.

■ pharmacological interventions: Refer to **Figures 5A.1, 5A.2,** and **5A.3** and **Table 5A.1, Types of Medications for the Treatment of Asthma** for the medications and algorithms recommended by NIH for the treatment of mild to moderate asthma in adults.

• Patients exhibiting severe symptoms or symptoms that persist after therapy need an immediate evaluation by a physician.

• Exercise-induced asthma: Use of the following medication(s) 15 minutes prior to exercise is often beneficial:
  –inhaled cromolyn (Intal®), 2 inhalations.
  –inhaled beta$_2$-adrenergic agent such as albuterol (Proventil®, Ventolin®), 2 inhalations.

NOTE: If moderate to severe symptoms characteristically accompany exercise, then these two medications can be combined 15 minutes prior to exercise (Wooley 1990).

• Nocturnal asthma: Use of the following medications may be beneficial:
  –inhaled beta$_2$-adrenergic agent such as albuterol (Proventil®, Ventolin®) at bedtime (Jenne 1984).
  –sustained release theophylline (Theo Dur®, Theolaire-SK®, Constant-T®, Uniphye®) 200 mg/p.o. taken between 6:00 p.m. and 8:00 p.m. (Arkinstall 1987).

NOTE: In patients with nocturnal asthma symptoms, a work-up should be considered to rule out the possibility of gastroesophageal reflux.

• Mild, chronic asthma: Use of beta$_2$-agonists for the treatment of patients with mild asthma is recommended because these agents act faster, have fewer adverse side effects, and achieve desired results at lower doses than do oral medications (Rivo and Malveaux 1992). The following medications can be prescribed:
  –albuterol (Ventolin®, Proventil®) 1 to 2 puffs every 3 to 4 hours as needed during the acute exacerbation of the asthma episode.
  –metaproterenol (Alupent®, Metaprel®) 1 to 2 puffs every 3 to 4 hours as needed during acute exacerbation of asthma episode.

Table 5A.1. TYPES OF MEDICATIONS FOR TREATMENT OF ASTHMA

Medication	Common Generic	Preps Available	Mechanism	Uses/Advantages	Disadvantages
Beta-adrenergic agonist:			Relax smooth muscles, and may modulate most cell release of medicator.	Efficacious; can be easily delivered to airways via nebulizer or metered dose inhaler.	Can produce systemic cardiovascular and skeletal effects, though less than methylxanthine.
Albuterol	Ventolin; Proventil	Oral/Inhaled/Nebulized			
Metaproterenol	Alupent; Metaprel	Oral/Inhaled			
Pirbuterol	Maxair	Oral/Inhaled			
Bitolterol	Tornalate				
Isoetharine		Oral/Inhaled			
Epinephrine		Inhaled/Sub q			High alpha adrenergic component seldom indicated
Terbutatine	Bretnaire; Bricanyl	Oral/Sub q			
Methylxanthine: Theophylline (Currently prolonged release most useful.)	Elizophyllin SR Slo-Bid Slo-Phyllin Theo-Dur	Oral	Bronchodilator; may have some anti-inflammatory response.	Mainstay for decades but highest rate of side effects. Sustained release useful for nighttime asthma. Can be added to β-agonists as second-line drug serum level can be monitored (desired level 10–20 µg/ml).	Significant β and some α adrenergic side effects, CV, muscle tremor, abdominal pain.
Anticholinergics: Ipratropium	Atrovent	Inhaled	Reduce vagal tone to airway.	Effective in status asthmaticus in conjunction with β-agonists.	Limited use outside emergency room.
Corticosteroids: Prednisone Solucortef, solumedrol		Oral Intravenous	Interrupt development and terminate ongoing inflammatory response.	Earlier treatment of severe asthma attack.	Appellate fluid retention, weight gain, moved alteration, increase BP, (fatal if varicella develops).
Beclomethasone Triamcinolone Flunisolide	Beclovent, Vanceril Azmacort AeroBid	Inhaled		Effective in controlling airway inflammation and safer. Primary drug in moderate/severe asthma in adults.	

NOTE: The need for the use of an inhaler on a daily basis or 3 to 4 times a day indicates the need for additional therapy (Rivo and Malveaux 1992).

- Moderate chronic asthma: Use of inhaled anti-inflammatory agents is indicated for patients with moderate asthma, characterized by exacerbations occurring more than twice a week, lasting a few days, and affecting the patient's sleep and/or daily living activities (Rivo and Malveaux 1992). The following agents can be prescribed:
  - cromolyn sodium (Intal®), 2 puffs QID.

  NOTE: A 4- to 6-week trial of this agent is necessary before its effectiveness can be determined.
  - beclamethasone (Becolovent®, Vanceril®) 42 ug/puff, 2-4 puffs BID.
  - triamcinolone acetonide (Azmacort®), 100 ug/puff, 2-4 puffs BID.
  - flunisolide (AeroBid®) 250 ug/puff, 2-4 puffs BID.

NOTE: Attaining maximum benefit from the above medications may require two to four weeks of therapy. Side effects of these agents include occasional coughing, dysphonia, and oral candidiasis. Use of a spacer device or having the patient rinse her mouth after use will reduce the incidence of side effects.

- If a patient's symptoms persist after the use of beta$_2$ agonists and inhaled cromolyn or corticosteroids at the above doses, consultation with a physician is indicated.
- Therapeutic options at this point include increasing the dosage of the inhaled corticosteroid, use of a longer-acting bronchodilator, or sustained-release theophylline.
- If theophylline is prescribed, the usual initial dose is 200 mg/p.o. BID with adjustments in the dose based on clinical symptoms and serum theophylline levels. (Obtaining serum theophylline levels after initiating therapy is indicated to determine if a therapeutic level (10 ug/ml to 20 ug/ml) has been attained. Toxicity occurs when the level is 20 ug/ml or greater but may occur in some patients with levels of at least 15 ug/ml. Theophylline toxicity often is manifested by nausea, vomiting, tachycardia, tachypnea, arrhythmias, hyperglycemia, hypokalemia, and seizures) (Rivo and Malveaux 1992; Stauffer 1994).
- Persistence of symptoms after initiation of maximum dosages of bronchodilators and inhaled steroids or cromolyn may require oral corticosteroids and referral to a physician for further evaluation and treatment.
  - If the patient smokes, she should be advised to stop.
  - Psychological evaluation and/or counseling may be indicated for patients exhibiting significant signs or symptoms of depression, anxiety, or other psychological sequelae associated with chronic disease.

CONSULTATION

→ Consultation with a physician is indicated in a patient exhibiting moderate to severe asthma symptoms, or in a patient who is having significant side effects associated with medications.

→ Physician consultation is indicated:
  - for a patient with a history of multiple emergency room visits, hospital stays, and symptoms that are atypical and raise questions about other diagnostic possibilities.
  - if diagnostic testing for allergens is indicated.
  - if there are complicating factors requiring special care (e.g., nasal polyps), or other

significant complications (e.g., pneumonia, suspected tension pneumothorax).

→ Any patient with chronic severe asthma should be referred to an asthma specialist.

→ As needed for prescriptions(s).

PATIENT EDUCATION

→ Educate the patient about asthma—the cause(s), clinical course, preventive measures, treatment options, possible complications, side effects of medications, and when to seek immediate medical care.

→ Educate the patient about the need to avoid triggering agents and prevent exacerbations.

→ If the patient smokes, discuss the need to stop smoking and refer to community programs.

→ Instruct the patient in the proper use of *metered-dose inhalers* (MDIs) and spacer devices for inhaled medications. The following instructions for the use of MDIs should be reviewed with the patient (Rivo and Malveaux 1992) (see **Figure 5A.5, Correct Use of a Metered-Dose Inhaler**):
  - make sure there is enough medicine in the canister. An easy way to determine this is to place the canister in a container of water: if it sinks to the bottom, it is full; if it floats on the surface (tipped sideways), it is empty.
  - hold the canister upright, remove the cap, and shake.
  - tilt head back slightly and breathe out.
  - open mouth, holding the inhaler one to two inches away from mouth.
  - press down on the top of the canister and breathe in slowly. Continue to breathe in slowly for three to five seconds.
  - after breathing in, hold breath for 10 seconds, allowing the medicine to reach lungs.
  - if repeat puffs are necessary, wait one minute between puffs so the medication can reach lungs.

→ Educate patient about medications, their proper use, possible side effects, and when to notify health care providers after initiating therapy (e.g., if expected response does not occur, if significant side effects).

→ Reinforce the use of peak flow meters for additional monitoring of pulmonary function, as recommended by physician consultants.

→ Educate the patient and her family regarding emergency measures (e.g., contacting emergency

Figure 5A.5.   CORRECT USE OF A METERED-DOSE INHALER*

Steps for checking how much medicine is in the canister
1. If the canister is new, it is full.
2. If the canister has been used repeatedly, it might be empty. (Check product label to see how many inhalations should be in each canister).
   To check how much medicine is left in the canister, put the canister (not the mouthpiece) in a cup of water.
   —If the canister sinks to the bottom; it is full.
   —If the canister floats sideways on the surface, it is empty.

Steps for using the inhaler
1. Remove the cap and hold inhaler upright.
2. Shake the inhaler.
3. Tilt the head back slightly and breathe out.
4. Position the inhaler in one of the following ways (A is optimal, but C is acceptable for those who have difficulty with A or B):

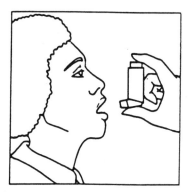   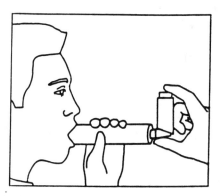   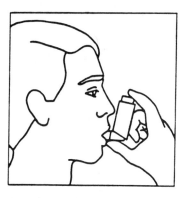

A. Open mouth with inhaler 1-2 inches away.   **B.** Use spacer (this is recommended especially for young children).   **C.** In the mouth.

5. Press down on inhaler to release medication as you start to breathe in slowly.
6. Breath in *slowly* (3-5 seconds).
7. *Hold* breath for 10 seconds to allow medicine to reach deep into lungs.
8. Repeat puffs as directed. Waiting 1 minute between puffs may permit second puff to penetrate the lungs better.
9. Spacers are useful for all patients. They are particularly recommended for young children and older adults and for use with inhaled steroids.

*Inhaled dry powder capsules require a different inhalation technique. To use a dry-powder inhaler, it is important to close the mouth tightly around the mouthpiece of the inhaler and to inhale rapidly.

Source: Reprinted with permission from *Guidelines for the diagnosis and management of asthma, executive summary.* June 1991. Bethesda, MD: National Asthma Education Program, National Institutes of Health. Publication No. 91-3042A.

care providers if patient does not respond to therapy).
→ Educate the patient about signs and symptoms of depression, anxiety, or other emotional/psychological sequelae associated with chronic disease.

FOLLOW-UP

→ The patient with stable, mild, chronic asthma should be seen at least every six months for evaluation.
   ▪ The patient should return more frequently if she experiences any exacerbation of symptoms.

→ If the patient experiences severe, acute symptoms, she should be seen immediately by a physician for evaluation and treatment.

→ If the patient is taking theophylline, she should return for serum theophylline levels as recommended by the consulting physician (usually every six months). She should also do so if she begins taking another medication that can alter theophylline serum levels (e.g., erythromycin), or if she experiences any signs or symptoms associated with theophylline toxicity.

→ Document in progress notes and problem list.

5-B

Bronchiectasis

Bronchiectasis is a condition characterized by permanent dilatation of the bronchi and destruction of bronchial wall tissue (Stauffer 1994; Stockley 1987). The pulmonary changes resulting in bronchiectasis can be a consequence of congential or acquired conditions (Stockley 1987). Patients usually present with a history of persistent or intermittent productive cough in the absence of contributing factors such as smoking or asthma (although these factors may also be reported by patients).

The actual incidence of bronchiectasis is unknown because in many patients the symptoms are often mild and intermittent, unless an exacerbation of pulmonary symptoms occurs secondary to bacterial infection. Recently, a decreased incidence of acquired bronchiectasis has been reported, probably as a result of more effective treatment of bronchopulmonary infections (Stauffer 1994).

The symptoms associated with bronchiectasis vary from mild to severe and are related to the pulmonary damage that has occurred. The pathophysiology of bronchiectasis involves minor to severe epithelial damage, hyperplasia of goblet cells, reduced connective tissue, bronchial dilatation, and inflammatory changes.

Such pulmonary damage, in turn, results in reduced mucociliary clearance with increased mucous retention and bacterial colonization (most commonly with *Hemophilus influenzae* [*H. influenzae*] or *Streptococcus pneumoniae* [*S. pneumoniae*]) which may be intermittent or continuous (Stauffer 1994; Stockley 1987). Bacterial colonization stimulates an increase in neutrophils in the pulmonary secretions which then contributes to further pulmonary damage and repair, and which is often responsible for an exacerbation of symptoms. Complications associated with bronchiectasis include right ventricular hy-

pertrophy, heart failure, amyloidosis, and the development of secondary abscesses at extrapulmonary sites (e.g., brain).

DATABASE

SUBJECTIVE

→ Predisposing factors may include (Stockley 1987):
- congenital conditions:
  - cystic fibrosis (50 percent of patients with bronchiectasis).
  - immunoglobulin deficiency.
  - immotile cilia syndrome.
  - alpha-1 antitrypsin deficiency.
- acquired conditions.
  - history of:
    - pulmonary infections (e.g., tuberculosis, pneumonia, fungal infections, lung abscess).
    - inflammatory disease (e.g., rheumatoid arthritis, inflammatory bowel disease).
    - pulmonary fibrosis.
    - heroin use.

→ Patient may report one or more of the following symptoms which can vary in intensity from mild to severe (Stauffer 1994; Stockley 1987):
- chronic cough producing copious amounts of mucus (often foul-smelling).
- hemoptysis.
- dyspnea (increasing with exertion).
- wheezing.
- fever (if coexistent bacterial infection).
- weight loss.

OBJECTIVE

→ Physical findings are often nonspecific but may include the following (Stauffer 1994; Stockley 1987):

- elevated temperature if superimposed bacterial infection.
- increased respiratory rate and pulse if significant pulmonary disease.
- auscultation of the patient's lungs revealing persistent bibasilar crackles.
- collection of sputum in a specimen cup revealing copious amounts of purulent mucus (often foul-smelling) that will separate into three distinct layers (Stauffer 1994).

ASSESSMENT

→ Bronchiectasis

→ R/O acute pulmonary infection (e.g., bronchitis, pneumonia, tuberculosis)

→ R/O COPD

→ R/O cor pulmonale

→ R/O immunoglobulin deficiency

→ R/O immotile cilia syndrome (rare).

PLAN

DIAGNOSTIC TESTS

→ CBC may be within normal limits or may demonstrate leukocytosis if secondary pulmonary infection coexists.

→ Gram stain of sputum may reveal an organism requiring antimicrobial treatment (see **Pneumonia** Protocol).

→ Sputum culture may reveal pathogenic organism requiring antimicrobial treatment (see **Pneumonia** Protocol).

→ In moderate to severe bronchiectasis, pulmonary function tests (PFTs) will reveal obstructive dysfunction including (see **Table 5D.2, Pulmonary Function Tests**, p. 5-21, for definitions of PFT tests):

- spirometry testing will demonstrate a normal or decreased FVC, and a decreased FEV_1, FEV_1/FVC, FEF_{25-75}, PEFR, and *maximum voluntary ventilation* (MVV).
- lung volume testing will demonstrate an increased *total lung capacity* (TLC), *functional residual capacity* (FRC), and *residual volume* (RV)/TLC.

→ Arterial blood gases will reveal hypoxemia in patients with severe bronchiectasis.

→ Chest x-ray will demonstrate peribronchial fibrosis and cystic spaces at the lung bases.

→ Tuberculosis skin testing will be negative.

→ Bronchoscopy may be indicated in patients to:

- evaluate the etiology of hemoptysis.
- rule out the possibility of an obstructing airway lesion, and/or
- remove retained secretions.

→ Consultation with a physician also would be indicated.

TREATMENT/MANAGEMENT

→ If evidence of pulmonary infection (based on gram stain or sputum culture results), initiation of specific antibiotic therapy is indicated. When a patient exhibits an acute exacerbation of symptoms without evidence of a specific pathogen, empiric antibiotic therapy may be initiated, with one of the following agents, for 10 to 14 days (Stauffer 1994):

- amoxicillin (Amoxil®, Trimox®) 500 mg p.o. TID.
- ampicillin (Principen®) 250 mg-500 mg p.o. QID.
- tetracycline (Achromycin V®) 250 mg-500 mg p.o. QID.
- trimethoprim/sulfamethoxazole (Septra DS®, Bactrim®) 160 mg/800 mg p.o. every 12 hours.

→ In patients with severe bronchiectasis and copious amounts of purulent sputum, alternating 2 or 3 of the above antibiotics with one another for up to 4 weeks may be necessary to resolve symptoms of an exacerbation (Stauffer 1994).

→ Pulmonary toilet (including chest physiotherapy, chest percussion, postural drainage) may be necessary on a daily basis for patients with symptoms of severe disease.

→ If moderate to severe symptoms are evident, bronchodilators should be prescribed (see **Chronic Obstructive Pulmonary Disease** Protocol).

→ Avoidance of situations that may aggravate bronchiectasis should be recommended (e.g., smoking, exposure to air pollutants).

→ Immunization with pneumococcal vaccine and influenza vaccine should be advised (see **Pneumonia** and **Influenza** protocols).

→ Occasionally, surgical resection is indicated in patients with localized bronchiectasis and adequate PFTs who are not responding to conservative management. Decisions and referrals would be the responsibility of the consulting physician.

CONSULTATION

→ Consultation is indicated in any patient with moderate to severe symptoms (e.g., hypoxemia), significant hemoptysis, or with symptoms persisting after appropriate conservative treatment.

→ Patient referral to a respiratory physical therapist—so she can be properly instructed in pulmonary toilet techniques—may be beneficial.

→ As needed for prescription(s).

PATIENT EDUCATION

→ Educate patient about bronchiectasis—the possible cause(s), clinical manifestations, ways to prevent exacerbation, signs and symptoms of complications, possible diagnostic tests required, and any indicated follow-up.

→ Discuss with patient prophylactic measures that are indicated and why such measures can be beneficial (e.g., pneumococcal and influenza vaccinations).

→ When appropriate, educate patient about the possible psychological sequelae (e.g., depression) of an obstructive pulmonary disorder, and provide her with referrals and resources.

→ Review any potential side effects of medications (see *Physicians' Desk Reference* [*PDR*] as needed). In women using long-term antibiotic therapy, education about possible vaginal candidiasis infections—signs, symptoms, preventive measures, treatment options—is essential (see **Vaginitis** Protocols).

FOLLOW-UP

→ Patients with evidence of acute pulmonary infection, who are treated as outpatients, should have a follow-up visit scheduled after completion of their antibiotic therapy. If symptoms persist or worsen in the course of antibiotic therapy, the patient should return for re-evaluation prior to finishing the antibiotics.

→ If there has been consultation/management with a physician, follow-up visits should be upon recommendation of the physician.

→ Document in progress notes and problem list.

Maureen Shannon, C.N.M., F.N.P., M.S.

5-C

Bronchitis—Acute

Acute bronchitis is an inflammation of the trachea and bronchi, usually occurring during the winter. It is a result of infection with a virus, mycoplasma, or bacteria.

In the majority of patients, the episode is self-limited, lasting one to two weeks, and requiring only symptomatic treatment. However, in patients with a history of COPD, acute bronchitis may require more pharmacological management. Use of such pharmacological treatment for acute bronchitis in healthy patients without a history of COPD is controversial (Billas 1990).

DATABASE

SUBJECTIVE

→ Predisposing factors may include a history of:
- recent upper respiratory infection (URI).
- smoking.
- recent influenza.

→ Patient may report one or more of the following symptoms:
- URI symptoms—headache, malaise, pharyngitis.
- low-grade fever.
- productive cough (mucoid to purulent in character).
- substernal chest discomfort.

OBJECTIVE

→ Physical examination may reveal:
- mild temperature elevation.
- pharyngeal erythema.
- rhonchi or crackles without consolidation revealed upon auscultation of the lungs.

ASSESSMENT

→ Acute bronchitis

→ R/O chronic bronchitis

→ R/O URI

→ R/O asthmatic bronchitis

→ R/O pneumonia

→ R/O influenza

PLAN

DIAGNOSTIC TESTS

→ The diagnosis of acute bronchitis is usually made based on the clinical presentation and physical examination findings. However, in patients with a history of COPD or severe symptoms, the following diagnostic tests can be ordered (Billas 1990):
- chest x-ray—usually within normal limits.
- sputum cultures—may reveal a pathogen such as *Mycoplasma pneumoniae*. However, common oropharyngeal contaminants are usually recovered and are of unknown significance in the presence of acute bronchitis symptoms.

TREATMENT/MANAGEMENT

→ Symptomatic treatment for acute bronchitis in patients without COPD includes rest, increased fluid intake, and the use of antipyretics (e.g., acetaminophen) as needed.

→ Cough suppression can be attempted through the use of over-the-counter medications containing dextromethorphan (Delsym®). The usual dose for dextromethorphan is 15 mg p.o. every 6 hours. In patients with severe coughing, a codeine preparation may be necessary.

→ If the patient is suspected of having coexistent influenza A, use of amantadine hydrochloride (Amantadine®, Symmetrel®) can be considered (see **Influenza** Protocol).

→ Antimicrobial therapy usually is not indicated because most acute bronchitis in healthy adults is caused by viruses.

▪ In elderly patients, patients with persistent or severe symptoms, or patients with significant medical problems (e.g., COPD, immuno-compromise), antimicrobial therapy may be indicated and include (Stauffer 1994):

▪ erythromycin (E-Mycin®, Ery Tab®) 250 mg p.o. QID for 7 to 10 days.
NOTE: Erythromycin provides a wide spectrum of coverage with limited cost and side effects.

▪ tetracycline (Achromycin®) 250 mg p.o. QID for 7 to 10 days.

▪ amoxicillin (Amoxil®, Trimox®) 500 mg p.o. TID for 7 to 10 days.

CONSULTATION

→ Consultation with a physician may be indicated in patients with COPD, severe symptoms, or significant underlying medical conditions.

→ As needed for prescription(s).

PATIENT EDUCATION

→ Educate the patient about acute bronchitis—the most common cause(s), usual symptomatic treatments, signs and/or symptoms of complications, and any follow-up that may be indicated.

→ If the patient requires antibiotic therapy, educate the patient about the need to take the medications as prescribed, and discuss any potential side effects.

→ If the patient smokes, educate her about the adverse effects of smoking (e.g., lung disease, cancer, heart disease), and possible ways to reduce or stop smoking (e.g. smoking cessation programs). See **Smoking Cessation** Protocol.

FOLLOW-UP

→ If physician consultation is indicated, follow up per physician recommendation.

→ Document in progress notes and problem list.

Maureen Shannon, C.N.M., F.N.P., M.S.

5-D

Chronic Obstructive Pulmonary Disease

Chronic obstructive pulmonary disease (COPD) is a condition characterized by expiratory airway obstruction. COPD is comprised of two diseases, *emphysema* (COPD Type A) and *chronic bronchitis* (COPD Type B). In most patients, elements of both these diseases coexist. Patients diagnosed with COPD as a result of chronic bronchitis have a somewhat better prognosis than those patients with COPD as a result of emphysema.

It is estimated that as many as 10 million people in the United States have COPD (Stauffer 1994). It is the fifth leading cause of death in the United States, with a higher death rate noted among elderly men. Additionally, there is significant morbidity associated with this condition including frequent pulmonary infections, cor pulmonale, and psychosocial sequelae associated with chronic disease (e.g., depression).

Emphysema

Emphysema is characterized by permanent enlargement of lung parenchyma distal to the terminal bronchioles, resulting in destruction and coalescence of alveolar walls. Emphysematous changes are thought to occur in response to excessive lysis of elastin by elastase and other enzymes produced by lung neutrophils, mononuclear cells, and macrophages (Stauffer 1994).

There are two types of emphysema: *panlobular*—which is characterized by destructive changes in the alveoli and alveolar sacs, and is a result of alpha-1 antitrypsin deficiency or idiopathic causes; and *centrilobular*—which is characterized by pathology in the respiratory bronchioles and is the result of chronic bronchitis (Littler and Momany 1990).

Chronic Bronchitis

Chronic bronchitis is a recurrent, chronic, productive cough, present for at least three months, annually for two consecutive years, in the absence of other causes for the symptoms (Billas 1990; Ruben 1989; Stauffer 1994; Thompson et al 1992). Although chronic bronchitis is not an active infection—but, instead, a condition involving airway obstruction and inflammation—it is associated with an increased incidence of acute respiratory infections (e.g., pneumonia).

It affects approximately 7.5 million Americans. General surveys indicate that among adults 25 years to 74 years of age, 31 percent of men and 12.9 percent of women are affected (Ruben 1989). It is estimated that the incidence of chronic bronchitis in women will increase as a result of the increase in the number of women who smoke (Ruben 1989). The etiology of chronic bronchitis includes pulmonary damage associated with cigarette smoking, air pollution, recurrent respiratory infections, and hereditary factors (Billas 1990).

DATABASE

SUBJECTIVE

The patient may report one or more of the following predisposing factors associated with COPD (Billas 1990):

→ history of cigarette smoking.

→ exposure to air pollution.

→ history of recurrent respiratory infections.

→ history of hereditary disorder associated with COPD (e.g., alpha-1 antitrypsin deficiency, immotile cilia syndrome, cystic fibrosis).

→ emphysema.
- Patients with emphysema usually report the onset of the following symptoms after age 50 years (Littler and Momany 1990; Stauffer 1994):
  • shortness of breath that becomes more severe and constant.
  • weight loss (usually noted in advanced disease).
  • minimal or no cough.
  • if cough present, associated with little or no mucous production. If mucous is reported, it is usually clear or mucoid, not purulent.

→ chronic bronchitis.
- Patients with chronic bronchitis usually report the onset of symptoms, after the age of 35 years, including (Littler and Momany 1990; Stauffer 1994):
  • persistent, severe cough producing copious amounts of purulent, often foul-smelling sputum. The cough is usually most intense in the morning.
  • mild, intermittent shortness of breath and dyspnea associated with increased exertion. As the disease progresses, moderate to severe shortness of breath and dyspnea are noted, even at rest.
  • hemoptysis (may be reported in association with aspirin intake).
  • patients often report weight gain.

OBJECTIVE

→ See **Table 5D.1, Comparison of Clinical Manifestations and Laboratory Findings**.
- Emphysema.
  • The following physical findings may be evident, depending on disease severity (Billas 1990; Littler and Momany 1990; Ruben 1989; Stauffer 1994):
    –vital signs—blood pressure and temperature will be within normal limits unless there is a coexisting condition (e.g., hypertension, infection). The respiratory rate and pulse may be within normal limits or increased depending on the level of respiratory distress the patient is experiencing.
    –patient may appear thin and wasted in advanced disease.

–examination of the chest will reveal an increased anteroposterior diameter ("barrel chest") and hypertrophied accessory respiratory muscles.
–palpation of the chest will reveal normal to decreased tactile fremitus.
–percussion of the chest will reveal hyper-resonance.
–auscultation of the lungs will reveal diminished breath sounds usually with few, if any, rhonchi, and no rubs, crackles, or wheezes.
- Chronic bronchitis.
  • Physical examination may reveal the following findings depending on disease severity (Billas 1990; Littler and Momany 1990; Stauffer 1994):
    –vital signs—blood pressure and temperature will be within normal levels unless there is a coexisting condition (e.g., hypertension, infection). The patient's respiratory rate and pulse may be within normal levels or increased, depending on the severity of the condition.
    –skin—may note plethora and, in advanced disease, central cyanosis.
    –examination of the chest will reveal a normal anteroposterior diameter.
    –palpation of the chest may reveal decreased tactile fremitus.
    –percussion of the chest may be normal to dull.
    –auscultation of the lungs may reveal normal to decreased breath sounds with diffuse wheezes and rhonchi.
    –examination of sputum will reveal copious amounts of mucopurulent or purulent sputum.

ASSESSMENT

→ COPD
→ Emphysema (COPD Type A)
→ Chronic bronchitis (COPD Type B)
→ R/O acute infection (e.g., pneumonia)
→ R/O asthmatic bronchitis
→ R/O bronchiectasis
→ R/O cor pulmonale
→ R/O central airway obstruction
→ R/O congestive heart failure

Table 5D.1.   COMPARISON OF CLINICAL MANIFESTATIONS AND LABORATORY FINDINGS

Characteristic Inspection	Emphysema	Chronic Bronchitis
Body	thin	stocky or obese (bloater)
Chest	hyperinflation (barrel chest)	normal
	hypertrophy of accessory muscles	increased use of accessory muscles
Breathing pattern	progressive dyspnea	variable
	labored (puffer)	normal
	retractions	normal
	decreased chest movements	normal
	decreased I/E ratio	decreased I/E ratio
Posture	orthopnea	variable
Cough	little	considerable
Sputum	little-mucoid	large-purulent
Color	normal (pink)	cyanosis (blue)
Palpation	normal to decreased fremitus	normal to decreased fremitus
Percussion	hyper-resonance	dull
Auscultation		
Breath sounds	decreased	normal to decreased
Rhonchi	little	episodic
Blood Gases		
PO_2 resting	slight decrease	moderate to severe decrease
PO_2 exercises	falls	stable
PCO_2	normal	increased
PCO_3	normal	increased
PFTs		
Spirometry	obstructive pattern	obstructive pattern
RV and TLC	increased	normal to decreased
Diffusion capacity	decreased	normal
Compliance	increased	normal
Hematocrit	<55%	≥55%
X-Ray		
Bronchovascular markings	decreased	increased
Hyperinflation	yes	no
Bullae/blebs	yes	no
Past History	normal	frequent respiratory infections
Life Span	normal (60-80 yrs)	decreased (40-60 yrs)
Cor Pulmonale	uncommon	common

Source: Reprinted with permission from Littler, J.E. and Momany, T. 1990. *The family practice handbook*, pp. 117–119. Chicago: Year Book Medical Publishers. Adapted from Oakes, D.R. 1988. *Clinical practitioner's pocket guide to respiratory care*. Chelmsford, MA: Old Town Health Educator Publications.

PLAN

DIAGNOSTIC TESTS

See **Table 5D.1, Comparison of Clinical Manifestations and Laboratory Findings**.

→ CBC may reveal an increased hematocrit (> 55%) secondary to polycythemia in advanced COPD due to chronic bronchitis (Littler and Momany 1990; Stauffer 1994).

→ Chest x-ray findings (Littler and Momany 1990; Stauffer 1994):
  ▪ emphysema.
   • Hyperinflation of the lungs with decreased bronchovascular markings.
   • Bullae (parenchymal) and blebs (subpleural) will be evident and are pathognomonic.
   • Diaphragm will be low and flat.
   • Heart will be normal size and vertical.
  ▪ chronic bronchitis.
   • Increased bronchovascular markings.
   • Diaphragm will be normal.
   • Heart size may be increased and horizontal.

→ Electrocardiogram can be ordered if heart disease is suspected. It will demonstrate right axis deviation, right ventricular hypertrophy, and "p" pulmonale in patients with severe chronic bronchitis secondary to cor pulmonale (Littler and Momany 1990; Stauffer 1994).

→ Pulmonary Function Tests (PFTs) will demonstrate the following (see **Table 5D.2, Pulmonary Function Tests**):
  ▪ emphysema:
   • spirometry will reveal an obstructive pattern.
   • TLC will be increased.
   • RV will be increased.
   • *static lung compliance* (SLC) will be increased.
   • *diffusing capacity* (DC) will be decreased.
  ▪ chronic bronchitis:
   • spirometry will reveal an obstructive pattern.
   • TLC will be normal to decreased.
   • RV will be normal to decreased.
   • SLC will be normal.
   • DC will be normal.

→ Blood gases are not routinely done unless indicated. If performed, the following results may be noted, depending on the severity of the patient's disease (Littler and Momany 1990; Stauffer 1994):
  ▪ emphysema:
   • resting PO_2—slight decrease.
   • exercise PO_2—decreased.
   • PCO_2—normal.
   • PCO_3—normal.
  ▪ chronic bronchitis:
   • resting PO_2—moderate to severe decrease.
   • exercise PO_2—stable.
   • PCO_2—increased.
   • PCO_3—increased.

→ Gram stain of sputum may reveal a pathogen (e.g., *Streptococcus pneumoniae, Hemophilus influenzae, Moraxella catarrhalis*) if there is a coexisting active infection.

→ Culture of sputum may identify a pathogen if there is a coexisting active infection.

TREATMENT/MANAGEMENT

→ In patients with evidence of significant symptoms or disease (e.g., respiratory distress, pneumonia), hospitalization may be required for effective treatment. In such patients, physician consultation and management is indicated.

→ In patients with mild to moderate symptoms, outpatient management is possible as long as their symptoms respond to conservative therapy.

→ An essential component of the patient's treatment is improving ventilation through reducing respiratory secretions (e.g., pulmonary toilet, deep breathing, coughing).
  ▪ In some patients, referral to a respiratory therapist for instruction in proper pulmonary toilet techniques may be necessary.

→ Patients need to maintain adequate hydration and nutritional intake.
  ▪ In those patients exhibiting weight loss, supplemental caloric intake is indicated.
  ▪ Referral of patients to a nutritionist for specific recommendations may be necessary.

→ If the patient smokes cigarettes, she must be advised to stop.
  ▪ Referral of the patient to community programs or support groups may be necessary.
  ▪ The use of nicotine chewing gum (2-mg piece chewed slowly over 30 minutes) or a nicotine patch may be helpful during her withdrawal from cigarettes (Stauffer 1994). See **Smoking Cessation** Protocol.

→ Reducing exposure to potential respiratory irritants and allergens is essential (e.g., air pollution, secondary smoke, toxic inhalants). Specific recommendations for each patient should be made based on individual circumstances.

Table 5D.2. PULMONARY FUNCTION TESTS (PFTS)—DEFINITIONS AND RESULTS IN OBSTRUCTIVE AND RESTRICTIVE PULMONARY DISEASE

Tests	Definition	Results in Obstructive[1] Pulmonary Disease	Results in Restrictive[1] Pulmonary Disease
Tests Derived from Spirometry			
Forced vital capacity (FVC) in liters	the volume of gas that can be forcefully expelled from the lungs after maximal inspiration.	N or ↓	↓
Forced expiratory volume in 1 second (FEV$_1$) in liters	the volume of gas expelled in the first second of the FVC maneuver.	↓	N or ↓
Forced expiratory flow from 25% to 75% of the vital capacity (FEF$_{25-75}$) in liters per second (L/s)	the maximal midexpiratory airflow rate.	↓	N or ↓
Peak expiratory flow rate (PEFR) in L/s	the maximal airflow rate achieved in the FVC maneuver.	↓	N or ↑
Maximum voluntary ventilation (MVV) in liters per minute (L/min)	the maximum volume of gas that can be breathed in 1 minute (usually measured for 15 seconds and multiplied by 4).	↓	N or ↓
FEV$_1$/FVC percentage	N/A	↓	N or ↑
Lung Volumes			
Slow vital capacity (SVC) in liters	the volume of gas that can be slowly exhaled after maximal inspiration.	N or ↓	↓
Total lung capacity (TLC) in liters	the volume of gas in the lungs after a maximal inspiration.	N or ↑	↓
Functional residual capacity (FRC) in liters	the volume of gas in the lungs at the end of a normal tidal expiration.	↑	N or ↓
Expiratory reserve volume (ERV) in liters	the volume of gas representing the difference between functional residual capacity and residual volume.	N or ↓	N or ↓
Residual volume (RV) in liters	the volume of gas remaining in the lungs after maximal expiration.	↑	N, ↓, or ↑
RV/TLC ratio	N/A	↑	N or ↑

[1]N = normal; ↓ = less than predicted; ↑ = greater than predicted

Source: Reprinted with permission from Stauffer, J.L. 1993. Pulmonary Diseases. In *Current medical diagnosis and treatment*, eds. L.M. Tierney, Jr., S.J. McPhee, M.A. Papadakis, and S.A. Schroeder, 32 ed., pp. 185-186. Norwalk, CT: Appleton & Lange.

→ Improving the patient's airway diameter—through the reduction of edema and inflammation, and relief of bronchospasm—may require pharmacological therapies, including beta-agonists, theophylline compounds, and corticosteroid agents.

■ Individualized therapeutic regimens may include one or more of the following agents (Stauffer 1994):

• bronchodilators indicated to partially reverse airway obstruction in patients with exacerbation of disease, wheezing, or asthmatic bronchitis including the following medications:

–ipratropium spray (Atrovent®), an anticholinergic bronchodilator, 2 inhalations every 6 hours (maximum dose 12 inhalations in 24 hours).

–metaproterenol (Alupent®, Metaprel®), a sympathomimetic bronchodilator, 1-4 inhalations every 3-4 hours (maximum dose 12 inhalations in 24 hours).

–albuterol (Proventil®, Ventolin®), a sympathomimetic bronchodilator with a slightly longer duration than that of metaproterenol, 1-4 inhalations every 4 to 6 hours.

–theophylline (Theo-Dur®) 400 mg-1000 mg/24 hours p.o. in 2 divided doses.

NOTE: Theophylline use in COPD generally is reserved for those patients who have failed to respond to or are intolerant of inhaled brochodilators, or who have sleep-related respiratory symptoms.

Careful monitoring of theophylline levels is recommended when adjusting doses. A baseline serum theophylline level should be obtained when initiating therapy. Additional theophylline levels should be obtained 3 to 5 days after initiating therapy. The therapeutic serum theophylline level is 10 mcg/ml-20 mcg/ml with toxic levels greater than 20 mcg/ml (Ellsworth et al. 1991; Stauffer 1994).

- corticosteroid therapy will reduce inflammation. Agents that may be prescribed include:
  - inhaled corticosteroids. Studies have demonstrated improvement in patients—especially those with chronic bronchitis—using these agents. Inhaled corticosteroids are most effective in COPD if administered several minutes after inhaling a bronchodilator. This is true especially if the patient remains "tight" or if both agents are being used (Ellsworth et al. 1991; Stauffer 1994).
    - ▸ Beclamethasone (Beclovent®, Vanceril®) 2 inhalations TID-QID.
    - ▸ Triamcinolone (Azmacort®) 2 inhalations TID-QID (maximum dose not to exceed 16 inhalations/24 hours).
    - ▸ Flunisolide (Aerobid®) 2-4 inhalations BID (maximum dose not to exceed 4 inhalations BID).

    NOTE: Instruct the patient to rinse her mouth after use to prevent oral candidiasis.
  - oral corticosteroid therapy may be necessary in patients with exacerbation of symptoms after use of conventional therapy. It can be especially beneficial in patients with eosinophils noted on their sputum or peripheral blood smears. The following dosages may be prescribed (Stauffer 1994):
    - ▸ prednisone (Deltasone®) 5 mg-40 mg p.o. every day or every other day.

    NOTE: Discontinue oral corticosteroids if there is no evidence of spirometric improvement after 2 to 4 weeks of therapy. Tapering of the dose should be done in increments of 5 mg-10 mg every 2 to 3 days.

→ Antibiotic therapy should be initiated in patients with evidence of acute infection.
- Ideally, such therapy should be based on the results of sputum gram stain or culture results.
- If acute exacerbation of symptoms is evident—especially in chronic bronchitis patients—empiric antibiotic therapy may be initiated with one of the following agents for 7 to 10 days (Stauffer 1994):

- amoxicillin (Amoxil®, Trimox®) 500 mg p.o. TID.
- ampicillin (Principen®) 250 mg-500 mg p.o. QID.
- tetracycline (Achromycin®) 250 mg-500 mg p.o. QID.
- trimethoprim/sulfamethoxazole (Septra DS®, Bactrim®) 160 mg/800 mg p.o. BID.

→ Prophylactic immunizations (e.g., yearly influenza vaccination, pneumococcal immunization) should be administered to patients with COPD and household members in close contact with COPD patients (see **Pneumonia** and **Influenza** protocols).

→ Home oxygen therapy may be necessary in certain patients with significant hypoxemia. If home oxygen therapy is being considered, consultation with a physician is indicated.

→ Patients should be carefully monitored for the development of any signs and symptoms of complications including cor pulmonale, respiratory infections, and psychosocial problems (e.g., depression).

→ In patients exhibiting signs or symptoms of depression, psychological evaluation and therapy should be recommended.

CONSULTATION

→ Consultation with a physician is warranted in any patient with moderate to severe symptoms or signs of COPD, with evidence of complications associated with COPD, or in patients not responding to conservative therapy.

→ As needed for prescription(s).

PATIENT EDUCATION

→ Educate the patient about COPD—the cause(s), clinical manifestations, recommended diagnostic tests, therapeutic interventions, prognosis, possible complications, and indicated follow-up.

→ Discuss ways in which the patient can prevent the development of further lung damage and complications (e.g., cessation of cigarette smoking, avoidance of inhalation of toxic substances and pollutants, immunizations).
- If the patient smokes cigarettes, referral to community resources and support groups for cessation of smoking may be beneficial (see **Smoking Cessation** Protocol).
- When appropriate, educate the patient about the possible psychological sequelae that she may experience as a result of COPD (e.g., depres-

sion) and provide her with referrals and resources.

■ Educate the patient about any potential side effects of medications that are prescribed (see the *PDR* as needed) and the need to report such side effects to her clinician.

FOLLOW-UP

→ Patients requiring hospitalization, consultation, or management of care by a physician should have follow-up evaluations per physician recommendation.

→ Follow-up evaluations of patients receiving outpatient care should be based on the severity of their symptoms before, during, and after therapeutic interventions. Patients without evidence of improvement in their symptoms should return as soon as possible for further evaluation.

→ Document in progress notes and problem list.

Maureen Shannon, C.N.M., F.N.P, M.S.

5-E

Epistaxis

Epistaxis (nosebleed), a common problem, occurs in approximately 60 percent of the population (Vitek 1991). The majority of epistaxis episodes are self-limited and associated with minimal blood loss. However, in approximately six percent of the population, the bleeding persists and requires medical evaluation and interventions (Vitek 1991). Most cases of epistaxis which require medical evaluation are successfully managed by conservative treatments (e.g., nasal packing, local chemical cautery, or electrocautery) (Erwin 1987).

In patients unresponsive to such treatments, a diagnosis of intractable epistaxis is made. Intractable epistaxis, although uncommon, can be life-threatening if the bleeding cannot be controlled. Hospitalization is necessary to stop the bleeding, determine and treat the underlying cause, and stabilize the patient in situations of significant blood loss (Jackson and Jackson 1988; Vitek 1991). Complications associated with intractable epistaxis include anemia, infection, hemorrhage, and, in severe cases, death.

There are two anatomic sites associated with epistaxis episodes. Anterior nasal bleeding occurs in the anterior portion of the nasal septum where a thin nasal mucous membrane covers a plexus of blood vessels. When exposed to dry air or minor trauma (e.g., finger picking), bleeding can occur. The most frequent type of epistaxis, anterior nasal bleeding, is responsible for most epistaxis occurring in children and young adults. Usually, anterior epistaxis is self-limited and does not require medical evaluation.

Posterior nasal bleeding originates in the area posterior to the middle turbinate, an area which is difficult to access for treatment. This type of epistaxis often is associated with older patients and patients with certain medical conditions (e.g., hypertension, bleeding disorders). Medical evaluation and interventions are usually necessary to treat this epistaxis episode and minimize blood loss (Erwin 1987; Jackson and Jackson 1988; Vitek 1991; Votey and Dudley 1989).

DATABASE

SUBJECTIVE

→ Predisposing factors may include:
- decreased ambient humidity.
- trauma.
- nasal infection.
- anatomic deviations (deviated nasal septum, septal spur).
- allergic rhinitis.
- hypertension.
- bleeding disorders.
- chronic, excessive alcohol intake.
- overuse of platelet-inhibiting medication (e.g., aspirin, nonsteroidal anti-inflammatory drug [NSAID]).
- severe liver disease.
- neoplasm.
- use of decongestants, nasal steroids.

→ Symptoms may include:
- nasal bleeding. May be unilateral or bilateral.
- symptoms associated with URI or allergic rhinitis.
- dizziness (if increased blood loss).
- lightheadedness (if increased blood loss).
- bleeding from other sites (if overuse of platelet-inhibiting medication, coagulopathy, or if severe liver disease).

- symptoms associated with severe liver disease (e.g., anorexia, jaundice).

OBJECTIVE

→ Patient may present with the following changes in vital signs:
  - blood pressure. Postural change in blood pressure may be observed if significant blood loss.
  - pulse may be increased if significant blood loss.
  - skin pallor may be observed if significant blood loss.

→ Direct observation with nasal speculum may reveal localized bleeding site in anterior portion of nasal vestibule. The bleeding site may not be visualized if bleeding site is located posterior to middle turbinate.

→ Crusting, inflammation, and ulceration may be observed if nasal mucosa has been traumatized.

ASSESSMENT

→ Epistaxis

→ R/O nasal trauma

→ R/O allergic rhinitis

→ R/O infection

→ R/O anatomic deviations

→ R/O hypertension

→ R/O bleeding disorders

→ R/O overuse of platelet-inhibiting medications

→ R/O chronic alcohol use

→ R/O liver disease

→ R/O neoplasm

PLAN

DIAGNOSTIC TESTS

→ If significant blood loss is suspected, the following tests may be ordered in consultation with a physician:
  - CBC. Decreased hemoglobin and hematocrit may be noted with significant blood loss.
  - platelet count. May be decreased in patients with idiopathic thrombocytopenia, severe liver disease.
  - prothrombin time (PT), Partial thrombolastin time (PTT). May be increased in patients with severe liver disease, anticoagulation therapy (e.g., warfarin sodium).

TREATMENT/MANAGEMENT

→ If the patient does not have history of prolonged epistaxis, and there is no evidence of excessive blood loss (e.g., postural changes), the patient should apply direct digital pressure—tightly compressing the soft nasal tip of the nose (not the bony portions of the nose) between the index finger and thumb—for at least 5 minutes.
  - During this time, the patient should be sitting with her head bent *slightly* forward to reduce the swallowing of blood (Jackler and Kaplan 1994).

→ After application of digital pressure, evaluate patient for cessation of bleeding.
  - If bleeding has stopped, attempt to visualize and identify the site of the epistaxis to rule out specific pathology.
  - Observe the patient for several minutes to ensure that bleeding will not resume.

→ If the bleeding recurs or continues despite application of digital pressure, the patient should be evaluated immediately by a physician for additional diagnostic and therapeutic interventions. Epistaxis can lead to severe blood loss and death if inadequately evaluated and treated, though this is a rare occurrence.

→ Treatment of underlying pathology (e.g., rhinitis, infection, hypertension, liver disease) is essential to reduce the likelihood of recurrence.

→ Patients with epistaxis caused by decreased ambient humidity should be educated about ways to increase ambient humidity (e.g., vaporizer use) and advised to avoid nasal mucosa trauma (e.g., finger picking).

CONSULTATION

→ Consultation with a physician is warranted in all instances of suspected intractable epistaxis, if visualization of the bleeding site is not accomplished, or when significant underlying medical conditions are suspected.

→ As needed for prescription(s).

PATIENT EDUCATION

→ Educate the patient about epistaxis—the most common cause, treatment, signs and symptoms of complications, preventive measures, and, if epistaxis recurs, the proper technique to use when applying direct pressure to the nostrils.

→ Educate the patient to avoid hot and spicy foods and tobacco since vasodilation may result from their ingestion/use (Jackler and Kaplan 1994).

→ When a patient requires hospitalization, education of the patient is the responsibility of the attending physician.

FOLLOW-UP

→ If there has been physician consultation, follow up per physician recommendation.

→ Document in progress notes and problem list.

5-F

Influenza

Influenza is a systemic illness caused by one of three types of orthomyxoviruses—types A, B, and C. Influenza epidemics are caused by types A and B. They usually occur in the fall or winter, and the two types are similar in their clinical presentations. Type C influenza infection is associated with an illness milder than types A and B.

The influenza viruses are capable of changing their envelope proteins in response to the development of immunity in populations exposed to the viruses. After such a change in the envelope proteins, persons previously immunized or infected with a type of influenza virus may again be susceptible to the virus (CDC 1992a; Littler and Momany 1990; Shandera and Gill 1994).

Viral shedding from nasal secretions is the method of transmission, with the individual most infectious 24 hours prior to the onset of symptoms. Cessation of viral shedding occurs by seven days after the onset of symptoms. The incubation period is one to four days.

Clinical illness usually lasts four to seven days after the onset of symptoms. The mortality rate associated with influenza is reportedly between one and four percent, with the highest rates associated with persons 65 years of age or older (CDC 1992b).

Complications associated with influenza may include otitis media, sinusitis, myositis, bronchitis, secondary bacterial pneumonia, and, rarely, pericarditis, myocarditis, and thrombophlebitis. Reye's syndrome is a rare but serious complication of influenza, occurring two to three weeks after symptom onset. It is usually reported in school-age children (Shandera and Gill 1994). Although the exact pathogenesis is unknown, the incidence of Reye's syndrome is associated with the ingestion of aspirin.

DATABASE

SUBJECTIVE

→ Patient may report exposure to an individual with similar symptoms.

→ Patient may report one or more of the following symptoms, with severity ranging from mild to severe (CDC 1992a; Shandera and Gill 1994):
  - sudden onset of high-grade fever.
  - chills and/or rigors.
  - malaise.
  - generalized myalgia.
  - headache.
  - cough—initially non-productive but may become productive.
  - nasal congestion.
  - sore throat.
  - conjunctivitis.
  - abdominal pain.
  - nausea.
  - vomiting.

OBJECTIVE

→ Physical examination may reveal the following:
  - elevated temperature.
  - weight loss and/or orthostasis if severe nausea and vomiting.
  - mild pharyngeal injection.
  - conjunctival erythema and/or discharge.
  - auscultation of the lungs may reveal basilar crackles or rhonchi if bronchitis or pneumonia.
  - auscultation of the heart may reveal a rub if pericarditis.

- change in mental status may be observed in patients with central nervous system (CNS) complications or Reye's syndrome (such signs and symptoms usually occur two to three weeks after the onset of illness if Reye's syndrome complicates influenza).

ASSESSMENT

→ Influenza (Type A, B, or C)

→ R/O URI

→ R/O otitis media

→ R/O sinusitis

→ R/O bronchitis

→ R/O pneumonia

→ R/O other viral infections (e.g., mononucleosis)

PLAN

DIAGNOSTIC TESTS

→ In a patient exhibiting moderate to severe symptoms, one or more of the following tests may be ordered after consultation with a physician:
  - CBC.
    - May demonstrate leukopenia.
  - Cultures of nasopharyngeal swabs or aspirates may be positive.
    - Cultures should be obtained within 72 hours of illness secondary to the rapid decline in quantity of virus after 72 hours.
    - Culture results require 2 to 6 days (Shandera 1993).
  - Immunofluorescence of nasopharyngeal specimens for influenza antigen may be positive (sensitivity is variable).
  - Acute and convalescent titers of serum will reveal a significant increase in titer.
  - Chest x-ray.
    - May reveal evidence of bronchitis or pneumonia in patients with these complications.
  - If Reye's syndrome is suspected, the following will be noted (Shandera and Gill 1994):
    - decreased blood glucose.
    - increased serum transaminase levels.
    - increased blood ammonia levels.
    - increased prothrombin time.

TREATMENT/MANAGEMENT

→ During the symptomatic phase of influenza, the patient should rest, increase fluid intake, and use acetaminophen for fever and myalgia (Littler and Momany 1990; Shandera and Gill 1994).
  - The patient should avoid contact with others—especially those most susceptible to possible complications from influenza (e.g., patients 65 years of age or older, immunocompromised patients).

→ In severely ill patients or patients at high risk for the development of complications, the use of amantadine hydrochloride (Amantadine®, Symmetrel®) should be considered.
  - This is an antiviral agent with an approximately 50 percent efficacy rate in reducing severe symptoms when used against influenza type A.
  - It is not effective when used against influenza type B.
  - Treatment should start immediately after symptoms begin and continue for 10 days.
  - The following dosages are recommended (Ellsworth et al. 1991, Shandera and Gill 1994):
    - amantadine hydrochloride (Amantadine®, Symmetrel®) 100 mg p.o. BID for 10 days.
    - in elderly patients, the dose is reduced to 50 mg p.o. BID for 10 days.

NOTE: Potential side effects associated with amantadine hydrochloride use include CNS symptoms (e.g., confusion, inability to concentrate, depression, hallucinations, jitteriness, insomnia, tremors) and nausea. Use of anticholinergics with this medicine will potentiate the side effects of amantadine hydrochloride (Ellsworth et al. 1991).

→ Immunization with polyvalent influenza virus vaccine (one 0.5 ml I.M. injection) during the fall provides partial immunity for up to 1 year.
  - Annual immunization is necessary because the antigenic configuration of the virus changes yearly.
  - Annual immunization is recommended for individuals at greatest risk of having serious complications associated with influenza or individuals who can transmit influenza to such high-risk groups as (CDC 1992a):
    - persons 65 years of age or older.
    - persons with chronic heart or lung disease.
    - residents of nursing homes or other chronic care facilities.
    - persons who required ongoing medical care or hospitalization during the previous year because of chronic medical diseases (e.g., diabetes mellitus), hemoglobinopathies, renal dysfunction, or immunosuppression (including

pharmacologically induced
immunosuppression).
- adolescents (and children) receiving long-term
aspirin therapy (and therefore at risk of
developing Reye's syndrome after influenza
infection).
- persons who are HIV-positive.
- pregnant women who have other medical
conditions which place them at risk of
complications associated with influenza
infection.
NOTE: Whenever possible, influenza vaccine
should be administered after the first
trimester.
- persons preparing to travel to foreign
countries. The risk of exposure depends upon
the destination, the season during which
arrival is planned, and whether or not the
person has received an influenza vaccination
during the previous fall or winter months. In
the tropics, influenza can occur throughout
the entire year; in the southern hemisphere
the peak influenza season is between April
and September.
- health care workers, nursing-home/chronic-
care facility employees, providers of home
care, or household members who have contact
with high-risk persons.
NOTE: Influenza vaccination should not be
administered to patients with a known
anaphylactic hypersensitivity to eggs or other
components of the influenza vaccine without
first consulting a physician.

CONSULTATION

→ Consultation with a physician is warranted for any
patient with suspected or diagnosed complications
associated with influenza, or prior to prescribing
amantadine hydrochloride for a patient.

→ As otherwise indicated.

→ As necessary for prescription(s).

PATIENT EDUCATION

→ Educate the patient about influenza—the cause,
clinical course, diagnostic tests that may be
necessary, treatment options, possible
complications, and any indicated follow-up.

→ Educate high-risk patients about preventive
measures to avoid influenza infection (e.g.,
influenza vaccination).

FOLLOW-UP

→ If consultation with a physician was necessary,
follow up as recommended by the physician.

→ If symptoms of complications develop, the patient
should return for re-evaluation.

→ Document in progress notes and problem list.

5-G

Otitis Externa

Otitis externa is an inflammation of the external auditory canal caused by pathogens which grow readily in moist environments (e.g., *Pseudomonas aeruginosa*, fungi). Usually, exposure to water followed by some type of trauma to the auditory canal (e.g., insertion of a cotton-tipped swab or hairpin) precedes the onset of symptoms (Amundson 1990).

Necrotizing (malignant) external otitis is a rare, but potentially lethal, infection that can occur in immunocompromised patients (e.g., older patients, diabetic patients). It is caused by *P. aeruginosa* and, occasionally, *aspergillus*. This infection is characterized by severe otalgia and persistent, foul aural discharge (Evans and Hoffman 1994).

DATABASE

SUBJECTIVE

→ Symptoms may include otalgia of affected ear (usually within hours after the trauma).

→ Patient may report a small amount of watery discharge or bleeding.

→ Patient may experience diminished hearing if significant edema.

→ Patient may report recent history of water exposure and trauma of auditory canal.

→ A patient with necrotizing external otitis will report severe otalgia unresponsive to analgesics, and a persistent foul aural discharge.

OBJECTIVE

→ Scant amount of discharge from affected ear may be observed.

→ Manipulation of the auricle of the affected ear will cause/increase pain.

→ Otoscopic examination of the auditory canal will reveal edema, erythema, and possibly discharge (purulent, bloody, serous). Insufflation of tympanic membrane (TM) will be within normal limits.

→ Pre- and post-auricular lymph node enlargement, with or without tenderness to palpation, may be noted.

→ If necrotizing otitis externa is suspected, examination of the cranial nerves may reveal palsies (cranial nerves VI, VII, IX, X, XI and/or XII).

ASSESSMENT

→ Acute otitis externa

→ R/O otitis media

→ R/O foreign body in external auditory canal

→ R/O necrotizing external otitis

→ R/O perforated tympanic membrane

PLAN

DIAGNOSTIC TESTS

→ Culture of discharge is rarely necessary since most cases readily respond to topical therapy.

→ Potassium hydroxide (KOH) 10% wet prep of discharge may reveal elements of hyphae and/or yeast buds in suspected cases of fungal infection.

TREATMENT/MANAGEMENT

(Amundson 1990; Ellsworth et al. 1991; Jackler and Kaplan 1993)

→ Cleansing of canal using gentle suction is recommended before beginning treatment.
  ▪ This also may result in better visualization of the TM if this has been a problem.
  ▪ Instillation of cerumenolytics and/or irrigation of the canal is not recommended.
→ Direct instillation of topical medications into the affected ear is the standard treatment.
  ▪ Otic preparations available for therapy include acid/alcohol solutions or antibiotic/steroid solutions/suspensions.
    • Acid/alcohol otic preparations reduce inflammation, and have a drying and an antifungal effect. Available preparations include:
      –acetic acid 2% solution (Vo-Sol®) instill 4 gtt in affected ear TID–QID for 7 to 10 days
      –hydrocortisone 1%, acetic acid 2% solution (Vo-Sol HC®) instill 4 gtt in affected ear TID–QID for 7 to 10 days.
    • Antibiotic/steroid otic preparations have an antimicrobial effect and reduce inflammation. Available preparations include:
      –hydrocortisone 1%, 5 mg neomycin sulfate, 10,000 units polymyxin B per ml suspension/solution (Cortisporin®) instill 4 gtt in affected ear TID–QID for 7 to 10 days.
      –hydrocortisone 1%, 3.3 mg neomycin sulfate, 3 mg colistin sulfate per ml suspension (Coly-Mycin®) instill 4 gtt in affected ear TID–QID for 7 to 10 days.

NOTE: Neomycin-containing solutions/suspensions may sensitize the patient and result in a more pronounced reaction to future use of neomycin preparations.

→ The affected ear canal should be protected from water exposure for at least 2 weeks.
→ For recurrent episodes of otitis externa, prophylactic treatment with boric acid 2.75% in isopropyl alcohol solution (Dri-Ear®, Swim Ear®) may be an option prior to swimming.
→ Systemic analgesic (e.g., NSAIDs) may be necessary for severe discomfort.

CONSULTATION

→ If necrotizing (malignant) external otitis is suspected, physician consultation is warranted.
→ For resistant, recurrent episodes.
→ As needed for prescription(s).

PATIENT EDUCATION

→ Educate the patient about otitis externa—the cause(s), treatment, and the importance of avoiding future trauma as a means of preventing future episodes.
→ If episodes occur after exposure to water (e.g., swimming), discuss the possibility of using an otic preparation (e.g., Dri Ear®, Swim Ear®) prior to swimming to reduce the possibility of recurrence. The patient should also use a hand-held hair dryer to facilitate drying of canal after water exposure.

FOLLOW-UP

→ If condition is resistant to treatment, or as recommended by physician after consultation.
→ Document in progress notes and problem list.

Maureen Shannon, C.N.M., F.N.P, M.S.

5-H

Otitis Media

Otitis media, an inflammation of the mucous membranes of the middle ear and the tympanic membrane (TM), is observed frequently in children, and found less commonly in adults. The pathophysiology of otitis media involves a combination of factors including eustachian tube dysfunction (secondary to mucous membrane edema, an obstruction, or an anatomic deformity); impaired ciliary function of the mucosa; barotrauma; and/or infection with a specific pathogen (e.g., bacteria or virus) (Kemp 1990).

Complications associated with otitis media include diminished hearing, mastoiditis, meningitis, brain abscess, subdural empyema, subperiosteal abscess, sinus vein thrombosis, suppurative labyrinthitis, and chronic perforation of the TM (Kemp 1990).

The most common pathogens isolated in adult otitis media are *S. pneumoniae, H. influenzae, Streptococcus pyogenes, M. catarrhalis (Branhamella catarrhalis),* and *S. aureus* (Celin et al. 1991; Jackler and Kaplan 1994). Beta-lactamase-producing organisms have been associated with approximately 25 percent of otitis media (Celin et al. 1991; Kemp 1990).

The terminology used to describe the spectrum of symptoms and clinical diagnosis associated with this pathology can be confusing. As a result, Kemp (1990, 267-268) suggests the following definitions as a means of clarifying and classifying otitis media and its sequelae:

→ *"Eustachian tube dysfunction* is any condition in which the ability of the eustachian tube to permit equilibration of ambient and middle ear pressure is impeded."

→ *"Acute otitis media* is rapid-onset inflammation (usually minutes or hours) of the mucous

membranes of the middle ear and tympanic membrane of less than three weeks duration, regardless of cause."

→ *"Subacute otitis media* is inflammation of the mucous membranes of the middle ear and tympanic membranes lasting longer than three weeks but less than three months."

→ *"Chronic otitis media* is inflammation of the mucous membranes of the middle ear and of the tympanic membrane that has been present for longer than three months."

→ *"Middle ear effusion* is the presence of fluid in the middle ear space (independent of character or duration). This effusion (or when perforations of tympanic membrane are present) may be further classified as purulent, serous, or mucoid."

DATABASE

SUBJECTIVE

→ Predisposing factors may include history of:
  ▪ recent URI.
  ▪ allergies.
  ▪ otitis media.

→ Patient may report one or more of the following symptoms:
  ▪ otalgia.
  ▪ fever.
  ▪ diminished hearing.
  ▪ tinnitus.
  ▪ otorrhea.
  ▪ sore throat (may be unilateral).
  ▪ temporomandibular joint (TMJ) pain.

- vertigo.
- anorexia.
- nausea.
- vomiting.

OBJECTIVE

→ Temperature may be elevated, but often is normal in adults.

→ External auditory canal may contain purulent discharge if TM perforation has occurred.

→ TM may be bulging or retracted, opaque, erythematous, bullous, or hyperemic. Air-fluid level or purulent fluid may be observed behind the TM. There may be distorted or absent TM landmarks and light reflex. TM may be immobile when insufflation is attempted.

→ Enlarged and tender pre- and post-auricular lymph nodes may be palpated.

→ Diminished gross hearing tests (e.g., wristwatch ticking, whispering) of affected ear may be evident.

ASSESSMENT

→ Otitis media (acute, subacute, or chronic)

→ R/O middle ear effusion

→ R/O URI

→ R/O otitis externa

→ R/O TM perforation

→ R/O barotrauma

→ R/O anatomic deformity

→ R/O foreign body in external auditory canal

→ R/O cerumen impaction

PLAN

DIAGNOSTIC TESTS

→ Audiometry testing may demonstrate diminished hearing in affected ear(s).

→ Tympanocentesis may reveal purulent discharge. If tympanocentesis is being considered, the patient should be referred to an otolaryngologist.

TREATMENT/MANAGEMENT

→ Initiate antibiotic treatment for otitis media with amoxicillin (Amoxil®, Trimox®) 500 mg p.o. TID for 10 days.

→ In patients who have a history of penicillin allergy and who are not responding to amoxicillin after 3 to 5 days of treatment, or who experience a recurrence of symptoms, therapy with one of the following should be initiated (Celin et al. 1991; Kemp 1990; Littler and Momany 1990):
- cefaclor (Ceclor®) 250 mg p.o. BID for 10 days.
- trimethoprim/sulfamethoxazole (Bactrim®, Septra DS®) 1 tablet p.o. BID for 10 days.
- erythromycin (Ery Tab®, E-Mycin®) 250 mg p.o. QID for 10 days.

→ Use of analgesics (e.g., aspirin, acetaminophen) may help diminish the otalgia associated with otitis media.

CONSULTATION

→ As indicated in otitis media that is unresponsive to therapy, associated with significant hearing loss, or if complications are suspected.

→ As needed for prescription(s).

PATIENT EDUCATION

→ Educate the patient about otitis media—the cause, treatment options and possible side effects, signs and symptoms of complications.

→ Educate the patient about non-pharmacological management of common side effects associated with antibiotic therapy (e.g., vaginal candidiasis, diarrhea).

→ Advise the patient to avoid activities that can aggravate the condition (e.g., traveling to high altitudes, scuba diving) until resolution of symptoms and completion of therapy.

FOLLOW-UP

→ If otitis media has been associated with hearing loss, consider repeating audiometry testing four to six weeks after completion of therapy to determine whether this problem has resolved.

→ If consultation with a physician was required, follow up as recommended by physician.

→ Document in progress notes and problem list.

Maureen Shannon, C.N.M., F.N.P., M.S.

5-1

Pharyngitis

Pharyngitis is an inflammation of the pharynx which can result from several etiological factors. In 50 percent of cases, the most common cause is a virus often associated with URI—adenovirus, respiratory syncytial virus, Epstein-Barr virus (EBV), coxsackievirus, influenza, and parainfluenza virus.

Although less common, *group A beta-hemolytic streptococcus* (GABHS) is the most common bacterial pathogen responsible for pharyngitis (10 percent to 40 percent). Other less frequent bacterial pathogens responsible for pharyngitis include non-group A *Streptococci, Neisseria gonorrhoreae, Hemophilus influenzae, Corynebacterium diptheriae, Mycoplasma pneumoniae,* and *Chlamydia trachomatis* (Rabinowitz 1990; Jackler and Kaplan 1994).

Environmental factors such as exposure to cigarette smoke, decreased levels or lack of humidity, and air pollution can also be responsible for pharyngitis symptoms (Loos 1990). Possible serious sequelae (e.g., acute rheumatic fever, glomerulonephritis) associated with GABHS are a major concern when evaluating and considering treatment of a patient with pharyngitis.

DATABASE

SUBJECTIVE

Viral

→ Symptoms may include:
- sore throat.
- dysphagia.
- fever (can be high).
- anorexia (often associated with coxsackievirus).
- rhinorrhea.
- cough.
- hoarseness.

GABHS

→ Patient may report recent exposure to person with GABHS.

→ Patients may present with minimal symptoms or experience all of the following:
- severe dysphagia.
- high fever.
- cervical lymphadenopathy.
- headache.
- lethargy.
- anorexia.
- abdominal pain.
- scarlatiniform rash with generalized distribution.

Gonococcal

→ Patient is usually asymptomatic, but can present with symptoms associated with pharyngitis.

→ Patient has history of orogenital sexual contact.

→ See **Gonorrhea** Protocol for other symptoms.

Diphtheria (rarely observed today in United States because of immunizations)

→ Patient has history of no or incomplete immunizations.

→ Symptoms may include:
- low-grade fever.
- sore throat.
- dysphagia.
- hoarseness.
- malaise.

- shortness of breath, if associated myocarditis.
- double vision, slurred speech, if associated neuropathy.

OBJECTIVE

Viral

→ Patient may present with:
- elevated temperature.
- mild erythema, edema of mucosa of pharynx.
- exudate on tonsils.
- small vesicles on tonsils, uvula and palate, palms and soles of feet (coxsackievirus).

→ See **Rhinitis** Protocol for additional physical findings.

GABHS

→ Patient may present with:
- elevated temperature.
- erythema, edema of tonsils and pharynx.
- exudate on tonsils and pharynx (70 percent of patients).
- palatal petechiae.
- enlarged, tender anterior cervical lymph nodes (40 percent to 50 percent of patients).
- scarlatiniform rash.

Gonococcal

→ Occasionally may observe exudative pharyngitis.

→ Cervical adenitis may be present.

→ See **Gonorrhea** Protocol for other physical findings.

Diphtheria

→ Patient may present with:
- elevated temperature.
- gray tenacious tonsillar/pharyngeal pseudomembrane.
- tachycardia (disproportionate to temperature elevation).

→ Cranial nerve testing may be abnormal (if neuropathy).

ASSESSMENT

→ Pharyngitis

→ R/O GABHS pharyngitis

→ R/O URI

→ R/O mononucleosis

→ R/O peritonsillar abscess

→ R/O coxsackievirus infection

→ R/O diphtheria (rare)

PLAN

DIAGNOSTIC TESTS

Viral

→ CBC with differential may reveal atypical lymphocytosis if EBV infection.

→ Heterophile Test—positive if EBV infection.

→ Throat cultures—negative.

GABHS

→ Because it is not possible to distinguish GABHS pharyngitis from other types of pharyngitis on clinical presentation, certain diagnostic tests are indicated to confirm the diagnosis.

→ Strategies vary regarding when certain tests should be done and are based on such factors as cost(s) of the test(s), sensitivity/specificity of the test(s), and time required to perform the test(s), as well as the incidence of pharyngitis *not* due to GABHS in the area—and patient follow-up.

→ Throat culture.
- Considered the gold standard with sensitivity of 90 percent and specificity of 100 percent.
- A cotton-tipped swab is used to obtain the specimen from the posterior pharynx and tonsils. This specimen is plated on sheep's-blood agar medium with a bacitracin disc; results are available 24 to 48 hours later.
- Positive culture indicates presence of beta-hemolytic streptococcus.
  - However, it will not distinguish between serologically infected patients (50 percent) versus GABHS carriers or group C and G streptococci infection (beta-hemolytic strains which may cause pharyngitis).

→ Rapid tests.
- *Latex agglutination* (LA) antigen tests and solid-phase *enzyme immunoabsorbent assays* (ELISA) are less costly than the throat culture and results are available within 1 to 2 hours. Sensitivity is 55 percent to 75 percent (Lieu, Fleisher, and Schwartz 1990) with a specificity of 95 percent (Loos 1990).
- Positive LA or ELISA indicates hemolytic streptococcus infection.

→ CBC.
- Leukocytosis may or may not be observed; usually not done for work-up of GABHS pharyngitis.

Gonococcal

→ Throat culture.
  ■ 2 or 3 swabs rubbed over posterior pharynx and tonsils for 10 to 20 seconds and plated on Thayer-Martin medium.
  ■ Positive result indicates gonococcal infection.

→ Obtain other tests to rule out presence of gonococcus at other sites (e.g., cervical, rectal cultures) and rule out coexistent sexually transmitted diseases (STDs) (e.g., chlamydia culture, VDRL). See **Gonorrheas** and *Chylamydia Trachomatis* protocols.

Diphtheria

→ Diagnosis usually made by clinical findings.

→ Throat culture.
  ■ Swab posterior pharynx and tonsils and plate on Loeffler's medium to confirm diagnosis.

TREATMENT/MANAGEMENT

→ Recommended for all episodes of pharyngitis are rest, increased fluids, use of analgesics (e.g., acetaminophen) as needed and warm saline gargles (¼ tsp. salt in 8 oz. warm water) TID to help alleviate symptoms.
  ■ Viral pharyngitis is usually a self-limited, benign condition, and requires no additional therapy.

→ GABHS antibiotic therapy is recommended as a means of preventing serious sequelae. Penicillin V (PenVee K®) 500 mg p.o. QID for 10 days should be initiated within 9 days of the onset of symptoms to prevent acute rheumatic fever.
  ■ Cefuroxime axetil (Ceftin®) 250 mg p.o. BID for 10 days is an alternative treatment that may result in better compliance for some patients (Jackler and Kaplan 1994).
  ■ If compliance with oral therapy is of concern, benzathine penicillin G 1.2 million units I.M. can be administered.
  ■ In penicillin-allergic patients, erythromycin (E-Mycin®, Ery-Tab®) 250 mg p.o. QID for 10 days may be substituted.

→ The treatment of gonococcal pharyngitis consists of ceftriaxone (Rocephin®) 250 mg I.M. or aqueous procaine penicillin G 4.8 million units I.M. in combination with probenecid (Benemid®) 1 gm p.o.
  ■ Treatment of any suspected or coexistent STDs also is indicated (see appropriate protocols).

→ If diphtheria is suspected, the treatment includes antitoxin administration with the dose dependent upon the severity/duration of disease.
  ■ Antitoxin is available through the Drug Service, Centers for Disease Control and Prevention (404/639-3670 during business hours, Monday through Friday; 404/639-2888 during nights, weekends, or holidays).
  ■ Antibiotic therapy also is indicated and includes penicillin (Pen Vee K®) 500 mg QID p.o. or erythromycin (E-Mycin®, Ery Tab®) 500 mg p.o. QID for 7 to 10 days.

→ In patients with severe odynophagia, hospitalization for hydration and antibiotic therapy may be necessary.

→ In β-lactamase-resistant cases of GABHS, alternative antibiotic therapy is necessary and may include:
  ■ cefuroxime axetil (Ceftin®) 250 mg p.o. every 12 hours for 10 days

  OR

  dicloxacillin (Dynapen®) 250 mg p.o. QID for 10 days

  OR

  amoxicillin with clavulanate acid (Augmentin®) 500 mg p.o. TID for 10 days.

→ Surgical intervention (i.e., tonsillectomy) is rarely indicated and should be considered only in patients with documented recurrent GABHS pharyngitis.

→ Symptomatic contacts of patients with GABHS should have throat cultures done with appropriate treatment initiated as indicated.

→ Sexual contacts of patients with gonococcal pharyngitis should be evaluated and treated as indicated. See **Gonorrhea** Protocol.

CONSULTATION

→ As indicated in recurrent pharyngitis, suspected peritonsilar abscess, or in patients with severe symptoms that may require hospitalization for treatment.

→ As needed for prescription(s).

PATIENT EDUCATION

→ Educate the patient about the cause of pharyngitis, the clinical course, treatment, possible complications, and any required follow-up.

→ Discuss the need for evaluation of symptomatic contacts (in non-gonococcal pharyngitis) and for evaluation and treatment of all sexual contacts in patients with gonococcal pharyngitis.

→ Advise the patient to call or return for evaluation of any signs/symptoms of complications (including antibiotic reactions).

FOLLOW-UP

→ Test of cure usually is not necessary in GABHS pharyngitis but should be obtained in patients with gonococcal pharyngitis.

→ Because gonococcal infections and diphtheria are state-mandated reportable diseases, a morbidity report must be filed with the local department of public health.

→ Document in progress notes and problem list.

Maureen Shannon, C.N.M., F.N.P, M.S.

5-J

Pneumonia

Pneumonia is an infection of the lung caused by various pathogens including bacteria, viruses, and fungi. Individuals may be exposed to the infecting organism by transmission from colonization in the upper respiratory tract, through hematogenous spread, or by inhaling infected droplets.

Many types of bacterial organisms are responsible for so-called "community-acquired" pneumonias including *Streptococcus pneumoniae* (*S. pneumoniae*), *Hemophilus influenzae* (*H. influenzae*), *Moraxella catarrhalis* (*M. catarrhalis*), *Mycoplasma pneumoniae* (*M. pneumoniae*), *Chlamydia pneumoniae* (*C. pneumoniae* [TWAR]), and *Legionella pneumophila* (*L. pneumophila*) (Griffith and Mazurek 1991; Littler and Momany 1990; Martin and Bates 1991; Musher 1991; Stauffer 1994).

Viral pneumonia is responsible for eight percent of community-acquired pneumonia in adults and often results in bacterial superinfection in 26 percent to 77 percent of patients (Greenberg 1991). The most common viral pathogens causing pneumonia in adults include influenza viruses type A and B (responsible for 50 percent of viral pneumonias), parainfluenza viruses, adenovirus, respiratory syncytial virus (RSV), and viruses associated with exanthems (e.g., measles, varicella zoster virus) (Greenberg 1991).

Nosocomial acquisition of pneumonia also can occur. Pathogens frequently—though not exclusively—associated with nosocomial infection include *Staphylococcus aureus* (*S. aureus*), *Klebsiella pneumoniae* (*K. pneumoniae*), *Escherichia coli* (*E. coli*), and *Pseudomonas aeruginosa* (*P. aeruginosa*), along with influenza viruses type A and B (Greenberg 1991; Littler and Momany 1990; Stauffer 1994; Toews 1987).

Pneumonia resulting from fungi (e.g., *Pneumocystis carinii, Cryptococcus neoformans, Aspergillus fumigatus, Histoplasma capsulatum,* and *Coccidioides immitis*) is rarely seen in individuals with competent immune systems, but is of concern in immunocompromised patients (e.g., HIV-positive patients, patients undergoing cytotoxic therapy) who are in advanced stages of immune dysfunction (Johnson and Sarosi 1991).

Complications associated with pneumonia are related directly to the infecting organism and the immune status of the patient. In most healthy adults, community-acquired pneumonias usually can be effectively treated with oral antibiotics on an outpatient basis, without the development of serious sequelae.

However, in patients with diminished immune responses (e.g., the elderly, alcoholics, malnourished patients, immune-deficient patients) or a history of preexisting pulmonary disease (e.g., COPD), there is an increased risk of complications which can include pleural effusion, bacteremia, lung abscesses, meningitis, or death (Greenberg 1991; Griffith and Mazurek 1991; Martin and Bates 1991; Musher 1991). In patients who are at increased risk of such complications, hospitalization is often indicated.

An in-depth presentation inclusive of all pathogens, clinical manifestations, and treatment modalities for the various types of pneumonia is beyond the scope of this protocol. This protocol will present information about selected pathogens associated with pneumonia, their clinical manifestations, and current treatment recommendations (see **Table 5J.1, Clinical Manifestations and Treatment of Selected Pneumonias,** for additional information).

Table 5J.1. CLINICAL MANIFESTATIONS AND TREATMENT OF SELECTED PNEUMONIAS

Pathogen	Predisposing Factors	Symptoms	Diagnostic Tests	Treatment

Streptococcus pneumoniae (*S. pneumoniae*, pneumococcus)	↑ incidence in very young and elderly, IDU, chronic alcohol use, immune deficiency, COPD.	Usually rapid onset of ↑ temperature (≥38°C/ 100.4°F), chills, cough productive of copious amounts purulent → blood-tinged mucus, chest pain. Elderly patients: more insidious onset.	• CBC: ↑ WBC (>13000 cells/mm³)
			• Serum bilirubin: ↑ (3-4 md/dL)
			• Serum LD: ↑ (>250 u/L)
			• Gram Stain: ↑ PMNs, gm + coccobacilli
			• Sputum culture: may be +
			• Chest x-ray: infiltrate, consolidation, pleural effusion, lung abscess (rarely)
				• Healthy adult patients may be treated as outpatients with one of the following:
				  −Penicillin 250 mg-500 mg p.o. QID x 10 days
				  −Erythromycin 500 mg p.o. QID x 10 days
				  −Amoxicillin 500 mg p.o. TID x 10 days
				  −Cephalexin 500 mg p.o. QID x 10 days
				  −Clindamycin 300 mg p.o. TID x 10 days
				• Hospitalization of some patients (especially those with ↓ immune functioning) may be necessary for initiation of parenteral therapy.

Hemophilus influenzae (*H. influenzae*)	↑ incidence in patients with immune deficiency (e.g., chronic alcohol use, neoplasm, HIV infection), COPD.	Usually sudden onset of fever, chills, cough producing copious amounts of sputum. COPD patients: less acute symptoms with gradual onset of ↑ cough, shortness of breath (SOB), ↑ sputum, low grade or no fever, myalgia, arthralgia.	• CBC: ↑ WBC
			• Gram stain: small gm—coccobacilli, pleomorphic
			• Sputum culture: may be +
			• Blood culture: may be + (usually non-typeable *H. influenzae*)
			• Chest x-ray: patchy bronchopneumonic disease; chronic interstitial changes in COPD patients
				• Initially patient can be treated with:
				  −Ampicillin 500 mg p.o. QID x 10 days
				  −Amoxicillin 500 mg p.o. TID x 10 days
				• Use of antibiotics effective against beta-lactamase-producing organisms may be necessary because of ↑ incidence of beta lactamase producing *H. influenzae* (15%-30% of strains) including:
				  −Amoxicillin and clavulanic acid 250 mg-500 mg p.o. TID x 10 days
				  −Trimethoprim (160 mg)/ Sulfamethoxazole (800 mg) (TMP/SMX DS) p.o. BID x 10 days

Moraxella catarrhalis (*M. catarrhalis*)	↑ incidence in COPD, malnourished or immune-deficient patients; seasonal variation noted (↑ October-May).	↑ COPD symptoms, ↑ cough, ↑ SOB, ↑ sputum production, malaise, pleuritic pain, chills.	• CBC: ↑ WBC
			• Gm. stain: ↑ PMNs, large kidney-bean-shaped gm—diplococci
			• Cultures: difficult to isolate organism from blood or pleural fluid. Organism is commonly isolated from lower respiratory tract secretions of COPD patients.
			• Chest x-ray: patchy infiltrate of single lobe; possible consolidation; pleural effusion (rare)
				• Reports indicate 80% to 90% of *catarrhalis* strains are beta-lactamase-producing, therefore antibiotic therapy should use agents effective against such strains including:
				  −Amoxicillin and clavulanic acid 500 mg p.o. TID x 10 days
				  −TMP/SMX DS 1 tablet p.o. BID x 10 days
				  −Ciprofloxacin 500 mg p.o. BID x 10 days
				  −Erythromycin 500 mg p.o. QID x 10 days
				  −Tetracycline 500 mg p.o. QID x 10 days
				• Hospitalization of patients may be necessary.

Legionella pneumophila (*L. pneumophila*, Legionnaires' disease)	↑ risk in COPD, smoking patients exposed to contaminated water sources.	Mild → severe fulminant disease, may have multi-organ involvement. Minimal cough producing blood-tinged mucus, malaise, myalgia, nausea, vomiting, diarrhea, ↑ fever (>40°C/104°F), headache, change in mental status, ataxia.	• CBC: ↑ WBC- ↓ Hct/Hgb ↓ platelets • Serum transaminase levels: ↑ • Serum sodium: ↓ (<130 mEq/L) • Gram stain: ↑ neutrophils few if any organisms	• Hospitalization of patients is necessary for initiation of parenteral erythromycin therapy followed by outpatient oral therapy for 21 days. • Prevention includes disinfection of water and soil contaminated with organism.

Continued

Table 5J.1. **CLINICAL MANIFESTATIONS AND TREATMENT OF SELECTED PNEUMONIAS** CONTINUED

Pathogen	Predisposing Factors	Symptoms	Diagnostic Tests	Treatment
			• Sputum cultures: + in 70% of patients; need special medium-charcoal yeast extract or CVE medium. • Chest x-ray: unilateral alveolar infiltrate; often cannot differentiate from other types of pneumonia • Serology: acute and convalescent antibody titers ↑ to 1:128 (diagnostic but requires 4-8 weeks)	
Mycoplasma pneumoniae (*M. pneumoniae*)	↑ incidence in school-age children, young adults, military recruits, individuals living in close quarters. ↑ incidence in summer and fall.	Gradual onset of symptoms including headache, malaise, low-grade fever, sore throat, sinusitis symptoms, enlarged cervical nodes, ear pain. Protracted, non-productive cough (90% to 100% of patients).	• CBC: ↓ Hct/Hgb (2° to cold agglutin production); seen in patients with ↑ IgM titers. • Complement fixation titer: will demonstrate a fourfold ↑ titer. • Gram stain: ↑ PMNs and monocytes, no bacteria • Cold agglutin titers: results ≥ 1:64 are suggestive of *M. pneumoniae* (usually become positive 7 days after infection; peak at 4 weeks after infection)	• Majority of patients recover from *M. pneumoniae* pneumonia within 2 to 6 weeks even without treatment. • Antibiotic therapy may reduce the duration of symptoms but prolonged therapy (2 to 3 weeks) is usually indicated including: —Erythromycin 250 mg-500 mg p.o. QID x 14 to 21 days —Tetracycline 250 mg-500 mg p.o. QID x 14 to 21 days
Chlamydia pneumoniae (TWAR)	10% of pneumonia cases; ↑ incidence in adolescence through early adulthood (up to 40s)	Fever, sore throat, laryngitis, severe pharyngitis (up to 50% patients with TWAR), sinusitis symptoms, cough with minimal production of mucus.	Diagnosis of TWAR pneumonia is difficult but the following tests may be helpful: • Complement fixation tests (nonspecific): will demonstrate ↑ titers to *Chlamydia* species but not specific to TWAR strain. • Micro-immunoflourescence antibodies (MIF): specific for TWAR —IgM + from 3 weeks to 2 to 6 months after onset of illness —IgG titer will demonstrate a fourfold ↑ ≥ 1:512 compared to acute titer (Do not obtain convalescent titer until 3 weeks after illness). • Gram stain: nonspecific • Chest x-ray: segmental infiltration, consolidation rarely noted.	• Personal hygiene measures to ↓ exposure • Antibiotic therapy including: —Tetracycline 500 mg p.o. QID x 14 days —Erythromycin 500 mg p.o. QID x 14 days
Viral (adenovirus, parainfluenza, RSV, influenza types A and B)	↑ incidence in persons with pulmonary or cardiac disease.	Usually associated with abrupt onset of fever, upper respiratory symptoms, nausea, diarrhea, possibly viral exanthem (if measles or varicella virus).	• CBC: may demonstrate ↑ WBC • Cultures (throat, sputum): may be + in symptomatic patients but results depend on collection and transport of specimens. • Serology: fourfold rise between acute and convalescent titer for particular viral pathogen. • Chest x-ray: similar findings noted with bacterial pneumonias.	• Symptomatic treatment • If influenza type A virus suspected may consider Amantadine therapy (see **Influenza** Protocol). • Antibiotic therapy has not been proven efficacious unless superimposed bacterial infection is suspected or documented through sputum culture.

Source: Adapted with permission from Stauffer, J.L. 1993. Pulmonary Diseases. In *Current medical diagnosis and treatment*, 32 ed., eds. Tierney, Jr., L.M.; McPhee, S.J., Papadakis, M.A., and Schroeder, S.A., pp. 208-209. Norwalk, CT: Appleton & Lange.

DATABASE

SUBJECTIVE

→ Patient may be elderly.

→ Patient may have a history of:
- cigarette smoking.
- COPD.
- splenectomy.
- chronic illness(es): diabetes mellitus, chronic liver or kidney disease, neoplasm, cardiac disease.
- substance abuse (e.g., alcohol, injection drug use).
- immune deficiency.
- malnutrition.
- recent URI, influenza, or viral exanthem (e.g., measles, varicella).
- recent hospitalization.

→ The symptoms, and their intensity, will vary depending upon the pathogen causing the pneumonia, as well as the patient's baseline health status.

Bacterial pneumonia (Griffith and Mazurek 1991; Littler and Momany 1990; Musher 1991; Stauffer 1994)
- Symptoms may include:
  - fever often > 38°C/100.4°F (especially in patients with pneumococcal pneumonia).
  - cough producing copious amounts of thick, purulent, and/or blood-tinged mucus.
  - chills.
  - chest pain.
  - dyspnea.
  - malaise.
  - headache (rare).
  - myalgia.
  - change in mental status (often noted in *L. pneumophila*).
  - nausea, vomiting, diarrhea (usually in association with *L. pneumophila*).
- Patients with COPD may report less significant symptoms and note only a gradual increased intensity of shortness of breath (SOB), increased cough, and, possibly, a low-grade temperature.
- Elderly patients often present with a minimal cough (usually nonproductive), dehydration, mental status changes, and no fever (Fein, Feinsilver, and Niederman 1991).

Viral pneumonia

→ The symptoms associated with viral pneumonia are similar to those noted by patients with bacterial pneumonias. However, the following symptoms may be reported as a result of the patient's underlying viral illness (Greenberg 1991):
- history of a viral exanthem that may indicate recent measles or varicella zoster virus infection (see **Measles [Rubeola]** and **Varicella Zoster Virus** protocols).
- history of symptoms that may indicate recent influenza infection including:
  - fever.
  - nausea.
  - vomiting.
  - myalgias.
  - malaise.
  - arthralgias.
  - headache.

Atypical pneumonia

→ The patient with *M. pneumoniae* or *C. pneumoniae* (TWAR) pneumonia may report a gradual onset of the following symptoms (Martin and Bates 1991):
- headache.
- malaise.
- low-grade fever.
- sore throat.
- enlarged cervical glands (if *M. pneumoniae*).
- persistent, nonproductive cough (especially if *M. pneumoniae*).
- chest muscle discomfort (not pleuritic pain).
- symptoms associated with sinusitis (see **Sinusitis—Acute** Protocol).
- CNS symptoms including stiff neck, problems with coordination, and diminished hearing (may occur in up to seven percent of patients with *M. pneumoniae* pneumonia).

OBJECTIVE

→ The following physical findings may be noted in patients with pneumonia (Griffith and Mazurek 1991; Littler and Momany 1990; Musher 1991; Stauffer 1994):
- may appear anxious, apprehensive, or confused, depending on level of hypoxia.
- vital signs.
  - Temperature may be elevated, normal, or decreased (usually noted in elderly patients).
  - Blood pressure may be normal or decreased in patients with shock (secondary to bacteremia/sepsis) or dehydration.
  - Pulse may be elevated (> 90 beats/minute).

- Respiratory rate may be normal or patient may be tachypnic or orthopnic.
- skin.
  - Color may be normal or grayish to cyanotic, depending on the patient's oxygen perfusion.
  - Poor tissue turgor may be evident if the patient is dehydrated.
  - Rash of viral exanthem may be evident in patients with a concomitant viral infection.
- examination of the chest may reveal diminished excursion of the thorax secondary to pain.
- palpation of the chest wall may reveal tenderness to palpation of intercostal muscles. Increased tactile fremitus may be noted in area(s) of consolidation.
- percussion of chest may reveal:
  - decreased diaphragmatic excursion on affected side if pleural fluid accumulation at the lung bases.
  - dullness in area(s) of consolidation.
- auscultation of the lungs may reveal:
  - presence of crackles.
  - presence of bronchial or tubular breath sounds (if consolidation).
  - presence of a pleural friction rub if pleural effusion.
  - diminished or absent vesicular breath sounds if pleural effusion.
  - increased bronchophony, egophony, and whispered pectoriloquy if consolidation or pleural effusion.
- auscultation of the heart may reveal a systolic murmur if endocarditis is present.
- neurological examination may reveal nuchal rigidity and/or altered mentation if CNS involvement.

ASSESSMENT

- → Pneumonia (bacterial, viral, atypical)
- → R/O bacteremia
- → R/O meningitis
- → R/O cardiac disease (e.g., congestive heart failure)
- → R/O COPD
- → R/O influenza infection
- → R/O tuberculosis
- → R/O adult respiratory distress syndrome
- → R/O pulmonary embolism and infarction

- → R/O neoplasm
- → R/O immune deficiency

PLAN

DIAGNOSTIC TESTS

- → A number of the following diagnostic tests may be ordered to determine the etiology of the patient's illness:
  - CBC.
    - Bacterial pneumonias (especially *S. pneumoniae*) will usually result in a leukocytosis (WBC count > 13,000 cells/mm^3) with a left shift present. However, up to 25 percent of patients may have a WBC count within normal limits (Musher 1991).
    - Hematocrit/hemoglobin (Hct/Hgb) may be decreased if hemolytic anemia associated with *M. pneumoniae* or *L. pneumophila* infections or other medical conditions (e.g., significant malnutrition, chronic alcohol abuse) (Martin and Bates 1991; Nguyen, Stout, and Yu 1991).
    - Decreased platelets may be noted when *L. pneumophila* infection (Nguyen, Stout, and Yu 1991).
  - serum chemistry panel may reveal elevated transaminases (alanine aminotransferase [ALT], aspartate aminotransferase [AST]) and decreased serum sodium (< 130mEq/L) in *L. pneumophila* infection (Nguyen, Stout, and Yu 1991).
  - increased serum bilirubin (> 3-4 mg/dL) and lactate dehydrogenase (LDH) (> 250 U/L) is often noted in *S. pneumoniae* infection (Musher 1991).
  - gram stain of sputum may reveal the organism if an adequate specimen is obtained.
    - A reliable sputum specimen must contain >25 *polymorphonuclear* cells (PMNs)/field and <10 squamous epithelial cells on low magnification to minimize the possibility of contamination from upper airway organisms (Hampson, Woolf, and Springmeyer 1991; Stauffer 1994).
  - specimens for culture.
    - Sputum culture to identify a specific organism may be positive if adequate specimen has been obtained.
      - If the patient is unable to produce an adequate specimen, sputum induction may be necessary.

- In patients presenting with significant symptoms, blood or pleural fluid specimens should be obtained for culture.
  - A positive culture result is considered diagnostic for the causative organism (e.g., *S. pneumoniae, H. influenzae,* influenza virus type A) (Stauffer 1994).
  - Cultures from urine and stool specimens may be obtained to identify possible pathogens (e.g., *cytomegalovirus* [CMV]).
- chest x-rays may demonstrate local or diffuse changes including infiltration, consolidation, pleural effusion, and abscess formation (the last, rarely).
  - In patients with COPD, chest x-ray findings may be subtle and may be considered indicative only of chronic lung disease (Griffith and Mazurek 1991).
- serum antibody titer(s).
  - Acute and convalescent serum antibody titers for viral pathogen, when suspected, may demonstrate a fourfold rise in titer indicating recent infection (e.g., CMV, herpes simplex virus [HSV], measles. See specific viral infection protocols).
  - IgM titer rise may indicate acute infection with viral pathogen (see specific viral infection protocols).
  - Cold agglutin titer ≥ 1:64 is suggestive of *M. pneumoniae* infection (50 percent of patients with *M. pneumoniae* infection will demonstrate such a rise in titer) (Martin and Bates 1991).

TREATMENT/MANAGEMENT

→ Patients with moderate to severe symptoms, with underlying medical conditions which may impair immune response (e.g., the elderly, or patients with chronic medical conditions, neutropenia, immune deficiency), or in whom a particularly virulent organism is suspected, should be hospitalized for parenteral therapy.

→ In a *healthy* adult patient with uncomplicated community-acquired pneumonia, outpatient therapy is possible. Empiric antibiotic treatment for suspected bacterial pneumonia includes the following (Stauffer 1994):
- *S. pneumoniae* infection:
  - penicillin G (Pentids®) or V (Pen Vee K®) 250 mg-500 mg p.o. QID for 7 to 10 days.
- *M. pneumoniae* infection:

  - erythromycin (E-Mycin®, Ery-Tab®) 250 mg-500 mg p.o. QID for 10 to 14 days.
- *M. catarrhalis* infection:
  - amoxicillin—clavulanic acid (Augmentin®) 250 mg-500 mg p.o. TID for 10 to 14 days.

→ If influenza virus type A infection is suspected because of evidence of an epidemic in the community, consider amantadine (Amantadine®, Symmetrel®) therapy (see **Influenza** Protocol).

→ Symptomatic treatment includes rest, increased fluid intake, adequate nutrition, use of antipyretics (e.g., acetaminophen), as needed.

→ If the patient smokes, she should be advised to stop to prevent exacerbation of symptoms and further damage to her lung tissue.
- If the patient does not smoke but lives in an environment in which she is exposed to secondary smoke, she should be advised to limit her exposure as much as possible.

→ Prevention strategies include immunization of individuals recommended to receive pneumococcal and influenza vaccinations.
- Pneumococcal vaccination is recommended for individuals at risk of pneumococcal disease and its complications including:
  - immune-competent individuals with chronic illnesses (e.g., diabetes mellitus, cardio-vascular disease, pulmonary disease, alcoholism, cirrhosis, or cerebrospinal fluid leaks).
  - individuals 65 years old and older.
  - immunocompromised adults (e.g., individuals with chronic renal failure, nephrotic syndrome, splenic dysfunction or anatomic asplenia, Hodgkin's disease, lymphoma, multiple myeloma, or conditions such as organ transplantation).
  - adults with HIV infection (both asymptomatic and symptomatic).
  - individuals living in environments or social settings with an identified increased risk of pneumococcal disease and its complications (e.g., members of certain Native American tribes) (CDC 1991).
- Administration of pneumococcal vaccine will afford protection against 23 strains of *S. pneumoniae* reportedly responsible for 88 percent of bacteremic pneumococcal disease.
  - Duration of immunity is unknown but has been documented in healthy adults for up to five years.

- Efficacy of pneumococcal vaccination in preventing pneumococcal bacteremia has been documented to range from 61 percent to 81 percent and is apparently related to the immune status of the patient, with higher efficacy rates noted in immune-competent individuals (CDC 1991).
  - Immunization, prior to discharge, of hospitalized patients who are considered at risk of pneumococcal disease and its complications should be considered.
    - This is because over 60 percent of patients with significant pneumococcal disease have a history of hospitalization within a 5-year period before the episode of pneumococcal disease (CDC 1991).
  - Influenza vaccination should be administered annually to individuals at risk of complications associated with this infection, as well as individuals who are care givers or have close household contact with persons at risk of complications of influenza infection (see **Influenza** Protocol).

NOTE: Pneumococcal vaccines and influenza vaccines reportedly can be given at the same time at different sites without an increase in side effects (CDC 1991).

CONSULTATION

→ Physician consultation is warranted in any patient with:
  - a history of complications of pneumonia (e.g., respiratory distress, CNS involvement, abscess).
  - an underlying medical condition which may impair immune response.
  - a poor response to initial therapy.

→ As needed for prescription(s).

PATIENT EDUCATION

→ If the patient's condition requires hospitalization for treatment, the physician responsible for the patient's care should discuss the treatment options and need for hospitalization with the patient.

→ Educate the patient about pneumonia—the causes, clinical course, diagnostic tests indicated, treatment options, possible complications, and need for follow-up.

→ Educate the patient regarding signs and symptoms of possible complications associated with pneumonia, and the need for medical evaluation if any occur.

→ Educate the patient about the need for compliance with treatment regimens to facilitate resolution of the pneumonia.

→ If the patient smokes, advise the patient to stop and provide her with information regarding smoking cessation programs and available community resources. See **Smoking Cessation** Protocol.

→ Educate the patient about the need for any immunizations as indicated (e.g., influenza, pneumococcal).

FOLLOW-UP

→ If the patient is hospitalized, follow-up visits should be as recommended by the physician responsible for her care.

→ Follow-up evaluation of any patient is indicated when there are persistent symptoms after initiation of appropriate therapy, in patients who may not be compliant with treatment regimens, or with patients who develop symptoms of complications.

→ Document in progress notes and problem list.

5-K

Rhinitis

Rhinitis is an inflammation of the nasal mucosa resulting in congestion and rhinorrhea. There are several causes of rhinitis including viral infection and allergic and vasomotor responses. Although many of the clinical manifestations of the various types of rhinitis are similar, there are differences in the clinical presentations that can help determine the type and indicated therapy for each.

Viral Rhinitis (common cold)

Viral rhinitis is an infection of the upper respiratory tract which can be caused by more than 200 different serological types of viruses. The most common types of viruses associated with rhinitis include *rhinovirus* (cause of 30 percent to 50 percent of colds), coronavirus, adenovirus, parainfluenza virus, respiratory syncytial virus, and influenza types A, B, and C (Rabinowitz 1990).

These viruses are transmitted by direct or close contact, entering the body via the ciliated epithelium of the nose. Exposure of ciliated epithelium to the virus causes edema and hyperemia of the nasal mucosa, resulting in increased secretion of the mucous glands responsible for the production of both serous and mucinous fluid.

The nasal obstructive symptoms that are associated with viral rhinitis are caused by the narrowing of the nasal passages, which, in turn, results from the edema of the mucous membranes (Jackler and Kaplan 1994; Rabinowitz 1990).

Although viral rhinitis is considered to be a benign infection, in the United States it is the leading cause of visits to health care providers (Jackler and Kaplan 1994; Rabinowitz 1990). On the average, adults experience two to four colds annually, while preschool children have a reported annual frequency of six to ten colds.

Susceptibility to viruses associated with the common cold varies, though there is an increased incidence during the fall, winter, and spring. The incubation period for most of the causative viruses is one to six days. The course of the infection is usually self-limited, with acute symptoms lasting up to seven days.

Complications associated with viral rhinitis are uncommon, with the majority of complications resulting from secondary bacterial infections. These include acute otitis media (2 percent of cases), acute sinusitis (0.5 percent of cases), and pneumonia (usually occurring in high-risk populations already infected with influenza virus) (Jackler and Kaplan 1994; Rabinowitz 1990).

Allergic Rhinitis

Allergic rhinitis is a chronic, recurrent inflammation of the mucous membranes of the nose, resulting in nasal congestion and discharge. It affects approximately 10 percent of Americans (Vogt 1990). Allergic rhinitis often occurs seasonally or perennially and is the result of an antigen-specific IgE response by the nasal mucosa, usually to an inhaled allergen (Vogt 1990).

The seasonal variation of symptoms can provide information about the type of allergen causing an individual's symptoms. Common allergens responsible for allergic rhinitis symptoms include grass (symptoms usually noted during summer), pollens (symptoms usually noted during spring), ragweed (symptoms usually noted during fall), and animal dander and dust (symptoms noted throughout the year) (Jackler and Kaplan 1994; Naclerio 1991).

Vasomotor Rhinitis

Vasomotor rhinitis is a nasal mucous membrane inflammation not associated with infection or allergy. Though its etiology is unknown, an autonomic imbalance resulting in vasodilatation, nasal congestion, and increased mucous secretion is one theory proposed (Vogt 1990).

Precipitating factors associated with vasomotor rhinitis include emotional stress, environmental factors (e.g., toxins, smoke), exercise, and recumbency. Rhinitis observed during pregnancy and in hypothyroid patients also is thought to be due to this vasomotor response (Vogt 1990).

DATABASE

SUBJECTIVE

Viral Rhinitis

→ Patient may report recent exposure to a person with viral rhinitis symptoms.

→ Patient may report one or more of the following symptoms:
  - nasal congestion.
  - sneezing.
  - rhinorrhea—usually watery but may be purulent if secondary bacterial infection.
  - "scratchy" sore throat.
  - nonproductive cough.
  - headaches.
  - low-grade fever.
  - malaise.
  - myalgia.
  - hoarseness.
  - lymphadenopathy.

Allergic Rhinitis

→ Patient may report history of one or more of the following:
  - asthma.
  - eczema.
  - other allergic reactions (e.g., urticaria).
  - nasal polyps.

→ Patient may report one or more of the following symptoms, usually in a seasonal or perennial pattern:
  - rhinorrhea:
    • usually watery.
  - sneezing:
    • usually in the morning.
  - recurrent nasal obstruction.
  - lacrimation.
  - itching of eyes, nose, and oropharynx.

- frequent sore throats:
  • usually secondary to nasopharyngeal dryness from mouth breathing.
- recurrent/persistent, nonproductive cough.
- frequent clearing of throat.
- halitosis.
- snorting (to attempt to clear nasal passages).

Vasomotor Rhinitis

→ Recent history may include:
  - emotional stress.
  - exercise.
  - exposure to smoke, odors, noxious fumes, and other environmental toxins.
  - recumbency.

→ Patient may report one or more of the following symptoms:
  - nasal congestion:
    • may be unilateral or bilateral, may alternate sides of nose.
  - rhinorrhea may or may not be reported.

OBJECTIVE

(Jackler and Kaplan 1994; Rabinowitz 1990; Vogt 1990)

Viral Rhinitis

→ Physical examination will reveal one or more of the following:
  - vital signs usually within normal limits (WNL), although a low-grade temperature may be observed.
  - erythema, edema of nasal mucosa.
  - nasal discharge:
    • may be thin and watery or thick and purulent.
  - mild erythema, edema of pharyngeal mucous membranes.
  - enlarged tonsillar and/or cervical lymph nodes may be palpated.
  - auscultation of lungs WNL.

Allergic Rhinitis

→ Physical examination may reveal one or more of the following:
  - edema of eyelids.
  - conjunctival erythema.
  - lacrimation.
  - bluish discoloration of the infraorbital area.
  - transverse crease of the nose.
  - pale, bluish discoloration of the nasal turbinates.
  - edema of nasal mucosa.
  - nasal discharge:
    • usually clear, thin, and watery.

- may be yellow in appearance (due to increased eosinophils).
- nasal polyps.
- gingival hypertrophy, halitosis, and/or enlarged adenoid or tonsillar lymphoid tissue (signs of chronic mouth breathing).

Vasomotor Rhinitis

→ Physical examination may reveal one or more of the following:
- nasal turbinate edema.
- nasal mucosa bluish to dark red in color.
- thin, clear nasal discharge.

ASSESSMENT

→ Rhinitis—viral, allergic, vasomotor

→ R/O influenza

→ R/O sinusitis

→ R/O otitis media, serous otitis

→ R/O nasal polyposis

→ R/O drug-induced rhinitis

→ R/O pneumonia

→ R/O eosinophilic non-allergic rhinitis

PLAN

DIAGNOSTIC TESTS

Viral Rhinitis

→ No specific diagnostic tests are indicated in cases of viral rhinitis.
- If secondary bacterial complications are suspected, then tests indicated for the diagnosis of such conditions may be ordered (see **Sinusitis—Acute, Sinusitis—Chronic,** and **Pneumonia** protocols).

Allergic Rhinitis

→ Specific diagnostic tests for allergic rhinitis should be ordered only as clinically indicated by the frequency and severity of a patient's symptoms.
- Tests may include:
  - WBC count and differential.
    - Increased eosinophils may be noted. However, absence of absolute eosinophilia does not rule out the presence of allergic rhinitis.
  - serum IgE levels—may be elevated, but are of limited usefulness because of a lack of sensitivity and specificity.

- smear of nasal secretions—can be air dried and prepared with Giemsa or Hansel's stain to demonstrate eosinophilia.
  - In acute allergic rhinitis, 10 percent to 100 percent eosinophils may be observed.
- allergy testing.
  - Various types of allergy tests are available including the prick test, the scratch test, intradermal testing, and in vitro tests.
  - These tests are done to determine the presence or absence of allergen-specific IgE antibodies.
  - These tests are not routinely done on all patients with allergic rhinitis. They must be used only according to a patient's severity of symptoms and history of allergy.
  - Patient referral to an allergist is indicated when such testing is being considered because of the cost, indicated treatment and follow-up, and possibility of anaphylaxis in some patients undergoing testing and treatment.

Vasomotor Rhinitis

→ No specific diagnostic testing is indicated for vasomotor rhinitis. (If allergy testing is done, the results will be negative.)

TREATMENT/MANAGEMENT

Viral Rhinitis

→ No specific treatment has been found effective in shortening or eliminating symptoms of the common cold.
- Prescribing antibiotics is unnecessary since they are ineffective in the treatment of the condition and will not prevent the development of associated complications.
- Antibiotics should be prescribed for patients who develop secondary bacterial infections (e.g., sinusitis, pneumonia).

→ Symptomatic treatment with simple home remedies should be recommended and includes:
- increased rest (especially if the patient is febrile).
- increased fluid intake (especially warm liquids).
- use of a steam vaporizer to help liquify secretions. **NOTE:** Warn patients about placement of steam vaporizers in hazardous areas where small children or other household members could be harmed if the steaming liquid is spilled.

■ use of acetaminophen every 4 to 6 hours as needed to reduce fever and alleviate generalized discomfort.
  NOTE: Aspirin should not be used because it may increase viral shedding, and in children and adolescents should be avoided because of the risk of Reye's syndrome.

→ There may be some relief of nasal congestion and sneezing with the use of systemic antihistamines.
  ■ Many OTC products with chlorpheniramine (an effective agent to relieve these symptoms) as their active ingredient are available.
    • The dose of chlorpheniramine (Chlor-Trimeton®) is 4 mg to 8 mg p.o. BID or TID (maximum daily dose ≤ 24 mg); or sustained release chlorpheniramine 8 mg to 12 mg p.o. once at bedtime or every 8 hours (maximum daily dose ≤ 24 mg).
    • Diphenhydramine (Benadryl®) is another common OTC antihistamine that can be used in a dose of 25 mg-50 mg p.o. TID or QID (maximum daily dose ≤ 300 mg).
    NOTE: Warn the patient of CNS effects associated with systemic antihistamines (e.g., drowsiness, dizziness).

→ Systemic decongestants also may reduce nasal congestion and sneezing.
  ■ Several OTC preparations, containing pseudoephedrine as their active ingredient, are available.
    • The dose of short-acting pseudoephedrine (Sudafed®) is 30 mg-60 mg p.o. every 4 to 6 hours (maximum daily dose ≤ 240 mg).
    • The dose of sustained-released pseudo-ephedrine is 120 mg every 12 hours (maximum daily dose ≤ 240 mg).
    NOTE: Patients with severe hypertension, heart disease, seizure disorders, hyper-thyroidism, or those taking monoamine oxidase (MAO) inhibitor medications should not be given preparations containing pseudo-ephedrine (Naclerio 1991). Consult *PDR* and clinical pharmacist as indicated for additional information.

→ In elderly patients, use short-acting systemic antihistamine or decongestant preparations prior to recommending sustained-release products. An increased sensitivity to CNS side effects has been noted in elderly patients (Ellsworth et al. 1991).

→ Antitussive preparations containing dextro-methorphan may help diminish the frequency of coughing episodes.

■ The usual dose for dextromethorphan is 10 mg-20 mg p.o. every 4 hours prn (maximum daily dose ≤ 120 mg).

→ Although expectorants (e.g., guaifenesin) often are recommended for the treatment of cold symptoms, they have not been shown to be any more effective than a placebo (Rabinowitz 1990).

→ Though topical decongestant sprays often provide patients with a sense of improved nasal patency, their use must be monitored carefully and be limited to 3 to 5 days to prevent rebound nasal hyperemia and tachyphylaxis (Ellsworth et al. 1991; Jackler and Kaplan 1994; Rabinowitz 1990).
  ■ Common OTC topical nasal decongestants include:
    • phenylephrine (Neosynephrine®, Nostril®, Sinex®) 0.125%-1.0% solutions. Apply 1 to 2 intranasal sprays every 4 hours prn (begin with ≤ 0.25% solutions).
    NOTE: Precautions and contraindications similar to those applying to the use of pseudoephedrine products apply also to the use of phenylephrine (see ''Treatment/Management'' section, ''Viral Rhinitis'') (Naclerio 1991).
    • oxymetazoline (Afrin®, Allerest 12 Hour®) 0.025% solution. Apply 2-3 intranasal sprays BID prn; or 0.05% solution, apply 2-3 drops BID prn.

→ If influenza type A is suspected because of a community epidemic and the patient is being seen within 48 hours of symptom onset, consider initiating amantadine therapy to shorten the symptomatic phase of the illness (see **Influenza** Protocol for indications for amantadine therapy).

Allergic Rhinitis

→ Maintaining an allergen-free environment is essential. The following steps may help reduce symptoms:
  ■ removal of dust-collecting household fixtures (e.g., drapes, carpets).
  ■ substitution of synthetic materials for animal products (e.g., wool).
  ■ covering mattresses, pillows, and cushions with plastic covers.

→ The use of an air purifier may help decrease allergen exposure.

→ The use of systemic antihistamines and decongestants may help reduce symptoms. Because they reduce allergic mechanisms, antihistamines are usually more effective than decongestants in relieving symptoms. See "Viral Rhinitis" for dosages and possible side effects.

→ Non-sedating antihistamines are preferable for patients unable to tolerate the CNS side effects associated with OTC antihistamine products. However, the former are available only by prescription and are more costly than OTC preparations.

■ Non-sedating antihistamine products include:
  • astemizole (Hismanal®) 10 mg p.o. every day or every other day.
    NOTE: Astemizole should be taken on an empty stomach.
  • terfenadine (Seldane®) 60 mg p.o. BID.
    NOTE: Terfenadine should not be taken with either erythromycin or ketoconazole because it can cause heart arrhythmias when used in conjunction with these medications.

→ Intranasal steroid sprays often are helpful. But patients need to be advised that improvement of symptoms may not be noted until after 2 weeks of proper use.

■ Intranasal steroid sprays include:
  • beclamethasone (Vancenase®, Beconase®) 2 intranasal sprays per nostril BID for 30 days.
    NOTE: Potential side effect is epistaxis (Ellsworth et al. 1991).
  • flunisolide (Nasalide®) 2 intranasal sprays per nostril BID–TID. Maximum dose = 8 sprays per nostril a day.
    NOTE: Potential side effects include nasal dryness, irritation, or stinging (Ellsworth et al. 1991).
  • intranasal cromolyn (Nasalcrom®) 4% spray, 2 intranasal sprays BID prior to exposure to allergen.

→ The use of systemic corticosteroids for allergic rhinitis is rarely necessary and if indicated should be done in consultation with a physician.

→ Immunotherapy (e.g., desensitization or hyposensitization) of patients with severe symptoms should be managed by an allergist.

Vasomotor Rhinitis

→ Whenever possible, avoiding precipitating factors will help reduce the symptoms associated with vasomotor rhinitis.

→ Symptomatic treatment of this condition may include the use of oral antihistamines and/or decongestants (see "Viral Rhinitis" section).

→ Intranasal saline drops may relieve symptoms in patients with nasal congestion. The usual dose is 2 drops in each nostril TID–QID.

CONSULTATION

→ As necessary, depending upon the severity of the patient's symptoms, evidence of complications (e.g., sinusitis, pneumonia with viral rhinitis), or the need for referral to a specialist (e.g., allergist) for additional diagnostic testing and/or treatment.

→ As needed for prescription(s).

PATIENT EDUCATION

→ Educate the patient about rhinitis (viral, allergic, vasomotor)—the cause(s), clinical course, treatment options, any potential side effects associated with medications, possible complications, preventive measures, and any indicated follow-up (see specific sections of protocol for all these educational components).

FOLLOW-UP

→ Follow-up evaluations usually are not indicated in most patients unless severe symptoms or complications develop. If a patient was referred to a physician for further diagnostic testing and/or treatment, then follow-up is per recommendation of the consulting physician.

→ Document in progress notes and problem list.

5-L

Sinusitis—Acute

Acute sinusitis is an infection of the mucosa of the paranasal sinuses which results from a combination of factors including edema of the nasal mucosa, causing narrowing of the sinus ostia; decreased (sinus) ciliary transport of mucous secretions; overprotection of mucous secretions; and a reduction in oxygen tension, which, in turn, promotes the growth of certain pathogens (Godley 1992; Herr 1991; Slavin 1988a; Slavin 1988b). Because the paranasal sinuses directly communicate with a nonsterile cavity, infection is a component of acute sinusitis.

In adults, the most common organisms associated with acute sinusitis are *S. pneumoniae, H. influenzae, S. aureus*, respiratory viruses, various anaerobes, and *M. catarrhalis (Branhamella catarrhalis)* (Herr 1991). It is estimated that 25 percent of sinusitis is caused by beta-lactamase-producing organisms that are resistant to standard antibiotic therapy (Loch, Alleva, and Paparella 1990).

Viral pathogens such as rhinovirus and influenza and parainfluenza viruses have been observed in 15 percent to 30 percent of studies investigating sinusitis, and fungi such as *Aspergillus* and *Candida albicans* have also been identified as etiologic pathogens (Loch, Alleva, and Paparella 1990).

Cellulitis, meningitis, abscess formation, subdural empyema, osteomyelitis, and cavernous sinus thrombosis are possible complications associated with untreated or inadequately treated acute sinusitis (Herr 1991).

DATABASE

SUBJECTIVE

→ Predisposing factors may include (Godley 1992; Herr 1991; Slavin 1988a):

- allergic rhinitis.
- URI.
- asthma.
- deviated nasal septum.
- environmental irritants.
- excessive topical decongestant use.
- nasal polyps, tumors, or foreign bodies.
- hypertrophied adenoids.
- swimming/diving.
- barotrauma.
- dental infection.
- nasal surgical packing.
- cystic fibrosis.
- bronchiectasis.
- immobile cilia syndrome.
- immune deficiency.

→ Symptoms may include (Godley 1992; Herr 1991; Slavin 1988a):

- fever (may not be documented in up to 65 percent of patients).
- chills (may not be documented in up to 65 percent of patients).
- headache.
- facial pain or facial fullness which is aggravated by coughing, straining, a head-down position, or an acute change in barometric pressure.
- malaise.
- nasal discharge (may be clear, mucoid, or purulent).
- post-nasal discharge.
- photophobia.
- anorexia.
- symptoms of an URI persisting beyond 10 days.

- chronic morning cough.
- halitosis.

OBJECTIVE

(Godley 1992; Herr 1991)

→ Patient may present with:
- temperature of 39°C/102.2°F or above (may not be documented in up to 65 percent of patients).
- discharge in the nasal meatus which may be thin or thick, clear, mucoid, or purulent.
- discharge observed in the posterior pharynx.
- tenderness to palpation over the frontal, periorbital, or subzygomatic regions of the head.
- conjunctivitis.
- edema of eyelid(s) and/or medial canthus.

→ Transillumination for frontal and maxillary opacification can be performed but generally is regarded as unreliable.

ASSESSMENT

→ Acute sinusitis

→ R/O chronic sinusitis

→ R/O allergy (allergic rhinitis, asthma)

→ R/O nasal obstruction (tumor, polyp, deviated septum, foreign body)

→ R/O dental infection

→ R/O overuse of topical nasal decongestants

→ R/O immobile cilia syndrome

PLAN

DIAGNOSTIC TESTS

→ Gram stain of nasal smear may reveal eosinophils or neutrophils, differentiating an allergic condition from an infectious rhinorrhea, and should be considered prior to initiating antibiotic therapy.

→ Sinus x-ray series may demonstrate air-fluid levels, mucosal thickening of 5 mm, or opacification of an infected sinus and will confirm the diagnosis of acute sinusitis.

→ Computerized tomography (CT) scan findings of thickened mucosa within the sinuses and stenosis of anatomic structures.
- CT scans are recommended in patients who are not responding appropriately to antibiotic therapy for acute sinusitis, to rule out spread of infection to the brain.
- If possible, the patient should be on antibiotics for 3 weeks prior to the scan.

- This will help reduce tissue edema and facilitate better visualization of the area during the scan.

→ Maxillary antrum aspiration for culture and sensitivity should be reserved only for patients failing antibiotic therapy, in patients with immunodeficiency (e.g., HIV-positive patients, patients with diabetes mellitus), or in patients with nosocomial infections.
- Patients requiring this procedure should be referred to an otolaryngologist.

TREATMENT/MANAGEMENT

→ Initiate antibiotic therapy (in patients without a history of penicillin allergy) with one of the following (Herr 1991; Jackler and Kaplan 1994):
- amoxicillin (Amoxil®, Trimox®) 500 mg p.o. TID for 10 to 14 days. First choice because it provides better sinus penetration than ampicillin.
- amoxicillin-clavulanate potassium (Augmentin®) 500 mg p.o. TID for 10 to 14 days (if beta-lactamase-positive organisms are suspected).

→ If the patient is allergic to penicillin, therapy can be initiated with one of the following (Littler and Momany 1990):
- trimethoprim/sulfamethoxazole (Bactrim®, Septra®) one double-strength (DS) tablet p.o. every 12 hours for 14 days.
- erythromycin (E-Mycin®, Ery Tab®) 250 mg-500 mg p.o. QID for 14 days.

→ If, after 72 hours, the patient is unresponsive to initial antibiotic therapy, then one of the following antimicrobials should be used:
- trimethoprim/sulfamethoxazole (Bactrim®, Septra®) one DS tablet p.o. every 12 hours for 14 days.
- cefaclor (Ceclor®) 500 mg p.o. QID for 14 days.
- amoxicillin-clavulanate potassium (Augmentin®) 500 mg p.o. TID for 14 days.

→ Oral decongestants may provide some symptom relief in simple sinusitis.
- If appropriate, the patient could initiate therapy with pseudoephedrine (Sudafed®) 30 mg-60 mg p.o. every 4-6 hours as needed (maximum daily dose not to exceed 240 mg).

NOTE: Pseudoephedrine is contraindicated in severe hypertension and/or coronary artery disease.

→ In simple sinusitis, limited use of a topical decongestant can be initiated with one of the following:
- oxymetazoline 0.05% (Afrin®) spray 1-2 sprays in each nostril every 8 hours prn for up to 3 days.
- xylometazoline 0.05%-0.1% (Otrivin®) spray 1-2 sprays in each nostril every 8 hours prn for up to 3 days.

→ Nasal saline spray may be useful in maintaining moist nasal mucosa and avoiding desiccation.

→ Humidification with warm, moist air helps clear sinus congestion and avoid desiccation.

CONSULTATION

→ Physician consultation is indicated in patients who are unresponsive to antibiotic therapy after 72 hours. Further evaluation, treatment, and/or possible referral to an otolaryngologist may be indicated.

→ As needed for prescription(s).

PATIENT EDUCATION

→ Educate the patient about sinusitis—the cause(s), clinical course, treatment options, possible complications and side effects of medications, and any indicated follow-up.

→ Educate the patient about the adverse effects on nasal mucosa of antihistamines and the overuse of topical decongestants.
- Antihistamines can cause desiccation of the mucosa, resulting in an increase in viscous secretions, and should be avoided.
- Topical nasal decongestants can cause ciliastasis and a decreased blood flow to the nasal mucosa, resulting in an inhibition of clearance of nasal secretions and a reduction in the amount of antibiotics delivered to the sinuses (Herr 1991).

FOLLOW-UP

→ See "Consultation" section.

→ Document in progress notes and problem list.

5-M

Sinusitis—Chronic

Chronic sinusitis is a prolonged infection of the paranasal sinuses resulting from interference with the normal transport and clearance of nasal mucous secretions. It is usually caused by a mechanical obstruction (anatomical or pathophysiological) of the osteomeatal unit, resulting in diminished mucociliary movement and an increased accumulation of mucous secretions. When mucous secretions continue to accumulate, there is a reduction in the oxygenation of the nasal mucosa, resulting in proliferation of pathogens.

Pathogens most commonly associated with chronic sinusitis are anaerobes, *S. aureus*, and beta-lactamase-producing *H. influenzae* or *M. catarrhalis* (*B. catarrhalis*) (Godley 1992; Loch, Alleva, and Paparella 1990; Maisel and Kimberley 1988).

DATABASE

SUBJECTIVE

→ Predisposing factors may include:
- history of recent sinus infection, allergic rhinitis, asthma.
- anatomic deviations of the nose (e.g., obstructed osteomeatal unit, deviated septum).
- nasal polyps, tumor, foreign body.
- immune deficiency.

→ Symptoms may include:
- dull ache or pressure of the midface.
- pressure between the eyes.
- morning headache aggravated by head movement.
- nasal congestion.
- post-nasal drip.
- otalgia.
- slight epistaxis.
- dental pain.
- halitosis.
- chronic cough:
  • usually most noticeable in the morning.
- bronchitis.
- fatigue.
- lightheadedness.
- dizziness.
- recurrent laryngitis.

OBJECTIVE

→ Patient may present with:
- purulent nasal discharge.
- nasal polyp.
- deviated septum.
- tenderness to palpation over involved sinuses.

ASSESSMENT

→ Chronic sinusitis

→ R/O failed therapy for acute sinusitis

→ R/O chronic rhinitis

→ R/O nasal polyposis

→ R/O dental infection

→ R/O migraine or tension headache

→ R/O temporal arteritis

→ R/O TMJ disorder

→ R/O asthma

PLAN

DIAGNOSTIC TESTS

→ In consultation with a physician, the following tests may be ordered to confirm the diagnosis of chronic sinusitis and rule out other significant conditions (e.g., abscess, neoplasm) (Jackler and Kaplan 1994; Littler and Momany 1990):

- nasal smear:
  - may reveal eosinophils or neutrophils, differentiating allergic from bacterial sinusitis.
- sinus series x-rays:
  - may reveal findings consistent with sinusitis (e.g., air fluid levels, opacification of an infected sinus) and eliminate the presence of an abscess.
- CT scan:
  - may identify osteomeatal unit disease.
  - three weeks of antibiotic therapy should be completed prior to a CT scan:
    - –to reduce tissue edema, allowing better visualization of anatomic structures during the scan.
- magnetic resonance imaging (MRI) is useful only in identifying soft-tissue masses.
- nasal cultures, if done, correlate poorly with bacteria causing infection of the sinuses because normal nasal flora often grow in such cultures.
- maxillary antrum aspiration may be necessary in resistant cases. If so, referral to an otolaryngologist is warranted.

TREATMENT/MANAGEMENT

→ When chronic sinusitis is suspected, antibiotic therapy should be initiated with an antimicrobial agent effective against beta-lactamase-producing organisms. Such agents include (Godley 1992; Loch, Alleva, and Paparella 1990):

- amoxicillin-clavulanate potassium (Augmentin®) 500 mg p.o. TID for 21 days
  OR
- trimethoprim/sulfamethoxazole (Bactrim®, Septra®) 1 double-strength tablet (DS) p.o. BID for 21 days
  OR
- cefaclor (Ceclor®) 500 mg p.o. QID for 21 days
  OR
- clindamycin (Cleocin®) 600 mg p.o. TID for 21 days.
  - This antibiotic will cover bacteroides, but patients must be monitored for pseudo-membranous colitis caused by *Clostridium difficile*.

→ When using prolonged antibiotic therapy in women or immune-deficient patients, consider prophylaxis for yeast infections (e.g., vaginal antifungal agents, oral candidiasis therapies) and review nonpharmacological methods to diminish the likelihood of a yeast infection. See **Vaginitis** Protocols.

→ Humidification with warm, moist air may help prevent desiccation.
- Other helpful measures include forcing fluids orally, use of a nasal saline spray, and the avoidance of physical or chemical irritants.

→ Use of oral decongestants (e.g., pseudoephedrine) may help reduce the edema of the nasal mucosa (see **Sinusitis—Acute** Protocol for doses).
- Since sleeplessness is a common side effect of such medications, this medication should be used in the morning and its use avoided during late afternoon or evening.

→ Topical steroid nasal sprays should be avoided during the initial acute phase of therapy because of the potential suppression of local immune response to the organism.
- However, their use to decrease the tissue edema observed in association with allergic or vasomotor rhinitis may be beneficial (see **Rhinitis** Protocol, "Allergic Rhinitis" or "Vasomotor Rhinitis").

CONSULTATION

→ Consultation with a physician is indicated in patients who do not respond to therapy within 72 hours, who may require maxillary antrum aspiration, or who have an underlying immunodeficiency.

→ As needed for prescription(s).

PATIENT EDUCATION

→ Educate the patient about chronic sinusitis—the cause(s), the therapeutic interventions (including possible side effects of medications), possible complications, and indicated follow-up. Discuss ways to prevent further episodes.

FOLLOW-UP

→ If symptoms are not ameliorated within 72 hours, patient should return for further evaluation, or as per recommendation of physician if consultation was required.

→ Document in progress notes and problem list.

5-N
Tuberculosis

Tuberculosis is an infection caused by a member of the *Mycobacterium* genus that includes *Mycobacterium tuberculosis, Mycobacterium bovis,* and *Mycobacterium africanum* (Des Prez and Heim 1990). Although illness in humans as a result of infection with *M. bovis* and *M. africanum* has been reported, such instances are rare (Des Prez and Heim 1990). The majority of illnesses associated with mycobacteria are a result of infection with *M. tuberculosis.*

M. tuberculosis is an aerobic, non-motile, non-spore-forming, slow-growing bacteria that is an obligate parasite. Though it infects humans primarily, other primates and mammalian species in close and fairly constant contact with humans (e.g., cats, dogs) can be infected, though these species are not reservoirs of the organism.

Almost every case of tuberculosis infection occurs through inhalation of small (1 μm-5 μm), infected respiratory droplets. Usually, prolonged exposure to an infectious person or environment is necessary for effective transmission to occur. Factors facilitating transmission also include a decreased natural resistance to the organism and crowded living conditions favoring airborne spread of the organism (Des Prez and Heim 1990).

Tuberculosis remains a major health problem worldwide with 10 million new cases reported each year. This disease is responsible for three million deaths annually, and six percent of total deaths worldwide. In the United States, there are 10 million to 15 million individuals with latent tuberculosis infection (CDC 1990a; CDC 1992c).

The annual new case rate for the United States is 9.4 cases/100,000 persons, with an overall annual death rate of 0.75 deaths/100,000 cases. There is an increased incidence of tuberculosis infection reported in urban areas with populations over 100,000 (20.7 cases/ 100,000) (Des Prez and Heim 1990).

Specific factors reportedly increasing the risk of tuberculosis infection within a population include lower socioeconomic status, non-Caucasian race, recent immigration, drug addiction, alcoholism, HIV infection, end-stage renal disease, homelessness, and residence in a long-term health care facility (Des Prez and Heim 1990). In addition, certain age groups are more likely to develop active disease once infected with tuberculosis, specifically, children younger than six years of age, adolescents, young adults, and the elderly.

The pathological features of tuberculosis result from the host's degree of hypersensitivity and the local concentration of the antigen. Once *M. tuberculosis* is inhaled, it is transmitted to the terminal airspaces where the organism is ingested by macrophages. At this point, the organism either dies or remains viable and multiplies.

The site of infection is usually in lung segments where greater airflow facilitates the deposition of the inhaled bacilli. The most commonly affected sites are the anterior segment of the upper lobes, and the middle lobe, lingula, and lower division of the lower lobes. Dissemination of the organism also can occur as a result of lymphohematogenous spread from the primary pulmonary site to extrapulmonary sites including the kidneys, bones, bone marrow, liver, spleen, ovaries, endometrium, and brain (Des Prez and Heim 1990).

In most individuals infected with tuberculosis, the cell-mediated immune response is adequate to limit multiplication of the bacilli, with effective encapsulation and calcification of the organism occurring. However, 10 percent of infected persons are unable to contain the organism effectively, thus developing active clinical disease. In 10 percent of these patients, active disease occurs within one year after infection. The remaining patients develop clinical disease one or more years after infection (CDC 1990a).

During the past five years, there has been an increased incidence of *multi-drug-resistant tuberculosis* (MDR-TB), with most cases reported in HIV-infected persons (CDC 1990b; CDC 1992c; CDC 1992d; Chawla et al. 1992).

The case-fatality rate associated with MDR-TB in these outbreaks has been extremely high, ranging from 72 percent to 89 percent (CDC 1990b). In the majority of cases, resistance to both isoniazid (INH) and rifampin (RFM) has been documented. Resistance to other anti-tuberculosis medications—including ethambutal (EMB), streptomycin (STM), kanamycin (KM), ethionamide, and rifabutin—has also been reported (CDC 1992c; CDC 1992d; Chawla et al. 1992).

DATABASE

SUBJECTIVE

→ High-risk factors include:
- history of close contact (e.g., sharing same household or enclosed environments) with a person with, or suspected of having, tuberculosis.

→ Persons with medical risk factors associated with an increased risk of active tuberculosis if infection occurs include patients with a history of:
- silicosis.
- gastrectomy.
- jejunoileal bypass.
- weight loss of 10 percent or more of ideal body weight.
- chronic renal failure.
- conditions requiring prolonged high-dose corticosteroid therapy and/or other immunosuppressive therapy.
- particular hematological disorders (e.g., leukemia, lymphoma).
- malignancies.
- persons with HIV infection.
- persons with abnormal chest x-ray demonstrating fibrotic lesions consistent with old, healed tuberculosis.
- positive tuberculin skin test within two years without evaluation for preventive therapy.

→ Patients infected with tuberculosis may be asymptomatic (latent infection) or may report one or more of the following symptoms (American Thoracic Society 1990; Des Prez and Heim 1990; Stauffer 1994):
- fever, often remittent, and occurring in the early afternoon.
- night sweats.
- malaise.
- keratitis or conjunctivitis.
- erythema nodosum—painful red nodules, commonly appearing on the anterior aspects of the legs.
- cough that may be productive of mucopurulent sputum.
- hemoptysis.
- anorexia.
- weight loss.
- intermittent chills.
- chest pain secondary to extension of infection into the pleura.
- pharyngeal and mouth ulcers (rare).
- hoarseness (rare, associated with laryngeal involvement).
- dysphagia (rare, associated with laryngeal involvement).
- enlarged, firm, tender cervical or supraclavicular lymph nodes that may soften, slough, and drain.
- if coexistent meningitis, possible CNS symptoms varying in intensity (e.g., headache, change in mentation, nuchal rigidity, confusion).
- if skeletal tuberculosis develops, possible red, painful joints (usually monoarticular, weight-bearing), with symptoms starting after a traumatic event.
- dysuria, gross hematuria, and flank pain if renal involvement present (70 percent of patients with renal tuberculosis report such symptoms).
- pelvic pain, abdominal pain, and/or menstrual disorders possible in women with genital tuberculosis infection.
  NOTE: In immunocompromised (e.g., HIV-infected) and elderly patients, the symptoms of tuberculosis often are subtle and atypical.

OBJECTIVE

→ Physical examination may be unremarkable or may reveal one or more of the following findings, depending on the extent of the infection and the immune status of the patient (Des Prez and Heim 1990; Stauffer 1994):
- vital signs:
  - WNL or
  - may demonstrate an elevated temperature (> 37.7°C/100°F), pulse, and respiratory rate, depending on the status of the patient.

- the patient's weight may be less than 10 percent of ideal body weight for height.
- skin:
  - may reveal pallor if patient has moderate to severe anemia (secondary to hematologic abnormalities associated with miliary tuberculosis).
  - elevated, erythematous nodules of the anterior aspect of the legs may be noted with erythema nodosum.
- eyes:
  - may be evidence of keratitis or conjunctivitis (see **Conjunctivitis** and **Keratitis** protocols).
- mouth:
  - may be ulcerations.
- lymphadenopathy:
  - usually palpation of a single, firm, enlarged, tender cervical or supraclavicular node (although, over time, the node may soften, slough, and produce drainage).
- palpation of the chest wall:
  - may reveal decreased tactile fremitus in the presence of pleural thickening or fluid.
- dullness to percussion of the chest wall.
- auscultation of the lungs may reveal:
  - increased tubular breath sounds and whispered pectoriloquy.
  - post-tussive rales (elicited after the patient takes several short coughs).
  - distant, hollow breath sounds ("amphoric" sounds noted over tuberculous cavities).
  - rubs (with pleural effusion).
- abdominal examination:
  - may reveal splenomegaly.
- examination of the extremities may reveal:
  - erythema nodosum and/or a single erythematous, tender weight-bearing joint.
- neurological examination may reveal:
  - confusion.
  - nuchal rigidity.
  - photosensitivity (with meningeal involvement).
- pelvic examination may reveal:
  - a granulomatous ulcerating cervical mass and/or
  - an enlarged, tender ovary or uterus.

ASSESSMENT

→ Tuberculosis infection (latent, active)
→ R/O MDR-TB
→ R/O meningitis
→ R/O pneumonia
→ R/O cancer
→ R/O immune deficiency (e.g., HIV infection)

PLAN

DIAGNOSTIC TESTS

→ Tuberculin skin tests.
- Though an important screening tool, such tests do not distinguish between past infection or current disease.
- There are 2 types of skin tests commonly used in the United States, the *multiple puncture devices* and the *Mantoux test*.
  - Multiple puncture devices (e.g., Tine Test) are often used to screen large, low-risk populations (e.g., school-age children without a history of risk factors).
    - The test is applied to the volar aspect of the patient's forearm and is read 48 to 72 hours after placement.
    - Various patterns of induration or vesicular eruptions may occur, with further evaluation indicated in patients demonstrating any abnormal result.
    - This test is not commonly used in adult populations (Des Prez and Heim 1990).
  - The Mantoux test is the best screening test for detecting tuberculosis infection.
    - The test consists of an intradermal injection of 0.1 ml solution containing 5 tuberculin units (TU) of purified protein derivative (PPD), using a #26 or #27 needle on the volar aspect of the patient's forearm.
    - If the PPD was placed correctly, a raised, blanched wheal will occur.
    - Injections deeper than the subdermal layer may result in the "washing out" of the PPD solution by vascular flow, thereby reducing the amount of antigen administered to the patient (Des Prez and Heim 1990).
    - The test should be read 48 to 72 hours after placement for any evidence of induration (not erythema) at the skin test site.
    - The transverse diameter of the induration should be measured in millimeters. A test is positive if the induration measured reaches the size required for specific risk groups as indicated below (American Thoracic Society 1990):
      - reaction ≥ 5 mm is considered positive if the patient is HIV-positive, a close contact

of a person with tuberculosis, or has evidence of old, healed tuberculosis on chest x-ray findings.

▸ reaction of ≥ 10 mm is considered positive if the patient is:
  – from a region with a high incidence of tuberculosis (e.g., Africa, Latin America, Asia).
  – an injection drug user known to be HIV-negative.
  – medically underserved, of lower socioeconomic status, or is a member of an ethnic minority (including African American, Hispanic, and Native American populations).
  – resident of a long-term care facility, correctional institution, or psychiatric institution.
  – reporting a history of medical conditions associated with an increased risk of active tuberculosis including: silicosis, weight 10 percent or more below ideal body weight, chronic renal failure, diabetes mellitus, gastrectomy, jejunoilieal bypass, prolonged high-dose cortico-steroid therapy or immunosuppressive therapy, malignancies, or certain hematological disorders (e.g., leukemia, lymphoma).

▸ reaction of ≥ 15 mm is considered positive in all other patients.

NOTE: When induration does occur, the amount of the reaction correlates with the likelihood of infection (e.g., a reaction of ≥ 20 mm is highly indicative of infection) (Des Prez and Heim 1990).

A negative PPD does not eliminate the possibility of tuberculosis infection. It takes 6 to 14 weeks after infection for the development of the tissue hypersensitivity response required for a positive test reaction to occur. False-negative results are estimated to be as high as 20 percent in persons with active tuberculosis infection and may be a result of malnutrition, general illness (e.g., intercurrent viral illnesses), corticosteroid therapy, and other causes of anergy (e.g., advanced HIV infection). False positive results can occur if there is infection with a non-tuberculous mycobacteria (Des Prez and Heim 1990).

Patients who received vaccination with *Calmette-Guerin bacillus* (BCG) will have a positive tuberculin test which is either in response to the vaccination or evidence of tuberculosis infection. In the United States, a patient with a history of BCG vaccination and a positive tuberculin test is considered to have tuberculosis infection and should be further evaluated to exclude the possibility of active infection.

→ Sputum specimens for diagnostic testing should be done to confirm active pulmonary tuberculosis infection.
  ▪ Sputum specimen collection for gram stain and *acid-fast bacilli* (AFB) culture should be done early in the morning.
    • Sputum acid-fast stain. Evidence of acid-fast bacilli is diagnostic of infection and indicates that the patient is highly infectious (Des Prez and Heim 1990). Acid-fast stains will be positive in 50 percent to 80 percent of patients with pulmonary tuberculosis (American Thoracic Society 1990).
    • Sputum for AFB culture. A positive result indicates tuberculosis infection and can reveal organisms resistant to antituberculosis drugs (American Thoracic Society 1990, 1994; Des Prez and Heim 1990).
  ▪ 3 to 5 early-morning, daily collections should be sufficient to obtain an adequate sample.
  ▪ In patients unable to produce adequate specimens in the morning, 24-hour collection can be attempted, though there is an increased chance of normal oral flora over growth in specimens obtained this way.
  ▪ Other options to obtain specimens include sputum induction and aspiration of gastric contents (rarely done today because of the success associated with sputum induction techniques).

→ CBC may be WNL or may reveal a decreased hemoglobin/hematocrit, an increased leukocyte count (10,000-15,000 cells/mm³), decreased platelets, and an increased monocyte count (in 10 percent of patients).

→ Serum chemistry panel should be ordered to rule out hepatic and/or kidney involvement, and may reveal:
  ▪ hyponatremia in advanced disease or if associated with Addison's disease.
  ▪ elevated liver function tests (ALT, AST) when there is hepatic involvement or in association with other medical conditions (e.g., substance abuse).

→ With associated renal involvement, a urinalysis may reveal pyuria, hematuria, and albuminuria (a rare finding usually associated with amyloidosis).

→ Chest x-ray should be ordered when a patient has a positive PPD or has signs and symptoms suggestive of tuberculosis infection.

▪ Certain chest x-ray findings are suggestive of pulmonary tuberculosis. The following may be evident (Des Prez and Heim 1990; Stauffer 1994):

• a patchy, nodular infiltrate in the apical or subapical posterior regions of the upper lobes or superior segment of the lower lobes.

• cavitation in the apical segment of the lower lobes (This finding may be obscured by the overlying heart shadow or dorsal spine.).

• air-fluid levels are commonly noted in lower-lobe cavities, but are uncommon in upper-lobe tuberculosis.

• evidence of bronchogenic spread may be demonstrated when multiple, discrete infiltrates adjacent to a cavity are observed.

• granulomatous and exudative lesions, fibrotic scars, and caseation may be noted.

• evidence of a pneumonic lesion with enlarged hilar nodes in any lobe of the lung is suggestive of primary tuberculosis infection.

• presence of a miliary infiltrate may be evident.

• in some patients, pleural effusion may be the only x-ray finding.

NOTE: In HIV-positive patients, chest x-ray findings may be subtle and atypical and can result in misdiagnosis.

→ Analysis of cerebrospinal fluid (CSF) in patients suspected of CNS involvement will reveal increased lymphocytes and polymorphonuclear cells, increased protein, and a decreased glucose level.

▪ AFB stain of CSF may be positive. CSF culture for AFB often is positive but it takes a number of weeks before results are obtained (Des Prez and Heim 1990).

→ If genital tuberculosis is suspected, AFB smears and cultures of tissue obtained during surgery,

Table 5N.1. RECOMMENDED DRUGS FOR INITIAL TREATMENT OF TUBERCULOSIS IN CHILDREN AND ADULTS

Drug	Dosage Forms		Daily Dose (mg/kg)		Maximum Daily Dose in Children and Adults	Twice-Weekly Dose (mg/kg)		Adverse Reactions
			Children	Adults		Children	Adults	
Isoniazid	Tablets	100 mg,*+ 300 mg	10-20 p.o. or I.M.	5 p.o. or I.M.	300 mg	20-40 (max 900 mg)	15 (max 900 mg)	Hepatic enzyme elevation, peripheral neuropathy, hepatitis hypersensitivity
	Syrup	50 mg/5 ml						
	Vials	1 gm						
Rifampin	Capsules	150 mg,*+ 300 mg	10-20 p.o.	10 p.o.	600 mg	10-20 (max 600 mg)	10 (max 600 mg)	Orange discoloration of secretions and urine; nausea, vomiting, hepatitis, febrile reaction, purpura (rare)
	Syrup Formulated from capsules	100 mg/ml						
	Vials	600 mg						
Pyrazinamide	Tablets	500 mg+	15-30 p.o.	15-30 p.o.	2 gm	50-70	50-70	Hepatotoxicity, hyperuricemia
Streptomycin	Vials	1 gm, 4 gm	20-40 I.M.	15& I.M.	1 gm&	25-30 I.M.	25-30	Ototoxicity, nephrotoxicity
Ethambutol	Tablets	100 mg 400 mg	15-25 p.o.	15-25 p.o.	2.5 gm	50	50	Optic neuritis (decreased red-green color discrimination, decreased visual acuity), skin rash

*Isoniazid and rifampin are available as a combination capsule containing 150 mg of isoniazid and 300 mg of rifampin.

+A combination of isoniazid, rifampin, and pyrazinamide in a single tablet is being introduced.

&In persons above age 60 years, the daily dose of streptomycin should be limited to 10 mg/kg with a maximum dose of 750 mg.

Source: Reprinted with permission from Mangura, B.T., Mangura, C.T., and Reichman, L.B. 1991. Tuberculosis and the atypical pneumonia syndrome. *Clinics in Chest Medicine* 12(2):356. Adapted from National Tuberculosis Training Initiative: Core Curriculum on Tuberculosis. Atlanta, Centers for Disease Control, and New York, American Thoracic Society, June 1990.

cervical biopsy, or endometrial scraping may be positive (Des Prez and Heim 1990).

→ CT scan or MRI may demonstrate focal lesions, basilar arachnoid meningitis, cerebral infarction, and/or hydrocephalus in patients with CNS involvement (Des Prez and Heim 1990).

TREATMENT/MANAGEMENT

→ The treatment options presented in this section will be limited to patients with uncomplicated latent or active pulmonary infection.

■ Documented MDR-TB infection, tuberculosis infection in severely immunocompromised patients, patients requiring hospitalization, and patients lacking appropriate response to therapy—all require consultation with specialists (e.g., pulmonologist, infectious disease specialist). Furthermore, health care providers inexperienced in the diagnosis and treatment of patients with tuberculosis infection should consider specialist consultation for all patients, since improper treatment can result in serious consequences for the patient and her close contacts.

→ The preferred standard drug regimen for active tuberculosis infection (both pulmonary and extrapulmonary) in patients who are not HIV-positive or at risk of HIV-infection combines the following medications and doses: (see **Table 5N.1, Recommended Drugs for Initial Treatment of Tuberculosis in Children and Adults,** and **Table 5N.2, Second-Line Anti-Tuberculosis Drugs:**

■ isoniazid (INH) 300 mg p.o. every day for 6 months.
■ rifampin (RIF) 600 mg p.o. every day for 6 months.
■ pyrazinamide (PZA) 15 mg/kg-30 mg/kg p.o. every day during first 2 months.
■ another option is the use of INH and RIF for 9 months without PZA. However, the use of three drugs to combat active tuberculosis is preferred over two-drug therapy by some authors (American Thoracic Society 1994; Mangura, Mangura, and Reichman 1991; Stauffer 1994).

NOTE: Both INH and RIF are bacteriocidal to all organisms and reach therapeutic levels in all tissues, including the subarachnoid space. PZA is bacteriocidal to intracellular organisms.

Hepatotoxicity is of concern with INH therapy, especially in elderly patients, alcoholics, cancer patients, uremic patients, and pregnant women. However, such toxicity is rarely observed in healthy patients younger than 20 years of age. Transient increases in transaminase levels are reported in 10 percent to 20 percent of patients using INH.

In addition to hepatotoxicity, INH has been associated with peripheral neuropathy. The addition of Vitamin B$_6$ (pyridoxine), 50 mg p.o. daily can prevent or ameliorate this symptom in some patients.

The use of RIF in combination with INH increases the risk of hepatotoxicity to four times that observed with INH therapy alone. Additionally, jaundice often is observed 1 to 3 weeks after the initiation of this combination therapy. If frank hepatitis develops, it is

Table 5N.2. SECOND-LINE ANTI-TUBERCULOSIS DRUGS*

Drug	Dosage Forms		Daily Dose+ (mg/kg)	Maximum Daily Dose+ (gm)	Principal Adverse Reactions	Recommended Regular Monitoring
Capreomycin	Vials	1 mg	15-30 I.M.	1	Auditory, vestibular, and renal toxicity	Vestibular function, audiometry, BUN and creatinine
Kanamycin	Vials	75 mg, 500 mg, 1 gm	15-30 I.M.	1	Auditory and renal toxicity; vestibular toxicity (rare)	Vestibular function, audiometry, BUN and creatinine
Ethionamide	Tablets	250 mg	15-20 p.o.	1	Hepatotoxicity, hypersensitivity, GI disturbance	Hepatic enzymes
Para-aminosalicylic	Tablets	500 mg, 1 gm	150 p.o.	12	GI disturbance, hypersensitivity, hepatotoxicity, sodium load	Acid
Cycloserine	Capsules	250 mg	15-20 p.o.	1	Psychosis, convulsions, rash	Mental status

*These drugs are more difficult to use than drugs listed in Table 5N.1. They should be used only when necessary and should be given and monitored by health providers experienced in their use.

+for both children and adults.

Source: Reprinted with permission from Mangura, B.T., Mangura, C.T., and Reichman, L.B. 1991. Tuberculosis and the atypical pneumonia syndrome. *Clinics in Chest Medicine* 12(2):357. Adapted from National Tuberculosis Training Initiative: Core Curriculum on Tuberculosis. Atlanta, Centers for Disease Control, and New York, American Thoracic Society, June 1990.

associated with a 6 percent to 12 percent chance of death.

Though PZA does not increase the hepatotoxicity of INH and RIF, it is associated with hyperuricemia and mild polyarthralgias. Elevated uric acid levels can occur, though they usually don't necessitate discontinuation of PZA. Discontinuation of INH and RIF is indicated in patients who develop frank hepatitis or who have transaminase elevations 5 times normal levels (Des Prez and Heim 1990).

→ If drug resistance is suspected or the patient exhibits symptoms of overwhelming infection, either ethambutol or streptomycin should be added to the drugs listed above in the following doses:
- Streptomycin (STM) 1gm I.M./day for at least 6 months.
- Ethambutol (EMB) 15 mg-25 mg/kg/day p.o. for at least 6 months.

NOTE: STM is associated with 8th cranial nerve damage and deafness, especially in patients older than 50 years of age. In patients 60 years of age or older, the dose of STM is 10 mg/kg/day with a maximum daily dose of 750 mg/day. EMB also is associated with hyperuricemia and optic neuritis (which appears to be dose-related) (Des Prez and Heim 1990; Mangura, Mangura, and Reichman 1991).

- intermittent (twice weekly), directly observed dosing of the standard drugs used for active tuberculosis may be necessary when non-compliance with medication regimens is of concern (e.g., homeless patients, substance-abusing patients).
  - Such regimens have been successful, with minimal toxicity and no increase in drug resistance reported thus far (Brausch and Bass 1993; Iseman, Cohn, and Sbarbaro 1993). The regimen for intermittent dosing for active tuberculosis is:
    –INH, RIF, and PZA standard daily dosing as above for 2 months followed by NH 900 mg p.o. and RIF 600 mg p.o. twice a week for a minimum of 4 months (American Thoracic Society 1994; Mangura, Mangura, and Reichman 1991).

→ In HIV-positive patients, chemotherapeutic agents for active tuberculosis should be administered for at least 6 months after conversion of sputum cultures to negative (American Thoracic Society 1990; Barnes et al. 1991).

→ In patients demonstrating documented INH resistance after the initiation of standard therapy, the use of RIF and EMB is recommended for a minimum of 12 months. In HIV-positive patients, RIF and EMB therapy is continued for 12 months after conversion of sputum cultures to negative or for 18 months after initiation of therapy (whichever is longer) (American Thoracic Society 1990, 1994).
- When documented INH resistance occurs, consultation with specialists is indicated.

→ Corticosteroid therapy may be necessary in a patient who exhibits severe constitutional symptoms or who is debilitated. Corticosteroid therapy will usually help resolve symptoms.
- Consultation with a physician is indicated if such therapy is being considered, since hospitalization often is necessary.
- The following dosing schedule is usually the one recommended (Des Prez and Heim 1990):
  - prednisone (Deltasone®) 30 mg-35 mg p.o. every day with tapering of the dose by 2.5 mg every 3 to 5 days.

→ Other therapeutic interventions include modified bed rest during symptomatic disease, and adequate nutrition and hydration.

→ Hospitalization of a patient is indicated if she has evidence of miliary tuberculosis (i.e., lympho-hematogenous spread) or significant debilitation, cannot care for herself, or is likely to expose susceptible individuals during the infectious stage of her disease (Des Prez and Heim 1990; Stauffer 1994).

→ Patient immunization with pneumococcal vaccine and yearly influenza vaccine is recommended (see **Pneumonia** and **Influenza** protocols).

→ Because of the high incidence of tuberculosis in HIV-infected individuals, offering HIV counseling and testing to any patient with active tuberculosis infection and unknown HIV status is recommended (CDC 1992c).

→ Patients with substance abuse problems should be referred for appropriate counseling and treatment.

→ Contacts of persons with infectious tuberculosis are at high risk of developing the disease. Therefore, contacts must be rapidly identified and evaluated for infection.
- Contacts who are at high risk of developing active disease if infected with tuberculosis should be considered for preventive therapy with INH.

- INH has proven to be more than 90 percent effective in preventing the development of active tuberculosis when taken as prescribed.
- The recommended regimen for INH preventive therapy is (American Thoracic Society 1994; CDC 1990b; Miller 1993):
  - INH 300 mg p.o. every day for 6 to 12 months in immunocompetent patients.
    NOTE: INH therapy for 6 months is the *minimum* length of time recommended for preventive therapy.
  - INH 300 mg p.o. every day for 12 months is recommended for HIV-positive patients and patients with chest x-ray findings consistent with past tuberculosis infection.
  - INH 900 mg p.o. twice a week for 6 to 12 months may be considered for patients requiring direct observation of medication administration.
→ Members of high-risk groups who should be considered for preventive therapy regardless of age include (American Thoracic Society 1994; CDC 1990b):
  - HIV-positive persons with tuberculin skin test ≥ 5mm, and persons with risk factors for HIV infection whose HIV status is unknown but who are suspected of being infected.
  - close contacts of persons newly diagnosed with infectious tuberculosis who have a tuberculin skin test ≥ 5 mm.
  - recent converters with a tuberculin skin test increase to ≥ 10 mm within a 2-year period if younger than 35 years of age; ≥ 15 mm increase if older than 35.
  - intravenous drug user (IDU) known to be HIV-negative with a tuberculin skin test ≥ 10 mm.
  - persons with abnormal chest x-rays indicating fibrotic lesions likely to represent healed tuberculosis.
  - persons with medical conditions associated with an increased risk of active tuberculosis (see "Subjective" section, "High-Risk Factors" of this protocol) who have a tuberculin skin test ≥ 10 mm.
  - children and adolescents with negative tuberculin tests (<5 mm)—who have been close contacts of infectious persons during the past 3 months—should be considered for preventive therapy until a repeat tuberculin test is done 12 weeks after contact with the infectious person.

→ In the absence of any risk factors already discussed, persons younger than 35 years of age and in any of the following high-incidence groups should also receive preventive therapy if their tuberculin skin test ≥ 10 mm (CDC 1990b):
  - foreign-born individuals from high-prevalence regions (e.g., Asia, Africa, Latin America).
  - medically underserved, low-income populations or ethnic minority populations (e.g., African American, Hispanic, Native American).
  - residents of long-term care facilities.

CONSULTATION

→ Consultation with a physician is indicated in any patient with tuberculosis or suspected of having tuberculosis.

→ Consultation with a physician specializing in the evaluation and treatment of tuberculosis is indicated in any patient with severe symptoms, evidence of concomitant debilitating disease, suspected drug-resistant tuberculosis, symptoms of toxicity associated with therapeutic agents, or suspected noncompliance with treatment regimens.

→ As needed for prescription(s).

PATIENT EDUCATION

→ Educate the patient about tuberculosis infection—the cause, clinical manifestations, clinical course, diagnostic tests, treatment options, need for strict compliance with treatment regimens, possible side effects/toxicity of therapeutic agents, prognosis, follow-up evaluations, and the need for testing of close contacts.

→ Educate the patient about ways to maintain health, including proper nutrition, rest, and hydration.

→ If the patient smokes cigarettes, discuss the adverse effects of smoking on immediate and long-term health, and provide resources and referrals for smoking cessation programs (see **Smoking Cessation** Protocol).

→ Patients requiring hospitalization should discuss with the physician responsible for their care the reasons for hospitalization and their plans.

→ Educate the patient regarding respiratory precautions when infectious tuberculosis is suspected or documented (i.e., evidence of tubercle bacilli on AFB sputum smear or significant colony count on AFB sputum culture).

- Usually, respiratory precautions are necessary during the first one to two weeks of therapy and involve the patient wearing a facial mask covering her nose and mouth.
- Additionally, it is essential to ventilate rooms to reduce the number of droplet nuclei within the environment and decrease the possibility of transmission to others (American Thoracic Society 1990; Des Prez and Heim 1990).

FOLLOW-UP

→ Patients being managed by a physician specialist should have follow-up as recommended by that physician.

→ Patients receiving INH therapy should have baseline transaminase levels done, with periodic monitoring throughout the course of treatment as indicated. In patients aged 35 years or older, monthly transaminase levels should be obtained (American Thoracic Society 1994).

→ Patients with active pulmonary tuberculosis should have monthly sputum examinations until they convert to negative. This is a means of evaluating the effectiveness of treatment.
- Patients with evidence of positive sputum results after three months of therapy should be evaluated for possible drug resistance or noncompliance with treatment regimens.

→ Patients who are experiencing any signs and symptoms of complications or adverse side effects of therapeutic agents should return for immediate evaluation.

→ Tuberculosis is a CDC-reportable disease and notification of the local public health department is mandated by law when a patient is diagnosed with tuberculosis.

→ Document in progress notes and problem list.

5-0
Bibliography

American Thoracic Society. 1990. Diagnostic standards and classification of tuberculosis. *American Review of Respiratory Diseases* 142:725–735.

———. 1994. Treatment of tuberculosis and tuberculosis infection in adults and children. *American Journal of Respiratory Critical Care Medicine* 149:1359–1374.

Amundson, L.H. 1990. Disorders of the external ear. *Primary Care* 17(2):213–231.

Arkinstall, W.W. 1987. Once-daily sustained-release theophylline reduces clinical variation in spirometry and symptomatology in adult asthmatics. *American Review of Respiratory Diseases* 135:316–321.

Barnes, P.F., Bloch, A.B., Davidson, P.T., and Snider, Jr., D.E. 1991. Tuberculosis in patients with human immunodeficiency virus infection. *New England Journal of Medicine* 324(23):1644–1650.

Billas, A. 1990. Lower respiratory tract infections. *Primary Care* 17(4):811–824.

Brausch, L.M., and Bass, J.B., Jr. 1993. The treatment of tuberculosis. *Medical Clinics of North America* 77(6):1277–1288.

Celin, S.E., Bluestone, C.D., Stephenson, J., Yilmaz, H.M., and Collins, J.J. 1991. Bacteriology of acute otitis media in adults. *Journal of the American Medical Association* 266(16):2249–2252.

Centers for Disease Control. 1990a. Screening for tuberculosis and tuberculosis infection in high-risk populations. Recommendations of the Advisory Committee for Elimination of Tuberculosis. *Morbidity and Mortality Weekly Report* 39(RR-8):1–8.

———. 1990b. The use of preventive therapy for tuberculosis infection in the United States. Recommendations of the Advisory Committee for Elimination of Tuberculosis. *Morbidity and Mortality Weekly Report* 39(RR-8):9–12.

———. 1991. Update on adult immunization. Recommendations of the Immunization Practices Advisory Committee. *Morbidity and Mortality Weekly Report* 40(RR-12):34–36, 42–44.

———. 1992a. Prevention and control of influenza. Recommendations of the Immunization Practices Advisory Committee. *Morbidity and Mortality Weekly Report* 41(RR-9):1–17.

———. 1992b. Influenza surveillance—United States, 1991-1992. *Morbidity and Mortality Weekly Report* 41(SS-5):35–46.

———. 1992c. Management of persons exposed to multidrug-resistant tuberculosis. *Morbidity and Mortality Weekly Report* 41(RR-11):61–70.

———. 1992d. National action plan to combat multidrug-resistant tuberculosis. *Morbidity and Mortality Weekly Report* 41(RR-11):6–48.

Chawla, P.K., Klapper, P.J., Kamholz, S.L., Pollack, A.H., and Heurich, A.E. 1992. Drug-resistant tuberculosis in an urban population including patients at risk for human immunodeficiency virus infection. *American Review of Respiratory Diseases* 146:280–284.

Des Prez, R.M., and Heim, C.R. 1990. Mycobacterial diseases. In *Principles and practice of infectious diseases*, 3rd ed., eds. G.L. Mandell, R.G. Douglas, Jr., and J.E. Bennett, pp. 1877–1906. New York:Churchill Livingstone.

Elborn, J.S., Finch, M.B., and Stanford, C.F. 1991. Non-arterial assessment of blood gas status in patients with chronic pulmonary disease. *Ulster Medical Journal* 60(2):164–167.

Ellsworth, A.J., Bray, R.F., Bray, B.S., and Geyman, J.P. 1991. *The family practice drug handbook*. St. Louis:Mosby Year Book.

Erwin S.A. 1987. Epistaxis:How to control the persistent nosebleed. *Postgraduate Medicine* 82(4):59–65.

Evans, P., and Hoffman, L. 1994. Malignant external otitis: A case report and review. *American Family Physician* 49(2):427–431.

Fein, A.M., Feinsilver, S.H., and Niederman, M.S. 1991. Atypical manifestations of pneumonia in the elderly. *Clinics in Chest Medicine* 12(2):319–336.

Godley, F.A. 1992. Chronic sinusitis: An update. *American Family Physician* 45(5):2190–2199.

Greenberg, S.B. 1991. Viral pneumonia. *Infectious Disease Clinics of North America* 5(3):603–621.

Griffith, D.E., and Mazurek, G.H. 1991. Pneumonia in chronic obstructive lung disease. *Infectious Disease Clinics of North America* 5(3):467–484.

Hampson, N.B., Woolf, R.A., and Springmeyer, S.C. 1991. Oral antibiotics for pneumonia. *Clinics in Chest Medicine* 12(2):395–407.

Herr, R.D. 1991. Acute sinusitis: Diagnosis and treatment update. *American Family Physician* 44(6):2055–2061.

Holmgren, D., and Sixt, R. 1992. Transcutaneous and arterial blood gas monitoring during acute asthmatic symptoms in older children. *Pediatric Pulmonary* 14(2):80–84.

Iseman, M.D., Cohn, D.L., and Sbarbaro, J.A. 1993. Directly observed treatment of tuberculosis. We can't afford not to try it. *New England Journal of Medicine* 328(8):576–578.

Jackler, R.K., and Kaplan, M.J. 1994. Ear, nose, and throat. In *Current medical diagnosis and treatment*, 33d ed., eds. L.M. Tierney, Jr., S.J. McPhee, M.A. Papadakis, and S.A. Schroeder, pp. 175–206. Norwalk, CT: Appleton & Lange.

Jackson, K.R., and Jackson, R.T. 1988. Factors associated with active, refractory epistaxis. *Archives of Otolaryngologic Head Neck Surgery* 114:862–865.

Jenne, J.W. 1984. Theophylline use in asthma: Some current issues. *Clinics in Chest Medicine* 5:645–658.

Johnson, P., and Sarosi, G. 1991. Current therapy of major fungal diseases of the lung. *Infectious Disease Clinics of North America* 5(3):635–645.

Kemp, E.D. 1990. Otitis media. *Primary Care* 17(2):267–287.

Lieu, T.A., Fleisher, G.R., and Schwartz, J.S. 1990. Cost-effectiveness of rapid latex agglutination testing and throat culture for streptococcal pharyngitis. *Pediatrics* 85(3):246–256.

Littler, J.E., and Momany, T. 1990. *The family practice handbook*. Chicago: Year Book Medical Publishers.

Loch, W.E., Alleva, M., and Paparella, M.M. 1990. Sinusitis. *Primary Care* 17(2):323–334.

Loos, G.D. 1990. Pharyngitis, croup, and epiglottitis. *Primary Care* 17(2):335–345.

Maisel, R.H., and Kimberley, B.P. 1988. Treatment of chronic sinusitis with open drainage and cefaclor. *American Journal of Otolaryngology* 9(1):30–33.

Mangura, B.T., Mangura, C.T., and Reichman, L.B. 1991. Tuberculosis and the atypical pneumonia syndrome. *Clinics in Chest Medicine* 12(2):349–362.

Martin, R.E., and Bates, J.H. 1991. Atypical pneumonia. *Infectious Disease Clinics of North America* 5(3):585–601.

Miller, B. 1993. Preventive therapy for tuberculosis. *Medical Clinics of North America* 77(6):1263–1275.

Musher, D.M. 1991. Pneumococcal pneumonia including diagnosis and therapy of infection caused by penicillin-resistant strains. *Infectious Disease Clinics of North America* 5(3):509–521.

Naclerio, R.M. 1991. Allergic rhinitis. *New England Journal of Medicine* 325(12):860–869.

National Institutes of Health. June 1991. *Guidelines for the diagnosis and management of asthma*. Executive Summary of the National Asthma Education Program (Publication No. 91-3042A). Bethesda, MD: NIH.

National Tuberculosis Training Initiative: Core Curriculum on Tuberculosis. Atlanta, Centers for Disease Control, and New York, American Thoracic Society, June 1990.

Nguyen, M.H., Stout, J.E., and Yu, V.L. 1991. Legionellosis. *Infectious Disease Clinics of North America* 5(3):561–584.

Oakes, D.R. 1988. Clinical practitioners guide to respiratory care. Chelmsford, MA: Old Town Health Educator Publications.

Rabinowitz, H.K. 1990. Upper respiratory tract infections. *Primary Care* 17(4):793–809.

Rivo, M.L., and Malveaux, F.J. 1992. Outpatient management of asthma in adults. *American Family Physician* 45(5):2105–2113.

Ruben, F.L. 1989. The prevention of severe lower respiratory infections in chronic bronchitis. *Seminars in Respiratory Infections* 4(4):261–264.

Schappert, S.M. 1993. *National ambulatory medical care survey: 1991 summary*. Advance data from vital and health statistics, No. 230. Hyattsville, MD: National Center for Health Statistics.

Shandera, W. 1993. Infectious diseases:Viral and rickettsial. In *Current medical diagnosis and treatment*, 32d ed., eds. L.M. Tierney, S.J. McPhee, M.A. Papadakis and S.A. Schroeder, pp. 1047–1048. Norwalk, CT: Appleton & Lange.

Shandera, W., and Gill, E.P. 1994. Infectious diseases: Viral and rickettsial. In *Current medical diagnosis and treatment*, 33d ed., eds. L.M. Tierney, Jr., S.J. McPhee, and M.A. Papadakis, pp. 1098–1128. Norwalk, CT: Appleton & Lange.

Slavin, R.G. 1988a. Sinusitis in adults. *Journal of Allergy and Clinical Immunology* 81(5):1028–1032.

———. 1988b. Sinusitis in adults and its relation to allergic rhinitis, asthma, and nasal polyps. *Journal of Allergy and Clinical Immunology* 82(5):950–956.

Stauffer, J.L. 1993. Pulmonary diseases. In *Current medical diagnosis and treatment*, 32nd ed., eds. L.M. Tierney, Jr., S.J. McPhee, M.A. Papadakis, and S.A. Schroeder, pp. 183–262. Norwalk, CT: Appleton & Lange.

———. 1994. Pulmonary diseases. In *Current medical diagnosis and treatment*, 33d ed., eds. L.M. Tierney, Jr., S.J. McPhee, and M.A. Papadakis, pp. 207–279. Norwalk, CT: Appleton & Lange.

Stockley, R.A. 1987. Bronchiectasis—new therapeutic approaches based on pathogenesis. *Respiratory Infections* 8(3):481–494.

Thompson, A.B., Mueller, M.B., Heires, A.J., Bohling, T.L., Daughton, D., Yancey, S.W., Sykes, R.S., and

Rennard, S.I. 1992. Aerosolized beclomethasone in chronic bronchitis. Improved pulmonary function and diminished airway inflammation. *American Review of Respiratory Diseases* 146:389–395.

Toews, G.B. 1987. Nosocomial pneumonia. *Respiratory Infections* 8(3):467–479.

Vitek J.J. 1991. Idiopathic intractable epistaxis: Endovascular therapy. *Radiology* 181:113–116.

Vogt, H.B. 1990. Rhinitis. *Primary Care* 17(2):309–322.

Votey S., and Dudley, J.P. 1989. Emergency ear, nose, and throat procedures. *Emergency Medicine Clinics of North America* 7(1):117–154.

Weiss, K.B., and Wagener, D.K. 1990. Changing patterns of asthma mortality: Identifying target populations at high risk. *Journal of American Medical Association* 264:1683–1687.

Wooley, M. 1990. Duration of protective effect of terbutaline sulfate and cromolyn sodium alone and in combination on exercise-induced asthma. *Chest* 97:39–45.

SECTION 6

Cardiovascular Disorders

Ellen Scarr, M.S.N., F.N.P.

6-A

Angina

Angina pectoris, commonly known as chest pain, is most often caused by atherosclerosis, or *coronary artery disease* (CAD), the result of localized deposits of fat and fibrous tissue (*plaque*) in the subintimal layer of the coronary arteries. Factors promoting the buildup of these deposits include excess intake of saturated fat, excess cholesterol intake, or altered metabolism of lipids.

Angina results from lack of oxygen to the myocardium. The coronary arteries, impeded by atherosclerotic changes, are unable to deliver adequate blood flow to the heart muscle. Often, angina is precipitated by exercise, which increases myocardial oxygen demand. With more extensive disease, angina results from decreased blood flow secondary to obstruction.

Angina also can develop from coronary artery spasm. Vasoconstriction of the artery leads to decreased blood flow, ischemia, and then chest pain. Usually seen with atherosclerosis, spasm also can occur in normal coronary arteries. *Prinzmetal's angina*, commonly found in women under the age of 50 years, develops at rest without precipitating factors, often waking the woman from sleep. The coronary arteries are usually without stenosis.

Cardiovascular disease is the leading cause of death for women in the United States, accounting for more than 500,000 deaths per year. Twice as many women die of cardiovascular disease as die from cancer (Keresztes and Dan 1992).

In the third and fourth decade of life, men have five times more cardiovascular disease than women do. Apparently, women in reproductive years benefit from the cardioprotective benefit of estrogen. In the Framingham Heart Study, no premenopausal women had myocardial infarcts or died of coronary artery disease (Nachtigall 1987).

After menopause, the incidence of CAD increases in women until the seventh decade, when women have the same rate as men. It is postulated that the effect of estrogen on lipid metabolism, particularly its ability to lower *low-density lipoprotein* (LDL) cholesterol—the main atherogenic lipoprotein—protects women from developing CAD. Estrogen also raises *high-density lipoprotein* (HDL), the lipoprotein that transports free cholesterol to the liver for excretion, thereby lowering serum cholesterol (Keresztes and Dan 1992).

Studies have looked at other cardiovascular risk factors in women, many of which are amenable to early intervention. Cigarette smoking, Type A personality, stress, high blood pressure, and diabetes have been identified as factors responsible for the development of CAD, particularly in premenopausal women (Burkman 1988; Perlman et al. 1988).

DATABASE

SUBJECTIVE

→ Symptoms may include:
- chest discomfort usually described as burning, squeezing, tightness, or pressure.
  - Localization of discomfort:
    - usually behind or slightly to left of midsternum.
    - often radiates to left shoulder, left arm.
    - occasionally radiates to jaw, neck, back, or right anterior chest.
  - Timing of chest pain:
    - usually begins with exertion, after meals, or with stress.

–as disease progresses, or if patient has spasm, can occur at night.
- Duration of chest pain:
  –usually lasts several minutes, often resolves after patient stops precipitating activity; resolves without residual pain.
  –persistent pain may be precursor of myocardial infarction (MI).
- Relieving factors:
  –decreases with rest.
  –decreases with nitroglycerin (NTG).

→ Past medical history may include:
- risk factors for coronary disease, including:
  - diabetes.
  - hypertension.
  - CAD.
  - coronary artery spasm.
  - hypercholesterolemia.
  - hypertriglyceridemia.
- conditions related to coronary disease, including:
  - cerebral vascular accident (CVA).
  - peripheral vascular disease.
  - thyroid disease. Patients with hyperthyroidism may present with chest pain.
  - obesity. Being more than 30 percent overweight increases coronary risk.

→ Social history:
- may include use of:
  - cigarettes. More than 10/day increases coronary risk.
  - alcohol.
  - caffeine.
  - drugs (includes recreational drugs).
- activity level. Sedentary patients at higher risk for coronary disease.

→ Family history may include:
- hypertension.
- coronary disease (especially sudden death or MI before 55 years old).
- hypercholesterolemia.

OBJECTIVE

→ If patient is asymptomatic at time of visit, physical assessment to include:
- vital signs.
- weight.
- fundoscopic examination to assess for hypertensive changes, diabetic retinopathy.
- cardiac examination to assess for murmurs, clicks, gallops, rubs.
- lung examination.

- extremity examination to assess for neuropathies, clubbing, edema, cyanosis.
- jugular vein distention.

→ If patient is having chest pain at time of examination, there may be changes in:
- vital signs (often see hypertension; may hear irregular heart rhythm or ectopy).
- cardiac examination (may hear gallop or murmur that is absent when asymptomatic).

→ Electrocardiogram (EKG):
- often normal in patient who is asymptomatic at time of examination. May observe:
  - old infarction.
  - nonspecific ST-T wave changes.
  - intraventricular conduction defects.
  - atrioventricular conduction defects.
  - left ventricular hypertrophy.
  - rhythm disturbances.
  - ectopy.
- if patient is having angina, EKG may demonstrate:
  - ST segment depression (horizontal or downsloping) which reverses as pain resolves.
  - ST segment elevation (with coronary artery spasm or infarction).

ASSESSMENT

→ Angina: acute versus unstable versus stable:
- R/O coronary artery disease
- R/O coronary spasm
- R/O other cardiac etiologies:
  - mitral valve prolapse
  - cardiomyopathy
  - myocarditis
  - pericarditis
  - aortic valve disease
- R/O metabolic etiologies
- R/O musculoskeletal etiologies:
  - costochondritis
  - intercostal neuritis
  - cervical spine disease
  - degenerative joint disease
- R/O gastrointestinal etiologies:
  - peptic ulcer disease
  - esophageal spasm
  - esophageal reflux
- R/O pulmonary etiologies:
  - pneumonia
  - pneumothorax
  - pulmonary embolism
- R/O aortic dissection

PLAN

DIAGNOSTIC TESTS

→ Laboratory data:
- cholesterol level.
- hematocrit.
- renal tests; electrolytes, blood urea nitrogen (BUN), creatinine.
- thyroid tests: TSH, FT4I, T_3.

→ EKG

→ Exercise treadmill test (ETT):
- looks for ischemia precipitated by exercise.
- confirms the diagnosis of angina.
- determines activity level/limitation.
- testing of asymptomatic patients indicated only for high-risk patients including:
  - patients with strong family history of CAD, especially early-onset.
  - patients with hyperlipidemia.
  - older patients beginning exercise program.
  - individuals in occupations involving potential risk to other people (e.g., airline pilots).
- positive test: ≥1 mm horizontal or downsloping ST depression.
  - 60 percent to 80 percent of those with CAD will have positive tests.
  - 10 percent to 20 percent false positives (can decrease this with 2 mm as criterion for ST depression).

→ Thallium scan:
- confirms positive ETT (useful when asymptomatic patient has positive ETT).
- localizes region of ischemia.
- distinguishes ischemia from infarction.
- assesses revascularized myocardium (after bypass surgery or angioplasty).
- also useful if EKG abnormalities make ETT difficult to interpret (intraventricular conduction defects, baseline ST-T wave changes).
- see **Congestive Heart Failure** Protocol.

→ Cardiac catheterization:
- localizes coronary atherosclerosis.
- determines need for revascularization or angioplasty.
- may demonstrate coronary artery spasm.

TREATMENT/MANAGEMENT

→ For patients with acute angina or a history suggesting unstable angina, monitored transport to the nearest acute care facility is indicated.

→ For patients with a history suggesting stable angina, begin risk-factor modification (see "Patient Education" section).

→ In consultation with physician, medication therapy should be started for symptoms suggesting stable angina as follows: (Lehne 1990; Massie and Sokolow 1992):
- NTG gr 1/150 (all patients): 1 tablet sublingually (SL) at onset of chest pain, may repeat 2 more times at 5-minute intervals. If chest pain persists after 15 minutes, advise patient to call 911 or initiate emergency care.
- longer-acting nitrate therapy:
  - isosorbide dinitrate (Isordil®): begin 5 mg p.o. QID; gradually increasing dosage over 1-2 weeks to maximum of 30 mg QID.
  - NTG ointment (2 percent): 1-2 inches every 4-8 hours.
  - NTG transdermal patch: 2.5 mg-15 mg every day.
  - Continuous nitrate blood levels are associated with development of nitrate tolerance. Patient needs certain periods of the day, depending on the level of her pain, when she is nitrate-free.
- Non-nitrate therapy:
  - beta blockers; see **Table 6D.1, Pharmacological Therapies for Hypertension**, pp. 6-19 and 6-20.
  - calcium Channel blockers: see **Table 6D.1**, pp. 6-19 and 6-20.
  - antiplatelet therapy: acetylsalicylic acid (ASA) 325 mg p.o. every day.

CONSULTATION

→ Consult with physician for persistent or worsening symptoms requiring modification of medication regime (increased dosage of single agent or addition of second agent such as beta blocker and long-acting nitrate or calcium channel blocker and long-acting nitrate).

→ Refer to cardiologist for cardiac catheterization when diagnosis of CAD is suspected given results of ETT and/or thallium scan.

→ Refer to cardiologist for angioplasty or to surgeon for bypass grafting, depending on anatomical lesion and location, age, symptoms, comorbid conditions (e.g., diabetes, hypertension, hypercholesterolemia, hypertriglyceridemia, peripheral vascular disease, obesity) and patient's preference.

→ As needed for prescription(s).

PATIENT EDUCATION

→ Advise patient to decrease aggravating factors including strenuous exercise, large meals, and emotional stressors.

→ Advise patient to premedicate with NTG (gr 1/150 SL) before activities known to precipitate angina (e.g., overexertion, large meals, stress, cold exposure).

→ Advise patient to modify risk factors by quitting smoking, lowering cholesterol (LDL <130), increasing exercise, and losing weight (if obese) (see **Hypercholesterolemia** Protocol).

→ Educate patient about medications used:
  ▪ NTG must be stored in dark bottle and discarded after six months.
  ▪ NTG ointment and patches should be applied over hairless skin, rotating site to minimize local irritation.
  ▪ long-acting nitrates must not be discontinued abruptly.

→ Discuss safety of sexual intercourse, giving individual guidelines to patient based on activity level, ETT results. Initiate discussion openly and directly because many patients may hesitate to do so.

→ Encourage patient to participate in cardiac exercise class, teaching isotonic exercises if patient has stable angina.

FOLLOW-UP

→ Maintain weekly contact with patient while initiating and maximizing medication therapy.

→ Once patient stabilized, visits three to four times per year are appropriate to discuss exercise tolerance, symptom control, medication side effects, and need for possible intervention.

→ Document in progress notes and problem list.

Ellen Scarr, M.S.N., F.N.P.

6-B

Congestive Heart Failure

Congestive heart failure (CHF) is a fall in cardiac output with a concomitant rise in pulmonary and systemic venous pressures, with resulting fluid retention (Goroll, May, and Mulley 1987).

CHF may result from an accumulation of excess fluid downstream from either ventricle, hence the terms, *right-sided* and *left-sided heart failure*. While right-sided heart failure will be more likely to present with jugular venous distention and ascites, and left-sided failure with dyspnea and pulmonary congestion, clinically it can be difficult to distinguish between the two. Despite the underlying etiology, prolongation of either right-sided or left-sided heart failure soon leads to overall heart failure.

There are numerous etiologies of CHF, the most common of which are hypertension, coronary artery disease (CAD), and valvular heart disease. However, the clinical manifestations and principles of management are fairly uniform.

The goal of therapy in CHF is to:

→ decrease preload:
  ▪ lower filling pressures in the heart, reduce venous return to the heart.

→ decrease afterload:
  ▪ lower systemic vascular resistance.

→ strengthen myocardial contractility:
  ▪ increase cardiac output.

Treatment modalities will reduce the symptoms of CHF, but diagnosis and treatment of the underlying disease process, if possible, are crucial.

DATABASE

SUBJECTIVE

→ Symptoms may include:
  ▪ initial presentation/mild cases:
    • easily fatigued.
    • dyspnea on exertion.
    • unexplained weight gain.
  ▪ progressive symptoms:
    • worsening fatigue, decreased exercise tolerance.
    • dyspnea on exertion or at rest.
    • orthopnea.
    • paroxysmal nocturnal dyspnea.
    • edema; lower extremity most common but may see edema of upper extremities and periorbitally.
    • palpitations, intermittent or constant.
    • chest pains, exertional and/or at rest.

→ Past medical history may include:
  ▪ cardiac disease:
    • arrhythmias.
    • hypertension.
    • CAD.
    • valvular heart disease.
    • pericarditis.
  ▪ pulmonary disease:
    • pulmonary embolism.
  ▪ thyroid disease.
  ▪ anemia.
  ▪ pregnancy.

→ Medications may include: negative inotropes—
  e.g., beta blockers, digitalis, verapamil.

→ Family history may include cardiac and pulmonary
  disease.

→ Social history:
  ▪ may include use of:
    • tobacco.
    • alcohol.
    • recreational drugs.
  ▪ dietary habits: intake of excess salt, highly
    processed foods.
  ▪ exercise. Exercise may precipitate CHF.
  ▪ stressors. Emotional stress may precipitate CHF.

OBJECTIVE

→ Vital signs may include:
  ▪ elevated temperature. Infection can precipitate
    CHF.
  ▪ increased pulse rate.
    • Tachycardia tries to compensate for decreased
      cardiac output but jeopardizes coronary artery
      filling during diastole.
  ▪ increase or decrease in blood pressure.
    • Initially elevated or maintained as a result of
      fluid retention and increased heart rate, but
      subsequently falls.
  ▪ increased respiratory rate.
    • Tachypnea results from pulmonary congestion
      and hypoxia.
  ▪ increased weight.
    • Provides parameter to measure efficacy of
      treatment or worsening of symptoms.

→ Physical examination to include:
  ▪ mental status examination to assess for
    decreased cerebral blood flow.
  ▪ ophthalmic examination to assess for retinal
    changes.
  ▪ pulmonary examination to assess for:
    • bibasilar rales.
    • bronchospasm.
    • tachypnea.
    • decreased oxygen saturation; assess SAO_2
      with pulse oximetry.
  ▪ cardiac examination to assess for:
    • rhythm/rate.
    • heaves, lifts, diffuse point of maximal impulse
      (PMI).
    • murmurs, especially mitral regurgitation or
      aortic stenosis.
    • gallops, especially S_3.

–Indicative of decreased ejection fraction, left
 ventricular dilatation, and increasing left
 atrial pressure.
  ▪ right-sided S_3.
    • Indicative of right ventricular failure.
  ▪ jugular venous distention.
  ▪ Abdominal examination to assess for:
    • ascites.
    • venous distention.
    • hepatojugular reflex.
    • hepatomegaly.
  ▪ Extremity examination to assess for:
    • edema.
    • cyanosis.

ASSESSMENT

→ Congestive heart failure
  ▪ R/O valvular heart disease
  ▪ R/O CAD
  ▪ R/O pericarditis
  ▪ R/O arrhythmias
  ▪ R/O hypertensive heart disease
  ▪ R/O hypertrophic cardiomyopathy
  ▪ R/O pulmonary embolism
  ▪ R/O alcoholic or postviral cardiomyopathy
  ▪ R/O chronic obstructive pulmonary disease
    (COPD)
  ▪ R/O infection (endocarditis, pneumonia)
  ▪ R/O liver disease
  ▪ R/O renal disease
  ▪ R/O venous insufficiency

PLAN

DIAGNOSTIC TESTS

→ The goal is to identify the underlying cause of
  CHF. Determination of appropriate therapy then
  follows.

→ Acute diagnostic work-up.
  ▪ Chest x-ray to assess for:
    • increased pulmonary vasculature.
    • increased interstitial markings
      (Kerley "B" lines and perihilar haziness).
    • enlarged heart size.
  ▪ EKG to assess for:
    • left ventricular hypertrophy (LVH).
    • "p" mitrale.
    • left atrial hypertrophy (LAH).
    • arrhythmias.
    • ST-T wave changes suggestive of ischemia.
  ▪ Labs may include:
    • CBC.

- electrolytes.
- renal function tests.
- liver function tests.
- thyroid function tests.
- arterial blood gases or pulse oximetry.

→ Other diagnostic tests (in consultation).
  - Echocardiogram:
    - R/O valvular disease.
    - R/O pericarditis.
    - assess LVH.
    - assess cardiac function—ejection fraction.
    - assess wall motion abnormalities.
  - Computerized tomography (CT) or magnetic resonance imaging (MRI).
    - Use determined by underlying etiology of CHF, echocardiogram findings, and need for further evaluation.
  - cardiac catheterization.
    - Left and right heart hemodynamics.
    - Assess cardiac function.
    - R/O ischemic CAD.
    - Assess hemodynamics in pericarditis.
  - Pulmonary ventilation/perfusion scan.
    - R/O pulmonary embolism.
  - Nuclear medicine wall motion study.
  - ETT.
    - If indicates ischemia, or if patient has arrythmias making it difficult to interpret EKG changes, may do ETT with thallium to indicate areas of cardiac hypoperfusion.
    - Newer technetium perfusion agents (with shorter half-lives) now available.
      - Sestamibil (Cardiolite®).
      - Teroroxine (Cardiotec®).
    - If patient unable to exercise, may use pharmacological agents to assess the myocardium under stress.
      - Dypyndamole (Persantine®).
      - Adenosine (Adenocard®).
      - Dobutamine (Dobutrex®).

TREATMENT/MANAGEMENT

→ Acute onset CHF.
  - May require hospitalization (in consultation) for:
    - oxygen.
    - diuretics.
    - vasoactive drugs.
    - correction of identified precipitating factors
      - infection/high fever.
      - severe anemia.
      - tachycardia.
      - pulmonary emboli.
        ‣ Anticoagulation.
        ‣ Surgical intervention.

→ Mild or chronic/stable CHF (see **Table 6D.1**, pp. 6-19 and 6-20).
  - Low-dose diuretics.
    - Reduce preload (by eliminating excess fluid).
    - Lower right- and left-heart filling pressures.
    - Improve dyspnea, orthopnea, edema.
    - Furosemide (Lasix®) as drug of choice: 20 mg-40 mg p.o. BID; may add thiazide drug if needed.
  - Nitrate therapy.
    - Reduce preload (by venodilation).
    - Improve coronary artery blood flow.
    - Begin with isosorbide dinitrate (Isordil®) 10 mg p.o. QID, increase as needed to maximum of 80 mg QID.
  - Vasodilators.
    - Arterial agents reduce afterload, thereby increasing cardiac output.
    - Venous agents decrease preload, thereby decreasing pulmonary fluid overload.
    - ACE inhibitors: captopril (Capoten®), enalapril (Vasotec®), lisinopril (Prinivil®, Zestril®), ramipril (Altace®).
      - Begin captopril: 25 mg p.o. BID, increase as tolerated to maximum of 100 mg TID–QID.
  - Inotropes.
    - Digitalis has been mainstay of therapy for years. In mild CHF, begin digoxin (Lanoxin®) 0.25 mg p.o. every day.
      - Useful with LVH, persistent S_3, severe aortic stenosis, rapid atrial fibrillation.
      - Symptoms of digitalis toxicity include nausea, vomiting, diarrhea, arrhythmias.
      - Newer oral sympathomimetic nonglycosides (perbuterol, prenalterol) and non-sympathomimetic agents (amrinone, milrinone) have proven disappointing in outpatient management of CHF.
    - Calcium channel blockers (see **Table 6D.1**, pp. 6-19 and 6-20).
      - Use cautiously. Negative inotrope effect may outweigh benefit.
      - Useful in cardiomyopathies, hypertension.
      - Improve exercise tolerance.
    - Beta blockers.
      - Usually contraindicated in CHF because of their negative inotropic effect, but may be used cautiously to treat the causative process (e.g., hypertension, angina).

CONSULTATION

→ For patients with acute-onset CHF, consult physician regarding initial work-up and treatment.

→ For patients with progressive CHF refractory to medication therapy, refer to cardiologist or internist for stabilization.

→ In consultation, treat underlying etiology of CHF (if possible):
- valvular heart disease/CAD/arrhythmias:
  - initiate medication per consultation.
  - cardiology/cardiothoracic surgery referral.
- hypertension:
  - initiate medication (see **Hypertension** Protocol).
  - consider underlying etiologies of hypertension.
- thyroid disease:
  - initiate medication per consultation (see **Thyroid Disorders** Protocol).
- pulmonary disease/pulmonary embolism:
  - referral for anticoagulation or pulmonary evaluation.
- infection:
  - treat underlying etiology as appropriate.

→ For patients with end-state CHF, referral to a physician is indicated.
- Cardiac transplantation may be considered.

→ As needed for prescription(s).

PATIENT EDUCATION

→ Educate patient and family regarding pathophysiology and treatment plan.
- Provide medication instructions including:
  - possibility of multiple medications.
  - avoidance of evening dosing of diuretics.
  - symptoms of drug toxicity.

→ Advise patients with symptoms of worsening CHF to:
- keep daily weight record before eating breakfast.
- call if gain of more than two to three pounds in one week.

→ Advise patient regarding dietary management including:

- avoiding salting foods at table or during cooking.
- avoiding foods with high sodium content.
- increasing dietary potassium—especially on diuretic therapy—with 10 oz. orange, pineapple, or grapefruit juice; one medium banana; two oranges; medium-sized baked potato (all include 15 mEq of potassium). If taking potassium supplements, may mix with any of the above juices.
- weight reduction if needed.
- fluid restriction if hyponatremic or in severe CHF.

→ Advise patient to schedule daily rest, but avoid prolonged bed rest, venous stasis.

→ Educate patient regarding stress reduction activities.

FOLLOW-UP

→ For patients on diuretic therapy:
- monitor serum potassium, BUN, and creatinine weekly until stabilized, then every two to three months as indicated.
- monitor postural vital signs to assess for hypovolemia.
- assess need for potassium supplementation, which usually is necessary when patient is on furosemide.
- if hypokalemia occurs, begin potassium chloride elixir, 20 mEq in one tablespoon (15cc) TID.

→ For patients on ACE-inhibitor therapy, monitor blood pressure, BUN, creatinine, and white blood-cell count weekly, then every two to three months.

→ For patients on digitalis therapy:
- monitor pulse rate, rhythm, BUN, creatinine, potassium, and serum digitalis level in one week after initiation, adjusting dose as necessary.
- digitalis levels should be monitored at least every three to four months.

→ Monitor exercise tolerance via patient report. Patient may note decreased symptoms at rest but not with activity. Adjust/maximize medications as indicated.

→ Document in progress notes and problem list.

6-C

Hypercholesterolemia

Hypercholesterolemia—defined as a serum cholesterol level of ≥ 200 mg/dl—is a strong predictor of coronary artery disease (CAD) (Castelli 1988). Most often, an elevated serum cholesterol is caused by excessive dietary intake. Other causes include an underlying disease state that results in hyperlipidemia or an inherited error in lipid metabolism.

The *total serum cholesterol* is the sum of the cholesterol concentrations of *very low-density lipoproteins* (VLDL), low-density lipoprotein (LDL), and high-density lipoproteins (HDL). (VLDL is calculated by dividing the fasting serum triglyceride level by 5.)

LDL cholesterol is known to cause atherosclerosis in the aorta and coronary arteries. Conversely, HDL is cardioprotective: the higher the HDL concentration, the lower the risk of coronary disease. Raised LDLs and lowered HDLs separately and jointly determine atherosclerosis, with HDLs being the more important predictor (Oliver 1992; Baron 1992).

Cholesterol levels increase with age, and men have higher levels than women until age 50 years. Women generally have higher concentrations of HDLs (Peters 1987). In the Framingham Heart Study, elevated triglyceride levels were found to be an independent predictor of increased risk for CAD in women (Castelli 1988).

Major primary prevention trials—including the Finnish Mental Hospital Study, the Lipid Research Clinics Coronary Prevention Trial, and the Helsinki Heart Study—clearly show that lowering of LDL and serum cholesterol will decrease the incidence of atherosclerosis in men (Oliver 1992). It is unclear exactly what impact hypercholesterolemia has in women, who do not develop extensive coronary disease until after menopause.

There have been no clinical trials for women only. Until such trials are performed, it seems prudent to extrapolate data on the effects of hypercholesterolemia in men.

DATABASE

SUBJECTIVE

→ Past medical history may include other conditions associated with hypercholesterolemia:
  ▪ hypertension.
  ▪ increased cholesterol/increased LDL.
  ▪ CAD.
  ▪ diabetes.
  ▪ cerebral vascular accident (CVA)/transient ischemic attack (TIA).
  ▪ peripheral vascular disease.

→ Family history may include:
  ▪ hypercholesterolemia.
  ▪ premature CAD (MI or sudden death before age 55 years in parent or sibling).

→ Social history may include:
  ▪ cigarette smoking.

→ Dietary history may include:
  ▪ high percentage of calories from fat on 24-hour diet recall. Ideally diet should contain less than 30 percent of calories from fat.
  ▪ budget restrictions influencing food purchases.

OBJECTIVE

→ Physical examination to include:
  ▪ weight.
  ▪ blood pressure.

- cardiovascular examination to assess for:
  - bruits.
  - signs of arterial insufficiency:
    - absent or decreased pulses.
    - pale color on extremity elevation; dusky red color when extremity is dependent.
    - cool skin temperature.
    - thin, shiny skin with absent hair.
    - thick, ridged finger nails.
→ Serum cholesterol (non-fasting).

ASSESSMENT

→ Hypercholesterolemia
  - R/O genetic hyperlipidemia

PLAN

DIAGNOSTIC TESTS
(Baron 1992; Knopp and Mishell 1988)

→ If non-fasting serum cholesterol is ≥240 mg/dl, obtain fractional levels (HDL, LDL, VLDL) after 12-hour fast. **NOTE**: Many clinicians obtain fractional levels if non-fasting cholesterol is ≥200 mg/dl to aid in early detection and enhance dietary modification and patient education.

→ If serum cholesterol is borderline high (200-239 mg/dl) and patient has CAD or 2 other risks for CAD (see **Angina** Protocol), obtain fractional levels.

→ Obtain 2 to 3 measurements, 1 to 8 weeks apart.

TREATMENT/MANAGEMENT

→ Determined by patient's LDL.

→ Use goals as minimums; the lower the level, the lower the risk.

→ Goals include:
  - LDL to <160 in low-risk patients.
  - LDL to <130 in high-risk patients.
  - LDL to <100 in patients with CAD.

→ If LDL ≥160 in low-risk patients, ≥130 in high-risk patients, or ≥100 in patients with CAD, initiate diet therapy.

→ If LDL borderline (130-160), initiate diet therapy if have CAD or two risk factors for CAD.

→ Dietary Therapy (Step 1):
  - saturated fat to <10 percent of calories.
  - total fat to <30 percent of calories.
  - dietary cholesterol to <300 mg/dl.
  - most benefit is achieved within 1 to 2 years.

- diet usually requires severe fat restriction to be effective.
- treatment of low-risk women (premenopausal women, women with elevated HDLs) probably not indicated.

→ Re-evaluation after 4 to 6 weeks of dietary therapy (Step 1) and again at 3 months:
  - if cholesterol is decreased to desired level (including LDL), continue Step 1 therapy and obtain total cholesterol 4 times in the first year, twice a year thereafter.
  - if desired cholesterol level not achieved, modify dietary therapy to Step 2 as follows:
    - saturated fat to <7 percent of calories.
    - dietary cholesterol to <200 mg/day and refer to registered dietitian. Obtain cholesterol in 4 to 6 weeks and at 3 months (total of 6 months of dietary therapy).
  - if desired level still not achieved, obtain LDL and consider drug therapy (National Cholesterol Education Program 1988).

→ Drug Therapy Guidelines (see **Table 6C.1, Pharmacological Therapies for Hypercholesterolemia**. Consult *PDR*.
  - Drugs are a supplement to ongoing dietary therapy.
  - If LDL is 160-189, and the woman is without CAD risks, implement maximal dietary modification and consider low-dose bile acid-binding resins.
    - Monitor CAD risk factors.
    - Obtain cholesterol yearly.
  - If the LDL is ≥190, or ≥160 in women with CAD or CAD risk factors, implement maximal dietary modification and initiate drug therapy (bile acid-binding resins with or without a second agent such as lovastatin).
    - Obtain LDL in 4 to 6 weeks and at 3 months.
      - If LDL has decreased, continue therapy, monitor cholesterol level every 4 months, and check LDL yearly.
      - If LDL remains elevated, consider another drug or combination drug therapy. Consider referral to lipid disorder specialist to assess for genetic disorder (National Cholesterol Education Program 1988).

CONSULTATION

→ Registered dietitian can facilitate dietary instruction and planning of meals.

→ Physician consultation if dietary modification unsuccessful and drug therapy being considered.

Table 6C.1. PHARMACOLOGICAL THERAPIES FOR HYPERCHOLESTEROLEMIA

Drug	Dosage	Actions	Side Effects/Comments
Bile Acid-Binding Resins+			

1. Cholestyramine (Questran®)
 	
2. Colestipol HCl (Colestid®)
	• 12 gm-16 gm/d in 2-4 divided doses*
	
	• 15 gm-30 gm/d in 2-4 divided doses*
		• Lowers LDL
		  –maximal reduction of approximately 20% achieved by one month.
			• Can raise VLDL level
			  –avoid in patients whose VLDL levels are already elevated.
			• Safest of lipoprotein-lowering drugs.
			• Can cause constipation (↓ with dietary fiber and fluids), bloating, indigestion, and nausea.
			• Can bind with thiazide diuretics, digitalis, anticoagulants, and some antibiotics; need to take these drugs either 1 hour before or 4 hours after taking bile acid-binding resins.

*Must be reconstituted with fluid before taking.			
Nicotinic Acid+			

(Many trade names)	• 2 gm-8 gm/d in 3 divided doses (with meals or immediately after meals)
	  –(Begin with 100 mg TID with meals and gradually ↑ dose)
		• Lowers VLDL 20%-80%.
		• Lowers LDL 10%-15%
		  –maximal effect takes 3-5 weeks.
		• When used with bile acid-binding resin, lowers LDL 40%-60%.
			• Frequent side effects
			  –skin reactions (flushing, itching).
			  –GI (nausea, vomiting, diarrhea).
			• Can ↓ flushing by taking ASA 30 minutes before nicotinic acid.
			• Can cause arrhythmias, jaundice, glucose abnormalities, gout. Use with caution in patients with heart disease, liver disease, diabetes, or gout.

+First-line drugs.			
HMG-COA Reductase Inhibitors			

1. **Lovastatin** (Mevacor®)
 	
2. **Simvastatin** (Zocor®)
 	
3. **Pravastatin** (Pravachol;®)
	• 20 mg/d-80 mg/d with meals (in single or divided doses)
	
	• 10 mg/d-40 mg/d
	
	• 20 mg/d-40 mg/d
		• Lowers LDL, VLDL, total cholesterol, and triglycerides
		  –maximal effect in 4 to 6 weeks.
		  –effect enhanced when used with bile acid-binding resins.
		• HDL unchanged or increased.
			• Best taken at night.
			• Transient, mild side effects:
			  –GI upset (nausea, constipation, diarrhea, cramping).
			  –headache.
			  –rash.
			• Rarer side effects:
			  –hepatotoxicity
			    –Check LFTs every 4 to 6 weeks during first year of therapy, periodically thereafter (every 3 to 6 months).
			    –Caution in patients with liver disease, alcohol abuse.
			  –myositis.
			• Contraindicated in pregnancy/breast-feeding.
			• Relatively new drugs, very effective. May soon be considered first-line. Data lack on long-term safety.

Continued

→ See additional consultation/referral in "Follow-Up," "Treatment/Management," and "Drug Therapy Guidelines" sections.

→ As needed for prescription(s).

PATIENT EDUCATION

→ Advise patient that hypercholesterolemia is a CAD risk factor that she can modify.

→ Educate patient regarding correlation between hypercholesterolemia and CAD.

→ Advise patient that many dietary aids are available to assist with planning low-cholesterol meals, including American Heart Association and other low-cholesterol cookbooks, cholesterol counters, and cholesterol and fat information available on most food labels.

→ Educate patient regarding specific dietary planning, incorporating food preferences and budgetary restrictions. See **General Nutrition Guidelines**.

→ Advise patient that regular aerobic exercise, quitting smoking (if applicable), and weight loss (if obese) can raise desirable HDLs.

→ If drug therapy is initiated, advise patient that maximal dietary modification still is necessary.

Table 6C.1.   PHARMACOLOGICAL THERAPIES FOR HYPERCHOLESTEROLEMIA CONTINUED

Drug	Dosage	Actions	Side Effects/Comments
Fibrates			

1. **Gemfibrozil***
 (Lopid®)
	600 mg BID (30 min. before breakfast and dinner)	• Lowers VLDL
		   –40% to 55% after one month of treatment.
		 • Increases HDL by 25%.
		 • Lowers triglycerides.
			• Variable effects on LDL levels.
			 • May cause gallstones.
			   –contraindicated in those with gall bladder disease.
			 • Increases anticoagulant drug effects.
			 • Should not be used concomitantly with lovastatin.

2. **Clofibrate***
 (Atromid-S®)
	2 gm/d in 2-4 divided doses	• Lowers VLDL
		   –20% decrease within one week.
		 • May lower LDL or, in some cases, raise LDL.
			• Decreasing in popularity
			   –serious side effects.
			   –lack of beneficial decrease in cardiovasular mortality.
			 • Side effects:
			   –flu-like syndrome.
			   –GI.
			   –gallstones.
			   –cardiovascular effects.
			    –arrhythmias.
			    –cardiomegaly.
			    –chest pain.
			    –pulmonary embolism.
			    –peripheral vascular disease.
			    –claudication.
			 • Increases effect of phenytoin and oral anticoagulants.
			 • Contraindicated in pregnancy and breast-feeding.

Probucol*
 (Lorelco®)
	500 mg BID with breakfast and dinner	Lowers LDLs and HDLs
		   –10% to 15% reduction in 1 to 3 months.
			• Long-term effects unknown.
			 • Lasts in body 6 months after discontinuation because of high lipid solubility.
			 • Mild side effects:
			   –GI upset.
			 • Causes arrhythmias in animals (not yet seen in humans).
			   –obtain baseline EKG and repeat in 6 months, then yearly.
			   –avoid in patients with ventricular arrhythmias or myocardial damage.

*Not considered major drugs for treatment of hypercholesterolemia.

→ If drug therapy is initiated, provide detailed information regarding side effects and specific measures to manage these side effects. See *PDR*.

FOLLOW-UP

→ Obtain serum cholesterol on all adults once every five years.

→ At every visit, encourage patients to continue with diet and pharmacological therapy as indicated.

→ Document in progress notes and problem list.

Ellen Scarr, M.S.N., F.N.P.

6-D

Hypertension

Hypertension (HTN), a significant health problem for American women, is a treatable, often preventable cause of cardiovascular morbidity and mortality. Coronary artery disease (CAD), angina, myocardial infarction (MI), and stroke are all directly related to hypertension, and account for the deaths of more than 500,000 women each year (Castelli 1988).

In the *Fifth Report of the Joint National Committee on Detection, Evaluation, and Treatment of High Blood Pressure* (1993), the classification of HTN was revised as follows:

	Systolic BP	Diastolic BP
Normal	< 130 mmHg	< 85 mmHg
High Normal	130-139	85-89
Hypertension		
Stage 1 (mild)	140-159	90-99
Stage 2 (moderate)	160-179	100-109
Stage 3 (severe)	180-209	110-119
Stage 4 (very severe)	≥ 210	≥ 120

If a woman's systolic and diastolic blood pressures fall into different stages, the higher category is used to classify the blood pressure status. The diagnosis of HTN is based on the average of two or more readings taken at each of two or more visits, after the initial screening. Optimal blood pressure with respect to a woman's cardiovascular risk is <120/<80.

Blood pressure is determined by cardiac output, heart rate, and vascular resistance, and is regulated by the renin-angiotensin-aldosterone system and the sympathetic nervous system. Multiple factors may contribute to the development of hypertension. In 95 percent of cases, no single cause can be identified, a condition known as *primary*, or *essential hypertension* (Massie and Sokolow 1993; Nachtigall 1987).

In the other approximately five percent of cases, there is an underlying cause of hypertension. These causes include:

→ oral contraceptive use:
- most common cause of secondary hypertension.
- reversible with discontinuation of pills.
- no known association between *post-menopausal estrogen therapy* and development of hypertension (Massie and Sokolow 1993).

→ pregnancy-induced hypertension:
- common cause in childbearing women.

→ renal vascular hypertension:
- disorders of the renal parenchyma.
- stenosis of the renal arteries.
- may respond to surgical or pharmacological therapy.

→ primary aldosteronism:
- rare etiology.

→ pheochromocytoma:
- rare etiology.

→ coarctation of the aorta:
- aortic narrowing, usually discovered in childhood or adolescence.

→ thyroid/parathyroid diseases.

→ hypercalcemia.

→ neurological disorders.

The treatment of hypertension in women remains controversial because of the lack of well-controlled studies. Studies of pharmacologically treated male hypertensives with mild HTN show prevention of stroke, of congestive heart failure (CHF), and of worsening HTN. But they do not conclusively demonstrate reduced cardiovascular mortality (Baron 1991). Studies suggest that comorbid conditions (e.g., diabetes, EKG abnormalities, smoking ten or more cigarettes per day, elevated LDL cholesterol, family history of early cardiovascular disease) as well as coexisting systolic HTN are predictive of cardiovascular mortality in men, and may determine need for earlier pharmacological intervention (rather than allowing for a trial of lifestyle modification) (Perez-Stable 1989).

It is unclear how these studies correlate to women. Further studies are needed. Treatment benefit determinations suggest postponing pharmacological intervention in white women until the diastolic BP (DBP) reaches 100, with lower DBP readings appropriate for black women (Browner 1988). Meanwhile, it seems prudent to adopt the most recent guidelines for the treatment of HTN for women.

The guidelines for the treatment of HTN, as presented by the Fifth Report of the Joint National Committee (JNC V), are outlined here:

Lifestyle modification is emphasized as initial therapy for patients with Stages 1 and 2 HTN, as well as ongoing therapy for those requiring pharmacological intervention. Lifestyle modifications include:

→ weight loss. Thirty percent of HTN cases are associated with obesity (Arakawa 1989). Excess caloric intake stimulates catecholamines, sympathetic activity, and insulin secretion, all of which may cause an increase in sodium retention, then an increase in renin-angiotensin-aldosterone activity. Weight loss can lower blood pressure and decrease left ventricular hypertrophy (LVH) (Graettinger and Weber 1992).

→ sodium reduction. The impact of sodium on HTN remains controversial. Studies suggest some hypertensives are "salt-sensitive," especially elderly and African American patients (Arakawa 1989; Baron 1991). For some patients, reduced-sodium diets are easier than weight loss and/or exercise, and most people lose their taste for salt (NaCl) after three months. Also, sodium restriction increases the efficacy of many antihypertensives, allowing a decrease in medication dosage (Lehne 1990).

→ decreased alcohol consumption. Many studies show an association between alcohol intake and HTN. This is true especially in those whose intake is three or more drinks per day. A study at Kaiser Permanente health maintenance organization demonstrated this relationship to be more common in whites and Asian Americans than in African Americans, greater in women than in men, and greater in the elderly (Baron 1991). The physiological mechanism appears to be the result of increased vascular resistance. Excessive alcohol intake also increases the risk of stroke, but not of CAD (Arakawa 1989).

→ increased exercise. Regular exercise has been shown to lower blood pressure, vascular resistance, LDL, and total cholesterol, and increase HDL cholesterol (Arakawa 1989; Baron 1991).

→ elimination of cigarette smoking. Nicotine has only a transient effect on blood pressure (Nachtigall 1987). However, studies show it increases the risk of coronary disease and MI in women over 50 years old, in addition to its clear association with lung cancer.

Other non-pharmacological interventions that may benefit hypertensive women are:

→ adequate calcium intake. Studies of calcium supplementation have shown inconsistent effects on blood pressure, possibly lowering systolic, but not diastolic (Baron 1991).

→ increased potassium intake. The usual diet contains 60 mmol of potassium. Some studies suggest a mild reduction in blood pressure with an additional 60 mmol of dietary potassium. Pharmacological potassium supplementation is not indicated as an initial, isolated approach to blood pressure reduction (Baron 1991).

→ stress reduction techniques. Some studies demonstrate mild reductions in blood pressure by decreasing sympathetic activity, especially in patients who respond to stress with increased heart rate and pulse (Arakawa 1989; Waddell 1986).

Pharmacological Treatment

If a woman with Stage 1 or Stage 2 HTN continues to have a blood pressure of >140/90 despite three to six months of lifestyle modification, the JNC V recommends the initiation of single-drug therapy. Diuretics or beta-blockers are the drugs of first choice. These are the only agents shown to reduce morbidity and mortality in long-term clinical trials (Alderman 1992).

Calcium channel blockers and ACE inhibitors have been deleted from the guidelines as agents of first choice. While these drugs do lower blood pressure and exert other potentially beneficial effects, they have not been shown to decrease morbidity and mortality in long-term studies. These agents are now reserved for those patients in whom diuretics or beta-blockers are ineffective, unacceptable, or contraindicated because of co-morbid conditions (JNC V 1993).

→ Diuretics:
  ▪ are widely used.
  ▪ are effective in all populations, especially elderly patients, African American patients, smokers, and obese patients.
  ▪ are safely used with other agents.
  ▪ work by decreasing the circulating blood volume (increase excretion of sodium and water), as well as decreasing vascular resistance (in long-term therapy).
→ Beta-blockers:
  ▪ are useful in younger patients, Caucasian patients, non-smokers (Medical Research Council trials showed no benefit of propranolol over placebo in smokers [Perez-Stable 1991]).
  ▪ are useful in patients with known CAD, prior MI, migraines, anxiety.
  ▪ work by decreasing heart rate, cardiac output, and renin release.

LVH has been shown to increase the risk of cardiovascular morbidity and mortality (Browner 1988; Graettinger and Weber 1992; Perez-Stable 1991). If present, certain antihypertensives (ACE inhibitors, calcium channel blockers, selected beta-blockers) can be utilized to stabilize or decrease LVH.

The efficacy of beta-blockers or ACE inhibitors in African American patients can be enhanced with concomitant use of a thiazide diuretic (Perez-Stable 1991).

DATABASE

SUBJECTIVE

→ Most patients are asymptomatic but may complain of headaches, blurred vision, dizziness, tinnitus, chest pain, shortness of breath, nausea, edema, and/or anxiety.
→ Past medical history may include:
  ▪ hypertension. Elicit information regarding:
    • type of therapy.
    • length of therapy.
    • efficacy of treatment.
    • side effects of pharmacological therapy.
  ▪ diabetes, hypercholesterolemia, hyper-triglyceridemia, CAD, cerebrovascular disease, renal disease, obesity.
  ▪ oral contraceptive use.

  ▪ menopause.
  ▪ estrogen therapy.
→ Medication history may include the following (especially those which can elevate blood pressure or interfere with anti-hypertensive medications):
  ▪ oral contraceptives.
  ▪ steroids.
  ▪ nonsteroidal anti-inflammatory drugs (NSAIDs).
  ▪ decongestants.
  ▪ appetite suppressants.
  ▪ tricyclic antidepressants.
  ▪ MAO inhibitors.
  ▪ cocaine.
  ▪ amphetamines.
  ▪ cyclosporine.
  ▪ erythropoietin.
→ Family history may include:
  ▪ hypertension.
  ▪ CAD.
  ▪ stroke.
  ▪ diabetes.
→ Social history:
  ▪ may include use of:
    • cigarettes.
    • alcohol.
    • caffeine.
    • recreational drugs.
      −quantify amounts.
  ▪ obtain information on:
    • activity level. Quantify amount of aerobic exercise per week.
    • ethnicity, food habits. Obtain description of usual diet, noting sodium intake, highly processed and fast-food intake, and total calories.
    • emotional stressors. Obtain description of stressors and coping mechanisms.
    • economic situation, occupation. Include information about job stress, ability to pay for health care and medicines.

OBJECTIVE

→ Physical examination to include:
  ▪ vital signs
    • including blood pressure in both arms, sitting and standing, three or more readings (over several weeks to months).
  ▪ neurological examination.
  ▪ fundoscopic examination to assess for spasm or thickening of arteriolar walls, silver wire arterioles, or copper wire arterioles.

- neck examination to assess for jugular vein distention, carotid bruits, enlarged thyroid.
- chest examination to assess for rales, rhonchi, and wheezes.
- heart examination to assess rate, rhythm, murmurs, gallops, rubs, thrills, heaves.
- abdomen examination to assess for aortic bruit, renal artery bruit, iliac bruit, hepatomegaly, hepatojugular reflex.
- extremity examination to assess for edema, clubbing, cyanosis, bilateral comparison of peripheral pulses.

→ Labs usually normal in uncomplicated cases of essential HTN.

→ EKG may show LVH or ST-T wave abnormalities.

→ Chest x-ray usually normal, though may show cardiomegaly, aortic dilatation or calcification, congestive heart failure; rarely, rib notching in coarctation.

ASSESSMENT

→ Hypertension:
- primary (essential)
- R/O secondary

PLAN

DIAGNOSTIC TESTS

→ Laboratory data.
- Prior to initiating pharmacological therapy, obtain baseline labs to rule out treatable causes of hypertension, evaluate other cardiovascular risks.
- CBC, urinalysis, renal function tests, electrolytes, fasting blood sugar, fasting lipid panel.

→ EKG.

→ Chest x-ray.
- As indicated; may defer in young, essentially healthy hypertensive.
- May see rib-notching if patient has coarctation of the aorta.

→ Echocardiography.
- Consider if there is evidence of LVH.

→ Further studies.
- Intravenous pyelogram, renal sonogram, thyroid tests warranted only if symptoms suggest secondary hypertension. Consult with physician.

TREATMENT/MANAGEMENT

→ Lifestyle modifications should be initiated for all patients with HTN.
- May avoid drug use and subsequent side effects.
- Safe, acceptable, cost-effective.
- Even those requiring earlier pharmacological intervention (moderate to severe hypertension, comorbid conditions) will benefit from non-pharmacological interventions to reduce risk factors.
- A single intervention intensively applied may be more successful than multiple interventions (Baron 1991).
- Weight loss.
  - Low calorie diet—1200 calories per day.
  - Very low-calorie diet, modified fast—less than 500 calories per day.
  - Aerobic exercise. Begin with 30 minutes 2 to 3 times per week, increasing as tolerated.
- Reduced sodium.
  - Restrict sodium intake to 2 gm/day (equivalent to 5 gm NaCl/day).
  - No salt added to cooking.
  - No salt on table.
  - Avoid heavily processed foods.
- Decreased alcohol consumption.
  - Limit alcohol to no more than 1 oz. of ethanol per day.
    - 1 ounce ethanol = 2 oz. 100-proof whiskey.
      - 8 oz. wine.
      - 24 oz. beer.
- Increased exercise.
- Cessation of cigarette smoking.
- Increased calcium intake.
  - At least 800 mg/day.
- Increased dietary potassium.
  - Fresh fruits, vegetables.
- Stress reduction techniques.
  - Breathing, deep muscle relaxation, meditation.
- Pharmacological Therapy (see **Table 6D.1**).
- Begin low-dose medication, choosing one of the agents now advisable for initial therapy:
  - diuretics.
  - beta-blockers.
- If blood pressure control is inadequate:
  - increase dose of initial medication, or,
  - substitute different (initial) medication, or,
  - add low dose of second medication to the first.

Table 6D.1. PHARMACOLOGICAL THERAPIES FOR HYPERTENSION

Drug	Dosage	Side Effects	Comments
DIURETICS			
1. Thiazides			
a. Chlorthalidone (Hygroton®)	25 mg-200 mg/day	— ↑ total cholesterol — ↑ LDL	• In men, a low-fat diet limited the effect of thiazides on lipid profile. Lipid effects thought to be short-term (≤1 year).
b. Chlorthiazide (Diuril®)	500 mg-2000 mg/day	— ↑ triglycerides — ↑ serum glucose ▲ especially diabetics	• Less effect on glucose if lower dosage used.
c. Hydrochlorothiazide (HCTZ)	12.5 mg-100 mg/day	—electrolyte imbalance ▲ ↓ K⁺ —dehydration	• Less effect on electrolytes if lower dosage used. • Use lowest effective dose to avoid dehydration.
d. Indapamide (Lozol®)	2.5 mg-5mg/day		• Inexpensive.
e. Metolazone (Zaroxolyn®)	2.5 mg-20 mg/day		• Convenient. • Well-tolerated and effective in mild to moderate HTN.
f. Quinethazone (Hydromax®)	50 mg-100 mg/day		• No effect on LVH. • Indapamide and metolazone may be effective in renal insufficiency.
2. Loop Diuretics			
a. Bumetanide (Bumex®)	0.5 mg-2 mg QOD	—dehydration —hypotension	• Potent drugs, reserved for patients requiring massive diuresis.
b. Ethacrynic Acid (Edecrin®)	50 mg-100 mg QD or QOD	—electrolyte imbalance —ototoxicity — ↑ glucose	—pulmonary edema. —congestive heart failure. —chronic renal failure.
c. Furosemide (Lasix®)	20 mg-80 mg 2-4 × /week	— ↑ uric acid	• No effect on LVH.
3. Potassium-Sparing Diuretics			
a. Amiloride (Midamor®)	5 mg-20 mg/day	—hyperkalemia —menstrual irregularities	• Usually used in conjunction with another diuretic.
b. Spironolactone (Aldactone®)	50 mg-200 mg/day	—nausea/vomiting —leg cramps —hirsutism	• No effect on LVH.
c. Triamterene (Dyrenium®)	200 mg-300 mg/day	—dizziness	
4. Combination Diuretics			
a. Amiloride (5 mg) with HCTZ (50 mg) (Moduretic®)	½-2 tablets/day	—See side effects listed for thiazide diuretics and potassium-sparing diuretics.	• Expensive • See comments listed for thiazide diuretics and potassium-sparing diuretics.
b. Triamterene (50 mg) with HCTZ (25 mg) (Dyazide®)	1-4 tablets QD or BID		
c. Triamterene (75 mg) with HCTZ (50 mg) (Maxzide®)	½-2 tablets/day		

Continued

Table 6.D.1. PHARMACOLOGICAL THERAPIES FOR HYPERTENSION CONTINUED

Drug	Dosage	Side Effects	Comments
BETA-BLOCKERS			
a. Acebutolol (Sectral®)	400 mg-1200 mg in 1-2 doses	—masks hypoglycemia —bradycardia, AV block, CHF —bronchoconstriction, worsening allergies —fatigue, insomnia, depression — ↓ HDL — ↑ triglycerides	• Avoid in insulin-dependent diabetes mellitus; caution in non-insulin-dependent diabetes mellitus.
b. Atenolol (Tenormin®)	25 mg-200 mg/day		• Avoid in second- and third-degree heart block, sick sinus syndrome, CHF.
c. Metoprolol (Lopressor®)	50 mg-200 mg in 1-2 doses		• Avoid in asthmatics.
d. Nadolol (Corgard®)	20 mg-160 mg QD		• Effects on cognitive function controversial.
e. Pindolol (Visken®)	5 mg-20 mg BID		• Tricyclic antidepressants inhibit beta-blockers.
f. Propranolol (Inderal®)	20 mg-160 mg BID		• Useful in hypertensives with ↑ sympathetic stimulation
g. Timolol (Blocadren®)	5 mg-20 mg BID		▲ tachycardia. ▲ palpitations.
BETA/ALPHA BLOCKERS			• ↓ LVH: atenolol, labetolol, metoprolol, nadolol, propranolol
a. Labetolol (Normodyne®, Trandate®)	100 mg-600 mg BID	—see side effects above —also postural hypotesion	• Beta one (cardioselective): acebutolol, atenolol, metoprolol
ACE INHIBITORS			
a. Captopril (Capoten®)	50 mg-300 mg in 2-3 doses	—cough (10% of patients) —hypotension —headache —dizziness — ↑ K⁺ in renal insufficiency —alterations in taste	• Expensive.
b. Enalapril (Vasotec®)	5 mg-40 mg in 1-2 doses		• Well-tolerated, few side effects
c. Lisinopril (Prinivil®, Zestril®)	10 mg-40 mg/day		• No adverse effect on lipid profile or glucose.
d. Ramipril (Altace®)			• May stabilize or decrease LVH.
CALCIUM CHANNEL BLOCKERS			
a. Diltiazem (Cardizem®)	120 mg-180 mg in 2-3 doses	—headaches —bradycardia —edema	• Expensive
b. Nifedipine (Procardia®, Adalat®)	20 mg-90 mg in 2-3 doses	—headaches —palpitations —edema	• ↓ side effects with sustained-release formulas.
c. Nicardipine (Cardene®)	20 mg-40 mg TID		• Negative inotropic effect. Use cautiously with CHF.
d. Nitrendipine	5 mg-20 mg BID		• May elevate glucose in some patients. Use cautiously with diabetes mellitus (not diltiazem).
e. Verapamil (Calan®, Isoptin®)	240 mg-480 mg QD or BID	—headaches —bradycardia —edema —constipation	• No adverse lipid effects. • Verapamil may ↓ LVH. • Nifedipine may ↓ atherosclerosis.

–two-drug therapy:
  ‣ diuretic and beta-blocker.
  ‣ diuretic and ACE inhibitor.
  ‣ diuretic and calcium channel blocker.
  ‣ calcium channel blocker and ACE inhibitor.

→ Refractory hypertension (in consultation).
  ■ Three-drug therapy:
    • diuretic and beta-blocker, and either a calcium channel blocker or vasodilator.
    • diuretic and ACE inhibitor, and either a calcium channel blocker or sympatholytic (or both).
    • calcium channel blocker and ACE inhibitor, and either a sympatholytic or beta-blocker (or both).

→ Goals of therapy.
  ■ Decrease blood pressure ≤140/90 mmHg.
    • In patients with mild diastolic hypertension, reduction of at least 10 points is optimal.
    • In elderly patients with systolic hypertension, a decrease in blood pressure to 150-160 may be adequate.
    • Patients with known coronary artery stenosis may need higher perfusion pressure (i.e., DBP ≥85 mmHg).
  ■ Minimize adverse effects of therapy.
    • Many patients who are asymptomatic at onset will discontinue medications because medication side effects have an impact on their quality of life (Dennis et al. 1991).
  ■ Any lowering of blood pressure can reduce risks associated with hypertension. It may be realistic to compromise between blood pressure and tolerable level of drug effects in order not to affect patient well-being adversely (Bulpitt and Fletcher 1988).

CONSULTATION/REFERRALS

→ Immediate referral is warranted with hypertensive emergencies:
  ■ SBP >240 mmHg and/or DBP >130 mmHg (asymptomatic).
  ■ SBP >200 mmHg and/or DBP >120 mmHg (symptomatic).
    • Associated with angina, CHF, headaches.

  ■ hypertensive encephalopathy.
    • Headache, irritability, confusion, altered mental status, +/− papilledema.
  ■ hypertensive nephropathy.
    • Hematuria, proteinuria, renal dysfunction.

→ Consultation or referral is indicated for refractory hypertension.

→ Consultation is recommended with suspected cases of secondary HTN.

→ As needed for prescription(s).

PATIENT EDUCATION

→ Educate patient regarding physiology of hypertension.

→ Provide patient detailed information on non-pharmacological ways to lower blood pressure to:
  ■ encourage active patient participation.
  ■ increase patient's sense of well-being.

→ Educate patient regarding medication side effects and importance of compliance.

FOLLOW-UP

→ Reassess blood pressure control and medication side effects within a time period—usually one to eight weeks—to be determined by patient reliability, compliance, severity of hypertension, and other medical problems.

→ Give patient with mild hypertension two- to three-month trial before adjusting drug regime.

→ If blood pressure control is inadequate, before changing drug therapy assess possible causes:
  ■ patient non-compliance.
  ■ sub-therapeutic dosage of medication.
  ■ use of other medications interfering with efficacy of antihypertensive.
  ■ unrecognized secondary hypertension.

→ In patients with good response to medication, consider trial of decreased dosage after six months to one year.

→ Document in progress notes and problem list.

Ellen Scarr, M.S.N., F.N.P.

6-E

Mitral Valve Prolapse

Mitral valve prolapse (MVP) is defined as the abnormal displacement of the mitral valve leaflets posteriorly and superiorly during systole (Quill, Lipkin, and Greenland 1988). This condition varies from minor prolapse of the mitral leaflets, without any subjective symptoms or objective findings on cardiac examination, to marked hemodynamic impairment with mitral insufficiency/regurgitation.

The Framingham Heart Study found an echocardiogram prevalence of MVP of 5 percent (Quill, Lipkin, and Greenland 1988). MVP is common in thin young women, and is usually idiopathic, although it is occasionally associated with connective tissue disease (e.g., Marfan's syndrome). Patients who are symptomatic may present with complaints of atypical chest pain, palpitations, dyspnea, or dizziness—symptoms that are common among the general population.

The prognostic significance of MVP is unclear. While it rarely progresses to hemodynamically significant mitral regurgitation, there is documentation in the literature of some association between MVP and arrhythmias, syncope, sudden death, transient ischemic attacks (TIAs), cerebral vascular accidents (CVAs), and bacterial endocarditis. However, patients with MVP who have little or no associated mitral regurgitation are probably at no increased risk for morbidity (Liberthson 1987; MacMahon, Devereux, and Schron 1987; Quill, Lipkin, and Greenland 1988).

DATABASE

SUBJECTIVE

→ Symptoms may include:
  ▪ palpitations.
  ▪ atypical chest pain, unrelieved with rest or nitroglycerin, poorly correlated with exercise.
  ▪ dyspnea on exertion.
  ▪ shortness of breath.
  ▪ dizziness.
→ Past medical history may include:
  ▪ cardiac disease—e.g., rheumatic heart disease, endocarditis, pericarditis.
  ▪ endocrine disorders—e.g., thyroid disorders.
  ▪ anemia.
→ Family history may include:
  ▪ cardiac disease, including sudden death.
→ Social history
  ▪ may include use of:
    • caffeine.
    • tobacco.
    • recreational drugs.
→ Inquire regarding diet. Assess for recent weight loss.

OBJECTIVE

→ Physical examination to include:
  ▪ vital signs.
  ▪ height and weight.
→ Cardiac examination may include mid-systolic click and late systolic murmur *(click/murmur syndrome)*.
  ▪ Maneuvers to elicit these findings:
    • click and/or murmur heard best with standing or the valsalva maneuver, measures which decrease left ventricular volume and increase mitral prolapse.

- conversely, squatting or isometric exercises, which increase left ventricular end-diastolic volume and decrease prolapse, will delay or even eliminate the click/murmur (Braunwald 1987).
→ If mitral regurgitation is present, the cardiac exam may include the following findings (Massie and Sokolow 1993):
  - prominent and hyperdynamic apical impulse to left of the midclavicular line (MCL).
  - forceful, brisk point of maximal impulse (PMI); systolic thrill over PMI.
  - mid-systolic click; prominent S_3.
  - blowing, high-pitched pansystolic murmur heard (maximally) at the apex; radiating into left axilla, infrascapular area, and occasionally the base.

ASSESSMENT

→ Mitral valve prolapse
→ R/O arrhythmias

PLAN

DIAGNOSTIC TESTS

→ Laboratory studies:
  - CBC to assess for anemia.
  - thyroid function studies to assess for hyperthyroidism (see **Thyroid Disorders** Protocol).
→ EKG:
  - highly sensitive and specific.
  - probably not necessary if patient has asymptomatic click/murmur syndrome.
  - useful in symptomatic patients for diagnosis and determination of need for therapy.

TREATMENT/MANAGEMENT

→ Rarely needed for arrhythmias (see **Palpitations** Protocol).
→ Infective endocarditis prophylaxis regimens (**NOTE:** The American Heart Association recommends prophylaxis only in MVP patients with evidence of mitral insufficiency [regurgitation].) (Massie and Sokolow 1993; Liberthson 1987):
  - dental/oral/upper respiratory tract procedures:
    - amoxicillin 3.0 grams p.o. 1 hour before procedure, then 1.5 grams p.o. 6 hours later (Dajani et al. 1990).

- if allergic to penicillin, may use erythromycin ethylsuccinate (E.E.S.®) 800 mg or erythromycin stearate (Filmtab®) 1.0 gram p.o. 2 hours before procedure, then ½ the dose 6 hours later, or clindamycin (Cleocin®) 300 mg p.o. 1 hour before procedure, then 150 mg p.o. 6 hours later (Dajani et al. 1990).
    - parenteral regimens may be used for high-risk patients (e.g., those with prosthetic heart valves or a previous history of endocarditis) and individuals unable to take oral medications (Dajani et al. 1990). Details of parenteral administration are beyond the scope of this protocol. Consult with physician.
  - gastrointestinal or genitourinary tract procedures:
    - parenteral prophylaxis—details of which are beyond the scope of this protocol—is recommended, especially in high-risk patients. Consult with physician.
    - oral prophylaxis is an alternative for low-risk patients: amoxicillin 3 grams p.o. 1 hour before the procedure, then 1.5 grams p.o. 6 hours later (Dajani et al. 1990).
  - see **Table 6E.1, Procedures for Which Infective Endocarditis Prophylaxis Is/Is not Recommended.**

CONSULTATION

→ Symptomatic patients with click/murmur syndrome should be referred to a cardiologist or managed in consultation with an internist.
→ Patients with findings of mitral regurgitation should be referred to a cardiologist or managed in consultation with an internist.
→ As needed for prescription(s).

PATIENT EDUCATION

→ Reassure asymptomatic patient that this is a common condition that most often remains benign.
→ Advise the asymptomatic patient that there is no need for medication, diet restriction, or limitation of activities.

FOLLOW-UP

→ Asymptomatic patient.
  - Yearly physical examination to assess for change in symptoms, need for further studies (e.g., echocardiogram).
→ Document in progress notes and problem list.

Table 6E.1.   Procedures for Which Infective Endocarditis Prophylaxis Is/Is not Recommended[1]

Endocarditis prophylaxis recommended

Dental procedures known to include gingival or mucosal bleeding, including professional cleaning
Tonsillectomy or adenoidectomy
Surgical operations that involve intestinal or respiratory mucosa
Bronchoscopy with a rigid bronchoscope
Sclerotherapy for esophageal varices
Esophageal dilation
Gall bladder surgery
Cystoscopy
Urethral dilation
Urethral catheterization if urinary tract infection is present[2]
Urinary tract surgery if urinary tract infection is present
Prostatic surgery
Incision and drainage of infected tissue
Vaginal hysterectomy
Vaginal delivery in the presence of infection[2]

Endocarditis prophylaxis not recommended[3]

Dental procedures not likely to induce gingival bleeding, such as simple adjustment of orthodontic appliances or fillings above the gum line
Injection of local intraoral anesthetic (except intraligamentary injections)
Shedding of primary teeth
Tympanostomy tube insertion
Endotracheal intubation
Bronchoscopy with a flexible bronchoscope, with or without biopsy
Cardiac catheterization
Endoscopy with or without gastrointestinal biopsy
Cesarean section
In the absence of infection: urethral catheterization, dilation and curettage, uncomplicated vaginal delivery, therapeutic abortion, sterilization procedures, or insertion or removal of intrauterine devices.

[1]This table lists selected conditions and is not meant to be all-inclusive.

[2]In addition to prophylactic regimen for genitourinary procedures, antibiotic therapy should be directed against the most likely bacterial pathogen.

[3]In patients who have prosthetic heart valves, a history of endocarditis, or surgically constructed systemic pulmonary shunts or conduits, physicians may chooose to administer prophylactic antibiotics even for low-risk procedures that involve the lower respiratory, genitourinary, or gastrointestinal tracts.

Source: Modified and reproduced with permission from Dajani, A.S. et al. 1990. Prevention of bacterial endocarditis. Recommendations by the American Heart Association. *Journal of the American Medical Association* 264:2919 (1990). Copyright © 1990 by the American Medical Association.

Ellen Scarr, M.S.N., F.N.P.

6-F

Palpitations

Palpitations is a frequent presenting complaint by patients seeking attention from a health care provider. An awareness of one's heartbeat is often frightening to a patient, and a careful history and physical, coupled with reassurance, are essential components in determining the appropriate work-up.

There are many causes of palpitations. These can often be determined by the characteristics of the palpitations.

→ Isolated Palpitations.
  ▪ *Premature atrial, junctional,* or *ventricular contraction* (PAC, PJC, or PVC).
  ▪ The premature beat may be felt, or the subsequent beat (with or without a compensatory pause) may be more perceptible because of an increase in stroke volume.
→ Palpitations characterized by rapid rate and regular rhythm.
  ▪ Catecholamine excess.
  ▪ Hypovolemia.
  ▪ Hyperthyroidism.
  ▪ Pheochromocytoma.
  ▪ Marked anemia.
  ▪ Drug use (e.g., insulin, theophyllines, sympathomimetics).
  ▪ Arrhythmias with constant block or 1:1 conduction.
    • Atrial flutter.
    • Paroxysmal atrial tachycardia.
    • Supraventricular tachycardia.
    • Wolff-Parkinson-White syndrome.
    • Torsade de pointes tachycardia.

→ Palpitations, characterized by rapid rate and irregular rhythm.
  ▪ Arrhythmias.
    • Atrial fibrillation.
    • Multifocal atrial tachycardia.
    • Atrial flutter with variable block.
    • Paroxysmal atrial tachycardia with variable block.
    • Supraventricular tachycardia with variable block.
    • Multiple PACs, PJCs, or PVCs.
→ Palpitations, characterized by variable rate and regular rhythm, due to:
  ▪ fever.
  ▪ anxiety/emotional stress.
  ▪ valvular disease.
  ▪ exercise.
  ▪ pregnancy.
  ▪ stimulants (e.g., caffeine, tobacco, recreational drugs).

DATABASE

SUBJECTIVE

→ Patient presents with complaint of palpitations. While many patients have difficulty being specific about their symptoms, an accurate history of the palpitations, including descriptors, may indicate the underlying etiology or narrow the differential diagnosis.
  ▪ When did the symptoms begin?
  ▪ How often do the palpitations occur?
  ▪ How long do the episodes last?
  ▪ How fast is the pulse?

- Is the pulse regular or irregular?
- Is the heart "pounding," "fluttering," "flopping"?
- Do the episodes occur with exercise, after medication or drug use, with stress, or at random?
- Are there any other associated symptoms with the palpitations?
- How does the episode resolve?

→ Associated symptoms may include:
- tremor.
- nervousness.
- chest pain.
- shortness of breath.
- dyspnea on exertion.
- syncope/lightheadedness.
- perspiration.

→ Precipitating events, if known, may include:
- exercise.
- stress.
- dehydration.
- drug use (e.g., decongestants, appetite suppressants, caffeine, marijuana, cocaine).

→ Past medical history may include:
- anemia.
- heart murmur.
- heart disease:
  - valvular.
  - coronary.
  - cardiomyopathy.
  - arrhythmias.
- pheochromocytoma.
- insulin-dependent diabetes.
- thyroid disease.

→ Medications may include:
- insulin/oral hypoglycemic agents.
- theophylline compounds.
- sympathomimetics.
- long-acting antihistamines.
- decongestants.
- appetite suppressants.
- psychoactive drugs.

→ Social history may include use of:
- caffeine.
- alcohol.
- tobacco.
- recreational drugs.

OBJECTIVE

→ Patient's general appearance exhibits:
- anxiousness.

- tremulousness.
- pallor.
- exophthalmus.

→ Vital signs should be assessed for:
- temperature, which may be elevated with infection.
- apical heart rate—regularity, character; comparison with radial pulse for deficit.
- blood pressure, including orthostatic measurements.
  - May be hypotensive if hypovolemic or low cardiac output.
  - Widened pulse pressure may be present.

→ Thyroid examination should assess for:
- nodules.
- goiter.
- tenderness.

→ Lung examination should assess for:
- adventitious sounds.
- respiratory rate and pattern.

→ Heart examination should assess for:
- rhythm characteristics.
  - Thready.
  - Bounding.
  - Regular.
  - Occasionally irregular (i.e., PACs, PVCs).
  - Irregularly irregular (i.e. atrial fibrillation, multifocal atrial tachycardia, atrial flutter with variable block).
  - Regularly irregular (i.e. bigeminy, trigeminy, quadrigeminy).
- murmurs.
  - Grade.
  - Systolic/diastolic.
- rubs.
- gallops
  - S_3.
  - S_4.
- heaves.
- thrills.
- PMI.

→ Extremity examination should assess for:
- color.
- warmth.
- cyanosis.
- clubbing.
- edema.

ASSESSMENT

→ Palpitations

→ R/O arrhythmias/heart disease

→ R/O systemic etiologies:
  - thyroid disease
  - anemia
  - pheochromocytoma
  - medication side effect
  - stimulant side effect

→ R/O anxiety

PLAN

DIAGNOSTIC TESTS

→ 12-lead EKG:
  - assessing for rate, arrhythmias, ectopy, ischemia.

→ Holter monitor:
  - useful if patient complains of syncope, dizziness.
  - questionable whether helpful in healthy patient with normal EKG.

→ Thyroid function tests (see **Thyroid Disorders** Protocol):
  - if symptoms suggest thyroid disease.

→ CBC:
  - to rule out anemia

→ Exercise treadmill test (ETT):
  - if symptoms occur with exercise, or,
  - if patient has history of heart disease, or,
  - if patient is very anxious.

TREATMENT/MANAGEMENT

→ If EKG is normal and symptoms are suggestive of stress or stimulant use, reassure patient that cardiac exam is normal and her symptoms are amenable to appropriate therapy (e.g., stress reduction, elimination of stimulants).

→ If work-up suggests underlying illness or disease, initiate appropriate evaluation (e.g., anemia [see **Anemia** Protocol], hyperthyroidism [see **Thyroid Disorders** Protocol]).

→ If EKG is normal and patient is moderately symptomatic (e.g., tachycardia, tremors), may begin low-dose beta-blocker therapy (e.g., propranolol [Inderal®] 40 mg p.o. BID, see **Table 6D.1,** pp. 6-19 and 6-20), for symptom control. Consider 24-hour Holter monitor prior to initiating drug to rule out significant underlying cardiac disease.

→ If EKG is normal and patient symptoms suggest situational stress, may begin (in consultation with physician) low-dose anxiolytic therapy (e.g., alprazolam [Xanax®] 0.25 mg p.o. BID) if appropriate (determined by patient reliability, clinic setting, follow-up).

CONSULTATION

→ Referral to a cardiologist is indicated for:
  - abnormal EKG—including arrhythmias, frequent ectopy, or ischemic changes.
  - palpitations associated with syncope.

→ As needed for prescription(s).

PATIENT EDUCATION

→ Teach patient to take radial or carotid pulse to assess for rate and regularity.

→ Advise patient that healthy patients can have palpitations.

→ Educate patient regarding stress reduction techniques to be used in reducing or eliminating palpitation:
  - a regular exercise routine—e.g., 30 minutes of aerobic exercise two to three times/week (in low-risk patient).
  - meditation and relaxation techniques useful for stress reduction.

→ Advise patient to decrease/eliminate stimulant use (e.g., cigarettes, alcohol, caffeine, recreational drugs).

→ Advise patient regarding regular use of stimulant medications including discontinuing medication or switching to another agent with fewer side effects. Patient may tolerate symptoms better after reassurance that palpitations are medication-related.

FOLLOW-UP

→ Re-evaluate patient in one to two months if no discernible cause is found.

→ Re-evaluate patient in two to three weeks if pharmacological therapy begun.

→ Document in progress notes and problem list.

6-G
Bibliography

Alderman, M.H. 1992. Which antihypertensive drugs first—and why! *Journal of the American Medical Association* 267(20):2786–2787.

Arai, A., and Greenberg, B. 1990. Medical management of congestive heart failure. *Western Journal of Medicine* 153(4):406–414.

Arakawa, K. 1989. Non-pharmacologic measures for lowering blood pressure. *Cardiovascular Drugs and Therapy* 3(6):847–852.

Baron, R. 1991. Non-drug treatment of hypertension. Course syllabus, Sixth Annual *Primary Care Medicine, Principles and Practice*. San Francisco: University of California, San Francisco.

———. 1992. Management of hypercholesterolemia: Time for new treatment guidelines. Course syllabus, Seventh Annual *Primary Care Medicine, Principles and Practice*. San Francisco: University of California, San Francisco.

Beanlands, D. 1990. Concepts in the management of congestive heart failure. *Canadian Journal of Cardiology* 6(suppl c):1c–3c.

Bonow, R., and Udelson, J. 1992. Left ventricular diastolic dysfunction as a cause of congestive heart failure. Mechanisms and management. *Annals of Internal Medicine* 117(6):502–510.

Braunwald, E. 1987. Valvular heart disease. In *Harrison's principles of internal medicine*, eds. E. Braunwald, K. Isselbacher, R. Petersdorf, J. Wilson, and A. Fauci. New York:McGraw Hill.

Browner, W. 1988. Controversies in hypertension. Course syllabus, Fourth Annual *Primary Care Medicine, Principles and Practice*. San Francisco: University of California, San Francisco.

———. 1989. Outpatient therapy of coronary artery disease. Course syllabus, Fifth Annual *Primary Care Medicine, Principles and Practice*. San Francisco: University of California, San Francisco.

Brunelli, C., Ghigliotti, G., Martini, U., and Caponnetto, S. 1991. New therapeutic strategies in the management of congestive heart failure. *European Heart Journal* 12(suppl G):53–57.

Bulpitt, C., and Fletcher, A. 1988. The importance of well-being to hypertensive patients. *The American Journal of Medicine* 84(18):40–46.

Burkman, R. 1988. Obesity, stress and smoking: Their role as cardiovascular risk factors in women. *American Journal of Obstetrics and Gynecology* 158(6):1592–1597.

Castelli, W. 1988. Cardiovascular disease in women. *American Journal of Obstetrics and Gynecology* 158(6):1553–1560.

Chatterjee, K. 1988. Pharmaco-therapeutic approach for chronic heart failure due to primary myocardial disease. Course syllabus, Fourth Annual *Primary Care Medicine, Principles and Practice*. San Francisco: University of California, San Francisco.

Cressman, M., and Gifford, R. 1989. Pharmacologic management of hypertension. *Postgraduate Medicine* 85(8):259–268.

Dajani, A.S., Bisno, A.L., Chang, K.J., Durack, D.T., Freed, M., Gerber, M.A., Karchmer, A.W., Millard, H.D., Rahimtoola, S., Shulman, S.T., Watanakunakorn, M.D., and Taubert, K.A. 1990. Prevention of bacterial endocarditis. Recommendations by the American Heart Association. *Journal of the American Medical Association* 264(22):2919–2922.

Dennis, K., Froman, D., Morrison, A., Holmes, K., and Howes, D. 1991. Beta-blocker therapy. Identification and management of side effects. *Heart & Lung: The Journal of Critical Care* 20(5):459–463.

Devereux, R., Kramer-Fox, R., Shear, M., Kligfield, P., Pini, R., and Savage, D. 1987. Diagnosis and classification of severity of mitral valve prolapse: Methodologic, biologic, and prognostic considerations. *American Heart Journal* 113(5):1265–1280.

Goroll, A., May, L., and Mulley, A., eds. 1987. *Primary care medicine.* Philadelphia: J.B. Lippincott.

———, eds. 1995. *Primary care medicine.* Philadelphia: J.B. Lippincott.

Graettinger, W., and Weber, M. 1992. Left ventricular hypertrophy and antihypertensive therapy. *American Family Physician* 42(2):483–491.

Holloway, J. 1991. Congestive heart failure mechanism and medical management. *Journal of the Arkansas Medical Society* 87(8):322–325.

Hulley, S. 1988. A national program for lowering high blood cholesterol. *American Journal of Obstetrics and Gynecology* 158(6):1561–1566.

Joint National Committee on Detection, Evaluation and Treatment of High Blood Pressure. 1993. The fifth report of the Joint National Committee on Detection, Evaluation and Treatment of High Blood Pressure. *Archives of Internal Medicine* 153(2):154–183.

Kahn, J. 1991. Progressive congestive heart failure: Ways to approach office management. *Postgraduate Medicine* 89(6):102–107.

Keller, K., and Lemberg, L. 1990. Changing concepts in the management of congestive heart failure. *Heart and Lung* 19(4):425–429.

Keresztes, P., and Dan, A. 1992. Estrogen and cardiovascular disease. *Cardiovascular Nursing* 28(1):1–6.

Kligfield, P., Levy, D., Devereux, R., and Savage, D. 1987. Arrhythmias and sudden death in mitral valve prolapse. *American Heart Journal* 113(5):1298–1307.

Knopp, R., and Mishell, D. 1988. Cholesterol treatment recommendations for adults: Highlights of the 1987 report from the National Cholesterol Education Program Adult Treatment Panel. *American Journal of Obstetrics and Gynecology* 158(6):1670–1673.

Kopp, D.E., and Wilber, D.J. 1992. Palpitations and arrhythmias: Separating the benign from the dangerous. *Postgraduate Medicine* 91(1):241–251.

Lehne, R. 1990. *Pharmacology for nursing care.* Philadelphia: W.B. Saunders.

Levy, D., and Savage, D. 1987. Prevalence and clinical features of mitral valve prolapse. *American Heart Journal* 113(5):1281–1290.

Liberthson, R. 1987. Management of acquired valvular heart disease. In *Primary care medicine,* eds. A. Goroll, L. May, and A. Mulley, pp. 145–153. Philadelphia: J.B. Lippincott.

Lobo, R. 1990. Cardiovascular implication of estrogen replacement therapy. *Obstetrics and Gynecology* 75(4):185–255.

MacMahon, S., Devereux, R., and Schron, E., eds. 1987. Clinical and epidemiological issues in mitral valve prolapse. American Heart Journal 113(5):1265–1331.

MacMahon, S., Roberts, J., Kramer-Fox, R., Zucker, D., Roberts, R., and Devereux, R. 1987. Mitral valve prolapse and infective endocarditis. *American Heart Journal* 113(5):1291–1298.

Massie, B., and Sokolow, M. 1992. The heart and great vessels. In *Current medical diagnosis and treatment,* eds. S.A. Schroeder, L.M. Tierney, S.J. McPhee, M.A. Papadakis, and M. Krupp. San Mateo, CA: Appleton & Lange.

———. 1993. Cardiovascular diseases. In *Current medical diagnosis and treatment,* eds. L.M. Tierney, S.J. McPhee, M.A. Papadakis, and S.A. Schroeder. Norwalk, CT: Appleton & Lange.

Murtagh, J. 1992. Palpitations. *Australian Family Physician* 21(4):475–482.

Nachtigall, L. 1987. Cardiovascular disease and hypertension in older women. *Obstetrics and Gynecology Clinics of North America* 14(1):89–105.

National Cholesterol Education Program. 1988. *Detection, evaluation, and treatment of high blood cholesterol in adults.* Bethesda, MD: National Institutes of Health, U.S. Department of Health and Human Services.

Oakley, C. 1992. Mitral valve palpitations. *Australian and New Zealand Journal of Medicine* 22(5):562–565.

Oliver, M. 1992. Cholesterol and coronary disease: Outstanding questions. *Cardiovascular Drugs and Therapy* 6(2):131–136.

Perez-Stable, E. 1989. Management of hypertension: Selection of an antihypertensive regime. Course syllabus, Fifth Annual *Primary Care Medicine, Principles and Practice.* San Francisco: University of California, San Francisco.

———. 1991. Pharmacologic management of hypertension: Current controversies. Course syllabus, Sixth Annual *Primary Care Medicine, Principles and Practice.* San Francisco: University of California, San Francisco.

Perlman, J., Wolf, P., Ray, R., and Lieberknecht, G. 1988. Cardiovascular risk factors, premature heart disease, and all-cause mortality in a cohort of Northern California women. *American Journal of Obstetrics and Gynecology* 158(6):1568–1574.

Perloff, J., and Child, J. 1987. Clinical and epidemiological issues in mitral valve prolapse: Overview and perspective. *American Heart Journal* 113(5):1324–1332.

Peters, W. 1987. Approach to the patient with hypercholesterolemia. In *Primary care medicine*, eds. A. Goroll, L. May, and A. Mulley. Philadelphia: J.B. Lippincott.

Petronis, K., and Anthony, J. 1989. An epidemiologic investigation of marijuana- and cocaine-related palpitations. *Drug and Alcohol Dependence* 23(3):219–226.

Quill, T., Lipkin, M., and Greenland, P. 1988. The medicalization of normal variants: The case of mitral valve prolapse. *Journal of General Internal Medicine* 3(3):267–276.

Rapaport, E. 1987. Modern management of congestive heart failure. Course Syllabus, Third Annual *Primary Care Medicine, Principles and Practice*. San Francisco: University of California, San Francisco.

Ringqvist, I., Jonason, T., Nilsson, G., and Khan, A. 1989. Diagnostic value of long-term ambulatory EKG in patients with syncope, dizziness or palpitations. *Clinical Physiology* 9(1):47–55.

Sanford, V. *Guide to antimicrobial therapy*. Dallas: Antimicrobial Therapy, Inc.

Waddell, D. 1986. Behavioral treatment of hypertension. Course syllabus, *Annual Review in Family Medicine: Controversies and Challenges in Primary Care*. San Francisco: University of California, San Francisco.

Wolf, P., and Sila, C. 1987. Cerebral ischemia with mitral valve prolapse. *American Heart Journal* 113(5):1308–1315.

SECTION 7

Gastrointestinal Disorders

Lisa L. Lommel, R.N., C., F.N.P., M.P.H.

7-A

Abdominal Pain

Abdominal pain is either acute or chronic and recurrent. If the pain is acute in onset and severity, the management goal is early diagnosis and timely referral to the appropriate specialist. In cases of chronic or recurrent pain, the goal is to provide an effective work-up to establish a diagnosis and treatment plan.

The major pathogenic mechanisms underlying abdominal pain include obstruction and perforation of the hollow viscus, peritoneal irritation, vascular insufficiency, mucosal ulceration/inflammation, altered bowel motility, capsular distention or inflammation, metabolic imbalance, nerve injury, abdominal wall injury, and referral from an extra-abdominal site. (Burkhart 1992; Richter 1995a).

Because the location of pain often does not coincide with the site of involvement, the provider should elicit a thorough history and physical examination and be familiar with areas where abdominal pain commonly is referred or perceived (see **Table 7A.1, Common Anatomical Pain Sites for Specific Disease States**).

DATABASE

SUBJECTIVE

→ Obtain a complete description of the abdominal pain—location, characterization (quality and quantity), progression, radiation, setting, duration, aggravating and alleviating factors, similar episodes, associated symptoms (nausea and vomiting, anorexia, bowel or urinary dysfunction, jaundice, gynecological symptoms).

→ A comprehensive medical and surgical history including recent travel, drug ingestion, family history, social history, psychological history, occupational history, and review of systems should be elicited.

→ In cases of acute abdominal pain or with a young or elderly patient, it may be difficult to elicit a complete history. A relative may be helpful in providing information.

→ The following are symptoms experienced in common pathogenic mechanisms of abdominal pain (Richter 1995a). See **Table 7A.1.**

Obstruction

→ Acute small bowel obstruction:
  ▪ history of abdominal surgery or hernia is common.
  ▪ rapid onset of cramping, intermittent, mid-abdominal pain.
  ▪ may be severe in proximal obstruction.
  ▪ patient may be comfortable between bouts of pain.
  ▪ pain steady with complete obstruction.
  ▪ flatus and small amounts of stool common at onset of obstruction; diarrhea with partial obstruction; stool passage absent with complete obstruction.
  ▪ distention is increased with a more distal obstruction.
  ▪ nausea, vomiting, weakness, anxiety.

→ Large bowel obstruction:
  ▪ more common in patients over 50 years of age; often preceded by constipation or change in bowel habits.

Table 7A.1. COMMON ANATOMICAL PAIN SITES FOR SPECIFIC DISEASE STATES

Right Upper Quadrant and Flank
Hepatitis
Pancreatitis
Gastritis
Duodenitis
Cholecystitis
Pyelonephritis
Nephrolithiasis
Choledocholithiasis

Duodenal ulcer
Penetrating or perforating ulcer
Intestinal obstruction
Inflammatory bowel disease
Retrocecal appendicitis
Gastric ulcer
Colon carcinoma

Epigastrium
Pancreatitis
Gastritis
Duodenitis
Gastroenteritis
Duodenal ulcer
Early appendicitis
Gastric ulcer
Colitis

Penetrating or perforating ulcer
Inflammatory bowel disease
Intestinal obstruction
Mesenteric adenitis
Mesenteric thrombosis
Colon carcinoma
Aneurysm

Left Upper Quadrant and Flank
Hepatitis
Gastritis
Pancreatitis
Splenic enlargement, rupture, infarction
Pyelonephritis

Nephrolithiasis
Diverticulitis
Intestinal obstruction
Inflammatory bowel disease
Colon carcinoma

Right Lower Quadrant and Flank
Appendicitis
Intestinal obstruction
Hernia
Nephrolithiasis
Pyelonephritis
Cholecystitis
Mittelschmerz
Salpingitis
Ovarian cyst/torsion
Diverticulitis

Inflammatory bowel disease
Penetrating or perforating ulcer
Endometriosis
Ectopic pregnancy
Abdominal wall hematoma
Psoas abscess
Leaking aneurysm
Mesenteric adenitis
Seminal vesticulitis

Umbilical
Early appendicitis
Gastroenteritis
Pancreatitis
Hernia
Mesenteric adenitis

Inflammatory bowel disease
Intestinal obstruction
Abdominal wall hernia
Aneurysm
Mesenteric thrombosis

Left Lower Quadrant and Flank
Diverticulitis
Intestinal obstruction
Hernia
Pyelonephritis
Nephrolithiasis
Mittelschmerz
Salpingitis
Ovarian cyst/torsion

Endometriosis
Appendicitis
Abdominal wall hematoma
Ectopic pregnacy
Leaking aneurysm
Psoas abscess
Seminal vesiculitis

Hypogastrium
Cystitis
Diverticulitis
Appendicitis
Prostatism
Salpingitis
Hernia
Ovarian cyst/torsion

Endometriosis
Nephrolithiasis
Inflammatory bowel disease
Intestinal obstruction
Ectopic pregnancy
Abdominal wall hematoma
Colon carcinoma

Source: Reprinted with permission from Hickey, M.S., Kiernan, G.J., and Weaver, K.E. 1989. Evaluation of abdominal pain. *Emergency Medicine Clinics of North America* 7(3):437-452.

- bloating, distention, cramping pain, obstipation, mild nausea and vomiting, diarrhea with partial obstruction.
→ Common bile duct obstruction:
  - usually presents with a history of biliary tract disease.
  - steady, acute pain—known as biliary "colic"—lasting hours after sudden onset in epigastric region/right upper quadrant; vomiting present.
→ Acute ureteral obstruction:
  - pain is crampy, beginning in the back and flank and radiating to the lower abdomen and groin; may have nausea, vomiting, anorexia.
  - see **Urinary Tract Disorders, Urinary Tract Infection** Protocol for other renal causes of abdominal pain.
→ Acute cholecystitis: See **Cholecystitis** Protocol.

Peritoneal irritation

→ Peritonitis:
  - localized injury from infection or chemical irritation may cause mild to severe, sharp, aching, or burning pain.
  - degree of pain and systemic reaction depends on severity of insult.
  - spread of the irritant may cause generalized abdominal pain. Pain increased with coughing, palpation, or movement.
  - patient tends to lie very still.
  - malaise, nausea, and vomiting may be present.
→ Acute pancreatitis:
  - gallstone pancreatitis more common in women.
  - alcoholic pancreatitis more common in men.
  - usual history of similar episodes. Epigastric pain with abrupt onset, steady and severe, worse when walking and supine, better sitting and leaning forward; radiating to the back or costal margins, usually constant, may vary in intensity from mild to severe.
  - severe pain more common in left upper quadrant.
  - nausea, vomiting, sweating, weakness (Beal 1983).
→ Chronic pancreatitis:
  - history of alcohol abuse.
  - episodes of epigastric pain, radiation to back.
  - anorexia, nausea, vomiting, constipation, flatulence, weight loss.
  - attacks may be two hours to two weeks long or become continuous.
→ See **Appendicitis, Cirrhosis** protocols.

Vascular disorders

→ Acute arterial insufficiency from atherosclerosis or mesenteric thrombus:
  - acute, sudden, periumbilical, or generalized abdominal pain.
  - atherosclerosis may be preceded by several days of mild, constant pain; with thrombus—severe, resistant, central abdominal pain.
  - may have history of myocardial infarction.
→ Chronic arterial insufficiency:
  - may precede acute episode of infarction.
  - cramping or dull mid-abdominal pain 15 to 30 minutes after a meal, lasting two to three hours.
  - symptoms are more extreme after a large meal.
  - may have large weight loss secondary to avoidance of eating.
→ Ruptured abdominal aortic aneurysm:
  - severe, acute abdominal pain radiating to back or genitalia; symptoms of shock.

Mucosal ulceration/inflammation

→ Upper gastrointestinal (GI) tract ulceration—see **Peptic Ulcer Disease, Gastroesophageal Reflux and Heartburn** protocols.

Alteration in bowel motility

→ See protocols for **Irritable Bowel Syndrome, Diverticular Disease,** and **Diarrhea.**
→ Psychiatric disorders—especially mood and anxiety disorders—are common in people with irritable bowel syndrome. The result is a broad spectrum of presentations including nausea, vomiting, dyspepsia, flatulence, and abdominal cramping.

Capsular distention

→ Hepatic capsular distention from hepatitis, congestive heart failure; fatty infiltration or subcapsular hematoma may cause aching pain in right upper quadrant.
→ Splenic capsular distention from blunt trauma may cause pain in left upper quadrant.

Metabolic disturbances

→ Lead poisoning may simulate bowel obstruction with pain that is cramping, wandering, poorly localized, and colicky. Rigid abdomen may be present.
→ Acute intermittent porphyria may present with moderate to severe abdominal pain, localized or generalized. Vomiting and diarrhea usually present. Proximal muscle pain may be present.

→ Ketoacidosis: may be associated with severe abdominal pain and vomiting. See **Type I Diabetes Mellitus, Type II Diabetes Mellitus** protocols.

Nerve injury

→ Abdominal pain may be secondary to mechanical obstruction or injury to an intra-abdominal nerve. For example, intra-abdominal cancers can invade pain-causing nerves. Pain can be of varying severity, character, and include a variety of symptoms associated with bowel dysfunction.

→ See also **Varicella Zoster Virus** Protocol.

Abdominal wall pathology

→ Traumatic injury to the abdominal wall may present with pain that is constant, aching, and exacerbated by movement.

→ Previous abdominal surgery with incision involving cutaneous nerve may cause burning, shooting pain at site of incision (Gallegos and Hobsley 1990). See **Hernia** Protocol.

→ Pain can be perceived as intra-abdominal but may be associated with nerve root irritation secondary to herpes zoster, especially before the rash appears. There is no associated bowel dysfunction and palpation does not increase pain. See also **Varicella Zoster Virus** Protocol.

Referred pain from extra-abdominal site

→ Pulmonary or cardiac disorders may be the primary site, with referral of pain to the (upper) abdomen. Nausea and vomiting may be present. Symptoms or cardiac or pulmonary disorders are also evident.

→ See **Dysmenorrhea, Ectopic Pregnancy, Endometriosis, Pelvic Inflammatory Disease, Pelvic Masses, Pelvic Pain—Acute, Pelvic Pain—Chronic,** and **Urinary Tract Disorders, Urinary Tract Infection** protocols.

OBJECTIVE

→ A complete physical examination should be done and include targeted assessment of general appearance, vital signs; and cardiac, pulmonary, abdominal, renal, pelvic, and rectal examinations.

→ Signs and symptoms of shock should be assessed in patients with suspected acute abdomen.
  ▪ Sequential vital sign assessment will assist in determining the pace of the work-up and need for referral.

→ The abdominal examination should include:

▪ inspection (presence of distention, visible peristalsis, jaundice, scarring, abdominal wall masses).
▪ auscultation (altered bowel sounds, hepatic rub, or bruit).
▪ percussion (delineate masses and free air).
▪ palpation (hepatosplenomegaly, masses, costovertebral angle (CVA) tenderness, external hernias) and
▪ assessment for involuntary guarding, cough, rebound tenderness, and special signs and maneuvers (see **Table 7A.2, Abdominal Palpation**).
  • Palpation should begin at the region away from the maximal area of pain.

→ abdominal examination may be difficult to complete in patients who have moderate to severe degrees of anxiety or pain.

Obstruction

→ Small bowel obstruction:
  ▪ inspect for previous scars or hernias.
  ▪ patient is restless during bouts of pain; temperature normal or mildly elevated.
  ▪ obstruction with or without perforation can cause postural changes in blood pressure and heart rate.
  ▪ tender, distended abdomen, especially with distal obstruction; high-pitched, hyperactive bowel sounds.
  ▪ a tender hernia may be present.
  ▪ stool guaiac negative.
  ▪ plain radiograph of the abdomen (kidneys/ureters/bladder [KUB] and upright) shows distention of loops of small bowel with air-fluid levels; absence of gas in the large bowel (distal to the obstruction).
  ▪ elevated white blood cell (WBC) count; elevated hematocrit with signs of dehydration.

→ Large bowel obstruction:
  ▪ progressive abdominal distention and tympany; hyperactive bowel sounds.
  ▪ rectal examination may present with positive stool guaiac. Mass may be present in cases of carcinoma (Beal 1983).

→ Common bile duct obstruction:
  ▪ right upper quadrant tenderness and jaundice; chills and spiking, intermittent fever with infection; positive Murphy's sign.
  ▪ elevated WBC count (20,000 to 30,000/mm) and mild hyperbilirubinemia may occur.

→ Acute ureteral obstruction:

Table 7A.2. ABDOMINAL PALPATION

Finding or Sign	Description	Clinical Occurrence
Bassler's sign	Sharp pain elicited by pinching the appendix between the thumb of the examiner and the iliacus muscle	Chronic appendicitis
Beevor's sign	Upward movement of the umbilicus	Paralysis of the lower portions of the recti abdominis muscles
Blumberg's sign	Transient abdominal wall rebound tenderness	Peritoneal inflammation
Ballance's sign	Presence of a dull percussion note in both flanks consistent on the left side but shifting with change of position on the right	Ruptured spleen
Carnetts' sign	Disappearance of abdominal tenderness to palpation when anterior abdominal muscles are contracted	Abdominal pain of intra-abdominal origin
Chandelier sign	Intense lower abdominal and pelvic pain upon manipulation of the cervix	Pelvic inflammatory disease
Charcot's sign	Intermittent right upper-quadrant abdominal pain, jaundice, and fever	Choledocholithiasis
Chaussier's sign	Severe epigastric pain in gravid female	Eclampsia
Claybrook's sign	Transmission of breath and heart sounds through the abdomen	Ruptured abdominal viscus
Courvoisier's sign	Palpable, non-tender gallbladder in the presence of clinical jaundice	Pancreatic or common bile duct malignancy
Cutaneous hyperesthesia	Increased abdominal wall sensation to light touch	Parietal peritoneal inflammation secondary to an inflammatory intra-abdominal pathology
Direct abdominal wall tenderness		Localized inflammation of the abdominal wall, peritoneum, or an intra-abdominal viscus
Fothergill's sign	Abdominal wall mass that does not cross the midline and remains palpable when the rectus muscle is tense	Rectus muscle hematoma
Iliopsoas sign	Elevation and extension of the leg against pressure of the examiner's hand causes pain	Appendictis (retrocecal) or an inflammatory mass in contact with the psoas
Kehr's sign	Left shoulder pain when the patient is supine or in the Trendelenburg position. (Note: The pain may occur spontaneously or following the application of pressure to left subcostal region.)	Free blood in the peritoneal space
Kustner's sign	Palpable mass anterior to the uterus	Dermoid cyst of the ovary
McClintock's sign	Postpartum heart rate >100/min	Postpartal hemorrhage
Murphy's sign	Palpation of the right upper abdominal quadrant during deep inspiration results in right upper-quadrant abdominal pain	Acute cholecystitis
Obturator sign	Flexion of right thigh at right angles to trunk and external rotation of the same leg in the supine position results in hypogastric pain	Appendicitis (pelvic appendix); pelvic abscess; an inflammatory mass in contact with muscle
Puddle sign	Alteration in intensity of transmitted sound in the intra-abdominal cavity secondary to percussion when the patient is positioned on all fours and the stethoscope is gradually moved toward the flank opposite the percussion	Free peritoneal fluid
Rovsing's sign	Pain is referred to McBurney's point on applying pressure to the descending colon	Acute appendicitis
Subcutaneous crepitance		Subcutaneous empyema or gas gangrene
Sumner's sign	Increased abdominal muscle tone upon exceedingly gentle palpation of the right or left iliac fossa	Early appendicitis; nephrolithiasis; ureterolithiasis; ovarian torsion
Toma's sign	Right-sided tympany and left-sided dullness in the supine position as a result of peritoneal inflammation and subsequent mesenteric contraction of the intestine to the right side of the abdominal cavity	Inflammatory ascites

Source: Reprinted with permission from Hickey, M.S., Kiernan, G.J., and Weaver, K.E. 1989. Evaluation of abdominal pain. *Emergency Medicine Clinics of North America* 7(3):437-452.

- diaphoretic; anxious; right- or left-sided, diffuse, flank, or groin tenderness. See **Urinary Tract Disorders, Urinary Tract Infection** Protocol for other renal causes of abdominal pain.

→ Acute cholecystitis: See **Cholecystitis** Protocol.

Peritoneal irritation

→ Peritonitis:
- rebound tenderness, tenderness to palpation or percussion; abdomen rigidly distended; bowel sounds reduced or absent.
- rectal and vaginal tenderness.
- patient usually lies very still due to increase in pain with movement.
- peritonitis can cause postural changes in blood pressure and heart rate as a result of blood loss; low-grade fever.

→ Acute pancreatitis:
- elevated temperature, tachycardia, hypotension pallor, jaundice.
- diffuse epigastric tenderness with varying degrees of guarding usually without rigidity or rebound; hypoactive or absent bowel sounds.
- moderate elevation in WBCs. Bilirubin, serum lipase, and amylase may be elevated. In severe pancreatitis, may present with hypotension, signs of shock, significant elevation of WBCs and hematocrit, and decreased calcium level (Beal 1983).

→ Chronic pancreatitis:
- tenderness over pancreas, mild guarding, steatorrhea.
- elevated serum amylase, serum lipase, and bilirubin. Normal amylase does not exclude diagnosis.

→ See **Appendicitis, Cirrhosis, Hepatitis—Viral,** and **Diverticulosis** protocols.

Vascular disorders

→ Acute arterial insufficiency from atherosclerosis or mesenteric thrombus:
- abdominal tenderness may be present but poorly localized. Early in disorder, pain may be out of proportion to clinical findings.
- diagnosis usually evident with signs of shock.
- specific to mesenteric thrombus, atrial fibrillation may be present and a tender mass may be felt in upper or mid-abdomen.

→ Chronic arterial insufficiency:
- abdominal tenderness may be present.

- diminished femoral pulsation and a bruit over the abdomen or back may be heard.
- diagnosis usually confirmed with arteriography.

→ Ruptured abdominal aneurysm:
- sudden onset of symptoms with clinical signs of shock from blood loss.

Mucosal ulceration

→ See **Peptic Ulcer Disease** Protocol. (Beal 1983, for perforated ulcer)

Alteration in bowel motility

→ See protocols for **Irritable Bowel Syndrome, Diverticular Disease,** and **Diarrhea.**

Capsular distention

→ Hepatic capsular distention: enlarged liver, jaundice, ascites, other signs of chronic liver disease.

→ Splenic distention: enlarged spleen.

Metabolic disturbances

→ Lead poisoning: hyperperistalsis, abdominal rigidity, encephalopathy, peripheral neuropathy, and anemia.

→ Acute intermittent porphyria: soft abdomen, fever, elevated WBCs, range of neuropsychiatric symptoms.

→ Ketoacidosis: elevated WBCs. See **Type I Diabetes Mellitus, Type II Diabetes Mellitus** protocols.

Nerve injury

→ A variety of objective findings may be associated with nerve injury depending on the etiology.

Abdominal wall pathology

→ Abdominal wall trauma may be evident or a mass may be palpated. There is also muscle spasm and exacerbation of pain with abdominal muscle contraction.

→ Carnett's sign (see **Table 7A.2.**) will distinguish intra-abdominal versus abdominal wall pain. Cutaneous nerve involvement will show impaired sensory function in area of nerve distribution.

→ With herpes zoster, minimal associated symptoms are present and a hallmark rash appears after several days. There is also pain in the dermatomal distribution and hyperesthesia.

→ See **Hernia** Protocol.

Referred pain from extra-abdominal site

→ Objective findings of cardiac or pulmonary disorders are evident, with pain radiating from these regions.

→ See **Dysmenorrhea, Ectopic Pregnancy, Endometriosis, Pelvic Inflammatory Disease, Pelvic Masses, Pelvic Pain—Acute, Pelvic Pain—Chronic,** and **Urinary Tract Disorders, Urinary Tract Infection** protocols.

ASSESSMENT

→ Abdominal pain

→ See **Table 7A.3, Conditions Simulating an Acute Abdomen**, for differential diagnoses.

PLAN

DIAGNOSTIC TESTS

→ Initial diagnostic studies should be used to help in the diagnosis of serious disorders that warrant immediate referral—e.g., obstruction, peritonitis, acute vascular insufficiency, metabolic disorders, and cardiac or pulmonary disease.

→ Complete blood count (CBC) with differential can be helpful in determining the presence of an acute infection.

- A markedly elevated WBC count—especially with a shift to the left—is indicative of an infection.
- A low WBC count may occur with a viral illness such as gastroenteritis.
- A low hematocrit may indicate the possibility of a GI malignancy or bleeding, especially with a positive stool occult blood.
- An elevated hematocrit may indicate dehydration.
- Because the CBC is a non-specific test, management must not rest on this result alone, but should consider the entire clinical picture.

→ Stool for occult blood should be done on all patients.

→ Stool examination for polymorphonuclear leukocytes, ova, and parasites, and bacterial cultures may be ordered in cases of diarrhea. Sudan red stain for fecal fat may also be ordered.

→ Urinalysis should be completed. Red cells in the urine, along with flank pain, suggest a ureteral stone. Bacteria and white cells suggest an inflammation of the urinary tract.

→ Serum electrolytes may be helpful with severe or persistent vomiting and diarrhea.

→ Tests for renal function (24-hour urine and serum samples for calcium, uric acid, blood urea nitrogen [BUN], creatinine, urine oxalate, citrate, electrolytes) and hepatic function (hepatitis screen, liver function studies) may be ordered if clinical findings are suspicious for renal or liver disorders.

→ Serum amylase should be ordered with suspicion of pancreatitis.

- Levels are elevated in other diseases, but usually not to the levels found in pancreatitis.

→ Chest x-ray and electrocardiogram (EKG) should be ordered in cases of upper abdominal pain, if clinical findings are suspicious for pulmonary or cardiac disease, or with acute abdominal pain.

→ Supine and upright plain films of the abdomen (KUB and upright) will assist in diagnosing a perforated viscus, small bowel obstruction, biliary or renal stone, abdominal aortic calcification suggesting an aneurysm, or pancreatic calcification due to pancreatitis.

- Plain films should be utilized in patients with moderate to severe abdominal pain when any of the above conditions are suspected.
- Only bowel obstruction and perforation can be accurately ruled out with plain films.

→ Barium enema will assist in the diagnosis of large bowel obstruction.

→ Upper GI series or endoscopy may be ordered with failure to respond to ulcer therapy, or with symptoms of melena, hematemesis, and weight loss.

→ Colonoscopy, barium enema, or sigmoidoscopy may be ordered in cases of lower abdominal pain with bleeding.

→ Intravenous pyelogram (IVP) may assist in diagnosing disease in the kidneys or ureters or in identifying a mass impeding these structures.

→ Ultrasound can be used to assess a variety of conditions.

- Renal ultrasound may assess for renal stone or dilatation.
- Pelvic ultrasound for uterine or ovarian mass.
- Abdominal ultrasound for biliary obstruction, intra-abdominal abscesses, appendicitis, pancreatic tumors, or enlargement (Richter 1995a).

Table 7A.3. CONDITIONS SIMULATING AN ACUTE ABDOMEN

Metabolic, Hematologic
A. Familial Metabolic
   1. Porphyria
   2. Familial Mediterranean fever
   3. Hemochromatosis
   4. Hereditary angioneurotic edema
B. Endocrine
   1. DKA
   2. Addisonian crisis
   3. Hyperthyroidism/hypothyroidism
   4. Hypercalcemia (hyperparathyroidism); hypokalemia
C. Hematologic
   1. Sickle cell crisis
   2. Acute hemolytic states
   3. Leukemia
   4. Coagulopathies
   5. Pernicious anemia

Inflammatory Conditions
A. Infectious
   1. Enteric infections
      a. Salmonella, typhoid fever
      b. Shigellosis
      c. Staphylococcal
      d. Yersinia
      e. Campylobacter
      f. Tuberculosis
      g. Viral enterocolitis
      h. Parasitic
   2. Spontaneous bacterial peritonitis
   3. Hepatitis
   4. Mesenteric lymphadenitis
   5. Infectious mononucleosis
   6. Measles
   7. Mumps
   8. Malaria
   9. Rocky Mountain spotted fever
   10. AIDS-related disorders
B. Non-infectious
   1. Acute rheumatic fever
   2. SLE
   3. Polyarteritis nodosa
   4. Henoch-Schönlein purpura
   5. Dermatomyositis
   6. Scleroderma
   7. Inflammatory bowel disease
      a. Crohn's disease
      b. Ulcerative colitis
   8. Pancreatitis

Drug- and Toxin-Related Conditions
A. Heavy metal poisoning
   1. Lead
   2. Arsenic
   3. Mercury
B. Mushroom ingestion
C. Staphylococcus toxin
D. Black Widow spider bite
E. Anticoagulants
F. Narcotic withdrawal

Referred: Extraperitoneal Causes
A. Pulmonic
   1. Pneumonia
   2. Pulmonary embolism
   3. Pleurisy
   4. Spontaneous pneumothorax
B. Cardiac
   1. Angina: acute myocardial infarction
   2. Pericarditis
   3. Myocarditis
   4. Congestive hepatomegaly
C. Urologic
   1. Pyelonephritis
   2. Pyonephrosis
   3. Perinephric abscess
   4. Renal infarct
   5. Urolithiasis
   6. Cystitis
   7. Prostatitis
   8. Testicular torsion
   9. Epididymitis
   10. Orchitis
D. Obstetric, gynecologic
   1. Nonpregnant
      a. Mittelschmerz
      b. Ovarian cyst
      c. Salpingitis; Fitz-Hugh-Curtis syndrome
      d. Dysmenorrhea
      e. Endometriosis
   2. First-trimester pregnancy
      a. Ectopic pregnancy
      b. Simple pregnancy
      c. Threatened/incomplete abortion
E. Neurologic; spinal
   1. Multiple sclerosis
   2. Tabes dorsalis; gastric crisis
   3. Thoracic nerve root dysfunction
   4. Herpes zoster
   5. Abdominal migraine
   6. Abdominal epilepsy
   7. Glaucoma
F. Abdominal wall—rectus sheath hematoma
G. Skeletal
   1. Thoracolumbar spine
      a. Trauma
      b. Arthritis/discitis
      c. Osteomyelitis
   2. Hip
      a. Trauma
      b. Arthritis
H. Adynamic ileus and pseudo-obstruction
   1. Uremia
   2. Hypokalemia
   3. Constipation
I. Spontaneous splenic rupture

Functional
A. Somatization disorders
B. Hypochondriasis
C. Munchausen syndrome
D. Malingering

Source: Reprinted with permission from Purcell, T.B. 1989. Nonsurgical and extraperitoneal causes of abdominal pain. *Emergency Medicine Clinics of North America* 7(3):721-720.

→ Computerized tomography (CT) or angiography, to assess for vascular disorders, may be ordered with physician consultation.
  - A pregnancy test should be considered in a reproductive-age woman.

→ See **Dysmenorrhea, Ectopic Pregnancy, Endometriosis, Pelvic Inflammatory Disease, Pelvic Masses, Pelvic Pain—Acute, Pelvic Pain—Chronic,** and **Urinary Tract Disorders, Urinary Tract Infection** protocols for additional diagnostic tests.

TREATMENT/MANAGEMENT

→ Patients with evidence of obstruction, peritoneal irritation, acute vascular insufficiency, metabolic disorders, and cardiac or pulmonary disease should be referred to a physician immediately.

→ Consultation and/or referral is warranted in cases:
  - of undiagnosed abdominal pain.
  - when signs and symptoms do not follow the usual course of disease or with impressive signs and symptoms—e.g., high fever, severe pain, elevated WBC count, other laboratory test abnormalities, or patient inability to eat or drink.

→ Repeated histories and examinations may offer new data and allow for appropriate diagnosis, referral, and treatment.

→ Analgesia should not be given until an adequate diagnosis is made so as not to obscure symptoms/ signs of disease progression.

→ See **Gastrointestinal Disorders, Genitourinary Disorders, Dermatological Disorders, Respiratory/Otorhinolaryngological Disorders, Cardiovascular Disorders, Hematological/**

Endocrine Disorders, Infectious Diseases, and **Behavioral Disorders** protocols for management of specific conditions.

CONSULTATION

→ Referral to a physician is warranted in patients with evidence of obstruction, peritoneal irritation, acute vascular insufficiency, metabolic disorders, and cardiac or pulmonary disease.

→ Consultation with a physician and/or referral is warranted in cases:
  - of undiagnosed abdominal pain.
  - when signs and symptoms do not follow the usual course of disease, or
  - with impressive signs and symptoms—e.g., high fever, severe pain, elevated WBCs, other laboratory test abnormalities, or patient inability to eat or drink.

→ Referral to a mental health provider is warranted in cases of severe psychogenic disorder, depression, neurosis, or hysteria.

→ As needed for prescription(s).

PATIENT EDUCATION

→ Patient education will depend on etiology of abdominal pain. Refer to appropriate protocol for patient education regarding specific etiologies.

FOLLOW-UP

→ When diagnosis is unclear and patient is not ill enough for immediate referral or admission, close follow-up is important. Chronic abdominal pain may require a methodical work-up and therapeutic trials.

→ Document in progress notes and problem list.

Lisa L. Lommel, R.N., C., F.N.P., M.P.H.

7-B

Anorectal Conditions

Anorectal complaints may result from traumatic, vascular, infectious, inflammatory, neurological, or malignant etiologies. Brief descriptions of the most common anorectal conditions follow.

Hemorrhoids

Hemorrhoids are the most common anorectal problem. This condition is the subject of a separate protocol.

Fissure

Fissure is a split in the anoderm in the anterior (10%) or posterior (90%) midline due to a tense anal sphincter subjected to trauma by passing of a hard stool. Recurrence can leave a chronic condition or repeated healing can leave an inelastic scar. Fissure is more common in young individuals.

Fistula-in-ano

Fistula is a communication between the anal canal and the perianal skin, possibly caused by a rupture or surgical drainage of a perirectal abscess, Crohn's disease, carcinoma, tuberculosis, radiation therapy, lymphogranuloma venereum, or anal fissures.

Perirectal abscess

This condition is an infection in the anal glands causing secretions to empty into the anal crypts, which eventually drain into the anal skin. A fistula-in-ano often results from the abscess.

Proctitis

Proctitis is an inflammatory disease of the rectum due to a variety of etiologies: trauma, radiation, or inflammatory bowel disease. Infectious proctitis commonly is caused by a bacteria, virus, or amebic disease and is most common in women who engage in rectal intercourse.

Pruritus ani

Chronic perianal itching is not a diagnosis but a symptom of a variety of conditions. These include fistulas, fissures, hemorrhoids, anogenital warts, gonococcal proctitis, scabies, pinworm, psoriasis, contact dermatitis, eczema, neurodermatitis, *candida* infections, lichen sclerosis, poor hygiene, early cancer, or secondary to local disease (e.g., trichomoniasis).

Carcinoma

Perianal or anorectal carcinoma is uncommon but should be considered, especially if blood is present in the stool of an older woman.

DATABASE

SUBJECTIVE

→ Fissure.
- Symptoms may include splitting pain or tearing sensation associated with or immediately after a bowel movement. Pain lingers after the bowel movement and progressively wanes.
- Discharge and itching may appear later.

- Bright red blood is intermittently present with the bowel movement (Smith 1990).
→ Fistula-in-ano.
  - Fistula-in-ano may be secondary to a perirectal abscess. Patient may have symptoms of an abscess (see following discussion) with the fistula, which is usually non-tender.
  - Symptoms may include:
    • itching, tenderness, or pain aggravated by bowel movements.
    • persistent, irritating drainage of blood, pus, or mucus.
→ Perirectal abscess.
  - Symptoms may include constant throbbing pain in perianal or rectal areas.
  - An external perianal mass may be palpable.
→ Proctitis.
  - Inflammatory proctitis will present with mucopurulent discharge, rectal bleeding, pain, tenesmus, and constipation.
  - Gonococcal proctitis may present with discharge and rectal discomfort.
  - Amebic infection presents with diarrhea.
  - Herpes simplex proctitis is extremely painful and presents with pain in the thighs and buttocks, anorectal vesicles, discharge, itching, fever, urinary retention, and constipation.
  - Primary syphilis may present with painless lesions in perianal area.
→ Pruritus ani.
  - Symptoms will depend on etiology. See p. 7-12 for etiologies and then refer to specific protocols.
  - Hallmark symptom is itching, most often nocturnal.
→ Carcinoma.
  - Usually painless until late in stage.
  - Pruritus, mucoid drainage, change in bowel habits, or perianal mass may occur.

OBJECTIVE
→ Fissure.
  - With gentle separation of the buttocks, and stretching of the perianal skin, an elliptical ulcer appears at the anus when acute.
  - In a chronic state, the fissure has white scarred margins and a white sphincter at its base (Smith 1990).
  - A fissure, hypertrophied anal papilla at the pectinate line, and a skin tag are hallmark signs.

- Rectal examination may be extremely painful in acute stages, and may be deferred until patient is more comfortable.
- Anoscopy will reveal a fissure, discharge, and/or inflammation.
→ Fistula-in-ano.
  - Patient presents with single or multiple external opening(s) with granulation, tissue bud, and seropurulent discharge.
  - Anoscopy can aid in visualization of the openings.
  - Uncommonly, an indurated cord of tissue is palpable, extending from the external opening toward the anal canal.
→ Perirectal abscess.
  - A mass may be seen externally or may be palpable internally during a digital examination.
→ Proctitis.
  - Patient with inflammatory proctitis may present with mucopurulent discharge and bleeding.
  - Patient with infectious gonococcal proctitis may present with discharge and inguinal lymphadenopathy.
  - Patient with amebic proctitis may present with signs of perianal skin erythema secondary to diarrhea.
  - Patient with herpes simplex proctitis may present with perianal ulcers, erythema, and inguinal lymphadenopathy. Anoscopy reveals friable mucosa, diffuse ulcerations, vesicles, and pustules.
  - Primary syphilis may reveal single or multiple painless chancres in perianal area, inguinal lymphadenopathy.
→ Pruritus ani.
  - Examination may be variable, from no skin reaction to erythema, fissuring, excoriation, inflammation, and lichenification.
  - Signs will depend on etiology. See p. 7-12 for etiologies, then refer to specific protocols.
→ Carcinoma.
  - In early presentation, patient presents with painless nodules or plaques.
  - In late presentation, patient has developed ulcerative, bleeding lesion.

ASSESSMENT

→ Anal fissure
→ Fistula-in-ano
→ Perirectal abscess

→ Proctitis, inflammatory or infectious

→ Pruritus ani

→ R/O carcinoma

PLAN

DIAGNOSTIC TESTS

→ Unless the patient has an acutely painful lesion, anoscopy should be performed to visualize canal and mucosa and obtain samples. Topical anesthetic may be necessary for examination.

→ Refer for sigmoidoscopy patients with rectal inflammation, fistulas, non-healing fissures, bleeding, or diarrhea.

→ Refer for biopsy patients with atypical fissures, masses, nodules, and ulcerations.

→ Stool for occult blood should be performed on patients with anorectal complaints.

→ Rectal cultures for *Chlamydia trachomatis*, *Neisseria gonorrhoeae*, herpes simplex, and samples for ova and parasites should be done on women who engage in rectal intercourse.

→ Serological test for syphilis should be done on women who engage in rectal intercourse.

→ On patients with anal/rectal itching, obtain anal scraping and observe for presence of pinworms.

→ Additional testing may be warranted, depending on patient's condition. See specific protocols. (For example, obtain blood glucose to rule out diabetes in patients with pruritus ani).

TREATMENT/MANAGEMENT

(Goroll 1995a)

→ Fissure.
  ▪ Bulk stool softener (methylcellulose, e.g., Metamucil®) and anal suppository (Anusol®) twice daily for 1 month, to allow for spontaneous healing, along with a diet containing adequate fiber and liquids. If no healing, consider referral to a physician for possible surgical intervention.
  ▪ Oral analgesies if pain is moderate to severe.

→ Fistula-in-ano.
  ▪ Refer to a physician for surgical repair.

→ Perirectal abscess.
  ▪ Refer to a physician for surgical drainage and antibiotic therapy.
  ▪ Hot sitz baths may speed the process of abscess localization (Knauer 1993a).

→ Proctitis.

▪ Inflammatory proctitis management is related to identification of specific etiology—e.g., eliminating trauma.
  • If proctitis is due to radiation therapy, benefits of therapy should be weighed against side effect of proctitis.
    –Alternative management would allow for proctitis healing between radiation treatments.
  • See **Inflammatory Bowel Disease** Protocol if due to this condition.
▪ See specific protocols for gonococcal, amebic, chlamydia, herpes simplex, and syphilis infections.

→ Pruritus ani.
  ▪ Management is dependent on etiology. See p. 7-12 for etiologies, then refer to specific protocols.
  ▪ Topical steroid ointment (0.5%-1.0% hydrocortisone) applied sparingly to anal area twice a day for 2 to 3 weeks may reduce itching (Bassford 1992).
  ▪ An oral antihistamine may be used to break the itch/scratch cycle (Bassford 1992).
  ▪ Witch hazel premoistened pads (e.g., Tucks®), ointment, or cream may offer relief.

CONSULTATION

→ Referral to a physician is warranted with inflammatory proctitis, fistula, non-healing or atypical fissure, bleeding, diarrhea, nodules, or ulcerations.

→ As needed for prescription(s).

PATIENT EDUCATION

→ Fissure.
  ▪ Advise patient regarding diet high in fiber and fluids to encourage soft, bulky stools. Bulk-forming product such as methylcellulose may be needed for a month to initiate healing.
  ▪ Advise regular exercise and toilet habits. Teach patient to maintain good hygiene and avoid excessive cleansing.
  ▪ Sitz baths to relieve pain and discomfort.

→ Proctitis.
  ▪ Inflammatory proctitis: depends on etiology.
  ▪ Infectious proctitis: see specific protocols.

→ Pruritus ani.
  ▪ See p. 7-12 for etiologies, then refer to specific protocols.
  ▪ Advise ways of preventing constipation (see **Constipation** Protocol).

- Advise patient to avoid spicy foods that can irritate anal mucosa.
- Advise patient to maintain careful perianal hygiene, making sure to keep the area dry, using a soft or moistened tissue after bowel movement and urination.
- Advise patient about the harmful effects of scratching.
- Advise patient to change underclothes daily.
- Sitz baths twice a day may relieve itching and discomfort.
- Patient should avoid applying talc or perfumed products to perianal area.

FOLLOW-UP

→ For patients where a rectal examination or anoscopy could not be performed because of severely painful fissures, allow for healing of the acute stage and reexamine.

→ See specific protocols.

→ Advise patients of American Cancer Society's recommendations for early detection of cancer in asymptomatic individuals (American Cancer Society [ACS] 1993):
- sigmoidoscopy: every three years beginning at age 50 years.
- stool guaiac: yearly beginning at age 50 years.
- digital rectal examination: yearly beginning at age 40 years.
  - ACS suggests a digital rectal examination of all women during their annual gynecological visit.

→ Document in progress notes and problem list.

7-C

Appendicitis

Appendicitis is one of the most frequently occurring causes of acute surgical abdomen. The peak incidence is evenly distributed between males and females in their 20s and 30s but is most common in males between 10 years and 30 years of age.

Obstruction of the appendiceal lumen by a fecalith, inflammation, foreign body, or neoplasm is thought to initiate appendicitis. Although mucosal ulceration has been identified as an antecedent to obstruction in many cases, it is not known whether the ulceration causes obstruction of the lumen by infection or swelling.

Once the obstruction occurs, there is inflammation and secretion of mucus which, in turn, distends the appendix, causing pain, necrosis, and, eventually, perforation. Perforation is a serious complication of appendicitis because it can soil the peritoneal cavity, causing intra-abdominal sepsis.

Appendicitis can be recurrent in nature or have an acute, rapid course.

DATABASE

SUBJECTIVE

→ Patient has negative history of appendectomy.

→ Progression of symptoms—beginning with epigastric or periumbilical mild, intermittent, cramping pain—is hallmark in diagnosis.

→ Early symptoms may be associated with urge to defecate or pass flatus and with vomiting, neither of which relieves the pain.

→ After two to twelve hours, the pain spreads to the right lower quadrant where it is constant, increasing in severity, and aggravated by cough or motion.

→ Anorexia, malaise, constipation, or, sometimes, diarrhea, nausea, and vomiting develop.

→ Patient can usually point to specific area of maximal tenderness.

→ Depending on location of appendix, other symptoms may occur:
  ■ appendix adjacent to the bladder—urinary frequency and dysuria.
  ■ retrocecal or pelvic appendix—minimal or absent abdominal tenderness and positive tenderness in flank or on rectal examination.

→ Obese or elderly patients may have a delay in appearance of abdominal signs and may not experience sharp localization of symptoms.

OBJECTIVE

→ Temperature normal or slightly elevated (37.2°C-38°C; 99°F-100.4°F).

→ Temperature above 38.3°C (101°F) may indicate perforation.

→ Tachycardia present with elevation of temperature.

→ Elevated WBC count to 10,000μl-20,000/μl with increase in neutrophils.

→ Microscopic hematuria and pyuria may be present.

→ Light palpation or percussion can identify a point of maximal tenderness in right lower quadrant.

→ Rebound tenderness and muscle rigidity in right lower quadrant.

→ Hyperesthesia of the skin in right lower quadrant.

→ Tenderness on right side of rectal wall.

→ Diminished or absent bowel sounds.

→ Rigidity and tenderness are increased as disease progresses.

→ Positive iliopsoas sign (rectocecal), obturator sign (pelvic appendix), Rovsing's sign, Sumner's sign (see **Table 7A.2,** p. 7-7).

→ Perforation rarely occurs in first eight hours.

→ Signs of perforation include:
- increasing pain, tenderness, and spasm of right lower quadrant followed by evidence of generalized peritonitis (see **Abdominal Pain** Protocol) or a localized abcess (tender mass in right lower quadrant).
- temperature, malaise, tachycardia, and WBC increase.

→ Demonstration of an enlarged and thick-walled appendix on ultrasound is diagnostic. If the appendix cannot be seen, appendicitis cannot be excluded.

ASSESSMENT

→ Acute appendicitis

→ R/O gastroenteritis

→ R/O mesenteric adenitis

→ R/O pelvic inflammatory disease (PID)

→ R/O ruptured graafian follicle or corpus luteum cyst

→ R/O acute diverticulitis

→ R/O perforated ulcer

→ R/O acute cholecystitis

→ R/O ruptured ectopic pregnancy

→ R/O twisted ovarian cyst

→ R/O mittelschmerz

→ R/O nephrolithiasis

PLAN

DIAGNOSTIC TESTS

→ Symptoms, clinical findings, and progression of disease over time is hallmark in diagnosing appendicitis.

→ Observation is often used for diagnosis. It entails close observation of the patient in the presence of the provider in the clinic, office, or hospital. The provider is assessing for progressive constellation of symptoms that are diagnostic for appendicitis. Diagnosis is assisted if there is localization of symptoms to the right lower quadrant within twelve hours of symptom onset.

→ Obtain CBC and differential:
- moderate elevation in WBCs is common during appendicitis attack.
- WBC count has low specificity for diagnosis of appendicitis.
- normal WBC count should not rule out possibility of acute appendicitis.
- WBCs > 20,000 /µl may indicate perforation.

→ Urinalysis is helpful in ruling out genitourinary symptoms that can mimic appendicitis.

→ Radiographic films and barium enema are not consistent in visualizing the appendix. These techniques are usually reserved to rule out suspicion of other pathology.

→ High-resolution, real-time ultrasound has an overall accuracy of 96 percent for the diagnosis of acute appendicitis.

→ During close observation, abdominal and rectal exams, WBC count, and differential should be repeated periodically for signs of disease progression (Hoffmann and Rasmussen 1989).

TREATMENT/MANAGEMENT

→ During close observation, patient should be resting, given nothing by mouth, and not prescribed laxatives or narcotics that will interfere with assessment for disease progression.

→ Once a strong suspicion or diagnosis of appendicitis is made, immediate referral to a surgeon is warranted.

CONSULTATION

→ Physician consultation may be sought in diagnosis.

PATIENT EDUCATION

→ Explain disease process, progression, and treatment plan.

→ Advise patient about the probability of surgery if diagnosis is made.

FOLLOW-UP

→ As indicated by surgical team.

→ Document in progress notes and problem list.

7-D

Cholecystitis

Cholecystitis is an inflammation of the gallbladder that occurs most often when a stone becomes lodged in the ampulla of the gallbladder or in the cystic duct. Inflammation and pressure develop behind the obstruction as a result of continued secretion. Chronic cholecystitis is secondary to continued inflammation of the gallbladder. An acute cholecystitis attack is usually preceded by a history of previous symptomatic episodes. Occasionally, the acute attack is the first episode of biliary tract disease (Knauer 1993b; Goroll 1995b).

Approximately 10 percent of cholecystitis is a result of vascular abnormalities of the bile duct or pancreas, or secondary to multiple small stones undetectable by screening methods. Gangrene of the gallbladder and perforation are complications of cholecystitis.

DATABASE

SUBJECTIVE

Chronic cholecystitis

→ Recurrent episodes of sudden onset, intermittent, or constant, right hypochondriac, or epigastric "colicky" pain, building to a maximum within one hour, lasting one to four hours, radiating to left or right scapula.

Acute cholecystitis

→ Sudden onset of severe, usually constant, right hypochondriac or epigastric pain, subsiding in 12 to 18 hours.

→ Nausea and vomiting may occur.

→ Dark urine, light, clay-colored stools may occur in acute and chronic cholecystitis.

→ Patient may be asymptomatic.

→ Though ingestion of fatty foods or large amounts of food with subsequent flatulence, epigastric heaviness, belching, heartburn, and upper abdominal pain was thought to be a precipitating factor in cholecystitis symptoms, studies show that association is probably incidental (Goroll 1995b).

OBJECTIVE

Chronic cholecystitis

→ Mild or absent right upper-quadrant tenderness.

→ Jaundice may be present.

Acute cholecystitis

→ Right upper-quadrant abdominal tenderness with guarding and rebound.

→ Gallbladder that is palpable (15 percent of cases).

→ Jaundice (25 percent of cases) and fever.

→ Moderately elevated WBC count, total serum bilirubin, serum transaminase, serum amylase, alkaline phosphatase.

→ Positive Murphy's sign (**see Table 7A.2,** p. 7-7).

→ Radiographic film of the abdomen may show gallstones (15 percent of cases) (Knauer 1993b).

→ HIDA (99m dimethylimino-diacetic acid imaging agent) scan may show obstructed cystic duct.

→ Ultrasound may show gallstones.

ASSESSMENT

→ Cholecystitis—acute or chronic
→ R/O peptic ulcer
→ R/O pancreatitis
→ R/O hepatitis
→ R/O appendicitis
→ R/O diverticulitis
→ R/O right lower-lobe pneumonia
→ R/O irritable bowel syndrome
→ R/O neoplasm of the stomach, pancreas, liver, or gallbladder
→ R/O angina
→ R/O Fitz-Hugh-Curtis Syndrome

PLAN

DIAGNOSTIC TESTS

→ WBC count.
→ Total serum bilirubin, serum transaminase, serum amylase, alkaline phosphatase, and liver function studies.
→ Radiographic film of the abdomen.
→ HIDA scan (rarely necessary).
→ Ultrasound of the abdomen.
→ EKG to rule out cardiac symptoms.
→ Chest x-ray to rule out pulmonary symptoms.

TREATMENT/MANAGEMENT

Chronic cholecystitis

→ Referral to a physician is warranted for decision regarding surgical or non-surgical treatment.
→ Non-surgical methods include:
  ▪ ursodeoxycholic acids: oral bile salts that cause dissolution of some cholesterol stones.
  ▪ effective only in patients with functioning gallbladders.
  ▪ may take up to two years for dissolution.
  ▪ stones recur at the rate of 15 percent per year. This suggests a role for chronic suppressive therapy (Goroll 1995b).
  ▪ lithotripsy; extracorporeal shock wave technique.

▪ effective in small number of patients. Concomitant use of ursodeoxycholic acid agents is recommended (Goroll 1995b).
▪ analgesics (e.g., meperidine) to control pain.

Acute cholecystitis

→ Referral to a physician is warranted for decision regarding surgical or non-surgical treatment.
  ▪ Surgery is warranted if patient is diabetic or shows evidence of gangrene or perforation (Knauer 1993b).
    • Laparoscopic cholecystectomies are becoming the technique of choice.
→ With patient taking oral contaceptives, advise to consider alternative form of birth control.
  ▪ Estrogen preparations and clofibrate should also be discontinued in patients with known gallstones.

Dyspepsia

→ Avoidance of high-fat foods has not been shown to improve dyspeptic symptoms. Avoidance of specific foods that precipitate symptoms may be of benefit.
→ Antacids can be used to treat dyspeptic symptoms (see **Dyspepsia** Protocol).
→ Surgical removal of the gallbladder may improve dyspeptic symptoms though not consistently.
→ Weight reduction may be of benefit to some patients.

CONSULTATION

→ Referral to a physician is warranted for decision regarding whether treatment is non-surgical or surgical.
→ As needed for prescription(s).

PATIENT EDUCATION

→ See "Treatment/Management" section.
→ Explain disease process and management plan.
→ Provide information regarding effective use of antacids (see **Dyspepsia** Protocol).
→ Counsel patient on weight-reduction diet (see **General Nutrition Guidelines** section).

FOLLOW-UP

→ As indicated by case presentation.
→ Document in progress notes and problem list.

7-E

Cirrhosis

Cirrhosis refers to chronic, irreversible hepatocellular injury that leads to fibrosis and nodular regeneration of the liver. The most common causes of cirrhosis are related to: 1) excessive alcohol ingestion; 2) cryptogenic, post-viral or post-necrotic disorders; 3) biliary tract disorders; 4) cardiac disorders; and 5) metabolic, inherited, and drug-related disorders. It is often difficult to establish the etiology of cirrhosis since most affected persons present with end-stage cirrhosis, allowing for only an educated guess.

A new classification system that characterizes the developmental process of cirrhosis rather than delineating separate diseases was introduced recently. (Knauer 1993b). It includes:

→ *micronodular cirrhosis*: regenerating nodules less than or equal to 1 mm diameter; thought to be associated with chronic alcohol abuse.

→ *macronodular cirrhosis*: larger nodules up to several centimeters; thought to be associated with post-necrotic cirrhosis.

→ *mixed (micro and macronodular) cirrhosis*: mixture of liver cell death, regeneration, deposition of fat and iron and fibrosis; seen in varied forms in all etiologies.

Alcoholic liver cirrhosis is the most common type of cirrhosis in North America, accounting for 65 percent of cases (Knauer 1993b). It is characterized by diffuse fine scarring, uniform loss of liver cells, and micronodules, though it may progress to macronodules. It remains unclear what level of alcohol ingestion is necessary and for how long to cause cirrhosis. These are the two factors that appear to be the most important determinants of liver injury.

Malnutrition, a common characteristic of alcoholic cirrhosis, is thought to increase the injurious effects on the liver. Women appear to experience alcohol-related liver injury at lower levels of consumption than do men (Podolsky and Isselbacher 1991).

The prognosis for alcoholic cirrhosis is related to severity of hepatic disease and whether alcohol ingestion continues. In one study, patients with biopsy-proven alcoholic cirrhosis who discontinued intake of alcohol had a five-year survival rate of 60 percent compared to 40 percent for those who continued drinking. The five-year survival rate was 30 percent for non-drinking patients who had developed jaundice and ascites (Goroll 1995c). The major causes of cirrhosis-related deaths are variceal bleeding, encephalopathy, and infection.

This protocol covers alcoholic liver cirrhosis.

DATABASE

SUBJECTIVE

→ Patient has history of excessive alcohol intake over a long period of time.

→ After initial onset of symptoms, symptoms progress slowly.

→ Symptoms present in varying degrees, depending on extent of disease:
- anorexia.
- weight loss.
- fatigue and increasing weakness.
- easy bruising, prolonged time to clot.
- loss of libido.
- patient may be asymptomatic.

→ Symptoms may progress to:

- jaundice.
- redness of palms and face.
- abdominal pain.
- enlarged abdomen.
- nausea and vomiting.
- menstrual irregularities.
- pain in and malalignment of finger joints.
- hematemesis.
- decreased urine output.

OBJECTIVE

→ Signs present in varying degrees depending on extent of disease:
  - firm, nodular, usually enlarged liver; left lobe may be predominant.
  - jaundice.
  - palmar erythema.
  - spider nevi of upper half of body.
  - telangiectases of exposed areas.
  - parotid and lacrimal gland enlargement.
  - glotitis and cheilosis (rare).
  - clubbing of fingers (rare).
  - splenomegaly.
  - muscle wasting.
  - signs of virilization.
  - Dupuytren's contracture (i.e., flexion contracture of the digits).
  - progressive signs include:
    - ascites.
    - dilated vasculature visible on abdomen and thorax.
    - worsening jaundice.
    - peripheral edema.
    - pleural effusion.
    - purpuric lesions.
    - severe complications include signs of esophageal hemorrhage, infection, coagulopathy, renal dysfunction, and encephalopathy.
    - abnormal lab tests, degree of abnormality depending on extent of disease including:
      –decreased hemoglobin and hematocrit, macrocytic anemia.
      –increased or decreased WBC.
      –prolonged prothrombin time.
      –elevated aspartate aminotransferase (AST).
      –elevated alanine aminotransferase (ALT).
      –elevated bilirubin.
      –elevated gamma globulin.
      –decreased serum albumin.
      –variety of other metabolic disorders that may be present—elevated glucose tolerance,

hypomagnesemia, hypophosphatemia, hyponatremia, hypokalemia, azotemia.
      –liver biopsy showing cirrhosis.

ASSESSMENT

→ Alcoholic liver cirrhosis

→ R/O viral-hepatitis-induced cirrhosis

→ R/O primary biliary cirrhosis

→ R/O drug-induced cirrhosis

→ R/O cholangitis

→ R/O hemochromatosis

→ R/O Wilson's disease

PLAN

DIAGNOSTIC TESTS

→ Diagnosis can be strongly suspected with history of prolonged and excessive alcohol intake and clinical manifestations of liver disease.

→ Tests to evaluate extent of liver involvement may include:
  - CBC.
  - ferritin, folic acid.
  - AST, ALT.
  - serum bilirubin.
  - prothrombin time.
  - gamma globulin.
  - serum albumin.
  - glucose.
  - serum magnesium, phosphatase, sodium, calcium, and protein.

→ Ultrasound to evaluate liver size, hepatic nodules, occult ascites.

→ Ultrasound and doppler studies may be helpful in evaluating patency of splenic and portal veins.

→ Splenoportography remains the "gold standard" in evaluation of splenic and portal vein patency.

→ Flat plate x-ray of the abdomen to assess liver and spleen size.

→ Liver biopsy may be indicated to:
  - confirm diagnosis of alcoholic cirrhosis.
  - evaluate for other etiologies of cirrhosis.
  - evaluate patients who have clinical manifestations of alcoholic liver disease but deny alcohol intake.

→ Additional tests may be indicated to rule out other causes of cirrhosis—e.g., ultrasound to evaluate for primary biliary cirrhosis.

→ Additional tests may be indicated to evaluate for complications of cirrhosis—e.g., upper gastro-intestinal tract barium studies to rule out esophageal varices.

→ Stool for occult blood.

TREATMENT/MANAGEMENT

→ Abstinence from alcohol.

→ No use of other hepatotoxic drugs and agents. Also avoid tranquilizers and sedatives.

→ Well-balanced diet of at least 2,000 kcal to 3,000 kcal per day with low protein in later stages of encephalopathy. Low sodium if ascities is present.

→ Daily multiple vitamin and mineral supplement including 1 mg of folic acid.

→ Correction of iron deficiency with diet and iron supplementation of 300 mg enteric-coated tablets 3 times a day after meals.

→ Check stools at each visit for presence of occult bleeding.

→ Periodic monitoring of prothrombin time, serum albumin, and bilirubin to assess severity and progression of disease (Goroll 1995c).

→ Continuous monitoring for signs and symptoms of disease progression and complications.

→ Immediate physician referral/management is warranted in cases of advanced disease and complications including:
- ascites and edema.
- encephalopathy.
- coagulopathy.
- variceal bleeding.

CONSULTATION

→ Physician consultation for management of early disease.

→ Physician referral for diagnostic liver biopsy.

→ Immediate physician referral and management of advanced disease and complications including ascites, encephalopathy, coagulopathy, and variceal bleeding.

PATIENT EDUCATION

→ See "Treatment/Management" section.

→ Teach pathophysiology and etiology of disease and management plan.

→ Include patient's family in patient education and treatment plan.

→ Provide supportive relationship for patient and family.

→ Be aware that depression is common with this disease and patients should be evaluated for clinical signs and symptoms with referral to appropriate resources if indicated.

→ Stress importance of abstinence from alcohol and hepatotoxic agents to lessen symptoms and improve prognosis.

→ Encourage rest during acute phase of disease.

→ Advise patient regarding a well-balanced diet (see **General Nutrition Guidelines** section).

→ Referral to appropriate twelve-step support group may be indicated for alcohol cessation (Alcoholics Anonymous, Al-Anon for family members).

→ See **Behavioral Disorders, Alcoholism and Other Drug Dependencies** Protocol.

FOLLOW-UP

→ General measures including diet, rest, and vitamin therapy should continue throughout any phase of cirrhosis.

→ Major factor in patient survival is abstaining from alcohol. Patient should be reminded of this and given support for abstinence.

→ Periodic monitoring of prothrombin time, serum albumin, and bilirubin to assess progression of disease.

→ Periodic stools for occult blood should be obtained.

→ Immediate physician referral for clinical manifestations of deterioration or complications.

→ See **Behavioral Disorders, Alcoholism and Other Drug Dependencies** Protocol.

→ Document in progress notes and problem list.

Lisa L. Lommel, R.N., C., F.N.P., M.P.H.

7-F

Constipation

Constipation is defined as infrequent or difficult defecation that is delayed for days, with stools that are unusually hard, dry, and difficult to express (Knauer 1993a).

DATABASE

SUBJECTIVE

→ Patient has history of decreasing frequency of bowel movements and/or hard, dry stools that are difficult to express.

→ Symptoms may include (Sammons 1990):
- emotional tension, inability to relax.
- abdominal cramping, distension, flatulence.

→ Patient may recite history of contributing factors (Knauer 1993a):
- dietary factors: low fiber intake, inadequate fluids.
- physical inactivity.
- pregnancy.
- advanced age.
- drug use— e.g., use of codeine analgesics, anesthetics, antacids with aluminum or calcium salts, anticholinergics, anticonvulsants, antidepressants, antihypertensives, diuretics, iron salts, muscle relaxants, opiates.
- metabolic abnormalities—i.e., hypokalemia, hyperglycemia, uremia, porphyria, amyloidosis.
- endocrine abnormalities—i.e., hypothyroidism, hypercalcemia, panhypopituitarism.
- abnormalities of the lower bowel—i.e., the colon, rectum, anus.
- neurological abnormalities—e.g., innervation disorders of the bowel wall, disorders of spanchic nerves, cerebral disorders.

- psychogenic disorders—including involuntary suppression of the urge to defecate.
- chronic use of enemas.

OBJECTIVE

→ Mass or fullness may be palpable over large intestine.

→ Patient may present with abdominal tenderness and/or distension.

→ Bowel sounds may be hyperactive or absent.

→ Dry, hard stool may be felt on rectal examination.

→ Hemorrhoids may be present and felt on rectal examination.

→ Signs of metabolic, endocrine, neurological, or psychogenic disorders may be present. See other protocols for objective signs of specific causative etiologies.

ASSESSMENT

→ Constipation

→ R/O pathological disorders contributing to constipation

→ R/O bowel obstruction

→ R/O fecal impaction

PLAN

DIAGNOSTIC TESTS

→ History is hallmark in diagnosing constipation.

→ If conservative measures do not relieve constipation, further diagnostic work-up for other causes is warranted.

→ Further work-up will depend on history, signs, and symptoms.

→ Obtain stool for occult blood.

→ See other protocols for work-up of specific causative etiologies.

TREATMENT/MANAGEMENT

→ See "Patient Education" section.

→ Diet (see **General Nutrition Guidelines** section):
- fluid intake: increase water intake to 6 to 8 glasses/day.
- high fiber: bran, whole grain products, raw fruits and vegetables.
- avoid constipating foods (e.g., milk, cheese).

→ Laxatives:
- should not be used in patients with undiagnosed abdominal pain or with possible intestinal obstruction or fecal impaction.
- should be used only on a temporary basis until re-establishment of regular bowel movements. Prolonged use interferes with normal bowel motility and can cause mucous membrane or nerve injury.
- stimulant laxatives (Knauer 1993a):
  - cascara sagrada aromatic fluid extract—mild agent, acts within 6-12 hours: 4 ml-8 ml p.o., 1 dose.
  - bisacodyl (Ducolax®, etc.)—mild to moderate agent, oral form acts within 6 hours, suppository form, 15-60 minutes.
    –Oral form: 10 mg-15 mg p.o.; rectal form: 1 dose or 1 suppository per rectum.
  - phenolphthalein (Dialose Plus®, Medilax®)—potent agent, acts in 4-10 hours: 60 mg-200 mg p.o., one dose.
  - glycerin suppository—acts within 30 minutes: 3 g suppository per rectum, 1 dose.
- bulk-forming agents (Knauer 1993a):
  - psyllium hydrophilic mucilloid and methylcellulose (Citrucel®, Hydrocil®, Konsyl®, Metamucil®)—mild agent: 14 g, 1 tsp.-2 tsp., 2-3 times daily after meals in full glass of water.
  - Unprocessed bran: ¼ cup daily.

- osmotic laxatives (Knauer 1993a):
  - milk of magnesia—mild-moderate agent, not to be used in patients with impaired renal function: 15 ml-30 ml p.o., 1 dose at bedtime.
  - citrate of magnesia—not to be used in patients with impaired renal function: 120 ml-240 ml p.o.
  - sodium phosphate: 4 g-8 g p.o., 1 dose in cold water before breakfast.
  - lactulose syrup: 15 ml-60 ml p.o. daily.
- wetting agents (Knauer 1993a):
  - docusate sodium (Colace®, Doximate®): 50 mg-350 mg p.o. per day.
- lubricants (Knauer 1993a):
  - liquid petrolatum (mineral oil): 15 ml-30 ml per rectum, 1 dose. Oral administration should be avoided due to risk of aspiration and possible interference with absorption of fat-soluble vitamins.
- enemas (Knauer 1993a):
  - saline enema: 500 ml-2000 ml of warm physiological saline per rectum, 1 dose.
  - warm tap water: 500 ml-1000 ml of warm tap water per rectum, 1 dose.
  - soapsuds enema: 75 ml of soap solution per 1000 ml of warm water per rectum, 1 dose.
  - Oil retention: 180 ml of mineral or vegetable oil instilled in the rectum in the evening, left in overnight, and evacuated in the morning.
- see **Hemorrhoids** and **Anorectal Conditions** protocols if necessary.
- complete resolution of constipation may not be possible without treatment of causative disorder. See other protocols for management of specific causative etiologies.

CONSULTATION

→ Physician consultation is warranted for obstruction, impaction, failure to respond to conservative treatment, or for certain causative disorders.

→ As needed for prescription(s).

PATIENT EDUCATION

→ Explain to the patient causes and treatment of constipation.

→ Advise regular toilet habits—on a daily basis, physiologically best after breakfast.

→ Advise patient to drink warm beverage (e.g., tea, coffee) upon rising.

→ Advise patient to maintain regular exercise program.

→ Advise patient to avoid reliance on laxatives and enemas.

→ Advise patient to avoid straining at stool or sitting on the toilet for prolonged periods.

→ Advise patient that during periods of lifestyle alteration (e.g., bed rest, travel), constipation can be avoided by engaging in prevention activities (e.g., increase in fluids, fiber in diet, exercise).

FOLLOW-UP

→ Assess bowel activity and related lifestyle habits in subsequent visits.

→ Advise/teach regarding American Cancer Society's recommendation for early detection of cancer in asymptomatic people (American Cancer Society 1993):

- sigmoidoscopy: every three years beginning at age 50 years.
- stool guaiac: yearly beginning at age 50 years.
- digital rectal examination: yearly beginning at age 40 years.
  - ACS suggests a digital rectal examination of all women during their annual gynecological visit.

→ Document in progress notes and problem list.

Lisa L. Lommel, R.N., C., F.N.P., M.P.H.

7-G

Diarrhea

Diarrhea is defined as an increase in frequency, fluidity (70 percent to 90 percent water), and volume (> 200 grams/day) of bowel movements. For the average daily stool, weight is 100-150 grams per day with a water content of 60 percent to 70 percent (Knauer 1993a; Wadle 1990).

The pathophysiological mechanisms of diarrhea include (Goldfinger 1991; Knauer 1993a):

→ *Osmotic diarrhea:* excess water-soluble molecules in bowel lumen causing increased non-absorbable intraluminal water—as seen in lactose deficiency, magnesium-containing cathartics.

→ *Secretory diarrhea:* increase secretion and decrease absorption of electrolytes—as caused by cholera, bile salt enteropathy.

→ *Exudative diarrhea:* impaired colonic absorption with intestinal loss of serum proteins, blood, mucus, or pus—as associated with ulcerative colitis, shigellosis.

→ *Anatomic rearrangement:* decreased absorption surface—as with subtotal colectomy, gastocolic fistula.

→ *Motility disturbances:* decreased contact time— as in hyperthyroidism, irritable bowel syndrome.

Acute diarrhea is defined as diarrhea with an abrupt onset, lasting for less than two weeks. The most common causes include infection, drug reactions, and alterations in diet. Chronic or recurrent diarrhea may last for weeks or months and has many associated factors.

DATABASE

SUBJECTIVE

→ Symptoms may include:
  - loose liquid stools.
  - blood, mucus, pus, or grease in stools.
  - urgency to defecate.
  - increase in frequency of stools.
  - abdominal pain.
  - cramping before, during, and/or after defecation.
  - increase in flatulence.
  - abdominal bloating.
  - fever.
  - nausea, vomiting.
  - weight loss.

→ Historical evidence and symptoms of common causes of diarrhea include (Knauer 1993a):
  - recent travel or exposure to others with diarrhea.
  - psychogenic factors.
    • Nervousness or anxiety.
  - drugs.
    • Ingestion of magnesium-containing antacids, laxatives, sorbitol, metoclopramide, chemotherapeutic agents; laxative habituation.
    • Pseudomembranous colitis develops when normal bowel flora is suppressed by broad-spectrum antibiotic use, allowing *C. difficile* to proliferate; mild to severe, profuse watery stools.

- infection.
  - Usually abrupt onset.
  - Associated symptoms: headache, anorexia, fever, nausea, vomiting, malaise, myalgia.
  - Diarrhea of viral etiology has incubation period of 48-72 hours and lasts one to three days; primarily enterovirus or Norwalk virus.
  - See **Diarrhea—Infectious** Protocol.
- dietary factors:
  - excessive intake of fruits or caffeine-containing foods, alcohol, herbal teas.
  - lactase deficiency with intolerance to milk.
    –bloating and cramping.
  - malnutrition.
  - food allergy.
    –diarrhea after ingestion of certain foods.
- other intestinal factors:
  - fecal impaction more common in elderly; suggested after period of absent stools.
  - symptoms of diarrhea may actually indicate incontinence.
  - malabsorption syndrome: malabsorption of carbohydrate or fats (steatorrhea).
- gastrointestinal surgery.
  - Dumping syndrome causes sweating, lightheadedness, tachycardia, and diarrhea following food ingestion.
- see protocols for **Inflammatory Bowel Disease, Irritable Bowel Syndrome, Diverticular Disease, Abdominal Pain, Cirrhosis, Type I Diabetes Mellitus, Type II Diabetes Mellitus, Thyroid Disorders, and Hepatitis—Viral.**

OBJECTIVE

→ Depending on extent of dehydration secondary to diarrhea, may induce postural vital sign changes, elevation in temperature, and weight loss.

→ Patient presents with:
- abdominal tenderness, guarding, rebound.
- increased bowel sounds (though may be decreased as in cases of fecal impaction).

→ Rectal examination indicated.

ASSESSMENT

→ Diarrhea

→ See **Table 7G.1, A Differential Diagnosis of Diarrhea**.

PLAN

DIAGNOSTIC TESTS

→ Usually no diagnostic testing is recommended if history and physical examination suggest viral illness.

→ For history and clinical findings suggestive of bacterial or parasitic infection, obtain:
- stool culture.
- stool for ova and parasites.
- stool examination for leukocytes.

→ Stool for occult blood.

→ Sigmoidoscopy is recommended when blood or pus is present, if unable to attribute diarrhea to acute bacterial infection.

→ Barium enema and upper GI series may be indicated.

→ Patients with recent history of antibiotic ingestion should have stools examined for *C. difficile* toxin.

→ Stool alkalinization test is indicated for suspected laxative abuse. Paper will turn pink in presence of phenolphthalein, a common ingredient in laxatives.

→ Sudan stain for evidence of fat in stool if fat malabsorption is present. If present, obtain a 72-hour quantitative stool-fat determination.

→ CBC and serum electrolytes may be indicated for evaluation of moderate to severe dehydration.

TREATMENT/MANAGEMENT

→ Acute diarrhea of short duration is managed by restriction of food (not fluid) intake for 24 hours.

→ Oral hydration should be encouraged with solutions rich in electrolytes and sugar—8 oz. of fruit juice, with pinch of table salt and teaspoon of honey or sugar taken every hour.

→ Non-diet cola drinks that have lost their carbonation may be ingested.

→ Include with above hydration measures, 8-oz. glass of water with ¼ teaspoon of baking soda.

→ Food can slowly be added as tolerated, starting with broth-based soups, gelatin, tea, toast, or crackers, moving to bananas, baked potato, rice, and applesauce. Slowly increase protein intake and, lastly, fats. Limit milk-product intake until complete recovery.

Table 7G.1.   A DIFFERENTIAL DIAGNOSIS OF DIARRHEA

Acute Diarrhea	Chronic or Recurrent Diarrhea
Viruses	**Protozoa** *Giardia lamblia* *Entamoeba histolytica* Cryptosporidiosis
Bacterial Toxins *Staphylococcus* *Clostridium*	**Inflammation** Ulcerative colitis Crohn's disease Ischemic colitis Pseudomembranous colitis
Bacteria *Salmonella* *Shigella* *Escherichia coli* *Camphylobacter* *Yersinia* *B. cereus* *Vibrio parahemolyticus* *Vibrio cholerae*	**Drugs** Laxatives Antibiotics Quinidine Guanethidine; other antihypertensive agents Caffeine Digitalis
Protozoa *Giardia lamblia* *Entamoeba histolytica*	**Functional** Irritable bowel syndrome Diverticulosis
Drugs Laxatives Antibiotics Caffeine Alcohol	**Tumors** Bowel carcinoma Villous adenoma Islet-cell tumors Carcinoid syndrome Medullary carcinoma of thyroid
Functional Anxiety	**Malabsorption** Sprue Intestinal lymphoma Bile-salt malabsorption Whipple's disease Pancreatic insufficiency Lactase deficiency Other disaccharidase deficiencies Alpha-beta lipoproteinemia
Acute Presentations of Chronic or Recurrent Diarrhea (See next column)	**Postsurgical** Postgastrectomy dumping syndrome Enteroenteric fistulas Blind loops Parasympathetic denervation Short bowel syndrome
	Other Cirrhosis Diabetes mellitus Heavy-metal intoxication Other neurogenic diarrheas Hyperthyroidism Addison's disease Pellagra Scleroderma Amyloidosis

Source: Reprinted with permission from Richter, J.M. 1995b. Evaluation and management of diarrhea. In *Primary care medicine*, eds., A.H. Goroll, L.A. May, and A.G. Mulley, pp. 287–299. Philadelphia: J.B. Lippincott.

→ In cases of chronic diarrhea, best management strategy is to treat underlying condition.
  ▪ Re-evaluate need for drugs causing diarrhea.
  ▪ Eliminate foods causing diarrhea—e.g., caffeine, milk products.
  ▪ Vitamin therapy for patients with malnutrition and steatorrhea.
  ▪ Malabsorption as a result of pancreatic insufficiency responds to enzyme supplements.
  ▪ Dumping syndrome may respond to small, frequent feedings.
  ▪ Pseudomembranous colitis responds to antibiotic therapy.
  ▪ Discontinuation of chronic laxative use.
  ▪ See protocols for **Inflammatory Bowel Disease, Irritable Bowel Syndrome, Diverticular Disease, Abdominal Pain, Cirrhosis, Type I Diabetes Mellitus, Type II Diabetes Mellitus, Thyroid Disorders,** and **Hepatitis—Viral.**

→ Chronic diarrhea of unknown etiology after extensive work-up may be treated with a trial of therapy for irritable bowel syndrome (Richter 1995b) (see **Irritable Bowel Syndrome** Protocol).

→ Diarrhea of psychogenic origin may be managed with psychotherapy.

→ Antidiarrheal agents:
  ▪ kaolin and pectin (Kaopectate®): over-the-counter drug, prescribe as directed on package.
  ▪ bismuth subsalicylate (Pepto-Bismol®): 30 ml p.o. or 2 tablets p.o. up to 8 doses per day for symptomatic relief (Knauer 1993a).
  ▪ side effects: black stools and tongue; remind patient agent contains salicylates.
    NOTE: These agents should be avoided with inflammatory bowel disease or with parasitic infection because of risk of toxic megacolon.

→ Narcotic analogs:
  ▪ diphenoxylate with atropine (Lomotil®): 2.5 mg p.o. 3 to 4 times daily as needed, up to 20 mg/day (Knauer 1993a).
    • Contraindications: avoid in cases of obstructive jaundice, pseudomembranous or endotoxin-induced colitis. Use with caution in patients with advanced liver disease, patients who are addiction-prone, or those taking sedatives. Use with MAO inhibitor may induce hypertensive crisis.
  ▪ loperamide (Imodium®): 4 mg p.o. initially, then 2 mg p.o. after each loose bowel movement (maximum dose 16 mg/day) (Knauer 1993a).
    NOTE: These agents should be avoided with infectious diarrhea, as they may worsen or

prolong course, and with conditions which increase risk of toxic megacolon.
→ Narcotics:
  ▪ paregoric: 4 ml to 8 ml p.o. after liquid movements as needed or with bismuth (Knauer 1993a).
  ▪ codeine phosphate: 15 mg to 60 mg orally or subcutaneously (if vomiting) every 4 hours as needed (Knauer 1993a).
    NOTE: These agents should be avoided with chronic diarrhea or when there is a possibility of acute surgical abdomen (especially diverticulitis, obstruction). Addiction risk should be assessed.

→ Anticholinergics are useful with diarrhea due to irritable bowel syndrome. See **Irritable Bowel Syndrome** Protocol.

→ Antibiotic therapy is appropriate for certain types of bacterial and parasitic infections. See **Diarrhea—Infectious** Protocol.

→ Viral gastroenteritis infections causing diarrhea are usually self-limiting and can be treated with rehydration, kaolin and pectin, or bismuth salicylate.

CONSULTATION

→ With acute severe diarrhea, when unable to maintain oral hydration, referral to a physician is warranted.

→ Consultation and/or referral to a physician is warranted with elderly patients or those with chronic or debilitating illnesses.

→ Consultation with a physician is warranted in cases of chronic diarrhea when unable to establish diagnosis.

→ As needed for prescription(s).

PATIENT EDUCATION

→ Teach patient regarding pathophysiology and management plan.

→ Advise patient to continue with hydration throughout recovery period.

→ Advise patients with possible contagious diarrhea to maintain good hygiene, i.e., wash hands with soap and water after using the bathroom.

→ To relieve perineal discomfort teach patient to:
  ▪ take two to three sitz baths/day.
  ▪ gently dry perineal area with absorbent cotton.
  ▪ avoid use of soap.
  ▪ clean perineal area with witch hazel pads (TUCKS®).

→ Advise patient that a short course of 0.5 percent to 1 percent hydrocortisone cream to perianal inflammation may be helpful.

→ Advise patient to avoid narcotic therapy in the treatment of diarrhea.

→ See protocols for **Inflammatory Bowel Disease, Irritable Bowel Syndrome, Diverticular Disease, Diarrhea—Infectious, Abdominal Pain, Cirrhosis, Type I Diabetes Mellitus, Type II Diabetes Mellitus, Thyroid Disorders,** and **Hepatitis—Viral.**

FOLLOW-UP

→ As indicated by case presentation.

→ Document in progress notes and problem list.

7-H

Diverticular Disease

Diverticula are created by the herniation of intestinal mucosa and submucosa from increased colonic pressure through the muscular bowel into the serosa. The colon is the most common site for diverticular disease in the gastrointestinal tract and the sigmoid accounts for 95 percent of cases.

The incidence of *diverticulosis* (presence of diverticula in the colon) increases with age and is equally distributed between males and females. It is estimated that 65 percent of the United States population will have this disease by age 65 years.

During the past century, there has been a tremendous increase in diverticular disease in the industrialized countries. This is thought to be due to changes from high-fiber to lower-fiber diets, as well as an increased consumption of other foods (e.g., protein, fat, and salt) (Rege and Nahrwold 1989).

Diverticulitis occurs when undigested food and bacteria get trapped in the thin-walled mucosa, compromising blood supply and causing infection and inflammation. It is estimated that 10 percent to 25 percent of individuals with diverticulosis will experience diverticulitis (Ertan 1990).

In addition to diverticulitis, other complications of this disease include fistula and abscess formation, perforation, obstruction, and bleeding.

DATABASE

SUBJECTIVE

→ Diverticulosis is usually asymptomatic and commonly discovered on barium enema for other indications.

→ Occasionally diverticulosis may present with:

- left lower-quadrant, crampy intermittent, or continuous ache.
- constipation.
- constipation alternating with diarrhea.
- abdominal tenderness.
- flatulence, bloating, nausea, vomiting, anorexia.

→ Symptoms of diverticulitis depend on disease severity.

- Left lower abdominal pain usually constant, may be crampy with radiation to back.
- Abdominal tenderness.
- Constipation.
- Mucus or blood in stool.
- Fever.
- Ten percent of patients will have urinary frequency and urgency caused by close contact of bladder with colon.

→ Symptoms of diverticular disease may be recurrent or chronic.

→ History of chronic renal failure contributes to higher incidence of colonic disease at a younger age.

OBJECTIVE

→ Commonly, clinical findings are absent with diverticulosis.

→ Signs of diverticulitis depend on disease severity.

- Fever.
- Abdominal tenderness, muscle spasm, left lower quadrant guarding.
- Sausage-shaped mass palpable on abdominal, rectal, or pelvic examination.
- Decreased bowel sounds.

▪ Elevated WBC and erythrocyte sedimentation rate (ESR).

ASSESSMENT

→ Diverticulosis

→ R/O diverticulitis

→ R/O appendicitis

→ R/O irritable bowel syndrome

→ R/O inflammatory bowel disease

→ R/O angiodysplasia

→ R/O ischemic bowel disease

→ R/O gynecological disorders

→ R/O carcinoma

→ R/O urinary tract disease

PLAN

DIAGNOSTIC TESTS

→ Asymptomatic diverticulosis usually diagnosed by barium enema or flexible sigmoidoscopy/colonoscopy indicated for other reasons.

→ For patients with symptoms, diagnosis is usually made on clinical grounds.

→ Barium enema may assist in confirming presence of diverticulosis.

→ Barium enema should not be performed during an acute attack, if a mass is present, or with signs of peritoneal irritation.

→ Colonoscopy or sigmoidoscopy indicated to rule out other pathology included in differential diagnosis—e.g., carcinoma, polyps, inflammatory bowel disease.
  ▪ Should not be performed during acute phase.
  ▪ Not indicated for evaluation of diverticular disease.

→ Plain abdominal x-ray or chest x-ray is indicated in acute attacks to evaluate for complications (e.g., pneumoperitoneum).

→ Ultrasonography may be used for evaluation of complications.

→ Computed tomography is the most sensitive and specific test for diagnosis of acute colonic involvement and for detection of extracolonic disease.

→ CBC.

→ Urinalysis.

→ Stool test for occult blood.

TREATMENT/MANAGEMENT

→ Treatment of asymptomatic diverticulosis is controversial. No evidence showing benefit of treatment (e.g., high-fiber diet) in preventing disease or reducing incidence of complications (Rege and Nahrwold 1989).
  ▪ Since high-fiber diet is not harmful (and may be beneficial), it is commonly recommended.

→ Uncomplicated diverticulosis may be managed with (Knauer 1993a):
  ▪ high-fiber, high-residue diet of unprocessed bran—¼ cup per day in juice or food—raw vegetables, and fruits.
    • If unable to tolerate bran, consider bulk additives such as psyllium hydrophilic or methylcellulose (see **Constipation** Protocol).

→ Mild diverticulitis without evidence of complications (i.e., temperature < 38.3°C/101°F, WBCs < 13,000-15,000) may be managed as outpatient after physician consultation (Goroll 1995e):
  ▪ rest and clear liquids to rest bowel.
  ▪ broad-spectrum antibiotic (consult with physician.)
  ▪ mild non-opiate analgesic for pain.
  ▪ monitor temperature, pain, abdominal examination for signs of peritonitis and WBC count for elevation.

→ Anticholinergic and antispasmodic use is controversial because of increased risk of constipation leading to complications (Goroll 1995e).

→ Acute diverticulitis warrants referral to a physician for hospitalization, antibiotic therapy, and evaluation for possible surgical intervention.

→ Recurrent attacks of diverticulitis or presence of perforation, fistula, or abscess require surgical intervention and referral.

CONSULTATION

→ Consultation for management of diverticulosis and mild diverticulitis.

→ Physician consultation for diagnosis of diverticular disease.

→ Consultation with nutritionist as indicated for diet plan.

→ Referral to appropriate specialist for diagnostic tests.

→ Referral to a physician for management of acute diverticulitis, recurrent disease, or complications.

→ As needed for prescription(s).

PATIENT EDUCATION

→ Explain pathophysiology, risk factors, and treatment plan.

→ Inform patients that flatulence and bloating caused by bran intake will subside with continued use.

→ Advise patient to avoid foods that may increase risk of obstruction, including nuts, seeds, corn, popcorn, cucumbers, tomatoes, figs, and strawberries.

→ Advise patients to avoid laxatives, enemas, and opiates because of risk of constipation.

→ Advise patient to call for temperature elevation, abdominal pain, or bleeding.

FOLLOW-UP

→ Patients with mild diverticulitis should be followed closely and monitored for increasing temperature, WBC count, pain, change in abdominal exam or signs of peritonitis. Consultation with physician should be considered if there is no improvement within 48 hours.

→ Document in progress notes and problem list.

7-1

Dyspepsia

Dyspepsia (indigestion) refers to a constellation of episodic or recurrent symptoms (abdominal pain or discomfort, bloating, heartburn, belching, anorexia, nausea, vomiting, regurgitation, early satiety) initiating from the upper gastrointestinal tract (Heading 1991; Zell and Budhraja 1989).

Dyspepsia caused by a disease process is called *organic dyspepsia*, a condition more common in the elderly. Common pathological findings include gastric and duodenal ulcer, gastroesophageal reflux, biliary tract disease, pancreatitis, gastric or colorectal cancer, malabsorption syndromes, ischemic heart disease, neuromuscular diseases, diabetes mellitus, and drug use (i.e., aspirin, nonsteroidal anti-inflammatory drugs [NSAIDs], steroids, digitalis, alcohol) (Richter 1991).

The majority of cases of dyspepsia occur in younger patients, with no identifiable disease process. This is known as *non-ulcer, functional, essential,* or *idiopathic dyspepsia*. Factors thought to play a role in the pathogenesis of non-ulcer dyspepsia include gastric acid secretion, motility disorder, duodenogastric reflux, gastrointestinal peptide hormones, gastritis, psychosocial factors and stress, environmental factors, diet, and genetic factors (Malagelada 1991; Nyren 1991; Richter 1991; Talley and Phillips 1988; Tytgat, Noache, and Rauws 1991).

DATABASE

SUBJECTIVE

→ See specific protocols as they relate to etiologies of organic dyspepsia.

→ Symptoms may include:

■ diffuse upper abdominal pain or discomfort, commonly after eating.
■ postprandial fullness and inability to finish a normal meal.
■ belching, flatulence, and bloating.
■ heartburn and regurgitation.
■ nausea, vomiting, and anorexia.
■ associated symptoms of postprandial drowsiness and headache.

→ Specific foods—i.e., fatty foods, lactose-containing foods—may worsen symptoms.

→ Patient has:

■ personal or family history of stress.
■ history of aspirin, NSAID use.

→ Symptoms rarely occur during the night.

→ Bowel function is usually normal.

OBJECTIVE

→ Non-ulcer dyspepsia has minimal clinical findings except for diffuse upper abdominal tenderness on palpation.

→ Physical examination should emphasize findings associated with organic disease processes. See specific protocols as they relate to etiologies of organic disease.

ASSESSMENT

→ Non-ulcer (functional, essential) dyspepsia
→ R/O peptic ulcer disease
→ R/O gastroesophageal reflux
→ R/O biliary tract disease

→ R/O pancreatitis

→ R/O gastric or colorectal cancer

→ R/O malabsorption syndrome

→ R/O ischemic heart disease

→ R/O neuromuscular disease

→ R/O diabetes mellitus

→ R/O drug use

PLAN

DIAGNOSTIC TESTS

→ The decision to treat empirically or obtain diagnostic tests should be made in consultation with the patient and a physician.

→ The objectives of diagnostic investigation are to determine:
- if there is an upper gastrointestinal tract lesion, and
- whether there is a disease outside the gastrointestinal tract that could be causing the symptoms.

→ Diagnostic tests are warranted if symptoms and clinical findings are suspicious for organic causes. See specific protocols as they relate to etiologies of organic dyspepsia.

→ Endoscopy is considered the first-line test in evaluation of dyspepsia that is not considered to be due to a disease outside the gastrointestinal tract.
- Endoscopy (with biopsy) can identify malignant, ulcerative, or inflammatory lesions which are the most common causes of dyspepsia.

→ Endoscopy is required immediately in patients at increased risk for pathology (Goroll 1995f):
- age over 50 years.
- unexplained weight loss.
- protracted symptoms.
- persistent nausea and vomiting.
- dysphagia.
- jaundice.
- abdominal mass.
- evidence of GI blood loss.

→ Literature suggests that elimination of endoscopy is reasonable in low-risk patients under age 40 years when:
- there is not a strong suggestion of malignancy or other disease process.
- recent onset of symptoms.
- symptoms are not refractory to empiric therapy.

- when aggressive therapy (i.e., histamine 2 [H_2] blockers) is not being considered.
- absence of weight loss, persistent vomiting, anemia, stool blood test positivity.
- there is an absence of psychological disorders or acute anxiety for which a confirmed absence of organic disease may help the patient consider the possibility of psychosomatic mechanism (Brown and Rees 1990; Goroll 1995f; Malagelada 1991; Nyren 1991).

→ Obtain fecal occult blood testing.

→ Subsequent endoscopic investigation of low-risk patients is reserved for those who (Goroll 1995f):
- fail to show some improvement after 7 to 10 days of full anti-ulcer therapy.
- do not clear after 6 to 8 weeks of empiric treatment.
- quickly relapse when treatment is discontinued.

TREATMENT/MANAGEMENT

→ In patients under age 40 years, where there is no suspicion or diagnosis of organic disease, a therapeutic trial may be initiated.

→ After evaluation and reassurance that symptoms are not caused by a serious disease, some patients may not desire drug therapy.

→ Drug therapy may reinforce somatic symptoms in patients with a psychosomatic disorder.

→ Antacids, H_2 blockers, sucralfate and omeprazole are used in anti-ulcer treatment with varying degrees of efficacy. Recommendations suggest that drugs should be given for only a limited time and discontinued if symptoms fail to resolve (Goroll 1995f). See **Peptic Ulcer Disease** Protocol for drug regimens.

→ Antacids are used as a first choice in a therapeutic trial. Treatment schedule is similar to that for peptic ulcer disease. See **Peptic Ulcer Disease** Protocol.

→ The empiric use of H_2 blockers is controversial. H_2 blockers may:
- mask symptoms by partially healing malignant gastric lesions.
- weaken value of subsequent endoscopy by partially healing lesions.
- lead to inappropriate long-term use and occasionally to serious drug side effects (Talley and Phillips 1988).

→ There should be an attempt to identify a specific anatomic abnormality before prescribing H_2 blockers (Goroll 1995f).

→ See "Patient Education" section.

CONSULTATION

→ Consider physician consultation when instituting a therapeutic trial.

→ Referral to a physician is warranted if endoscopy is indicated.

→ Consultation with a physician is warranted if symptoms persist after eight weeks of therapeutic trial.

→ Consultation or referral to a mental health professional may be indicated.

→ As needed for prescription(s).

PATIENT EDUCATION

→ See "Treatment/Management" section.

→ Explain physiology and treatment regimes.

→ Provide reassurance, when indicated, as many patients have fear of malignancy.

→ Assist patient in cessation of alcohol intake and smoking with referral to appropriate support services (i.e., Alcoholics Anonymous, Nicotine Anonymous, and American Cancer Society). See **Alcoholism and Other Drug Dependencies** and **Smoking Cessation** protocols.

→ Advise patient to restrict intake of coffee, tea, and caffeinated colas.

→ Advise discontinuing use of products that increase gas—e.g, carbonated beverages, chewing gum, beans, and certain whole grains and fruits.

→ Limit intake of sorbitol (found in sugarless gums).

→ Consider an empiric trial of a lactose-free diet.

→ Encourage small, frequent meals eaten slowly.

→ Advise increased intake of high-fiber foods (see **General Nutrition Guidelines**).

→ Advise patient to avoid eating immediately before bedtime and not to lie down after a meal.

→ Assist patient in measures for stress reduction (see **Stress Management** Protocol).

FOLLOW-UP

→ Re-evaluate patient after four weeks of treatment. If no response, a second trial with another drug may be considered.

→ Therapeutic trials should last for no longer than eight weeks, at which time re-evaluation should occur. If symptoms persist, even partially, further investigation is warranted.

→ Advise patient regarding American Cancer Society's recommendation for early detection of cancer in asymptomatic people (American Cancer Society 1993):
  ▪ sigmoidoscopy: every three years beginning at age 50 years.
  ▪ stool guaiac: yearly beginning at age 50 years.
  ▪ digital rectal examination: yearly beginning at age 40 years.
    • ACS suggests a digital rectal examination of all women during their annual gynecological visit.

→ Document in progress notes and problem list.

Lisa L. Lommel, R.N., C., F.N.P., M.P.H.

7-J

Gastroesophageal Reflux and Heartburn

Gastroesophageal reflux results from regurgitation of gastric contents into the esophagus. The mechanisms involved in reflux are the result of a permanently or intermittently incompetent lower esophageal sphincter, frequency and duration of reflux, and inability of the esophagus to generate peristaltic wave action that would prevent acid and pepsin from coming into contact with the mucosa (Knauer 1993a).

A variety of factors—including hormonal, neural, anatomic, and dietary—are involved in the function of the lower esophageal sphincter. Many individuals will experience gastrointestinal symptoms but the frequency and duration will distinguish physiological reflux from gastroesophageal reflux disease.

Heartburn is the most common symptom of gastroesophageal reflux, as well as other disorders (see **Peptic Ulcer Disease** Protocol.) It presents as a retrosternal burning sensation caused by irritation from reflux of stomach acid into the esophagus.

Reflux esophagitis refers to inflammation of the esophagus secondary to injury of the mucosa by refluxed acid, pepsin, or bile. Complications can include pain, bleeding, ulcers, and strictures.

DATABASE

SUBJECTIVE

→ Heartburn characterized by retrosternal, intermittent aching, burning 30 to 60 minutes after eating.
  ▪ Symptoms more evident after a large meal.
  ▪ Radiation upward toward the throat and into the back.

▪ Increased symptoms when lying down, bending over, or exercising.
▪ Symptoms awaken patient at night.
▪ Can mimic cardiac ischemia with chest heaviness, pressure.
▪ Relieved by drinking water, milk, or taking antacids.

→ Gastroesophageal reflux characterized by regurgitation of food or fluid, especially at night.
  ▪ May awaken with coughing or strangling sensation.
  ▪ Soiling of pillow by regurgitation or water brash (i.e., regurgitation and increased saliva).

→ Use of anticholinergics, theophylline, meperidine, and calcium channel blockers induce symptoms by decreasing lower esophageal sphincter tone.

→ Tobacco, alcohol, chocolate, peppermint, citrus fruits, coffee, tea, colas, and foods with high fat or carbohydrate content induce symptoms by decreasing lower esophageal sphincter tone.

→ Pain or difficulty swallowing usually indicates long-term reflux with inflammation and/or stricture.

→ Pregnancy will increase symptoms, primarily because of decreased lower esophageal sphincter pressure related to increased levels of estrogen and progesterone.

→ Hiatal hernia, recurring or persistent vomiting, obesity, ascites, tight binders, or girdles may increase symptoms.

→ History of scleroderma or diabetes mellitus may predispose to reflux.

→ Hoarseness, morning laryngitis can be caused by severe reflux.

→ Hematemesis and melena.

→ History of adult-onset asthma—especially when associated with nocturnal coughing, wheezing, or dyspnea—may be caused by pulmonary aspiration of gastric contents (Lieberman 1991).

OBJECTIVE

→ Physical examination is unremarkable.

→ Special attention should be given to assessing for the possible presence of an abdominal mass.

→ Decreased hematocrit and hemoglobin may be present with bleeding.

ASSESSMENT

→ Gastroesophageal reflux

→ Heartburn

→ R/O peptic ulcer disease

→ R/O dyspepsia

→ R/O ischemic heart disease

→ R/O esophageal spasm

→ R/O esophageal infection in immunocompromised host

→ R/O cholelithiasis

→ R/O scleroderma

→ R/O diabetes mellitus

→ R/O anemia

PLAN

DIAGNOSTIC TESTS

→ CBC as indicated.

→ Stool for occult blood as indicated.

→ Diagnosis of reflux usually made, if symptoms are typical, with absence of clinical findings for other diseases.

→ Endoscopy with biopsy should be considered to assess extent of damage resulting from esophageal disease or if symptoms are not improved with therapeutic trial.

→ Endoscopy, barium swallow, or upper GI is indicated for suspicion of:
- other causative disorders (e.g., peptic ulcer, dyspepsia).
- dysphagia.
- significant weight loss.
- occult blood loss.

→ 24-hour pH probe recordings determine esophageal reflux and acid clearing time.
- Most sensitive and specific test, though expensive and not universally available.
- Helpful in assessing:
  - non-cardiac chest pain to determine if reflux episodes are associated with typical pain.
  - patients presenting with pulmonary or ear, nose, and throat symptoms.

→ Acid-perfusion test will reproduce symptoms if they are due to esophagitis.

→ Manometry studies assess ability to clear refluxed acid and the presence of dysmotility. They are indicated for patients who do not respond to medical therapy as a preliminary to surgery.

→ Esophageal reflux pain can mimic cardiac symptoms with a possibility of concomitant cardiac disease.
- Diagnostic tests for cardiac disease should be obtained if cardiac disease suspect (e.g., sequential EKGs, enzyme determinations, observation).
- See **Cardiovascular Disorders** Protocols.

TREATMENT/MANAGEMENT

→ In absence of suspicion of other disorders, therapeutic trial is appropriate in patients with suspected reflux.

→ Begin treatment with conservative measures including the following (Richter 1995c):
- avoid foods high in fats or carbohydrates.
- avoid large meals in evening or late-night snacks.
- avoid lying down after meals.
- elevate head of bed up to six inches.
- avoid cigarettes, alcohol, coffee, colas, peppermint, citrus, and spicy foods.
- assess necessity of drugs that promote reflux—e.g., anticholinergics, theophylline, meperidine, calcium channel blockers.
- assess necessity of drugs that may injure esophageal mucosa—e.g., tetracycline, quinidine, wax matrix KCl tablets, NSAIDs.
- reduce excess weight.
- avoid tight belts, girdles, bending over, heavy lifting.
- antacid trial (see **Peptic Ulcer Disease** Protocol for description of antacids.).

→ In patients who are not relieved of symptoms by preceding measures, or for those with mild to moderate symptoms consider:

- rantidine (Zantac®) (only H_2 receptor blocker approved for peptic esophagitis) 150 mg p.o. twice a day or 300 mg p.o. once every day.
  - Side effects: diarrhea, dyspepsia, loss of libido, dizziness, and mental confusion (Knauer 1993a).
- metoclopramide (Reglan®) (promotility agent increases rate of gastric and esophageal emptying) 10 mg-20 mg p.o. at bedtime (Knauer 1993a).
  - Side effects: agitation, drowsiness, fatigue, extrapyramidal effects; rarely hyperprolactinemia, galactorrhea.

→ In patients who are not relieved of symptoms by above measures or those who have severe symptoms consider:
- omeprazole (Prilosec®) (proton pump inhibitor, inhibits basal and stimulated gastric secretion, relapse rate after discontinuation high. Federal Drug Administration [FDA]-approved for only 8-week trial) 20 mg p.o. before first meal of the day (Knauer 1993a).

→ With moderate to severe symptoms, higher doses of these drugs may be appropriate. Consider physician consultation.

→ If therapeutic trial does not improve symptoms, or with moderate to severe symptoms, consider endoscopy to rule out malignancy or stricture and to determine extent of esophagitis.

→ Anti-reflux surgery may be indicated in patients with stricture, bleeding, pulmonary aspiration, or severe refractory symptoms.

CONSULTATION

→ Consultation with a physician may be sought when patient's symptoms are not relieved by conservative measures.

→ Consultation with a physician is warranted for atypical symptoms and if therapeutic trial does not improve symptoms.

→ Consultation or referral to a physician for evaluation of relapse of symptoms.

→ Referral to a physician is warranted for suspicion of organic disorders.

→ Referral to a physician is warranted for endoscopy.

→ As needed for prescription(s).

PATIENT EDUCATION

→ See "Treatment/Management" section.

→ Explain the pathophysiology of reflux, the chronic and recurrent nature of the disease, aggravating factors, and necessity of following conservative measures.

→ Advise patient to continue with medication as prescribed, even after symptoms have subsided.

→ Advise patient regarding a nutritious diet (see **General Nutrition Guidelines**.)

→ Advise patient to avoid straining at stool.

→ Assist patient in cessation of alcohol intake and smoking with referral to appropriate support services (Alcoholics Anonymous, Nicotine Anonymous, American Cancer Society). See **Alcoholism and Other Drug Dependencies** and **Smoking Cessation** protocols.

→ Instruct patient in methods of stress reduction (see **Stress Management** Protocol.)

FOLLOW-UP

→ Re-evaluate patient in four to six weeks after initiation of treatment.

→ Pharmacological therapy should be maintained for 12 weeks (Bennett 1991).

→ At every visit, reinforce adherence to conservative measures.

→ Withdraw one pharmacological agent at a time to assist in determination of minimum maintenance treatment.

→ Up to 45 percent of patients relapse after discontinuation of medication.
- Some patients may require a maintenance dose of a particular drug.
- It is unknown whether long-term pharmacological therapy is superior to surgery for symptom control (Lieberman 1991).

→ Advise patient regarding American Cancer Society's recommendation for early detection of cancer in asymptomatic people (American Cancer Society 1993):
- sigmoidoscopy: every three years beginning at age 50 years.
- stool guaiac: yearly beginning at age 50 years.

- ■ digital rectal examination: yearly beginning at age 40 years.
  - • ACS suggests a digital rectal examination of all women during their annual gynecological visit.
- → Document in progress notes and problem list.

7-K

Gastrointestinal Bleeding

Gastrointestinal (GI) bleeding is defined as bleeding originating from the upper GI tract and/or the lower GI tract.

The primary causes of upper GI bleeding include (Knauer 1993a):

→ gastroduodenal erosions or ulcers caused by NSAIDs, aspirin, or alcohol.

→ peptic ulcers resulting from duodenal, gastric, or esophageal lesions.

→ esophagitis.

→ Mallory-Weiss syndrome.

→ esophageal or gastric varices.

→ neoplasms such as leiomyomas or cancer.

→ vascular lesions such as Dieulafoy's erosions or angiodysplasia.

→ drugs such as warfarin or heparin.

The primary causes of lower GI bleeding include (Knauer 1993a):

→ anal lesions such as fissures or hemorrhoids.

→ neoplasms such as polyps or cancer.

→ inflammatory disorders such as bacterial or parasitic infections or inflammatory bowel disease.

→ diverticulosis.

→ vascular disorders such as angiodysplasia, bowel ischemia, colonic varices, aortenteric fistula, hereditary telangiectasias.

→ coagulopathies associated with anticoagulation therapy, blood dyscrasias.

→ upper GI source such as peptic ulcer, neoplasms, and esophageal varices.

DATABASE

SUBJECTIVE

→ Patient may present with history and symptoms of common cause of GI bleeding.

■ See **Peptic Ulcer Disease, Cirrhosis, Abdominal Pain, Diarrhea, Gastroesophageal Reflux and Heartburn, Anorectal Conditions, Hemorrhoids, Inflammatory Bowel Disease, Irritable Bowel Syndrome,** and **Diverticular Disease** protocols.

→ Symptoms usually found in upper GI bleeding include:

■ coffee-ground hematemesis (blood in contact with hydrochloric acid).

■ bright red hematemesis.

→ Symptoms usually found in lower GI bleeding include:

■ bright red blood per rectum (usually found on toilet tissue).

■ black, tarry stools *(melena)* may also present with upper GI bleeding.

→ Depending on extent and severity of bleeding, patient may experience:

■ postural symptoms.

■ weakness.

■ shortness of breath.

■ shock.

OBJECTIVE

→ Patient may present with clinical signs of common causes of GI bleeding.

- See **Peptic Ulcer Disease, Cirrhosis, Abdominal Pain, Diarrhea, Gastroesophageal Reflux and Heartburn, Anorectal Conditions, Hemorrhoids, Inflammatory Bowel Disease, Irritable Bowel Syndrome,** and **Diverticular Disease** protocols.
- Hemoccult-positive stools.
→ Depending on extent and severity of bleeding, patient may present with:
  - paleness.
  - weakness.
  - tachypnea.
  - tachycardia.
  - mild to severe hypotension.
  - postural signs.
  - increased bowel sounds.
→ Nose and pharynx are negative for signs of bleeding.
→ External examination of the anus and anoscopy may show evidence of bleeding hemorrhoid or fissure.

ASSESSMENT

→ Upper GI bleeding (see "Subjective," "Objective" sections for common causes)
→ Lower GI bleeding (see "Subjective," "Objective" sections for common causes)
→ R/O epistaxis
→ R/O respiratory tract bleeding

PLAN

DIAGNOSTIC TESTS

→ Approximate bleeding location can usually be determined by history of site of blood loss.
→ CBC.
→ Serum electrolytes.
→ BUN/creatinine ratio (increased BUN may indicate increased level of blood in GI tract, especially with normal creatinine).
→ Urinalysis.
→ Liver functions studies if appropriate.
→ Prothrombin time (PT), partial prothrombin time (PTT), and platelet count if suggestive of coagulation disorder (will confirm normal platelets if taking NSAIDs or aspirin).
→ Clot to blood bank if transfusion is needed.
→ Nasogastric aspiration and rectal examination to confirm presence of blood.

→ Hemoccult stool testing (**NOTE:** False positive hemoccult may occur with ingestion of red meat).
→ Endoscopy may be indicated if upper GI bleeding diagnosis is unclear.
→ Anoscopy and/or colonoscopy may be indicated for suspicion of lower GI bleeding.
→ If patient is 50 years of age or older, with rectal bleeding, further studies are indicated to rule out possibility of GI cancer, e.g., sigmoidoscopy, colonoscopy, and/or and barium enema.
→ See **Peptic Ulcer Disease, Cirrhosis, Abdominal Pain, Diarrhea, Gastroesophageal Reflux and Heartburn, Anorectal Conditions, Hemorrhoids, Inflammatory Bowel Disease, Irritable Bowel Syndrome,** and **Diverticular Disease** protocols.

TREATMENT/MANAGEMENT

→ Primary management strategy is to treat underlying cause of GI bleeding.
  - See **Peptic Ulcer Disease, Cirrhosis, Abdominal Pain, Diarrhea, Gastroesophageal Reflux and Heartburn, Anorectal Conditions, Hemorrhoids, Inflammatory Bowel Disease, Irritable Bowel Syndrome,** and **Diverticular Disease** protocols.
→ Mild to moderate decrease in hematocrit can be managed with diet high in iron-containing foods and iron sulfate ($FeSO_4$) 300 mg p.o. 3 times a day (see **Anemia** Protocol).
→ Discontinue NSAID or aspirin if suggestive of ulceration or gastritis.
→ Patients on heparin or warfarin treatment usually have underlying pathology causing bleeding.

CONSULTATION

→ Consultation with a physician is warranted for patients with stable chronic or acute mild blood loss.
→ Immediate referral to a physician is warranted in cases of acute hemorrhage, chronic unstable bleeding, dramatic decrease in hematocrit, or hemodynamic instability.
→ As needed for prescription(s).

PATIENT EDUCATION

→ Educate patient regarding pathophysiology and management plan for GI bleeding.
→ Educate patient regarding signs of worsening blood loss or volume depletion.

FOLLOW-UP

→ Monitor patient with acute mild or chronic stable bleeding with periodic hemoccult testing and hematocrits.

→ Document in progress notes and problem list.

Lisa L. Lommel, R.N., C., F.N.P., M.P.H.

7-L

Hemorrhoids

Hemorrhoids are a very common condition and affect males and females equally. In the United States, it is estimated that 58 percent of people over age 40 years of age have hemorrhoids (Dennison et al. 1989).

Traditionally, hemorrhoids were thought to be distended veins, like varicose veins, but, recently, there has been considerable doubt regarding this definition. The etiology of hemorrhoids is also unclear. Factors such as portal hypertension, carcinoma, straining at defecation, pregnancy or pelvic masses, hormonal fluctuations, anal corpus cavernosum, ampullary pump, anal cushions, elevation of anal pressure, and the process of aging, with accompanying fragmentation of supportive connective tissue, have been implicated in the etiology of hemorrhoids. And many of these factors have been disputed (Dennison et al. 1989; Smith 1990).

There are two major types of hemorrhoids, named because of their anatomic position and vascular origin. An *internal hemorrhoid* is an exaggerated vascular cushion with engorged venous plexus located above the dentate line and covered with mucous membrane (Cocchiara 1991).

Internal hemorrhoids are further classified into four groups which describe the relationship of the anatomic position of the hemorrhoid to the dentate line. A *first-degree hemorrhoid* does not prolapse. A *second-degree hemorrhoid* prolapses with bowel movements but reduces spontaneously. A *third-degree* prolapses readily with bowel movements and sometimes with exertion and requires manual reduction. A *fourth-degree* is a permanently prolapsed hemorrhoid (Cocchiara 1991; Smith 1990).

The *external hemorrhoid* is the second type of hemorrhoid. It involves the inferior hemorrhoidal plexus and is located below the dentate line. It is covered with squamous epithelium. Large hemorrhoids usually consist of an internal and external component.

A major complication of hemorrhoids is a thrombosis, which can involve both an internal and external hemorrhoid. Anal fissures, perianal hematomas, skin tags, and mucosal prolapse are more frequent in patients with hemorrhoids (Dennison et al. 1989).

DATABASE

SUBJECTIVE

→ Uncomplicated hemorrhoids may produce no symptoms.

Internal hemorrhoids

- Patient may experience prolapse with defecation, with or without spontaneous reduction, or permanent prolapse (second-, third-, or fourth-degree).
- Bright red, painless bleeding during bowel movement noticed in toilet water or on toilet tissue. With prolapse, the bleeding can be dripping or squirting.
- Pain is not common with internal hemorrhoids unless prolapse is trapped outside anal sphincter. Reduction will stop pain.
- If prolapse is extensive, pruritus, burning, and discharge may be present.

External hemorrhoids

- Patient may feel external anal mass.
- When thrombosed, the mass becomes large and very painful, especially during defecation.
- Skin tag may be present in later stages.

OBJECTIVE

Internal hemorrhoids

- These may be palpable on digital examination of anal canal.
- Prolapsed tissue present at anal canal. In fourth-degree, mucosa may be keratinized.
- Low hematocrit may be seen with bleeding.

External hemorrhoids

- These present as masses of varying sizes at anal opening. In later stages, a skin tag may be present.
- When thrombosed, a large, painful, firm mass is present.

ASSESSMENT

→ Hemorrhoid—internal: first-, second-, third-, or fourth-degree

→ Hemorrhoid—external: thrombosed

→ R/O anal fissure

→ R/O condylomata acuminata

→ R/O abscess

→ R/O carcinoma

→ R/O anal fissure

→ R/O proctitis

PLAN

DIAGNOSTIC TESTS

→ Rectal examination and anoscopy is warranted for diagnosis.

→ For patients over 40 years old, sigmoidoscopy or colonoscopy should be performed to rule out carcinoma.

→ Stool guaiac testing is recommended to confirm presence of blood.

→ Hemoglobin/hematocrit to rule out anemia if bleeding has been sustained.

→ Rectal cultures as indicated.

TREATMENT/MANAGEMENT

→ The decision for management/treatment is based on symptoms. If the patient has no major symptoms and does not notice the hemorrhoid, no treatment is necessary.

→ Hemorrhoids that cause minimal symptoms may be managed with methods at reducing constipation/straining and reducing local irritation.

→ All patients, regardless of severity or treatment choice, should be on a high-fiber diet. See **General Nutrition Guidelines**.

→ Psyllium products in powder or tablet may be used to increase fiber (see **Constipation** Protocol).

→ Stool softeners may be used initially to reduce constipation (see **Constipation** Protocol).

→ Laxatives should be avoided because they don't allow smooth evacuation.

→ OTC creams and suppositories (Anusol®, Preparation-H®) can be used but may be harmful to anal mucosa with prolonged use.

- Anusol® suppositories: insert 1 per rectum every morning, at bedtime, and post-bowel movement (BM).
- Anusol® ointment: apply freely and gently rub into anal area every 3-4 hours prn.
- Anusol® ointment with 1% hydrocortisone: apply freely and gently rub into anal area every 3-4 hours prn.
- Preparation-H® suppositories: insert 1 per rectum prn (3-5 per day, especially every morning, at bedtime, and post-BM).
- Preparation-H® ointment: apply freely to affected area (3-5 times per day, especially every morning, at bedtime, and post-BM).

→ Anusol® ointment with 2.5% hydrocortisone is available with prescription: apply freely and gently rub into anal area 2-4 times a day.

→ Astringent compresses (witch hazel pads, Tucks®).

→ If patient is experiencing severe pain or discomfort, referral to a physician is warranted. Treatment may include rubber-band ligation, sclerotherapy, cryotherapy, infrared photocoagulation, bipolar diathermy, laser treatment, or surgery.

→ A thrombosed external hemorrhoid is usually in the healing process after 48 to 72 hours. Then the hemorrhoid can be managed with warm sitz baths, stool softeners, and analgesics.

→ For an early thrombosed hemorrhoid (<48-72 hours), referral to a physician may be warranted for evacuation (Smith 1990).

→ Thrombosed internal hemorrhoids are usually always associated with extension to the external hemorrhoid. Immediate referral to a physician is warranted to prevent the possibility of gangrene (Smith 1990).

CONSULTATION

→ Referral to a physician is warranted:
- if symptoms are severe and not reduced with non-surgical intervention.
- for early acute (<48-72 hours) thrombosed hemorrhoid, and
- for thrombosed external and internal hemorrhoids presenting together.
- as needed for prescription(s).

PATIENT EDUCATION

→ Advise patient to avoid straining at stool or sitting on the toilet for prolonged period.

→ Advise regular toilet habits.

→ Advise patient to eat a high-fiber diet including bran, fresh fruits, and vegetables (see **General Nutrition Guidelines**).

→ Advise patient to increase fluid intake to six to eight glasses per day.

→ Warm sitz baths daily. Prolonged bathing should be avoided.

→ Epsom salts added to bath water, or ice packs may reduce swelling of edematous hemorrhoids.

→ Advise patient to maintain a regular exercise program.

→ If appropriate, advise patient to discontinue anal intercourse at least until the symptoms are under control and to use a generous amount of lubrication with penetration.

FOLLOW-UP

→ In two weeks, re-evaluate patients with moderate to severe symptoms to assess management plan. If symptoms not improved, consider referral for surgical treatment.

→ Re-evaluate patient with thrombosed hemorrhoid in one week.

→ Advise patient regarding American Cancer Society's recommendation for early detection of cancer in asymptomatic people (American Cancer Society 1993):
- sigmoidoscopy: every three years beginning at age 50 years.
- stool guaiac: yearly beginning at age 50 years.
- digital rectal exam: yearly beginning at age 40 years.
  - ACS suggests a digital rectal examination of all women during their annual gynecological visit.

→ Document in progress notes and problem list.

7-M

Hernia

A *hernia* is an abnormality in the musculofascial integrity of the abdominal wall that allows for the protrusion of structures through the defect (Margolies 1995). It is often not clear whether a hernia is a result of a congenital defect or secondary to trauma or injury. A hernia that presents after trauma may be due, in part, to a previously asymptomatic congenital defect.

Factors that increase the intra-abdominal pressure may predispose an individual to a hernia. These include coughing, heavy lifting, obesity, multiparity, and cirrhosis with ascites. The most common type of hernias in women are the indirect *inguinal, femoral,* and *umbilical hernias.*

The indirect inguinal hernia passes through the internal abdominal inguinal ring into the inguinal canal and exits through the external inguinal ring. It is thought to be a congenitally acquired hernia.

The femoral hernia passes through the femoral canal inferior to the inguinal ligament and becomes cutaneous in the fossa ovalis (Margolies 1995). Strangulation is common with femoral hernias.

The umbilical hernia passes through the umbilical ring and is considered to be a congenitally acquired hernia. Since large bowel is frequently involved, strangulation and incarceration are more common with this type of hernia.

An irreducible hernia (contents cannot be placed back into the abdomen by manipulation) can lead to complications including incarceration and strangulation.

DATABASE

SUBJECTIVE

→ Patients:
- often are asymptomatic.
- are noticed as a swelling or bulge over corresponding anatomical site.

→ Reducible hernias:
- usually present when standing or with increased intra-abdominal pressure via coughing or Valsalva's maneuver.
- mass disappears when supine.
- may have varying degrees of intermittent pain with radiation, when mass is present.
- pain aggravated by physical exertion.

→ Irreducible or incarcerated hernia may present with mass while supine; associated with higher levels of pain.

→ Strangulated hernia may present with colicky abdominal pain, nausea, vomiting, and symptoms of obstruction (see **Abdominal Pain** Protocol).

Indirect inguinal

→ Mass, tenderness over the deep inguinal ring.

Femoral

→ Mass, tenderness in femoral region.

Umbilical

→ Mass, tenderness at umbilicus.

OBJECTIVE

→ Examine in supine and standing position.

→ Examine while patient is doing Valsalva's maneuver.

→ Reducible hernias are evident when standing and reduce when supine.

Indirect inguinal

→ Examination of external inguinal ring difficult in women.

→ Visible and/or palpable mass over inguinal ring.

Femoral

→ Difficult to distinguish between femoral and indirect inguinal, especially with incarceration or a large sac.

→ Visible and/or palpable mass in femoral region.

Umbilical

→ Difficult to evaluate with large amount of subcutaneous fat.

→ Visible and/or palpable mass at umbilicus.

→ Ask the patient to lift her head from the examination table and bear down while lying supine.

→ An irreducible hernia may present with tenderness, discoloration, edema, fever, and signs of bowel obstruction (see **Abdominal Pain** Protocol), difficult to distinguish from incarceration or strangulation.

ASSESSMENT

→ Hernia
  - indirect inguinal
  - direct inguinal
  - femoral
  - umbilical
  - incisional

→ R/O enlarged lymph node

→ R/O intra-abdominal mass

PLAN

DIAGNOSTIC TESTS

→ None warranted.

TREATMENT/MANAGEMENT

→ Consultation with a physician and/or surgeon is warranted for evaluation regarding surgery for any type of hernia.

→ Asymptomatic reducible inguinal hernias (depending on size) may be managed expectantly. See "Patient Education" section.

→ Symptomatic reducible inguinal hernias should undergo elective repair to relieve symptoms and prevent strangulation.

→ Reducible femoral hernias should undergo elective repair because of high incidence of strangulation.

→ Umbilical hernias without protrusion may be managed expectantly.

→ Umbilical hernias with protrusion should undergo elective repair because of the high incidence of strangulation.

→ Any hernia presenting with evidence of irreducibility, incarceration, or strangulation should undergo repair.

→ Factors contributing to the occurrence of a hernia should be managed appropriately—e.g., coughing caused by smoking should be managed by advising smoking cessation.

CONSULTATION

→ Consultation with a general practitioner and/or surgeon is warranted in all cases of hernia.

→ Referral to a surgeon is indicated for surgery.

PATIENT EDUCATION

→ Patients who are managed expectantly should be advised to seek care for signs of incarceration or strangulation—e.g., tenderness, discoloration, edema, fever, signs of bowel obstruction (see **Abdominal Pain** Protocol).

→ Education should be provided for factors that may be contributing to the occurrence of a hernia—i.e., coughing caused by smoking—and a referral to the American Cancer Society or Nicotine Anonymous for smoking cessation should be made.

FOLLOW-UP

→ Patients who are being managed expectantly and who are knowledgeable about signs and symptoms of complications can be followed routinely.

→ Follow-up may be indicated for factors contributing to the occurrence of a hernia.

→ Document in progress notes and problem list.

7-N

Inflammatory Bowel Disease

Inflammatory bowel disease (*IBD*) refers to any intestinal inflammatory condition that is chronic in nature. The two most common inflammatory conditions are *ulcerative colitis* and *Crohn's disease*. Similarities between these conditions include: 1) clinical presentation, 2) average age at onset of between 15 years and 40 years, 3) higher incidence in Caucasians (particularly Jewish Caucasians) in developed western countries, 4) slightly higher incidence in females, and, 5) family clustering (Cooke 1991).

The cause of IBD is unknown. Factors thought to be involved in its pathogenesis include autoimmune factors, collagen disorders, genetic factors, infections, psychogenic factors, environmental factors, drugs, and weakened gastrointestinal defenses (Kirsner 1991).

Ulcerative colitis affects the mucosal and submucosal layers of the distal colon and rectum. It is characterized by ulcer lesions lining the entire colon tissue. The most common extracolonic manifestations of ulcerative colitis include arthritis, skin and eye lesions, and liver disease. Complications of ulcerative colitis include hemorrhage, pericolitis, toxic dilatation, perforation, and colon cancer.

Crohn's disease affects all layers of the mucosa and can occur anywhere in the gastrointestinal tract, from the buccal mucosa to the perineum. The terminal ileum, perineum, and distal colon are most commonly affected. It is characterized by areas of healthy tissue interspersed with affected tissue, a phenomena known as *skip lesions*. Extraintestinal manifestations include arthritis (more common with colonic disease), ankylosing spondylitis, skin and eye lesions, and an increase risk of cholelithiasis and nephrolithiasis.

Major complications of Crohn's disease include stenosis, enteric and perianal fistulas, abdominal and perianal abscess, perforation, and perineal suppuration. Patients with multiple bowel resections because of Crohn's disease are at risk for malabsorption of fat, bile acids, and deficiencies of zinc, calcium, magnesium, and Vitamins B_{12} and D (Kirsner 1991).

DATABASE

SUBJECTIVE

Ulcerative colitis

→ In mild cases, symptoms include:
- one to four semi-formed stools.
- minimal blood in stools.
- no systemic symptoms.

→ In moderate to severe cases, symptoms include:
- frequent liquid stools.
- blood and/or pus in stools.
- abdominal cramping.
- nocturnal diarrhea.
- mild fever during exacerbations.
- weight loss.
- symptoms of dehydration to varying degrees.

→ Patient has history of intolerance to dairy products.

→ Constipation, tenesmus, and anal incontinence may be present when only the rectum is involved.

→ Symptoms characterized by exacerbations and remissions. Remissions may last from months to years.

→ Variable symptoms of associated manifestations may be present for arthritis, skin and eye lesions, and liver disease (see appropriate protocols).

→ Variable symptoms of complications may be present for hemorrhage, pericolitis, toxic dilatation, perforation, and carcinoma (see appropriate protocols).

Crohn's disease

→ Symptom onset is subtle. May notice associated manifestations (weight loss) before GI symptoms.

→ Symptoms may include:
- diarrhea.
- lesions in mouth, soft palate, or perianal area.
- abdominal cramping and tenderness.
- steatorrhea in cases of bile salt malabsorption.

→ Symptoms not usually associated with passage of blood.
- If small bowel is involved:
  - fatigue.
  - fever (higher than in ulcerative colitis).
  - right lower-quadrant cramping pain (more severe than in ulcerative colitis).
  - nausea and vomiting.
  - weight loss and undernutrition.

→ Variable symptoms of associated manifestations may be present for arthritis, ankylosing spondylitis, skin and eye lesions, cholelithiasis, and nephrolithiasis (see appropriate protocols).

→ Variable symptoms of complications may be present for stenosis, enteric or perianal fistulas, abdominal or perianal abscess, perforation, and perianal suppuration (see appropriate protocols).

OBJECTIVE

Ulcerative colitis

→ Clinical findings depend on severity of illness.

→ In mild cases, patient may present with:
- slightly tender or normal abdominal examination.
- colonoscopy revealing loss of normal vascular pattern and mild to moderate diffuse inflammation.
- normal laboratory values.

→ In moderate to severe cases, patient may present with:
- abdominal tenderness, especially along course of colon.
- rectal examination revealing irritation, hemorrhoids, fissures, and spasm.
- signs of dehydration and undernutrition of varying degrees.
- fever.

- colonoscopy revealing continuous, granulomatous, superficial ulcerations.

→ Laboratory findings reflect severity of disease:
- decreased hemoglobin and hematocrit reflecting amount of blood loss.
- WBC count and ESR elevated in severe cases and with complications.
- electrolytes reflect severity with decrease in potassium, magnesium, and sodium.
- decreased albumin, calcium, and total protein in severe cases.
- abnormal liver function studies in severe cases.
- positive blood in stool.
- stool negative for bacteria and parasites.

→ Patient may present with enlarged lymph nodes.

→ Variable clinical findings of associated manifestations may be present for arthritis, skin and eye lesions, and liver disease (see appropriate protocols).

→ Variable clinical findings of complications may be present for hemorrhage, pericolitis, toxic dilatation, perforation, and carcinoma (see appropriate protocols).

Crohn's disease

→ Clinical findings depend on severity of illness.

→ Patient may present with:
- aphthoid ulcers in mouth, soft palate, or perianal area.
- anal fissures, fistulas, hemorrhoids, or abscesses.
- rectovaginal fistulas.
- enlarged lymph nodes.
- fever.
- if small bowel is involved:
  - mid-abdominal and right lower-quadrant tenderness.
  - right lower-quadrant fullness or mass reflecting adherent loops of bowel.
- varying degrees of undernutrition depending on severity.

→ Colonoscopy reveals deep, ulcerated fissures not continuous with areas of normal mucosa.

→ Laboratory findings reflect severity of disease:
- macrocytic anemia (Vitamin B_{12} malabsorption).
- decreased hemaglobin and hematocrit.
- normal or elevated WBC.
- elevated ESR.

- decreased total protein and albumin in severe cases.
- positive or negative blood in stool.
- stool negative for bacteria or parasite.
→ Variable clinical findings of associated manifestation may be present for arthritis, ankylosing spondylitis, skin and eye lesions, cholelithiasis, and nephrolithiasis (see appropriate protocols).
→ Variable clinical findings of complications may be present for stenosis, enteric or perianal fistulas, abdominal or perianal abscess, perforation, and perianal suppuration (see appropriate protocols).

ASSESSMENT

→ Inflammatory bowel disease
→ R/O ulcerative colitis
→ R/O Crohn's disease
→ R/O infectious colitis (bacterial, viral, fungal, parasitic)
→ R/O drug-induced colitis
→ R/O diverticular disease
→ R/O irritable bowel syndrome
→ R/O carcinoma

PLAN

DIAGNOSTIC TESTS

→ Ulcerative colitis diagnosis usually made by clinical presentation and sigmoidoscopy and confirmed by biopsy. Colonoscopy may determine extent of disease.
→ Crohn's disease diagnosis usually made by clinical presentation and contrast x-ray of large and small bowel. Pregnancy should be ruled out before initiation of x-ray.
→ Ultrasonography or computed tomographic scan of abdomen may detect abdominal mass, abscess, or obstruction.
→ CBC.
→ ESR.
→ Depending on severity of disease:
  - electrolytes.
  - total protein, albumin.
  - liver function studies.
→ Stool culture.
→ Stool for ova and parasites.
→ Stool for occult blood.

→ Additional testing may be warranted to rule out extra-intestinal manifestations of the disease.
→ Additional testing may be warranted to rule out complications of the disease.

TREATMENT/MANAGEMENT

→ Hospitalization is warranted for moderate to severe disease or major complications.
→ Majority of patients with mild disease can be managed on outpatient basis.
→ Diet should be altered during exacerbations and may be of benefit as a general measure:
  - trial elimination of lactose-containing foods (i.e., dairy products).
  - low-residue diet eliminating raw fruits and vegetables, fruit juices.
  - low-fiber diet with Crohn's disease to reduce risk of obstruction by eliminating nuts, seeds, tough meat, cole slaw.
  - patients with steatorrhea should have low-fat diet (< 80 gm/day).
  - fish oil intake for ulcerative colitis is under evaluation (Kirsner 1991).
  - undernourished patients should have balanced high-calorie (2,500 kcal/day to 3,000 kcal/day) and high-protein (120 g/day to 150 g/day) diet.
  - multivitamin with iron, calcium, and magnesium to aid in decreased absorption of fat-soluble vitamins. Megavitamin therapy not advised.
  - folic acid supplementation (1 mg/day) is warranted when intake of green leafy vegetables and fresh fruits is poor or when sulfasalazine therapy is being taken.
  - parenteral Vitamin B_{12} therapy as indicated.
  - parenteral iron therapy as indicated. Oral therapy not well-tolerated.
  - with severe exacerbations, elemental supplements (Ensure®, Vivonex®) or total parenteral alimentation may be warranted to rest the bowel. Home parenteral nutrition is widely available as an alternative to hospitalization.
→ Pharmacological therapy.

Ulcerative colitis (mild to moderate disease)

→ Sulfa antibiotic and 5-aminosalicylic acid (Sulfasalazine®): reduces frequency and severity of recurrent ulcerative colitis.
  - 25 percent of patients experience intolerable side effects.

- Alternate preparations (Mesalamine® and Olsalazine®) associated with increased efficacy and less side effects.
  - Can be taken during pregnancy.
- Recommend 1 mg/day folate supplementation when using this drug (Linn and Peppercorn 1992).
- Begin 500 mg/day p.o. QID with meals and increase dosage as tolerated over several days to 4 g/day. Then decrease to smallest dosage that maintains symptom control (usually 2 g/day) and continue for at least 1 year to maintain remission (Ruymann and Richter 1995).
  - Gastric side effects can be reduced by using enteric-coated tablets and taking them with food.
  - Mild allergic reactions can be managed through desensitization, i.e., give low daily dose of 10 mg-250 mg, increasing slowly every 3 to 7 days to therapeutic level (Cooke 1991).
- Side effects: headache, dyspepsia, anorexia, fever, rash, hemolytic anemia, leukopenia, folate deficiency, exacerbation of colitis, reversible male infertility caused by effects on spermatogenesis. See *PDR*.
- Contraindications: pregnancy at term, history of severe allergy to sulfa drugs.

→ If Sulfazalazine® fails to achieve control or in acute cases,

ADD:

→ Prednisone®:
- 40 mg/day p.o. in divided doses with round-the-clock symptoms, then change to A.M. dosage for 7 to 10 days or when control is achieved. Then decrease by 5 mg-10 mg every 2 weeks and taper off if possible, depending on disease activity.
  - Prednisone® is not effective in maintaining remission (Linn and Peppercorn 1992).
  - Side effects: dose-related—adrenal suppression, bone thinning, mood alterations, weakened resistance to infection, impaired glucose tolerance, cushingoid appearance. See *PDR*.

Ulcerative colitis (moderate to severe disease)

→ Refer to a physician for management.

Mild ulcerative proctitis (disease confined to rectosigmoid)

→ 5-aminosalicylic acid enema (Mesalamine®):
- 3 g/100 cc enema per rectum at bedtime for 2 to 6 weeks.
  - Foam preparation is easier to retain but more expensive.
  - Administer in left lateral position and retain overnight if possible.
  - Relapse is almost 100 percent after discontinuation. Recommend taper to every other or every third night.
- Found to be more effective than prednisone® enemas (Linn and Peppercorn 1992).
- Side effects: similar to oral preparation, but to varying degrees also anal irritation and mucosal sensitivity. See *PDR*.

→ Prednisone® enema:
- 1 cc-60 cc (100 mg hydrocortisone) enema per rectum at bedtime for 14 nights.
  - Foam preparation available.
  - Administer in left lateral position and retain overnight if possible. Taper to every other or every third night (Cooke 1991).
- side effects: systemic absorption and associated side effects with prolonged use—adrenal suppression, bone thinning, mood alteration, weakened defense against infection, impaired glucose tolerance, cushingoid appearance. See *PDR*.

→ If mild diarrhea persists during ulcerative colitis remission, consider trial of:
- psyllium hydrophilic colloid 1 tsp. in 8 oz. water p.o. every day or BID (Ruymann and Richter 1995).

→ For relief of mild to moderate diarrhea in patient with ulcerative colitis consider short course of:
- loperamide (Imodium®) 2 mg-4 mg p.o. with meals and at bedtime.
- codeine sulfate 15 mg-30 mg p.o. with meals and at bedtime.
- paregoric 4 ml-8 ml p.o. with meals and at bedtime.
- deodorized tincture of opium 5 drops-10 drops TID to QID.
- avoid prolonged use of all four drugs; can lead to narcotic dependence. Avoid use in severe disease (high risk of toxic dilatation) with ulcerative colitis (Kirsner 1991).

→ Surgery may be indicated with ulcerative colitis in cases unresponsive to medical therapy, or cases involving intractable bleeding, unresponsive toxic megacolon, disabling strictures, or carcinoma (Cooke 1991).

Crohn's disease (mild to moderate disease of small bowel)

→ Prednisone®:
- 60 mg/day p.o. in divided dose with round-the-clock symptoms. Then change to A.M. dose and continue until symptoms controlled (may be as long as four months). An every-other-day dose may be sufficient.
  - Taper by decreasing 5 mg-10 mg every few weeks. Not effective in maintaining remission (Linn and Peppercorn 1992).
- side effects: dose-related—adrenal suppression, bone thinning, mood alteration, weakening defense against infection, impaired glucose tolerance, cushingoid appearance. See *PDR*.

Colonic Crohn's disease

→ Begin Sulfasalazine® 500 mg/day p.o. QID with meals and increase as tolerated over several days to 4 g/day. Continue 4 to 8 weeks.
- See indications, side effects, and contraindications as per ulcerative colitis treatment.
- Will not prevent relapse in Crohn's disease (Ruymann and Richter 1995).

→ If no response to Sulfasalazine®

SWITCH TO:

→ Metroridazole (Flagyl®):
- 10 mg-20 mg/kg/day p.o. (e.g., 250 mg-500 mg TID) and continue for a 4-week trial. If there is satisfactory response, continue for 4 to 6 months, then stop if symptoms have ceased (Ruymann and Richter 1995).
- side effects: altered taste, paresthesia of hands and feet, peripheral neuropathy, epileptic seizures, abdominal complaints. Ingestion of alcohol may produce Antabuse® affect. Considered mutagenic. See *PDR*.

→ If inadequate response to Metronidazole

SWITCH TO:

→ Prednisone® as per "Small Bowel Disease Treatment" (Ruymann and Richter 1995).

Perianal Crohn's disease

→ Metronidazole (Flagyl®):
- 15 mg-20 mg/kg/day p.o. May be increased up to 50 mg/kg/day if necessary (Cooke 1991). Relapse occurs following discontinuation.

- side effects: altered taste, paresthesia of hands and feet, peripheral neuropathy, epileptic seizures, abdominal complaints. Ingestion of alcohol may produce Antabuse® affect. Considered mutagenic. See *PDR*.

→ For relief of mild to moderate diarrhea in patients with ulcerative colitis or Crohn's disease, consider short course of:
- loperamide (Imodium®) 2 mg-4 mg p.o. with meals and at bedtime.
- codeine sulfate 15 mg-30 mg p.o. with meals and at bedtime.
- paregoric 4 ml-8 ml p.o. with meals and at bedtime.
- deodorized tincture of opium 5 drops-10 drops p.o. TID to QID.
- avoid prolonged use of all four drugs; can lead to narcotic dependence. Avoid use in severe disease (high risk of toxic dilatation with ulcerative colitis) (Kirsner 1991).

→ Surgery may be indicated with Crohn's disease in cases of intestinal obstruction, abscess formation, bladder or vaginal fistula, or intractable bleeding, or diarrhea. There is a high recurrence rate (70 percent after 15 years) after surgery for Crohn's disease (Cooke 1991).

CONSULTATION

→ Consultation with a physician for management of mild to moderate disease.
→ Referral to a gastrointestinal specialist for diagnosis and to evaluate extent of disease.
→ Referral to a physician is warranted for surgical indications, conditions unresponsive to medical therapy, or moderate to severe disease.
→ Referral to a physician is warranted for colonoscopy and x-ray procedures.
→ Referral to a psychotherapist as indicated for anxiety or depression.
→ Consultation or referral to a nutritionist for education.
→ Referral to appropriate specialist for evaluation of extraintestinal manifestations.
→ As needed for prescription(s).

PATIENT EDUCATION

→ See "Treatment/Management" section.
→ Explain pathogenesis, treatment plan, chronicity, and course of disease. Include family in education.

→ Discuss concerns regarding conception, pregnancy, and childbearing.

→ Women with ulcerative colitis should be counseled to postpone pregnancy until remission of about one year.

→ Advise women considering pregnancy that there is an increased risk of pre-term delivery and low birth weight. Approximately 30 percent to 50 percent of women have exacerbations during pregnancy and postpartum.
  ▪ Sulfasalazine® and Prednisone® are relatively safe.
  ▪ IBD is not associated with risk of fetal defects (Podolsky 1991).

→ Discuss concerns regarding incontinence, cancer, and social isolation.

→ Provide supportive relationship and observe for signs of depression from chronic illness.

→ Advise patient regarding nutritious diet. See special indications under "Treatment/ Management."

→ Advise regular exercise program.

→ Encourage small, regular, frequent meals.

→ Advise elimination of caffeine-containing foods.

→ Advise cessation of smoking and alcohol intake. Refer to appropriate support services if indicated (American Cancer Society, Nicotine Anonymous, Alcoholics Anonymous). See **Alcoholism and Other Drug Dependencies** and **Smoking Cessation** protocols.

→ Patients can be taught to adjust their medications within a prearranged set of guidelines and limits, allowing them a more active role in their own care.

→ Refer patient to the Crohn's and Colitis Foundation of America (CCFA) to provide education and support services to patients and families. Toll-free number: 800-932-2423.

FOLLOW-UP

→ Patient should be followed closely during exacerbations.

→ During remission, evaluations are warranted every three to six months to document:
  ▪ number of exacerbations (if any).
  ▪ weight.
  ▪ proctoscopy or sigmoidoscopy.
  ▪ hemoglobin, ESR, and albumin (Jenner 1991).

→ Increased incidence of colorectal cancer after seven to ten years with ulcerative colitis involving the entire colon.
  ▪ Five to ten years post-diagnosis colonoscopy with directed biopsy should be performed every two years.

→ In Crohn's disease of the colon, cancer risk increases with increasing area of involvement and longer duration. In small bowel disease, risk increases with longer duration.
  ▪ Upper GI and small bowel x-ray with colonoscopy should be performed every two years.

→ Testing for occult blood in stool as an indicator of malignancy is inappropriate since many patients with IBD experience blood loss.

→ Document in progress notes and problem list.

7-O

Irritable Bowel Syndrome

Irritable bowel syndrome is a disturbance of bowel motor activity characterized by constipation and/or diarrhea, abdominal pain, hypersecretion of colonic mucus, dyspeptic symptoms, and varying degrees of anxiety or depression (Knauer 1993a). Nonpropulsive colonic contractions and slow-wave myoelectric activity predispose to constipation and discomfort. Diarrhea is a result of the increased contraction of the small bowel and colon and decreased activity in the large colon causing a pressure gradient.

Psychological stress is thought to be a major component in this syndrome, with affected individuals experiencing more severe colonic symptoms at times of stress than non-affected individuals. Diet is also suspected in the pathogenesis of this disorder. A low-residue diet or intolerance to lactose or sugar may predispose some individuals.

Irritable bowel syndrome is the most common gastrointestinal complaint for which patients seek medical care (Drossman 1989). It is referred to by many names, including *nervous indigestion, functional dyspepsia, irritable colon, spastic colitis, mucous colitis,* and *intestinal neurosis.*

DATABASE

SUBJECTIVE

→ A detailed history is hallmark in diagnosis, attempting to identify the symptom complex consistent with irritable bowel syndrome.

→ Patient has long-term history of symptoms, symptoms not steadily progressive.

→ History common for headaches, joint pain, allergies, lack of mental concentration, fatigue,

anxiety, depression, nervousness, or emotional disturbances.

→ Patient may have history of cathartic and enema use.

→ Symptoms may include:
  - varying degrees of bloating, nausea, vomiting, flatulence, anorexia, foul breath, heartburn, weakness, palpitations.
  - constipation alternating with diarrhea.
  - passage of mucus with or without stool.
  - episodic or continuous abdominal pain of varying degrees.
  - abdominal pain associated with urge to defecate or passage of flatus. Pain is relieved when passage is completed.
    • Pain may radiate to left chest or arm (gas in splenic flexure).
  - exacerbated by ingestion of large or fatty meals, foods that produce gas (beans, cabbage), stimulant foods (containing caffeine), medication, hormonal changes that occur at menses, and psychological stress.
  - absent nocturnal symptoms.

OBJECTIVE

→ Patient may appear anxious or depressed.

→ Patient may present with abdominal tenderness, especially along the course of the colon, to varying degrees.

→ Sigmoidoscopy may show increased spasm and mucus in the colonic lumen.

→ Radiographic study may show altered gastrointestinal motility without other evidence of abnormality.

ASSESSMENT

→ Irritable bowel syndrome

→ R/O inflammatory bowel disorder

→ R/O gastroenteritis

→ R/O lactase deficiency

→ R/O thyrotoxicosis

→ R/O psychological disorder

→ R/O other causes of chronic diarrhea

PLAN

DIAGNOSTIC TESTS

→ Diagnosis is commonly made by identifying symptom complex as consistent with irritable bowel syndrome and excluding other abnormalities.

→ CBC.

→ Stool for occult blood.

→ Stool examination for ova and parasites.

→ Stool examination for bacteria.

→ Consider serum electrolytes, liver and thyroid function studies.

→ Sigmoidoscopy or radiographic study of gastrointestinal system may be indicated to rule out other disorders.

TREATMENT/MANAGEMENT

→ No specific diet will prove helpful to all patients.
- Consider eliminating certain food when there is a suspicion of intolerance—i.e., lactose foods (milk and milk products)—on a trial basis for 1 to 2 weeks and evaluate for symptom improvement.
- Increase dietary fiber (grains, vegetables, fruits). Psyllium or methylcellulose may be of benefit (see **Constipation** Protocol).
- Reduce fat intake and intake of gas-producing foods.
- Avoidance of food stimulants—e.g., caffeine-containing products.

→ Psychotherapy may benefit individuals with signs of psychiatric conditions (see **Anxiety Disorders** and **Depression** protocols). Patients on antidepressive drugs (e.g., amitriptyline, doxepin)

may notice gastrointestinal symptom improvement due to the anticholinergic effects of the drug.

→ Hypnotherapy, biofeedback, or other structured relaxation techniques may be helpful.

→ Drug therapy may be indicated if there is no relief of symptoms with conservative measures. Prescribe short courses of these drugs and assess for drug dependence.
- Anticholinergic drugs may help reduce colonic spasm and relieve pain associated with constipation. Dicyclomine (Bentyl®), 10 mg-20 mg p.o. before meals (Knauer 1993a).
- Opiate derivatives may reduce diarrhea. Loperamide (Imodium®), 1 tablet p.o. BID, prn (Goroll 1995f). Prescribe only a 2- to 5-day supply.

CONSULTATION

→ Physician consultation may be needed for irritable bowel syndrome treatment plan.

→ Physician referral warranted for sigmoidoscopy or radiographic studies.

→ Physician referral may be indicated for disabling symptoms or refractory diarrhea.

→ Referral to a psychotherapist for patients with serious psychopathology.

→ Referral for hypnotherapy or biofeedback as indicated.

→ As needed for prescription(s).

PATIENT EDUCATION

→ Explain pathophysiology, etiology, and management plan.

→ Explain that the disorder is chronic and recurring. The management plan is to identify and modify factors that exacerbate symptoms (Drossman 1989).

→ Provide a supportive relationship with the patient. Acknowledge symptoms, address patient fears and provide reassurance.

→ Discuss psychological and environmental factors that predispose patient to symptoms or exacerbate them. Assist the patient in reducing these factors.
- Advise patient to keep a diary of daily factors that appear to exacerbate symptoms.
- Assist the patient in stress- and anxiety-reducing measures (see **Anxiety Disorders, Stress Management** protocols).

→ Encourage a nutritious diet, high in fiber and with reduced food stimulants.

→ Advise patient to discontinue all non-essential medications that affect bowel function, especially laxatives or enemas.

→ For patients with constipation, see **Constipation** Protocol.

FOLLOW-UP

→ Patient evaluation at regular intervals will assist in providing a supportive relationship and recognizing periods of increased stress.

→ Document in progress notes and problem list.

Lisa L. Lommel, R.N., C., F.N.P., M.P.H.

7-P

Peptic Ulcer Disease

Peptic ulcer disease refers to a group of related ulcerative disorders of the upper gastrointestinal tract. These are *duodenal ulcer* (80 percent of peptic ulcer disease), *gastric ulcer*, and *Zollinger-Ellison syndrome*.

Approximately 95 percent of duodenal ulcers occur in the duodenal bulb or cap. The remainder are between this area and the ampulla. Duodenal ulcers are two to three times more common than gastric ulcers. The majority of gastric ulcers are found within 6 cm of the pylorus at or near the lesser curvature on the posterior wall of the stomach.

Peptic ulcer disease is thought to be the result of an imbalance between the acid/pepsin secretion and mucosal defenses. Gastric acid and pepsin secretion, elevated in individuals with duodenal ulcers, is relatively normal in individuals with gastric ulcers. Gastric emptying is also accelerated in individuals with duodenal ulcers, causing greater acid exposure of the duodenal mucosa before neutralization of the acid can occur (Goroll 1995g).

Mucosal defense mechanisms are important in protecting the upper gastrointestinal tissue from excess secretions. Specifically, mucus secretion, bicarbonate production, mucosal blood flow, and cellular repair mechanisms are factors in mucosal defense. Prostaglandin E_2 is important in mucus production and bicarbonate secretion and repair. Prostaglandin E_2 has been found to be decreased in individuals with active ulcer disease (Debas and Mulholland 1989).

Peptic ulcer results when the protective factors of the mucosal defense mechanisms are outweighed by the aggressive factors of acid/pepsin. Mucosal defense is thought to play a larger role in gastric ulcer development than hypersecretion (Knauer 1993a).

Zollinger-Ellison syndrome causes peptic ulcer disease because of the effects of gastrin-releasing tumors (*gastrinomas*) which are usually located in the pancreas.

Various factors have been implicated in the cause or aggravation of ulcer disease. These include (McGuigan 1991; Goroll 1995g):

→ heredity. First-degree relatives are at increased risk.

→ cigarette smoking, which decreases mucosal defense, decreases response to therapy, increases duodenal ulcer mortality.

→ *Helicobacter pylori* colonization. There is high incidence in duodenal ulcer patients; uncertain whether it is contributing factor or commensal association (Tytgat and Rauws 1990).

→ stress of unconfirmed association.

→ alcohol and coffee ingestion. Association unconfirmed.

→ glucocorticosteroids. Association unconfirmed.

→ NSAIDs; especially prevalent in the elderly (Agrawal 1991).

Complications of peptic ulcer disease include refractoriness to therapy, perforation, obstruction, and hemorrhage. There is a greater incidence of malignancy and mortality—as a result of hemorrhage—with gastric ulcers than there is with duodenal ulcers.

DATABASE

SUBJECTIVE

→ History may include:
  ■ symptoms that are chronic and/or recurrent.

- high stress level.
- large-volume alcohol or coffee ingestion, or glucocorticosteroid or NSAID use.
- family member with ulcer disease.

→ Peptic ulcer disease rarely occurs during pregnancy.

Duodenal ulcer

→ Symptoms may include:
- recurrent, episodic, epigastric pain occurring 90 minutes to three hours after food ingestion.
  - Pain is sharp, gnawing, burning, or aching with abdominal pressure or "hunger sensation."
  - May radiate below costal margins to back.
  - Relieved within a few minutes by food, antacids, or vomiting.
    - Nausea and vomiting of small quantities of highly acidic gastric juices.

→ Symptoms are usually absent before breakfast, worsening over the day.

→ Patient is most symptomatic from 12:00 midnight to 2:00 A.M.

→ Change in character of pain or symptoms may indicate complication:
- pentration may produce:
  - constant pain, not relieved by food or antacid, and
  - radiation to back or either upper quadrant.
- obstruction may produce:
  - accentuated pain, not relieved by food.
  - epigastric fullness, and vomiting of undigested food after meals.
- perforation may produce:
  - acute onset of epigastric pain, radiating to shoulder or right lower quadrant.
    - Sometimes with nausea and vomiting.
    - Pain lessens after a few hours (see **Abdominal Pain** Protocol).
- Hemorrhage may produce sudden onset of:
  - weakness, faintness, dizziness.
  - chills.
  - moist skin.
  - desire to defecate.
  - red or tarry stools.
  - hematemesis.

Gastric ulcer

→ Symptoms may be atypical, vague, or absent.

→ Pain is gnawing, burning, aching, described as "hunger pangs" referred to left subcostal region.

→ Pain occurs 45 to 60 minutes after a meal or may be precipitated by a meal.

→ In contrast to duodenal ulcer, antacids less consistently helpful in relieving symptoms.

→ Nausea and vomiting are common.

→ Weight loss and fatigue secondary to food aversion.

→ Symptoms may come and go over time. May recur with ingestion of aspirin or NSAIDs.

OBJECTIVE

→ Epigastric tenderness and muscle guarding common with peptic ulcers.

→ Perforation may produce rigid abdomen, rebound tenderness, and initially hyperactive bowel sounds (progressing to hypoactive then absent), fever, leukocytosis, tachycardia.

→ Hemorrhage may produce postural hypotension/tachycardia, mucosal pallor, and positive occult blood in stools. Anemia may be present, although considered a late sign.

ASSESSMENT

→ Peptic ulcer disease
→ R/O duodenal ulcer
→ R/O gastric ulcer
→ R/O ulcer perforation
→ R/O hemorrhage
→ R/O gastritis
→ R/O gastric carcinoma
→ R.O irritable bowel syndrome
→ R/O pancreatitis
→ R/O biliary tract disease
→ R/O liver disease
→ R/O pneumonia
→ R/O cardiac disease

PLAN

DIAGNOSTIC TESTS

→ Diagnosis is most often made on clinical findings.

→ Management can proceed from clinical findings except in individuals:
- with suspicion of complication (bleeding, perforation, obstruction), refer to physician.
- over 40 years of age with increased risk of carcinoma, an endoscopy or barium-contrast radiography is recommended.

→ Endoscopy should also be considered in patients:
- whose symptoms persist after 7 days of empiric therapy.
- with early satiety.
- with weight loss.
- whose stools test positive for blood.
- after 14 days of therapy with a known duodenal ulcer (Feldman et al. 1992; Goroll 1995g).

→ Endoscopy with at least six biopsies is indicated in patients over age 50 years with a gastric ulcer (Feldman et al. 1992).

→ Barium-contrast radiography is most common initial diagnostic measure; can demonstrate duodenal ulcer in 50 percent to 70 percent of cases (Knauer 1993a) and gastric ulcer in up to 90 percent (McGuigan 1991).

→ Fiberoptic endoscopy of the upper gastrointestinal tract can facilitate diagnosis of peptic ulcers when not demonstrated radiographically.
NOTE: Because of false positive and false negative errors, radiographic appearance should not be used as sole criterion for determination of benign or malignant gastric ulcer. Endoscopy with at least 6 biopsies should be obtained.

→ Endoscopy with biopsy can also assess for presence of *H. pylori*.

→ CBC to evaluate for anemia.

→ Obtain stool occult blood tests.

TREATMENT/MANAGEMENT

→ Antacids: relieve pain by neutralizing acid, inactivating pepsin, bindings of bile salts, stimulation of gastric bicarbonate secretion (Freston 1990).
- Since gastric ulcers are not primarily caused by hypersecretion, antacid dose is approximately half that required in duodenal ulcer disease.
  - Prescribe amounts sufficient to provide 140 mEq/dose for treatment of duodenal ulcer and 70 mEq/dose for gastric ulcer.
  - Liquid form is superior to tablet form.

→ Dosages listed below are for duodenal ulcer treatment (Goroll 1995g). See **Tables 7P.1, Characteristics of Major Liquid Antacids,** and **7P.2, Characteristics of Major Antacid Tablets.**
- Aluminum hydroxide/magnesium hydroxide mixtures (Maalox® TC, Delcid®, Mylanta® II, Gelusil® II).
  - Dose: 30 ml p.o. 2 hours after meals and at bedtime.
  - Side effects: Aluminum may cause constipation, phosphate deficiency, and osteoporosis. Magnesium may cause diarrhea and should not be used in patients with renal insufficiency. Use combination preparations or alternate preparations to manage gastrointestinal symptoms.

Table 7P.1. CHARACTERISTICS OF MAJOR LIQUID ANTACIDS

Preparation	Neutralizing Capacity (mEq/ml)	Volume for 140 mEq/ml	Sodium Content (mg/5ml)	Buffers
Maalox TC	4.2	33	<1.0	Al/MgOH$_2$
Titralac	4.2	33	11.0	CaCO$_3$
Delcid	4.1	34	1.5	Al/MgOH$_2$
Mylanta II	3.6	39	1.0	Al/MgOH$_2$
Camalox	3.2	44	2.5	Al/MgOH$_2$, CaCO$_3$
Gelusil II	3.0	47	1.3	Al/MgOH$_2$
Basaljel ES	2.9	48	23.0	AlCO$_3$
Riopan	2.7	50	<1.0	Magaldrate
Mylanta	2.5	55	<1.0	Al/MgOH$_2$
Alternagel	2.4	60	2.0	AlOH$_2$
Maalox Plus	2.3	61	1.0	Al/MgOH$_2$
Maalox	2.3	61	1.0	Al/MgOH$_2$
Gelusil	2.2	64	<1.0	Al/MgOH$_2$
Riopan Plus	1.8	78	0.7	Al/MgOH$_2$
Di-Gel	1.8	80	15.0	Al/MgOH$_2$
Amphogel	4.0	100	7.0	AlOH$_2$

Source: Reprinted with permission and adapted from Goroll, A.H. 1995. Management of peptic ulcer disease. In *Primary care medicine*, eds. A.H. Goroll, L.A. May, and A.G. Mulley, p. 386. Philadelphia: J.B. Lippincott.

Table 7P.2. CHARACTERISTICS OF MAJOR ANTACID TABLETS

Preparation	Neutralizing Capacity (mEq/ml)	Volume for 140 mEq/ml	Sodium Content (mg/5ml)	Buffers
Canalox	16.7	8	1.5	$Al/MgOH_2$
Basaljel	15.4	9	2.0	$AlCO_3$
Mylanta II	11.0	13	1.3	$Al/MgOH_2$
Tums	10.5	13	2.7	$CaCO_3$
Alka II	10.5	13	2.0	$CaCO_3$
Riopan Plus	10.0	14	0.3	$Al/MgOH_2$
Titralac	9.5	15	0.3	$CaCO_3$
Gelusil II	8.2	17	2.1	$Al/MgOH_2$
Rolaids	6.9	20	53.0	$AlCO_3$
Maalox Plus	5.7	25	1.4	$Al/MgOH_2$
Digel	4.7	30	10.6	$Al/MgOH_2$, $MgCO_3$
Amphogel	2.0	70	7.0	$AlOH_2$

Source: Reprinted with permission and adapted from Goroll, A.H. 1995. Management of peptic ulcer disease. In *Primary care medicine*, eds. A.H. Goroll, L.A. May, and A.G. Mulley, p. 386. Philadelphia: J.B. Lippincott.

- Calcium carbonate alone (Tums®, Titralac®, Alka® II) is not recommended for treatment because of its calcium-induced gastric hypersecretion. A mixture of aluminum hydroxide, magnesium hydroxide, and calcium carbonate (Camalox®) is recommended.
  - Dose: 15 ml-30 ml p.o. 1 and 3 hours after meals and at bedtime.
- Sodium bicarbonate is not recommended in treatment of peptic ulcer disease because of its high sodium content.
→ Histamine H_2-receptor antagonists: potent inhibitors of basal and stimulated gastric acid secretion.
- Cimetidine (Tagamet®): inhibits gastric secretion stimulated by food, gastrin, histamine, and caffeine. Avoid taking at same time as antacids. Separate them by at least 1 to 2 hours.
  - Dose: 300 mg p.o. QID, before meals and at bedtime

    OR

    400 mg p.o. BID

    OR

    800 mg p.o. daily after dinner.
  - Side effects: rare effects of gynecomastia; galactorrhea; impotence; skin rashes; leukopenia; agranulocytosis; hepatitis; elevated serum creatinine; and interactions with warfarin, propranolol, benzodiazepines, phenytoin, theophylline compounds, and other drugs metabolized by hepatic microsomes (potentiates their effects); mental confusion in the elderly (Knauer 1993a). See *PDR*.

- Ranitidine (Zantac®): more potent than cimetidine and interferes less with other drugs.
  - Dose: 150 mg p.o. every 12 hours

    OR

    300 mg p.o. after dinner.
  - Side effects: diarrhea, dyspepsia, loss of libido, dizziness, and mental confusion (Knauer 1993a).
- Famotidine (Pepcid®): more potent than cimetidine or ranitidine.
  - Dose: 40 mg p.o. after dinner (Knauer 1993a).
- Nizatidine (Axid®): similar effectiveness to other H_2 antagonists.
  - Dose: 300 mg p.o. after dinner (Knauer 1993a).
→ Sucralfate (Carafate®): a mucosal protective agent that adheres to areas of duodenal and gastric ulcers; as effective with duodenal ulcers as antacids and H_2 antagonists.
- Dose: 1 g 30 to 60 minutes p.o. before meals and at bedtime

    OR

    2 g p.o. 30 to 60 minutes before breakfast and dinner. Antacids can be used concomitantly but not within 1 hour of sucralfate.
- Side effects: constipation, inhibits absorption of digoxin, tetracycline, phenytoin, and cimetidine (Freston 1990).
→ Omeprazole (Prilosec®): a proton pump inhibitor, inhibits basal and stimulated gastric secretion.
- Dose: 20 mg p.o. every day for 8 to 12 weeks only. See *PDR*.

→ Begin treatment with antacid and/or H_2-receptor antagonist based on patient preference, capacity for compliance, affordability, and potential for interaction with other drugs (Goroll 1995g).

→ Begin sucralfate if patient unable to tolerate antacids or H_2-receptor antagonists, but avoid if compliance or constipation is a problem (Goroll 1995g).

→ Omeprazole should be used for refractory ulcers. If patient has failed a course of H_2 blockers or sucralfate after 4 weeks of therapy, endoscopy with biopsy should be performed before initiating omeprazole (Feldman et al. 1992).
NOTE: Omeprazole should not be used as maintenence therapy for treatment of duodenal ulcer.

→ Patients with biopsy-proven *H. pylori* may be treated with triple treatment.
  ▪ Dose: Metronidazole (Flagyl®) 500 mg p.o. TID for 1 month
AND
Tetracycline (Achromycin®, Sumycin®) 500 mg p.o. QID for 1 month
AND
Bismuth subcitrate (Pepto Bismol®) 2 tabs chewed QID for 1 month (Feldman et al. 1992).

→ Diet has not been shown to be a factor in the incidence or healing of ulcers (Knauer 1993a).

→ Patient should cease smoking and alcohol consumption.

→ Discontinue or limit use of aspirin, NSAIDs, and steroids.

→ Patient should restrict caffeine intake, including coffee, tea, and cola beverages—regular or decaffeinated.

→ Management by a physician is warranted in cases of obstruction, sub-acute bleeding, and perforation.

→ Hemorrhage and acute perforation constitute a medical emergency. Referral to an emergency service and physician is warranted.

CONSULTATION

→ Physician consultation may be sought for management of typical symptoms of duodenal ulcer disease.

→ Referral to a physician may be warranted:
  ▪ with suspicion of gastric ulcer for diagnostic radiography and/or endoscopy.

  ▪ when there is no improvement of duodenal or gastric ulcer symptoms with medical management.
  ▪ with recurrent disease.
→ Immediate referral is warranted in cases of obstruction, and acute hemorrhage or perforation.
→ As needed for prescription(s).

PATIENT EDUCATION

→ Explain risk factors, chronic and recurrent nature of the disease, physiology, treatment regimes, and consequences of inadequate treatment.

→ Advise patient to continue with medication as prescribed, even after symptoms have subsided.

→ Advise patient not to take antacids with meals.

→ Advise patient not to take cimetidine at the same time as antacids.

→ Encourage patient to get adequate rest and sleep.

→ Advise patient regarding a nutritious diet (see **General Nutrition Guidelines**) and regular meal intake. A bland or milk diet is not necessary.

→ Encourage limiting only those foods that cause discomfort.

→ Advise patient to avoid eating immediately before bedtime, possibly helping eliminate nocturnal discomfort.

→ Encourage patient to restrict intake of coffee, tea, and cola beverages.

→ Assist patient in discontinuing alcohol and smoking with referral to appropriate support services if necessary (Alcoholics Anonymous, Nicotine Anonymous, and American Cancer Society). See **Alcoholism and Other Drug Dependencies** and **Smoking Cessation** protocols.

→ Assist patient in stress reduction. See **Stress Management** Protocol.

FOLLOW-UP

→ Re-evaluate patient in four to six weeks after initiation of treatment.

→ Most duodenal ulcers will heal in four to six weeks of treatment. Recommended period of treatment of active disease is four to eight weeks or until symptoms resolve. Then switch to maintenance therapy for another four to eight weeks.

→ Consider endoscopy with duodenal ulcer if:
  ▪ patient has more than two recurrences in six months, or three recurrences in one year, or

- if bleeding, perforation, vomiting, early satiety, or anemia occurs (Feldman et al. 1992).

→ For patients with recurrences or refractory duodenal or gastric ulcer disease, consider checking for *H. pylori* by endoscopy or breath test.

→ For refractory disease unresponsive to treatment for *H. pylori*, perform endoscopy to rule out malignancy.

→ Recommended treatment for gastric ulcer is until healing has been demonstrated, *not* just until symptoms have subsided.

→ Endoscopy is recommended with gastric ulcer after 12 weeks of therapy to document healing and rule out gastric cancer (Feldman et al. 1992).

→ If a gastric ulcer shows no healing at 12 weeks, patient should be referred to a physician. If the ulcer is smaller, therapy should continue (Feldman et al. 1992).

→ Total healing of gastric ulcer should be documented to rule out cancer (Feldman et al. 1992).

→ Recurrence of symptoms is common. Rate of recurrence is reduced if patient stops smoking and remains on therapy for a year (Knauer 1993a).

→ Traditionally, maintenance is recommended for the following patients:
  - those with three or more ulcer recurrences in a year, all treated with full doses of H_2 blockers.
  - those with complications such as bleeding, perforation, or obstruction, and

- elderly patients, whose ulcer complications may be life-threatening (Feldman et al. 1992).

→ Recommended dosages follow (Feldman et al. 1992):
  - cimetidine (Tagamet®) 400 mg p.o. at bedtime.
  - ranitidine (Zantac®) 150 mg p.o. at bedtime.
  - nizatidine (Axid®) 150 mg p.o. at bedtime.
  - famotidine (Pepcid®) 20 mg p.o. at bedtime.
               OR
  - sucralfate (Carafate®) 1 g or 2 g p.o. at bedtime.

→ Maintenence therapy for one year is often used for both duodenal and gastric ulcers, although data on preventing recurrence of the latter is much less extensive than data for the former (Feldman et al. 1992).

→ Teach patient regarding American Cancer Society's recommendation for early detection of cancer in asymptomatic people (American Cancer Society 1993):
  - sigmoidoscopy: every three years beginning at age 50 years.
  - stool guaiac: yearly beginning at age 50 years.
  - digital rectal examination: yearly beginning at age 40 years.
    - ACS suggests a digital rectal examination of all women during their annual gynecological visit.

→ Document in progress notes and problem list.

7-Q

Bibliography

Agrawal, N. 1991. Risk factors for gastrointestinal ulcers caused by nonsteroidal anti-inflammatory drugs (NSAIDs). *The Journal of Family Practice* 32(6):619–624.

Alper, S.L., and Lodish, H.F. 1991. Disorders of the kidney and urinary tract. In *Principles of Internal Medicine* 12th ed., eds. J.D. Wilson, E. Braunwald, K. Isselbacher, R.G. Petersdorf, J.B. Martin, A.S. Fauci, and R.K. Root, pp. 696–713. New York: McGraw-Hill.

American Cancer Society. 1993. *Summary of American Cancer Society recommendations for the early detection of cancer in asymptomatic people.* Professional Education Publications. Philadelphia: J. B. Lippincott.

———. 1994. *Cancer facts and figures, 1994.* Atlanta: the Author.

Bassford, T. 1992. Treatment of common anorectal disorders. *American Family Physician* 45(4):1787–1794.

Beal, J.M. 1983. How to diagnose the acute abdomen. *Contemporary OB/GYN* 21 (Special Issue):13–30.

Bennett, J.R. 1991. Heartburn and gastro-oesophageal reflux. *British Journal of Clinical Practice* 45(4):273–277.

Brown, C., and Rees, W.D. 1990. Dyspepsia in general practice. *British Medical Journal* 300:829–830.

Burkhart, C. 1992. Guidelines for rapid assessment of abdominal pain indicative of acute surgical abdomen. *Nurse Practitioner* 17(6):39–49.

Cocchiara, J.L. 1991. Hemorrhoids. *Postgraduate Medicine* 89(1):149–152.

Cooke, D.M. 1991. Inflammatory bowel disease: Primary health care management of ulcerative colitis and Crohn's disease. *Nurse Practitioner* 16(8):27–39.

Debas, H.T., and Mulholland, M.W. 1989. *Drug therapy in peptic ulcer disease.* Chicago: Year Book Medical Publishers.

De Dombal, F.T. 1991. *Diagnosis of acute abdominal pain.* London: Churchill Livingstone.

Dennison, A.R., Whiston, R.J., Rooney, S., and Morris, D.L. 1989. The management of hemorrhoids. *The American Journal of Gastroenterology* 84(5):475–481.

Drossman, D.A. 1989. Irritable bowel syndrome. *American Family Physician* 39(6):159–164.

Ertan A. 1990. Colonic diverticulitis. *Postgraduate Medicine* 88(3):67–77.

Feldman, M., Maton, P.N., McCallum, R.W., and McCarthy, D.M. 1992. Treating ulcers and reflux: What's new? *Patient Care* 26(13):53–72.

Freston, J.W. 1990. Overview of medical therapy of peptic ulcer disease. In *Gastroenterology Clinics of North America,* ed., R.H. Hunt. 19(1):121–140.

Gallegos, N.C., and Hobsley, M. 1990. Abdominal wall pain: An alternative diagnosis. *British Journal of Surgery* 77:1167–1170.

Goldfinger, S.E. 1991. Constipation and diarrhea. In *Principles of internal medicine,* 12th ed., eds. J.D. Wilson, E. Braunwald, K. Isselbacher, R.G. Petersdorf, J.B. Martin, A.S. Fauci, and R.K. Root, pp. 256–259. New York: McGraw-Hill.

Goroll, A.H. 1995a. Approach to the patient with anorectal complaints. In *Primary care medicine,* eds. A.H. Goroll, L.A. May, and A.G. Mulley, pp. 372–379. Philadelphia: J.B. Lippincott.

————. 1995b. Management of asymptomatic and symptomatic gallstones. In *Primary care medicine*, eds. A.H. Goroll, L.A. May, and A.G. Mulley, pp. 394–398. Philadelphia: J.B. Lippincott.

————. 1995c. Management of cirrhosis and chronic liver failure. In *Primary care medicine*, eds., A.H. Goroll, L.A. May, and A.G. Gulley, pp. 407–412. Philadelphia: J.B. Lippincott.

————. 1995d. Approach to the patient with constipation. In *Primary care medicine*, eds. A.H. Goroll, L.A. May, and A.G. Mulley, pp. 369–372. Philadelphia: J.B. Lippincott.

————. 1995e. Management of diverticular disease. In *Primary care medicine*, eds. A.H. Goroll, L.A. May, and A.G. Mulley, pp. 434–436. Philadelphia: J.B. Lippincott.

————. 1995f. Approach to the patient with functional gastrointestinal disease. In *Primary care medicine*, eds. A.H. Goroll, L.A. May, and A.G. Mulley, pp. 425–434. Philadelphia: J.B. Lippincott.

————. 1995g. Management of peptic ulcer disease. In *Primary care medicine*, eds. A.H. Goroll, L.A. May, and A.G. Mulley, pp. 382–393. Philadelphia: J.B. Lippincott.

Heading, R.C. 1991. Definitions of dyspepsia. *Scandinavian Journal of Gastroenterology* 182:1–6.

Hickey, M.S., Kiernan, G.J., and Weaver, K.E. 1989. Evaluation of abdominal pain. *Emergency Medicine Clinics of North America* 7(3):437–452.

Hoffmann, J., and Rasmussen, O.O. 1989. Aids in the diagnosis of acute appendicitis. *British Journal of Surgery* 76:774–779.

Jenner, C. 1991. Inflammatory bowel disease. *The Practitioner* 235:256–261.

Johnson, P.C., and Ericsson, C.D. 1990. Acute diarrhea in developed countries. *The American Journal of Medicine* 88(suppl. 6A):6A-5S-6A-9S.

Kirsner, J.B. 1991. Inflammatory bowel disease: Part II: Clinical and therapeutic aspects. *Disease-a-Month* 37(10):679–746.

Knauer, C.M. 1993a. Alimentary tract. In *Current medical diagnosis and treatment*, eds. L.M. Tierney, S.J. McPhee, M.A. Papadakis, and S.A. Schroeder, pp. 451–502. Norwalk, CT: Appleton & Lange.

————. 1993b. Liver, biliary tract and pancreas. In *Current medical diagnosis and treatment*, eds. L.M. Tierney, S.J. McPhee, M.A. Papadakis, & S.A. Schroeder, pp. 503–537. Norwalk, CT: Appleton & Lange.

Lieberman, D. 1991. Diagnosis and treatment of gastroesophageal reflux disease. *Comprehensive Therapy* 17(4):43–50.

Linn, F.V., and Peppercorn, M.A. 1992. Drug therapy for inflammatory bowel disease: Part I. *The American Journal of Surgery* 164:85–89.

Malagelada, J.R. 1991. When and how to investigate dyspeptic patient. *Scandinavian Journal of Gastroenterology* 182:71–73.

Margolies, M.N. 1995. Approach to the patient with an external hernia. In *Primary care medicine*, eds. A.H. Goroll, L.A. May, and A.G. Mulley, pp. 379–381. Philadelphia: J.B. Lippincott.

Marks, R.D., and Richter, J.E. 1991. Gastroesophageal reflux disease. In *Peptic ulcer disease and other acid-related disorders*, eds. D. Zakim and A.J. Dannenberg, pp. 247–314. New York: Academic Research Associates.

McGuigan, J.E. 1991. Peptic ulcer and gastritis. In *Principles of internal medicine*, 12th ed., eds. J.D. Wilson, E. Braunwald, K. Isselbacher, R.G. Petersdorf, J.B. Martin, A.S. Fauci, and R.K. Root, pp. 1229–1247. New York: McGraw-Hill.

Nyren, O. 1991. Therapeutic trial in dyspepsia: Its role in the primary care setting. *Scandinavian Journal of Gastroenterology* 182:61–69.

O'Toole, M. 1990. Advanced assessment of the abdomen and gastrointestinal problems. *Nursing Clinics of North America* 25(4):771–776.

Podolsky, D.K. 1991. Inflammatory bowel disease. *The New England Journal of Medicine* 325(14):1108–1016.

Podolsky, D.K., and Isselbacher, K.J. 1991. Cirrhosis of the liver. In *Principles of internal medicine* 12th ed., eds. J.D. Wilson, E. Braunmald, K. Isselbacher, R.G. Petersdorf, J.B. Martin, A.S. Fauci, and R.K. Root, pp. 1340–1350. New York: McGraw-Hill.

Purcell, T.B. 1989. Nonsurgical and extraperitoneal causes of abdominal pain. *Emergency Medicine Clinics of North America* 7(3):721–740.

Rege, R.V., and Nahrwold, D.L. 1989. Diverticular disease. *Current Problems in Surgery* 26(3):139–189.

Richter, J.M. 1991. Dyspepsia: Organic causes and differential characteristics from functional dyspepsia. *Scandinavian Journal of Gastroenterology* 182:11–15.

————. 1995a. Evaluation of abdominal pain. In *Primary care medicine*, eds. A.H. Goroll, L.A. May, and A. G. Mulley, pp. 325–334. Philadelphia: J.B. Lippincott.

————. 1995b. Evaluation and management of diarrhea. In *Primary care medicine*, eds. A.H. Goroll, L.A. May, and A.G. Mulley, pp. 357–368. Philadelphia: J.B. Lippincott.

————. 1995c. Approach to the patient with heartburn and reflux. In *Primary care medicine*, eds. A.H. Goroll, L.A. May, and A.G. Mulley, pp. 344–348. Philadelphia: J.B. Lippincott.

Ruymann, F.W., and Richter, J.M. 1995. Management of inflammatory bowel disease. In *Primary care medicine*, eds. A.H. Goroll, L.A. May, and A.G. Mulley, pp. 416–425. Philadelphia: J.B. Lippincott.

Sammons, L.N. 1990. Constipation. In *Ambulatory obstetrics: Protocols for nurse practitioners/nurse midwives*, 2nd ed., eds. W.L. Star, M.T. Shannon, L.N. Sammons, L.L. Lommel, and Y. Gutierrez, pp. 53–55. San Francisco: University of California, San Francisco School of Nursing.

Schuster, M.M., and Whitehead, W.E. 1986. Physiologic insights into irritable bowel syndrome. *Clinics in Gastroenterology* 15(4):839–853.

Smith, L.E. 1990. Anal fissures. *Netherlands Journal of Medicine* 37:S33–S36.

Talley, N.J., and Phillips, S.F. 1988. Non-ulcer dyspepsia: Potential causes and pathophysiology. *Annals of Internal Medicine* 108(6):865–879.

Tytgat, G.N.J., Noache, L.A., and Rauws, A.J. 1991. Is gastroduodenitis a cause of chronic dyspepsia? *Scandinavian Journal of Gastroenterology* 182:33–39.

Tytgat, G.N.J., and Rauws, E.A.J. 1990. *Campylobacter pylori* and its role in peptic ulcer disease. *Gastroenterology Clinics of North America* 19(1):183–196.

Wadle, K.R. 1990. Diarrhea. *Nursing Clinics of North America* 25(4):901–908.

Weinstein, D.F., and Richter, J.M. 1995 Evaluation of gastrointestinal bleeding. In *Primary care medicine*, eds. A.H. Goroll, L.A. May, and A.G. Mulley, pp. 352–357. Philadelphia: J.B. Lippincott.

Zell, S.C., and Budhraja, M. 1989. An approach to dyspepsia in the ambulatory care setting: Evaluation based on risk stratification. *Journal of General Internal Medicine* 4:144–150.

SECTION 8

Musculoskeletal Disorders

Diane C. Putney, R.N., C., M.N., N.P.

8-A

Common Disorders of the Musculoskeletal System— Introduction

Orthopedic problems account for an estimated 10 percent of all visits to primary care providers (Fields et al. 1992). Often, however, because of either patient demand or limited diagnostic sagacity on the part of the clinician, the patient receives perfunctory consideration of her complaint, followed by a prompt referral to the orthopedic surgeon.

The tendency to consider musculoskeletal disorders to be within the exclusive purview of the orthopedist is unfortunate and can often result in unnecessary delays in treatment, as well as an increased financial burden for the patient. Most musculoskeletal problems do not require surgical intervention, and conservative treatment usually can be successfully initiated and managed by the primary care provider.

In orthopedic practice, the focus is specifically on joint pathology, or the portion of the extremity manipulated by that joint. One author has proposed that a joint be defined as an organ, the function of which is to allow motion with low friction under high load (Radin et al. 1991).

Typical musculoskeletal problems with which women present to the primary care provider include one or more of the following clinical entities: osteoarthritis/ degenerative joint disease, rheumatoid arthritis, tendini-tis, bursitis, intra-articular cartilage problems, nerve compression, and overuse syndromes. The more common clinical presentations of orthopedic problems affecting the major joints is the primary focus of this protocol.

The author assumes that the majority of primary care/subspecialty care providers using this text have not received specific training in the administration of cortisone injections, which are frequently administered for musculoskeletal disorders. Instruction on methods of soft tissue and tendon injections is beyond the scope of this protocol. Therefore, the recommendation to refer a patient who requires such treatment is made in the appropriate protocols, as indicated.

Orthopedic evaluation of joint pathology requires a basic but precise knowledge and understanding of musculoskeletal anatomy and function. Palpable bony prominences often serve as landmarks for the underlying involved bursa, tendons, and ligaments, the locations of which are crucial when administering treatment such as cortisone injections. A brief anatomical description of the joints or extremities under specific consideration will precede each related clinical presentation.

Diane C. Putney, R.N., C., M.N., N.P.

8-B
Osteoarthritis

Osteoarthritis (OA) is the most common musculoskeletal disease in people over age 50 years. It may affect approximately one-third of all adults and 90 percent of individuals over age 65 years (Beary III, Christian, and Johanson 1988). When all age groups are considered, men and women are affected equally. Osteoarthritis is one of the most frequent causes of disability in the elderly and affects approximately 12.1 percent of adults between ages 25 years and 74 years (Liang and Fortin 1991; McAlindon and Dieppe 1990).

Osteoarthritis is classified into both primary and secondary entities, each involving at least one and usually two general pathological processes: degeneration of intra-articular cartilage as evidenced by joint space narrowing, and the formation of new bone at the base of the cartilage and in the joint margins, the latter being commonly referred to as *osteophytes* or *spurs*.

The precise physiology of OA is not known; however, the combined factors of aging, wear and tear, genetics, and biomechanics appear to converge in varying degrees to foster its development. Secondary OA results from damage to joint spaces by mechanical trauma or various physiological processes, including inflammation and neuropathic diseases such as diabetes, endocrinopathies, and metabolic disorders. Unlike *rheumatoid arthritis* (RA), OA tends to become symptomatic in fewer joints and is generally not as disabling (Altman 1990). The goals of treatment for all arthritic conditions are to decrease pain and maintain function.

DATABASE

SUBJECTIVE

→ This condition commonly occurs in patients:
  - over 40 years of age.
  - with a history of previous trauma to affected joint.
  - with a history of obesity.

→ Symptoms include:
  - pain and swelling in affected joint, aggravated by weight-bearing activity and going up and down stairs.
  - pain at rest.
  - decreased range of motion (ROM) and buckling of the knee in the affected joint as the disease advances.

→ Most commonly affected sites include the:
  - distal interphangeal (DIP) and first carpal metacarpal (CMC) joints of the hand.
  - first metatarsolphalangeal (MTP) joint of the foot.
  - wrist.
  - acromioclavicular joint.
  - hip.
  - lumbar and cervical spine.
  - knee, which is the most frequently involved joint of all (Altman 1990).

OBJECTIVE

→ Patient may present with:
- swelling of the affected joint.
- decreased ROM.
- painful ROM.
- joint line tenderness.
- crepitus.
- joint deformity.
- joint subluxation.
- muscle atrophy in the involved extremity.

ASSESSMENT

→ Osteoarthritis

→ R/O rheumatoid arthritis

→ R/O systemic lupus erythematosus (SLE)

→ R/O intra-articular cartilage tear

→ R/O gout

→ R/O tendinitis

→ R/O bursitis

→ R/O nerve compression syndrome

→ R/O chondrocalcinosis

→ R/O osteonecrosis

PLAN

DIAGNOSTIC TESTS

→ X-rays of affected joint (see sections on individual joint problems for specific views). Findings characteristic of the osteoarthritic joint may involve variations of the following: joint space narrowing, osteophytes, subchondral sclerosis, subchondral cysts, and subluxation (Quinet 1986).

→ Bone scan, computerized tomographic (CT) scan, magnetic resonance imaging (MRI) per physician consultation.

→ Laboratory studies: erythrocyte sedimentation rate (ESR), uric acid, rheumatoid factor (RF), anti-nuclear antibody (ANA), complete blood count (CBC), HLA-B27 as indicated.

→ Synovial fluid analysis for glucose, cell count and differential, culture and sensitivity, crystals, and cytology as indicated.

TREATMENT/MANAGEMENT

→ Initial treatment consists of maintenance nonsteroidal anti-inflammatory drugs (NSAIDs) for 4 to 6 weeks.

- The response to NSAIDs is idiopathic; if the patient has unpleasant side effects from one NSAID, or fails to experience amelioration of symptoms within 2 weeks, a different NSAID should be prescribed.
- NSAIDs must be prescribed with caution for patients with a history of peptic ulcer disease, gastrointestinal bleeding, and/or idiopathic sensitivity reactions; diabetics who may have renal insufficiency, and asthmatics in whom the use of NSAIDs has been observed to induce bronchospasm (see **Table 8-M, Anti-Inflammatory Agents,** p. 8-50).

→ Aspirin or enteric-coated aspirin is also an effective anti-inflammatory medication but it requires more frequent dosing and generally is no longer the treatment of choice.

→ The judicious use of mild analgesics such as propoxyphene and acetaminophen (Darvocet-N-100®) and hydrocodone (Vicodin®) may be helpful when symptoms are acute, and these drugs are used in conjunction with NSAIDs. But such use is discouraged in all forms of chronic musculoskeletal disorders.

→ Physical therapy to increase muscle strength and ROM is recommended.

→ Periodic steroid injections into joints and surrounding bursa may be helpful.
- General rule of thumb is not to exceed 3 per year or one every 4 months.

→ Application of ice 3 to 4 times a day for 20 to 30 minutes, unless the patient is diabetic or has peripheral vascular disease, may be helpful.

→ Bracing and splinting as indicated to provide rest, prevent deformity, and relieve spasm.

→ Prosthesis as indicated.

→ Cane, walker, or crutches as indicated.

→ Any weight loss may require dietary counseling.

CONSULTATION

→ Orthopedic consultation, if conservative measures of treatment have failed, for consideration of the following:
- joint replacement.
- osteotomy.
- arthroscopic debridement and/or lavage of joints.
- joint fusion.
- arthroplasty.

→ Physician consultation if conservative management of arthritic condition may interfere or compromise treatment of the patient's other medical problems—e.g., diabetics with nephropathies.

→ As needed for prescription(s).

PATIENT EDUCATION

→ Educate the patient regarding facets of osteoarthritis.

→ Weight loss and dietary counseling may be indicated. Refer the patient to the appropriate services and/or a nutritionist. See **General Nutrition Guidelines**.

→ Encourage a regular exercise regimen to increase muscle strength in extremities of involved joints.
  ▪ Encourage non-weight-bearing forms of exercise—e.g., swimming, bicycling, stretching, and weight-resistance training.

→ Icing is advisable for 15 to 20 minutes before and after engaging in potentially aggravating activities.

→ Educate patient regarding the appropriate use of canes, crutches, walkers, orthotics, braces, and splints.

→ Proper dosage, indications, actions, and potential side effects of NSAIDs should be understood by the patient.

→ Advise patient to avoid lifting heavy objects.

→ Patient should work in a sitting rather than standing position when possible.

FOLLOW-UP

→ The patient should return for a follow-up visit four to six weeks after conservative treatment is initiated.

→ Serum creatinine, blood urea nitrogen (BUN), and liver function studies should be monitored routinely—in consultation with the patient's internist—when the patient is maintained indefinitely on NSAIDs.

→ The patient is encouraged to seek medical follow-up when she fails to experience adequate sustained relief of symptoms.

→ Document in progress notes and problem list.

Diane C. Putney, R.N., C., M.N., N.P.

8-C

Rheumatoid Arthritis

Rheumatoid arthritis (RA) is an inflammatory systemic musculoskeletal disease which affects three times as many women as men, and approximately two percent of the United States population as a whole (Smith and Arnett 1990). Rheumatoid arthritis can occur at any age, although people in the third through sixth decade of life are those most often affected.

The exact etiology of RA is not well understood. However, the onset is usually insidious and the characteristic inflammatory changes in the synovia—that eventually result in body, cartilage, and tendon erosions—and nerve compression syndromes occur over a period of several months (Barker, Burton, and Zieve 1982; Bucholz et al. 1984).

The diagnosis of RA is formulated on the basis of seven criteria, four of which must be met:

→ at least one hour of morning stiffness involving the joints.

→ simultaneous swelling of three or more target joints that may include wrists, elbows, knees, ankles, MTP, proximal interphalangeal (PIP), and metacarpophalangeal (MCP) joints.

→ swelling in at least one wrist, MCP, or PIP.

→ symmetric swelling simultaneously at right and left target joints.

→ subcutaneous rheumatoid nodules.

→ positive RF.

→ radiographs that demonstrate joint erosions or unequivocal bony decalcifications (Persselin 1991).

People with RA also can present with a myriad of constitutional systems such as fever, myalgia and ex-

treme fatigue, which can even lead to a compromised cardiorespiratory status (Semble, Loeser, and Wise 1990). The resultant decreased physical endurance sets the stage for the significant muscle atrophy, limited ROM, and poor posture so characteristic of the rheumatoid patient. Both genetic and immunological factors are thought to contribute to the pathogenesis of RA.

Treatment of the person with RA demands a multidisciplinary approach for which medical management is the mainstay (Bucholz et al. 1984). Although the overall medical management of patients with RA is best conducted by a rheumatologist or the primary care giver, these individuals sometimes require orthopedic consultation with reference to specific joint pathology. Therefore, RA must often be considered in the differential diagnosis of musculoskeletal problems in women.

DATABASE

SUBJECTIVE

→ Patient most likely between 30 years to 60 years of age.

→ Symptoms may include:
  ▪ three or more months of persistent nontraumatic joint pain and swelling, most often involving the hands and feet.
  ▪ extreme fatigue, weight loss, depression, fever, and general malaise.

OBJECTIVE

→ Positive RF is present in 80 percent of people with RA; considered significant if titer is ≥1:160.

→ Patient may present with:

- elevated ESR indicating degree of inflammation.
- swelling of individual joints—e.g., wrists, hands, knees, and feet.
- ulnar deviation of the fingers.
- thickening and triggering of flexor tendons in the fingers.
→ Rheumatoid nodules are present in 20 percent of patients.

ASSESSMENT

→ Rheumatoid arthritis
→ R/O SLE
→ R/O OA
→ R/O seronegative spondylarthropathies
→ R/O gout
→ R/O polymyalgia rheumatica
→ R/O lyme disease
→ R/O infection

PLAN

DIAGNOSTIC TESTS

→ See **Osteoarthritis** Protocol.

TREATMENT/MANAGEMENT

→ Proposed treatment for RA in this protocol will be limited to that which could be generally implemented and managed by the primary provider. See **Osteoarthritis** Protocol. Omit instructions to apply ice to affected joints.

CONSULTATION

→ Rheumatologist.
- Especially with chronic, multi-joint involvement when patient experiences inadequate or poorly sustained relief from NSAIDs and injections.
→ Orthopedist.
- When the patient fails all means of conservative treatment and demonstrates intolerable pain or significant loss of function in a joint or extremity.
→ Internist.
- Regular consultation with the patient's internist or primary care provider regarding the ongoing management of the patient's constitutional symptoms as indicated.
→ As needed for prescription(s).

PATIENT EDUCATION

→ See **Osteoarthritis** Protocol.
→ Discuss importance of adequate rest periods to decrease joint inflammation.
→ Reassure patient that aerobic exercise will not exacerbate the disease process.

FOLLOW-UP

→ There is no clinical usefulness in following an RF once a positive result has been established.
→ See **Osteoarthritis** Protocol.
→ Document in progress notes and problem list.

Diane C. Putney, R.N., C., M.N., N.P.

8-D

Bursitis and Tendinitis

Bursitis and *tendinitis* are generic terms that until recently frequently were used to refer to a variety of clinical inflammatory processes involving the musculoskeletal system.

A *bursa* is an enclosed, fluid-filled sac lined with a synovial membrane situated over a bony prominence and between various tendons, muscles, and skin (Barker, Burton, and Zieve 1982). The basic function of a bursa is to inhibit friction between bone and tendon structures, improving their gliding motion (Reilly and Nicholas 1987).

Bursitis is defined as inflammation of the bursa. It can result from overuse, direct trauma, or an underlying systemic disorder such as RA (Baum 1989; Beary III, Christian, and Johanson 1988; Taylor 1989). Although the body contains well over 160 bursae, very few actually lead to a distinct clinical entity. The forms of bursitis that remain deserving of this diagnostic label mainly include olecranon in the elbow, prepatellar and pes anserine in the knee, and trochanteric and iliopsoas in the hip.

Clinicians' tendency to use the word bursitis as a catch-all diagnostic term to characterize the likes of all musculoskeletal aches and pains has seen its day.

Tendinitis refers to either the inflammation of a tendon sheath (*tenosynovitis*) or the tendon itself. Tendinitis is thought to result from microtrauma, with the decreased vascularity of the tendon as well as repetitive motion being two of the major associated factors (Beary III, Christian, and Johanson 1988).

Perhaps because of their close proximity in the involved structure, the terms tendinitis and bursitis are frequently used interchangeably. They present with sim-

ilar signs and symptoms, and, generally, comparable treatment modalities and follow-up are indicated.

DATABASE

SUBJECTIVE

→ These conditions are more common in middle-aged and elderly people.

→ Symptoms may include:
- localized aching-type pain, usually aggravated by use; sometimes painful at night.
- swelling, particularly when the prepatellar or olecranon bursa is involved.

→ Patient may present with history of:
- SLE, gout, or RA.
- minor trauma.
  - Often as a consequence of athletic or work-related activity requiring repetitive, forceful, gross motor movements of the upper and lower extremity.

OBJECTIVE

→ The objective findings on physical examination are generally mediated by the involved joint.
- Pain with specific movements as directed by the examiner, with and without applied resistance, is perhaps the most important indicator of the involved bursa or tendon.
- There is occasional warmth, swelling, and erythema of the affected joint.
- Localized tenderness is almost always present.

- There is decreased ROM and pain at the extremes of flexion and extension of the involved extremity.
- In patients with chronic or inadequately treated conditions, muscle atrophy may be present.

ASSESSMENT

→ Tendinitis

→ Bursitis

→ R/O tendon or intra-articular cartilage tear

→ R/O degenerative joint disease

→ R/O radiculopathy

→ R/O infection

→ R/O nerve compression syndrome

→ R/O gout

PLAN

DIAGNOSTIC TESTS

→ X-rays of the symptomatic joint are the most important studies; may reveal calcifications in the involved tendon and bursae, as well as osteophytes visible on bony prominences.

→ Laboratory: if symptoms are chronic, more than one joint is involved, or infection is suspected, the following are indicated:
  - CBC.
  - ESR.
  - ANA.
  - RF.
  - uric acid.

→ If gout or a septic joint is being considered, joint aspiration is advised for crystals, glucose, gram stain, and culture and sensitivity.

→ Electromyograms (EMGs) and nerve conduction studies if a nerve entrapment is suspected.

→ MRI, bone scans, CT scans, and arthrograms may be necessary.

TREATMENT

→ A 4- to 6-week course of NSAIDs would be appropriate for conditions that:
  - do not involve significant loss of joint motion.
  - have endured for less than 3 weeks. and
  - have not appreciably interfered with the person's activities of daily living or livelihood (see **Table 8-M**, p. 8-50).

→ Injection of corticosteroids in conjunction with local anesthetic usually affords considerable and dramatic relief from symptoms.
  - A person's response to corticosteroids is highly individualized, however, and sometimes it can take the better part of 2 weeks for discomfort in the affected extremity to resolve.

→ Physical therapy is generally indicated if there is loss of ROM and muscle weakness.

→ Temporary immobilization of the affected joint with braces, splints, slings, casts, and crutches as indicated.

→ Phonophoresis, a technique that uses ultrasound to administer cortisone transdermally, is sometimes effective (Hunter and Poole 1987).

→ Regular applications of ice—usually 4 times a day for 15 minutes, especially before and after engaging in aggravating activity—are very important in reducing inflammation and pain, unless the patient has a compromised peripheral vascular system or an underlying rheumatological disorder.

CONSULTATION

→ Referral to an orthopedist for surgical consultation is indicated when the patient has had no significant or sustained relief from conservative treatment. It may also be necessary to refer the patient who requires a cortisone injection for relief of symptoms.

→ Consultation from a neurologist or physiatrist may be important when nerve entrapment or compression syndromes are being considered.

→ The patient should be referred to a rheumatologist when the condition is chronic, involves multiple joints, and an underlying rheumatological condition has been established or is suspected.

→ The younger, competitive athlete may benefit from consultation with a sports medicine clinician when training techniques appear to be the cause of chronic musculoskeletal problems.

→ As needed for prescription(s).

PATIENT EDUCATION

→ Educate the patient regarding bursitis or tendinitis.

→ Education regarding the proper use of NSAIDs is essential in maintaining the patient's compliance.
  - The fact that NSAIDs are anti-inflammatory agents and not narcotic "pain pills" requires

emphasis as patients often express concern about becoming dependent on medication.

- This is especially important in light of the fact that four- to six-week courses of treatment with NSAIDs are the usual recommendation for musculoskeletal disorders, and non-compliance with treatment can be high.

→ Activity modification is essential and is determined by the joint involved, aggravating factors, and the patient's response to treatment.

→ Emphasize importance of complying with prescribed physical therapy or rehabilitation programs.

→ Discuss proper use of orthopedic appliances.

→ The patient for whom a cortisone injection is proposed must be instructed on the indications, actions, and potential side effects of cortisone.

- Steroid abuse in the athletic community, and indiscriminate use of steroids in some medical practices, has created a tremendous amount of apprehension and often results in the unnecessary, unfortunate prolongation of the patient's symptoms.

- The judicial use of standard doses of cortisone administered with local anesthetics such as lidocaine and marcaine is sometimes the first treatment of choice, and can often produce a prompt and dramatic resolution of the patient's symptoms.

FOLLOW-UP

→ Follow-up with the primary care provider would be appropriate at three to four weeks after a cortisone injection, and four to six weeks after a course of anti-inflammatory medication or physical or occupational therapy.

→ Orthopedic appliances may require modification, adjustment, or discontinuation.

→ The patient is encouraged to seek medical follow-up when conservative treatment has failed to adequately relieve symptoms, or the condition worsens.

→ Document in progress notes and problem list.

Diane C. Putney, R.N., C., M.N., N.P.

8-E

Shoulder Pain

The *shoulder*, the point of attachment between the upper extremity and the axial skeleton, is composed of the sternoclavicular, glenohumeral (GH), and the much smaller acromioclavicular (AC) joint (Lewis 1988). The shoulder joint is supported by a strong fibrous capsule. The portion that attaches to the scapula is the glenoid labrum. The thick, fibrous hood formed by the four tendons known collectively as the rotator cuff overlies the joint capsule. Their main function is to stabilize the glenohumeral joint (Nirschl 1989). The subacromial or subdeltoid bursa lies between the deltoid muscle and the rotator cuff tendons (Farin et al. 1990).

The shoulder is capable of wide ROM, and is relatively unstable as a result. The inherent instability of the shoulder complex predisposes this joint to frequent irritation and injury (Burns and Turba 1992). Thus, shoulder pain is one of the more common patient complaints.

Shoulder problems are classified in the literature as either extrinsic, in which pain originating in another location is referred to the shoulder, or intrinsic, in which the pain is related to the shoulder complex (Fu, Harner, and Klein 1991). Intrinsic shoulder lesions, which are the predominant focus of this section, become painful with both active and passive shoulder motion and primarily involve the rotator cuff. Rotator cuff problems may account for about 70 percent of shoulder pathology (Chard et al. 1991).

The most frequent type of rotator cuff problem encountered by the primary care provider is known as *impingement syndrome*. This term defines a number of shoulder problems, almost all of which involve the impingement of the supraspinatus tendon on the coricoacromial arch and subsequent inflammation (Craig and

Kuang-Chi 1992). The normal aging process, repetitive microtrauma, and acute trauma each contribute in varying degrees to the development of this condition (Brier 1992).

The pathophysiology of impingement syndrome is generally a progressive phenomenon that begins with edema and hemorrhaging within the rotator cuff, followed by fibrosis and tendinitis. Finally, if refractory to treatment or left unchecked, tendon degeneration results in a tendon tear (Hooke 1991; Zuckerman et al. 1991).

DATABASE

→ The main focus of history-taking and physical exam of the individual with shoulder pain is to:
  ■ recognize referred pain.
  ■ assess the integrity of the rotator cuff tendons and joint capsule.
  ■ identify point tenderness.
  ■ delineate malalignment or dysfunctional AC and GH joints (Smith and Campbell 1992).

SUBJECTIVE

→ Patient may present with history of occupations that require repetitive overhead motions and heavy lifting.

→ Patient usually athletic individual in her 20s or 30s whose sports involve repetitive overhead motions (e.g., swimmers, volleyball players).

→ Symptoms may include:
  ■ pain with overhead motions, often the predominant complaint.
  ■ pain when reaching behind one's back.

- pain occurring at night. Pain mostly occurring at night is suggestive of a rotator cuff tear or labral lesion.
- painful, limited ROM.
- pain usually located in the anterior portion of the shoulder, often radiating to the deltoid insertion.
- pain that is initially aggravated by activity, but becomes more constant with disease progression.
- sudden neck pain, referred to the scapular region, shoulder, and arm with associated numbness and weakness indicating cervical radiculopathy.
- weakness of the upper extremity, possibly the consequence of a progressive condition of impingement, but a rotator cuff tear should always be suspected.

→ Patient may present with:
- history of acute trauma—e.g., fall on an outstretched arm or a forcible pulling of the upper extremity into forward flexion; should heighten the clinician's suspicion of a possible rotator cuff tear.
- insidious onset of symptoms without history of related trauma, history of diabetes, recent cardiac surgery or immobilization of the affected extremity, in which ROM is severely restricted, suggesting adhesive capsulitis (Rizk, Pinals, and Talaiver 1991). Middle-aged women are most often affected.

→ Usual course of symptoms is one to two years.
→ Labral lesion should be considered, especially in young, athletic patients who give a history of forceful external rotation and abduction of the arm, often resulting in a tear of the glenoid labrum.
- Patient may complain of numbness and tingling in the shoulder that radiates distally.

→ Sometimes the patient will characterize symptoms as shoulder pain, while pointing more specifically to either side of the neck, or the trapezius area.

OBJECTIVE

→ Full neck examination should always precede the shoulder examination to ensure that any pain reproduced with neck ROM does not constitute the patient's chief complaint of shoulder pain (and which would indicate cervical disk disease).

→ Positive impingement signs become evident when pain is produced with:

- passive abduction of the affected arm to 90° with external rotation.
- passive elevation of the patient's arm to maximum forward flexion.

→ Positive impingement test.
- The subacromial bursa is infiltrated with 10 ml of lidocaine 2 percent using a 23-gauge, 1½-inch needle.
- The test is positive if, when the patient's ROM is retested, the majority of pain is alleviated.
- Unless the practitioner is trained in the administration of injections commonly used in the treatment of musculoskeletal disorders, the patient may require referral to an orthopedic clinic.

→ Limited ROM in forward flexion, abduction, and internal rotation.

→ Positive Spurling's sign.
- The patient complains of severe neck pain radiating into the arm with paresthesia and reflex changes, and indicates cervical radiculopathy.

→ Pain elicited with resisted forward flexion with arms tested in both pronation (supraspinatus tendon) and supination (biceps tendon).

→ Tenderness elicited by palpating the anterior acromion process, the greater tuberosity on the humeral head, and the supraspinatus tendon insertion.

→ Subacromial crepitus may be palpated by placing the examiner's hand over the affected shoulder and gently internally and externally rotating the extremity through internal and external rotation with the shoulder at 90° of abduction.

→ Patient may have a positive "drop sign," the patient's arm is actively or passively elevated to 180°.
- If, when lowering the arm to 90° of abduction, the patient experiences sudden weakness and pain with a concurrent drop of the arm by 40°, the test is considered positive, and a rotator cuff tear highly suspected.

→ An isolated bicipital tendinitis is rare:
- but can be confirmed with point tenderness over the long head of the biceps tendon in the bicipital groove; anterior shoulder pain with resisted forward flexion of the fully extended and supinated arm; impingement tests are negative (Post and Benca 1989).

→ Calcific tendinitis should be suspected if:

- shoulder pain is of sudden onset and severe.
- occasional distinct swelling over the humeral head is present.
- pain occurs with all resisted shoulder movements.
- diagnosis is confirmed on x-ray.

→ Adhesive capsulitis must be considered if:
- glenohumeral range of motion is severely restricted, both passively and actively, below 70°.
- poorly localized tenderness is present.

→ "Clicking" or "clunking" sensation with external rotation and abduction of the arm can usually be reproduced with examination and will reveal one or more positive posterior, anterior, and inferior drawer signs—suggests labral lesion.

→ AC joint synovitis must be considered as the origin of shoulder pain if:
- firm palpation directly over the AC joint produces severe pain.
- the patient's pain can be reproduced by fully adducting the arm across the chest.

→ Supraspinatus muscle atrophy may be present.

ASSESSMENT

→ Impingement syndrome of the rotator cuff

→ R/O rotator cuff tear

→ R/O bicipital tendinitis

→ R/O calcific tendinitis

→ R/O adhesive capsulitis

→ R/O shoulder instability

→ R/O AC joint synovitis

→ R/O degenerative joint disease of the glenohumeral joint (can be determined by radiographs)

→ R/O degenerative disk disease of the cervical spine

→ R/O cervical radiculopathy

→ R/O Paget's disease (can be suggested by radiographs)

PLAN

DIAGNOSTIC TESTS

→ Radiographs.
- The standard shoulder x-ray series should generally include three views: anterior-posterior scapula, axillary, and y-views.

- Additional "special" views may at times be indicated when considering the various etiologies of shoulder pain.

→ MRI of the affected shoulder is rapidly becoming the standard presurgical test for the confirmation of rotator cuff tears, labral lesions, and chronic impingement syndrome of the rotator cuff.
- MRI also is used to document the existence of cervical disk disease.

→ Arthrograms confirm the diagnosis of complete tears of the rotator cuff.
- Many orthopedic surgeons still consider this test the most reliable confirmation of a complete rotator cuff tear.

→ CT scans with double-contrast medium are still used to evaluate certain types of shoulder lesions, particularly those involving the labrum.

→ EMGs can be helpful in differentiating a neurological problem from the parasthesias sometimes associated with shoulder instability.

TREATMENT/MANAGEMENT

→ NSAIDs. A 4- to 6-week course of maintenance treatment is the general rule (see **Table 8-M,** p. 8-50).

→ Physical therapy is almost always indicated and generally consists of rotator cuff strengthening exercises and stretching routines. In the case of adhesive capsulitis, long-term and aggressive physical therapy is the mainstay of treatment.

→ The importance of daily application of ice packs, either 4 times a day for 15 to 20 minutes or 3 times a day for 30 minutes, cannot be over-emphasized.
- This is especially true for individuals who cannot tolerate NSAIDs or are otherwise experiencing modest or no relief from any medication.

→ The patient is discouraged from engaging in activities that require overhead lifting and repetitive external rotation and abduction of the arm until her discomfort resolves.

→ Occasionally, immobilizing the shoulder in a sling for not more than 2 weeks may be indicated, and usually only if there is a history of acute strain or trauma.
- This measure should not be implemented without orthopedic consultation.

CONSULTATION

→ Consultation from an orthopedist should be solicited in the following instances:
  ▪ complete or partial rotator cuff tear is suspected on examination or confirmed with an MRI or arthrogram.
  ▪ the patient presents with a history of long-standing symptoms—i.e., ≥6 months—and is losing full ROM in the affected extremity.
  ▪ the patient fails to respond adequately to a six-week course of NSAIDs and may require a steroid injection.
  ▪ the use of NSAIDs are contraindicated, and the patient would best benefit from a cortisone injection.

→ If an orthopedic referral is indicated, a prior consultation regarding the ordering of additional diagnostic studies will make for a more complete and expeditious evaluation of the patient's problem.

→ Immediate orthopedic consultation must be sought if plain shoulder radiographs indicate tumors or acute fractures and dislocations.

→ Referral to a neurologist or neurosurgeon is indicated:
  ▪ if the patient's clinical presentation is more consistent with a cervical spine lesion.

→ Referral to a rheumatologist is indicated if:
  ▪ the patient's shoulder problem exists as one of many sites of chronic musculoskeletal pain.
  ▪ the problem is poorly controlled with conservative treatment and.
  ▪ an underlying rheumatological condition is suspected.

→ As needed for prescription(s).

PATIENT EDUCATION

→ Explain the patient's etiology of shoulder pain to help elicit and maintain cooperation with treatment recommendations.

→ Instruct the patient on the proper dosage, administration, actions, and potential side effects of NSAIDs. See *Physicians' Desk Reference* (*PDR*).

→ When treatment with steroid injections is indicated, advise the patient that cortisone can weaken the surrounding soft-tissue structures in the shoulder for up to four weeks after administration.
  ▪ Caution the patient, therefore, to avoid strenuous and vigorous use of the affected upper extremity for this time period following injection.
    • This can include otherwise routine household chores such as vacuuming.
  ▪ Other potential side effects of steroid injection (e.g., lightening of skin pigment, rotator cuff tears, and post-injection soreness) should be explained to the patient.

→ Encourage the patient to ice the affected shoulder before and after engaging in unavoidable activities that may exacerbate symptoms.
  ▪ Unless contraindicated by a vascular or rheumatological condition.

FOLLOW-UP

→ The patient should return for re-evaluation four to six weeks after conservative therapy is initiated, unless, of course, she has been referred to the orthopedist or rheumatologist.

→ The patient should be instructed to seek clinical re-evaluation if symptoms persist beyond six months, or become progressively disabling.

→ Document in progress notes and problem list.

Diane C. Putney, R.N., C., M.N., N.P.

8-F

Elbow Pain

From the catalogue of various syndromes resulting in *elbow pain*, no other condition emerges more consistently and frequently than that of *lateral epicondylitis*, or, "tennis elbow." Although lateral epicondylitis afflicts approximately three percent of all adults, less than five percent of these individuals are actually avid tennis players (Chop 1989). Lateral epicondylitis, for the most part, is an overuse syndrome, which can be defined in general terms as tendinitis of the proximal forearm extensors at the origin of the extensor carpi radialis brevis (Leach and Miller 1987; Gellman 1992).

The annual incidence of work-related lateral epicondylitis has been estimated at 59 per 10,000, and is most frequent in the 35- to 55-year-old age group (Gellman 1992). It commonly afflicts the dominant arm of a middle-aged female (Corrigan and Maitland 1989).

Lateral epicondylitis occasionally can result from direct trauma to the elbow (Chop 1989). Present theory advances the hypothesis that repetitive gripping motions coupled with rotations of the elbow result in inflammation around the insertion of extensor carpi radialis brevis, progressing to microtears of this tendon, soft-tissue adhesions, and finally fibrosis (Chop 1989; Leach and Miller 1987; Beary III, Christian, and Johanson 1988). The result is a chronically inflamed and painful elbow, sometimes incapacitating and often resistant to the most conservative means of treatment. The majority of lateral epicondylitis cases can be treated conservatively, however, and initial treatment usually begins with the primary care provider.

Because elbow pain caused by lateral epicondylitis can be stubborn and disabling, individuals will fare better prognostically when treatment begins shortly after the initial onset of symptoms. As with most overuse syndromes involving the musculoskeletal system, treatment is focused on control of inflammation, promotion of healing, conditioning exercise, and modification of abusive force loads (Chop 1989).

DATABASE

SUBJECTIVE

→ Patient is between the ages of 30 years and 50 years.

→ Patient reports history of occupational tasks involving repetitive grabbing motions, elbow extension, and supination and pronation (Chop 1989; Corrigan and Maitland 1989).

→ Pain often is exacerbated by clutching heavy objects or even shaking hands.

→ Pain is located on the lateral side of the elbow, and frequently present at night.

→ Onset of pain is gradual and often radiates into the forearm.

→ Patient complains of weakness in the affected extremity; weakness often attributed to the limitations imposed because of severe pain.

→ Infrequently, the patient reports a history of precipitating trauma, such as bumping the elbow against a wall.

OBJECTIVE

→ Patient may present with:
  ▪ full range of flexion and extension with pain at the extreme of extension (180°).
  ▪ extreme point tenderness over the lateral epicondyle.

- occasionally, swelling over the lateral epicondyle.
- pain intensified when the examiner has the patient resist wrist extension and supination (Chop 1989).
- decreased grip strength in the affected extremity.
- loss of full extension of the elbow evident in cases which have been long standing and refractory to treatment.
- tenderness over the medial epicondyle at the site of insertion for the wrist flexors and forearm pronator suggesting medial epicondylitis (Corrigan and Maitland 1989).
- radial tunnel syndrome.
  - Compression of the posterior interosseous nerve in the proximal forearm should be considered with all resistant cases of "lateral epicondylitis."
  - Associated pain of this syndrome is located more internally and distally than in lateral epicondylitis.
→ Positive tennis elbow test—Pain over the lateral epicondyle intensifies when the examiner places his or her hand over the dorsal side of the patient's fully extended hand and instructs the patient to extend the middle finger against resistance supplied by the examiner's index finger.
→ Cervical nerve/root radiculopathy—should be suspected with complaints of medial elbow pain coupled with neck and shoulder pain (McPherson and Meals 1992).
→ Cubital tunnel syndrome (entrapment of the ulnar nerve at the elbow)—should be suspected with complaints of aching discomfort in the medial side of the elbow and the proximal forearm, in addition to complaints of shooting pains in the ring and small fingers; numbness, tingling, and a cold sensation (McPherson and Meals 1992).
→ Compression of the median nerve by the pronator teres as it crosses the elbow, or pronator syndrome—should be considered if pain is more localized to the proximal volar aspect of the forearm (Thorson and Szabo 1992).

ASSESSMENT

→ Lateral epicondylitis
→ R/O medial epicondylitis
→ R/O radial tunnel syndrome
→ R/O cervical nerve/root radiculopathy
→ R/O cubital tunnel syndrome

→ R/O pronator syndrome
→ R/O olecranon bursitis
→ R/O degenerative joint disease. This less typical condition can be determined by radiographs.

PLAN

DIAGNOSTIC TESTS

→ Radiographs: anterior/posterior, lateral and oblique views are standard.
  - X-rays are usually normal.
  - Soft-tissue calcifications may be noted over the lateral epicondyle approximately 25 percent of the time (Leach and Miller 1987).
→ ANA, RF, uric acid levels, ESR, CBC:
  - should consider ruling out underlying metabolic or rheumatological conditions in patients who have bilateral and chronic lateral epicondylitis, especially if the condition coexists with other multiple upper-extremity aches and pains.
→ Synovial fluid analysis should be obtained if septic olecranon bursitis is suspected.
→ EMGs and nerve conduction studies:
  - should be ordered when nerve compression syndromes are being considered as a cause of the patient's pain.
    - These studies will be normal in lateral epicondylitis (Leach and Miller 1987).

TREATMENT/MANAGEMENT

→ When patient seeks treatment with not more than a 3-week history of symptoms, treatment can begin by:
  - resting the affected elbow.
  - applying a force-counter-force splint, and
  - applying ice at least 4 times a day (Chop 1989; Gellman 1992; Leach and Miller 1987; Beary III, Christian, and Johanson 1988; Corrigan and Maitland 1989).
→ NSAIDs can be prescribed during any stage of the condition; a 4- to 6-week course of maintenance therapy as indicated. See **Table 8-M, p. 8-50.**
→ **When the symptoms of lateral epicondylitis are severe, incapacitating, long-standing, or resistant to the treatment methods described above, a local injection of cortisone is the recommended treatment.**
  - This may require referral to an orthopedist or other qualified clinician.

8

→ Conditioning exercises or rehabilitation are always prescribed and initiated when the acute phase of the condition has subsided.
- Exercises consist of repetitions of wrist flexion, extension, supination, and pronation performed with the wrist suspended off the edge of a table (Gellman 1992).
  - Initially the patient's other hand can be used to supply a traction force on the fingers of the affected extremity.
- The patient is then instructed to progress to 1- or 2-pound hand-held dumbbells.
- The goals of this regimen are to increase strength and flexibility of the wrist extensor tendons (Chop 1989).

→ Occasionally, the application of a short-arm fiberglass or plaster cast, which immobilizes the wrist extensors for 2 to 3 weeks, can help alleviate discomfort.
- The use of a removal sling is helpful during the acute phase of symptoms.

→ Phonophoresis requires referral to a physical therapist.

CONSULTATION

→ Referral to an orthopedist or other qualified clinician for a cortisone injection as indicated.

→ Referral to an orthopedic surgeon for further consultation if the patient:
- has been symptomatic for at least 1 year and
- has had no adequate sustained relief from conservative treatment which should have included NSAIDs, physical therapy, and a minimum of three cortisone injections.
  - The estimated number of cases eventually requiring surgery is about 10 percent (Chop 1989).

→ Referral to a physical therapist may be required for conditioning treatments, including exercises and phonopheresis.

→ Consultation with a rheumatologist may be necessary if:
- chronic lateral epicondylitis coexists with an underlying rheumatological condition, and
- no sustained adequate relief is derived from conservative treatment.

→ As needed for prescription(s).

PATIENT EDUCATION

→ Educate the patient regarding the causes of elbow pain.

→ Instruct the patient on activities to avoid: pushing, pulling, and heavy lifting (Gellman 1992).

→ Instruct the patient on proper application of a force-counter-force brace (this may vary with the actual type of brace prescribed).
- Educating the patient about the purpose and actions of the brace (i.e., the control of internally generated muscular forces, thereby decreasing the force of muscle contraction and stress on the lateral epicondyle) is an essential factor in maintaining compliance (Gellman 1992).

→ Instruct the patient to apply ice before and after engaging in potentially aggravating activities.

→ Instruct the patient to lift with the forearm supinated as opposed to pronated.

→ When the cause of the patient's condition can be attributed to involvement in racquet sports, instruct as to modification of technique and equipment used.
- This may include, for example, the selection of a racquet with a large head, as opposed to a small head, as well as one composed of materials which inhibit vibratory forces, such as graphite (Leach and Miller 1987).

FOLLOW-UP

→ A follow-up appointment should be made for four weeks after the initiation of conservative treatment.

→ When the patient's condition remains chronic and when it can be directly attributed to occupational demands, an environmental occupational consultant may be required to suggest necessary alterations in the patient's physical work environment.

→ The patient should be encouraged to seek medical re-evaluation if symptoms continue for one year or more.
- At this point, the practitioner has an obligation to refer the patient for surgical consultation.

→ Document in progress notes and problem list.

8-G

Wrist, Hand, and Finger Pain

Protocols for evaluation and treatment of *wrist, hand,* and *finger pain* in the primary care setting will be presented together because their integral relationship so often obfuscates the patient's perception of the true origin of discomfort and, therefore, the focus of the practitioner's examination. The individual with a related presenting complaint frequently uses the terms wrist, hand, or thumb interchangeably, and it is the responsibility of the practitioner to elucidate the precise location, if not always the etiology, of the patient's discomfort through careful history taking and proper examination techniques.

The clinical entities which best exemplify common and logical presentations of wrist, hand, and finger pain are *carpal tunnel syndrome* (CTS), *de Quervain's stenosing tenosynovitis, osteoarthritis of the basilar joint of the thumb,* and *stenosing flexor tenosynovitis,* or *trigger finger.*

Carpal Tunnel Syndrome

Carpal tunnel syndrome (CTS), which is often associated with a number of other medical conditions, has, over the past decade, become one of the most prevalent clinical entities identified as a work-related injury (Shellenbarger 1991; Schenck 1989; Siebenaler 1992). It is the single most common nerve compression syndrome (Weiss and Akelman 1992).

Although it remains a subject of intense debate among hand surgeons, current research indicates that as many as 47 percent of all cases of carpal tunnel syndrome can be attributed to occupational demands (Baker and Ehrenberg 1990). The majority of carpal tunnel syndrome cases, however, still are considered idiopathic (Greenspan 1988). Once it has been established that a

compression of the median nerve exists at or distal to the wrist, determining the predisposing factors, whether they be metabolic, anatomical, or occupational, becomes equally important (Szabo and Madison 1992). Theoretically, any process that structurally alters the carpal tunnel can cause symptoms of CTS (Mascola and Rickman 1991).

It is generally understood that in CTS the portion of the median nerve that passes through the carpal tunnel becomes irritated and produces symptoms of CTS (Spinner, Bachman, and Amadio 1989). The decrease in blood flow to the nerve and resultant tissue anoxia cause vessel dilation and edema. This process contributes to greater compression of the median nerve within the carpal tunnel, a rigid fibro-osseous structure formed by the eight carpal bones of the wrist (Corrigan and Maitland 1989; Spinner, Bachman, and Amadio 1989). The inevitable decrease in volume of the carpal tunnel can, by and large, be attributed to the inflammation and swelling of the sheaths covering the nine flexor tendons (*tenosynovitis*) which accompany the median nerve as it courses through the carpal tunnel (Corrigan and Maitland 1989; Spinner, Bachman, and Amadio 1989).

Underlying medical conditions which can predispose individuals to chronic tenosynovitis in the hands and wrist, resulting in CTS, are pregnancy, menopause, diabetes, collagen-vascular disorders such as SLE, RA, hypothyroidism, obesity amyloidosis, and infection (Lluch 1992; Mascola and Richman 1991; Spinner, Bachman, and Amadio 1989). It is also thought that women, who have anatomically smaller carpal tunnels, are at an increased risk of developing CTS (Shellenbarger 1991). Osteoarthritis in the wrist as well as the presence of ganglion cysts within the tunnel cause structural changes leading to CTS (Corrigan and Maitland 1989; Spinner, Bachman, and Amadio 1989).

The extent to which occupations mediate the pathogenesis of CTS is the subject of controversy. The common elements of the involved work-related tasks most frequently identified are repetitiveness, force (particularly gripping and pinching), mechanical stresses, posture, vibration, and temperature.

The putative causes of CTS which may—alone, or in combination—contribute to its etiology are matched in magnitude by the array of various symptoms each person with CTS can manifest. However, pain, numbness, and tingling in the thumb and index, long, and ring fingers—usually more intense at night and temporarily relieved by vigorous shaking of the hands—continue to reign as the cardinal symptom complex in the patient with CTS (Ireland 1986; Spinner, Bachman, and Amadio 1989). CTS can be bilateral, but most often symptoms are more severe in the dominant hand (Corrigan and Maitland 1989; Greenspan 1988; Cho and Cho 1989).

DATABASE

SUBJECTIVE

→ Patient is most likely between ages 40 years and 60 years.

→ Patient has history of obesity, diabetes, thyroid disease, RA, SLE, alcoholism, pregnancy, menopause, and present oral contraceptive use. Persons with end-stage renal disease may be more susceptible (Nakano 1991; Spinner, Bachman, and Amadio 1989).

→ Patients most likely have occupations requiring repetitive forceful grasping and pinching and use of vibrating hand-held tools.
  ▪ Examples include seamstresses, butchers, grocery clerks, typists and word processors, musicians, meat packers, cooks, carpenters, and mechanics (Baker and Ehrenberg 1990; Szabo and Madison 1992; Shellenbarger 1991).

→ Gradual onset of symptoms typical, although persons with volar wrist ganglion cysts often present with acute onset.
  ▪ Onset of symptoms precipitated by activities such as driving, holding a phone receiver, and reading (Carragee and Hentz 1988).

→ Symptoms may include complaints of:
  ▪ numbness and stiffness in the wrist, hands, and fingers (Spinner, Bachman, and Amadio 1989).
    • Numbness is either intermittent or ongoing (Carragee and Hentz 1988).

  ▪ Numbness is present in the thumb and index, middle, and ring fingers (Baker and Ehrenberg 1990).
  ▪ decreased fine motor coordination—e.g., dropping objects and feeling that the hands are "useless" (Greenspan 1988; Harter 1989).
  ▪ swelling in the hands and fingers (Greenspan 1988).
  ▪ decreased grip strength.

OBJECTIVE

→ Patient may present with:
  ▪ abnormal hand posture (Carragee and Hentz 1988).
  ▪ muscle atrophy over the thenar eminence of the palm.
  ▪ decreased grip and pinch strength.
    • In specialized settings such as orthopedics, this is usually objectively quantified with the use of a dynamometer and pinch meter.
  ▪ swelling over the volar aspects of the wrist, dorsum of the hand, and in the fingers sometimes noted.
  ▪ decreased sensation over the median nerve distribution of the hand as measured by two-point discrimination or the "stroke test"—i.e., the examiner gently strokes the palm or surface of the index and small finger tips. If the patient reports decreased sensation on the index fingertip, the test is positive.
  ▪ presence of volar wrist ganglion, sometimes a cause of "acute" CTS.

→ Positive Tinel's sign.
  ▪ Patient complains of tingling, usually in the index, middle, and ring fingers, when the examiner percusses the volar aspect of the patient's wrist with a reflex hammer or the index and middle fingers.

→ Positive Phalen's test.
  ▪ Patient develops parasthesias in the median nerve distribution of the hands within 60 seconds of palmar flexing the wrist while the forearms remain vertical (Szabo and Madison 1992).
    • With 80-percent specificity, this is the most sensitive and reliable test (Carragee and Hentz 1988; Greenspan 1988).
    • The shorter the amount of time it takes for the patient to develop paresthesia, the more significant the result.

→ Patient has full ROM of the wrists and often complains of discomfort with pain at the extreme point of wrist flexion.

→ Pain in the radial side of the wrist, without parasthesias, is the predominant complaint in the person with de Quervain's stenosing tenosynovitis.
  ▪ Patient is very tender over the radial styloid; often coexists with CTS (Ireland 1986).

→ When the patient's primary complaint is pain at the base of the thumb and in the thenar eminence—which increases with forceful use of the hand—osteoarthritis of the basilar joint of the thumb is suggested (Pellegrini 1992).

→ Cervical radiculopathy suggested if patient complains of neck pain and parasthesias radiating down the arm with passive extension of the neck and lateral flexion toward the affected side (Spinner, Bachman, and Amadio 1989).

ASSESSMENT

→ Carpal tunnel syndrome

→ R/O ulnar tunnel syndrome (parasthesias in the small and ulnar half of the ring finger) (Harter 1989)

→ R/O cubital tunnel syndrome (pain in the medial aspect of the elbow as well as parasthesias in the ring and small fingers and progressive weakness in the hand)

→ R/O de Quervain's stenosing tenosynovitis

→ R/O osteoarthritis of the basilar joint of the thumb

→ R/O cervical radiculopathy

PLAN

DIAGNOSTIC TESTS

→ Nerve conduction studies (NCSs):
  ▪ measure the motor and sensory responses of the median nerve (Harter 1989).
  ▪ EMG records electrical nerve potentials from active and relaxed muscles (Harter 1989).

→ Laboratory: RF, ANA, fasting blood sugar (FBS), thyroid screen if indicated by the patient's physical examination and history, but are not ordered routinely.

→ X-rays.
  ▪ Anterior-posterior, lateral, oblique, and scaphoid views of the wrist may be taken if the diagnosis

is uncertain or onset of symptoms is acute and preceded by trauma.
  ▪ X-rays generally not necessary or helpful in making the diagnosis of CTS (Carragee and Hentz 1988).

→ Patients who are diabetic and complain of persistent numbness in their fingers and who have decreased sensation over the planar surface of their hands should have EMGs and NCSs to help differentiate carpal tunnel syndrome from peripheral neuropathies.

TREATMENT

→ Initial treatment if the patient's symptoms are mild, intermittent, and not disabling consists of:
  ▪ splinting the wrists in neutral at bedtime.
  ▪ avoiding potentially aggravating activities.
  ▪ administration of pyridoxine (Vitamin B$_6$) 200 mg/day (Carragee and Hentz 1988, Greenspan 1988, Harter 1989, Szabo and Madison 1992).

→ The usual course of this initial treatment is 4 to 6 weeks.

→ Although current literature is riddled with suggestions to prescribe NSAIDs, their effectiveness in the treatment of CTS has not been statistically significant (Weiss and Akelman 1992).

→ The use of diuretics, especially in menopausal women, is of questionable benefit.

CONSULTATION

→ The following individuals should be referred to an orthopedic surgeon for surgical consultation or steroid injection:
  ▪ patients who have failed to respond adequately to conservative measures after a period of six weeks.
  ▪ patients who complain of ongoing, as opposed to intermittent, numbness and tingling over the median nerve distribution of the hand.
  ▪ patients who demonstrate evidence of thenar atrophy.

→ Patients with complaints of pain and swelling involving multiple sites in the upper extremities and who have a positive ANA or RF should be referred to a rheumatologist for further consultation and management.

→ Consultation with a neurologist may be indicated in patients with peripheral neuropathies.

→ As needed for prescription(s).

PATIENT EDUCATION

→ Educate the patient regarding the cause(s) of pain.

→ Patients with CTS must be instructed on the purpose of wrist splints and that applying them at night prevents compression of the median nerve at the wrist.

→ Patients for whom Vitamin B$_6$ is prescribed must be cautioned not to increase their dosage beyond 200 mg as hypervitaminosis, ataxia, and peripheral neuritis have been identified with dosages exceeding 1000 mg/day (Carragee and Hentz 1988).

→ Individuals whose CTS symptoms appear to be aggravated by work-related activities are advised to avoid repetitive wrist motions and to wear their wrist splints during such activities when possible.

→ Patients should be advised to try to optimize body mechanics/work site ergonomics.

→ Patients need to be firmly advised that inadequately treated CTS may result in eventual permanent nerve damage.
  ■ Persons often delay or refuse treatment because of their intense and generally unwarranted anxiety regarding cortisone injections and surgical carpal tunnel release, both highly successful methods of alleviating symptoms.

FOLLOW-UP

→ It needs to be emphasized to CTS patients that the goal of treatment is to prevent damage to the median nerve.

→ It is essential that these individuals seek follow-up if the following conditions exist:
  ■ no resolution of the progression of symptoms after an adequate trial of conservative treatment, generally considered to be six weeks.
  ■ numbness and tingling in the fingers which become persistent and unremitting.
  ■ decreased sensation in the fingertips or weakness in the thumb.

→ Patients who are diabetic must be instructed to monitor their blood glucose levels judiciously because poorly controlled levels may exacerbate symptoms.

→ Document in progress notes and problem list.

De Quervain's Stenosing Tenosynovitis

When the adult female patient complains of wrist pain, usually in the absence of parasthesias, a relatively common condition known as *de Quervain's stenosing tenosynovitis* must always be considered. Sometimes referred to as de Quervain's disease, de Quervain's stenosing tenosynovitis develops from the inflammation of the tendon sheaths of the abductor pollicus longus (APL) and the extensor pollicus brevis (EPB) in the first dorsal wrist compartment (Murtagh 1989; Strickland, Idler, and Creighton 1990a).

Potential causes of de Quervain's may include recurrent mild trauma, especially in individuals who engage in tasks requiring forceful grasping with ulnar, or lateral, deviation of the wrist or repetitive use of the thumb (Kiefhaber and Stern 1992). Although de Quervain's traditionally has been considered an affliction of middle-aged women, it presently is associated with certain occupations and may develop in athletes of both sexes (Kiefhaber and Stern 1992; Thorson and Szabo 1992).

The typical patient remains, however, a woman between the ages of 30 and 50 years (Strickland, Idler, and Creighton 1990a). Pregnant and postpartum women are susceptible to the development of de Quervain's disease, and the condition is often misdiagnosed as CTS, the cause of wrist discomfort most frequently associated with pregnancy.

When the individual with de Quervain's disease fails to demonstrate adequate sustained relief from treatment, an underlying metabolic predisposition must be considered. The likely systemic conditions include diabetes, RA, hypothyroidism, gout, and SLE (Stern 1990; Strickland, Idler, and Creighton 1990a; Thorson and Szabo 1992).

In approximately 30 percent of the cases of de Quervain's, there will be involvement of both wrists. The associated conditions of trigger fingers, or stenosing flexor tenosynovitis, and CTS in individuals with de Quervain's disease have been well documented (Stern 1990; Strickland, Idler, and Creighton 1990a; Thorson and Szabo 1992; Witczak, Maseur, and Meyer 1990). In persons whose symptoms were preceded by trauma, scaphoid and intra-articular fractures of the trapeziometacarpal joint are common (Stern 1990).

Wrist pain—generally characterized as severe—on the radial side of the wrist, and not infrequently described by the patient as "thumb pain," is the typical chief complaint of the person with de Quervain's (Kiefhaber and Stern 1992; Murtagh 1989; Stern 1990; Strickland, Idler, and Creighton 1990a). The pain is described as being aggravated by lifting objects or by any grasping movements. In addition, the patient may complain of swelling at the painful sight, as well as the presence of a lump which may be a ganglion cyst or a more characteristic nodularity of the tendon which is caused by the fibrous thickening associated with this condition (Kiefhaber and Stern 1992).

De Quervain's disease is most often successfully managed with conservative measures, especially in the absence of one of the associated subclinical entities. Early recognition and prompt initiation of treatment or appropriate referral to an orthopedist by the primary care provider can save the patient weeks and often months of needless and sometimes incapacitating wrist pain.

DATABASE

SUBJECTIVE

→ Patient is:
- primarily, an adult female of any race, most frequently in the third through sixth decade of life. Among patients, female to male ratio 10:1.
- pregnant or within a year postpartum without history of trauma.

→ Patient has history of:
- acute or recurrent wrist strain or trauma.
- RA, diabetes, hypothyroidism, CTS, gout, and SLE.

→ Symptoms may include:
- severe wrist pain, most often unilateral, on the dorsal-radial aspect of the wrist, exacerbated by forceful grasping movements.
- swelling over the wrist, or a painful lump.

→ Patient usually denies parasthesias in the hand.

OBJECTIVE

→ Involved wrist may appear swollen in the snuff box area, or just distal to the radial styloid (Kiefhaber and Stern 1992, Murtagh 1989).

→ Wrist is extremely tender to palpitation over the radial styloid.

→ A palpable thickening of the tendon sheath with nodularity may be discerned.

→ Mild crepitus may sometimes be present.

→ Mild erythema in the snuff box area can be noted.

→ Positive Finklestein's test.
- The examiner instructs the patient to make a fist with the thumb adducted, then passively pulls the wrist into ulnar deviation to produce severe pain (Kiefhaber and Stern 1992; Lewis 1988; Murtagh 1989; Strickland, Idler, and Creighton 1990a; Thorson and Szabo 1992).

- This test is generally considered to be the most pathognomonic for de Quervain's.
  • However, the maneuver may similarly induce discomfort in persons with osteoarthritis of the basilar joint of the thumb or in persons with an entrapment condition of the superficial branch of the radial nerve known as Wartenberg's syndrome (Thorson and Szabo 1992).

ASSESSMENT

→ De Quervain's stenosing tenosynovitis
→ R/O osteoarthritis of the basilar joint of the thumb
→ R/O CTS
→ R/O RA of the wrist
→ R/O carpal fractures
→ R/O Wartenberg's syndrome
→ R/O gout

PLAN

DIAGNOSTIC TESTS

→ Radiographs.
- A/P, lateral, scaphoid, and oblique views are routinely obtained, but are usually normal in the absence of a fracture, or a rheumatoid or osteoarthritic condition.

→ Laboratory: RF, ANA, uric acid level if underlying rheumatological or metabolic conditions are suspected.

→ Finklestein's test as previously described in "Objective" section.

TREATMENT/MANAGEMENT

→ A steroid injection into the first dorsal wrist compartment is generally considered to be the initial treatment of choice.
- Often provides dramatic and immediate relief of symptoms (Corrigan and Maitland 1989; Kiefhaber and Stern 1992; Thorson and Stern 1992).
- Steroid injection has been known to provide permanent relief 80 percent of the time (Harvey, Harvey, and Horsley 1990).

→ Alternately, when treatment commences within 2 weeks after the onset of symptoms, rest, anti-inflammatory medicine, and immobilization in a thumb-spica removal splint or non-removable cast can provide relief in approximately 25 percent to

70 percent of patients (Corrigan and Maitland 1989; Kiefhaber and Stern 1992; Witt, Pess, and Gelberman 1991).

- An adequate treatment trial utilizing these measures, however, is considered to be 4 to 6 weeks. See **Table 8-M**, p. 8-50.
- Application of ice compresses 3 to 4 times a day for 20 to 30 minutes may be helpful.

CONSULTATION

→ Unless the patient strenuously objects, she is best served by prompt referral to an orthopedist or other qualified clinician for the administration of a steroid injection.

→ Referral to a hand surgeon for consideration of a surgical release of the first dorsal wrist compartment would be appropriate if the patient presents with a chronic history of de Quervain's and inadequately sustained relief from conservative treatment.

- However, surgical treatment for de Quervain's disease is not a guaranteed remedy. Post-operative complications are of concern (Stern 1990; Thorson and Szabo 1992).

→ Referral to a rheumatologist may be indicated if the patient's symptoms are chronic, bilateral, and associated with multiple aches and pains in the upper extremities, or the overall presentation is one of an underlying rheumatological condition.

→ As needed for prescription(s).

PATIENT EDUCATION

→ Educate the patient regarding the cause(s) of pain.

→ Emphasize the importance of resting the involved wrist.

→ Instruct the patient to apply a thumb-spica splint for two to four weeks following the resolution of symptoms and when engaged in activities requiring wrist strain (e.g., carrying heavy suitcases).

FOLLOW-UP

→ If the patient declines referral to an orthopedist for injection or surgical consultation, have patient make a follow-up appointment with the primary provider four to six weeks following the initiation of more conservative treatment.

→ See "Consultation" section.

→ Document in progress notes and problem list.

Osteoarthritis of the Basilar Joint of the Thumb

Osteoarthritis of the basilar or carpometacarpal (CMC) joint of the thumb should always be considered in the differential diagnosis of a woman who complains of thumb or "wrist pain." Osteoarthritis of the first CMC joint is the most common site of premature joint degeneration in women, and women are ten to 15 times more likely to be afflicted than men (Wolock, More, and Weiland 1989). There is evidence the dominant hand is involved more often with both basilar joints of the thumbs being affected in more than 25 percent of cases (Strickland, Idler, and Creighton 1990b).

Like other forms of degenerative joint disease, osteoarthritis of the basilar joint of the thumb results from a combination of biomechanical and biochemical insults on the joint surfaces. The daily repetitive forces on the joint complex cause eventual ligamentous instability of the CMC, thus predisposing the individual to clinical symptomatology (Pellegrini 1992; Wolock, Moore, and Weiland 1989). Young women presenting with an almost identical clinical picture, with the exception of discernible degenerative changes on x-rays, may have a generalized joint hypermobility (Pellegrini 1992).

Previous trauma, most notably a Bennett's fracture, can predispose individuals of both sexes to osteoarthritis of the first carpometacarpal joint (Corrigan and Maitland 1989; Pellegrini 1992; Wolock, Moore, and Weiland 1989). Finally, anatomical construction of the first CMC, dysplastic joint surfaces, hormonal factors known to cause ligamentous laxity, and occupational endeavors requiring repetitive, forceful pinching can all contribute to eventual manifestations of osteoarthritis of the basilar joint of the thumb (Pellegrini 1992).

DATABASE

SUBJECTIVE

→ Patients are primarily post-menopausal woman.

→ More than 35 percent of patients with RA have CMC arthrosis.

→ Initial complaints consist of pain and weakness in the base of the thumb with certain tasks—e.g., opening jars, turning keys.

→ As the condition progresses, the patient is likely to complain of constant aching in the joint, which is often incapacitating and involves deterioration of fine motor coordination and grip strength.

OBJECTIVE

→ Positive "shoulder sign"—prominence of base of the thumb resulting from dorsal subluxation of the joint (Pellegrini 1992).

→ The first CMC joint and thenar eminence are very tender with direct palpation (Pellegrini 1992; Wolock, Moore, and Weiland 1989).

→ Decreased web space between the thumb and index finger may be noted.

→ Positive thumb abduction stress test (AST)—have the patient attempt to abduct the thumb against resistance supplied by the examiner's thumb; if this maneuver elicits severe pain in the first CMC, the test is considered positive.

→ Positive grind test—axial loading with simultaneous rotation of the thumb produces pain and crepitus in the first CMC (Pellegrini 1992).

→ Decreased pinch grip.

→ Swelling at the base of the thumb.

ASSESSMENT

→ Osteoarthritis of the basilar joint of the thumb

→ R/O carpal tunnel syndrome

→ R/O de Quervain's stenosing tenosynovitis

→ R/O old scaphoid fracture

→ R/O palmar or dorsal ganglion cyst

PLAN

DIAGNOSTIC TESTS

→ The existence of osteoarthritis of the basilar joint of the thumb can be confirmed on radiographs which should include an A/P, lateral, oblique, and scaphoid views of the CMC.

TREATMENT/MANAGEMENT

→ Initial treatment consists of immobilizing the first CMC with a removal thumb-spica splint and a 4-to 6-week course of NSAIDs. **See Table 8-M**, p. 8-50.

→ Patient may benefit from thenar muscle strengthening exercises, generally initiated in consultation with an occupational or hand therapist.

CONSULTATION

→ Patients who fail to respond adequately to splinting and NSAIDs should be referred to an orthopedist or other qualified clinician for a

steroid injection directly into the first CMC, as well as evaluation for surgery if indicated.

→ As needed for prescription(s).

PATIENT EDUCATION

→ Patient education emphasizes the general teaching principles of almost all osteoarthritic conditions with emphasis on the proper application and use of splints, compliance with NSAIDs, and hand therapy.

FOLLOW-UP

→ The patient should follow up with the primary care provider four to six weeks after the initiation of NSAIDs and splinting.

→ Patients are encouraged to solicit medical follow-up if conservative treatment has failed to alleviate symptoms or is no longer effective.

→ Document in progress notes and problem list.

Trigger Fingers

Stenosing flexor tenosynovitis of the thumb or fingers, or trigger fingers may well constitute the most common complaint associated with finger pain in the primary ambulatory care setting. Surprisingly, however, the condition is often misdiagnosed as an injury or tendinitis.

Triggering of digits usually results from the idiopathic thickening of the proximal part of the flexor tendon sheath (Kiefhaber and Stern 1992). Mechanical irritation from compressive and sheer forces in the tendon results in inflammation, swelling, and pain at the level of the A-1 pulley on the palmar surface of the MCP joint. Most often occurring in the thumb and middle or small fingers, the painful snapping of the digit is caused by the discrepancy between the thickened tendon sheath and the A-1 pulley.

The nodular thickening becomes trapped under the MCP ligament in the flexed finger, making subsequent extension of the digit painful and difficult, often requiring manual, passive manipulation (Corrigan and Maitland 1989).

Trigger digits affect persons of all ages, including the presence of trigger thumbs in neonates. Although, again, the condition is most likely to present in a woman, usually in the fifth decade (Freiberg, Mulholland, and Levine 1989; Thorson and Szabo 1992).

Trigger fingers and thumbs can be associated with underlying endocrine disorders such as hypothyroidism and diabetes, RA, CTS, SLE, and de Quervain's disease (Newport et al. 1992). Only rarely is the condition precipitated by a traumatic event (Thorson and Szabo 1992).

There is a general preponderance of trigger digits in the dominant hand (Thorson and Szabo 1992). Multiple trigger fingers may exist in the same person and be evident in both hands.

DATABASE

SUBJECTIVE

→ Symptoms may include:
  ▪ a painful "snapping" or "locking" of the affected digit, usually more apparent upon arising.
  ▪ pain on the palmar surface of the MCP joint radiating to the proximal interphalangeal joint of the affected finger.
  ▪ swelling of the affected digit with difficulty flexing or extending the finger from a flexed position.
→ Patient may report a history of diabetes, RA, or SLE.

OBJECTIVE

→ The affected thumb or finger may be mildly edematous.
→ The examiner can palpate a tender nodule or thickening on the palmar surface of the metacarpal just proximal to the palmar digital crease.
→ The patient can usually reproduce the snapping or locking of the digit at will. Otherwise, the examiner may have the patient flex all fingers into a fist.
  ▪ The patient is then instructed to extend the unaffected digits while the examiner holds the trigger finger in flexion, then releases the finger into extension.

ASSESSMENT

→ Trigger thumb or finger
→ R/O flexor tenosynovitis
→ R/O osteoarthritis of the basilar joint of the thumb
→ R/O de Quervain's stenosing tenosynovitis
→ R/O ganglion of the flexor tendon sheath of the finger.

PLAN

DIAGNOSTIC TESTS

→ X-rays are indicated only in the event of a precipitating trauma.
→ RF and ANA should be ordered if a rheumatological condition is suspected, especially in persons with multiple trigger fingers.

TREATMENT/MANAGEMENT

→ Although several authors have reported a 73 percent to 77 percent "success" rate when treating trigger fingers by splinting them in extension, their patients were individuals with mild symptoms that had been apparent for less than 6 months. An average of 3 to 9 weeks of splinting was required (Patel and Bassini 1992).
→ A steroid injection into the flexor tendon sheath of the affected digit provides resolution of symptoms, usually within 2 weeks, and is successful more than 80 percent of the time (Newport et al. 1992).

CONSULTATION

→ The patient should be promptly referred to an orthopedist or other trained practitioner for the steroid injection.
→ Patient should be referred to an orthopedist for surgical consultation when there is inadequate sustained relief from conservative treatment or in cases where the affected digit is locked in flexion.
→ Diabetics with trigger digits who complain of stiffness in the affected fingers, despite resolution of pain and snapping with treatment, may benefit from physical therapy as prescribed by a hand or occupational therapist.

PATIENT EDUCATION AND FOLLOW-UP

→ Education and follow-up are based on the treatment prescribed—generally either steroid injection or surgical trigger finger release.
→ Unless the patient has RA, the patient should be encouraged to submit to surgical treatment when symptoms are recurrent, as surgery constitutes a quick and minor procedure which almost always provides permanent relief.
→ Document in progress notes and problem list.

Diane C. Putney, R.N., C., M.N., N.P.

8-H

Low Back Pain

The majority of complaints from patients regarding back pain involve the low back, defined as the area of the back and spine inferior to the thoracolumbar junction (T12 to L1) and the costophrenic angles (Beary III, Christian, and Johanson 1988). For the most part, low back complaints may involve the entire lumbar spine as well as the sacrum.

Given that most people in the general population have experienced *low back pain* at some time in their lives, it is an encouraging fact that approximately 85 percent will be symptom-free within three months. (Manders 1989; Nachemson 1992). It is, actually, the mere five percent of persons with low back pain persisting more than three months which accounts for 80 percent of the financial burden incurred from the disease, estimated to be as high as $50 billion annually (Nachemson 1992).

Low back pain is second only to headaches as the most common cause of pain, as well as disability, in adults under age 45 years (Chase 1991). A review of the current literature indicates that the consequences of lumbar disk degeneration account for the majority of low back and leg pain complaints (Brown 1992).

However, in Nachemson's (1992) recent critique of this epidemic problem, the outcomes of the multiple epidemiological studies which underscore the importance of psychosocial factors are given new emphasis. These factors may include anything from specific dissatisfaction with one's job to more general states of psychological depression. Additional factors which contribute to the problem of low back pain include smoking, body weight, and tall build (Frymoyer and Cats-Biril 1991; Heliovaara et al. 1991).

It is important that the clinician establish whether the patient's discomfort is acute in nature—i.e., present for three to six months—or chronic and enduring for more than six months (Bucholz et al. 1984).

One suggested diagnostic strategy is to assign the patient's low back pain complaint to one of the following diagnostic groups:

→ benign etiologies such as osteoarthritis, mechanical back pain, and bulging disk;

→ radiculopathies or sciatica, caused by either tension or compression in the lumbar nerve roots;

→ spinal stenosis, which occurs with circumferential constriction of the lumbar nerve roots;

→ behavioral disorders which encompass the spectrum of psychogenic pain disturbances often observed in patients with liability claims and depression (Brown 1992). These first four categories are generally characteristic of chronic low back pain syndromes (Bucholz et al. 1984).

Conditions with more acute clinical presentations are manifested in a fifth category of serious underlying disorders which include cauda equina syndrome resulting from massive lumbar disk prolapse, neoplasms, disk space infection, and pathological fractures (Brown 1992). Low back pain resulting from underlying gynecological, hip, and sacroiliac joint problems, referred pain from the abdomen and the retroperitoneal space, syndromes which can be attributed to peripheral vascular and nerve lesions seen in diabetics and alcoholics—all must be considered in the process of diagnosing low back pain (Lewis 1988; Manders 1989).

Despite the well-documented histories of the clinical characteristics and progression of low back pain syndromes, in the majority of cases it is not known what specific pathophysiological mechanisms surrounding the lumbar nerves constitute the actual sources of pain (Nachemson 1992). It is known, for example, that in the early stages of disk degeneration in the lumbar spine, the motion segment unit becomes destabilized. However, it only can be assumed that the pain occurs because the disk displacement stimulates the free nerve endings in the posterior longitudinal ligament and annulus fibrosis (Brown 1992).

One suggestion is that the clinician direct the patient to delineate the location and type of discomfort on a "pain drawing" (Brown 1992; Bucholz et al. 1984; Manders 1989). Studies employing this technique suggest a series of patterns which, in a general sense, correspond to the five diagnostic categories discussed previously.

For example, patients with benign sources of low back pain mark the areas of the drawing on the lower back specifically. Those with herniated lumbar disks and spinal stenosis indicate the mid-aspect of the posterior leg, lateral aspect of the thigh and calf, and anterior thigh and lower leg respectively.

Individuals with underlying disease processes characteristically mark the lower thoracic and upper lumbar spine. Finally, persons whose complaints are primarily motivated by psychogenic phenomenon and behavioral disorders are inclined to make indiscriminate markings over both sides of the entire diagram (Brown 1992).

It is important to keep in mind that multiple joint involvement with a chief complaint of low back pain, particularly in the hips and knees, could indicate a spondylarthropathy such as ankylosing spondylitis (Bucholz et al. 1984). While spondylarthropathies are a more common source of low back pain in the younger adult, mechanical low back pain, prolapsed intervertebral disk, and spondylolisthesis presents routinely in both young and middle-aged persons. Osteoarthritis and rheumatoid arthritis, spinal stenosis, and Paget's disease afflict middle-aged individuals with regularity. Spinal metastasis is diagnosed more frequently in middle-aged and elderly populations (McRae 1990).

The scope and complexities of the problem of low back pain are enormous. Individual protocols for every syndrome within the general context of this discussion would only serve to confuse the reader. The vast majority of patients with low back pain have symptoms which are self-limiting and they recover with relatively standard and conservative treatment measures. This protocol is divided into two sections: "Acute Low Back Pain" and "Chronic Low Back Pain."

Acute Low Back Pain

DATABASE

SUBJECTIVE

Categories of low back pain may be delineated as follows:

Herniated Disk

→ Patients from all adult age groups; most common cause of acute low back pain in the patient who presents in an urgent-care setting (Anderson and Burchiel 1991; Brown 1992).

→ Pain:
  ▪ radiates from proximal to distal in the sciatic femoral nerve distribution (Brown 1992).
  ▪ radiates from the buttocks to the ankle (Torg, Welsh, and Shepard 1990).
  ▪ made worse by straining and relieved with rest (Corrigan and Maitland 1989).
  ▪ pain on coughing possible complaint (Walk 1989).

Myofascial Sprains, Strains, and Tendinitis

→ Symptoms may include: pain and tenderness of a gradual onset with a specific history of trauma.

→ Presents at either side of the midline of the lower back.

→ Most common type of lower back problem in athletes (Torg, Welsh, and Shepard 1990).

Cauda Equina Syndrome

→ Patient presents with acute onset of excruciating low back pain, bilateral leg pain, inability to stand or void.

Tumor

→ Symptoms may include:
  ▪ gradual onset of constant pain which worsens with recumbency.
  • Pain can be associated with weight loss and fever (Bucholz et al. 1984; Corrigan and Maitland 1989; McCowin, Borenstein, and Weisel 1991).

→ Patient may associate onset of pain with trauma.

Infection

→ Symptoms may include:
  ▪ pain over involved region.
  • Pain may be intermittent or constant (McCowin, Borenstein, and Wiesel 1991).
  ▪ limited ROM.
  ▪ fever.

Spondylarthropathy

→ Patients age at onset less than 40 years.

→ Symptoms may include:
  ▪ low back pain associated with large joint involvement, particularly the hips and knees, and gastrointestinal (GI) problems (Bucholz et al. 1984).
  ▪ frequent morning stiffness (Baron and Zendel 1989).
  ▪ bilateral heel pain.

Pathological Fractures

→ Symptoms may include:
  ▪ sudden onset of pain which may follow physical exertion or minor trauma.
    • Pain increases with movement; can be described as dull and aching and is frequently worse at night (Corrigan and Maitland 1989).

Referred Pain

→ Most often involves the genitourinary, vascular, and GI systems (McCowin, Borenstein, and Weisel 1991).

→ Usually described as sharp, deep, and well-localized; unrelated to activity.

OBJECTIVE

→ An examination of the patient whose chief complaint is low back pain should be comprehensive and ongoing, and include the acquisition of additional studies which may be required to rule out any number of underlying medical, orthopedic, and neurological conditions.

→ When evaluating the source of low back pain, active rather than passive musculoskeletal movements on the part of the patient provide the most useful information (Corrigan and Maitland 1989). Therefore, the examination begins the moment the clinician enters the examination room, with general inspection of the patient's gait and/or posture.

Objective clinical findings in the patient with acute low back pain can present as the following:

Herniated Disk

→ Patient has difficulty bearing weight on the affected leg and an antalgic gait.

→ Patient has tendency to posture herself with back held rigid and knees somewhat flexed.

→ Pain and limitation increased on forward flexion with normal lateral movement, but may be limited on one side.

→ Affected spinal vertebrae are often tender on the same side as the disk prolapse over the sciatic notch (Corrigan and Maitland 1989).

→ Ankle or knee jerk reflexes may be absent or decreased on the affected side (McRae 1990).

→ Patient sometimes has diminished sensation on the lateral aspect of the foot in the affected leg.

→ Complaints of low back pain with straight leg raising suggest center disk prolapse.

Myofascial Sprains, Strains, and Tendinitis

→ Patient has limited ROM of the lower spine in all spheres.

→ Patient has cautious, rigid gait in a slightly forward flexed position (Torg, Welsh, and Shepard 1990).

Cauda Equina Syndrome

→ Patient presents with varying degrees of neurological and sensory deficits in legs and perianal areas, and urinary retention.

Tumor

→ Patient presents with muscular spasm and resultant scoliosis, swelling, and erythema of skin surrounding tumor.

→ Diffuse bone tenderness, fever, pallor, and purpura can indicate multiple myeloma (McCowin, Borenstein, and Wiesel 1991).

→ Laboratory findings are usually within normal limits.

Infection

→ Patient may have decreased motion in the lumbar spine with paraspinal muscular spasm.

→ Fever may be present.

→ Patient may have an elevated white blood cell (WBC) count and ESR.

Spondylarthopathy

→ Patient presents with:
  ▪ minimal tenderness over sacroiliac joints.
  ▪ decreased lateral mobility of spine.

→ X-ray may be normal (Baron and Zendel 1989); positive HLA-B27.

Pathological Fractures

→ Diagnosis is confirmed on x-ray.

→ See "Diagnostic Tests" section.

Referred Pain

→ Pain referred to the lower back may be associated with reflex muscle contraction and hyperalgesia.

→ Patients with a ruptured abdominal aneurysm present with severe pain, circulatory shock, and an expanding mass (McCowin, Borenstein, and Wiesel 1991).

ASSESSMENT

→ Acute low back pain

→ R/O herniated disk

→ R/O myofascial sprain, strain, or tendinitis

→ R/O cauda equina syndrome

→ R/O tumor

→ R/O infection

→ R/O spondylarthropathy

→ R/O pathological fractures

→ R/O referred pain

PLAN

DIAGNOSTIC TESTS

→ X-rays:
  - standing anteroposterior, lateral, and occasionally oblique views of the lumbar-sacral spine are the standard views obtained.
  - can reveal degenerative disk disease and destructive lesions, such as tumors, infections, and pathological fractures.
  - A/P and lateral views of the hip and sacroiliac joints when indicated.

→ MRI, in consultation with physician, is becoming the study of choice for confirming disk displacement, spinal tumors, and infectious processes (Brown 1992).

→ CT scan of the lumbar-sacral spine can be obtained to rule out spinal stenosis.

→ Bone scan, in consultation with physician, can be obtained to identify sites of potential stress fractures, inflammation, and lytic lesions of the spine.

→ Laboratory.
  - CBC, ESR, blood cultures, alkaline phosphatase, calcium, phosphorus, Bence-Jones proteins, protein electrophoresis as indicated to evaluate the presence of a tumor or infection.
  - The cause of pathological fractures which result from underlying bone disease can be investigated with serum calcium levels, alkaline

phosphatase, and urinary hydroxyproline excretion.

→ While EMGs can help determine the level of nerve root involvement, their utility in the overall diagnostic evaluation of low back pain is not well-recognized.

TREATMENT/MANAGEMENT

→ Advise bed rest for 5 days on a firm mattress with a bed board.

→ When herniated disk is likely, advise bed rest with the hips and knees slightly flexed on pillows to reduce stretch on the sciatic nerve.

→ A 4- to 6-week maintenance course of NSAIDs is advisable. See **Table 8-M**, p. 8-50.

→ Muscle relaxants and analgesics are prescribed with caution.

→ Applications of ice packs to the lower back may be helpful—for 30 minutes at least 4 times a day for mechanical low back pain and disk prolapse.

→ When symptoms of low back pain begin to improve, physical therapy focusing on spinal manipulation and rehabilitation techniques should begin.
  - Acute nerve root irritation and muscle spasm require a period of passive therapy *before* active physical therapy is initiated (Torg, Welsh, and Shepard 1990).

→ Transcutaneous electrical nerve stimulation (TENS) can be utilized for short-term pain control (Torg, Welsh, and Shepard 1990).

→ *Cauda equina syndrome* is an orthopedic emergency which results from massive disk prolapse and requires surgical decompression (Brown 1992; Corrigan and Maitland 1989).

CONSULTATION

→ Referral to an anesthesiologist for an epidural steroid injection may be indicated with acute radicular symptoms.

→ Consultation with an orthopedist is warranted when the patient's clinical presentation and history of low back pain indicate infection, fractures, and the presence of a tumor or metastatic bone lesion.

→ Immediate evaluation by a neurologist and an orthopedist is required when cauda equina syndrome is suspected.

→ Patients require referral to an orthopedist when conservative measures have failed and the patient's symptoms become disabling, especially if progressive neurological dysfunction is evident.

- Sometimes painful trigger points and sacroiliac joints may benefit from steroid injections by an orthopedist.

→ Consultation with an internist, surgeon, or appropriate specialist is warranted when the source of the patient's pain is referred.

→ As needed for prescription(s).

PATIENT EDUCATION

→ Educational instruction for the person with acute low back pain is proscribed by diagnosis of the underlying cause.

→ During the acute phase of low back pain, excluding situations deemed to be surgical emergencies and possibly tumor or infection, the following general principles require emphasis:

- detailed explanations of the patient's structural disorder and how it is causing pain.
- importance of early mobilization, as prolonged bed rest (more than five days) can have debilitating catabolic effects on the patient's musculoskeletal system, as well as a detrimental impact on psychological well-being and rehabilitative potential (Torg, Welsh, and Shepard 1990).
- compliance with medication regimen, use of ice packs, and physical therapy regimen (which includes posture analysis, flexion, and extension exercises) depend in large part on how successfully the patient is educated.
- it is especially important to emphasize to the athletic patient that although early treatment is recommended, 90 percent of all acute low back pain resolves within three months without any treatment at all (Torg, Welsh, and Shepard 1990).
- educating patients beyond the initial phase of acute low back pain will be addressed in more detail in the protocol on managing chronic low back pain.

FOLLOW-UP

→ When the cause of the patient's low back pain has been determined to be mechanical or sciatic in nature, it is advisable to continue with conservative treatment for four to six weeks. The patient should schedule a follow-up visit for re-evaluation of her progress at that time.

→ Patients should be instructed to seek immediate follow-up if their symptoms include the onset of

bowel and bladder problems, fevers, weight loss, or other suspicious symptoms of neurological dysfunction, infection, and/or metastasis.

→ Document in progress notes and problem list.

Chronic Low Back Pain

DATABASE

SUBJECTIVE

The person with chronic low back pain usually has complaints of low back pain for at least six months. Chronic low back pain may be attributed to any of the following:

Degenerative Disk Disease (Spondylosis)

→ Most common cause of low back pain in persons over 50 years of age.

→ Pain described as diffuse dull ache in the lower back.

- Pain may be either relieved or exacerbated by posturing of the back, punctuated by episodes of more severe pain and muscle spasm (Corrigan and Maitland 1989).

Spinal Stenosis

→ Patient who is over age 60 years with medical history which includes peripheral vascular disease or a medical condition such as diabetes is at increased risk.

→ Patient may have a history of smoking (Brown 1992).

→ Pain occurs in the lower back and lower extremities upon activity and is relieved by rest. (Brown 1992).

→ Symptoms may include vague backache, morning stiffness (McRae 1990).

→ Pain is more proximal. Patient reports great difficulty walking upright.

- flexing spine relieves pain (Brown 1992).

→ Patient reports weakness in both legs with a need to sit down immediately (Corrigan and Maitland 1989).

Spondylolisthesis

→ More common in women.

→ Patient complains of low back pain:

- made worse by standing, eased by sitting (Corrigan and Maitland 1989).
- which radiates into the buttocks without paresthesia (McRae 1990).

Prolapsed Disk

→ Radicular pain (sciatica) is usually aggravated by coughing and sneezing and improves with rest (Beary III, Christian, and Johanson 1988).

→ Patient reports:
  ▪ severe pain with nagging quality and paresthesia in the buttocks and thighs.
  ▪ sciatic pain and paresthesia, muscle weakness, sensory impairment (McRae 1990).

→ Patient presents with leg pain which was preceded by low back pain with paresthesia, leg cramps, and weakness.

Psychogenic Pain

→ History is inconsistent and clinical findings do not correlate with the patient's symptoms.

Mechanical Low Back Pain

→ Patient is 20 years to 45 years old.

→ Patient reports:
  ▪ dull backache aggravated by activity.
  ▪ no radiation of pain.
  ▪ history of recurring episodes of low back pain, precipitated by mechanical stress or episodes of trauma (Brown 1992).

Ankylosing Spondylitis

→ Rare in women (10 percent of cases); age of onset younger than 40 years.

→ Onset is insidious.

→ Symptoms may include:
  ▪ morning stiffness which improves with exercise.
  ▪ heel pain (Baron and Zendel 1989; Corrigan and Maitland 1989).
  ▪ back pain often radiating to thighs, buttocks, and groin, but neurological symptoms are absent.

→ Initial presentation may be peripheral joint involvement, constitutional symptoms such as weight loss, fever, and generalized aches and pains.

Infection

→ See "Acute Low Back Pain" section.

Metabolic Bone Disease

→ Patient may report pain in the lumbar spine, usually of sudden onset and often occurring after heavy physical exertion.

→ Patient may report diminished height.

→ Patients with history of Paget's disease (rare under the age of 60 years) complain of dull aching pain which is worse at night.

Referred Pain

→ See "Acute Low Back Pain" section.

OBJECTIVE

Objective clinical findings in the individual with chronic low back pain are generally consistent with the following:

Degenerative Disk Disease

→ X-rays reveal disk space narrowing with osteophyte formation (Lewis 1988).

→ Patients are often obese (McRae 1990).

Spinal Stenosis

→ Patient presents in a "simian stance"—i.e., flexion of the lumbar spine, hips, and knees (McRae 1990).

Spondylolisthesis

→ Patient may present with:
  ▪ back pain with tight hamstring and back extensor muscles.
  ▪ increased lumbar lordosis.
  ▪ bilateral extensor muscle spasm.
  ▪ limited spinal extension (Corrigan and Maitland 1989).

→ Spondylosis, ankylosing spondylitis, osteoporosis: elderly patient with lumbar kyphosis.

→ Restricted ROM in all directions commonly observed in persons with muscle spasm, spondylosis, ankylosing spondylitis.

Prolapsed Disk

→ Positive tension signs—i.e., straight leg raises (Bucholz et al. 1984) are evidenced.

→ Patient presents with limited forward flexion.

→ Thickening of soft tissue in the interspinous spaces is common in chronic disorders.

→ Scoliosis is present when patient is standing or when the lumbar spine is flexed.

→ Affected spinal level in disk prolapse is usually tender to palpation (Corrigan and Maitland 1989).

→ Unilateral decreased ankle and knee jerk reflexes are evidenced.

→ Flattening or reversal of normal lumbar lordosis: prolapsed intervertebral disk, osteoarthritis, spinal infections, and ankylosing spondylitis (McRae 1990).

→ Patient presents with:
- positive straight leg raises and sciatic notch tenderness (Beary III, Christian, and Johanson 1988).
- muscle wasting in buttock or leg.

Psychogenic Pain

→ Patient presents with:
- exaggerated back stiffness.
- pain with an acutely flexed back.
- bizarre gait.

Mechanical Low Back Pain

→ Usually, ROM of the lumbar spine is normal with no positive neurological findings (McRae 1990).

Ankylosing Spondylitis

→ Patient presents with:
- large joint involvement, particularly the knee and the hip, or
- peripheral joint involvement—i.e, tenderness at the Achilles tendon insertion on the plantar surface of the heel.
- limited lateral flexion, bilateral muscle spasm.
- limited chest expansion.

→ Positive HLA-B 27 test results in 83 percent to 96 percent of cases (Baron and Zendel 1989).

Tumors

→ Diagnosis is usually radiographic.

→ Lower spine is a common site of metastasis.

→ Alkaline phosphatase is often elevated (Lewis 1988).

→ See also "Acute Low Back Pain" section.

Infection

→ See "Acute Low Back Pain" section.

Metabolic Bone Disease

→ See "Acute Low Back Pain" section.

Referred Pain

→ See "Acute Low Back Pain" section.

ASSESSMENT

→ Chronic low back pain

→ R/O degenerative disk disease

→ R/O spinal stenosis

→ R/O spondylolisthesis

→ R/O prolapsed disk

→ R/O psychogenic low back pain

→ R/O mechanical low back pain

→ R/O ankylosing spondylitis

→ R/O tumor

→ R/O infection

→ R/O metabolic bone disease

→ R/O referred pain

PLAN

DIAGNOSTIC TESTS

→ See "Acute Low Back Pain" section.

→ Laboratory.
- HLA-B27 should be ordered if ankylosing spondylosis is suspected.
- RF and ANA as indicated to determine the presence of an underlying rheumatological disorder.
- Serum calcium, phosphate, alkaline phosphate, urinary calcium or hydroxyproline as indicated to rule out metabolic bone disease.

TREATMENT/MANAGEMENT

→ See protocol for "Acute Low Back Pain" section for initial phase of treatment.

→ Maintenance program of protective back care are necessary and should be, formulated in consultation with a physical therapist, is essential (Torg, Welsh, and Shepard 1990).

→ Bed rest is contraindicated for individuals with chronic mechanical back pain only aggravated by specific movements (Torg, Welsh, and Shepard 1990).

→ Braces and back supports are beneficial in restricting painful movements and poor posturing which exacerbate painful episodes.

→ In the patient with persistent radicular pain, epidural steroid injection is the treatment of choice (Saal 1989).

→ Weight resistance training, aerobic conditioning, and, especially, swimming are important elements of back care maintenance programs.

→ Physical therapy generally focuses on a combination of spinal flexion and extension exercises, abdominal strengthening exercises, postural analysis, and stretching. Back extension exercises are contraindicated if they cause peripheralization of the patient's pain, or the patient continues to present with a lumbar list (Saal 1989).

→ The use of tricyclic antidepressants may be beneficial in the treatment of chronic low back pain syndromes. Consult with a physician.

→ Metabolic bone disorders require treatment of the underlying metabolic disorder, calcium and Vitamin D supplementation for osteoporosis, spinal orthotics (Bucholz et al. 1984).

CONSULTATION

→ See "Acute Low Back Pain" section.

→ When a behavioral disorder or psychogenic cause of chronic low back pain appears to be the most likely cause, consultation with a psychiatrist is recommended.

→ Other than in the event of a surgical emergency or serious underlying disorder, consultation with a physiatrist can be invaluable and is indicated for patients who do not respond adequately to conservative measures, who are not surgical candidates, and for whom the diagnosis may be in question.

→ As needed for prescription(s).

PATIENT EDUCATION

→ Findings of recent studies suggest that a patient's consistent failure to derive benefit from physical therapy regimens is due to a lack of physical effort on her part (Torg, Welsh, and Shepard 1990).

→ Advise patient that active treatment, or physical therapy, should be initiated as soon as symptoms permit.
  - Patients should be instructed to participate in a level of activity that will not increase their pain and radicular symptoms.

→ Instruct patient that passive treatment measures (e.g., medication and physical modalities) have no curative value; they only relieve pain (Torg, Welsh, and Shepard 1990).

→ Recommend the benefits of thermal therapy which include resolution of edema and muscle relaxation.

→ Advise patient that use of heavy lumbosacral supports with rigid stays is to be avoided (Manders 1989).

→ Patients should be instructed to avoid prolonged periods of sitting and, when sitting, should use straight-backed chairs.

→ The importance of weight reduction in the obese patient with chronic low back pain must be emphasized as an essential part of treatment.

→ Explain to patient the value of acupuncture and acupressure, which is based on theories regarding the release of endorphins, has not been fully established (Torg, Welsh, and Shepard 1990).

→ Patients should be instructed to participate in a level of activity that will not increase their pain and radicular symptoms.

→ Patients with chronic low back pain syndromes often inquire as to whether they would benefit from treatment by a chiropractor. **The patient should not undergo chiropractic treatment until an underlying medical condition or serious underlying pathological process, such as tumor or infection, has been firmly excluded.**

FOLLOW-UP

→ See "Acute Low Back Pain" section.

→ Document in progress notes and problem list.

Diane C. Putney, R.N., C., M.N., N.P.

8-1

Hip Pain

A patient presenting with a chief complaint of *hip pain* may use this description to characterize pain anywhere from the groin, thigh, buttock, and lateral sacrum. Even common clinical entities involving the hip may present a real diagnostic challenge for the primary care provider.

The most frequent cause of hip pain in the adult is, in fact, that which is referred from a prolapsed intervertebral disk (McRae 1990). The majority of true hip pain is usually secondary to degenerative joint disease, inflammation, and trauma (Bucholz et al. 1984).

The hip, which consists of a ball and socket-type joint, is one of the more stable weight-bearing joints in the body (Lewis 1988). Situated between the gluteus medius tendon, which inserts into the greater trochanter, and the tensor fascia lata is the trochanteric bursa.

Trochanteric bursitis, if not specifically the genuine cause of the majority of hip pain, may well be the most popular "working diagnosis" utilized to characterize an identified hip lesion. In trochanteric bursitis, the bursa becomes inflamed by its repetitive slipping back and forth across the trochanter of the tensor fascia lata. Overuse, acute trauma, low-grade inflammatory processes, and pyogenic infections constitute the pathophysiological factors culminating in the onset of trochanteric bursitis (Haller et al. 1989; Torg, Welsh, and Shepard 1990). Tightness of the iliotibial band and its contributing muscles also has been implicated as a causal factor (Clancy 1989).

Typically, the patient with trochanteric bursitis will complain of an extended period of hip pain with varying intensity, exacerbations of which are usually induced by increased physical activity (Corrigan and Maitland 1989). Approximately 70 percent to 90 percent of patients who have trochanteric bursitis experience

resolution of their symptoms following injection of a local anesthetic into the bursa (Handell 1990). When the patient fails to respond adequately to a diagnostic or therapeutic injection, then other sources of hip pain must be considered.

OA is the most common form of hip disease (Corrigan and Maitland 1989). Osteoarthritis of the hip must be considered as a cause of hip pain, particularly in middle-aged and elderly individuals. The main causes of osteoarthritis of the hip are trauma, inflammation, infection, degenerative joint disease, avascular necrosis, and conditions which cause a structural defect in the joint (Bucholz et al. 1984; Croft et al. 1992).

Avascular necrosis (AVN) of the hip, which invades the subchondral osteolysis and eventually causes necrosis of the femoral head, is the fourth leading cause of hip pain (Bucholz et al. 1984). Avascular necrosis should be considered in young as well as middle-aged and elderly persons who have a history of medical conditions requiring chronic treatment with oral steroid preparations, alcoholism, and hip dislocation. Avascular necrosis is frequently misdiagnosed as trochanteric bursitis because plain x-rays are often normal in the early stages of the disease process.

DATABASE

SUBJECTIVE

→ Patient most likely:
- athletic person who engages in running and cutting sports, gymnastics, and dancing.
- middle-aged.
- obese.

→ Patient may have history of RA, ankylosing spondylitis, degenerative joint disease (DJD) of the lumbar spine, hips, or knees (Collee, Dijkmans, and Vanddenbruucke 1991).

→ The patient with trochanteric bursitis reports pain in the lateral aspect of the buttock or thigh (Beary III, Christian, and Johanson 1988; Bucholz et al. 1984).

→ Pain is aggravated by hip movements such as climbing stairs (Corrigan and Maitland 1989).

→ Patient may complain of not being able to sleep on the affected side.

→ Complaints of deep-seated buttock pain may indicate gluteus bursitis.

→ Anterior thigh pain aggravated by activity suggests psoas tendinitis.

→ Anterior hip pain may indicate iliopsoas bursitis.

→ Hip pain, often referred to the knee, associated with weight bearing and relieved by rest, suggests osteoarthritis (Corrigan and Maitland 1989; McRae 1990).

→ Groin pain or pain over the greater trochanter of a sudden or insidious onset, with a history of medical conditions requiring treatment with oral steroids, alcohol abuse, prior history of hip trauma, or failure to respond to conservative treatment, should increase the clinician's suspicion for AVN.

OBJECTIVE

→ Tenderness on palpation well-localized over the greater trochanter (Corrigan and Maitland 1989).

→ Tenderness of the iliotibial tract.

→ Pain with flexion and external rotation of the hip while the patient is lying supine (Corrigan and Maitland 1989).

→ Pain may be reproduced when the patient resists hip abduction while lying on the unaffected side (Corrigan and Maitland 1989).

→ Lumbar spine motion should be normal in an isolated trochanteric bursitis (Bucholz et al. 1984).

→ Deep tendon reflexes and straight leg raises should be normal.

→ Gait may be antalgic (Bucholz et al. 1984).

→ Inguinal mass, tenderness just below the inguinal ligament that is aggravated by hip extension suggests iliopsoas bursitis (Toohey et al. 1990).

→ Fixed flexion and adduction contractures, limited external rotation, an antalgic gait, and quadriceps and gluteal muscle wasting are common clinical findings in the patient with osteoarthritis of the hip (Corrigan and Maitland 1989).

→ Plain x-rays of the pelvis and hip will reveal the presence of degenerative changes associated with osteoarthritis.

→ A positive "crescent sign" on an x-ray is diagnostic of AVN of the hip.
  ▪ However, its presentation frequently does not coincide with the relevance of the patient's complaint. MRI is generally used to either confirm or rule out the diagnosis.

ASSESSMENT

→ Trochanteric bursitis

→ R/O gluteal bursitis

→ R/O lumbar disk problem, piriformis syndrome, or sciatica

→ R/O iliopsoas bursitis

→ R/O psoas tendinitis

→ R/O OA of the hip

→ R/O AVN of the hip

PLAN

DIAGNOSTIC TESTS

→ Laboratory:
  ▪ ESR, protein electrophoresis, uric acid, HLA-B27, and RF as indicated (Bucholz et al. 1984).

→ X-rays: anterior-posterior views of the affected hip and pelvis, usually normal; calcifications in the bursa are noted in 20 percent of cases (Corrigan and Maitland 1989).

→ X-rays of the lumbar sacral spine may be indicated to rule out spinal pathology.

→ MRI to rule out or confirm the diagnosis of AVN.

TREATMENT/MANAGEMENT

→ Rest from aggravating activity is a priority.

→ NSAIDs for 4 to 6 weeks are instituted. See **Table 8-M**, p. 8-50.

→ Applications of ice packs to the hip for 30 minutes 3 times a day may be helpful.

→ Physical therapy is recommended for hip stretching exercises.

→ Patient should use a cane until weight-bearing is no longer painful.

→ See also **Osteoarthritis** Protocol for treatment of OA of the hip.

CONSULTATION

→ The patient should be referred to an orthopedist or other qualified clinician for the administration of a local steroid injection if the following conditions exist:

- failure to respond adequately to conservative measures.

- NSAIDs contraindicated by allergy or additional medical history.

- Patient's complaints are long-standing and severe.

→ Referral to an orthopedist, neurologist, or physiatrist should be considered to rule out other sources of pathology in patients who present with a long-standing history of hip pain and have failed to experience adequate sustained relief from treatment for "bursitis."

→ Patients with OA of the hip who have constant pain unrelieved by conservative treatment should be referred to an orthopedist to evaluate the need for a total hip replacement or arthroplasty.

→ Patients with AVN should be referred to an orthopedist.

→ As needed for prescription(s).

PATIENT EDUCATION

→ Discuss the identified etiology of hip pain.

→ As with all soft tissue inflammatory processes involving the musculoskeletal system, the principles of rest, NSAIDs, icing, and stretching must be elucidated.

→ Vigorous exercises involving the hip and extended periods of ambulation are contraindicated until the patient's symptoms have resolved for at least two weeks.

→ Teach the patient that early mobilization preserves muscle tone and ROM of the hip.

→ See **Osteoarthritis** Protocol for management of OA of the hip.

FOLLOW-UP

→ The patient should have a follow-up visit with the primary provider four to six weeks after treatment is initiated.

→ The patient is instructed to seek medical consultation if she fails to experience adequately sustained relief from treatment, or if symptoms progress.

→ Document in progress notes and problem list.

Diane C. Putney, R.N., C., M.N., N.P.

8-J

Knee Pain

Persons of all age groups with a presenting complaint of *knee pain*, will comprise a substantial part of the primary care provider's practice. The knee joint, which is the largest synovial joint in the body, is structurally comprised of the articulation of the femur against the proximal surface of the tibia, a surface which carries about 75 percent of the body's weight (Lewis 1988). The second articulation is between the patella and the femur.

The knee depends on the strength and tone of the quadriceps and hamstring muscles, the four major knee ligaments, and menisci for its stability. The ligaments include the medial and lateral collateral, and anterior and posterior cruciate ligaments. The articulation between the tibia and femur is buffered by both the medial and lateral menisci which serve as the main "shock absorbers" as well as stabilizing structures of the knee (Krinsky et al. 1992). Important bursae surrounding the knee include the suprapatellar pouch, and prepatellar, infrapatellar, semimembranous, and pes anserinus bursae.

The knee is primarily a weight-bearing joint subjected to repetitive stresses involving complex movements performed during activities of daily living and vigorous athletic endeavors. It remains a site vulnerable to trauma and chronic, progressive disease states, and is the most commonly involved joint in OA (McAlindon and Dieppe 1990). Fortunately, complete history taking, comprehensive physical examination, and current technology all serve to contribute to an appropriate clinical diagnosis of the patient's problem.

There are a number of clinical syndromes, both chronic and acute and involving the various structures of the knee which can afflict individuals of all ages. Referred knee pain can result from hip pathology, as well as intervertebral disk prolapse at L3 and L4. But knee-specific pathology produces pain within the knee itself (Corrigan and Maitland 1989).

The most common syndromes which trouble young, middle-aged, and elderly women will receive the major emphasis in this protocol.

The patella is a large sesamoid bone situated in the quadriceps mechanism and, therefore, subjected to all the extensor forces of the quadriceps, as well as patellar tendon pain.

Patellofemoral pain syndromes, which comprise the majority of complaints of knee pain in young and middle-aged women (O'Neill, Micheli, and Warner 1992), were until recently, diagnosed most often as chondromalacia patellae. However, true chondromalacia patellae, or softening of the articular cartilage of the patellae, is only rarely the cause of knee pain (Macnicol 1986).

The majority of persons with complaints of patellofemoral pain (PFP) cannot recall a precipitating traumatic event. Rather, the discomfort which constitutes the chief complaint generally follows activity which increases the mechanical overload on the patella, such as walking up and down stairs, or running and cutting activities (Milgrom et al. 1991).

Quadriceps inflexibility is thought to be the most probable cause of abnormal patellar pressures (Torg, Welsh, and Shepard 1990). Malalignment syndromes causing chronic patellar subluxation, include a valgus gait, excessive tibial torsion, and pes planus (Torg, Welsh, and Shepard 1990). Abnormalities present within the femoral condylar groove, hormonal influences, ligamentous laxity, occupational factors, and overuse syndromes in athletic persons can each contribute to the development of patellofemoral pain (Macnicol 1986). Direct trauma, in addition to any other abnormality in the patellofemoral joint complex, can cause damage to the intra-articular cartilage (Corrigan and Maitland 1989).

When evaluating the patient with PFP, it is important for the clinician to determine, first, if the pain is articular or retinacular, and, second, whether the person has patella subluxation, subluxation and patellar tilt, patella tilt only, or no malalignment problem (Fulkerson et al. 1992). With the exception of the various degrees of activity modification mediated by the age, health, occupational demands, and recreational pursuits of each individual, the vast majority of patients with PFP can be successfully managed by standard conservative means.

OA is the major cause of patella femoral pain in elderly persons. Degenerative changes within the knee leading to OA can be apparent in middle-aged and even young adults, but is a major cause of pain and disability in the elderly (McAlindon and Dieppe 1990). After the age of 60 years, OA of the knee becomes more common in women (Altman 1991).

OA usually affects the medial compartment of the knee. The progressive feature of joint space narrowing heralds the development of a varus gait, which further hastens the degenerative process (Lewis 1988). The destructive degenerative joint disease is a major cause of meniscal tears in persons over the age of 40 years, thus increasing the patient's level of pain and disability.

Patellofemoral Pain Syndromes

DATABASE

SUBJECTIVE

→ Patient most likely female adult age 40 years or younger who complains of unilateral or bilateral knee pain with a traumatic onset.

→ Patient has history of:
- recreational or competitive athletic endeavors.
- acute dislocation of the patella.
- relatively minor trauma—e.g., a fall or acute onset of pain while weight-training.
- obesity, particularly when the weight gain was sudden.
- occupations that require frequent squatting, kneeling, and lifting heavy objects.

→ Patient complains of:
- patellofemoral joint aching after repetitive use—such as walking—which is exacerbated by ascending and descending stairs.
  - Pain usually described as deep-seated and localized around the retropatellar and peripatellar area.

- Pain not usually present after rest (Corrigan and Maitland 1989).
- sensation of giving way, locking, popping, catching, and swelling (Corrigan and Maitland 1989; Bucholz et al. 1984; Beary III, Christian, and Johanson 1988).
  - A similar history is given by patients with meniscal or ligament tears, with the usual inclusion of a precipitating traumatic event.

OBJECTIVE

→ Patient presents with:
- increased "Q" angle of more than 20°, caused by increased femoral anteversion with compensatory external tibial torsion, knee valgus, and lateral displacement of the tibial tubercle (Bucholz et al. 1984; Fulkerson et al. 1992).
- wasting of the vastus medialis muscle.
- patellofemoral tenderness.
- pain with squatting, duckwalking, and hopping.

→ Patella may tilt to the side and can best be observed during the final phase of knee extension.

→ Retropatellar crepitus more commonly found on the medial surface.

→ Positive patellar apprehension test with recurrent subluxation of the patella.
- The patient experiences pain and apprehension when the examiner pushes the patella to the side while the knee is in 30° of flexion (Keene 1989).

→ A tender thickening of fold of synovial tissue—particularly around the medial suprapatellar and mediopatellar portion of the knee—suggests plica syndrome (Blauvelt and Nelson 1990).

→ Patella is excessively mobile in recurrent patellar subluxation.

→ Normal range of motion and ligamentous stability is demonstrated.

→ Tibial rotation tests—including McMurray's for meniscal tears, as well as anterior drawer and Lachman's to test ligamentous stability—are normal.

ASSESSMENT

→ Patellofemoral pain syndrome

→ R/O meniscal tear

→ R/O ligament injury

→ R/O degenerative joint disease

→ R/O plica syndrome

→ R/O osteochondritis dissecans

→ R/O fracture

→ R/O neuroma

PLAN

DIAGNOSTIC TESTS

→ X-rays:
  - anterior-posterior and lateral views of the affected knees and merchant's view of both knees can demonstrate a subluxed or laterally displaced patella(s).

→ Laboratory:
  - RF, ANA, ESR, CBC, aspiration of synovial fluid when indicated by examination and history.

→ Bone scans are helpful to rule out fractures, inflammatory processes, and osteochondral lesions.

→ MRI, if indicated:
  - when an anterior or posterior cruciate ligament, meniscal tear, or plica syndrome is highly suggested.

→ Bone scans (not routinely ordered) can detect presence and location of degenerative joint disease.

TREATMENT/MANAGEMENT

→ Rest from running and cutting activities for 6 weeks is recommended for the competitive or recreational athlete.

→ Physical therapy is recommended, emphasizing quadriceps strengthening (particularly the vastus medialis), hamstring strengthening, and stretching.

→ Stationary biking and swimming excellent ways to increase muscle strength without having to bear weight on the knees.

→ Regular applications of ice for 30 minutes, 4 times a day are encouraged.

→ Semi-rigid orthotics which correct overpronation of the feet are very helpful.

→ NSAIDs for 4 to 6 weeks are prescribed when pain is severe and inhibits the patient's normal activities of daily living. (See **Table 8-M**, p. 8-50.)

→ Weight reduction in obese persons is essential for establishing eventual pain control.

→ Use of patellofemoral supports can be beneficial, especially for sporting activities and when they do not restrict normal ROM.

CONSULTATION

→ Referral to an orthopedic surgeon is indicated:
  - if a meniscal or ligament tear or plica is highly suspect.
  - when patients with patellofemoral pain syndrome have not responded adequately to a minimum of six months of conservative treatment and
  - clinical and radiographic evidence have clearly established a mechanical disorder (Fulkerson et al. 1992).

→ Consultation with a rheumatologist is indicated if the patient has an underlying rheumatological condition.

→ Dietary consultation is essential for the obese patient.

→ As needed for prescription(s).

PATIENT EDUCATION

→ Discuss the etiology of patellofemoral pain syndrome.

→ Intruct the patient to continue a maintenance program of quadriceps strengthening at least three times a week, even after the acute phase of pain and disability has resolved.
  - Patients need to be informed that prevention of subluxing patellas and patella tracking problems depends upon the increased strength of the quadriceps muscles.

→ Advise athletic patients involved in running and cutting sports about cross-training techniques that do not stress the patellofemoral joint.
  - These are confined to non-weight-bearing activities such as biking and swimming.

→ Instruct weight trainers that they must avoid the leg extension machine, deep squatting, and forward lunging.

→ Emphasize the proper use of NSAIDs, icing, and, especially, the maintenance of optimal body weight.

→ Instruct patient on activity modification with respect to occupational demands.

→ Advise patient to avoid going up and down stairs when given the choice to do otherwise.

FOLLOW-UP

→ Patients with PFP should receive routine follow-up approximately six weeks after the initial evaluation.

→ Patients should be encouraged to seek medical consultation as needed, when symptoms are persistent, progressive, and increasingly disabling.

→ Document in progress notes and problem list.

Osteoarthritis of the Knee

DATABASE

SUBJECTIVE

→ Patient is age 40 years or more.

→ Patient often obese. (It has been estimated that 40 percent of women with OA of the knee are obese [Felson 1992].)

→ Patient has previous history of knee trauma.

→ Pain described as aching, low-grade, and localized:
  ▪ increases with activity initiated after prolonged sedentary activity.
  ▪ relieved by rest (Altman 1991).

→ Patient complains of morning stiffness, usually not lasting more than 30 minutes.

→ Persons with advanced disease may have knee instability.

OBJECTIVE

→ Varus gait is common and frequently antalgic.

→ Crepitus can be palpated when passively extending the knee.

→ Medial and lateral joint line tenderness is common.
  ▪ May also indicate a meniscal tear.

→ Patient evidences pain with tibial rotation.

→ Knee flexion can be painful and limited.

→ Medial collateral ligamentous laxity can be apparent in advanced disease.

→ Positive McMurray's test, joint line tenderness, and effusion should increase the examiner's suspicion of a meniscal tear, whether or not there is a history of trauma.

→ Patient may be morbidly obese.

ASSESSMENT

→ Degenerative joint disease/Osteoarthritis of the knee

→ R/O meniscal tear

→ R/O chondrocalcinosis

→ R/O RA

→ R/O PFP syndrome

→ R/O osteonecrosis

→ R/O loose body

→ R/O pes anserinus bursitis

PLAN

DIAGNOSTIC TESTS

→ X-rays:
  ▪ anterior-posterior view of both knees standing; lateral view of the affected knee(s); merchant's view of both knees when indicated.
  ▪ degenerative joint disease, chondrocalcinosis, lateral subluxation of the patella, osteochondral lesions, and loose bodies usually are readily discernable on radiographs.

→ MRI as indicated to evaluate meniscal pathology and confirm presence of osteonecrotic lesions and loose bodies.

→ Bone scans can rule out inflammatory processes involving the various knee compartments, which may not be apparent on plain radiographs.

→ Laboratory: See section on "PFP syndrome."

TREATMENT/MANAGEMENT

→ See section on "PFP syndrome."

→ See **Osteoarthritis** Protocol.

→ Prompt referral to an orthopedist or other qualified clinician for the administration of a steroid injection is indicated when an adequate trial of NSAIDs has failed or NSAIDs are contraindicated by the patient's history.

→ Use of a cane to inhibit weight-bearing on affected knee is encouraged.

CONSULTATION

→ See section on "PFP syndrome."

→ Referral to an orthopedic surgeon is indicated when the patient:
  ▪ presents with advanced degenerative joint disease.
  ▪ reports that conservative treatment is no longer adequate and complains of knee instability and constant pain.

→ Referral to an orthopedic surgeon also is indicated for:
  ▪ arthroscopy to remove a loose body
  ▪ meniscal injuries, or
  ▪ treatment of osteochondritis.

→ Referral to a rheumatologist is sometimes helpful, especially when there is multiple joint involvement.

PATIENT EDUCATION

→ See section on "PFP syndrome."

→ See **Osteoarthritis** Protocol.

→ Instruct patients not to put pillows under the knees (may cause flexion contractures) (Quinet 1986).

→ Advise that well-cushioned footwear is important.

→ Advise patient to work in seated rather than standing position when permitted.

FOLLOW-UP

→ See section on "PFP syndrome."

→ See **Osteoarthritis** Protocol.

→ Document in progress notes and problem list.

8-K

Ankle Pain

Ankle injuries comprise an estimated 30 percent of all musculoskeletal trauma (Miller and Hergenroeder 1990) and constitute the most common joint injury in the athletic population from grade school through professional level (Lassiter, Malone, and Garrett 1989; Hergenroeder 1990; De Maio, Paine, and Drez 1992a, 1992b). These statistics acquire added significance for the primary care provider who is involved in treating the most frequent ankle injury, the *sprain* (Stanley 1991).

Approximately 85 percent of all ankle sprains involve the three lateral ligaments that support the ankle (Diamond 1989; Hergenroeder 1990; Lassiter, Malone, and Garrett 1989; Ruda 1991; Stanley 1991). The majority of ankle sprains occur when the person is weight-bearing and the foot is supinated or adducted while in plantar flexion (De Maio, Paine, and Drez 1992a, 1992b). The usual biomechanics of ankle sprains are often characterized as *inversion sprains*, with the anterior talofibular ligament and capsule sustaining the most frequent injury (De Maio, Paine, and Drez 1992a; 1992b; Diamond 1989).

The ankle sustains the entire weight of the body with ambulation and, because of the dearth of muscle mass, relies almost entirely on its mechanical and ligamentous structure for stability. Limited support also is derived from the peroneal tendons on the lateral side and tibial tendons medially (Lewis 1988; Lassiter, Malone, and Garrett 1989). The actual ankle, which is a hinge joint, is comprised of three bones which include the talus, distal fibula, and distal tibia (Ryan et al. 1989; Brand 1992).

An *ankle sprain*, in the most general terms, can be defined as the overstretching of a ligament which does not involve the total disruption of the integrity of its fibers or avulsion from its bony attachments (Diamond 1989). When physiological loading of the ankle joint is exceeded during unanticipated forces, and the surrounding supporting structures fail to respond rapidly enough to maintain joint integrity, a sprain will result (Lassiter, Malone, and Garrett 1989).

Evaluation of the injured ankle with a positive diagnosis of inversion sprain involves the grading or classification of the sprain based on its severity. Although the traditional method of classification remains fraught with controversy and debate, it is the system still cited routinely in the current literature.

Grade I sprains indicate minimal functional loss or tearing of ligament fibers, and they are characterized by mild effusion and local tenderness with normal ROM. Grade II sprains present with moderate functional loss, joint effusion, and diffuse tenderness. Grade III sprains are significantly more disabling and imply a complete disruption of the ligament. There is usually a marked decrease in ROM with swelling, severe pain and hemorrhage (Hergenroeder 1990; Lassiter, Malone, and Garrett 1989; Ruda 1991; Ryan et al. 1989; Stanley 1991).

The examiner should consider the means of injury, which will indicate the structures most likely involved. Establishing whether there is a history of previous ankle sprains is also essential (De Maio, Paine, and Drez 1992a, 1992b).

Although the majority of ankle sprains involve ligaments alone, more serious sprains can be associated with a host of other injuries. These injuries may include osteochondral fractures of the talus; avulsion fractures of the tibia, fibula, talus, and base of the fifth metatarsal; epiphyseal injuries in children; talofibular syndesmosis injuries; peroneal tendon subluxation; deltoid ligament sprains; Achilles tendon ruptures; and peroneal and tibial nerve injuries (De Maio, Paine, and Drez 1992a, 1992b; Hergenroeder 1990; Oden 1987; Plattner 1989; Ryan et al. 1989).

The probability that ankle sprains are more likely to be undertreated than adequately treated is only speculative. However, the primary care provider called upon to evaluate the patient with an ankle injury is cautioned to avoid minimizing the implications of the diagnosis by characterizing the problem as "just a sprain" (Lassiter, Malone, and Garrett 1989; Stanley 1991).

DATABASE

SUBJECTIVE

→ Ankle sprains most common in a person under 35 years of age who is a recreational or competitive athlete.

→ Patient has history of:
  ▪ previous ankle injuries.
  ▪ diabetes, polio, arthritis, arthropathy (De Maio, Paine, and Drez 1992a, 1992b).

→ Patient reports a history of injury involving the turning under or turning in of the ankle, often when the foot is plantar flexed and strikes a fixed or uneven surface (Hergenroeder 1990, Ruda 1991).

→ Patient reports pain and swelling over area of ligament damage.

→ Patient recalls "popping" or "tearing" sensation at the time of injury; more common in grade II and III sprains (Ruda 1991).

→ Eversion injury with swelling and inability to bear weight may indicate deltoid ligament sprain, fracture, or syndesmosis injury (De Maio, Paine, and Drez 1992a, 1992b).

→ Complaints of numbness and tingling can indicate neurological damage (Ruda 1991).

OBJECTIVE

→ Patient presents with:
  ▪ tenderness to palpation along the sprained lateral ankle.
  ▪ swelling and ecchymosis.
  ▪ severe edema and tenderness with crepitus and an inability to bear weight, possibly indicating an ankle fracture.

→ If active and passive ROM (including plantar and dorsiflexion, inversion and eversion) is markedly decreased, the sprain is grade II or III.

→ Pain is increased with inversion stress.

→ Varus posture of the hindfoot can be present in lateral ankle sprains.

→ Positive anterior drawer test—performed by pulling the heel forward while pushing the tibia posteriorly with the other hand—indicates a tear of the anterior talofibular ligament (Ryan et al. 1989).
  ▪ Sometimes not apparent in an acute state due to muscle spasm (Hergenroeder 1990).

→ Positive talar tilt test, determined when the head of the talus can be felt laterally as the examiner attempts to invert the heel on the tibia (Ryan et al. 1989) indicates a complete tear of the anterior talofibular ligament and calcaneofibular ligament.

→ Point tenderness over a bone indicates a fracture (Hergenroeder 1990).

→ Tenderness posterior to the lateral malleolus and along the peroneal tendons suggests peroneal tendon subluxation (Hergenroeder 1990).

→ Egg-shaped swelling over the lateral malleolus is common in complete ligament tears (McRae 1990).

→ Weak plantar flexion or a positive Thompson squeeze test—determined by the absence of plantar movements when the calf muscles are squeezed just distal to the point of maximal girth—indicates an Achilles tendon rupture (Plattner 1989).

ASSESSMENT

→ Ankle inversion sprain

→ R/O eversion ankle/syndesmotic sprain (accounts for approximately 10 percent of ankle sprains) (Boytim, Fisher, and Newman 1991; Stanley 1991)

→ R/O avulsion fractures of the malleoli, tarsal bones, epiphysis, calcaneus, and base of fifth metatarsal

→ R/O stress fractures of the foot, tibia, and fibula

→ R/O sprain of the midfoot, longitudinal arch

→ R/O Achilles tendon rupture

→ R/O bony disorder, including accessory navicular, tarsal coalition, subtalar instability, osteochondritis desiccans

→ R/O peroneal or tibial tendon injuries

PLAN

DIAGNOSTIC TESTS

→ X-rays: anterior-posterior, lateral, and mortise views are standard.
  - Stress and weight-bearing views in consultation with physician may be indicated to assess stability, joint space narrowing, and alignment, when given a history of chronic ankle sprains.

→ CT scans, bone scans, and MRI to determine the existence of loose bodies, fractures, stress fractures, tendinitis, tendon ruptures, in consultation with physician.

→ EMGs to rule out peroneal and tibial nerve injuries.

TREATMENT/MANAGEMENT

→ Early treatment generally includes the RICE principles: <u>R</u>est, <u>I</u>ce, <u>C</u>ompression and <u>E</u>levation.
  - *Rest*—may require crutches or cane if weight-bearing increases pain.
  - *Ice*—Begin immediately.
    - Apply every 2 to 3 hours for 20 minutes for 2 to 4 days or until swelling has ceased.
    - Contraindicated in patients with PVD or rheumatoid conditions (Diamond 1989; Hergenroeder 1990).
  - *Compression*—Controls fluid from entering the joint space.
    - Methods may include the following devices:
      –air stirrup.
      –strapping with nonelastic adhesive tape.
      –laced stabilizers.
      –elastic ankle guards.
  - *Elevation*—Affected extremity should be elevated when possible until swelling has stabilized.

→ Casting for uncomplicated ankle sprain is usually indicated only if the patient is unable to manage with crutches when required for painful ambulation.
  - Casting generally should not exceed 2 weeks (Hergenroeder 1990).

→ Physical therapy includes the following:
  - ROM with active dorsiflexion and eversion should begin immediately.
    - Avoid inversion initially (Ruda 1991).
  - Achilles tendon stretching.
  - after 48 hours, patient may start "drawing the alphabet" with the foot.
  - toe/heel walking when normal ambulation is no longer painful.
  - proprioceptive training.

CONSULTATION

→ Indications for immediate referral to an orthopedist:
  - fracture.
  - obvious deformity.
  - signs of neurovascular compromise.
  - penetrating wound into the joint space.
  - locking of the ankle joint.
  - high index of suspicion of grade III sprain.
  - syndesmotic injury (Hergenroeder 1990).

→ Referral to an orthopedist should be made if the patient has a history of recurrent ankle sprains.

PATIENT EDUCATION

→ Discuss the mechanics of ankle sprain and the extent of the injury.

→ Advise the patient that ice should remain on the injured site three to five minutes after the area becomes numb (Diamond 1989).

→ For the athletic patient, the best "bracing" combination to prevent re-injury of the ankle is the use of low-top shoes with a lace-up ankle stabilizer (Miller and Hergenroeder 1990).

→ Advise that repair of a torn ligament may take as long as a year.
  - Therefore, the use of external ankle supports are encouraged during weight-bearing athletic activities for 12 months after injury (De Maio, Paine, and Drez 1992a, 1992b).
  - If the patient is casted, instruct regarding signs and symptoms of tightness: increased pain and swelling, numbness, and tingling (Ruda 1991).
  - Recommend heel cord stretching—prevents re-injury to the ankle (Lassiter, Malone, and Garrett 1989).

FOLLOW-UP

→ Patients should be scheduled for a follow-up visit two to four weeks following an acute sprain, depending on the clinical findings noted during the initial evaluation.

→ Patients are encouraged to seek medical consultation if they have recurrent ankle sprain or are experiencing symptoms indicative of complications of ankle sprains—e.g., persistent snapping in osteochondral lesions, progressive flat foot in tibial tendon ruptures, and constant giving way.

→ Document in progress notes and problem list.

Diane C. Putney, R.N., C., M.N., N.P.

8-L

Foot Pain

When the patient presents with a chief complaint of *foot pain*, more often than not careful history taking and a precise and perfunctory examination will culminate in a timely diagnosis of *plantar fasciitis*, sometimes referred to as *painful heel syndrome*.

The plantar fascia's main function is to preserve the integrity of the longitudinal arch (Warren 1990). The plantar fascia consists of multiple bundles of collagen and fibroblasts, and originates from the medial calcaneal tuberosity. Running the length of the foot, the plantar fascia inserts into the proximal phalanges (Dreeben and Mann 1992).

Plantar fasciitis is a clinical entity for which there exists any number of contributing factors and no one clearly established cause. The predominant symptom of plantar fasciitis is severe heel pain on the plantar surface of the foot, which is thought to result from inflammation at the site of the plantar fascia attachment to the medial plantar surface of the calcaneal tuberosity (Dreeban and Mann 1992; Warren 1990).

Repetitive strain from relatively normal use can cause microtearing of the plantar fascia, which results in inflammation and pain (Torg, Welsh, and Shepard 1990). An inferior calcaneal spur may be the incidental byproduct of periosteal detachment, hemorrhage, and osteoblastic activity (Warren 1990). Patients with heel pain tend to characterize the problem as "heel spurs," even before existence of the condition has been established by the appropriate radiograph. The incidence of spurs in heel pain syndromes is present in only 50 percent of persons with plantar fasciitis (Dreeban and Mann 1992).

Plantar fasciitis plagues both men and women throughout adulthood. The patient with the presenting complaint of heel pain usually does not recount a specific precipitating traumatic event. Rather, plantar fasciitis appears to result from the cumulative effects of biomechanical abnormalities of the foot, such as excessively high arches or rigid flat feet, over use syndromes in the athlete, inadequate running shoes, excessive body weight, and underlying systemic disorders, as well as occupations which require prolonged periods of standing and walking (Kibler, Goldberg, and Chandler 1991; Hill 1989; Bucholz et al. 1984; Gormley and Kuwada 1992).

Plantar fasciitis most often involves one extremity. Even though there is a 15 percent incidence in both heels, other potential causes of pain, such as fat pad atrophy and spondylarthropathies, must be given careful consideration when the symptoms are bilateral and chronic (Dreeban and Mann 1992).

The patient with plantar fasciitis frequently experiences a transience in symptoms with varying degrees of intensity over a protracted period of weeks and months and consequent delays seeking medical treatment. Once the patient presents to the clinician for evaluation of heel pain, the pain often is described as an agonizing, sometimes incapacitating phenomenon. Since the diagnosis of plantar fasciitis usually is made readily and within minutes, it is essential to reassure the patient of the benign and ubiquitous nature of the condition, and discuss the high rate of success with conservative treatment.

DATABASE

SUBJECTIVE

→ Patients of all ages, most frequently 40- to 50-year-olds.

→ Patient has history of:

- diabetes, gout, PVD, RA, SLE.
- obesity, often with a history of *sudden* weight gain.
- occupations which require prolonged standing—e.g., security guard, grocery checkers.

→ Patient reports recent change in shoe wear—e.g., deciding to wear flat shoes, ironically, "for comfort."

→ Athletes whose main sport is running sometimes report sudden onset, often precipated by change in running routines, increasing mileage.

→ Patient reports gradual onset of symptoms.

→ Symptoms include severe heel pain usually localized on the medial plantar fascia of the calcaneal tuberosity.

→ Pain most severe upon arising in the morning and after prolonged periods of sedentary activity; often abates during the day with normal ambulation, only to return at the end of the day; exacerbated by walking and stair climbing.

→ If patient reports sudden onset of pain with a painful tearing or popping sensation, rupture of the plantar fascia should be considered.

→ Poorly localized pain extending throughout the arch may indicate distal plantar fasciitis.

OBJECTIVE

→ Patient may present with:
- most often excessively high arches, or pes cavus; sometimes a rigid flat foot, pes planus.
- normal skin color, usually without the presence of edema.
- severe tenderness to palpation over the medial plantar aspect of the calcaneal tuberosity, which is the most important finding.
- pain sometimes elicited along the more proximal fascia with passive dorsiflexion of the toe or eversion of the heel and pronation of the forefoot.
- tight Achilles tendon as assessed by dorsiflexing the foot.
- diffuse tenderness along the mid-portion of the plantar fascia, a less frequent complaint.
- excessive pronation of the foot.
- valgus position of the heel.

→ Positive Tinel's sign, when the foot is percussed over the tarsal tunnel just posterior and distal to the tip of the medial malleolus, suggests tarsal tunnel syndrome.

ASSESSMENT

→ Plantar fasciitis

→ R/O heel pad atrophy

→ R/O ruptured plantar fascia

→ R/O tarsal tunnel syndrome

→ R/O Achilles tendinitis

→ R/O ankylosing spondylosis if complaints are bilateral

→ R/O gout

→ R/O retrocalcaneal bursitis

→ R/O calcaneal fracture (with a precipitating history of trauma)

→ R/O calcaneal stress fracture

PLAN

DIAGNOSTIC TESTS

→ X-rays.
- Lateral and calcaneal views of the affected heel are usually adequate when the symptoms and signs are confined to that area.
  - Demonstrate presence of inferior calcaneal spur 50 percent of the time.

→ Bone scan may confirm fractures or an inflammatory process when the diagnosis is in question.

→ Laboratory.
- CBC, ESR, ANA, RF and HLA B27; uric acid as indicated when considering underlying systemic condition.

TREATMENT/MANAGEMENT

→ NSAIDs for 4 to 6 weeks may be employed. See **Table 8-M,** p. 8-50.

→ Cortisone injection into the plantar fascia is rapidly effective and has an overall superior degree of therapeutic efficacy.

→ Daily heel cord stretching recommended.

→ Heel supports—which may include heel cushions and full-length semi-rigid orthotics—e.g., Spenco Tri-Tec Heel Supports or Spenco Semi-Rigid Orthotics—may be helpful in individuals with medial longitudinal arch pain and flat feet.

→ Short-leg walking cast for 4 to 6 weeks is recommended if NSAIDs fail or are contra-indicated by the patient's medical condition, of if patient refuses to submit to a cortisone injection.

→ Ice massage for 20 minutes, several times a day may be helpful.

→ Occasionally, referral to a physical therapist for the administration of phonophoresis is helpful, especially if the patient refuses an injection and has exhausted other treatment options.

CONSULTATION

→ The patient should be referred to a nurse practitioner or physician—not necessarily an orthopedist—who is skilled in administering a cortisone injection into the plantar fascia attachment when the patient requests this method of treatment, or when other means of treatment have failed and the symptoms are severe and disabling.

→ Orthopedic consultation is warranted when conservative treatment has failed for a year and a plantar fascia release is indicated.

→ Referral to a rheumatologist is indicated if an underlying rheumatological condition is determined to be the main cause of the patient's symptoms.

→ Since surgery (although relatively successful), is considered a last resort for treatment of plantar fasciitis, it is worthwhile to consider consultation with a physiatrist before sending the patient for evaluation for surgical plantar fascia release.

→ As needed for prescription(s).

PATIENT EDUCATION

→ Teach the patient the biomechanical and pathophysiological mechanisms of plantar fasciitis, and inform the patient that relief of symptoms may be only temporary.

→ Advise the obese patient that weight loss is imperative.

→ Instruct the patient to avoid weight-bearing exercise and athletics while the heel pain is resolving and for approximately four weeks after resolution of the pain.

→ Advise the patient to avoid ambulating while barefoot.

→ Advise avoidance of shoes with either too high or too flat an arch.

→ Advise the patient that assiduous compliance with daily heel cord stretching is essential.

→ Instruct patient in appropriate use of orthotic devices.

→ Educate the patient about the potential side effects of NSAIDs and cortisone injections into the plantar fascia—e.g., plantar fascia rupture and heel pad atrophy.

FOLLOW-UP

→ The patient should have a follow-up visit approximately six weeks after treatment is initiated.

→ Patients are encouraged to seek medical consultation if symptoms remain intractable and recurrent over the course of a year.

→ Document in progress notes and problem list.

Table 8-M. ANTI-INFLAMMATORY AGENTS

Drug	Anti-Inflammatory Dose	Side Effects	Comments
Acetylsalicyclic Acid			
ASA	4 gm-5 gm/day in 3-4 divided doses (12-16 tablets); JRA begin 80-90 mg/kg/d up to 100-120 mg/kg/d	Tinnitus; epigastric distress, gastric erosions/ulcers; bronchospasm; urticaria; angioedema	Buffered and enteric-coated preps available. Combination preps abound. Zero order release (Zorprin) available
NSAIDs			
Phenylbutazone (Butazolidin®) [100 mg]	100 mg TID–QID; load 1st 800 mg (1st 24 hrs), 600 mg (2nd 24 hrs)	Bone marrow depression; gastric irritation; fluid retention, rashes, parotitis	Use in gout, ps gout, spondyloarthritis; occas. tendinitis; not for RA or OA generally; potentiates coumadin, demerol, MS and oral hypoglycemics
Indomethacin (Indocin®) [25/50/75 mg SR]	25 mg BID–50 mg QID	Gastritis, ulcers; headaches, dizziness, drowsiness, depersonalization	Use in gout, ps gout, OA, spondyloarthritis, tendinitis, RA at bedtime; will increase lithium levels
Ibuprofen (Motrin®, Rufen®) [200/300/400/600/800 mg]	1600 mg–3200 mg (in 3–4 divided doses); ≤1600 mg analgesic but not anti-inflammatory	Gastritis, bleeding, nausea; fluid retention; rashes; toxic hepatitis, and aseptic meningitis—rare	Use in OA, RA; analgesic safe, effective first-line therapy
Tolmetin (Tolectin®) [200/400 mg DS]	1200 mg-1600 mg (in 3-4 divided doses); JRA 15-30 mg/kg/d	Dyspepsia, gastritis, ulcer bleeding; fluid retention; headache, dizziness; rashes, anaphylactic reactions; interstitial nephritis—renal impairment	Use in OA, RA, JRA; analgesic
Fenoprofen (Nalfon®) [200/300/600 mg]	1200 mg-2400 mg (in 3-4 divided doses)	Interstitial nephritis—renal failure; dyspepsia, gastritis, ulcer, constipation; headaches, somnolence; rashes; fluid retention	Do not use in renal impairment; administer 30 min. before or at least 2 hrs. after meals unless GU symptoms
Naproxen (Naprosyn®) [250/375/500 mg 125 mg/5 ml]	250 mg-500 mg BID; JRA 10 mg/kg/d in 2 divided doses	Nausea, gastritis, bleeding; fluid retention; rare: rashes	Use in OA, RA, JRA; gout, spondylitis, tendinitis; analgesic (Anaprox); benemid increases naproxen levels; offers no real advantage over ibuprofen other than inter-patient variation
Sulindac (Clinoril®) [150/200 mg]	150 mg-200 mg BID	Dyspepsia, gastritis, ulcer, constipation; hypersensitivity reaction; rare: liver dysfunction, rashes	Use in OA, RA, gout, spondylitis, tendinitis; does not affect platelet aggregation; prob. *NSAID with least effect on renal function*
Meclofenamate (Melclomen®) [50/100 mg]	100 mg TID-QID	Diarrhea, GI pain, nausea; rash; dizziness	Use in RA, OA; potentiates coumadin; ASA lowers meclofen levels; may take up to 7 days to show significant effect and up to 14 days to show maximal benefit
Piroxicam (Feldene®) [10/20 mg]	10 mg-20 mg every day	Very high incidence of GI upsets: epigastric distress, bleeding, ulcers, rashes	Use in OA, RA, spondylitis; cautiously use with coumadin in the elderly
Diflunisal (Dolobid®) [250/500 mg]	500 mg BID	GI symptoms; rash; headache; tinnitus	Use as analgesic; also in OA, RA
Ketoprofen (Orudis®) [50/75 mg]	75 mg-100 mg TID	GI symptoms; CNS symptoms (HA, dizziness, drowsiness); tinnitus, rashes; renal	Use in RA, OA; reduce dose by ½ - ⅓ in elderly and with impaired renal function; careful with hypoalbuminemia
Diclofenac (Voltaren®) [25/50/75 mg]	100 mg-200 mg total daily dose	GI symptoms; CNS symptoms (HA, dizziness); ↑ LFTs	OA up to 150 mg/d RA up to 200 mg/d (divided doses) AS up to 125 mg/d (divided doses)
Flurbiprofen (Ansaid®) [50/100 mg]	200 mg-300 mg total daily dose	GI symptoms (diarrhea, etc); CNS symptoms (HA, anxiety, etc); GU (UTI) symptoms	For RA and OA use up to 300 mg/d (divided dose)

Continued

Table 8M. ANTI-INFLAMMATORY AGENTS (CONTINUED)

Drug	Anti-Inflammatory Dose	Side Effects	Comments
Non-Acetylated Salicylates			
Salsalate (Disalcid®/Salflex®) [500/750 mg]	1500 mg BID 1000 mg BID	salicylism (tinnitus, ↓ hearing, vertigo); rash; GI symptoms	less GI and renal toxicity than ASA and NSAIDs; less effect on PGs and coag. Use OA/RA analgesia
Mg Salicylate (Magan®) [500 mg]	2 tabs TID	as above	as above
Choline Mg Trilisate (Trilisate®) [500/750/1000 mg 500 mg/5 ml]	750 mg TID to 1500 mg BID children: 50 mg/kg/d	as above	as above

NOTE: Providers are encouraged to refer to the *Physicians' Desk Reference (PDR)* prior to prescribing above medications.

Sources: Adapted from Scopelitis, E. 1992. *Anti-inflammatory agents.* As presented in a lecture by Wilma Wooten, M.D., M.P.H., at the Sixth Annual Sports Medicine Conference: A Practical Approach for the Primary Care Physician, July 27-31. University of California, San Diego. NSAID Algorithm for Orthopedics; internal document 1992. Kaiser Permanente Medical Center, South San Francisco, CA.

8-N
Bibliography

Altman, R.D. 1990. Osteoarthritis: Differentiation from rheumatoid arthritis, causes of pain, treatment. *Postgraduate medicine* 87:66–78.

———. 1991. Classification of disease: Osteoarthritis. *Seminars in Arthritis and Rheumatism* 20:40–47.

Anderson, B.J., and Burchiel, K.J. 1991. Surgical treatment of low back pain. *Neurology Clinics of North America* 2:921–931.

Baker, E.L., and Ehrenberg R.L. 1990. Preventing the work-related carpal tunnel syndrome: Physician's reporting and diagnostic criteria. *Annals of Internal Medicine* 12:317–319.

Barker, L.R., Burton, J.R., and Zieve, P.D. 1982. *Principles of ambulatory care medicine.* Baltimore: Williams & Wilkins.

Baron, M., and Zendel, I. 1989. HLA-B27 testing in ankylosing spondylitis: Analysis of the pretesting assumptions. *Journal of Rheumatology* 16:631–636.

Baum, J. 1989. Joint pain: It isn't always arthritis. *Postgraduate Medicine* 85:311–316.

Beary III, J.F., Christian, C.L., and Johanson, N.A. 1988. *Manual of rheumatology and outpatient orthopedic disorders: Diagnosis and treatment;* 2d ed. Boston: Little, Brown and Company.

Blauvelt, C.T., and Nelson, F.R.T.C. 1990. *A manual of orthopedic terminology,* 4th ed. St. Louis: C.V. Mosby.

Boytim, M., Fischer, D. A., and Neuman, L. 1991. Ankle sprains. *The American Journal of Sports Medicine* 19:294–298.

Brand, R.L. 1992. Ligamentous injuries to the lateral aspect of the ankle: The ankle sprain. *Journal of the Medical Association of Georgia* 81:293–295.

Brier, S.R. 1992. Rotator cuff disease: Current trends in orthopedic management. *Journal of Manipulative Physiotherapy* 15:123–128.

Brown, M.D. 1992. The pathophysiology and diagnosis of low back pain and sciatica. *Instructional Course Lectures* 41:205–215.

Bucholz, R.W., Lippert, F.G., Wenger, D.R., and Ezaki, M. 1984. *Orthopaedic decision making.* Philadelphia: B.C. Decker.

Burns, T.P., and Turba, J.E. 1992. Arthroscopic treatment of shoulder impingement in athletes. *The American Journal of Sports Medicine* 20:13–16.

Carragee, E.J., and Hentz, V.R. 1988. Repetitive trauma and nerve compression. *Orthopedic Clinics of North America* 19:157–164.

Chard, M.D., Hazelman, B.L., King, R.H., and Reiss, B.B. 1991. Shoulder disorders in the elderly: A community survey. *Arthritis and Rheumatism* 34:766–769.

Chase, J.A. 1991. Spinal stenosis: When arthritis is more than arthritis. *Nursing Clinics of North America* 26:53–65.

Cho, D.S., and Cho, M.J. 1989. The electrodiagnosis of the carpal tunnel syndrome. *South Dakota Journal of Medicine* July:5–8.

Chop, W.H. 1989. Tennis elbow. *Postgraduate Medicine* 86:301–307.

Clancy, W.G. 1989. Specific rehabilitation for the recreational runner. *Instructional Course Lectures* 38:483–486.

Collee, G., Dijkmans, B.A., and Vandenbruucke, J.P. 1991. Greater trochanteric pain syndrome (trochanteric bursitis) in low back pain. *The Scandinavian Journal of Rheumatology* 20:262–266.

Corrigan, B., and Maitland, G.D. 1989. *Practical orthopaedic medicine.* Boston: Butterworths Company.

Craig, E.V., and Kuang-Chi, H. 1992. Shoulder problems in the weekend athlete. *Orthopaedic Review* 21:155–167.

Croft, P., Cooper, C., Wickham, C., and Coggon, P. 1992. Is the hip involved in generalized osteoarthritis? *British Journal of Rhematology* 31:325–328.

DeMaio, M., Paine, R., and Drez, D. 1992a. Chronic lateral ankle instability—inversion sprains: Part I. *Orthopedics* 15:87–96.

———. 1992b. Chronic lateral ankle instability—inversion sprains: Part II. *Orthopedics* 15:241–248.

Diamond, J.E. 1989. Rehabilitation of ankle sprains. *Clinics in Sports Medicine* 8:877–891.

Dreeban, S.M., and Mann, R. 1992. Heel pain: Sorting through the differential diagnosis. *The Journal of Musculoskeletal Medicine* 9:21–37.

Farin, P.U., Jaroma, H., Harjn, A., and Suimakallio, S. 1990. Shoulder impingement syndrome: Sonographic evaluation. *Radiology* 176:845–849.

Felson, D.T. 1992. Obesity and osteoarthritis of the knee. *Bulletin on the Rheumatic Diseases* 41:6–7.

Fields, K.B., Rasco, T., Kramer, J.S., and Cates, R. 1992. Rehabilitation exercises for common sports injuries. *American Family Physician* 45:1233–1243.

Freiberg, A., Mulholland, R.S., and Levine, R. 1989. Treatment of trigger fingers and thumbs. *The Journal of Hand Surgery* 14A:553–558.

Frymoyer, W., and Cats-Biril, W.L. 1991. An overview of the incidences and costs of low back pain. *The Orthopedic Clinics* 22:264.

Fu, F., Harner, C.O., and Klein, A.H. 1991. Shoulder impingement syndrome: A critical review. *Clinical Orthopaedics and Related Research* 269:162–173.

Fulkerson, J.P., Kalenak, A., Rosenberg, T.D., and Cox, J.S. 1992. Patellofemoral pain. *Instructional Course Lectures* 41:57–71.

Gellman, H. 1992. Tennis elbow (lateral epicondylitis). *Orthopedic Clinics of North America* 23:75–82.

Gormley, J., and Kuwada, G.T. 1992. Retrospective analysis of calcaneal spur removal and complete fascial release for the treatment of chronic heel pain. *The Journal of Foot Surgery* 31:166–169.

Greenspan, J. 1988. Carpal tunnel syndrome: A common but treatable cause of wrist pain. *Postgraduate Medicine* 84:34–43.

Haller, C.C., Coleman, P.A., Estes, W.C., and Grisolia, A. 1989. Traumatic trochanteric bursitis. *Kansas Medicine* (January):17–22.

Handell, B.F. 1990. Avascular necrosis of the femoral head presenting as trochanteric bursitis. *Annals of Rheumatic Diseases* 49:730–733.

Harter, B.T. 1989. Indications for surgery in work-related compression neuropathies of the upper extremity. *Occupational Medicine* 4:485–495.

Harvey, F.J., Harvey, P.M., and Horsley, M.W. 1990. De Quervain's disease: Surgical or nonsurgical treatment? *The Journal of Hand Surgery* 15A:87.

Heliovaara, M., Makela, M., Knekt, P., Impivaara, O., and Aromaa, A. 1991. Determinants of sciatica and low back pain. *Spine* 16:608–614.

Hergenroeder, A.C. 1990. Diagnosis and treatment of ankle sprains. *Sports Medicine* 85:153–163.

Hill, J.J. 1989. Heel pain and body weight. *Foot and Ankle* 9:254–256.

Hooke, N.L. 1991. Diagnosis and treatment of shoulder injuries in the athlete. *Sports Nursing* 26:199–209.

Hunter, S.C., and Poole, R.M. 1987. The chronically inflamed tendon. *Clinics in Sports Medicine* 6:371–389.

Ireland, D.C.R. 1986. The hand: Part one. *Australian Family Physician* 15:1162–1171.

Iversen, L.D. and Clawson, D.K. 1987. *Manual of acute orthopaedic therapeutics*, 3rd ed. Boston: Little, Brown and Company.

Kaiser Permanente Medical Center. NSAID algorithm for orthopedics. South San Francisco: the Author.

Keene, J.S. 1989. Diagnosis of undetected knee injuries. *Postgraduate Medicine* 85:153–163.

Kibler, W.S., Goldberg, C., and Chandler, T.J. 1991. Functional biomechanical deficits in running athletes with plantar fasciitis. *American Journal of Sports Medicine* 19:66–71.

Kiefhaber, T.R., and Stern, P.J. 1992. Upper extremity tendinitis and overuse syndromes and tendon injuries. *Hand Clinics* 6:467–476.

Krinsky, M.B., Abdenour, T.E., Strakey, C., Albo, R.A., and Chu, D.A. 1992. Incidence of lateral meniscus injury in professional basketball players. *The American Journal of Sports Medicine* 20:17–19.

Lassiter, T.E., Malone, T.R., and Garrett, W.E. 1989. Injury to the lateral ligaments of the ankle. *Orthopedic Clinics of North America* 4:629–640.

Leach, R.E., and Miller, J.K. 1987. Lateral and medial epicondylitis of the elbow. *Clinics in Sports Medicine* 6:259–272.

Lewis, R.C. 1988. *Primary care orthopedics*. New York: Churchill Livingstone.

Liang, M.H., and Fortin, P. 1991. Management of osteoarthritis of the hip and knee. *The New England Journal of Medicine* 325:125–127.

Lluch, A.L. 1992. Thickening of the synovium of the digital flexor tensions: Cause or consequence of the carpal tunnel syndrome. *The Journal of Hand Surgery* 17B:209–212.

Macnicol, M.F. 1986. *The problem knee: Diagnosis and management in the younger patient.* Rockville, MD: Aspen Publishers.

Mandell, B.F. 1990. Avascular necrosis of the femoral head presenting as trochanteric bursitis. *Annals of Rheumatic Disease* 49:730–732.

Manders, K.L. 1989. Lumbar disorders: When and when not to operate. *Seminars in Neurology* 9:186–192.

Mascola, J.R., and Rickman, L.S. 1991. Infectious causes of carpal tunnel syndrome: Case report and review. *Reviews of Infectious Diseases* 13:911–917.

McAlindon, T., and Dieppe, P. 1990. The medical management of osteoarthritis of the knee: An inflammatory issue. *British Journal of Rheumatology* 29:471–473.

McCowin, P.R., Borenstein, D., and Wiesel, S. 1991. The current approach to the medical diagnosis of low back pain. *Orthopedic Clinics of North America* 22:315–325.

McPherson, S.A., and Meals, R.A. 1992. Cubital tunnel syndrome. *Orthopedic Clinics of North America* 23:111–123.

McRae, R. 1990. *Clinical orthopaedic examination,* 3rd ed. New York: Churchill Livingstone.

Miller, E.A., and Hergenroeder, A.L. 1990. Prophylactic ankle bracing. *Pediatric Clinics of North America* 37:1175–1185.

Milgrom, Z., Einkerem, J., Finestone, A., Eldad, A., and Shlamkovitch, N. 1991. Patellofemoral pain caused by overactivity. A prospective study of risk factors in infantry recruits. *The Journal of Bone and Joint Surgery* 73(7):1041–1043.

Murtagh, J. 1989. De Quervain's tenosynovitis and Finkelstein's test. *Australian Family Physician* 18:1552.

Nachemson, A.L. 1992. Newest knowledge of low back pain: A critical look. *Clinical Orthopaedics and Related Research* 279:8–20.

Nakano, K.K. 1991. Peripheral nerve entrapments, repetitive strain disorder, occupation-related syndromes, bursitis, tendinitis. *Current Opinion in Rheumatology* 3:226–239.

Newport, M.L., Lane, L.B., Manhasser, N.Y., and Stuchin, S.A. 1992. A treatment of trigger finger by steroid injection. *The Journal of Hand Surgery* 17A:748–750.

Neviaser, R.J., and Neviaser, T.J. 1990. Observations on impingement. *Clinical Orthopaedics and Related Research* 254:60–63.

Nirschl, R.P. 1989. Rotator cuff tendinitis: Basic concepts of pathoetiology. *Sports Medicine: Instructional Course Lectures* 386:439–455.

Oden, R.R. 1987. Tendon injuries about the ankle resulting from skiing. *Clinical Orthopaedics and Related Research* 216:63–69.

O'Neill, D.B., Micheli, L.J., and Warner, S.P. 1992. Patellofemoral stress: A prospective analysis of exercise treatment in adolescents and adults. *The American Journal of Sports Medicine* 20:151–156.

Patel, H.R., and Bassini, L. 1992. Trigger fingers and thumb: When to splint, inject, or operate. *The Journal of Hand Surgery* 17A:110–113.

Pellegrini, V.D. 1992. Osteoarthritis at the base of the thumb. *Orthopedic Clinics of North America* 23:83–102.

Persselin, J.E. 1991. Diagnosis of rheumatoid arthritis: Medical and laboratory aspects. *Clinical Orthopaedics and Related Research* 265:73–82.

Plattner, P.F. 1989. Tendon problems of the foot and ankle. *Postgraduate Medicine* 86:155–169.

Post, M., and Benca, P. 1989. Primary tendinitis of the long head of the biceps. *Clinical Orthopedics and Related Research* 246:117–125.

Quinet, R.J. 1986. Osteoarthritis: Increasing mobility and reducing disability. *Geriatrics* 41:36–50.

Radin, E.L., Burr, D.B., Caterson, B., Fyhrie, D., Brown, T.D., and Boyd, R.D. 1991. Mechanical determinants of osteoarthrosis. *Seminars in Arthritis and Rheumatism* 21:12–21.

Reilly, J.P., and Nicholas, J.A. 1987. The chronically inflamed bursa. *Clinics in Sports Medicine* 6:345–371.

Rizk, T.E., Pinals, R.S., and Talaiver, A.S. 1991. Corticosteroid injections in adhesive capsulitis: Investigation of their value and site. *Archives of Physical Medicine and Rehabilitation* 72:20–22.

Ruda, S.C. 1991. Common ankle injuries in the ankle. *Nursing Clinics of North America* 26:167–181.

Ryan, J.B. Hopkinson, W.J., Wheeler, J.H., Arciero, R.A., and Swain, J.H. 1989. Office management of the acute ankle sprain. *Clinics of Sports Medicine* 8:477–495.

Saal, J.A. 1989. Nonoperative treatment of herniated lumbar intervertebral disc with radiculopathy: An outline study. *Spine* 14:431–437.

Schenck, R.R. 1989. Carpal tunnel syndrome: The new "industrial epidemic." *AAOHN Journal* 37:226–230.

Scopelitis, E. 1992. *Anti-inflammatory agents.* Sixth Annual Sports Medicine Conference: A Practical Approach for the Primary Care Physician, July 27-31. University of California, San Diego.

Semble, E.L., Loeser, R.F., and Wise, C.M. 1990. Therapeutic exercise for rheumatoid arthritis and osteoarthritis. *Seminars in Arthritis and Rheumatology* 20:32–40.

Shellenbarger, T. 1991. When you're asked about carpal tunnel syndrome. *RN* 54(7):40–42.

Siebenaler, M.J. 1992. Carpal tunnel syndrome: Priorities for prevention. *AAOHN Journal* 40:62–70.

Smith, C.A., and Arnett, F.C. 1990. Epidemiological aspects of rheumatoid arthritis: Current immunogenetic approach. *Clinical Orthopaedics and Related Research* 265:23–35.

Smith, D.L., and Campbell, S.M. 1992. Painful shoulder syndromes: Diagnosis and management. *Journal of General Internal Medicine* 7:328–339.

Spinner, R.J., Bachman, J.W., and Amadio, P.C. 1989. The many faces of carpal tunnel syndrome. *Mayo Clinic Procedures* 64:829–836.

Stanley, K.L. 1991. Ankle sprains are always more than "just a sprain." *Postgraduate Medicine* 89:251–255.

Stern, P.J. 1990. Tendinitis, overuse syndromes, and tendon injuries. *Hand Clinics* 6:467–476.

Strickland, J.W., Idler, R.S., and Creighton, J.C. 1990a. De Quervain's stenosing tenosynovitis. *Indiana Medicine* 83(5):340–341.

———. 1990b. Osteoarthritis of the carpometacarpal joint of the thumb. *Indiana Medicine* 83(11):828–830.

Szabo, R.M., and Madison, M. 1992. Carpal tunnel syndrome. *Orthopedic Clinics of North America* 23:103–109.

Taylor, P.W. 1989. Inflammation of the deep infrapatellar bursa of the knee. *Arthritis and Rheumatism* 32:1312–1314.

Thorson, E., and Szabo, R. M. 1992. Common tendinitis problems in the hand and forearm. *Orthopedic Clinics of North America* 23:65–74.

Toohey, A.K., Lasalle, T.L., Martinez, S., and Polisson, R.P. 1990. Iliopsoas bursitis: Clinical features, radiographic findings, and disease associations. *Seminars in Arthritis and Rheumatism* 20:41–46.

Torg, J.S., Welsh, R.P., and Shepard, R.J. 1990. *Current theory in sports medicine*. Philadelphia: B.C. Decker.

Walk, L. 1989. Pain on coughing and numbness in sciatica: What exactly do these symptoms mean? *Archives of Surgery* 124:751.

Warren, B.L. 1990. Plantar fasciitis in runners: Treatment and prevention. *Sports Medicine* 10:338–345.

Warren, R.F., and O'Brien, S.J. 1989. Shoulder pain in the geriatric patient: Part II: Treatment options. *Orthopaedic Review* 18:248–263.

Watson, M. 1989. Rotator cuff function in the impingement syndrome. *The Journal of Bone and Joint Surgery* 3:361–366.

Weiss, A.P., and Akelman, E. 1992. Carpal tunnel syndrome: A review. *Rhode Island Medicine* 75:303–306.

Witczak, J.W., Maseur, V.R., and Meyer, R.D. 1990. Triggering of the thumb with de Quervain's stenosing tendovaginitis. *The Journal of Hand Surgery* 15A:265–268.

Witt, J., Pess, G., and Gelberman, R.H. 1991. Treatment of de Quervain's tenosynovitis. *The Journal of Bone and Joint Surgery* 73-A:219–222.

Wolock, B.S., Moore, R.J., and Weiland, A.J. 1989. Arthritis of the basal joint of the thumb: A critical analysis of treatment options. *The Journal of Arthroplasty* 4:65–78.

Zimmer, T.J. 1991. Chronic and recurrent ankle sprains. *Clinics in Sports Medicine* 3:653–659.

Zuckerman, J., Mirabello, S.C., Newman, D., Gallagher, M., and Cuomo, F. 1991. The painful shoulder: Part II: Intrinsic disorders and impingement syndrome. *American Family Physician* 43:497–512.

SECTION 9

Neurological Disorders

9-A

Bell's Palsy

Bell's palsy (idiopathic facial paralysis) is an acute paralysis of the seventh cranial nerve, the facial nerve. According to Adour (1982), there also can be dysfunction of the other cranial nerves such as the fifth, eighth, ninth, and tenth, and even the second cervical nerve. Thus, Bell's palsy can be considered a cranial polyneuritis. A viral etiology for Bell's palsy has been postulated in the literature. Adour (1991) states that an autoimmune reactivation of the herpes simplex virus (HSV) is the most likely cause.

The incidence of Bell's palsy has been estimated at ten to thirty cases per 100,000, occurring mostly in those between 15 years and 45 years of age (Petruzzelli and Hirsch 1991). However, persons of any age may be affected.

Females and males are affected approximately equally. In women, there is a higher incidence in the third trimester of pregnancy and early postpartum period. Hilsinger Jr., Adour, and Doty (1975) report a 3.3 times higher risk in pregnant women than in non-pregnant women. Also, they noticed 65.5 percent of their Bell's palsy patients reported the onset during the first half of their menstrual cycles, with the peak at day one. There is a small familial predisposition for Bell's palsy.

Diabetics are 4.5 times more likely to have Bell's palsy, and this can be the presenting symptom of diabetes (Adour, Wingerd, and Doty 1975). Diabetics are also more likely to get recurrent Bell's palsy.

The left and right side of the face are affected equally. There is a less than one percent incidence of bilateral Bell's palsy and a ten percent incidence of recurrence, either ipsilateral or contralateral (Adour 1991).

With an understanding of the anatomy of the facial nerve, the signs and symptoms of Bell's palsy are more easily comprehended (see **Figure 9A.1, Distribution of the Facial Nerve**). The motor facial nerve begins at the pons, and with the nervus intermedius (the sensory and parasympathetic part of the facial nerve), enters the facial canal through the internal auditory canal. There, the fibers branch off to the lacrimal glands, the stapedius muscle in the ear, anterior two-thirds taste fibers of the tongue, and sublingual and submandibular salivary glands. After the motor facial nerve exits through the stylomastoid foramen, motor fibers go through the parotid gland to the facial muscles. Motor fibers and sensory fibers also go to the auditory canal, the pinna, and the mastoid area behind the ear (McArthur 1990).

The patient with Bell's palsy presents with an acute unilateral partial or complete facial paralysis. Frequently, paralysis is preceded by a viral syndrome. Other common complaints are facial or retroauricular pain in 60 percent, dysgeusia in 57 percent, hyperacusis in 30 percent, and decreased tearing in 17 percent (Adour 1982). Adour (1982) also reports that there often is hypesthesia or dysesthesia of the trigeminal nerve or glossopharyngeal nerve. Also, there sometimes may be hypesthesia of the second cervical nerve or a vagal motor weakness. While in some patients there may be decreased tear production, in others there may be increased tearing secondary to irritation because the eyelids are not able to close completely.

The course of Bell's palsy is favorable. Seventy-five to 90 percent recover satisfactorily without treatment (Pruitt 1987). Most people begin to recover in three weeks, and all begin to recover within six months (Hughes 1990). The longer it takes to begin to recover, the poorer the prognosis for complete recovery.

Figure 9A.1. DISTRIBUTION OF THE FACIAL NERVE

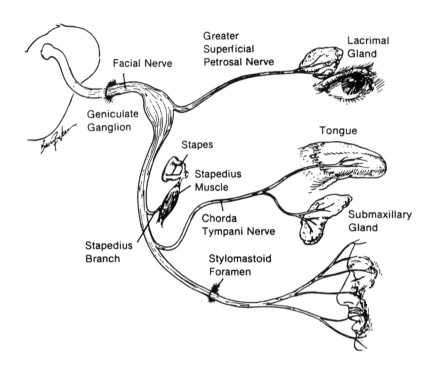

Source: Reprinted with permission from Alford, B.R., Jerger, J.E., Coats, A.C., Peterson, C.R., and Weber, S.C. 1973. Neurophysiology of facial nerve testing. *Archives of Otolaryngology* 97:215.

Complications arise from faulty nerve regeneration. They may consist of contractures, *synkinesis* (voluntary movement in one set of muscles which causes involuntary movement in others), facial spasms, and, uncommonly, crocodile tears. (Eating can cause large tear formation.) Those at highest risk for poor recovery are patients over age 55 years, diabetics, hypertensives, and patients with symptoms of hyperacusis, decreased tearing, ear pain, facial pain, and psychiatric disorders (Adour 1982; Ohye and Altenberger 1989).

Before a diagnosis of Bell's palsy is made, other causes of facial paralysis should be ruled out. The literature commonly mentions *Ramsay Hunt syndrome* (facial paralysis caused by the herpes zoster virus), diabetic neuropathy, trauma, tumors of the cerebellar pontine angle (CPA), primary parotid malignancy, Lyme disease, human immunodeficiency virus (HIV), and disorders of the ear such as otitis media and cholesteatoma. For a more complete list, see **Table 9A.1, Causes of Facial Paralysis.**

Although other cranial nerves can be affected in Bell's palsy, concern is heightened if there is more than a mild dysfunction. A parotid or CPA tumor should be suspected if the paralysis is progressive, if partial paralysis does not resolve in three to six weeks, or if complete paralysis lasts three to five months. Recurrent unilateral

Table 9A.1. CAUSES OF FACIAL PARALYSIS

Traumatic
Facial injuries
Birth trauma
Surgical trauma—e.g., parotid
  surgery

Infectious
Ramsay Hunt syndrome (herpes
  zoster)
Otitis media, otitis externa,
  mastoiditis
Mononucleosis
Tuberculosis
Lyme disease
Human immunodeficiency virus
  (HIV)
Syphilis
Polio
Mumps
Leprosy
Influenza
Botulism
Coxsackie virus
Cat scratch fever

Metabolic
Diabetes
Hyperthyroidism
Hypertension

Neoplastic
Cholesteatoma
Glomus jugulare tumor
Leukemia
Cerebellar pontine angle tumor
  (such as acoustic neuroma)
Parotid tumors, benign or
  malignant
Metastatic tumors from breast,
  lung, kidney, colon, skin

Neurological
Brain stem (pontine)
  (cerebrovascular accident
  [CVA])
Multiple sclerosis
Guillain-Barré syndrome
Myasthenia gravis (primarily
  bilateral paralysis)

Other
Pregnancy
Tetanus
Bell's palsy (infectious origin is
  suspected but not proven)

facial paralysis may be caused by a tumor and is of more concern than a recurrent contralateral paralysis.

DATABASE

SUBJECTIVE

→ Determine time of onset including:
  - prior episodes.
  - viral prodrome.
  - rate of progression.
  - area (side of paralysis).
  - associated Bell's palsy symptoms:
    • numbness.
    • pain.
    • eye irritation/tearing.
    • changes in hearing.
    • change in taste.
  - associated symptoms linked with other etiologies:
    • rash, change in vision, change in speech, swallowing difficulty, extremity weakness, numbness in extremities, ear pain, discharge, tinnitus, vertigo, joint pain, fever.

→ Present/past medical history:
  - recent immunizations, Lyme disease, HIV infection, herpes zoster, diabetes, tumors/malignancies, ear problems (including surgical trauma), last menstrual period, and, if pregnant, which trimester (see **Table 9A.1**).

→ Family history:
  - facial paralysis, diabetes, hypertension, hyperthyroidism.

→ Social history:
  - occupation, outdoor activities, history of alcohol/drugs, HIV risk factors.

OBJECTIVE

→ Check:
  - vital signs
  - blood pressure.
  - skin:
    • observe for vesicular facial rash.

→ Physical examination should include:
  - eyes:
    • tearing, redness, epiphora (drooping lower lid), Bell's phenomenon (when trying to close eyelids, the eyeballs roll upward and outward—a normal finding).
  - ears:
    • gross hearing, Weber and Rinne, canal for redness, discharge, swelling, tympanic

membrane for redness. A purple small mass may indicate a glomus tumor.
  - parotid:
    • a mass presenting with facial paralysis may be malignant.
  - mouth:
    • patient may be drooling.
    • inspect oral cavity for lesions.
  - neck:
    • nodes, salivary glands, thyroid gland, bruits.

→ Neurological examination should be performed with emphasis on cranial nerves.
  - Note especially if the patient has any facial movement which would indicate a partial paralysis and a better prognosis for Bell's palsy.
  - Observe whether there is forehead movement since preservation of forehead movement may be seen with a central brain lesion.
  - Note symmetry of the face at rest and with movement, ability to close eyes, corneal reflex, and ability to puff out cheeks.

ASSESSMENT

→ Bell's palsy
→ See **Table 9A.1** for differential diagnoses

PLAN

DIAGNOSTIC TESTS

→ Laboratory tests should include:
  - complete blood count (CBC).
  - fasting blood sugar if possible.
  - thyroid function tests.
  - Lyme titer if indicated.
  - HIV test if indicated.

→ If available, the Schirmer's test, which is 60 percent sensitive in Bell's palsy patients, is helpful in assessing lacrimation and, thus, prognosis (Hughes 1990). (See **Face Pain** Protocol.)

→ An audiogram is indicated, since decreased hearing is associated with tumors affecting the acoustic nerve.

→ A specialist may obtain an electrical stimulation test to assess prognosis.

→ Computerized tomography (CT) scan or magnetic resonance imaging (MRI) may be ordered for suspicion of a secondary cause for the paralysis.

TREATMENT/MANAGEMENT

→ The use of steroids has been controversial in the literature, but most sources say that prednisone may prevent denervation, shorten the course, slow the progression, and lessen sequelae (Stankiewicz 1983).

■ Adour (1991) states that prednisone greatly reduces pain and recommends using 1 mg/kg a day by mouth in divided doses for 5 days.
• If there is a partial paralysis, medication can be tapered over the next 5 days.
• If the progression is uncertain, the dosage should remain the same for the next 5 days with a gradual taper over 5 more days.
• The prednisone must be started within 3 weeks of onset (Hughes 1990).
• Contraindications to short-term prednisone are diabetes, uncontrolled hypertension, and peptic ulcer disease.
• Use in pregnancy should be determined by individual institutional protocols. See also *Physicians' Desk Reference (PDR)*.

→ In a recently completed study, Adour et al. (1992) found that acyclovir plus prednisone had a better outcome than prednisone alone.

■ They recommended the addition of acyclovir, 200 mg-400 mg by mouth, 5 times a day to a 10-day course of prednisone, tapered after the fifth day. (It remains to be seen which dose of acyclovir is preferred and if this regimen will be more widely accepted.)
• Acyclovir should be used with caution in patients with decreased renal function and pre-existing neurological dysfunction.
• Gastrointestinal disturbances are the most common side effects (see *PDR*).

→ Eye care is crucial to prevent corneal injury.
■ Sterile moisturizing drops should be used during the day and ointment such as Lacrilube® at night.
■ Sunglasses should be worn outside.
■ In the literature, there are different recommendations as to whether the eyes should be taped, patched, or a moisture chamber used. Rarely is lid tarsorrhaphy performed for eye protection.

→ Electromyographic (EMG) biofeedback, botulinum toxin injection, and surgical reanimation procedures have been investigated as ways to improve facial function after facial nerve paralysis, but studies are limited (May, Croxon, and Klein 1989).

→ Surgical techniques are used for acute cases of lagopthalmus to prevent exposure keratis. Upper lid problems are treated by gold implant, spring implant, and suture tarsorrhaphic techniques. Lower lid ectropion can be resolved with lateral canthoplasty (W. Barber, personal communication, April 1993).

→ Various surgical procedures have been incorporated to provide either facial symmetry at rest (dynamic slings, browlift) or physiological animation of the face (VII → XII cross-grafting procedure). In general, the rare cases of Bell's palsy that do not resolve spontaneously can be rehabilitated in some patients for aesthetic and functional improvement (W. Barber, personal communication, April 1993).

CONSULTATION

→ A physician should be consulted in all cases of facial paralysis, with referral as indicated.

PATIENT EDUCATION

→ Bell's palsy patients are naturally distressed over their appearance. Listen to the patient's concerns and offer reassurance that in most cases the prognosis is very good for return of facial appearance and function.

→ Since there is decreased taste and decreased motor control, nutrition may suffer. The patient and family should be encouraged to prepare well-seasoned food. Nutritional guidelines should be offered, and referral to a nutritionist may be indicated.

FOLLOW-UP

→ Referrals should be made promptly. Encourage the patient to follow through with appointments.

→ Document in progress notes and problem list.

Jacqueline W. Wasserman, R.N., C., M.S., F.N.P.

9-B

Dizziness/Vertigo

Dizziness is a broad term used to describe disorders of equilibrium. That includes normal bodily sensations, hyperventilation, presyncope, or vertigo. It refers to unsteadiness, without movement, motion, or spatial disorientation (Murtagh 1990).

Vertigo, more specifically, is a sensation of rotation or movement of one's self or of one's surroundings. It indicates a dysfunction of a specific organ system. The majority of dysfunctions are benign (Edmeads 1990). Most often the cause is within the inner ear. Eighty-five percent of individuals may have peripheral vestibular disorders and 15 percent have central disorders (Paparella, Alleva, and Bequer 1990). (See **Table 9B.1, Dizziness.**)

The following helpful mnemonic can outline potential causes of dizziness, including vertigo (Hanson 1989, with permission):

S **S**ystemic (e.g., cardiac disease, multiple sensory deficits).

N **N**eurological (e.g., multiple sclerosis, degenerative disease, migraine, vascular disorders).

O **O**phthalmological (e.g., refractive errors).

O **O**tolaryngological (e.g., labyrinthitis, trauma, tumor).

P **P**sychogenic (e.g., hyperventilation, hysteria).

See **Table 9B.1** for a subdivision of dizziness into categories and possible causes.

DATABASE

SUBJECTIVE

→ In determining the cause of dizziness, it is important to elicit the client's understanding of

Table 9B.1. DIZZINESS

VERTIGO		PSEUDOVERTIGO	
Peripheral Disorders			
■ *The most common causes:*	**Fainting or Syncopal Episodes**		**Disequilibrium**
• Benign positional vertigo	• Cardiogenic		• Neurogenic origins
• Vestibular neuronitis	• Postural hypotension—drug-induced		
• Acute viral labyrinthitis	• Vasovagal		
■ *Other causes:*	**Lightheadedness/Giddiness**		
• Ménière's disease	• Psychoneurotic		
• Drugs	• Hyperventilation		
• Trauma	• Postural hypotension		
• Acoustic neuroma	• Post head injury		
Central Disorders			
• Vertebro basilar insufficiency			
• Infarction			
• Degeneration			
• Tumors			

Source: Adapted with permission from Murtagh, J. 1991. Dizziness (vertigo). *Australian Family Physician* 20(10):1485-1486.

the symptom, including associated symptoms, frequency of symptoms, and precipitants as follows:

- sensation of uncertainty or ill-defined lightheadedness (giddiness).
- sensation of impending fainting or loss of consciousness (syncope).
- loss of balance or instability without any associated sensations of spinning.
- a symptom pattern that:
  - is paroxysmal or continuous.
  - effects position or changes posture.
- aural symptoms:
  - tinnitus.
  - deafness.
  - history of middle ear disease.
- visual symptoms:
  - double vision.
  - loss of vision.
- neurological symptoms:
  - history of central nervous system disease.
- associated nausea and vomiting.
- symptoms of psychoneurosis.
- history of recent upper respiratory infection.
- history of drugs taken:
  - alcohol.
  - marijuana.
  - hypertensives.
  - psychotropics.
  - other.

OBJECTIVE

→ Ear examination should include:
  - auroscopic examination:
    - checking for wax.
    - tympanic membrane assessment.
  - hearing test.
  - Weber and Rinne tests.
→ Eye examination should include:
  - visual acuity.
  - test movements for nystagmus (see "Diagnostic Tests" section).
→ Cranial nerves examination should include, in particular:
  - second (optic)—visual fields (bitemporal abnormality indicative of lesion).
  - fifth (trigeminal)—corneal reflex (sign of intracranial disease).
  - seventh (facial nerve)—facial strength.
  - eighth (auditory).
→ Neck examination should include:
  - cervical spine.
  - thyroid.

→ Cardiovascular examination should include:
  - blood pressure: supine, standing, sitting.
  - cardiac dysrhythmias.
  - evidence of atherosclerosis.
→ Cerebellar examination should include:
  - gait.
  - coordination.
  - reflexes.
  - Romberg test.
  - finger-nose test.

ASSESSMENT

Types of dizziness

→ Vertigo
  - Peripheral causes:
    - R/O benign positional vertigo
    - R/O vestibular neuronitis/labyrinthitis
    - R/O Ménière's disease
    - R/O motion sickness
    - R/O drug use
    - R/O local ear dysfunction
  - Central causes:
    - R/O brain stem ischemia
    - R/O cerebellar ischemia
    - R/O acoustic neuroma
    - R/O multiple sclerosis
    - R/O basilar artery migraine
    - R/O temporal lobe seizure
    - R/O posterior fossa tumor
→ Presyncope
  - R/O arrhythmias
  - R/O vasovagal reflex
  - R/O orthostatic hypotension
  - R/O aortic stenosis
  - R/O low cardiac output states
  - R/O anemia
  - R/O hypoglycemia
  - R/O hypoxemia
→ Disequilibrium
  - R/O cerebellar disease
  - R/O Parkinsonism
  - R/O drug use
  - R/O altered visual input
→ Lightheadedness (giddiness)
  - R/O anxiety
  - R/O depression
  - R/O panic disorders
  - R/O hyperventilation
  - R/O drug use

PLAN

DIAGNOSTIC TESTS

→ For benign dizziness no specific lab tests are indicated.

→ When indicated, the following tests may be considered, depending on the presentation of symptoms and history:
  - CBC.
  - blood sugar.
  - electrocardiogram (EKG)—Holter monitor.
  - audiometry.
  - hyperventilation.
  - caloric tests.
  - electronystagmography (ENG), when unable to differentiate between peripheral and central causes.
  - rotational tests.
  - Romberg and tandem gait tests.
  - radiology:
    • chest x-ray.
    • CT scan.
  - Nylen-Bárány Test.
  - orthostatic blood pressure movement.
  - see **Table 9B.2, Initial Evaluation Tests for Vertigo, Presyncope, Disequilibrium, and Lightheadedness.**

TREATMENT/MANAGEMENT

→ When the cause of dizziness has been established, an effective treatment plan can be developed.

→ For vertigo, several classes of drugs are effective in reducing symptoms.

- Drug therapy may be used to control the autonomic symptoms of nausea and vomiting or to suppress the vestibular system. (See **Table 9B.3, Drugs of Choice for Vertigo.**)

- For presyncope, identify the precipitating factor (e.g., vasovagal attacks), avoid the inciting factor, or correct the cause by correcting the underlying disorder.

- For disequilibrium, treatment is determined by cause (e.g., someone with multiple sensory deficits may find eyeglasses, a cane, or a walker helpful).

- For dizziness related to psychological disorders, counseling as well as antidepressants may be advised.

- See "Patient Education" section.

CONSULTATION

→ Consultation with a physician is recommended when an underlying pathological condition is suspected or when severe symptoms are not responsive to palliative treatment.

→ Referral to a physician as appropriate when complex pathology is present.

→ As needed for prescription(s).

PATIENT EDUCATION

→ Explain cause of dizziness based on examination findings.

→ Reassure patient that dizziness may be a temporary manifestation of viral illness and is usually benign.

Table 9B.2.   INITIAL EVALUATION TESTS FOR VERTIGO, PRESYNCOPE, DISEQUILIBRIUM, AND LIGHTHEADEDNESS

VERTIGO:

Nylen-Bárány Test. This test, if positive, will confirm the diagnosis of benign positional vertigo (Warner et al. 1992). Rotate the client's head to one side. Gradually lower head and body below the horizontal position (thirty degrees to forty-five degrees), so the head hangs over the edge of the table. An attack is triggered when the affected ear is in the downward position. Within a few seconds, nystagmus and vertigo occur. The vertigo diminishes in 30 seconds. The nystagmus is rotatory and, when the client sits up, changes direction. (**NOTE:** The ability to reproduce symptoms with repeated maneuvers is reduced.)

Caloric Testing. Caloric testing can be done as part of the electronystagmography. It is an accurate and reproducible measure of vestibular sensitivity. The client should be supine with the head elevated 30 degrees. Each ear is irrigated with 240 ml of water, first at 30°C (86°F) and then at 44°C (110°F). The resulting nystagmus is monitored with the client looking straight ahead.

PRESYNCOPE:

Orthostatic Blood Pressure Measurement. Check the blood pressure in the supine position, ideally after the client rests for fifteen minutes. Then check the blood pressure at one-minute intervals for five minutes with the client standing. Record the pulse and presence of symptoms while the client is standing.

DISEQUILIBRIUM:

Romberg and tandem gaits.

LIGHTHEADEDNESS:

Hyperventilation. Deliberate hyperventilation can reproduce recognizable symptoms.

Table 9B.3. DRUGS OF CHOICE FOR VERTIGO

ANTIHISTAMINES	DOSAGES	COMMON SIDE EFFECTS
Meclizine (Antivert)®	25 mg-50 mg po q 6 h	Anticholinergic effects
Dimenhydrinate (Dramamine)®	50 mg po q 6 h	
Promethazine (Phenergan)®	25 mg-50 mg po q 6 h	
ANTICHOLINERGIC		
Scopolamine (Transderm Scop®)	0.5 mg transdermally q 3 d	Blurred vision, dry mouth
PHENOTHIAZINE		
Prochlorperazine (Compazine)®	10 mg po q 6 h or	Extrapyramidal effects
	25 mg suppository q 12 h	
BENZODIAZEPINES		
Diazepam (Valium)®	2 mg-10 mg po q 6 h	Drowsiness

Source: Adapted with permission from Warner, E.A., Wallach, P.M., Adelman, H.A., and Sahlin-Hughes, C. 1992. Dizziness in primary care patients. *Journal of General Internal Medicine* 7(4):454-463.

→ Recommend bed rest in a darkened room, with no reading or watching television.

→ Advise patient to reduce unnecessary stimuli as indicated.

→ Advise patient to avoid excessive intake of salt, because of fluid balance in inner ear.

→ Advise patient to avoid caffeine and nicotine, which can aggravate dizziness.

→ Advise patient to avoid alcohol.

→ Advise patient to reduce movements that may exacerbate dizziness.

→ Discuss medication side effects as indicated.

→ If a psychological component is present, provide counseling and reassurance as indicated.

→ Discuss safety measures to take during the course of dizziness, involving family members in the plan.

FOLLOW-UP

→ Re-evaluate medication/management response within one to two weeks.

→ If not responsive to the therapeutic plan, provide additional evaluation and consultation.

→ Document in progress notes and problem list.

9-C

Face Pain

Face pain is a problem that clients frequently present with in a primary care setting. Therefore, the clinician needs to be familiar with several different causes of face pain. This protocol will review some of the most common ones. Conditions covered in other protocols will be mentioned but not discussed at length.

Neurological

Trauma, disease, or other conditions affecting the neurological system can contribute to face pain. The trigeminal nerve, which is the largest cranial nerve, carries sensation from structures in the face, scalp, and neck. The pain fibers of the sensory nuclei descend down to the fourth segment of the spinal cord. There are three major branches of the trigeminal nerve—the ophthalmic, maxillary, and mandibular nerves. There are sensory nuclei that convey pain, touch, pressure, and proprioception. There is also a motor component to the muscles of mastication. Sympathetic and parasympathetic fibers connect with portions of the trigeminal nerve.

Migraines often cause face pain (see **Headache** Protocol, "Migraine Headache"). Key questions to ask concern family history of migraines, timing around menstruation, typical triggers, and associated symptoms of nausea, vomiting, photophobia, phonophobia, and scotoma.

There are a variety of neuralgias that cause facial pain. The quality of pain is typically described as sharp, lancinating, or electric-like. Trigeminal neuralgia is first seen about age 40 years, with the average age of occurrence over 60 years of age.

Trigeminal neuralgia is characterized by paroxysms of pain, primarily over the second and third division of the trigeminal nerve. Triggers for these attacks consist

of touch—such as applying make-up, brushing teeth—the wind, and movements such as chewing and talking (Green and Shenen 1991). Bilateral trigeminal neuralgia in a younger patient should arouse suspicion of multiple sclerosis. Although a conclusive cause for trigeminal neuralgia has not been found, arterial compression of the nerve near the pons usually is cited.

Atypical trigeminal pain that is more constant, progressive, and associated with neurological deficits should alert the clinician to the possibility of a tumor of the cerebellar pontine angle. Aneurysms of the posterior cerebral artery may have similar symptoms.

Herpes zoster is a common cause of facial pain. The pain can precede the skin lesions by one week, so the initial picture can be confusing. Post-herpetic neuralgia can be quite difficult to treat (see **Varicella Zoster Virus** Protocol).

Diabetic neuropathy occasionally has a pain-causing facial distribution. Trauma, including surgical and dental, may irritate the pain-sensitive nerves. Neuromas also can develop in traumatized nerves and cause pain.

Greater occipital neuralgia is another common cause of facial pain. The greater occipital nerve comes off the second cervical nerve and can cause radiating pain over the posterior scalp, the vertex, the frontal region, the retro-orbital region, and the face (Burchiel and Burgess 1989).

The lesser occipital nerve and greater auricular nerve are fed by the second and third cervical nerves. Neuralgia from the lesser occipital nerve causes pain at the posterior border of the sternocleidomastoid muscle, superior lateral neck, upper auricle, and adjacent scalp, while from the greater auricular nerve, pain can be located at the sternocleidomastoid muscle, parotid gland, posterior inferior face, mastoid process, and lower auricle (Mitchell 1983). Thus, in examining a patient who has facial pain, it is important to palpate over the scalp and under and behind the ear for trigger points that will reproduce the pain (see **Figure 9C.1, A. Radicular Cutaneous Field/B. Peripheral Cutaneous Field**).

Atypical facial pain does not follow any characteristic neurological pattern and is present even though no organic pathology can be found. The pain frequently is achy and can vary in duration. Women over age 50 years are affected most often. Psychological components often are found in these patients. There may be associated insomnia, gastrointestinal complaints, fatigue and dizziness, and bizarre sensory and motor complaints (Kessler 1989).

Ophthalmological

Ophthalmological conditions—such as acute glaucoma, iritis, optic neuritis, and corneal abrasion (due to factors including herpes simplex and foreign body)—can cause face pain. It is usually obvious that the primary problem is with the eye. However, optic neuritis may present with a normal examination except for symptoms of visual acuity and color vision loss (see **Ophthalmological Disorders** Protocols).

Otolaryngological

Sinusitis is a common producer of face pain. Frontal sinusitis presents with focal localized pain near the supraorbital region. In maxillary sinusitis, there is malar tenderness. Pain in sphenoid sinusitis is located in the vertex and occipital regions. Ethmoid sinusitis presents with periorbital and nasal bridge discomfort. Other conditions can be confused with sinusitis. Tension headache, cervical headache, and myofascial pain can create pain in the sinus region (see **Sinusitis—Acute, Sinusitis—Chronic** protocols).

Pain-causing salivary gland inflammation is primarily due to stasis of the salivary flow. Calculi are a common cause of stasis, which can lead to infection. The submandibular glands are the most susceptible to stone formation. Most frequently, *Staphylococcus aureus* is the infectious organism. The parotid glands most often are affected by viruses such as mumps, cytomegalovirus, (CMV) Coxsackie virus, or Epstein-Barr virus (EBV). Pain due to salivary gland inflammation becomes worse with eating.

Autoimmune disorders such as Sjögren's syndrome are associated with salivary inflammation. Sjögren's is characterized by dry eyes, dry mucous membranes, and salivary gland swelling. The syndrome may occur on its own or in association with other autoimmune diseases such as rheumatoid arthritis (RA). A painless, firm swelling may be indicative of benign or malignant tumors, although occasionally salivary gland cancer can present with a painful swelling. In women, alcohol consumption causes a 5.5-fold increased risk of salivary cancer (Shemen 1991).

Other ominous causes of facial pain are oral, nasopharyngeal, and sinus malignancies. The patient may complain of pain in the throat, dysphasia, hoarseness, the sense of a lump in the throat, trismus, ear pain, or facial pain. Cranial nerves may be affected. Risk factors are heavy alcohol use and smoking. Even though men are affected more than women, these cancers also occur in women.

Dental

Dental origins of facial pain are sometimes overlooked, but they need to be included in the differential diagnosis. Pulpitis, periapical abscess, an impacted tooth, and tooth fracture can cause diffuse and sometimes severe pain to the cheek, jaw, throat, or ear. Initial decay, which may not be picked up on a dental x-ray, can cause face pain. Patients may complain of heat or cold sensitivity, with heat sensitivity having a poorer prognosis for the tooth. There also may be a sensitivity to sweets and pain with chewing. Mandibular lesions such as fractures, osteomyelitis, and tumor also should be ruled out when face pain is the complaint.

Vascular

In the older population, temporal arteritis needs to be ruled out as a cause of face pain because it can have serious consequences, such as loss of vision and stroke. Patients often complain of a throbbing headache and jaw claudication (pain with chewing). They also may have the constitutional symptoms of polymyalgia rheumatica, such as fatigue and stiffness of the neck, shoulders, and hips. There often is pain and swelling of the temporal artery. With rare exceptions, the erythrocyte sedimentation rate (ESR) is elevated. Temporal artery biopsy may be done for diagnostic purposes, but there may be a false negative result due to patchy distribution of vasculitis in the artery (see **Headache** Protocol, "Temporal Arteritis").

Angina must also be kept in mind when a patient with cardiac risk factors complains of pain over the lower face and mandible which is aggravated with exercise.

Carotodynia occasionally can be seen in a primary care setting. It is a self-limited condition where

Figure 9C.1.   A. RADICULAR CUTANEOUS FIELD. B. PERIPHERAL CUTANEOUS FIELD.

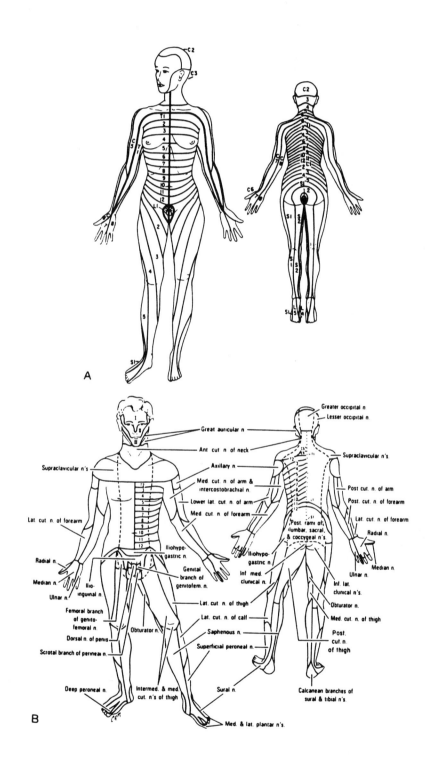

Source: Reprinted with permission from Wiederholt, W.C. 1988. Review of clinical neuroanatomy. *Neurology for non-neurologists*, p. 7. Orlando, FL: W.B. Saunders.

there is tenderness and sometimes swelling over the carotid artery. Pain can radiate to the face.

Musculoskeletal

Temporomandibular disorder and myofascial pain are discussed in the **Temporomandibular Disorder** Protocol.

Cervicogenic

Cervical headache tends to be underdiagnosed as a cause for headache and facial pain. Cervical pain typically is unilateral and often is triggered or aggravated by neck movement or palpation of the cervical spine. The pain can radiate to the temporal or supraorbital area, and occasionally pain can be referred to the contralateral side of the head (Wright and Wright 1992). Associated symptoms may include ipsilateral lacrimation, photophobia, ipsilateral tinnitus, phonophobia, and blurred vision (Wright and Wright 1992). One explanation is that pain from the cervical area may be referred through the trigeminal distribution. (Proximity of the two systems was mentioned earlier.)

Other causes of cervical headaches include cervical root irritations and inflammation of the joints—particularly the facet joints. Myofascial trigger points from the neck muscles can also be referred to the head and face. There may be a history of neck trauma, chronic awkward posture, or osteoarthritis (OA).

DATABASE

SUBJECTIVE

→ Symptom history should include:
  - side of pain.
  - duration of symptoms.
  - how did symptoms start? Make sure to ask about:
    · trauma, including whiplash.
    · dental examination/nerve block.
    · stress.
  - quality of the pain (e.g., achy, burning, throbbing, sharp).
  - specific pain triggers and exacerbators, including pain with:
    · chewing.
    · opening mouth.
    · hot or cold foods.
    · talking.
    · exercise.
    · neck movement.
  - other aggravating factors (e.g., stress, position, job, school, weather).

  - associated symptoms, including:
    · neck pain.
    · ear symptoms, such as pain, plugging, tinnitus.
    · headache.
    · tooth pain.
    · sinus discomfort/drainage.
    · eye disturbance—vision change (blurred vision, double vision, visual field loss, scotoma, photophobia, pain, redness).
    · numbness.
    · weakness.
    · rash.
  - jaw function, including:
    · locking—open or closed.
    · joint noise.

→ Medical history should include:
  - trauma, including:
    · motor vehicle accident (MVA).
    · surgery or dental work.
    · domestic violence.
  - dental problems, including:
    · braces.
    · bridge work and dentures (loose fit may contribute to bruxism).
    · tooth extraction, root canal.
    · splint.
    · clencher/grinder—when and if associated with stress.

→ other medical problems, particularly:
  - diabetes.
  - hypertension.
  - thyroid disorder.
  - sleep disorder.
  - psychiatric disorder such as depression/anxiety.
  - connective tissue disorder/joint laxity.
  - heart disease.
  - headaches.
  - arthritis.
  - vasculitis.

→ Ascertain any family history of:
  - connective tissue disease.
  - headache.

→ Ascertain degree of substance use, including use of:
  - alcohol.
  - tobacco.
  - street drugs, particularly stimulants.
  - caffeine.

→ Ascertain medication use, including:

- over-the-counter (OTC) medications.
  - Overuse of OTCs and prescription medications can cause an analgesic rebound headache in patients with a primary headache problem (Mathew, Kurman, and Perez 1990; Rapoport 1988).
    - –This is commonly seen in headache clinics.
    - –It is important to monitor the pain medication intake of patients with headaches and to counsel them before a secondary headache problem emerges.
- decongestants.
  - These act as stimulants and can cause poor sleep and bruxing.
- prescription medications, including birth control pills.
→ Ask patient about social factors, such as:
- occupation:
  - including shift work (irregular circadian rhythms can exacerbate migraines).
- home life:
  - especially stressors and faulty coping mechanisms.
- hobbies:
  - including sports that cause clenching or activities that cause poor posture.

OBJECTIVE

→ Include portions of the physical examination appropriate to the symptoms:
- blood pressure.
- skin.
  - Look for vesicular rash.
- facial symmetry.
- eyes.
  - Snellen, visual fields, color chart, lid inflammation, conjunctival redness, pupil size and reactivity, disc margins and color, and fluorescein stain, if pain and photophobia.
- ears.
  - Gross hearing; Weber, Rinne; ear canal for swelling, redness, and discharge; tympanic membrane.
- throat.
  - Include tongue, palate, buccal mucosa (linea alba on the buccal mucosa can indicate bruxism, as can a scalloped tongue).
    - –Observe for mucosal lesions.
- salivary glands.
  - Note size, consistency, pain.
  - A ductal stone may be palpated, or purulent drainage may be seen.

- teeth.
  - Observe for missing teeth, wear marks, state of repair, tooth pain with percussion or biting gauze (The latter may indicate fracture).
- mandible abnormalities.
  - Such as malocclusion, mandible asymmetry, retrognathia, prognathia, mandible pain.
- temporomandibular joint (TMJ):
  - palpate for pain, open and closed, and crepitance.
  - Range of motion (ROM) (note deflection to the side):
    - –intercisal opening (normal range 35 mm-50 mm).
    - –laterotrusion (normal range 8 mm-10 mm).
    - –protrusion (normal range 8 mm-10 mm)— This is difficult to measure. Look for deflection with movement. Deflection on one side may indicate joint dysfunction on the same side.
  - Joint noises (with and without stethoscope):
    - –click/pop.
      - ▸ It is difficult to ascertain the exact cause of the click or pop on physical examination. These noises can be caused by fossa/disc/condyle incoordination or structural bony and soft-tissue irregularities.
      - ▸ Note the timing, coordination, and consistency in opening and closing. Early open clicks and pops have a better prognosis than late open noises.
    - –crepitance.
  - Joint loading.
    - –Have client bite with molars on two tongue blades. Pain on the opposite side is a positive test and can indicate joint pathology.
- neck:
  - posture.
  - pain with palpation and ROM.
  - ROM.
  - radicular symptoms with movement.
  - thyroid.
  - carotid arteries—pain, swelling, bruits.
- neurological:
  - symmetry of facial muscles.
  - facial sensation.
  - symmetry of tongue.
  - symmetry of palate.
  - gag reflex.
  - greater auricular nerve and greater occipital nerve.
  - other cranial nerves, as appropriate.

■ muscle screening examination:
  • masseters.
  • temporalis.
  • suboccipitals.
  • trapezius.
  • sternocleidomastoid.
  • For more complete evaluation of muscles, including intraoral muscles, refer to photographs in reference books.
→ Obtain past laboratory work records or x-rays pertaining to face pain.

ASSESSMENT

→ A number of causes need to be ruled out when a patient presents with face pain. The more common ones are listed below.
■ Neurological:
  • R/O trigeminal neuralgia
  • R/O herpes zoster and post-herpetic neuralgia
  • R/O post-traumatic neuralgia
  • R/O migraine
  • R/O cluster headache (uncommon among women)
  • R/O atypical face pain
  • R/O diabetic neuropathy
  • R/O occipital neuralgia
  • R/O greater auricular neuralgia
  • R/O tumor of the cerebellar pontine angle
  • R/O multiple sclerosis
  • R/O Bell's palsy
  • R/O optic neuritis
■ Ophthalmological:
  • R/O acute glaucoma
  • R/O iritis
  • R/O optic neuritis
  • R/O corneal abrasions
  • R/O foreign body
■ Otolaryngological:
  • R/O sinusitis
  • R/O salivary gland disorder due to conditions such as:
    –bacterial infection
    –viral infection
    –calculus
    –tumor
    –autoimmune syndrome (e.g., Sjögren's syndrome)
  • R/O oropharyngeal cancer
  • R/O nasopharyngeal cancer
■ Dental:
  • R/O dental caries
  • R/O pulpitis

• R/O periodontal lesions
• R/O periapical abscess
• R/O tooth fracture
• R/O impacted tooth
• R/O mandibular lesions due to:
  –osteomyelitis
  –tumor
  –fracture
■ Vascular:
  • R/O temporal arteritis
  • R/O angina
  • R/O carotodynia
■ Musculoskeletal:
  • R/O temporomandibular disorder (TMD)
  • R/O myofascial pain
  • R/O cervicogenic headache

PLAN

DIAGNOSTIC TESTS

→ Laboratory tests should include:
■ sedimentation rate for patients over 50 years and for patients with suspected connective tissue disease.
■ for suspected Sjögren syndrome A and B, serum test (SSA and SSB), and the Schirmer test.
  • On the Schirmer test, less than 5 mm wetness on a filter paper strip is positive, 15 mm is negative, in between is equivocal. (A lip biopsy is diagnostic.)
■ viral titers for mumps and CMV, EBV, as indicated for bilateral parotiditis.
■ blood sugar to check diabetic control or if diabetes is suspected.
■ thyroid function tests if indicated.
→ X-rays:
■ see **Temporomandibular Disorder** Protocol for TMJ and mandible.
■ sinus x-rays as appropriate. A CT scan may be more accurate and is occasionally done. Consult with physician.
■ cervical spine x-rays, MRI of cervical spine (consult with physician for the latter), as indicated.
■ MRI when tumor of the cerebellar pontine angle (CPA) is suspected. Consult with physician.

TREATMENT/MANAGEMENT

→ General principle—Narcotic analgesics should be avoided in treating chronic pain syndromes.
→ Neurological:

- migraine and cluster headaches—see appropriate protocols.
- trigeminal neuralgia:
  - carbamazepine (Tegretol®) is the most effective medication but can have significant side effects, such as hepatitis, blood dyscrasias, fatigue, diplopia, dizziness, ataxia, nausea, rash (e.g., Stevens-Johnson syndrome), and pneumonitis.
    - –Get baseline serum glutamic oxaloacetic transaminase (SGOT) and CBC; repeat in 1 month and 3 months later.
    - –Carbamazepine may decrease the effectiveness of theophylline and may increase the metabolism of warfarin.
      - ▸ Start dosage at 100 mg p.o. BID and, as needed, work up to 200 mg p.o. TID for maintenance. Do not use more than 1200 mg per day.
  - phenytoin (Dilantin®)—300 mg p.o. at bedtime.
    - –See **Seizures** Protocol.
    - –Phenytoin has numerous drug interactions. Refer to *PDR*.
  - baclofen (Catrofen®, Lioresal®).
    - –This is a muscle relaxant and antispasmodic.
    - –The most common side effect is drowsiness and other central nervous system (CNS) effects.
    - –Use with caution with other CNS-depressant drugs and tricyclics.
    - –Baclofen may raise the blood sugar; if patient is diabetic, regular glucose monitoring should be performed.
    - –Dosage is 5 mg p.o. TID which can be increased to 20 mg p.o. TID.
  - divalproex sodium (Depakote®).
    - –250 mg 1 pill BID. Can slowly increase to 2 pills BID.
    - –Get baseline CBC and serum glutamic pyruvic transaminase (SGPT) and recheck every 3 to 6 months.
    - –The most common adverse effects are liver inflammation and blood dyscrasias.
    - –Avoid in pregnancy and in patients with liver dysfunction.
    - –May cause drowsiness, decrease the effectiveness of birth control pills, and produce a false positive test for ketones in the urine.
  - capsaicin (Zostrix®) is a topical analgesic which is a component of red pepper.

  - –Fusco and Alessandri (1992) found it to be effective in their patients with trigeminal neuralgia. Clinicians are beginning to use this drug.
    - –Refer to *PDR*.
  - acupuncture may be helpful.
- herpes zoster—See **Varicella Zoster Virus** Protocol.
- diabetic neuropathy.
  - Good diabetic control may be helpful in improving nerve conduction (Troni et al. 1984).
  - The following also may be helpful:
    - –vitamin B_6 50 mg p.o. TID was found to be useful in decreasing pain and improving diabetic control in one study (Bernstein and Lobitz 1988).
    - –tricyclics are the most effective medication (see **Appendix 9C.1, Tricyclics and Pain Syndromes**, p. 9-20).
    - –phenytoin can be helpful.
- a typical facial pain:
  - tricyclics are the medications of choice (see **Appendix 9C.1**, p. 9-20).
  - baclofen can be used as well.
  - carbamazepine has been used.
- occipital and greater auricular neuralgia:
  - nerve blocks can be helpful for diagnostic purposes and for treatment (refer to physician).
  - medications used for other neuropathies can be used.
  - nonsteroidal anti-inflammatory drugs (NSAIDs) are used for milder cases.
    - –See **Temporomandibular Disorder** Protocol.
  - acupuncture has been helpful in some cases.
  - physical therapy may be helpful.

→ Ophthalmological (see **Ophthalmological Disorders** Protocols).

→ Otolaryngological:
- sinusitis (see **Sinusitis—Acute, Sinusitis— Chronic** protocols).
- sialoadenitis (bacterial infection of the salivary gland):
  - dicloxacillin (Dynapen®): 500 mg p.o. QID for 10 days.

    OR
  - cephalexin (Keflex®): 500 mg p.o. QID for 10 days.

    OR
  - erythromycin (E-Mycin®): 250 mg p.o. QID for 10 days.

- apply heat, massage gland, and recommend sour lozenges. Increase fluids. Re-evaluate the patient in 5 days to 1 week.

→ Dental:
- penicillin V Potassium (Pen-Vee® K): 250 mg p.o. QID for 10 days.

        OR
- erythromycin (E-Mycin®): 250 mg p.o. QID for 10 days. If there appears to be a dental infection, these can be used while the patient is waiting for a dental appointment.
- short-term pain medication: Acetaminophen with codeine: 1 to 2 tablets p.o. every 4 hours.

        OR
- hydrocodone with acetaminophen (Vicodin®)— 1 to 2 tablets p.o. every 4 hours.

→ Vascular:
- temporal arteritis (see **Headache** Protocol, "Temporal Arteritis").
- angina (see **Angina** Protocol).
- carotodynia.
  - NSAIDs may be helpful.

→ Musculoskeletal:
- TMD (see **Temporomandibular Disorder** Protocol).
- myofascial pain. The treatment consists predominantly of physical modalities. Examples are:
  - spray and stretch with Fluori-Methane® spray.
  - trigger point injections.
  - ultrasound.
  - transcutaneous electrical nerve stimulation (TENS).
  - acupressure.
  - acupuncture.
  - biofeedback.
  - a program of posture improvement and stretching.
  - medications such as NSAIDS, tricyclics, or muscle relaxants are sometimes useful.

→ cervicogenic face pain:
- medications, including:
  - NSAIDS.
  - acetaminophen.
  - tricyclics.
  - muscle relaxants.
- physical modalities that have been used:
  - heat/cold, massage.
  - posture instruction.
  - cervical traction.
  - mobilization.

- cervical pillows.
- facet injections.

CONSULTATION

→ Physician consultation for face pain is recommended when:
- the diagnosis is unclear.
- diagnostic tests, such as CT scans or MRIs, or invasive studies may be indicated.
- the disorder could have serious consequences.
- the medication to be used has potentially serious side effects or drug interactions.
- the patient has other significant medical problems that may be affected by the facial pain problem or the treatment.

→ Patients with facial pain frequently need referrals to other health care providers, including:
- neurologists for patients with neuralgias such as trigeminal neuralgia, cluster headaches, or complicated migraines.
- otolaryngologists for patients with:
  - severe ear pain or face pain when the diagnosis is unclear.
  - painless unilateral salivary gland swelling.
  - painful salivary gland swelling when the patient is toxic.
  - a calculus that has been palpated.
  - atypical oral lesions, including tongue lesions.
  - a strong history of alcohol use or smoking.
  - also refer if the patient is elderly, if the patient has not responded to a week of antibiotics, or if the patient is an Asian male.
    - Asian males have a higher incidence of oral pharyngeal cancer and nasal pharyngeal cancer.
- oral surgeons or otolaryngologists for patients with mandibular lesions.
- physical therapists when face pain may be related to musculoskeletal causes.
- rheumatologists for Sjögren syndrome.
- dentists for obvious dental problems.
- mental health professionals for patient with chronic pain syndromes.
- if all other measures fail, chronic pain programs to improve day-to-day mood and functioning.

→ As needed for prescription(s).

PATIENT EDUCATION

→ Advise regarding regular exercise to promote general conditioning and improve depression and pain.

→ Advise regarding posture, muscle stretching and strengthening, and use of heat/cold.

→ Advise regarding nutrition, especially if chewing or swallowing aggravates symptoms.
- A soft, nutritionally sound diet is helpful. Fiber and multivitamins may need to be added.

→ Advise regarding environmental and food triggers. This is very important in migraine patients.

→ Advise regarding stress management techniques and provide basic counseling.

→ Provide support to families.

FOLLOW-UP

→ Determine guidelines for follow-up at individual practice settings. Individual follow-up measures have been mentioned in the "Treatment/ Management" section.

→ Document in progress notes and problem list.

Wendy L. Berk, C.A.N.P.

Appendix 9C.1

Tricyclics and Pain Syndromes

Tricyclics are commonly used for pain syndromes though usually not at the dosage level used for depression. It is advised to start at 10 mg by mouth one hour before bedtime and to slowly increase by 10 mg each week until 50 mg are reached, if needed. When there is a significant underlying depression or insomnia, this can be increased to 150 mg with psychiatric guidance. Tricyclics should be used with caution in patients with glaucoma, diabetes, thyroid disease, seizure disorder (it may decrease the seizure threshold), and renal or hepatic disease. Tricyclics may interfere with cardiac conduction. Desipramine and nortriptyline have the fewest cardiac effects. Barbiturates and smoking may decrease tricyclic effectiveness. Birth control pills and beta blockers may increase tricyclic blood levels. The patient needs to be told that tricyclics are not pain medications, but work on pain receptors to prevent pain. Thus, it can take a month to reach a full effect. It is important to reassure patients that tricyclics are used for pain syndromes since they may be confused by reading the package insert, which states that they are antidepressant medications.

COMPARISON OF TRICYCLICS COMMONLY USED IN PAIN SYNDROMES

	Sedation	Orthostatic Hypotension	Anticholinergic Effects
Amitriptyline	+ + + +	+ + → + + + +	+ + +
Desipramine	+	+ → + +	+ + → + + +
Doxepin	+ + + → + + + +	+ + + → + + + +	+ + +
Imipramine	+ + → + + +	+ + → + + +	+ + +
Nortriptyline	+ + → + + +	+	+ +

Key: + = weak; + + = mild; + + + = moderate; + + + + = strong

Source: Adapted with permission from Krishnan, K. R. R., and France, R. D. 1989. Antidepressants in chronic pain syndromes. *American Family Physician* 39:235.

Jacqueline W. Wasserman, R.N., C., M.S., F.N.P.

9-D

Headache

Headache is one of the most common complaints in the general population. Each year, 80 million people in the United States have at least one acute headache. Forty-five million have chronic headaches, and 16 to 18 million of those are diagnosed as having migraines (Diamond 1992).

A headache is a diffuse pain that can occur in different areas of the head. The major mechanisms are inflammation of vessels and meninges, vascular dilatation, excessive muscle contraction, and traction on pain-sensitive structures. More than one mechanism may occur simultaneously, and an individual may have more than one type of headache (Goroll 1987).

Headaches can be classified into three major groups, according to information recently updated and specified by the International Headache Society (IHS) in 1988. There are psychological or functional headaches—the most prevalent types—which include tension-type headaches; vascular headaches, which include migraine headaches; and organic headaches, which include headaches caused by brain tumors and arteritis.

There are others in the field of headache research who have classified headaches into similar categories but have identified the categories differently. Diamond (1992) describes three categories: vascular types, which include migraine; tension types, which include psychological factors; and traction and inflammation types, which include tumors and arteritis (see **Table 9D.1, Types of Headaches**).

This section will include discussion of the most common types of headaches, and their treatment and management. These include the migraine and cluster forms of vascular headaches; tension-type headaches, specifically the muscle contraction headache; and the tem-poral arteritis form of traction and inflammation headache. Each category of pathological traction and inflammation headache should be ruled out before a headache can be classified as benign (see **Table 9D.1**).

The vast majority of headaches are not associated with life-threatening disease. Some guidelines for determining when a work-up is not necessary include:
- history of previous identical headaches.
- alertness and cognition are intact.
- neurological examination is normal.
- neck is supple.
- vital signs are normal.
- observation reveals continual improvement (Edmeads 1990).

Headaches that require a more extensive work-up and follow-through may present as:
- most severe headache ever experienced.
- onset noted with exertion.
- any abnormality on examination.
- cognition or alertness decreased.
- neck not completely supple.
- observation reveals no improvement or worsening (Edmeads 1990).

The following general database is for reference when the presentation is headache and no diagnosis has yet been reached.

DATABASE

SUBJECTIVE

→ Age and circumstance of onset:
- certain headache disorders are common to particular phases of life—e.g., migraine frequently begins in childhood.

Table 9D.1. TYPES OF HEADACHES

Vascular	Tension Type	Traction and Inflammation
Migraine	Anxiety	Mass lesions
With aura (classic)	Cervical osteoarthritis	Diseases of the ear, eye, nose, throat, and teeth
Without aura (common)	Chronic myositis	Arteritis, phlebitis, cranial neuralgias
Complicated		Temporomandibular joint disease
Hemiplegic	Psychogenic	
Ophthalmoplegic	Depressive	Occlusive vascular disease
Basilar artery	Conversion reactions	Atypical face pain
Benign exertional		Infection
Cluster (histamine or migrainous neuralgia)		
Toxic vascular		
Hypertensive		
	Mixed Headache	

Source: Adapted with permission from Diamond, S. 1992. Acute headache. Differential diagnosis and management of the three types. *Postgraduate Medicine* (Spec Rep), Aug 3:21-29.

- circumstances surrounding onset are significant—e.g., headaches prior to or during menstruation or ovulation, or headaches during pregnancy are often migrainous (Saper 1983).

→ Location and laterality:
- important clues to the type of headache are revealed by the location—e.g., cluster, migraine, and temporal arteritis headaches characteristically are unilateral; muscle contraction pain is typically generalized and bilateral (Diamond 1992).

→ Prodromal events:
- warning symptoms prior to onset such as aura, fluid retention, malaise, personality change, or sleep disturbance provide clues to the type of headache.
- migraine headaches characteristically present with prodromal events.

→ Precipitating factors:
- menstruation, alcohol consumption, oral contraceptives, or missed meals can be triggers for migraines.
  - Alcohol often can provoke vascular headaches, but may relieve tension-type headaches (Saper 1983).

→ Time of onset and duration:
- nocturnal awakening often is associated with vascular headache.
- morning headaches may be migraine or muscular (due to jaw clenching, for example). Morning-associated headaches also may be due to withdrawal from caffeine, analgesics, or ergot preparations (Murtagh 1990).

→ Quality of the pain:

- pulsating, throbbing pain usually is related to vascular headaches.
- band-like pain usually is a symptom of muscle contraction headaches.
- intense, burning, boring, searing pain is associated with cluster headaches (Saper 1983).

→ Frequency:
- muscular headaches often last the majority of a day and may happen daily.
- migrainous headaches usually occur once or twice a month at ovulation and/or menstruation (Murtagh 1990).

→ Accompanying symptoms:
- specific headache syndromes have specific symptoms (see discussions of specific types of headaches).

→ Relieving factors:
- vascular headaches can be relieved with the application of cold.
- muscular headaches respond to heat.
- determining what relieves the pain (e.g., two cups of coffee) can be a diagnostic indicator (Saper 1983).

OBJECTIVE

→ Physical examination is usually normal since benign headaches are not associated with structural abnormalities.
- Vital signs, including temperature; should be taken.
- Head and neck examination should include:
  - check for craniocervical bruits over the eyes, carotid, and vertebral arteries.

- palpation for painful areas, rigidity, masses, or signs of trauma in the scalp, sinuses, and temporal arteries.
- Eye examination should include:
  - check for glaucoma, optic atrophy, papilledema, impaired vision, subhyaloid hemorrhage.
- Nose, mouth, and dentition examination should include:
  - check for tenderness, jaw ROM, and the TMJ.
- Neurological examination should include:
  - cranial nerves.
  - gait, deep tendon reflexes, meningeal signs, cerebellar, Romberg.
  - mental status examination as indicated by history.
  - any neurological abnormalities will necessitate consultation/referral.

ASSESSMENT

→ To be ruled out depending on the presentation and history:
- for vascular and tension-type headaches (see discussions of specific types of headaches).
  - R/O sinusitis
  - R/O post-traumatic causes
  - R/O post-lumbar puncture
  - R/O psychogenic causes
  - R/O trigeminal neuralgia (see **Facial Pain** Protocol.)
- for secondary headaches:
  - R/O pseudotumor
  - R/O temporal or giant cell arteritis (see "Temporal or Giant Cell Arteritis."
  - Protocols)
  - R/O TMJ (see **Facial Pain** Protocol)
  - R/O cervical spondylosis
  - R/O eye disease
  - R/O meningitis
  - R/O subdural hematoma
  - R/O tumor
  - R/O hypertension
  - R/O subarachnoid hemorrhage

PLAN

DIAGNOSTIC TESTS

→ Diagnostic testing in the majority of individuals with benign headaches is of limited value. However, when indicated by the history and physical, order the following diagnostic tests:

- baseline laboratory tests:
  - CBC, ESR.
  - urinalysis.
  - blood chemistry profile.
- sinus x-rays.
- cervical spine x-rays.
- tonometry.
- lumbar puncture (LP).
- skull series.
- brain scan, tomography, CT scan.
- EEG.

→ For more details on pertinent diagnostics, see discussions of specific types of headaches).

TREATMENT/MANAGEMENT

→ First-line approaches are:
- establish good rapport with client.
- pay attention to precipitating factors.
- provide psychological support.
- discuss relaxation therapy.

→ If the pain is quite severe and simple treatment measures have failed, medication can be given for:
- symptomatic relief of an acute episode.
- abortive therapy to prevent a headache after warning signs have appeared.
- prophylaxis to reduce frequency, particularly if symptomatic therapy has failed. Prophylaxis guidelines:
  - 2 or more incapacitating episodes per month.
  - unresponsive to abortive therapy.
  - complicated migraine with significant defects (Gallagher 1991).

CONSULTATION

→ Consultation with a physician is indicated for any presentation of headache that does not fall within parameters of clinician's experience, or if there is a question about the diagnosis/treatment.

→ As needed for prescription(s).

PATIENT EDUCATION

→ Provide reassurance that most headaches do not represent a serious disease.

→ Include patient participation in the treatment plan. This is essential to ensure success.

→ Advise patient that because the best treatment may require several trials, patience is necessary.

→ Advise patient that triggering factors and stresses may contribute to the headache.

→ Discuss the possibility of relaxation training, biofeedback, hypnosis, acupuncture, or meditation as adjuncts to the treatment plan or as the main mode of treatment.

→ Explore lifestyle choices in work and domestic life to evaluate possible modifications to reduce stress.

→ Recommend possibility of psychotherapy.

→ Discuss medications and side effects.

FOLLOW-UP

→ While developing a treatment approach—such as medication, lifestyle changes, and adjunct therapy—follow-up should be frequent to evaluate management as determined by practitioner and client.

→ Document in progress notes and problem list.

Migraine Headache

Migraine headaches afflict five to ten percent of all adults. They occur four times as often in women and may begin or terminate with menopause. With pregnancy, migraine often lessens, but occasionally may worsen (Goroll 1987). The cranial arteries of individuals with migraines tend to be particularly reactive, provoked by various stimuli. In young women in particular, the problem may be of unusual intensity and complexity (Dalessio 1987).

Considerable evidence links estrogen with migraine headache. Sixty percent of those with migraine attacks are menstruating women. Consequently, these headaches are called *menstrual migraines*. Oral contraceptive initiation may stimulate the first migraine attacks. These may worsen, improve, or show no change. With advancing age, all types of migraines tend to decrease in number. However, hormone replacement therapy can exacerbate the condition (Silberstein 1992).

Previously, migraines were classified as either *classic* or *common*. The new IHS nomenclature distinguishes between migraine *with* or *without aura*. Neurological warning signs define a migraine with an aura. These signs often are visual and may occur one to two hours before the onset of a migraine attack. The prodrome may consist of photopsia (flashing lights and colors), teichopsia (shimmering, wavy lines), fortification spectrum (zigzag patterns), scotoma (blind spot), hemianopia (partial visual-field loss), and metamorphopsia (illusions of distorted size or shape) (Diamond 1992).

More severe, less common forms of migraine are *hemiplegic* and *ophthalmoplegic*. A hemiplegic migraine is considered to be linked with the vascular reactions of migraine with an aura. An inherited instability of vascular control has been suggested. Long-lasting ischemia of brain tissue can occur (Dalessio 1987). Hemiplegic migraine may begin suddenly with hemiplegia or hemiparesis accompanied by confusion and aphasia. A contralateral throbbing headache develops, with symptoms persisting sometimes for days (Barrigan-Hornibrook and Rich 1987).

An ophthalmoplegic migraine involves structures associated with the third cranial nerve and ocular palsy. The dilated and edematous wall of the internal carotid artery and its branches puts pressure on the nerve (Dalessio 1987). The symptoms resemble a carotid aneurysm with ocular muscle weakness, pupillary changes, ptosis, and extraocular paralysis on the same side. It begins with focal head pain around the eye, nausea and vomiting, and photophobia. Symptoms last hours to days to weeks. Onset occurs in childhood (Barrigan-Hornibrook and Rich 1987).

DATABASE

SUBJECTIVE

→ Patient may have:
- positive family history.
- history of cyclic vomiting.
- history of motion sickness.
- onset in early A.M.; headache lasts two to twelve hours.
- onset in late childhood, early adolescence.
- onset occurring after alcohol consumption.

→ Symptoms may include:
- photophobia.
- nausea, often with vomiting.
- throbbing pain across forehead, behind the eyes.

→ Sleep or resting in a dark room often terminates the attack.

→ Stress or the relaxation period after stress can increase the number of attacks.

→ Provoking factors may include:
- bright light, noise, alcohol, tension.
- an aura (often a transient visual disturbance).

OBJECTIVE

→ Physical examination is usually normal since benign headaches are not associated with structural abnormalities.
- Vital signs, including temperature, should be taken.
- Head and neck examination should include:
  - check for craniocervical bruits over the eyes, carotid, and vertebral arteries.
  - palpation for painful areas, rigidity, masses or signs of trauma in the scalp, sinuses, and temporal arteries.

- Eye examination should include:
  - check for glaucoma, optic atrophy, papilledema, impaired vision, subhyaloid hemorrhage.
- Nose, mouth, and dentition examination should include:
  - check for tenderness, jaw ROM and the TMJ.
- Neurological examination should include:
  - cranial nerves.
  - gait, deep tendon reflexes, meningeal signs, cerebellar, Romberg.
  - mental status examination as indicated by history.
- Neurological examination is typically normal.
  - Transient neurological deficits may be detected during an attack (Day 1990).
    -Any neurological abnormalities will necessitate consultation/referral.

ASSESSMENT

→ Migraine headache (with or without aura).

→ R/O tension-type headache

→ R/O cluster headache

→ R/O organic lesion

PLAN

DIAGNOSTIC TESTS

→ Laboratory studies not routinely recommended.

→ Radiological studies unnecessary in typical cases.

TREATMENT/MANAGEMENT

→ Non-pharmacological measures (see "Treatment/ Management" section of **Headache** Protocol):
  - investigate family and social circumstances for stress or psychological conflict in anticipation of stress reduction recommendations.
  - Recommend activities that reduce stress:
    - exercise.
    - relaxation techniques.
    - biofeedback.
    - acupuncture.
    - meditation.
    - supportive counseling.
    - a dark room, cold packs, and sleep to alleviate pain.

→ Pharmacological measures for an acute attack:
  - ergotamine tartrate (Ergostat®) (2 mg sublingually):
    - at first sign of attack, 1 tablet under tongue; take subsequent doses at 30-minute intervals;

take no more than 3 tablets in 24 hours and no more than 10 mg/week.
    - a caffeine-containing preparation may help quicken the action (e.g., Cafergot®). Repeat every hour until relieved or up to a maximum of 6 mg-8 mg in 24 hours or 12 mg per week.
    - ergotamine therapy is contraindicated in individuals with coronary artery disease (CAD), severe hypertension (HTN), acute infection, renal or hepatic dysfunction, significant peripheral vascular disease (PVD), Raynaud's phenomenon, and pregnancy (Diamond 1992).
    - side effects include nausea, vomiting, cramping, and paresthesias.
  - medihaler® ergotamine inhalation (aerosol):
    - start with 1 inhalation and repeat if not relieved in 5 minutes; space additional inhalations 5 minutes apart; take no greater than 6 inhalations in 24 hours or 15 inhalations/week.
  - dihydroergotamine (DHE):
    - 0.5 mg-1 mg intraveneously or 1 mg subcutaneously or I.M.
    - DHE is contraindicated in individuals with CAD, PVD, transient ischemic attacks (TIAs), pregnancy, and sepsis.
  - codeine sulfate:
    - 30 mg-60 mg p.o. every 4 hours, if unresponsive to ergotamine (Goroll 1987).
  - isometheptene-mucate with dichloraphenazone and acetaminophen (Midrin®):
    - take 2 capsules p.o. initially, and 1 capsule repeated hourly up to 5 capsules.
    - midrin is contraindicated during pregnancy, or in individuals with CAD, liver or kidney dysfunction, PVD, glaucoma, severe HTN, or if taking a monoamine oxidase (MAO) inhibitor (Diamond 1992).
    - side effect is dizziness.
  - mild analgesics:
    - NSAIDs:
      -ibuprofen (Motrin®), 400 mg-2400 mg p.o. day (treatment of choice for menstrual migraine).
    - aspirin—600 mg p.o. every 4 hours.
    - acetaminophen—600 mg p.o. every 4 hours.
  - antiemetics:
    - chlorpromazine (Thorazine®): 10 mg-25 mg p.o. every 4 to 6 hours.
    - prochlorperazine (Compazine®): 5 mg-10 mg p.o. TID–QID.

- narcotic analgesics (to be used with caution secondary to risk of habituation, and for severe persistent headache when ergotamine therapy is not possible):
  - meperidine HCL (Demerol®) 75 mg-100 mg I.M.
  - morphine sulfate: 10 mg I.M.
  - hydromorphone (Dilaudid®): 4 mg orally or I.M.
- parenteral corticosteroids may provide relief for status migrainosus:
  - dexamethasone (Decadron®) 8 mg (Gallagher 1991).
- sumatriptan (Imitrex®)—serotonin receptor (5-HT₁ specific) agonist (Kaiser Foundation Hospital 1993):
  - new drug.
  - mode of action includes vasoconstriction and reduction of plasma protein extravasation into perivascular space.
  - patient must have an accurate diagnosis of migraine.
  - used for acute treatment, *not* prophylaxis.
  - administer 16 mg subcutaneously at onset of symptoms.
    - Can be administered in office/emergency room or patient can be instructed in self-administration with autoinjection device.
    - Maximum dosage is 12 mg (2 injections, minimum of 1 hour apart) during 24 hours.
    - Observe for side effects prior to discharging patient.
      - ▸ Side effects include taste disturbance, tingling, warm-hot sensations, dizziness, tightness/heaviness/pressure in neck and chest; injection reaction.

NOTE: Due to its short half-life, patients may get rebound headaches from use of this drug.
  - precautions—Do not administer to patients:
    - taking ergotamine within past 24 hours.
    - taking MAO inhibitors (e.g.; Marplan®, Nardil®, Parnate®).
    - taking selective serotonin reuptake inhibitors (e.g., Prozac®, Zoloft®).
    - taking lithium.
    - with cardiovascular disease, HTN (BP > 150/90 at time of injection), renal disease, diabetes, asthma.
  - refer to *PDR* or drug package insert for further information. Consult physician prior to use.

→ Non-pharmacological measures for migraine prophylaxis: See "Treatment/Management" section of **Headache** Protocol.
→ Pharmacological measures for migraine prophylaxis:
  - beta-adrenergic blocking agents:
    - propranolol (Inderal®): 20 mg p.o. BID up to 240 mg/day.
    - atenolol (Tenormin®): 50 mg-150 mg p.o./day.
    - nadolol (Corgard®): 40 mg-240 mg p.o./day.
    - side effects include drowsiness, nightmares, insomnia, depression.
  - methysergide (Sansert®): 2 mg-8 mg p.o./day:
    - despite its effectiveness, a second line agent because of retroperitoneal, pleuropulmonary, and valvular fibrosis with prolonged use. Contraindicated with PVD, CAD, and severe HTN.
    - side effects include nausea, muscle cramps, abdominal pain, weight gain.
  - calcium channel blockers:
    - verapamil (Calan®): 240 mg-720 mg p.o./day.
    - nifedipine (Procardia®): 30 mg-180 mg p.o./day.
    - diltiazem, HCL (Cartizem®): 120 mg-360 mg p.o./day.
    - prophylactic effect takes 10-14 days with a full response in 2-4 weeks.
    - side effects include hypotension, edema, headache, constipation, nausea.
  - tricyclic antidepressants:
    - nortriptyline HCL (Pamelor®): 25 mg-100 mg p.o./day.
    - doxepin (Sinequan®): 25 mg-100 mg p.o./day.
    - desipramine (Norpramin®): 100 mg-200 mg p.o./day.
    - side effects include nausea, flu-like symptoms, jitteriness, dry mouth, sedation (Schulman and Silberstein 1992).
  - other antidepressants:
    - fluoxetine HCL (Prozac®): 20 mg-80 mg p.o./day.

CONSULTATION

→ Consultation with a physician is indicated in the following instances:
  - for migraine headache unresponsive to treatment.
  - if there is uncertainty about diagnosis.
  - for complicated presentation of migraine.

- for complex pharmacological regimens and narcotic use.
→ As needed for prescription(s).

PATIENT EDUCATION

→ See "Patient Education" section of **Headache** Protocol.

→ Explain causes of migraines. Reassure as to benign nature.

→ Advise patient to avoid factors that trigger headaches:
  - exogenous:
    • foods—chocolate, oranges, cheese, tomatoes, citrus fruits.
    • alcohol—especially red wine.
    • drugs—vasodilators, estrogens, monosodium glutamate, nitrites.
    • glare or bright lights.
    • emotional stress.
    • minor head trauma.
    • allergens.
    • climatic change.
  - endogenous:
    • physical exhaustion.
    • oversleeping.
    • stress, relaxation after stress.
    • exercise.
    • hormonal changes:
      –puberty.
      –menstruation.
      –climacteric.
      –pregnancy.
    • hunger (Day 1990).

→ Educate about signs of impending attack so can start treatment plan as soon as possible, if necessary.

→ Instruct on medication usage.

→ Instruct about side effects of drugs and which medications may be habit-forming.
  - Ergot agents should not be used on the second, third, or fourth days of migraine attack because of risk of rebound phenomenon (Diamond 1992).

FOLLOW-UP

→ Until a successful regimen is established to control headaches, frequent follow-up is recommended.

→ Document in progress notes and problem list. Note known trigger factors and successful treatment plan.

Cluster Headache
(Histamine headache, Horton's headache, Migrainous neuralgia)

A cluster headache is a vascular-type headache with such specific features that often history can be enough to make a diagnosis. The pain occurs around the area of the eye, temples, neck, and face and may extend into the shoulder on the same side. The pain is of a burning, boring, high-intensity nature, lasting usually 30 minutes to two hours. It tends to end suddenly. Associated with the pain is a profuse watering and congestion of the conjunctiva, rhinorrhea, nasal obstruction, and increased perspiration.

Sufferers of cluster headache are very sensitive to alcohol, aged cheeses, vasodilating agents, and drugs such as histamine or nitroglycerin (Dalessio 1987). Cluster headache occurs more often in older men than in women (6:1), with the onset later in life (20 years to 50 years old).

The headaches occur in clusters lasting six to twelve weeks and may recur a few months or a year later, often at the same time of year (Eckel 1985). The course of a cluster headache, unlike other headaches, does not appear to be affected by menstruation, pregnancy, or the puerperium (Manzoni et al. 1988).

DATABASE

SUBJECTIVE

→ Symptoms include: intense, non-throbbing, sharp, boring, stabbing, or lancinating pain.
  - Lasts 30 minutes to two hours and begins abruptly.
  - May occur daily, often at the same time of day.
  - Occurs commonly in the evening, within two hours of falling asleep.

→ Symptoms may also include:
  - associated ipsilateral conjunctival injection, eye tearing, and nasal stuffiness.
  - sweating or reddening of affected side of face.

→ There is no aura.

OBJECTIVE

→ Physical examination is usually normal since benign headaches are not associated with structural abnormalities.
  - Vital signs, including temperature, should be taken.
  - Head and neck examination should include:
    • check for craniocervical bruits over the eyes, carotid, and vertebral arteris.

- palpation for painful areas, rigidity, masses, or signs of trauma in the scalp, sinuses, and temporal arteries.
- Eye examination should include:
  - check for glaucoma, optic atrophy, papilledema, impaired vision, subhyaloid hemorrhage.
- Nose, mouth, and dentition examination should include:
  - check for tenderness, jaw ROM, and the TMJ.
- Neurological examination should include:
  - cranial nerves.
  - gait, deep tendon reflexes, meningeal signs, cerebellar, Romberg.
  - mental status examination as indicated by history.
- Any neurological abnormalities will necessitate consultation/referral.

ASSESSMENT

- → Cluster headache
- → R/O migraine
- → R/O trigeminal neuralgia (see **Facial Pain** Protocol).
- → R/O organic lesion (if no periodicity of remission and failure to respond to treatment)

PLAN

DIAGNOSTIC TESTS

- → Diagnostic testing in the majority of individuals with benign headaches is of limited value. However, when indicated by history and physical, order the following diagnostic tests:
  - baseline laboratory tests:
    - CBC, ESR
    - urinalysis.
    - blood chemistry profile.
  - sinus x-rays.
  - cervical spine x-rays.
  - lumbar puncture.
  - skull series.
  - brain scan, tomography, CT scan.
  - EEG.
- → For more details on pertinent diagnostics, see specific headache protocols.

TREATMENT/MANAGEMENT

- → Abortive measures:
  - inhaled oxygen: 100% O_2 at 8-10 liters/minute for 10 minutes (preferred treatment).

- ergotamine tartrate (Ergostat®): 2 mg sublingual or oral (see "Migraine Headache").
- lidocaine HCL: 4% nasal drops.
- cocaine HCL in saline solution (less preferred treatment because of potentially addictive properties).
- sumatriptan (Imitrex®): See "Migraine Headache."

- → Prophylactic measures:
  - for clients with episodic cluster, start early in the cluster period and continue until headache-free for at least 2 weeks (Marks and Rapoport 1992).
    - Prednisone: 40 mg-60 mg p.o./day, tapered after 2 weeks; relief within 24 hours.
    - Calcium channel blockers (see "Migraine Headache" for side effects).
      - Verapamil (Calan® SR): 240 mg-480 mg p.o./day (combine with ergotamine for preferred treatment of choice).
      - Nifedipine (Procardia®): 30 mg-60 mg p.o./day.
    - Oral ergotamine (Ergostat®): Taken 1-2 hours before bedtime (1 mg p.o. every day–BID to prevent nocturnal attacks).
    - Lithium carbonate (600 mg-1200 mg p.o./day): Will require a full week before response. Blood lithium levels must be monitored.
    - Valproic acid (Depakene®): 250 mg p.o. QID. Side effects limit usefulness. These include drowsiness, tremor, nausea and vomiting, hair loss, weight gain (Marks and Rapoport 1992).
    - Methsergide maleate (Sansert®): 2 mg-8 mg p.o./day (see "Migraine Headache" for side effects).
  - indomethacin (Indocin®): 25 mg p.o. TID.
- → See "Patient Education" section.

CONSULTATION

- → As necessary if unresponsive to treatment regimen.
- → As needed for prescription(s).

PATIENT EDUCATION

- → See "Patient Education" section of **Headache** Protocol.
- → Advise patient to avoid trigger factors.
- → Advise patient to seek treatment at the first sign of a headache.

→ Advise patient to be aware of possible side effects of medications.

FOLLOW-UP

→ At intervals, if being treated for chronic cluster headache.

→ As necessary, if no relief with treatment regimen.

→ Document in progress notes and problem list.

Tension-Type Headache

Tension-type headaches are the most common types of benign headaches, amounting to 70 to 80 percent of all headaches. They result from chronic contraction of muscles around the head and neck due to emotional conflict or tension (Dalessio 1987). They begin in early adulthood and are more common in women (3:1) (Smith 1988).

DATABASE

SUBJECTIVE

→ Symptoms may include:
  ▪ ache, sensation of tightness, pressure, or constriction in the head, usually in the suboccipital or bifrontal area.
    • May experience hatband-like sensation.
  ▪ associated tightness in neck and/or shoulders.
  ▪ tenderness of upper border of the trapezius and other posterior shoulder, neck, and scalp muscles.
  ▪ neck muscles taut and contracted.
  ▪ associated nausea, photophobia, and photopsia.

→ Headache usually bilateral; rarely unilateral as in migraine.

→ Pain may be mild to incapacitating.

→ Pressure on tender muscles may increase headache intensity.

→ Headache lasts hours to days; in chronic form may persist months to years.

→ Headache often related to stress, depression, or anxiety.

→ There is positive family history in 40 percent of clients.

→ Symptoms can overlap with those of migraine without aura (common migraine).

OBJECTIVE

→ Physical examination is usually normal since benign headaches are not associated with structural abnormalities.

▪ Vital signs, including temperature, should be taken.
▪ Head and neck examination should include:
  • check for craniocervical bruits over the eyes, carotid, and vertebral arteries.
  • palpation for painful areas, rigidity, masses, or signs of trauma in the scalp, sinuses, and temporal arteries.
▪ Eye examination should include:
  • check for glaucoma, optic atrophy, papilledema, impaired vision, subhyaloid hemorrhage.
▪ Nose, mouth, and dentition examination should include:
  • check for tenderness, jaw ROM, and the TMJ.
▪ Neurological examination should include:
  • cranial nerves.
  • gait, deep tendon reflexes, meningeal signs, cerebellar, Romberg.
  • mental status examination as indicated by history.
▪ Any neurological abnormalities will necessitate consultation/referral. Neurological examination typically will be negative.

ASSESSMENT

→ Tension-type headache

→ R/O migraine without aura

→ R/O mass lesion

PLAN

DIAGNOSTIC TESTS

→ There are no diagnostic tests for this type of headache.

→ See "Diagnostic Tests" section of **Headache** Protocol if work-up is deemed necessary.

TREATMENT/MANAGEMENT

→ A supportive client/clinician relationship is significant for the most therapeutic benefit in treatment.

→ Non-pharmacological:
  ▪ massage.
  ▪ heat.
  ▪ acupuncture/acupressure.
  ▪ biofeedback.
  ▪ relaxation training.
  ▪ social support.
  ▪ exercise.
  ▪ yoga.

- stress reduction exercises (visualization/guided imagery).
- counseling.
→ Pharmacological:
  - abortive:
    • NSAIDs.
      –ibuprofen (Motrin®): 400 mg-2400 mg p.o./ day.
      –naproxen (Naprosyn®): 500 mg p.o. BID– TID.
      –naproxen sodium (Anaprox®): 275 mg p.o. BID–TID.
    • aspirin: 600 mg p.o. QID.
    • acetaminophen: 600 mg p.o. QID.
    • analgesic combinations:
      –try after other treatments and only if client is not addiction-prone. For short-term use only.
      –ASA 325mg/caffeine 40 mg/butalbital 50 mg (Fiorinal®): 1-2 tablets p.o. immediately; maximum 6 per attack.
      –Acetaminophen 325 mg with caffeine and butabital (Fioricet®): 1-2 tablets p.o. immediately, maximum 6 per attack.
  - prophylactic:
    • NSAIDs (see "Abortive" above).
    • muscle relaxants (short-term use only):
      –cyclobenzaprine (Flexeril®) 10 mg-40 mg p.o./day in divided doses.
      –diazepam (Valium®): 2 mg-10 mg p.o./day.
    • tricyclic antidepressants (most effective for frequent or daily headaches):
      –amitriptyline (Elavil®): 25 mg-100 mg p.o./ day.
      –trazodone (Desyrel®): 50 mg-150 mg p.o./ day.
    • other antidepressants:
      –fluoxetine (Prozac®): 20 mg-80 mg p.o./day
  - other migraine drugs may be tried (see "Migraine Headache").

CONSULTATION

→ Consultation with a physician is indicated for headaches:
  - unrelieved with non-pharmacological or common pharmacological treatment.
  - requiring addition of analgesic combinations, antidepressants, or muscle relaxants.
→ As needed for prescription(s).

PATIENT EDUCATION

→ See "Patient Education" section of **Headache** Protocol.

FOLLOW-UP

→ See "Follow-Up" section of **Headache** Protocol.
→ Document in progress notes and problem list.

Temporal or Giant Cell Arteritis

Temporal arteritis has the characteristics of an autoimmune process and is a vasculitic disorder of unknown origin. An inflammatory process occurs, predominantly in the cranial arteries, and tends to be segmental (Goroll 1987). The headache is localized to the affected temporal arteries. It affects individuals over age 50 years and is more common in females by a ratio of two to one (2:1). Irreversible blindness in one or both eyes occurs in 50 percent or more of untreated cases (Diamond 1992).

DATABASE

SUBJECTIVE

→ Symptoms may include:
  - severe, unilateral, throbbing pain localized to the scalp, often noticed when brushing hair.
  - pain experienced with chewing (i.e., jaw claudication), with possible resultant weight loss.
  - low-grade fever.
  - joint pain (polymyalgia rheumatica).
  - decreased vision (may have diplopia).
  - night sweats.
→ Symptoms may be:
  - exacerbated by exposure to cold.
  - of recent onset (Marks and Rapoport 1992)
→ Patient may be asymptomatic.

OBJECTIVE

→ Vital signs, including temperature, should be taken.
→ Head and neck examination should include:
  - check for craniocervical bruits over the eyes, carotid, and vertebral arteries.
  - palpation for painful areas, rigidity, masses, or signs of trauma in the scalp, sinuses, and temporal arteries.
→ Eye examination should include:
  - check for glaucoma, optic atrophy, papilledema, impaired vision, subhyaloid hemorrhage.
→ Nose, mouth, and dentition examination should include:
  - check for tenderness, jaw ROM, and the TMJ.
→ Neurological examination should include:

■ cranial nerves.

■ gait, deep tendon reflexes, meningeal signs, cerebellar, Romberg.

■ mental status examination as indicated by history.

→ Any neurological abnormalities will necessitate consultation/referral.

→ Specific objective components of temporal arteritis may include:

■ tender temporal arteries.

■ reddened temple area.

■ low-grade fever.

■ myalgias.

■ elevated ESR.

ASSESSMENT

→ Temporal arteritis

→ R/O other causes of headache

PLAN

DIAGNOSTIC TESTS

→ ESR: If greater than 40 mm/hr a temporal artery biopsy should be performed (Marks and Rapoport 1992).

TREATMENT/MANAGEMENT

→ Immediate, urgent treatment is required to prevent blindness.

→ Prednisone 40 mg-60 mg p.o./day (1mg/kg/day):

■ should be started before biopsy results are received. Tapering begins when the sedimentation rate has been significantly reduced and symptoms are controlled.

→ Corticosteroid treatment may be required for as long as several years.

→ Monitor ESR periodically.

→ Observe for improvement in headache symptoms. (Marks and Rapoport 1992)

CONSULTATION

→ Co-management with a physician is recommended.

→ Consultation with a rheumatologist is recommended if the temporal artery biopsy is negative but the presentation suggests temporal arteritis.

→ Referral to a physican is recommended for cases that do not respond to steroid therapy.

→ As needed for prescription(s).

PATIENT EDUCATION

→ Inform patient of symptoms of arteritis.

→ Instruct patient to report symptom occurrence immediately.

→ Discuss need for prednisone on a daily basis to promote compliance.

→ Discuss side effects of steroids.

→ Involve family in care as appropriate.

FOLLOW-UP

→ Close follow-up is recommended for steroid tapering and reduction of symptoms.

→ Document in progress notes and problem list.

Jacqueline W. Wasserman, R.N., C., M.S., F.N.P.

9-E

Seizures

Seizures result when an abnormally active group of neurons discharge in an excessive and hypersynchronous pattern. A focal or partial seizure results when this pattern of discharge is localized in a cortical area. A generalized seizure results when localized in deeper brain structures. (Eckel 1985).

Approximately two million people in the United States have epileptic seizures, the majority of whom (70 to 80 percent) experience their first seizure before age 20 years. The frequency is variable. In women, episodes may be more frequent prior to menses. In pregnancy, the frequency may increase or decrease. (Barrigan-Hornibrook and Rich 1987).

Seizures are classified according to the focus of onset, clinical manifestations, and EEG changes. There are two major categories: partial (focal) seizures and generalized seizures (Eckel 1985).

Partial seizures can be simple or complex. If consciousness is not impaired, the seizure is considered a *simple partial seizure.* If consciousness is impaired, the seizure is considered a *complex partial seizure.* Complex seizures can involve complex motor behavior, chewing, swallowing, spoken words, or emotional mimicry. A partial seizure is characterized by a warning or aura before the attack (Eckel 1985).

Generalized or *grand mal* seizures often begin without warning, with a sudden generalized onset of rigid tonic muscle tone. There may be associated incontinence and an epileptic cry. These generalized tonic-clonic seizures have a tonic phase, lasting one to two minutes, and then a clonic phase of generalized jerking movements of the extremities, usually lasting no more than five minutes. During the following postictal phase—lasting up to one to two hours—the individual is unarousable, then stuporous and confused (Eckel 1985).

Identifiable causes of seizures can be linked to symptomatic or acquired epilepsy, including congenital malformation, maternal infection, prematurity, alcohol and drug use, and perinatal problems that result in birth trauma and asphyxia, causing brain damage and then seizures.

Epileptic lesions develop in two percent of previously neurologically normal children after febrile convulsions. In adults and adolescents, head trauma and brain tumors (in eight percent to ten percent of adults) are major causes of acquired seizures, as well as meningitis, encephalitic infections, and brain abscesses. However, in 50 percent of individuals, there are no specific structural or biochemical abnormalities and, therefore, the cause is considered idiopathic. A genetic predisposition is found in individuals with idiopathic epilepsy (Barrigan-Hornibrook and Rich 1987).

DATABASE

SUBJECTIVE

→ Patient may have history of:
- any kind of seizure activity including:
  - sudden loss of consciousness accompanied by staring and blinking; immediate regaining of consciousness.
  - brief jerks in arms or legs.
  - sudden loss of muscle tone causing a fall and subsequent head injuries.
  - initial cry, respiratory arrest, cyanosis, tonic-clonic convulsions, relaxation followed by deep sleep.

- incontinence.
- postictal confusion.
- presence of aura before seizure.
- alcohol use.
- drug use.
- sleep deprivation.
- closed head trauma (Seizures may develop within a two-year time period).
- open head trauma (Seizures may develop at any time after injury).
- cardiac arrhythmias.
- mitral or aortic valve disease.
- malignancy or stroke.

→ Patient may have family history of seizures.

OBJECTIVE

→ Assess vital signs for symptoms, including postural changes in blood pressure and pulse.

→ Complete neurological examination should be done for focal findings that localize central nervous system disease.

→ Assess for:
- head trauma.
- papilledema.
- carotid disease.
- cardiac dysrhythmias or valvular problems.
- manifestations of alcohol or drug use.

ASSESSMENT

→ Seizure disorder

→ R/O disorders that mimic seizures:
- transient ischemic attacks (TIA)
- migraine
- nerve compression

→ R/O syncopal attacks from:
- cardiac arrhythmias
- TIA
- severe hypoglycemia
- hypotension

→ R/O infection

→ R/O underlying disease

→ R/O neoplasm

→ R/O drug/alcohol withdrawal

→ R/O trauma

→ R/O CVA

PLAN

DIAGNOSTIC TESTS

→ Routine blood tests—including CBC, electrolytes, glucose, calcium, magnesium, kidney and liver functions, VDRL or RPR are indicated.

→ EEG is indicated.

→ Toxicology screen of blood and urine is recommended if drug/alcohol use is suspected.

→ CT scan of the head or MRI indicated if acute brain injury, new seizures, or a significant change in the pattern of seizures (Eckel 1985). Otherwise, not immediately required (Pruitt 1987).

→ Lumbar puncture recommended if CT scan has ruled out a mass lesion or hydrocephalus.
- Lumbar puncture can establish the diagnosis of encephalitis, meningitis, cerebrospinal fluid infiltration of tumor, or CNS syphilis (Eckel 1985).

TREATMENT/MANAGEMENT

→ Therapy for seizure disorders focuses on suppressing seizures and assisting the client in living with the disorder.
- This approach is established after any treatable underlying cause of seizures has been ruled out (e.g., brain tumor or encephalitis).
- Treatment is not recommended after a single seizure.
- Treatment recommendations should be based on drug side effects in addition to information on the potential psychological, vocational, and physical consequences of further seizures (Scheuer and Pedley 1990).

→ Accurate diagnosis of the type of seizure, once established, will determine the choice of anticonvulsant drug(s) (ACDs).
- See **Table 9E.1, Six Most Frequently Used Anticonvulsant Drugs.**
- In choosing ACDs, consider that:
  - rarely is there a ''best'' drug for a seizure type.
  - a given client may not tolerate a particular drug.
  - often, a combination of 2 ACDs is necessary, as 1 ACD may not provide optimal control.

→ Factors involved in choosing ACDs:
- age.
  - Chronic effects in young adults make some choices less desirable.

Table 9E.1.   SIX MOST FREQUENTLY USED ANTICONVULSANT DRUGS

Drug	Dose	Indications (Types of Seizures)	Common Side Effects
Phenytoin (Dilantin®)	300 mg-600 mg p.o./day	Simple and complex partial Secondarily generalized Primary generalized	Ataxia, dysarthria, gingival hypertrophy, hirsutism, acneiform eruption, liver failure, osteomalacia
Carbamazepine (Tegretol®)	600 mg-1200 mg p.o./day	Simple and complex partial Secondarily generalized Primary generalized	Drowsiness, blurred vision, diplopia, disequilibrium, leukopenia, liver failure
Phenobarbital (Luminal®)	90 mg-180 mg p.o./day	Simple and complex partial Secondarily generalized Primary generalized	Sedation, depression, loss of concentration, mental dulling, hyperactivity
Primidone (Mysoline®)	750 mg-1500 mg p.o./day	Simple and complex partial Secondarily generalized	Sedation, dizziness, nausea, ataxia, depression
Valproic acid (Depakene®)	1000 mg-3000 mg p.o./day	Primary generalized	Gastrointestinal upset, weight gain, hair loss, tremor, thrombocytopenia, liver failure, pancreatitis
Ethosuximide (Zarontin®)	750 mg-1500 mg p.o./day	Absence Atonic	Gastrointestinal, mood changes, lethargy, hiccups, headache

Source: Adapted with permission from Scheurer, M.L., and Pedley, T.A. 1990. The evaluation and treatment of seizures. *The New England Journal of Medicine* 323(21):1471-1472.

- sex.
  - Some ACDs induce the metabolism of steroid hormones which may lessen the effectiveness of low-dose oral contraceptives, and present potential risks during pregnancy and lactation.
- compliance.
  - Tailor to individual needs and schedule.
- cost.
  - Some drugs are not covered by third-party payers.
→ Individuals who are seizure-free for 2 years may be considered for discontinuation of drug therapy.
  - This must be done gradually, especially with barbiturates (Bleck 1990).
→ ACDs should be introduced slowly to minimize side effects.
→ Regular serum levels are helpful to establish a baseline for therapeutic level, as well as detect noncompliance or other causes of lowered serum drug levels, should seizures recur.
  - The serum drug level should be checked during the steady state.
  - After a client has been medicated for 5 half-lives of a drug, a steady state is usually achieved (Eckel 1985).

CONSULTATION

→ Medical and neurological consultation is recommended, particularly during the initial evaluation and the development of a treatment plan. If seizures continue to occur after three months, care should be assumed by a neurologist. When the client is stable, primary management can be resumed.

→ As needed for prescription(s).

PATIENT EDUCATION

→ Explain possible restrictions that may be placed on lifestyle, e.g., driving.
  - Laws vary from state to state, but generally one must be seizure-free for one year before one may reapply for a driver's license.
→ Educate regarding seizure disorders and possible societal stigmas. Allay fears and maintain dialogue regarding client concerns.
→ Explain signals that may indicate when a seizure may occur—e.g., headache, malaise, or some other vague symptom.
→ Stress importance of taking medications.
→ Educate family members and client of signs and symptoms of drug toxicity:
  - anorexia.
  - visual symptoms (double vision).
  - numbness of extremities.
  - dizziness.
  - behavioral problems.
  - fever.
  - drowsiness.
  - rash.

- ataxia.
- irritability.
- gastric distress (Barrigan-Hornibrook and Rich 1987).

→ Advise as to routine for checking drug levels at regular intervals.

→ Educate family members for emergency measures during a seizure:
  - protect head.
  - place person on bed or floor.
  - avoid objects in the mouth.
  - do not forcibly restrain.
  - remove eyeglasses and loosen clothing around head and neck.

→ Educate regarding measures after the seizure:
  - turn the person on the side to allow saliva, etc., to drain.
  - allow person to rest undisturbed.
  - call for help if an injury occurs, if the person does not start breathing, or if the person passes from one seizure to another without regaining consciousness (Barrigan-Hornibrook and Rich 1987).

→ Recommend abstention from drugs and alcohol and avoidance of certain stimulants such as coffee and tobacco.

→ Stress importance of adequate and regular meals.

→ Encourage getting adequate rest.

→ Encourage regular exercise, such as swimming, biking, jogging.

→ Advise avoiding dangerous sports (e.g., scuba diving, mountain climbing, hang gliding, or snow sports) where momentary loss of consciousness could be fatal.

→ Avoid jobs involving the operation of heavy machinery, underground or underwater work, or other potentially dangerous work.

→ Advise genetic counseling when one or both partners have epilepsy and desire children.
  - Six percent of children with one epileptic parent and 10 percent to 12 percent of children with two epileptic parents will develop the disorder (Barrigan-Hornibrook and Rich 1987).

→ Advise women of childbearing age of the slightly higher risk of maternal complications during pregnancy and delivery. Also advise that ACDs contribute to the risk of fetal abnormalities.

→ Inform about the availability of additional information from the following organizations:

American Epilepsy Society
Department of Neurology
Reed Neurological Research
   Center
710 Westwood Plaza
Los Angeles, CA 90024
(213) 825-5745

Epilepsy Foundation of America
4351 Garden City Drive
Landover, MD 20781
(301) 459-3700

FOLLOW-UP

→ Evaluate the stability of the client's status based on the number and frequency of seizures.

→ Monitor serum drug levels as needed.

→ Follow up more frequently if drug levels and symptoms are poorly controlled.

→ Refer as indicated under "Consultation" section.

→ Note seizure disorder on problem list and treatment regimen in progress notes.

Wendy L. Berk, C.A.N.P.

9-F

Temporomandibular Disorder

Temporomandibular disorder (TMD), formerly known as temporomandibular joint (TMJ) syndrome, is a common problem encountered in primary care. It is important to recognize it so patients may be advised and managed appropriately. However, it should not be overdiagnosed, thereby delaying treatment of an underlying problem.

It has been estimated that 75 percent of the population has at least one sign of jaw dysfunction and 25 percent has at least one symptom. Most cases are mild and self-limited. A small minority actually need treatment. Recent studies report a 6:1 to 8:1 ratio of females to males who present with TMD in health care settings (McNeill 1991). The majority of women are between the ages of 15 years to 40 years (Graff-Radford 1990).

The TMJ is a complex synovial joint located between the temporal and mandibular bones. It is surrounded by a highly innervated fibrous capsule. Separating the joint into upper and lower compartments is the disc, which is a fibrous structure (see **Figure 9F.1, Illustration of TMJ Joint**). Its purpose is to cushion and stabilize the joint. The posterior attachment of the disc to the fossa, the retrodiscal tissue, is well vascularized and innervated. This can be the location of pain when there is TMJ dysfunction.

Two movements are characteristic of the TMJ. The first is a rotation movement for 12 mm between incisors followed by a gliding translation. The disc and the condyle normally move together. Dysfunction and pain can occur when there is incoordination between the condyle and disc (see **Figure 9F.2, TMJ Condyle/Disc Dynamics**).

Patients may complain of the mouth locked in the closed position (closed lock) caused by blocking by a displaced disc and/or muscle trismus. The mouth locked in an open position (open lock) may occur when the condyle gets stuck in front of the disc or beyond the articular eminence.

Subluxation, degenerative joint changes, and connective tissue disease such as rheumatoid arthritis (RA), osteoarthritis (OA), psoriatic arthritis, or gout can affect the TMJ. The jaw joint is very adaptable, however, and many people function well with significant structural abnormalities, even when the disc is displaced.

Muscular pain is the major symptom of TMD. The major muscles that cause movement of the TMJ are the temporalis, masseters, and medial pterygoids for closing the jaw and the lateral pterygoids and digastrics for opening the jaw.

Myofascial pain from masticatory and cervical muscles is considered a major cause of TMD-related muscular pain. Myofascial pain is described as pain from trigger points located in muscles and tendons. The pain can be local or referred.

The exact mechanism that causes myofascial pain is unknown. Myofascial pain may be caused by muscle overuse or disuse, although emotional factors, fatigue, and various illnesses may be part of the etiology (Tanaka 1989). The trigger points are stimulated by normal muscle activity. Counterstimulation, muscle stretching, and postural correction have been used to treat myofascial pain (Fricton 1991). The references listed contain detailed illustrations of trigger points.

There has been much debate about predisposing factors for TMD. Parafunctions are universally accepted as contributing to dysfunction. These include bruxism (clenching and grinding), lip biting, nail chewing, and tongue thrusting.

Figure 9F.1.   ILLUSTRATION OF TMJ JOINT

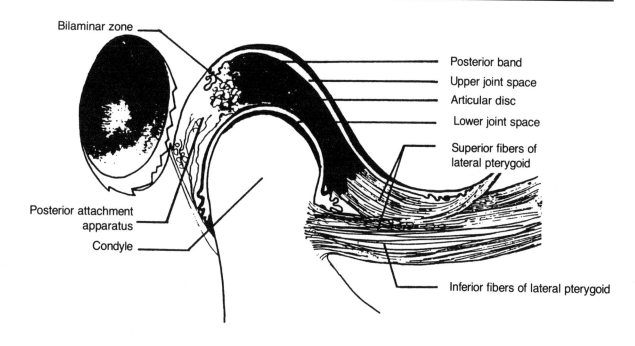

Reprinted with permission from Tanaka, T.T. *A diagnostic and therapeutic approach for TMJ disorders for restorative dentists and other health professionals,* 4th ed., p. K. Copyright © 1989 by Clinical Research Foundation, San Diego.

Bruxism is common but frequently unrecognized by patients unless they are asked to observe for it. Bruxism is thought to be more common in children, although they tend to grow out of it in time. Stress and problems with occlusion are thought to be common etiological factors. Bruxism frequently occurs during the transition from deeper to lighter sleep. Bruxism is more common during an exacerbation of allergic rhinitis or asthma. Severe bruxism can lead to enamel damage, tooth loosening, and muscle tension. When patients complain of morning headaches, bruxism should be entertained as a possible cause (Leung and Robson 1991).

Dysfunction of the cervical area—e.g., poor posture, degenerative changes, muscle tightness, and active trigger points—can cause referred pain to the jaw and changes in occlusion. Ligament laxity has been postulated as a predisposing factor, but studies to date have been inconclusive.

The role of malocclusion has been quite controversial, but recently, most TMD research centers are downplaying it as a causative factor. Apart from gross structural deformities, malocclusion may aggravate the ongoing condition. Malocclusion may need to be addressed if conservative measures fail. Lack of posterior teeth can cause abnormal loading of the TMJ and contribute to pain and dysfunction.

Trauma has been acknowledged as a contributor to TMD. Occasionally, TMD symptoms can begin after a dental appointment where the mouth is held open for a long time. It also is not uncommon to obtain a history of traumatic family violence. However, the patient often will not admit to current battery. It may be unclear if the physical violence would have initiated the symptoms or if stress would be the major contributing factor.

Car accidents and the role of whiplash are controversial. Whiplash has been commonly thought to precipitate TMD symptoms. However, Heise, Laskin, and Gervin (1992) studied whiplash patients and found that in their population the incidence of joint noises and pain initially and on follow-up was very low. The role of secondary gain must be considered. It is crucial to find out if litigation is pending. There is a sizeable monetary award for TMD, and symptoms may not improve until settlement is made.

Anxiety and depression have been associated with TMD. However, with chronic pain, it is difficult to sort out the physical and psychological symptoms. The clinician needs to be alert for abuse of prescription pain medications and muscle relaxants in chronic pain patients. Also, caffeine and stimulant abuse can increase muscle tension and worsen TMD symptoms.

Figure 9F.2. TMJ CONDYLE/DISC DYNAMICS

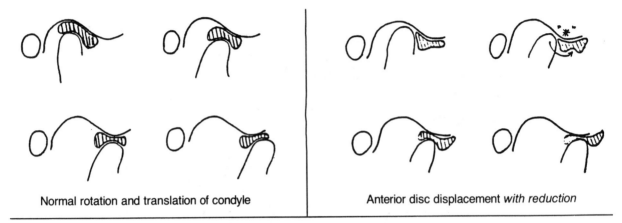

Normal rotation and translation of condyle

Anterior disc displacement *with reduction*

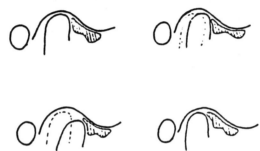

Anterior disc displacement without reduction (closed lock)

Reprinted with permission from Tanaka, T.T. *A diagnostic and therapeutic approach for TMJ disorders for restorative dentists and other health professionals*, 4th ed., p. K-18a. Copyright © 1989 by Clinical Research Foundation, San Diego.

Since TMD affects mainly young women, new onset of jaw pain in a patient over 50 years of age should alert the clinician to the possibility of another cause such as temporal arteritis, tumor, angina, or connective tissue disease (see **Face Pain** Protocol).

The key to treatment of TMD is conservatism. Treatment should be focused on relieving pain, reducing inflammation, and restoring function. A multidisciplinary approach is very useful. A team approach can help quality control, facilitate communication, and avoid the use of unnecessary tests and treatments.

DATABASE

SUBJECTIVE

→ Symptom history should include:
- side of pain.
- duration of symptoms.
- how did symptoms start? Make sure to ask about:
  - trauma, including whiplash.
  - dental examination/nerve block.
- stress.
- quality of the pain (e.g., achy, burning, throbbing, sharp).
- specific pain triggers and exacerbators, including pain with:
  - chewing.
  - opening mouth.
  - hot or cold foods.
  - talking.
  - exercise.
  - neck movement.
- other aggravating factors (e.g., stress, position, job, school, weather).
- associated symptoms, including:
  - neck pain.
  - ear symptoms, such as pain, plugging, tinnitus.
  - headache.
  - tooth pain.
  - sinus discomfort/drainage.

- eye disturbance—vision change (blurred vision, double vision, visual field loss, scotoma, photophobia, pain, redness).
- numbness.
- weakness.
- rash.
- jaw function, including:
  - locking—open or closed.
  - joint noise.

→ Medical history should include:
- trauma, including:
  - MVA.
  - surgery or dental work.
  - domestic violence.
- dental problems, including:
  - braces
  - bridge work and dentures (a loose fit may contribute to bruxism).
  - tooth extraction, root canal.
  - splint.
  - clencher/grinder.
    - –when and if associated with stress.

→ Other medical problems, particularly:
- diabetes.
- hypertension.
- thyroid disorder.
- sleep disorder.
- psychiatric disorder such as depression/anxiety.
- connective tissue disorder/joint laxity.
- heart disease.
- headaches.
- arthritis.
- vasculitis.

→ Ascertain family history, including:
- connective tissue disease.
- headache.

→ Ascertain level of substance use, including:
- alcohol.
- smoking.
- street drugs, particularly stimulants.
- caffeine.

→ Ascertain medication use, including:
- OTC medications.
  - Overuse of OTCs and prescription medications can cause an analgesic rebound headache in patients with a primary headache problem (Mathew, Kurman, and Perez 1990; Rapoport 1988). This is commonly seen in headache clinics.
  - It is important to monitor the pain medication intake of patients with headaches and to

counsel them before a secondary headache problem emerges.
- decongestants.
  - These act as stimulants and can cause poor sleep and bruxing.
- prescription medications, including birth control pills.

→ Social factors, such as:
- occupation—including shift work (irregular circadian rhythms can exacerbate migraines).
- home life—especially stressors and faulty coping mechanisms.
- hobbies—including sports that cause clenching or activities that cause poor posture.

OBJECTIVE

→ Include portions of the physical examination appropriate to the symptoms:
- blood pressure.
- skin:
  - look for vesicular rash.
- facial symmetry.
- eyes:
  - Snellen, visual fields, color chart, lid inflammation, conjunctival redness, pupil size and reactivity, disc margins and color, and fluorescein stain, if pain and photophobia.
- ears:
  - gross hearing; Weber and Rinne; ear canal for swelling, redness, and discharge; tympanic membrane.
- throat:
  - include tongue, palate, buccal mucosa (linea alba on the buccal mucosa can indicate bruxism, as can a scalloped tongue).
  - observe for muscosal lesions.
- salivary glands:
  - note size, consistency, pain. A ductal stone may be palpated, or purulent drainage may be seen.
- teeth:
  - observe for missing teeth, wear marks, state of repair, tooth pain with percussion or biting gauze (the latter may indicate fracture).
- mandible abnormalities:
  - e.g., malocclusion, mandible asymmetry, retrognathia, prognathia, mandible pain.
- TMJ:
  - palpate for pain, open and closed, and crepitance (crackling noise).
  - ROM (note deflection to the side):

–intercisal opening (normal range 35 mm-50 mm).

–laterotrusion (normal range 8 mm-10 mm).

–protrusion (normal range 8 mm-10 mm).

▸ This is difficult to measure. Look for deflection with movement. Deflection on one side may indicate joint dysfunction on the same side.

- joint noises (with and without stethoscope):

–click/pop.

▸ It is difficult to ascertain the exact cause of the click or pop on physical examination. These noises can be caused by fossa/disc/condyle incoordination or structural bony and soft tissue irregularities. Note the timing, coordination, and consistency in opening and closing. Early open clicks and pops have a better prognosis than late open noises.

–crepitance.

- joint loading:

–have client bite with molars on two tongue blades. Pain on the opposite side is a positive test and can indicate joint pathology.

▪ neck:

- posture.
- pain with palpation and ROM.
- ROM.
- radicular symptoms with movement.
- thyroid.
- carotid arteries—pain, swelling, bruits.

▪ neurological:

- symmetry of facial muscles.
- facial sensation.
- symmetry of tongue.
- symmetry of palate.
- gag reflex.
- greater auricular nerve and greater occipital nerve.
- other cranial nerves, as appropriate.

▪ muscle screening examination:

- masseters.
- temporalis.
- suboccipitals.
- trapezius.
- sternocleidomastoid.
- for more complete evaluation of muscles, including intraoral muscles. Refer to photographs in reference books.

→ Past laboratory work or x-rays pertaining to face pain.

ASSESSMENT

→ Temporomandibular dysfunction—in all instances—includes the following symptoms:

- pain with jaw movement
- pain with palpation
- limitation of jaw movement if pain is minimal

→ Temporomandibular dysfunction also may present with these symptoms:

- joint noises
- jaw movement, limitation, or deflection
- history of locking
- headache
- ear discomfort/tinnitus

→ Causes of TMD (may be a mixture of these):

- muscle activity causing myofascial pain
- bruxism joint dysfunction such as disc displacement
- connective tissue disease
- significant skeletal abnormality

→ See **Face Pain** Protocol for differential diagnoses

PLAN

DIAGNOSTIC TESTS

→ Laboratory:

- ESR for patients over 50 years old.
- ESR, RF, anti-nuclear antibody (ANA), uric acid, if appropriate for TMJ crepitance.

→ Radiology:

- x-rays should be done if there is significant trauma or if significant joint pathology is suspected.
- panorex.
  - If accessible, this is inexpensive and is very helpful in visualizing mandibular tumors, fractures, dental abnormalities, the maxillary sinuses, and, grossly, the TMJ. Plain TMJ films and mandible films are not as good.
- TMJ tomograms.
  - This is best for arthritic findings.
  - It also can visualize the position of the condyle in the fossa.
- MRI.
  - This is a very expensive test which best visualizes soft tissue, such as the disc.
  - It should only be used if surgery is contemplated, with the recommendation of the oral surgeon.

TREATMENT/MANAGEMENT

→ Non-TMD disorders—treat or refer appropriately.

→ TMD and jaw-related disorders:
- joint noises as isolated findings do not need further treatment or follow-up.
  - reassure patients that this will not lead to arthritis.
- local applications of heat or cold, massage, acupressure may be helpful.
- anti-inflammatory drugs such as aspirin or NSAIDs.
  - Avoid NSAIDs in patients with peptic ulcer disease and bleeding problems.
  - Use with caution in patients with asthma, decreased renal function, gastric reflux, uncontrolled hypertension.
- tricyclics—See **Appendix 9C.1, Tricyclics and Pain Syndromes**, in **Face Pain** Protocol, p. 9-20.
- non-narcotic analgesics as appropriate.
- muscle relaxants as appropriate, such as:
  - cyclobenzaprine (Flexiril®), 10 mg p.o. at bedtime.
  - carisoprodol (Soma®), 350 mg p.o. QID.

NOTE: Advise patients that muscle relaxants can cause drowsiness and to avoid using them with other central nervous system depressants. Also advise patients of their addiction potential (Elder 1991). Cyclobenzaprine is similar to tricyclics and may cause similar side effects.

- Advise patient to avoid of caffeine and stimulants such as cocaine and amphetamines.
- Treatment of nasal congestion, since mouth breathing can cause the mandible to protrude slightly.
- For bruxers:
  - recommend relaxation training/biofeedback.
  - splint as appropriate, especially if grinding is damaging the teeth.
    - Splints are clear acrylic devices that are fitted on the maxillary teeth or occasionally over the mandibular teeth.
    - Splints help prevent bruxing, decompress the TMJ joint, decrease muscle tension, and stabilize the joint.
    - Splint therapy can be used for bruxers, myofascial pain, open locking, mild to moderate closed locks, and protection of inflamed joints.
    - Splints are worn all the time except for eating. Night bruxers and patients with milder symptoms may wear them only while sleeping.
    - The cost to the patient must be considered before a referral is made to the dentist.
      ‣ In the San Francisco Bay Area, splints can cost $300-$500 (G. A. Hong, personal communication, October 6, 1992). This is excluding the cost of fitting, x-rays and adjustment.
    - Athletic bite guards are not recommended since they can change occlusion over time.
  - medication:
    - tricyclics may be helpful.
  - education and awareness training.
  - re-evaluate medication usage—e.g., prescription medications such as neuroleptics, stimulants.
  - evaluate if bruxing is secondary to psychiatric problem and then refer as appropriate.

→ Surgery is rarely indicated.
- Braun (1989) mentions studies that report a 2.7 percent to 4.1 percent incidence of TMD patients who went on to surgery.
  - Osteotomies can correct mandibular deformities like retrognathia.
  - Arthroscopy and, more recently, arthrocentesis are used to break up adhesions and improve mobility.
  - Arthroplasty is used if all else fails for arthritic conditions.

→ In very severe cases when all appropriate treatments have been attempted, chronic pain programs can teach patients how to live satisfactory lives with their pain.

CONSULTATION

→ Consult a physician when the patient does not exhibit typical symptoms and signs, and the diagnosis is unclear.

→ Refer to otolaryngology for patients over age 60 years with new onset of symptoms.

→ Physical therapy is very useful in the treatment of TMD.
- Therapy can improve the mobility of the joint, and therapists can perform upper-cervical soft-tissue techniques, demonstrate proper posture, teach a home exercise program, and utilize various modalities to reduce inflammation and spasm.

→ Mental health professionals are very helpful to patients who present an emotional component.

- Besides initial assessment and psychotherapy, they can teach relaxation training, such as biofeedback and self-hypnosis.
- Stress management classes are useful.
- Occasionally, referral to a social worker or child protection services for family violence is indicated.

→ Refer to rheumatologist if there is significant connective tissue disease.

→ For prolonged open lock, refer to the emergency room or to a dental consultant who can manipulate the jaw back to the proper position.

→ Refer to dentist for splint.

→ Refer to a maxillofacial surgeon for:
- progressive closed lock without pain.
- major mandible deformities.
- patients who have already had TMJ surgery.

- continued pain and decreased functioning unrelieved by six months of splint therapy.
- jaw pain and progressively decreasing function with connective tissue disease.
- acute new closed lock that is not primarily myofascial. These patients are candidates for arthrocentesis.

→ As needed for prescription(s).

PATIENT EDUCATION

→ See **Appendix 9F.1, Patient Instructions for Jaw Pain**, p. 9-43.

FOLLOW-UP

→ Mild cases can be followed easily in a primary care setting. For moderate to severe cases, a team approach is preferred.

→ Document in progress notes and problem list.

APPENDIX 9F.1

Patient Instructions for Jaw Pain

1. Stick to a soft diet. Cut up your food. Do not eat chewy foods such as french bread, bagels, licorice, or tough meat. Avoid crunchy food such as nuts, raw vegetables, and corn nuts. If you are experiencing a lot of pain, grind foods in a blender. Protect your jaw joint as you would other joints in your body.

2. Never chew gum. Also avoid chewing ice.

3. Do not bite your lower lip or nails, or chew on pens or pencils.

4. Avoid tongue protrusion, e.g., licking ice cream cones.

5. Do not grind or clench your teeth. Try to keep your teeth apart with your tongue gently resting against the roof of your mouth as it does when you say the word "no."

6. Do not open your mouth wide when you yawn or eat large sandwiches.

7. Maintain good posture. Protrusion of the jaw and neck will change the position of your bite. Avoid resting your jaw in your hand.

8. Sleep on your back or on your side if this doesn't cause pain. Stomach sleeping will put additional strain on the jaw and neck.

9. Avoid caffeine, which increases muscle tension. Also avoid cigarette smoking, which causes your jaw to protrude and creates facial muscle tightness.

10. Do not cradle the phone between your jaw and shoulder or carry uneven loads, such as heavy purses.

11. Wear sunglasses to prevent squinting of the facial muscles.

12. Exercise regularly, especially walking and swimming, to help reduce pain. Avoid exercise that causes clenching such as weight lifting and scuba diving. Also avoid the jarring of horseback riding.

13. When pain occurs, notice which activities worsen your symptoms.

14. Learn and then practice relaxation techniques. It is well known that these can lessen pain. A stress management class can be very useful.

By Wendy L. Berk, C.A.N.P. Permission is granted to reproduce for patients as needed.

9-G
Bibliography

Adour, K.K. 1982. Diagnosis and management of facial paralysis. *The New England Journal of Medicine* 307(6):348–351.

———. 1991. Medical management of idiopathic (Bell's) palsy. *Otolaryngologic Clinics of North America* 24: 663–673.

Adour, K.K., Santos, D.Q., Ruboyiances, J.M., Von Doersten, P.G., Byl, F.M., Trent, C.S., and Hitchcock, T. 1992. *Bell's palsy treatment study.* Manuscript submitted for publication.

Adour, K.K., Wingerd, J., Bell, D.N., Manning, J.J., and Hurley, J.P. 1972. Prednisone treatment for idiopathic facial paralysis (Bell's palsy). *The New England Journal of Medicine* 287:1268–1972.

Adour, K.K., Wingerd, J., and Doty, H.E. 1975. Prevalence of concurrent diabetes mellitus and idiopathic facial paralysis (Bell's palsy). *Diabetes* 24:449–451.

Alford, B.R., Jerger, J.F., Coats, A.C., Peterson, C.R., and Weber, S.C. 1973. Neurophysiology of facial nerve testing. *Archives of Otolaryngology* 97:214–219.

Barrigan-Hornibrook, J., and Rich, E. 1987. Central nervous system and hormone control. In *Handbook of Adult Primary Care*, ed. C.S. Greene, pp. 949–951. New York: John Wiley & Sons.

———. 1987. Central nervous system and hormone control. In *Handbook of Adult Primary Care*, ed. C.S. Green, pp. 929–934, 981–985. New York: John Wiley & Sons.

Bernstein, A.L., and Lobitz, C.S. 1988. A clinical and electrophysiologic study of the treatment of painful diabetic neuropathies with pyrodoxine. *Current Topics of Nutritional Disease* 19:415–423.

Bleck, T.P. 1990. Convulsive disorders: The use of anticonvulsant drugs. *Clinical Neuropharmacology* 13(3):198–209.

Braun, T. 1989. Temporomandibular joint surgery: Surgical management of internal derangement. *Selected Readings in Oral and Maxillofacial Surgery* 1(3):1–36.

Burchiel, K.J., and Burgess, J.A. 1989. Differential diagnosis of orofacial pain. In *Handbook of chronic pain management*, ed. C.D. Tollison, pp. 275–287. Baltimore: Williams & Wilkins.

Cohen, N.L. 1991. The dizzy patient. Update on vestibular disorders. *Medical Clinics of North America* 75(6):1251–1260.

Dalessio, D.J., ed. 1987. *Wolff's headache and other head pain*, 5th ed. New York: Oxford University Press.

Day, T.J. 1990. Migraine and other vascular headaches: An overview of diagnosis and management. *Australian Family Physician* 19(12):1797–1804.

Diamond, S. 1992. Prolonged benign exertional headache: Its clinical characteristics and response to indomethacin. *Headache* 22:96–98.

———. 1992. Acute headache. Differential diagnosis and management of the three types. *Postgraduate Medicine* (Spec Rep) Aug 3:21–29.

Eckel, R.W. 1985. Headache: Evaluation and treatment. In *Manual of clinical problems in adult ambulatory care*, eds. L. Dorbrand, A. Hoole, R. Fletcher, and C.G. Pickard, Jr., pp. 401–411. Boston: Little, Brown & Co.

———. 1985. Seizures: Evaluation. In *Manual of clinical problems in adult ambulatory care*, eds. L. Dorbrand, A. Hoole, R. Fletcher, and C.G. Pickard, Jr., pp. 411–420. Boston: Little, Brown & Co.

Edmeads, J. 1990. Understanding dizziness. How to decipher this nonspecific symptom. *Postgraduate Medicine* 88(5):255–258, 263–268.

———. 1990. Challenges in the diagnosis of acute headache. *Headache* 30(Suppl. 2):537–540.

Elder, N.C. 1991. Abuse of skeletal muscle relaxants. *American Family Physician* 44:1223–1226.

Fricton, J.R. 1991. Clinical care for myofascial pain. *Dental Clinics of North America* 35(1):1–25.

Fusco, B.M., and Alessandri, M. 1992. Analgesic effect of capsaicin in idiopathic trigeminal neuralgia. *Anesthesia and Analgesia* 74:375–377.

Gallagher, R.M. 1991. Headache diagnosis and treatment. *Journal of the American Academy of Nurse Practitioners* 3(1):3–10.

Goroll, A.H. 1987. Evaluation of a headache. In *Primary care medicine*, eds. A.H. Goroll, L.A. May, and A.G. Mulley, Jr., 2nd ed., pp. 714–720. Philadelphia: J.B. Lippincott.

———. 1987. Managment of migraine and other vascular headaches. In *Primary care medicine*, eds. A.H. Goroll, L.A. May, and A.G. Mulley, Jr., 2nd ed., pp. 749–752. Philadelphia: J.B. Lippincott.

———. 1987. Management of temporal arteritis and polymyalgia rheumatica. In *Primary care medicine*, eds. A.H. Goroll, L.A. May, and A.G. Mulley, Jr., 2nd ed., pp. 704–706. Philadelphia: J.B. Lippincott.

Graff-Radford, S.B. 1990. Oromandibular disorders and headache: A critical appraisal. *Neurologic Clinics* 8(4):929–945.

Green, M.W., and Selman, J.E. 1991. Review article: The medical management of trigeminal neuralgia. *Headache* 31:588–592.

Hanson, M.R. 1989. The dizzy patient. A practical approach to management. *Postgraduate Medicine* 85(2):99–102, 107–108.

Headache Classification Committee of the International Headache Society. 1988. Proposed classification and diagnostic criteria for headache disorders, cranial neuralgias, and facial pain. *Cephalgia* (Suppl 7):9–96.

Heise, A.P., Laskin, D.M., and Gervin, A.S. 1992. Incidence of temporomandibular joint symptoms following whiplash injury. *Journal of Oral Maxillofacial Surgery* 50:825–828.

Hilsinger, R.L., Jr., Adour, K.K., and Doty, H.E. 1975. Idiopathic facial paralysis, pregnancy, and the menstrual cycle. *Annals of Otolaryngology* 84:433–442.

Hughes, G.B. 1990. Practical management of Bell's palsy. *Otolaryngology—Head and Neck Surgery* 102:658–663.

International Study Group, Subcutaneous Sumatriptan. 1991. Treatment of migraine attacks with sumatriptan. *New England Journal of Medicine* 325:316–321.

Kaiser Foundation Hospital. 1993. *Sumatriptan (Imitrex®) for treatment of acute migraine headache: Prescribing guidelines*, Internal document. Redwood City, CA: Kaiser Foundation Hospital.

Kessler, J.T. 1989. Neurologic causes of head and face pain. In *Management of facial, head, and neck pain*, eds. B.C. Cooper and F.E. Lucente, pp. 23–51. Philadelphia: W.B. Saunders.

Krishnan, K.R.R., and France, R.D. 1989. Antidepressants in chronic pain syndromes. *American Family Physician* 39:233–237.

Leung, A.K.C., and Robson, W.L.M. 1991. Bruxism: How to stop tooth grinding and clenching. *Postgraduate Medicine* 89(8):167–171.

Manzoni, G.C., Micici, G., Granella, F., Martignoni, E., Farina, S., and Nappi, G. 1988. Cluster headache in women: Clinical findings and relationship with reproductive life. *Cephalgia* 8(1):37–44.

Marks, D.R., and Rapoport, A.M. 1992. Cluster headache syndrome. *Postgraduate Medicine* 91(3):96–104.

Mathew, N.T., Kurman, R., and Perez, F. 1990. Drug induced refractory headache—Clinical features and management. *Headache* 30:630–638.

May, M., Croxon, G.R., and Klein, S.R. 1989. Bell's palsy: Management of sequelae using EMG rehabilitation, botulinum toxin, and surgery. *The American Journal of Otology* 10(3):220–229.

McArthur, J. 1990. Bell's palsy: Diagnosis and treatment. *Hospital Practice* 3:81–92.

McNeill, C. 1991. Temporomandibular disorders: Guidelines for diagnosis and management. *CDA Journal* 19(6):15–26.

Mitchell, G.A.G. 1983. Nerve plexus and peripheral nerves. In *The CIBA collection of medical illustrations: Vol. 1, Nervous system, Part 1, Anatomy and physiology*, ed. A. Brass, pp. 113–128. West Caldwell, NJ: Ciba-Geigy.

Murtagh, J. 1990. Common problems: Headache. *Australian Family Physician* 19(2):1854–1857.

———. 1991. Dizziness (vertigo). *Australian Family Physician* 20(10):1483–1486, 1490.

Ohye, R.G., and Aitenberger, E.A. 1989. Bell's palsy. *American Family Physician* 40(2):159–166.

Paparella, M.M., Alleva, M., and Bequer, N.G. 1990. Dizziness. *Primary care: Clinics in office practice* 17(2):299–308.

Petruzzelli, G.J., and Hirsch, B.E. 1991. Bell's palsy: A diagnosis of exclusion. *Postgraduate Medicine* 90(2):115–127.

Poletti, C.E. 1991. C_2 and C_3 pain dermatomes in man. *Cephalgia* 11:115–159.

Pruitt, A.A. 1987. Management of Bell's palsy. In *Primary care medicine*, eds. A.H. Goroll, L.A. May, and A.G.

Mulley, Jr., 2nd ed., pp. 760–761. Philadelphia: J.B. Lippincott.

———. 1987. Approach to the patient with seizures. In *Primary care medicine*, eds. A.H. Goroll, L.A. May, and A.G. Mulley, Jr., 2nd ed., pp. 739–745. Philadelphia: J.B. Lippincott.

Rapoport, A.M. 1988. Analgesic rebound headache. *Headache* 28:662–665.

Saper, J.R. 1983. *Headache disorders, current concepts, and treatment strategies*. Boston: John Wright, PSG Inc.

Scheurer, M.L., and Pedley, T.A. 1990. The evaluation and treatment of seizures. *The New England Journal of Medicine* 323(21):1471–1472.

Schulman, E.A., and Silberstein, S.D. 1992. Symptomatic and prophylactic treatment of migraine and tension-type headache. *Neurology* 42(Suppl 2):16–21.

Shemen, L.J. 1991. The salivary glands: Benign and malignant disease. In *Essential otolaryngology: Head/neck surgery*, ed. K.J. Lee. New York: The Medical Examination Publishing Co.

Silberstein, S.D. 1992. The role of sex hormones in headache. *Neurology* 42(Suppl 2):37–42.

Smith, L.S. 1988. Evaluation and management of the muscle contraction headache. *Nurse Practitioner* 13(1):20–27.

Stankiewicz, J.A. 1983. Steroids and idiopathic facial paralysis. *Otolaryngology: Head and Neck Surgery* 91:672–677.

Tanaka, T.T. 1989. *A diagnostic and therapeutic approach for TMJ disorders for restorative dentists and other health professionals*, 4th ed. San Diego: Clinical Research Foundation.

Troni, W., Carta, Q., Cantello, R., Caselle, M.T., and Rainero, I. 1984. Peripheral nerve function and metabolic control in diabetes mellitus. *Annals of Neurology* 16:178–183.

Warner, E.A., Wallach, P.M., Adelman, H.A., and Sahlin-Hughes, C. 1992. Dizziness in primary care patients. *Journal of General Internal Medicine* 7(4):454–463.

Wiederholt, W.C. 1988. Review of clinical neuroanatomy. In *Neurology for non-neurologists*, ed. W.C. Wiederholt, pp. 3–22. Philadelphia: Grune & Stratton.

Wright, P.D., and Wright, B.D. 1992. Cervicogenic headache: A report on success in diagnosis and treatment. *Headache Quarterly* 3:290–294.

SECTION 10

Hematological / Endocrine Disorders

Michelle M. Marin, R.N., M.S., A.N.P.

10-A
Anemia

Anemia can be defined as an inappropriately low hemogloblin (Hgb), given the individual's oxygen supply and ⌐emand. The World Health Organization (WHO) laboratory definition, based upon a population mean, is adult male's Hgb less than 13 g/dl, menstruating female's Hgb less than 12 g/dl, and pregnant female's Hgb less than 11 g/dl. Given that the Hgb varies with age, sex, race, the altitude at time of blood sampling, and hydration status, the mean may not reflect the individual's true anemic status.

Anemia is a sign of disease, not a separate disease entity itself. In most individuals, the most significant clinical symptoms and signs reflect the underlying illness responsible for the anemia rather than the anemia itself.

Correct identification of the underlying etiology is essential and treatment must be specific to the cause.

Anemia classification is based on pathogenesis: 1) excessive red blood cell (RBC) loss, 2) inadequate or ineffective RBC production, 3) abnormal RBC destruction, or 4) morphological characteristics. For this protocol, morphological characteristics are used. **Table 10A.1, Classification of Anemia Based on Morphology of RBCs,** lists the common causes of anemia according to this classification.

Table 10A.1. CLASSIFICATION OF ANEMIA BASED ON MORPHOLOGY OF RBCS

Microcytic/Hypochromic MCV <80 fl	Normocytic/Normochromic MCV 80–100 fl	Macrocytic MCV >100 fl
→ Iron deficiency	→ Acute hemorrhage	→ Megaloblastic
→ Thalassemia	→ Acute hemolysis	▪ Vitamin B_{12} deficiency
→ Sideroblastic	→ Early iron deficiency	▪ Folate deficiency
→ Hemoglobinopathies	→ Anemia of chronic disease:	▪ Drug-induced
→ Anemia of chronic disease (some types)	▪ chronic inflammation	▪ Inherited disorder of DNA synthesis
→ Lead poisoning	▪ chronic infections	→ Reticulocytosis
	▪ chronic metabolic diseases	▪ Intense RBC stimulation due to acute hemolysis or hemorrhage
	▪ neoplasms	→ Chronic liver disease
	→ Alcoholic liver disease	→ Myelodysplastic syndromes, bone marrow failure, or infiltration
	→ Endocrinopathies	→ Endocrinopathies
	→ Marrow failure or infiltration	→ Post splenectomy
	→ Pregnancy	

Source: Adapted with permission from McPhee, S.J., and Hughes, E.F. 1991. Anemia. In *Current practices of emergency medicine*, 2nd ed., ed. M.L. Callahan, p. 779. Philadelphia: B.C. Decker.

Table 10A.2. MICROCYTIC/HYPOCHROMIC ANEMIA LABORATORY REVIEW
N = normal, I = increased, D = decreased

	RDW	MCV	Retic	Iron	TIBC	% SAT	FER/FEP	Smear
Fe deficiency	I	<80	D	D	I	D	D, FEP-I	aniso- and poikilocytosis
Beta Thalassemia	N	<80	I	N	N	N	N, FEP-NL	basophilic stippling, target cells
Alpha Thalassemia	N	<80	N	N	N	N	N, FEP-N	
Sideroblastic	I	<80	I	I/N	N/D	I/N	N, FEP-I	dimorphic population
Chronic disease	N	N/D	D	D	D	N	N/I, FEP-I	

Source: Adapted with permission from Esposito, N.W. 1992. Thalassemias: Simple screening for heredity anemias. *The Nurse Practitioner* 17, 53. Copyright © 1992 by Elsevier Science Publishing Co.

Microcytic/Hypochromic Anemia
(See Table 10A.2, Microcytic/Hypochromic Anemia Laboratory Review)

Iron-deficiency anemia, the most common anemia worldwide, occurs when the iron supply to the bone marrow falls short of that required for RBC production. Other factors contributing to its development are increased requirements during infant and adolescent growth spurts and pregnancy; inadequate dietary intake, notably among impoverished and elderly people, vegetarians, and alcoholics; decreased absorption due to chronic intestinal malabsorption, atrophic gastritis, or gastrectomy; or blood loss through menstruation, gastrointestinal bleeding, regular blood donation, or chronic hemoglobinuria (Brittenham 1991; Bunn 1991).

Usually developing insidiously, a characteristic, dynamic sequence of changes occurs in the body as iron requirements exceed the available stored or absorbed iron. Iron stores deplete without compromising erythropoiesis; therefore, initially only the serum ferritin is decreased. As the process continues, serum total iron binding capacity gradually rises and serum iron levels and saturation fall.

Eventually, iron reserves are depleted, resulting in inadequate iron supply for RBC development. Iron-deficiency anemia develops and the mean corpuscular volume (MCV) gradually falls (MCV correlates with degree of anemia). The RBCs become microcytic and hypochromic and progressively more distorted in shape (*poikilocytosis*), correlating with the restricted hemogloblin production. (see **Table 10A.3, Iron-Deficiency Anemia: A Continuum of Change in Iron Stores and Distribution**).

Iron deficiency is the only microcytic/hypochromic anemia with absent mobilizable iron stores (Brittenham 1991). Iron deficiency exclusively responds to iron replacement, a factor that differentiates it from other microcytic anemias.

Thalassemias, the most common inherited hemoglobinopathies worldwide, are a diverse group of autosomal recessive disorders in which there is a defect in synthesis of either alpha or beta globin chains of Hgb. The severity of the anemia depends on the degree of reduction in number of these globin chains and its associated mild hemolysis (Waterbury 1991).

In normal inheritance, each parent contributes a genetic code for the production of the various chains that comprise hemoglobin. It is the combination of these chains that produces the different types of hemogloblin. Hgb A, making up 98 percent of adult Hgb, is made of two alpha and two beta chains. Hgb A2, making up one percent to two percent of Hgb, is made of two alpha and two delta chains. Hgb F, the major fetal Hgb that comprises less than one percent of normal adult Hgb, is made of two alpha and two gamma chains.

Normally, four genes code for the production of alpha globin changes. In alpha thalassemia syndromes, either one, two, three, or four of these genes are missing.

In the most severe form of alpha thalassemia, *alpha thalassemia major*, no genes for alpha globin chains are inherited. This causes a condition known as hydrops fetalis, which is incompatible with life. The red blood cells only contain Hgb Barts (four gamma chains).

In *Hgb H disease*, when an individual inherits only one gene for alpha globin chain production, a moderate to severe hemolytic anemia occurs and splenomegaly develops. Usually individuals with this disorder are hematologically stable except when hemolysis is increased by infection or exposure to oxidative drugs.

In people with alpha thalassemia trait, two genes for alpha globin chain synthesis are inherited. These individuals are clinically stable and may have a mild anemia with significant microcytosis. Asians with alpha thalassemia trait should be referred for genetic counseling (Esposito 1992). This group is at increased risk for pro-

Table 10A.3. IRON-DEFICIENCY ANEMIA: A CONTINUUM OF CHANGE IN IRON STORES AND DISTRIBUTION

	Iron Overload	Positive Iron Balance	Normal	Early Negative Iron Stores	Iron Depletion	Iron-Deficient Erythropoiesis	Iron-Deficiency Anemia
Marrow iron stores	4+	3+	2+	1+	0 to trace	0	0
Iron µg/dl	200	>150	115 +/− 50	<115	<115	<60	<40
Ferritin µg/dl	>250	>250	100 +/− 60	<25	<20	10	<10
TIBC µg/dl	<300	<300	300 +/− 30	330 − 360	360	390	410
Transferrin saturation %	>60	>50	35 +/− 15	30	<30	<15	<10
FEP µg/dl RBC	30	30	30	30	30	100	200
Erythrocyte	Normal	Normal	Normal	Normal	Normal	Normal	Microcytic hypochromic

Adapted with permission from Herbert, V. 1988. Anemias. In *Clinical nutrition*, 2nd ed., ed. D.M. Paige, p. 593. St. Louis: C.V. Mosby.

ducing children with the most severe forms of alpha thalassemia because of the location of the gene deletions on the chromosome. Alpha thalassemia-1, with three out of four genes inherited, is an asymptomatic silent carrier state with no RBC microcytosis.

Alpha thalassemia syndromes are seen more commonly in people from China and Southeast Asia and less commonly in black people. In general, alpha thalassemia has a wider racial distribution than does beta thalassemia (Waterbury 1991).

Beta thalassemia major, also called *Cooley's anemia*, is the complete absence or partial deficiency of the beta globin chain. Affected individuals, usually of Mediterranean descent (especially Greeks and Italians) and less commonly Asians and blacks, appear healthy until about the age of six months when Hgb switches from Hgb F to A (Linker 1992). Severe anemia develops along with other clinical problems such as bony deformities, jaundice, and hepatosplenomegaly. Death usually occurs between the ages of 20 years and 30 years due to transfusional iron overload. In *thalassemia intermedia*, individuals comfortably survive without regular transfusions but they may develop complications similar to those encountered with Cooley's anemia.

Beta thalassemia minor or trait results from one abnormal beta chain. Individuals have lifelong asymptomatic mild anemia 1 gl/dl to 2 gl/dl lower than normal people of the same age and sex (Schwartz and Benz 1991). Only during pregnancy may these individuals require supportive transfusions due to the iron deficiency compounding the initial anemia.

Sideroblastic anemia is a congenital but usually acquired anemia that results in reduced hemoglobin synthesis and secondary iron accumulation. The primary acquired forms are frequently myelodysplastic disorders (Desnick and Anderson 1991). The secondary acquired

sideroblastic anemias arise from toxic affects to the bone marrow by chronic alcohol use, medications (e.g., isoniazid), lead poisoning, chronic infection, or inflammation.

The hallmark of this diagnosis is ringed sideroblasts in the bone marrow; however, it is suggested by an anemia with normal or low RBC indices, increased serum iron concentration and transferrin saturation, increased free erythrocyte protoporphyrin (FEP), and a dimorphic population of red cells on a peripheral smear (McPhee and Hughes 1991).

Anemia of chronic disease (ACD) is associated with chronic infection or inflammation such as tuberculosis, rheumatoid arthritis (RA), malignancy, and acquired immunodeficiency syndrome (AIDS). The classic definition rests on identifying the chronic disorder, a low serum iron and transferrin, and a normal serum ferritin level (Mohler 1992). However, ACD is a diagnosis of exclusion and a bone marrow aspirate will confirm adequate iron stores (Berliner and Duffy 1991). Decreased red cell survival, bone marrow function, and erythropoietin level contribute to this moderate anemia.

Normocytic/Normochromic Anemia

Hemolysis is defined as an RBC life less than 120 days, either continuously or episodically. Anemia appears when the bone marrow's compensation is less than the rate of hemolysis, due either to the bone marrow's impaired function or the red cell's extremely short survival. When bleeding is excluded, reticulocytosis with a falling or stable hematocrit (Hct) suggests hemolysis, which can appear acutely with a rapidly developing anemia or develop gradually in an asymptomatic form (Schwartz, Berkman, and Silberstein 1991).

The causes of hemolysis are many, and include inherited and, more commonly, extrinsic etiologies. Individuals at higher risk for hemolytic anemia include: blacks in whom G6PD deficiency and hemoglobinopathies (e.g., sickle cell disease and related syndromes) are more common; people with certain infections, severe burns, or uremia; pregnant women; people with liver disease, lymphoproliferative diseases, connective tissue disorders and vasculitis, or prosthetic heart valves; people taking certain drugs known to precipitate hemolysis; and individuals with a family history of anemia (McPhee and Hughes 1991).

Macrocytic Anemia

Megaloblastic anemias are disorders caused by impaired DNA synthesis and are suggested by MCV greater than 115 fl. Most megaloblastic anemias are due to Vitamin B_{12} or folic acid deficiency. Vitamin B_{12} is found in all food products of animal origin and is stored in the liver. As a consequence of Vitamin B_{12} stores and small daily loss, even a diet devoid of all animal products would not result in Vitamin B_{12} deficiency for several years (Waterbury 1991). Thus, dietary Vitamin B_{12} deficiency is extremely rare.

The most common cause of Vitamin B_{12} deficiency is *pernicious anemia*. With this hereditary disease, a defect in the gastric mucosa results in a deficient formation of intrinsic factor, a substance that binds ingested Vitamin B_{12} and allows its absorption in the terminal ileum (Waterbury 1991). This disease rarely manifests itself before age 35 years. It is seen mostly in descendants of Scandinavian or northern European ancestry and to a lesser degree in blacks and Hispanics. Other causes of Vitamin B_{12} deficiency include malabsorption secondary to gastrectomy or ileal resection, chronic severe diarrhea, blind loop syndrome, or fish tapeworm *Diphyllobothrium latum*.

Individuals with an inadequate intake of folate-rich foods are likely to develop folate deficiency. Folic acid is present in most fruits and vegetables and daily requirements usually are met by the diet. Body folate stores are adequate for about four months (Antony 1991). Individuals with intestinal mucosal abnormalities may malabsorb folate, as well as iron, exacerbating the anemia (Antony 1991). In addition, individuals who have increased need for folate due to an exfoliative skin disease, pregnancy, or chronic hemolysis or because they are taking drugs that either inhibit DNA synthesis or are folate antagonists, may also require folate replacement.

DATABASE

SUBJECTIVE

→ Symptoms may include:
- dyspnea on exertion, palpitations, chest pain.
- dizziness, postural faintness, headache, tinnitus.
- fever, weight loss, malaise, enlarging lumps, poorly healing sores, night sweats.
- bleeding:
  - vaginal bleeding, hematochezia, melena, hematemesis, hematuria, hemoptysis, epistaxis, ecchymosis, and bleeding secondary to trauma may cause iron-deficiency anemia.
- pallor, brittle nails and hair, cheilosis, dysphagia, nonspecific gastrointestinal complaints (e.g., anorexia, nausea, belching, and constipation).
- pica, or compulsive eating of various things such as ice, soil, or clay.

→ With insidious onset, symptoms may not develop until Hgb and Hct are less than or equal to 50 percent of normal.

→ Marked fatigue and decreased exercise tolerance may be the earliest symptoms. Individuals with occlusive vascular diseases are prone to ischemic symptoms such as angina or claudication (Damon 1992a).

→ Rapid onset of anemia may lead to dyspnea, palpitations, and faintness on arising from a sitting or lying position before the Hgb and Hct are less than or equal to 50 percent of normal.

→ Weakness, glossitis, and constant symmetrical paresthesias are the classic presentations for megaloblastic anemia.
- However, skin changes (e.g., diffuse brownish pigmentation or lemon-yellow coloring), gastrointestinal symptoms (e.g., anorexia, belching, indigestion, and diarrhea) and central nervous symptoms (e.g., headache, ataxia, vertigo), mental disturbances (e.g., irritability, personality changes, and confusion), and loss of vibratory sense may also occur.
- Sensory changes usually occur before motor symptoms.

→ Mild icterus, dark urine, and episodic weakness may suggest hemolytic episodes.
- Fever, rash, skin bruising, decreased urine output, enlarging abdominal size, and enlarged lymph nodes may also be associated with autoimmune hemolytic anemia.

→ Past history:
  ▪ notable for recurrent episodes of anemia.
  ▪ past use of hematinics such as iron, folate, Vitamin B_{12}.
  ▪ surgeries such as splenectomy, ileal resection, cardiac valve replacement, or gastrectomy.
  ▪ chronic disorders (e.g., kidney and heart disease, gastritis).
  ▪ chronic infections (e.g., tuberculosis, parasitic infestations).
  ▪ inflammatory diseases (e.g., collagen vascular diseases).
  ▪ malabsorptive disorders (e.g., colitis) or autoimmune disorders (e.g., Hashimoto's disease or systemic lupus).
  ▪ closely spaced pregnancies.
→ Family history notable for sickle cell anemia or other hemoglobinopathies, thalassemia, G6PD deficiency, sideroblastic anemia, pernicious anemia, splenectomy, gluten sensitivities.
→ Current medications may include nonsteroidal anti-inflammatory drugs (NSAIDs), oral contraceptives, steroids, sulfa compounds, anticonvulsants, cancer chemotherapy, zidovudine, quinine, quinidine, primaquine, penicillin, methyldopa, hydralazine.
  ▪ Current use of hematinics such as iron, folate, Vitamin B_{12}, health food products, and combination vitamin supplements.
→ Social history/habits may include:
  ▪ diet inadequate in iron or folate-rich foods, or dairy and animal products.
  ▪ alcohol and recreational drug use.
  ▪ toxic exposures through occupation, home environment, or hobbies.
  ▪ travel.
  ▪ long-distance running and regular blood donation, HIV risks.

OBJECTIVE

→ Identify any recent weight loss, orthostatic blood pressure changes, rapid pulse and respiratory rate, fever.
→ Skin/nails:
  ▪ patient may present with:
    • pallor (decreased number of RBCs, but degree not correlated to pallor), petechiae (thrombocytopenia, leukemia), telangiectasia and spider angiomas (liver disease), jaundice (hemolytic or megaloblastic anemias), diffuse brownish pigmentation greatest in the skin crease or blotchy tanning areas (megaloblastic anemia), koilonychia, decreased elasticity of skin, brittle nails and hair (longstanding anemia, especially iron deficiency).
→ Mucous membranes:
  ▪ patient may present with:
    • pallor, cheilosis, and stomatitis (vitamin deficiency), smooth tongue, and atrophic glossitis (leukemia, pernicious anemia, or severe iron deficiency).
→ Lymph nodes:
  ▪ patient may present with:
    • lymphadenopathy (infectious mononucleosis, leukemia, lymphoma, HIV).
→ Eyes:
  ▪ patient may present with:
    • increased vessel tortuosity (sickle cell anemia), hemorrhage, exudate (leukemia, uremia, aplastic anemia, bacterial endocarditis).
→ Cardiorespiratory:
  ▪ patient may present with:
    • tachycardia, loud murmurs, increased point of maximal impulse (PMI), dyspnea, pedal edema, gallop (severe anemia), functional murmurs (mild anemia, pregnancy).
→ Abdomen:
  ▪ patient may present with:
    • splenomegaly, hepatomegaly, or hepatic tenderness (leukemia, lymphoma, hemolytic anemia, liver disease, autoimmune disease).
→ Central nervous system (CNS):
  ▪ patient may present with:
    • decreased vibratory/position sense and fine motor coordination, hyporeflexia or hyper-reflexia, decreased memory or confusion (pernicious anemia).
→ Skeletal:
  ▪ patient may present with:
    • bone tenderness (hematological disease, for example, leukemia, myeloma).
→ Pelvic:
  ▪ patient may present with:
    • abnormal bleeding (menses, spontaneous abortion, ruptured ectopic pregnancy, malignancy).
→ Rectal:
  ▪ patient may present with:
    • quaiac + stool, dark/tarry stool, or bright red blood per rectum (gastrointestinal bleeding).

ASSESSMENT

→ Anemia
- R/O microcytic/hypochromic anemia
- R/O normocytic/normochromic anemia
- R/O macrocytic anemia

PLAN

DIAGNOSTIC TESTS

→ Based on the history and physical exam, *consider screening* target populations for anemia:
- CBC or Hct/Hgb for women with heavy menses.
- CBC, Hgb electrophoresis with quantitative Hgb A2 and F for those at risk for thalassemias or hemoglobinopathies.
- G6PD prior to beginning oxidant medications, such as antimalarials (primaquine or dapsone), in blacks, and individuals of Mediterranean descent.
  - G6PD can be normal during the acute hemolytic episode.
- stool guaiac × 3 for individuals over the age of 40 years.

→ Evaluation of Anemia:
- initial evaluation: CBC with indices and differential, cell count, platelet count, peripheral blood smear stained with Wright's stain, reticulocyte count.
- after obtaining the initial laboratory evaluation, classify the anemia by the MCV, the direct measurement of the RBC size (Waterbury 1991).
  - This classification narrows the search for the etiology. See **Table 10A.1**.
    - microcytic <80 fl.
    - normocytic 80 fl − 100 fl.
    - macrocytic >100 fl.
- analyze the reticulocyte count.
  - The reticulocyte count expresses the appropriateness of the bone marrow's response to the anemia, differentiating RBC under-production from hemolysis. The normal bone marrow responds by increasing commensurately with its erythropoietic activity (Kaplan 1988).
  - Normally expressed in a percent of the individual's RBC count, the reticulocyte count alone does not adequately mirror the degree of marrow compensation and must be adjusted to the level of anemia.
    - This adjustment is called the *reticulocyte index*.

- The reticulocyte index is calculated as:

$$\text{Index} = \text{Reticulocyte count} \times \frac{\text{actual Hct}}{\text{normal Hct}}$$

- the reticulocyte index should then be divided by the maturation index, based on the Hct. See the chart below. This number is normally 1: Any deviation from this value represents the percent increase or decrease over the basal RBC production.

Hct	Maturation Index
45	1
35	1.5
25	2.0
15	2.5

- this corrected reticulocyte index should be greater than 1 percent for an Hct less than 45 (e.g., a normal bone marrow would increase its daily production of reticulocytes to 2 percent when the Hct has dropped to 35 percent).
- an elevated reticulocyte count signifies increased erythropoietic activity, as a normal response to bleeding or to hematinic use or hemolysis.

- Analyze these laboratory values and decide whether or not the anemia is appropriate for the individual's history. Base further tests on the clinical picture and results of initial evaluation.
  - Keep in mind the multifactorial causes of anemia.
  - See **Appendix 10A.1, Evaluation of the Common Anemias**, p.10-12 for instructions for further evaluation of the anemia.

TREATMENT/MANAGEMENT

Iron-Deficiency Anemia

→ Evaluate contributing factors.
- Chronic blood loss in adult males and postmenopausal women warrants a gastrointestinal evaluation (Berliner and Duffy 1991, Waterbury 1991).

→ Document Hgb/Hct and reticulocyte count prior to therapy.

→ Begin ferrous iron replacement with a daily total of 150 mg to 200 mg of elemental iron.

- Simple ferrous salts absorbed most efficiently:
  - ferrous gluconate 320 mg (39 mg elemental iron) 1 tablet 5 times a day.
  - ferrous sulfate 325 mg (65 mg elemental iron) 1 tablet 3 or 4 times a day.
  - ferrous fumarate 200 mg (66 mg elemental iron) 1 tablet 3 times a day.
  - for patients who have achlorhydria or have had a gastrectomy, liquid iron therapy may prevent iron malabsorption (ferrous sulfate elixir 220 mg/5 ml supplies 44 mg of elemental iron).

NOTE: Iron is absorbed best if taken on an empty stomach 1 hour before or 1 to 2 hours after meals. Absorption is decreased by 50 percent when taken with meals (Waterbury 1991) and by 90 percent when taken with milk or tea. Antacids and sucralfate, when taken with iron, may also decrease absorption. There is a 15 percent incidence of nausea within one hour after ingestion; diarrhea and abdominal cramping may also occur when iron is first started. To avoid these side effects, begin with a suboptimal dose and increase gradually, or advise the patient to take iron with a small amount of food. It may be necessary to switch to another preparation with less elemental iron per dose and prolong therapy (can titrate dose with liquid preparation if necessary) (Waterbury 1991).

→ If moderate to severe anemia, precipitous drop in Hgb, or in patients with evidence of organ dysfunction such as angina, consider transfusion. Watch for congestive heart failure due to volume expansion.

→ Assess the reticulocyte count in 1 week.
  - It increases within 5 to 10 days and will be directly proportional to the severity of the anemia.

→ When the anemia is not severe, assess the Hgb in one month. Hgb level increases by at least 2 gl/dl within 3 weeks (Brittenham 1991).

→ Continue therapy for 4 to 6 months after Hgb is normal to replace bone marrow iron stores (Continue iron until ferritin serum is greater than 50 μg/l) (Brittenham 1991).
  - Women with large menstrual blood losses may benefit from continued, intermittent therapy (1 week per month) or 1 tablet a day for maintenance (McPhee and Hughes 1991).

→ With failure to respond, consider: poor compliance, poor absorption, concurrent infection, malignancy or inflammatory process, concurrent lead poisoning, thalassemia, Vitamin B_{12} or folate deficiencies, wrong diagnosis (as in anemia of chronic disease), or continued bleeding greater than the rate of erythropoiesis.

→ If oral ferrous sulfate is ineffective, consider iron dextran intramuscularly or referral for intravenous iron dextran treatment. Parenteral therapy should be used only in clinically significant anemia after oral therapy has failed (Waterbury 1991).

Thalassemia Anemia

→ Document HgbA, HgbA2, and HgbF levels by Hgb electrophoresis. If concurrent iron-deficiency anemia is suspected or documented, iron stores may need to be replete before the HgbA2 levels will be elevated on electrophoresis.

→ HgbA, HgbA2, and HgbF levels will be normal in alpha thalassemia. Thus, this is a diagnosis of exclusion.

→ No treatment is required if patient is hematologically stable.

→ Asians with alpha thalassemia trait require genetic counseling (Esposito 1992).

Sideroblastic Anemia

→ May need to treat the inherited form with transfusions, but some individuals may benefit from phlebotomy to reduce the iron stores (Desnick and Anderson 1991).

→ Withdraw the offending agents in cases of secondary sideroblastic anemia.

→ Treat the associated underlying illness or coexisting anemias.

→ Vitamin B_6 (pyridoxine) 50 mg to 200 mg daily for 2 to 3 months should be tried in acquired idiopathic sideroblastic anemia (Bunn 1991).
  - Reassess the reticulocyte count or Hgb level. Symptoms may resolve but the anemia may not completely reverse (Desnick and Anderson 1991; McPhee and Hughes 1991).

→ Instruct the patient to avoid iron or iron-containing vitamins due to the risk of iron overload (McPhee and Hughes 1991).

Anemia of Chronic Disease

→ Diagnosis of exclusion—exclude associated deficiencies as iron, folate, Vitamin B_{12} (McPhee and Hughes 1991).

→ Treat the underlying condition.

→ If the diagnosis is unclear despite an evaluation, consider a trial of iron therapy. If no hematological response occurs within two months, stop the iron therapy.

→ Erythropoietin therapy is now available and may be appropriate in some cases (e.g., transfusion-dependent cases of chronic renal failure, AIDS) (Damon 1992a).

Hemolysis

→ Identify the etiology—inherited or extrinsic. Treatment depends on symptoms, rapidity of illness, and etiology (Schwartz, Berkman, and Silberstein 1991).

Pernicious Anemia

→ Requires lifelong treatment.

→ Initial therapy is intramuscular cyanocobalamin (B_{12}) 100 μg every day for 1 week, then twice weekly for 1 week, then once a week for a month to replenish stores (stores last 3 to 5 years); then 100 μg monthly (Antony 1991).

- Monitor reticulocyte count and potassium in first 10 days, and the Hgb in several months. Symptomatic improvement as well as white blood cell and platelet recovery occurs within 2 to 3 days, peak reticulocytosis occurs between 7 and 10 days, and hematological correction occurs at the rate of 4 to 5 percentage points a week with complete correction within 2 months regardless of the initial degree of anemia (Antony 1991, Waterbury 1991).

→ CNS symptoms and signs are reversible if they are of less than 3 months duration (Antony 1991). "Megaloblastic madness" dramatically clears, but the peripheral neuropathies and dorsal column (vibratory/position sense) damage recover more slowly, with maximal response taking 6 months (Antony 1991, Waterbury 1991). Cortical spinal tract signs are less amenable to treatment (Waterbury 1991).

→ Initially, serum potassium, lactic dehydrogenase (LDH), bilirubin, and iron may drop. The hypokalemia may be significant if the anemia is severe. Consider supplemental potassium if potassium levels are borderline or low prior to therapy (Antony 1991).

→ Evaluate any neurological sign suggestive of Vitamin B_{12} deficiency, even in the absence of anemia or macrocytosis.

→ Watch for increased incidence of atrophic gastritis, gastric cancer, autoimmune diseases (e.g., IgA deficiency, RA, and Graves' disease),

and iron deficiency in individuals with pernicious anemia.

Folate Deficiency

→ Prior to beginning treatment, it is important to assess for Vitamin B_{12} deficiency.

→ 1 mg to 5 mg folate daily orally for 4 to 5 weeks is usually adequate to replenish body stores (stores last 4 to 6 weeks). Patients with severe malabsorption may require parenteral therapy initially.

- Assess the reticulocyte count 5 to 10 days after beginning folate therapy or reassess the CBC and RBC folate level several months after beginning treatment. If underlying cause of the deficiency has not been reversed—as in patients with chronic liver disease, renal dialysis, sickle cell anemia, or malabsorption—continue 1 mg folic acid a day indefinitely. In patients with drug-induced folate deficiency, withdraw the offending drug if possible. If the drug needs to be continued (such as with oral contraceptives and dilantin), folate will reverse the anemia. Once the anemia has resolved, therapy can usually be discontinued without relapse (Antony 1991; McPhee and Hughes 1991).

CONSULTATION

→ Consultation with a physician is indicated for:
- a transfusion.
- hospitalization:
  - severe anemia of unknown etiology (Hct less than 20 percent to 25 percent, Hgb less than 7 gl/dl). Be particularly concerned about elderly patients or those with congestive heart failure or angina pectoris.
  - pancytopenia suggesting potential aplastic anemia.
  - rapidly developing anemia and active bleeding.
  - thrombotic microangiopathies associated with microangiopathic hemolysis with thrombo-cytopenia and extremely high LDH may be life-threatening.

→ When the assessment, diagnosis, or treatment plan is in question.
- As needed for prescription.

PATIENT EDUCATION

→ See "Treatment/Management" section.

→ Discuss the underlying etiology of anemia and importance of participation in the treatment plan.

Include family members in management plan as necessary.

→ Discuss the importance of consistent follow-up.

→ Discuss medications: indications, regimens, side effects. Refer also to *Physicians' Desk Reference* (*PDR*).

Iron-Deficiency Anemia/Folate-Deficiency Anemia

→ Discuss importance of nutritionally sound diet high in iron or folate. See **Appendixes 10A.2, Patient-Education Handout: Dietary Iron**, p. 10-16 and **10A.3, Patient-Education Handout: Dietary Folate**, p. 10-17.

→ ; refer to nutritionist as indicated. See also **General Nutrition Guidelines** section.

→ Iron replacement—Advise patient that:
- iron tablets may cause nausea, abdominal cramping, diarrhea. If unable to tolerate on an empty stomach, advise ingestion with a small amount of food (best if it is high in Vitamin C).
- iron will cause black stools.
- iron elixir may stain teeth.

- Advise taking drug through a straw and then rinsing mouth immediately afterwards (Bushnell 1992).
- iron may be hazardous to small children. Ensure proper storage.

Sideroblastic Anemia

→ Instruct the patient to avoid iron or iron-containing vitamins due to the risk of iron overload (McPhee and Hughes 1991).

Vitamin B$_{12}$ Deficiency

→ Advise patient that lifelong treatment and regular follow-up visits every six months are necessary to ensure maintenance of hematopoiesis and early diagnosis of other diseases commonly associated with pernicious anemia (Antony 1991).

FOLLOW-UP

→ See "Treatment/Management" section for specific anemias.

→ Referral for genetic counseling as indicated.

→ Referral to nutritionist as indicated.

→ Document in progress notes and problem list.

APPENDIX 10A.1

Evaluation of the Common Anemias

Based upon the initial data, RBC morphology and reticulocyte index, and clinical picture, proceed in an orderly manner through the anemia evaluation.

Microcytic/Hypochromic

→ In addition to the initial laboratory evaluation, check iron studies–serum iron, total iron binding capacity, and ferritin or FEP. Calculate Mentzer index (MCV/RBC) to help differentiate between thalassemia and iron deficiency.
   - Mentzer > 13 suggests iron deficiency anemia.
   - Mentzer < 13 suggests thalassemia.
   - See **Table 10A.2**.
   - Review **Table 10A.3** if indicated. Low ferritin is a more specific test than serum iron or TIBC for iron deficiency. However, it may be inappropriately normal or elevated with liver disease, acute inflammation or infection, leukemias, and recent iron replacement.
   - Suspect thalassemia when the MCV is out of proportion to the anemia with normal iron studies. Check quantitative Hgb electrophoresis for HgbA2, HgbF levels for thalassemia and other hemoglobinopathies.

Normocytic/Normochromic

→ Etiologies can be distinguished by the reticulocyte index.

Increased Reticulocyte Index

   - Rule out hemorrhage first: most common causes include trauma, gastrointestinal bleeding.

   - Evaluate for spleen sequestration.
     • Enlarged spleen on examination.
   - Consider hemolysis by clinical history and peripheral blood smear. Hemolysis is suggested by polychromatophilia, spherocytes, poikilocytes, schistocytes, or sickle cells on peripheral blood smear and red-brown blood plasma.
   - If suspect hemolysis: check indirect bilirubin, LDH, haptoglobin, and plasma-free Hgb (bilirubin and LDH will be increased, haptoglobin decreased). Then consider checking direct antiglobulin test (Coomb's test) to rule out autoimmune hemolysis, drug-induced autoimmune hemolytic anemia, transfusion reactions, G6PD; indirect antiglobulin test; hemosiderin in the urine.

Normal/Decreased Reticulocyte Index

→ Check serum iron, transferrin saturation, total iron binding capacity, and ferritin or FEP. Evaluate for underlying causes:
   - anemia of chronic disease—mild to moderate anemia with Hemogloblin 7 to 11 g/dl, possibly hypochromia, associated with subacute chronic illness. Acute infections and inflammation also can cause a similar picture, but over a shorter time line.

Figure 10A.1.   EVALUATION OF MICROCYTIC ANEMIA

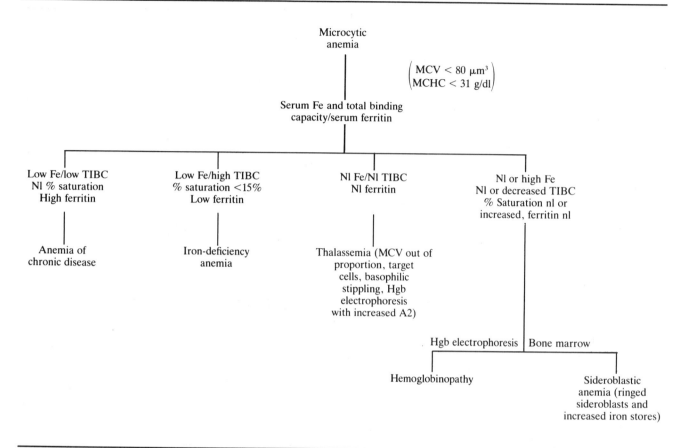

Source: Adapted with permission from Baker, W.F. 1993. The clinical evaluation of the patient with anemia. In *Hematology: Clinical and laboratory practice*, ed., R.L. Bick, p. 203. St. Louis: C.V. Mosby.

- end organ failure:
  - chronic renal failure—primarily hypoerythropoietinemia with "hemostat" reset for hematocrit 20 percent to 25 percent. The degree of anemia and the level of serum creatinine may not correlate. Consider checking an erythropoietin level.
  - endocrine/metabolic disorders such as hypothyroidism, Addison's disease, panhypopituitarism, hypogonadism. Do careful history and laboratory screening as appropriate.
  - chronic liver failure—multiple contributing factors possibly including iron and folate deficiency, spur cell hemolysis. Check liver function tests.

Markedly Decreased Reticulocyte Index

→ Requires a bone marrow biopsy to rule out hypoplastic anemia, marrow infiltrative disorder such as leukemia, myeloma, myelofibrosis, or cancer metastasis.

NOTE: The evaluation of this anemia may be complicated, as microcytic and macrocytic anemias may present in the early stages as normocytic anemia. A mixture of microcytic and macrocytic anemia also may appear as a normocytic anemia. Consider anemia of mixed etiologies when:

- iron studies are not classic for iron deficiency or anemia of chronic disease (i.e., treatment of iron deficiency may unmask an underlying thalassemia or anemia of chronic disease).
- with treatment of an identifiable cause of anemia, the MCV changes in the wrong direction (i.e., treatment of iron deficiency leads to macrocytosis due to a folate or Vitamin B_{12} deficiency).

Figure 10A.2. EVALUATION OF NORMOCYTIC ANEMIA

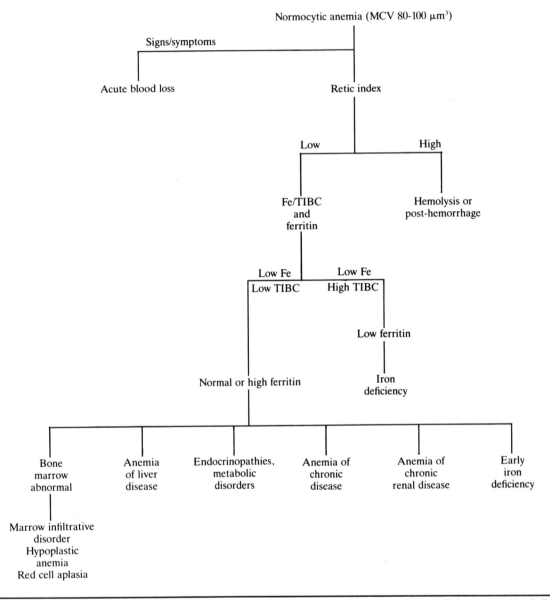

Adapted with permission from Baker, W.F. 1993. The clinical evaluation of the patient with anemia. In *Hematology: Clinical and laboratory practice*, ed., R.L. Bick, p. 204. St. Louis: C.V. Mosby.

- with treatment of identifiable cause of anemia, the anemia does not fully correct (i.e., treating iron deficiency) (Damon 1992b).

Macrocytic

→ After the initial laboratory evaluation, look first for megaloblastosis. Then use the reticulocyte index to further direct the evaluation.

Megaloblastic anemia

→ MCV >115 with oval macrocytes, anisocytosis, poikilocytosis combined with hypersegmented polymorphonuclear neutrophils with more than five lobes to the nucleus on the peripheral blood smear.

- Reticulocyte index will be low and may see pancytopenia with increase in serum LDH and bilirubin.

Figure 10A.3.   EVALUATION OF MACROCYTIC ANEMIA

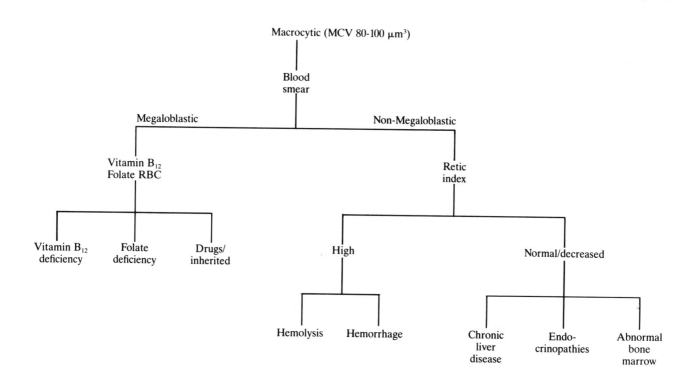

- Check serum RBC folate and serum Vitamin B_{12}.
  - Vitamin B_{12} deficiency—vitamin B_{12} < 200 pg/ml is abnormal. RBC folate level should be normal.
  - Vitamin B_{12} level may be spuriously low with folate deficiency.
- If Vitamin B_{12} is abnormal, check a two-staged Schilling test, which is best delayed for several weeks after replacement therapy has begun. Also check a serum anti-intrinsic factor antibody, which is specific for pernicious anemia. The blood must not be drawn within 48 hours of Vitamin B_{12} injection (Carmel 1993).
- Consider pernicious anemia with a normal MCV, especially in blacks or Hispanics, because they may also have alpha thalassemia trait, which will hide a megaloblastic MCV.

- Folate deficiency is diagnosed by low RBC folate level, <150 ng/ml, and a normal Vitamin B_{12} level.

Nonmegaloblastic anemia

→ MCV < 115 fl.

→ Separate etiologies by reticulocyte index.
- Increased reticulocyte index:
  - consider hemorrhage and hemolysis.
- Normal reticulocyte index:
  - chronic liver disease—check liver function. Peripheral blood smear will show target cells. The anemia may be multifactorial to include iron and folate deficiency.
  - hypothyroidism—check thyroid function test.
  - myelodysplastic syndrome—peripheral blood smear finds may be subtle. If normal liver function tests, thyroid function tests, vitamin B_{12} and RBC folate levels, a bone marrow exam should be done.

Michelle M. Marin, R.N., M.S., A.N.P.

APPENDIX 10A.2

Patient-Education Handout: Dietary Iron*

Iron is essential to the formation of hemoglobin (Hgb), which carries oxygen in the blood. When body iron stores are low, there are no physical symptoms. But as there is less iron to produce healthy red blood cells, iron-deficiency anemia appears. Symptoms of this anemia are weakness, pale skin, shortness of breath, and sometimes craving things that are not food, such as ice, clay, or soil.

→ Most balanced diets contain an adequate supply of iron unless you are in one of these groups:
  ▪ menstruating women, especially if bleeding heavily. Blood loss increases the need for iron.
  ▪ pregnant women, who have increased iron needs to support a growing fetus.
  ▪ dieters, who may not eat enough iron-containing foods.
  ▪ strict vegetarians, if adequate amounts of legumes, dried fruits, leafy greens, or enriched cereals are not eaten.
  ▪ endurance athletes, especially marathoners.
  ▪ infants and children with rapid growth.

→ The type of iron found in meat and other animal products, called *heme* iron, is better absorbed by the body than the *nonheme* iron found in plant foods. Nonheme iron found in grains and vegetables is better absorbed when eaten at meals with foods high in Vitamin C or with a small amount of heme-containing food.

→ Individuals with iron-deficiency anemia should cook in iron pots and pans when possible. In such

pots, the iron content of food can be increased from 2.4 times the amount for a three-minute cooking time to 29 times the amount for a three-hour cooking time.

→ Minimum daily requirement for iron: 10 mg to 15 mg.

→ Minimum daily requirement for Vitamin C: 60 mg.

Below are selected food items with their iron or Vitamin C amounts to assist in meal planning.

mg	Iron Source	Quantity	mg	Vit. C Source	Quantity
28.0	clams, cooked	3½ oz.	85	brussel sprouts	1 cup
12.4	bran flakes	1 cup	80	strawberries	1 cup
10.5	prune juice	1 cup	60	orange juice	½ cup
10.0	soybeans	1 cup	50	spinach, cooked	1 cup
7.5	rice bran	¼ cup	48	broccoli	1 cup
7.5	beef liver	3 oz	45	cantalope	¼ cup
6.7	oysters	7-10 med.	43	cabbage	1½ cup
6.0	pinto beans	1 cup	40	cranberry juice	1 cup
5.4	scotch barley	1 cup	21	watercress	1 cup
4.0	spinach, cooked	1 cup	20	tomato juice	½ cup
4.0	black beans	1 cup	18	carrots, raw	3 large
4.0	croissant	1 whole	16	green beans, cooked	1 cup
4.0	almonds, whole	¾ cup	12	peach, dried	5 halves
3.8	peach, dried	5 halves			
3.7	pumpkin seeds	¾ cup			
3.2	blackstrap molasses	1 tbsp.			
3.1	roast beef	3 oz			
3.0	chickpeas	1 cup			
2.3	tomato juice	1 cup			
2.0	raisins	½ cup			
2.1	butternut squash, baked	1 cup			
1.0	brussel sprouts, steamed	8			

*This handout may be reproduced for patient use.

APPENDIX 10A.3

Patient-Education Handout: Dietary Folate*

Folate, or folacin, is an important vitamin for tissue growth and red blood cell production. Most people get an adequate amount of folacin because it is plentiful in foods, but some people should be more careful to consume enough of this vitamin in the diet.

→ Populations at risk for folate-deficiency anemia include:
  ▪ pregnant and lactating women.
  ▪ women taking birth control pills.
  ▪ persons with certain medical conditions such as hyperthyroidism, tropical sprue, chronic hemolytic anemia, and psoriasis.
  ▪ persons with poor diets or heavy alcohol consumption.

→ Folate-rich foods include:
  ▪ dark green, leafy vegetables.
  ▪ citrus fruits and juices.
  ▪ beans and other legumes.
  ▪ wheat bran and other whole grains.
  ▪ pork, chicken, and shellfish.

This handout may be reproduced for patient use.

10-B

Thyroid Disorders

The primary function of the adult *thyroid* gland is to synthesize and secrete *L-thyroxine* (T$_4$) and *3,5,3'-triiodo thyronine* (T$_3$), active hormones that contribute to the regulation of an array of metabolic processes. This function is orchestrated by a number of intrathyroidal and extrathyroidal influences (e.g., contributions from the hypothalamus and pituitary). Thus, when an individual presents with signs and symptoms suggestive of an altered circulation of thyroid hormones or enlargement of the gland (goiter), extrathyroidal factors/pathology should be suspected in addition to intrinsic thyroid gland pathology.

The three thyroid conditions that the primary care provider is most likely to encounter in ambulatory care settings are:

Primary hypothyroidism

→ A condition caused by insufficient hormone secretion from the thyroid gland.

→ The most common causes of hypothyroidism are (Goroll, May, and Mulley 1995):
- radioiodine-induced or surgically induced hypothyroidism.
- idiopathic thyroid atrophy.
- thyroid inflammatory diseases (e.g., chronic [Hashimoto's] thyroiditis, postpartum [subacute lymphocytic] thyroiditis, and subacute thyroiditis).
  - The initial presentation of thyroiditis, however, often is consistent with a diagnosis of hyperthyroidism.

Hyperthyroidism

→ A condition resulting from excessive secretion of thyroid hormone.

→ The most common causes of hyperthyroidism are:
- diffuse toxic (hyperfunctioning) goiter (Graves' disease).
- toxic multinodular goiter.
- toxic uninodular goiter.
- thyroid inflammatory diseases (e.g., Hashimoto's thyroiditis, postpartum thyroiditis, and subacute thyroiditis).

Thyroid nodules

→ May be benign or malignant.

Primary hypothyroidism, a condition in which there is a loss of thyroid function secondary to pathology within the gland itself, accounts for 95 percent of all cases of hypothyroidism (Wartofsky and Ingbar 1991). The prevalence of primary hypothyroidism for the general population has been estimated to be 0.8 percent (Meek 1990). In the geriatric female population, however, the prevalence of primary subclinical hypothyroidism may be as high as 16 percent (Ross 1991b).

The most common cause of primary thyroid deficiency is radioiodine-induced or surgically induced hypothyroidism. Idiopathic thyroid atrophy also accounts for a significant number of cases. In addition, a number of thyroid inflammatory disorders, as part of the illness trajectory, may cause a longstanding hypothyroidism (e.g., people with chronic [Hashimoto's] thyroiditis and a few women with postpartum thyroiditis) or a self-limiting hypothyroidism (e.g., most women with postpartum thyroiditis and the vast majority of individuals with subacute thyroiditis). Many thyroid inflammatory conditions reflect an underlying autoimmune thyroid disease. Subacute thyroiditis, for example, may be linked to an underlying viral infection (Woolf 1990).

Hyperthyroidism—hyperfunctioning of the thyroid gland—can result from a variety of diseases. The most common diseases that cause ongoing overproduction of thyroid hormones are Graves' disease, toxic multinodular goiter, and toxic uninodular goiter. Thyroid inflammatory diseases such as Hashimoto's thyroiditis, postpartum thyroiditis, or subacute thyroiditis, may produce a transient form of hyperthyroidism. Although the exact prevalence of these disorders is not known, conditions are found more often in women than in men (Goroll, May, and Mulley 1995).

In diffuse toxic goiter (Graves' disease), extrathyroidal autoimmune processes stimulate excessive hormonal synthesis in the thyroid gland. This disorder usually occurs in women in their 30s or 40s (Wartofsky and Ingbar 1991).

Toxic multinodular goiter is a disease of the older adult, which often evolves from a longstanding simple goiter (thyroid enlargement without any clinical or laboratory manifestations of hypothyroidism or hyperthyroidism) (Wartofsky and Ingbar 1991). In addition, an autonomously functioning single thyroid nodule (toxic uninodular goiter) is another relatively common disorder that may occur at any age but is more often noted in the older population.

A variety of thyroid inflammatory diseases cause a transient and often mild form of hyperthyroidism. Due to rapid destruction of thyroid tissue, a sudden release of thyroid hormones ensues, thus causing signs and symptoms consistent with hyperthyroidism. Except for Hashimoto's thyroiditis, many thyroiditis syndromes reflect self-limiting conditions. After an individual proceeds through the cycles of hyperthyroidism and hypothyroidism, respectively, she recovers and returns to a euthyroid state (normal thyroid status). But most people with Hashimoto's thyroiditis and a few women with postpartum thyroiditis eventually develop a permanent form of hypothyroidism (Woolf 1990).

Thyroid nodules are extremely common entities (37 percent to 57 percent prevalence rate via autopsy surveys) that often go undetected by the clinician because the nodules may be very small or located in a posterior region of the gland or because the clinician's physical examination was limited (Ross 1991b).

Thyroid nodules may be functional (e.g., toxic uninodular goiter) or nonfunctional (e.g., benign follicular adenomas). The incidence of thyroid nodules, single and multiple, increases as one ages. Although these neoplasms are usually benign, a malignancy should be suspected, particularly if only one nodule is noted in an individual without any manifestations of an altered hormone status.

DATABASE

SUBJECTIVE

Primary hypothyroidism

→ Signs and symptoms:
- early manifestations include fatigue, a modest weight gain, dry skin, constipation, arthralgias/ myalgias, heavy menses or amenorrhea (although hypothyroidism menorrhagia is a more common presentation than amenorrhea), and/or cold intolerance.
- as the condition progresses, an individual will present with ongoing weight gain, notable dry skin, coarse hair, and/or hoarseness.
- characteristic myxedematous presentations (severe and exaggerated hypothyroidism) include the presence of lethargy, flat affect, daytime somnolence, continued weight gain, puffy and doughy skin, hair loss, dysphagia, dysarthria, exaggerated hoarseness, decreased hearing, dyspnea, chest pain, severe constipation, joint complaints, hand pain and paresthesias (carpal tunnel syndrome), depressed mood, and/or an ataxic gait (rare presentation).

→ Past health history may include (Wartofsky and Ingbar 1991):
- thyroid surgery.
- radioiodine therapy.
- neck irradiation.
- thyroiditis.
- autoimmune disorders that may coexist with primary hypothyroidism (e.g., diabetes mellitus, pernicious anemia, systemic lupus erythematosus [SLE], and rheumatoid arthritis [RA]).
- neuroendocrine conditions (e.g., pituitary or hypothalamic tumors or disorders) so as to rule out secondary/extrathyroidal hypothyroidism.
- ingestion of medications that affect hormone synthesis (e.g., para-aminosalicylic acid or lithium).
- iodide administration.

→ Patient may have family history of thyroid disease.

→ Personal/social and occupational/environmental health history may include:
- iodine-deficient diet (now uncommon due to iodination programs in most communities where there is iodine-deficient soil).
- work-related exposure to radiation or radioactive iodine.

Hyperthyroidism

→ Signs and symptoms:
  ▪ the most common manifestations are increased appetite, weight loss, generalized weakness, excessive perspiration, frequent bowel movements, irregular menses or amenorrhea, heat intolerance, insomnia, nervousness, and/or tremors.
  ▪ in the elderly population, the usual clinical presentation is generalized weakness, weight loss, dyspnea, chest pain, palpitations, and/or apathy (Goroll, May, and Mulley 1995).

→ Past health history may include:
  ▪ thyroid disorders, including thyroid cancer and postpartum thyroiditis.
  ▪ neuroendocrine conditions (e.g., pituitary tumors).
  ▪ thyroid surgery.
  ▪ antithyroid drug use (e.g., propylthiouracil or methimazole).
  ▪ radioiodine therapy.
  ▪ ingestion of thyroid hormone supplements.
  ▪ ingestion of iodine.

→ Patient may have family history of thyroid diseases.

→ Personal/social and occupational/environmental health history may include:
  ▪ a diet that is relatively high in iodine content (particularly for individuals who previously consumed an iodine-deficient diet due to geographic location [e.g., some regions of South America]).

Thyroid nodules

→ Signs and symptoms:
  ▪ if the nodular gland is hypofunctional, the individual may have signs and symptoms consistent with primary hypothyroidism (see previous discussion of "Primary Hypothyroidism").
  ▪ if the nodule(s) are autonomously functioning, the individual will often demonstrate signs and symptoms of hyperthyroidism (see previous discussion of "Hyperthyroidism").
  ▪ if the nodule(s) are nonfunctional, the individual will be without signs and symptoms of an altered thyroid status (euthyroid).
  ▪ if surrounding suprathyroidal structures have been invaded by the nodule(s), either malignant or benign, the individual may present with complaints of hoarseness and/or dysphagia.

→ Past health history may include:

  ▪ head and neck irradiation.
  ▪ goitrous thyroid conditions (e.g., Graves' disease).
  ▪ thyroid surgery.
  ▪ intake of certain goiter-producing medications (e.g., lithium).
  ▪ past health historical data specific for hypothyroidism or hyperthyroidism. If the patient demonstrates signs and symptoms for these respective thyroid conditions, then elicit pertinent past health data consistent with hypothyroidism or hyperthyroidism.

→ Patient may have family history of goitrous thyroid conditions and/or thyroid cancer.

→ Personal/social and occupational/environmental history may include:
  ▪ regular intake of dietary goitrogens—e.g., turnips or beets.
  ▪ iodine-deficient or excessively rich diet.

OBJECTIVE

Primary hypothyroidism

→ The following findings may be noted on physical examination:
  ▪ hypothermia if the individual is myxedematous.
  ▪ slight to moderate weight gain (usually no more than about 2 kilograms to 4 kilograms).
  ▪ flat or blunted facial expressions.
  ▪ dry skin in early stages of hormonal depletion to pale, rough, and doughy skin with advanced depletion.
  ▪ coarse hair that tends to fall out or be brittle.
  ▪ periorbital swelling and loss of outer one-third of the eyebrows in myxedema.
  ▪ decreased auditory acuity with advanced disease.
  ▪ enlarged tongue with advanced disease.
  ▪ symmetrically enlarged and smooth thyroid gland or an enlarged multinodular gland or a nonpalpable thyroid gland.
  ▪ bradycardia.
  ▪ signs of congestive heart failure (e.g., S_3, S_4, and jugular venous distention) with advanced disease.
  ▪ decreased bowel sounds.
  ▪ diminished tendon reflexes or a prolonged relaxation phase.
  ▪ depressed affect and poor attention span and/or somnolence.

→ Results from commonly ordered diagnostic studies include:

- altered blood tests:
  - altered thyroid function tests (see **Table 10B.1, Common Thyroid Tests**).
  - hyponatremia in severe disease.
  - increased serum cholesterol.
  - mild anemia.
- usually negative to a slight uptake of radioisotopes, in comparison to normal tissue, via thyroid scintigraphy (see **Table 10B.1**).
- electrocardiogram (EKG) changes secondary to a hypometabolic state.
- abnormal EKG consistent with congestive heart failure that has resulted from a pericardial effusion.

Hyperthyroidism

→ Common findings on physical examination include (Wartofsky and Ingbar 1991, Woolf 1990):

- restlessness.
- warm and moist skin.
- pretibial myxedema with Graves' disease.
- fine and silky hair.
- ocular signs from sympathetic hyperstimulation:
  - diminished blinking.
  - lid lag.
  - inability to furrow the eyebrows on upward gaze.
- exophthalmus with Graves' disease.
- thyroid bruit.
- abnormal thyroid gland on palpation:
  - diffusely enlarged with Graves' disease.
  - irregularly enlarged and multinodular gland with toxic multinodular goiter.
  - symmetrically enlarged tender or painless thyroid with thyroid inflammatory diseases.
  - single nodule with toxic uninodular goiter.

Table 10B.1. COMMON THYROID TESTS

Test	Definition	Clinical Implications	Comments
Serum-free T_4 (FT$_4$)	Measurement of the metabolically active T_4 (unbound to thyroid-binding globulin)	Assists with the diagnosis (dx) of hypothyroidism, hyperthyroidism, or other causes of thyrotoxicosis.	May be increased by various drugs or conditions in individuals who are clinically euthyroid.
Free T_4 Index (FT$_4$I)	Indirect measurement of FT$_4$	Assists with the dx of hypothyroidism, hyperthyroidism, or other causes of thyrotoxicosis. Aids with the dx of conditions related to altered thyroid-binding globulins but with unaltered thyroid hormone secretion.	May be increased by various drugs or conditions in individuals who are clinically euthyroid.
Serum T_3	Measurement of bound and free serum levels of T_3	Aids with the diagnosis of T_3 toxicosis.	May be increased by various drugs or conditions in individuals who are clinically euthyroid.
Highly sensitive thyroid-stimulating hormone (TSH)	Measurement of TSH: an anterior pituitary hormone that stimulates growth and function of thyroid cells	Sensitive and specific test for initial assessment of hypo- and hyperthyroidism.	Values may be altered by certain drugs (e.g., aspirin and lithium).
Serum antithyroid antibodies	Measurement of antithyroglobulin antibodies or antimicrosomal antibodies	High levels of antibodies are seen in autoimmune disorders, such as chronic thyroiditis and Graves' disease.	thyroid antibodies = $102 antimicrosomal antibodies = $56
Radioactive iodine uptake (RAIU)	Measurement of thyroid function via uptake of radioactive iodine (^{123}I)	Helps to confirm the dx of hyperthyroidism and with the assessment of the functional activity of an enlarged gland.	Variety of medications and conditions may interfere with ^{123}I uptake. Contraindications: —allergy to iodine —pregnancy and lactation.
Thyroid scintigraphy	Visualization of the thyroid gland via scintillation camera after the administration of a radioactive isotope (e.g. ^{123}I)	Assists with assessment of the size and functional status of thyroid nodules. Hyperfunctional/"hot" nodules are rarely malignant. A non-functional/"cold" nodule is suspicious for being malignant although unlikely to be cancerous.	Variety of medications and conditions may interfere with radiosotope uptake. Contraindications: —allergy to employed radiosotope —pregnancy and lactation.
Thyroid ultrasonography	Ultrasonic visualization of the thyroid gland	Assists with the assessment of neck masses with questionable thyroid origin.	Not an accurate screening tool for determining status of nodules (benign versus malignant).

Sources: Adapted from Kee, J.L. 1990. *Handbook of laboratory and diagnostic tests with nursing implications.* Norwalk, CT: Appleton & Lange and Wartofsky, L., and Ingbar, S.H. 1991. Diseases of the thyroid. In *Harrison's principles of internal medicine*, 12th ed., eds. J.D. Wilson, E. Braunwald, K.J. Isselbacher, R.G. Petersdorf, J.B. Martin, A.S. Fauci, and R.K. Root, vol. 2, pp. 1692-1712. New York: McGraw-Hill.

- tachycardia.
- systolic murmur.
- signs of congestive heart failure (e.g., S_3, S_4, and jugular venous distention).
- increased bowel sounds.
- fine tremor of the tongue and hands and/or increased tendon reflexes.

→ Results from commonly ordered diagnostic studies include:
- altered thyroid function tests (see **Table 10B.1**).
- elevated erythrocyte sedimentation rate (ESR) with some of the thyroid inflammatory disorders (e.g., subacute thyroiditis).
- elevated white blood cell (WBC) count in some of the thyroid inflammatory diseases (e.g., subacute thyroiditis).
- usually negative uptake of radioisotopes, in comparison to the adjacent normal thyroid tissue, for diffuse toxic goiter, toxic multinodular goiter, and most thyroid inflammatory disorders via thyroid scintigraphy (see **Table 10B.1**).
- usually positive uptake of radioisotopes for toxic uninodular goiter via thyroid scintigraphy (see **Table 10B.1**).
- atrial fibrillation on EKG.
- chest x-ray and echocardiographic changes consistent with congestive heart failure in the elderly population or in persons with underlying heart disease.

Thyroid nodules

→ Findings on the physical examination are determined by the functional status of the thyroid gland.
- Thus, if the individual has a multinodular hypofunctioning gland (e.g., chronic [Hashimoto's] thyroiditis), the individual will have objective findings of hypothyroidism (see "Objective" section, "Hypothyroidism.")
- On the other hand, if the person has a toxic uninodular goiter then the individual will have physical findings consistent with hyperthyroidism (see "Objective" section, "Hyperthyroidism"). If the patient has one or more thyroid nodules that are afunctional, the patient will be euthyroid.

→ Results from commonly ordered diagnostic procedures include:
- altered thyroid function tests if the thyroid gland is hypo- or hyperfunctioning (see **Table 10B.1**).
- positive radioisotope uptake (a "hot" nodule) via thyroid scintigraphy in autonomously

functioning nodules which are almost always benign (see **Table 10B.1**) (Ross 1991a).
- negative to a slight radioisotope uptake, which represents "cold" or "warm" nodularity, respectively, in nonfunctioning or hypofunctioning nodular glands.
  • These nodules are also usually benign.
  • However, more definitive diagnostic procedures (e.g., fine-needle aspiration [FNA]) should be used for ruling out a malignancy, particularly if there is only one dominant nodule, because malignant nodules are more likely to be cold than hot (see **Table 10B.1**).
- malignant, benign, nondiagnostic, or indeterminate/suspicious biopsy results via cutting needle biopsy or FNA (Ross 1991a).
- alterations in other blood tests, the chest x-ray, EKG, and/or echocardiogram if the individual demonstrates signs and symptoms consistent with hypothyroidism or hyperthyroidism (see respective "Objective" sections).

ASSESSMENT

→ Hypothyroidism (primary)

→ Hyperthyroidism

→ Thyroid neoplasms (benign or malignant)

→ Rule out other possible causes for the patient's presentation:
- pituitary disease
- hypothalamic disease
- cardiac disease
- psychiatric conditions
- nonthyroidal malignant neoplasm

PLAN

DIAGNOSTIC TESTS

(See **Table 10B.1**, for a description of the following thyroid tests and **Table 10B.2**, **Suggested Approach for the Assessment of Thyroid Dysfunction**.)

→ Diagnostic thyroid studies include, but are not limited to: the serum free T_4, Free T_4 Index, Serum T_3, highly sensitive thyroid-stimulating hormone (TSH), serum antithyroid antibodies, radioactive iodine uptake, thyroid scintigraphy, and/or thyroid ultrasonography.

→ FNA biopsy is warranted if the patient has a solitary thyroid nodule or a multinodular gland suspected of having a cancerous nodule due to a

Table 10B.2.   SUGGESTED APPROACH FOR THE ASSESSMENT OF THYROID DYSFUNCTION

If the patient has signs and symptoms and/or findings suggestive of thyroid disease, order the highly sensitive thyroid-stimulating hormone (TSH) test:

→ Normal TSH—clinically euthyroid.

→ Increased TSH—order a Free T_4 Index (FT_4I):
- Decreased FT_4I—primary hypothyroidism.
- Increased FT_4I—pituitary (TSH-induced) hyperthyroidism.
- Normal FT_4I—subclinical hypothyroidism.
  - Normal FT_4I—order antithyroid antibodies to rule out compensated chronic thyroiditis and consult with a physician to determine the necessity for a thyrotropin-releasing hormone (TRH) stimulation test (a test for assessing hypothalamic-pituitary function).

→ Decreased TSH—order a Free T_4 Index (FT_4I):
- Decreased FT_4I—secondary hypothyroidism.
- Increased FT_4I—hyperthyroidism.
  - Increased FT_4I—order antithyroid antibodies to distinguish between autoimmune thyroiditis syndromes and other forms of thyroiditis (e.g., subacute thyroiditis). (The clinician may need to consider ordering thyroid-stimulating immunoglobulbins, another antibody test, if the diagnosis of Graves' disease is not supported by the previously mentioned antithyroid antibody results.) Consult with a physician to detemine the need for ordering thyroid-stimulating immunoglobulbins and thyroid scinitigraphy.
- Normal FT_4I—subclinical hyperthyroidism or a rare form of hyperthyroidism called T_3 toxicosis.
  - Normal FT_4I—consult with a physician to determine the necessity for a serum T_3 or a TRH stimulation test.

Sources: Adapted from Schectman, J.M., and Pawlson, G. 1990. The cost-effectiveness of three thyroid function testing strategies for suspicion of hypothyroidism in a primary care setting. *Journal of General Internal Medicine* 5(1):8-15 and Wartofsky, L., and Ingbar, S.H. 1991. Diseases of the thyroid. In *Harrison's principles of internal medicine*, 12th ed., eds. J.D. Wilson, E. Braunwald, K.J. Isselbacher, R.G. Petersdorf, J.B. Martin, A.S. Fauci, and R.K. Root, vol. 2, pp. 1692-1712. New York: McGraw-Hill.

history of neck irradiation or a rapid growth of part of the gland.

TREATMENT/MANAGEMENT

Primary hypothyroidism

→ Discontinue medications/exposures with an antithyroid effect (e.g., lithium).

→ Initiate oral hormone replacement with L-thyroxine in consultation with a physician:
- initial dosing:
  - young patients without underlying cardiac conditions: 50 micrograms (μg) per day.
  - elderly patients and/or patients with heart disease: 25 μg per day.
- increase dosing gradually:
  - 25μg to 50 μg every 2 to 3 weeks until the highly sensitive TSH is within normal limits.

→ Maintain full replacement of L-thyroxine, which is usually 100 μg and 150 μg per day.

→ Hospital management is indicated when there is associated severe respiratory compromise, unstable angina, and/or congestive heart failure.

→ Monitor highly sensitive TSH annually or as needed to assess adequacy of treatment (Goroll, May, and Mulley 1987; Wartofsky and Ingbar 1991).

Hyperthyroidism

→ Decrease iodine intake if thought to be contributing to hyperthyroidism.

→ Initiate use of beta-blocking agents (e.g., propanolol [Inderal®] 20 mg QID) to control signs and symptoms related to hyperthyroidism (e.g., nervousness, palpitations, tremor, and heat intolerance) in consultation with a physician (Goroll, May, and Mulley 1987).
- Beta-blockers are generally contraindicated in patients with heart failure.

→ Refer to a physician for use of antithyroid agents (e.g., methimazole, propylthiouracil, or iodide) and/or ablative therapy, such as radioactive iodine (^{131}I) or subtotal thyroidectomy.

→ Hospital management is indicated when there is associated severe respiratory compromise, unstable angina, and/or congestive heart failure.

→ Monitor free T_4 Index and/or serum T_3 after the individual is in remission—annually or as needed—to assess adequacy of treatment (Goroll, May, and Mulley 1987).

Thyroid nodules

→ Discontinue goiter-producing medications.

→ If the patient has a solitary nodule or a distinct nodule within a multinodular gland, refer the patient to a physician for consideration of fine-needle biopsy/cutting-needle biopsy, thyroid scintigraphy, and/or surgical and/or medical (L-thyroxine-suppressive or replacement therapy) treatment.

→ If the patient has a hypofunctioning multinodular goiter (e.g., chronic thyroiditis), use the hypothyroidism treatment guidelines (see "Treatment/Management" section, "Hypothyroidism").

→ If the patient has a toxic mulitnodular goiter, use the hyperthyroidism treatment guidelines (see "Treatment/Management" section, "Hyperthyroidism").

CONSULTATION

Hypothyroidism

→ Physician consultation is indicated when:
  ▪ considering invasive/uncommon diagnostic studies (e.g., thyrotropin-releasing hormone stimulation test).
  ▪ initiating oral thyroid replacement therapy.

→ Consultation with an occupational health provider (nurse practitioner or physician) is indicated if the hypothyroidism is suspected to be associated with a work-related exposure.

→ Physician referral is indicated for individuals who:
  ▪ require hospitalization.
  ▪ are myxedematous.
  ▪ have secondary hypothyroidism.
  ▪ are not responding to conventional medical management.

Hyperthyroidism

→ Physician consultation is indicated when:
  ▪ considering invasive/uncommon diagnostic studies (e.g., thyrotropin-releasing hormone stimulation test and thyroid-stimulating immunoglobulins, respectively).
  ▪ initiating beta-blocking agents.

→ Physician referral is indicated for the administration of antithyroid agents and/or ablative therapy.

Thyroid nodules

→ Physician referral is indicated for the diagnostic evaluation and treatment of all patients who have a solitary nodule or a distinct nodule within a multinodular gland.

→ See "Hypothyroidism" and "Hyperthyroidism," in "Consultation/Referral" section for recommendations for individuals with hypofunctioning multinodular goiters and toxic multinodular goiters, respectively.

→ For all thyroid disorders, as needed for prescription(s).

PATIENT EDUCATION

→ Explain to the patient:
  ▪ the disease process (signs and symptoms and underlying etiologies).
  ▪ diagnostic studies (preparation, procedure(s), after-care, cost).
  ▪ management/treatment (action, use, adverse effects, cost).
  ▪ need for adhering to long-term management recommendations.

→ Address patient's and significant others' concerns and feelings regarding the disease process and/or management of the respective thyroid condition.

→ Provide a referral to a community agency if indicated, for example:

Thyroid Foundation of America, Inc.
630 Ambulatory Care Center
Massachusetts General Hospital
Boston, MA 02114

FOLLOW-UP

→ Emphasize need for ongoing care for the respective thyroid condition.

→ Document thyroid condition in progress notes and problem list.

Elisabeth O'Mara, R.N., M.S., A.N.P., C.D.E.

10-C

Type I Diabetes Mellitus

Diabetes mellitus is one of the most common endocrine conditions characterized by hyperglycemia due to the absolute or relative lack of insulin and/or insulin resistance. The American Diabetes Association (ADA) diagnoses for glucose tolerance include the following:

Type I diabetes mellitus, also known as *insulin dependent diabetes mellitus* (IDDM) and previously known as juvenile onset diabetes, usually occurs before the age of 30 years but can occur at any age. Onset of symptoms are frequently abrupt and ketosis is common. Genetics and environmental and autoimmune factors contribute to the etiology. Treatment consists of insulin, dietary management, and an exercise program (Schuman 1988).

Type II diabetes mellitus, also known as *non-insulin dependent diabetes mellitus* (NIDDM), previously known as maturity onset or adult onset, usually occurs after the age of 40 years but may occur at any age. Approximately 75 percent to 80 percent of people with NIDDM are obese. Frequently, the patient does not develop symptoms and may have the disease for years before an overt symptom occurs or a diagnosis is established. Ketosis is rare, but a condition called *hyperglycemic hyperosmolar nonketotic coma* (HHNKC) can occur in these patients. The etiology of NIDDM is considered multifactorial. Heredity plays a large role, predisposing the patient to beta cell dysfunction and insulin resistance. Treatment consists of diet alone, diet and oral medication, or diet and insulin.

Gestational diabetes mellitus (GDM), a condition of hyperglycemia recognized during pregnancy, places the fetus at greater risk for abnormalities at birth, such as macrosomia, hypoglycemia, hypocalcemia, and hyperbilirubinemia and at greater risk for intrauterine death and neonatal mortality (Metzger 1991). Diagnosis is established with an oral glucose tolerance test during weeks 24 through 28 of gestation. The majority of women with GDM can maintain normal glucose levels through diet alone (Star 1990).

Impaired glucose tolerance (IGT) was previously known as subclinical, latent, or chemical diabetes. The range in glucose levels is between normal and the level at which a diagnoses of diabetes mellitus is established. The person with IGT may develop diabetes mellitus or may return to normal, especially with appropriate dietary intervention. (See **Table 10D.1, Criteria for Diagnosis of Diabetes Mellitus,** p. 10-33.)

Approximately 10 percent of individuals with diabetes mellitus have Type I DM. Genetics plays a role in the development of this disease. Human lymphocyte antigen (HLA) haplotype DR_3 or DR_4 is usually detected in people with Type I DM (Ratner 1992). An identical twin whose sibling has developed Type I DM has a 50 percent chance of developing the disease (Tattersall and Pyke 1972).

Active autoimmunity is another factor in the development of the disease whereby the body attacks the islet cells of the pancreas. Ninety percent of the beta cells may be destroyed before overt symptoms of diabetes develop. The immunological dysfunction may be triggered by an environmental insult (or many insults) such as coxsackie virus, rubella, mumps, or others. The above stages in the development of overt Type I diabetes mellitus may take months or years (Ratner 1992).

All newly diagnosed Type I diabetes mellitus patients should be started on human insulin (White and Campbell 1992). Human insulin is produced from *E. coli* or yeast and is considered less antigenic than beef or pork insulin (White and Campbell 1992). The onset, peak, and duration of insulin varies between animal and human insulin (see **Table 10D.2, Insulin Action Curves,** p. 10-34).

The number of injections can vary depending on the blood sugar goals and results and the patient's lifestyle and compliance (see **Table 10D.3, Insulin Treatment Plans,** p. 10-35). Soon after the diagnosis of IDDM is established and insulin and dietary therapy is prescribed, it is not uncommon for the individual to go through a "honeymoon period" during which little or no insulin is required. This honeymoon period may last from months to a year (Ratner 1992).

Acute complications of IDDM include diabetic ketoacidosis (DKA) and hypoglycemia (blood sugar < 60 mg/dl). Diabetic ketoacidosis occurs when there is a lack of insulin and the body starts to use fat and protein for energy. DKA may result from undiagnosed IDDM, illness, undetected infections, stress, failure to take medication, or, rarely, too much food. DKA may be life-threatening and requires referral to a physician for hospitalization. The mortality rate with DKA is less than 5 percent (CDC 1991b).

Hypoglycemia may result from too much insulin, not enough food, or too much exercise. It is treated with immediate ingestion of sugar. If it is untreated and symptoms progress, the patient may become unconscious and may die (see **Table 10D.4, Hypoglycemia, or Insulin Reaction,** p. 10-36). Frequent severe episodes of hypoglycemia place the patient at risk for permanent neurological changes.

Chronic complications of IDDM include retinopathy, neuropathy, nephropathy, and cardiovascular disease. The risk of these complications is associated with family history, hypertension, hyperlipidemia, smoking history, and (many experts in the field believe) poor glycemic control. The National Institutes of Health—Diabetes Control and Complications Trial demonstrated that good glycemic control decreases the complications of retinopathy, neuropathy, and nephropathy in patients with insulin-dependent diabetes (Diabetes Control and Complications Trial Research Group 1993) (see **Table 10D.5, Biochemical Indices of Metabolic Control: Top Limits,** p. 10-38).

DATABASE

SUBJECTIVE

→ People at risk for IDDM include those with a positive family history of IDDM.

→ Classic symptoms include increased thirst (polydipsia), frequent urination (polyuria), hunger (polyphasia), frequent infections, difficulty healing or resolving infections, fatigue, blurred vision, abrupt weight loss, labored breathing.

→ More advanced symptoms may include fruity odor to the breath, abdominal pain, vomiting, dehydration, labored breathing.

→ Elements of a comprehensive medical history of particular concern in patients with diabetes include (American Diabetes Association 1991):

- dietary habits, nutritional status, and weight history; growth and development in children.
- details of previous treatment programs, including diabetes education.
- current treatment of diabetes, including medications, diet, and results of glucose monitoring.
- exercise history.
- frequency, severity, and cause of acute complications such as ketoacidosis and hypoglycemia.
- prior or current infections, particularly skin, foot, dental, and genitourinary.
- symptoms and treatment of chronic complications associated with diabetes: eye, heart, kidney, nerve, sexual function, peripheral vascular, and cerebral vascular.
- other medications that may affect blood glucose concentration.
- risk factors for atherosclerosis: smoking, hypertension, obesity, hyperlipidemia, and family history.
- psychosocial and economic factors that might influence the management of diabetes.
- family history of diabetes and other endocrine disorders.
- gestational history: hyperglycemia, delivery of an infant weighing more than 4000 g, toxemia, stillbirth, polyhydramnios, or other complications of pregnancy.

OBJECTIVE

→ Elements of a comprehensive physical examination of particular concern in patients with diabetes include (American Diabetes Association 1991):

- height and weight measurement (and comparison to norms in children).
- sexual maturation staging.
- blood pressure determination (with orthostatic measurements).
- ophthalmoscopic examination, if possible with dilation.
- thyroid palpation.
- cardiac examination.

- evaluation of pulses (with auscultation).
- foot examination.
- skin examination (including insulin-injection sites).
- neurological examination.
- dental and periodontal examination.

→ If DKA is not present:
- may have a few of the classic findings as listed previously.

→ If DKA is present, findings may include:
- weight loss.
- fruity odor to the breath.
- warm, dry skin.
- dry mucous membranes.
- poor skin turgor.
- tachycardia.
- hypotension.
- tender abdomen.
- diminished or absent bowel sounds.
- hypothermia.
- hyperreflexia.
- somnolence.
- impaired consciousness.

ASSESSMENT

→ Type I diabetes mellitus

→ R/O Type II diabetes mellitus

→ R/O IGT

→ R/O chronic pancreatitis

→ R/O hemochromatosis

→ R/O Cushing's syndrome

→ R/0 acromegaly

→ R/O pheochromcytoma

→ R/O glucagonoma

→ R/O drug-induced diabetes

→ Assess for acute severe stress (Foster 1980)

PLAN

DIAGNOSTIC TESTS

→ Laboratory tests to include:
- random blood glucose for diagnostic purposes; fasting plasma glucose for known diabetes.
- white blood cell (WBC) count.
- sodium.
- potassium.
- creatinine.
- serum ketones.
- bicarbonate.

- pH.
- cholesterol.
- triglycerides.
- low-density lipoprotein (LDL).
- high-density lipoprotein (HDL).
- thyroid function tests; T_4 or TSH.

→ Obtain urine to assess for:
- ketones.
- glucose.
- protein.

→ EKG.

TREATMENT/MANAGEMENT

→ If there is no evidence of DKA, individual may be managed on outpatient basis.
- If no ketosis is present, the diagnosis between Type I and Type II diabetes mellitus may be unclear and some clinicians may start the patient on a trial of an oral agent and diet.

→ Initiate insulin therapy.
- Total daily dose of insulin is calculated as 0.3 units/kg/day to 0.5 units/kg/day.
- There are many different insulin regimens (see **Table 10D.3**, p. 10-35).
  - BID injection: before breakfast and before dinner with split, mixed dose; short-acting (regular) and intermediate-acting (NPH) in a ratio 2:1.
  - TID injection: split mixed dose before breakfast; regular before dinner and NPH at bedtime.
  - QID injection: regular before each meal and NPH at bedtime (Hollander et al. 1990).
- Adjust insulin dose, depending on self blood glucose monitoring (SBGM) results (see **Table 10D.5**, p. 10-38).
- Prescribe glucagon kit (per physician's consultation).

→ Referral to dietitian to initiate/instruct ADA dietary goals.
- The amount of carbohydrate should be 55 percent to 60 percent of total caloric intake.
- The amount of daily protein should be 0.8g/kg body weight.
- Fat intake should be less than 30 percent of total caloric intake.
- Total cholesterol should be less than 300 mg/day.
- Total caloric intake is calculated to achieve and maintain ideal body weight (ADA 1991-1992).
- Alcohol is advised in moderation only.

- May inhibit liver production of glucose during the fasted state and increase the hypoglycemia effect of oral medication and insulin (Heins and Beeke 1992).
- Limit intake to 1 to 2 drinks, 1 to 2 times per week (ADA 1991-1992).

→ Prescribe exercise program.
  - Consult with physician regarding ordering treadmill (ADA [1991-1992] recommends stress EKG in patients older than 35 years).
  - Recommend warm-up exercises for 5 to 10 minutes followed by aerobic exercise (50 percent to 70 percent of patient's maximum oxygen uptake) 3 times per week for 20 to 45 minutes; cool down period for 5 to 10 minutes (ADA 1991-1992).

→ SBGM (see "Patient Education" section).

CONSULTATION

→ Physician referral required for DKA.
→ Physician consultation required for initiation of insulin therapy and adjustments of insulin dose.
→ Physician consultation required during or after loss of consciousness due to hypoglycemia.
→ Referral to nutritionist for instruction on ADA diet.
→ Referral to appropriate specialist(s) when indicated (i.e., cardiologist, neurologist, nephrologist, ophthalmologist, podiatrist, perinatologist).
→ Referral to social services when appropriate.

PATIENT EDUCATION

→ SBGM.
  - Instruct on use of meter, including check strip, cleaning, and memory. Choose a meter that is easy to use, has fewer steps, and that you know is reliable (e.g., One Touch II by Lifescan).
    - Advise patient to bring meter to all appointments. Recheck technique each visit.
  - Instruct on use of finger-sticking device and lancets.
    - Choose any finger.
      –Use sides of fingers and tips (avoid finger pads) and rotate sites.
    - Wash hands with soap and warm water.
      –Avoid using alcohol (unless in dirty environment) as it toughens skin.
    - Hang hand at side for 30 to 60 seconds to obtain blood sample more easily.

- Instruct on how to record blood glucose results in record book (see **Appendix 10C.1, How to Obtain Patient-Education Handouts**, p. 10-31).
  - Advise patient to bring record book to all appointments.
  - Advise patient what her target blood sugar range should be.

→ Instruct on urine testing for ketones.
  - Advise testing for ketones when blood glucose is over 240 mg/dl or when patient is ill.
  - Advise patient to call if ketones are moderate or large.
  - Advise patient to drink extra water if ketones are small.

→ Instruct on insulin administration.
  - Instruction regarding insulin to include types, source, dose, onset, peak, and duration (see **Table 10D.2**, p. 10-34).
  - Instruct on technique for drawing, measuring, and injecting insulin (see **Appendix 10C.1**, p. 10-31 for information on how to obtain patient handout on drawing and injecting insulin).
    - Do not aspirate prior to injecting.
  - Instruct patient on sites rotation (see **Appendix 10C.1**, p. 10-31 for information on how to obtain patient handout on site selection and rotation).
    - Abdomen has best absorption, followed by arms, thighs, buttocks.
    - Stay in same region, same time of day.
    - Avoid injections in exercising muscle.
    - Change site by one inch each time.
    - Do not use same site more than once every three to four weeks.
  - Advise patient to re-use needles if patient has good personal hygiene, has no acute illness or ongoing problems with infection, and is physically capable of safely recapping a syringe. Needles may be re-used until they become dull or bent (ADA 1991-1992).
    - If needle is re-used, recap after each use (ADA 1992).
  - Use needle clipper device to dispose of needle. Discard syringe and lancets in a hard plastic or needle container.
    - Check local county policy for syringe take-back program.
  - Advise on insulin storage.
    - Keep bottles currently in use at room temperature, out of sunlight for up to one month, then discard. If stored, store in door of

refrigerator and discard bottle after three months.

- Review symptoms, causes, treatment, and prevention of hypoglycemia with patient and family (see **Table 10D.4**, p. 10-36).
- Advise patient to obtain medical alert bracelet and explain purpose of bracelet.
- Instruct patient and family members on use of glucagon kit.
- Advise patient to call if blood sugar is less than 60 mg/dl on daily or weekly basis.

→ Review symptoms, causes, treatment, and prevention of hyperglycemia, including DKA.

→ Describe importance of following prescribed meal plan to improve blood sugar control.
- Encourage patient to check blood sugars one to two hours after meals occasionally to see the effects of different foods on blood glucose.

→ Teach patient about proper sick day management (e.g., colds, flu, infection):
- explain that illness, stress, infection may raise blood sugar.
- advise patient never to stop taking insulin, unless advised by provider or if experiencing severe hypoglycemia.
- advise patient to check blood sugar and urine ketones every four hours.
- advise patient to call if blood sugar remains over 300 mg/dl or less than 60 mg/dl or if the patient has trouble breathing or is vomiting (may be sign of DKA).
- advise patient to drink extra liquids (such as water, diet soda, and tea) ½ to ¾ cup every ½ hour to one hour.
- advise patient to weigh herself daily and if more than five-pound loss to call her provider.
- advise patient to check her temperature and to call if temperature is greater than 101°F (38.3°C).
- advise patient to call if she is having trouble breathing (may be a sign of DKA).

→ advise patient to have ophthalmological examination yearly.

→ Teach patient about proper foot care (see **Appendix 10C.2, Patient-Education Handout: Foot Care**, p. 10-32).

→ Recommend dental examination every six months.

→ Review local community resources.

→ Instruct patient regarding effects of smoking, alcohol, and drugs on diabetes. Counsel on lifestyle modification techniques when indicated.

→ Provide education for family on all aspects of diabetes care.

FOLLOW-UP

→ Number of visits depends on blood glucose control, change in treatment program, and presence of complications.

→ May need to contact patient weekly to check on SBGM results.

→ See patient within several weeks or one month if major changes in insulin dose are made.

→ See patient every three to six months if in good control.

→ The interim history should include:
- frequency, causes, and severity of hypoglycemia or hyperglycemia.
- results of regular glucose monitoring.
- adjustments by the patient of the therapeutic regimen.
- problems with adherence.
- symptoms suggesting development of the complications of diabetes.
- psychosocial status.
- other medical illnesses, and
- current medications.

→ Physical examination should include:
- yearly physical examination.
- check weight, blood pressure, and feet every visit.
- ophthalmological examination yearly if patient has IDDM five years or more.
- women planning pregnancy should have eye examination before pregnancy and during first trimester. Referral to a perinatologist for pre-pregnancy counseling is strongly advised.

→ Diagnostic tests should include:
- HgbA$_{1C}$ quarterly.
- cholesterol, HDL, triglycerides yearly.
- creatinine, urinalysis yearly; after five years of diabetes mellitus, obtain microalbuminuria (Haire-Joshu 1992).

→ Patient education should include a review of:
- diet; reasons for success or failure.
- exercise program; reasons for success or failure.
- SGBM; technique and results; interpret results with patient.
- hypoglycemic/hyperglycemic problems, symptoms, treatment, causes, and prevention.
- medications.
- birth control and family planning issues.

- advise three months of normal HgbA$_{1C}$ prior to conception.
  - foot care, dental care (CDC 1991a).
  - habits: smoking, alcohol, drugs.
  - psychological adjustment (CDC 1991a).
  - complications.

→ See "Treatment/Management" section.

→ Document in progress notes and problem list.

APPENDIX 10C.1

How to Obtain Patient-Education Handouts

Blood Glucose Testing Diary
    Becton Dickinson Consumer Products
    Becton Dickinson and Company
    Franklin Lakes, NJ
    07417-1883
    Part E1-0052-1   Cat. 9942

Drawing and Injecting Insulin
    Becton Dickinson Consumer Products
    Becton Dickinson and Company
    Franklin Lakes, NJ
    07417-1883
    Part E1-003-1   Cat. 9902

Site Selection and Rotation
    Becton Dickinson Consumer Products
    Becton Dickinson and Company
    Franklin Lakes, NJ
    07417-1883
    Part E1-005-1   Cat. 9904

APPENDIX 10C.2

Patient-Education Handout: Foot Care*

Being a diabetic means that you always have to think about your medications, diet, and exercise, as well as your other problems. The last thing you need is to worry about your feet. This handout gives you guidelines for daily foot care so that your feet won't become a worry.

As you may have heard, many people with diabetes have problems with their feet. However, this usually occurs with neglecting to take proper care of their feet.

With long-term diabetes (a period of many years), the blood flow to the feet may become poor. This prevents normal nourishment and will slow healing of injuries such as blisters, cuts, and scrapes. If an infection occurs, it will take longer to stop. This may be prevented by following your doctor's orders, properly using your medication, and carefully monitoring your blood sugar.

Occasionally, with long-term diabetes (here again, many years), the nerves that give feeling to the feet may not work properly. When this occurs, the person may not be aware of a problem because she cannot feel it. This is easily prevented by looking closely at your feet on a daily basis. If you see problems, please seek help from your internist, nurse practitioner, or podiatrist promptly. Starting good foot care habits now will insure lifelong healthy feet.

Foot Care

1. **Daily Inspection:** Look at your feet very carefully every day. Look for cuts, blisters, scratches, or irritations. Any break in the skin is a potential area of infection and should be treated with care. Bathe the area with mild soap and *warm* (not hot) water. Apply a mild antiseptic (Neosporin) and cover with a clean bandage (e.g., Band-Aid or gauze). If the area becomes inflamed or infected, seek medical help *immediately*.

2. **Daily Wash and Dry:** Poorly cleaned feet can lead to infection. Wash your feet daily with *warm* water and a mild soap. Check the water temperature with your hand. Dry well, particularly between the toes, but do not rub hard. Apply a bland lubrication cream (e.g., Nivea, Alpha Keri, baby lotion) if your skin is dry. A nonmedicated powder between the toes may help if this area stays moist.

3. **Care of Toenails:** Use clean nail *clippers*, not scissors or key chain cutters. Never tear your nails! Cut your nails straight across and never dig into the corners. If redness occurs, soak your toes in *warm*, salty water *three* times a day for fifteen minutes. Seek professional care if infection occurs.

4. Avoid wet feet, wet socks, and wet shoes. Never wear tennis shoes without socks. Don't walk with the shoelaces untied as this increases rubbing and friction, which causes blisters and abrasions.

5. Inspect the insides of your shoes for foreign objects, nail points, or torn linings. Any object that creates pressure may cause a break in the skin which is an opening for infection.

6. Never walk barefoot outside because stepping on rocks, stickers, broken glass, or hot sand may cause injury. Be careful walking barefoot inside the house.

7. Avoid extremes of temperature, too hot or too cold. Never sunburn your feet.

8. The only *safe* way to trim corns and calluses is to rub them gently with a pumice stone. Do *not* use chemical agents for this purpose. Painful skin problems need your doctor's care.

9. Do *not* smoke or chew tobacco. Nicotine in tobacco shrinks the blood vessels and slows the blood flow to your feet.

10. Do not listen to your friends and neighbors for foot care advice. Follow these guidelines and seek professional care promptly.

Healthy feet that will last a lifetime can be yours if you pay attention to them. Don't neglect your feet and they won't fail you.

*This handout may be reproduced for patient use.

Elisabeth O'Mara, R.N., M.S., A.N.P., C.D.E.

10-D

Type II Diabetes Mellitus

Diabetes mellitus is one of the most common endocrine conditions characterized by hyperglycemia due to the absolute or relative lack of insulin and/or insulin resistance. The ADA diagnoses for glucose tolerance include the following:

Type I diabetes mellitus, also known as *insulin-dependent diabetes mellitus* (IDDM) and previously known as juvenile-onset diabetes, usually occurs before the age of 30 years but can occur at any age. Onset of symptoms are frequently abrupt and ketosis is common. Genetics and environmental and autoimmune factors contribute to the etiology. Treatment consists of insulin, dietary management, and an exercise program (Schuman 1988).

Type II diabetes mellitus, also known as *non-insulin-dependent diabetes mellitus* (NIDDM), previously known as maturity-onset or adult-onset diabetes, usually occurs after the age of 40 years but may occur at any age. Approximately 75 percent to 80 percent of people with NIDDM are obese. Frequently, the patient does not develop symptoms and may have the disease for years before an overt symptom occurs or a diagnosis is established. Ketosis is rare, but a condition called *hyperglycemic hyperosmolar nonketotic coma* (HHNKC) can occur in these patients.

The etiology of NIDDM is considered multifactorial. Heredity plays a large role, predisposing the patient to beta cell dysfunction and insulin resistance. Treatment consists of diet alone, diet and oral medication, or diet and insulin.

Gestational diabetes mellitus (GDM), a condition of hyperglycemia recognized during pregnancy, places the fetus at greater risk for abnormalities at birth—including macrosomia, hypoglycemia, hypocalcemia, and

Table 10D.1. CRITERIA FOR DIAGNOSIS OF DIABETES MELLITUS

1. Elevation of random blood glucose ($\geq$200 mg/dl) and classic symptoms of diabetes, including polydipsia, polyuria, polyphagia, and weight loss.

2. Fasting blood glucose >140 mg/dl on two occasions.

3. Fasting blood glucose >140 mg dl and two (75g) oral glucose tolerance tests (OGTT) with the two-hour glucose $\geq$200 mg/dl and one intervening value $\geq$200 mg/dl.

Source: Adapted from ADA 1991-1992 Clinical practice recommendations. *Diabetes Care* 15(2): 474.

hyperbilirubinemia—and at greater risk for intrauterine death and neonatal mortality (Metzger 1991). Diagnosis is established with an oral glucose tolerance test during weeks 24 through 28 of gestation. The majority of women with GDM can maintain normal glucose levels through diet alone (Star 1990).

Impaired glucose tolerance (IGT) was previously known as subclinical, latent, or chemical diabetes. The range in glucose levels is between normal and the level at which a diagnoses of diabetes mellitus is established. The person with IGT may develop diabetes mellitus or may return to normal, especially with appropriate dietary intervention. (See **Table 10D.1, Criteria for Diagnosis of Diabetes Mellitus**).

Type II diabetes mellitus is also known as NIDDM which is confusing for the layperson as well as the professional, because appproximately 30 percent of the people with NIDDM are taking insulin. The etiologies are varied and include poor beta cell response to hyperglycemia, and insulin resistance at the level of the liver, fat, and muscle (Ratner 1992). Heredity plays a greater role in NIDDM than in IDDM. An identical twin whose sibling has NIDDM has an approximately 90 percent chance of developing the disease (Tattersall and Pyke 1972).

Individuals with Type II diabetes may be asymptomatic at the time of diagnosis through a routine urinalysis or random blood glucose (see **Table 10D.1**). In other cases, patients may present with long-term complications of diabetes mellitus before diagnosis is established. When typical symptoms of polyuria, polydipsia, and polyphagia do occur, they are usually much less acute than those seen in patients with Type I diabetes, and ketosis is rare (Schuman 1988).

Treatment of NIDDM is varied. Initially, if the patient is symptomatic and has a fasting blood sugar (FBS) >250-300 mg/dl, insulin and diet may be initiated until glycemic control is achieved (White and Campbell 1992). After that, insulin may be discontinued and sulfonylurea agents may be started to control hyperglycemia (in addition to diet therapy). If sufficient weight reduction occurs, the disease may be controlled with diet alone. Thirty percent of individuals with NIDDM control the disease solely by diet.

If the patient is not symptomatic, exhibits small ketonuria, and blood glucose is below 300 mg/dl, a trial of diet alone may be initiated. If after the trial period (which can vary from weeks to months) glycemic control has not been achieved, oral sulfonylureas will be added to the treatment regimen. There is no difference in efficacy between the sulfonylureas (White and Henry 1992). However, diabinase is usually not recommended for the elderly because long duration puts the patient at greater risk of hypoglycemia.

Secondary failure to sulfonylurea agents can be related to altered absorption during hyperglycemia and insulin deficiency (Groop 1992). Combination therapy using oral agents and insulin is controversial and found to be effective in only half the patients studied (Groop, Groop, and Stenman 1990; Peters and Davidson 1991). If diet and oral agents fail in glycemic control, then insulin and diet is the next step.

Type II diabetes mellitus patients starting on insulin should be started on human insulin (White and Campbell 1992). Human insulin is produced from *E. coli* or yeast and is considered to be less antigenic than beef or pork insulin (White and Campbell 1992). The onset, peak, and duration of insulin varies between animal and human insulin (see **Table 10D.2, Insulin Action Curves**). The number of injections can vary depending on the blood sugar goals and results and the patient's lifestyle and compliance (see **Table 10D.3, Insulin Treatment Plans**).

Acute complications in NIDDM include hyperglycemic hyperosmolar nonketotic coma (HHNKC) and

Table 10D.2. INSULIN ACTION CURVES

Insulin	Onset (hours)	Peak (hours)	Duration (hours)	Maximum Duration (hours)
Animal				
Regular	½-2	3-4	4-6	6-8
NPH	4-6	8-14	16-20	20-24
Lente	4-6	8-14	16-20	20-24
Ultralente	8-14	Minimal	24-36	24-36
Human				
Regular	½-1	2-3	3-6	4-6
NPH	2-4	4-10	10-16	14-18
Lente	3-4	4-12	12-18	16-20
Ultralente	6-10	?	18-20	20-30

Source: Reprinted with permission from Hollander, P., Castle, G., Joynes, J.O., and Nelson, J. 1990. *Intensified insulin management for you*, p. 13. Minneapolis: DCI Publishing.

hypoglycemia. HHNKC is typically characterized by severe hyperglycemia (>600-800 mg/dl), hyperosmolarity, severe dehydration, and altered mental status (CDC 1991b, White and Henry 1992). Ketosis is rarely seen. HHNKC may occur in individuals that are more than 60 years old who have NIDDM that is untreated or undiagnosed. Chronic illness with mild renal insufficiency, acute illness, recent surgery, or use of drugs may precipitate HHNKC. Immediate referral to a physician for hospitalization is required because the mortality rate has been reported to be as high as 50 percent (CDC 1991b).

Hypoglycemia (blood glucose level below 60 mg/dl) is an acute complication of NIDDM when the individual is on oral agents or insulin. It may result from too much medication (either oral agents or insulin), not enough food, or too much exercise. Symptoms vary from mild sweating, tremors, and hunger, to more severe symptoms characterized by confusion, seizures and coma. Hypoglycemia is treated with immediate ingestion of sugar (see **Table 10D.4, Hypoglycemia, or Insulin Reaction**).

Long-term complications of NIDDM include retinopathy, nephropathy, neuropathy, and cardiovascular disease. Epidemiological studies have suggested that poor glycemic control may increase the onset and progression of these complications. The Diabetes Control and Complications Trial demonstrated that good glycemic control decreases the onset and progression of retinopathy, nephropathy, and neuropathy in insulin-dependent diabetes patients. (The Diabetes Control and Complications Trial Research Group 1993). Many authorities believe that the results of this study can be applied to Type II diabetes mellitus patients. Most authorities recommend good glycemic control while avoiding hypoglycemia. Screening for NIDDM with a FBS is advised for people with one or more diabetic risk factors (ADA 1991-1992) (see "Subjective" section for risk factors).

Table 10D.3. INSULIN TREATMENT PLANS

The most commonly prescribed insulin plan is Regular and NPH given before breakfast and before supper.

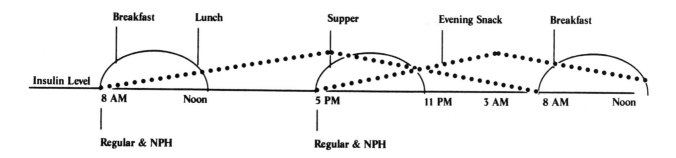

A common three-injection regimen is Regular and NPH before breakfast; regular before lunch, and NPH at evening snack.

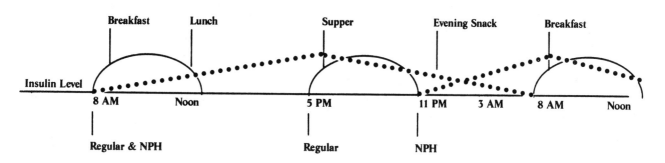

An additional insulin plan involves giving NPH as a basal insulin before evening snack. Bolus doses of Regular are given before breakfast, lunch, and supper.

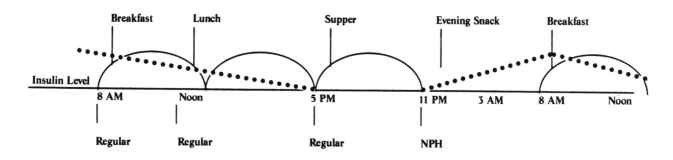

Source: Reprinted with permission from Hollander, P., Castle, G., Joynes, J.O., and Nelson, J. 1990. *Intensified insulin management for you*, pp. 14-15. Minneapolis: DCI Publishing.

Table 10D.4. HYPOGLYCEMIA, OR INSULIN REACTION

Symptoms	Treatment

Initial
  Mood change (irritability)
  Nausea and vomiting
  Weakness
  Shakiness
  Sweating
  Pale skin
  Hunger
  Excitability
  Dizziness
	Quick Sugar
	  Fast-acting sugar
	
	  10 gm-15 gm carbohydrate, same as one fruit exchange
	
	  If not better in 10-15 minutes, repeat.
	
	  Examples: ½ c orange juice ½ c regular soda pop
	                   2-4 lg sugar cubes 4-6 sm sugar cubes
	                   7 Life Savers 2 tsp. honey or corn syrup
	                   3 glucose tablets

Intermediate
  Confusion
  Poor coordination
  Headache
  Restlessness
  Double vision
	Glucose
	  Concentrated glucose, available without prescription at most pharmacies.
	  Lemon-lime flavor.
	  Squeeze ⅓ bottle between teeth and cheek.
	  It will be swallowed by reflex and absorbed through stomach wall.
	  Can be carried on trips, to school.
	  Stores indefinitely.
	  May also be used as one fruit and one starch exchange.

Advanced
  Unconscious
  Convulsions
	Glucagon
	  Glucagon is a hormone that acts on the liver to release stored glucose.
	  Must be administered by another person.
	
	  If no response in 15 minutes, repeat dose or call emergency personnel. Inform physician of reactions.
	
	  Cannot be taken orally. Note expiration date.
	
	  Occasional side effects are nausea and vomiting.
	
	  Feed immediately after regaining consciousness (unless vomiting)—crackers, 7-Up, etc. Follow with ½ meat sandwich, glass of milk.
	
	  Review instructions periodically.

Source: Reprinted with permission from Hollander, P., Castle, G., Joynes, J.O., and Nelson, J. 1990. *Intensified insulin management for you*, p. 71. Minneapolis: DCI Publishing.

DATABASE

SUBJECTIVE

→ Risk factors for NIDDM include:
  ▪ African American, Hispanic, and Native American origin.
  ▪ family history of NIDDM.
  ▪ obesity (>20 percent over ideal body weight) (ADA 1991-1992).
  ▪ gestational diabetes mellitus or delivery of baby > 4000 g (ADA 1991-1992).
  ▪ previously identified individuals with impaired glucose tolerance (ADA 1991-1992).
  ▪ hypertension and hyperlipidemia (> 240 mg/dl) (ADA 1991-1992).

→ Patient may be asymptomatic.

→ Symptoms may include frequent urination (polyuria), thirst (polydipsia), weight loss, blurred vision, frequent infection.

→ Presenting symptoms of numbness, paresthesias, or visual problems may be chronic complications secondary to undiagnosed hyperglycemia.

→ Elements of a comprehensive medical history of particular concern in patients with diabetes include (American Diabetes Association 1991):
  ▪ dietary habits, nutritional status, and weight history; growth and development in children.
  ▪ details of previous treatment programs, including diabetes education.
  ▪ current treatment of diabetes, including medications, diet, and results of glucose monitoring.
  ▪ exercise history.
  ▪ frequency, severity, and cause of acute complications such as ketoacidosis and hypoglycemia.
  ▪ prior or current infections, particularly skin, foot, dental, and genitourinary.
  ▪ symptoms and treatment of chronic complications associated with diabetes: eye, heart, kidney, nerve, sexual function, peripheral vascular, and cerebral vascular.
  ▪ other medications that may affect blood glucose concentration.

- risk factors for atherosclerosis: smoking, hypertension, obesity, hyperlipidemia, and family history.
- psychosocial and economic factors that might influence the management of diabetes.
- family history of diabetes and other endocrine disorders.
- gestational history: hyperglycemia, delivery of an infant weighing more than 4000 g, toxemia, stillbirth, polyhydramnios, or other complications of pregnancy.

(American Diabetes Association 1991)

OBJECTIVE

→ Elements of a comprehensive physical examination of particular concern in patients with diabetes include (American Diabetes Association 1991):
- height and weight measurement (and comparison to norms in children).
- sexual maturation staging.
- blood pressure determination (with orthostatic measurements).
- ophthalmoscopic examination, if possible with dilation.
- thyroid palpation.
- cardiac examination.
- evaluation of pulses (with auscultation).
- foot examination.
- skin examination (including insulin-injection sites).
- neurological examination.
- dental and periodontal examination.

ASSESSMENT

→ Type II versus Type I diabetes mellitus (depends on age, risk factors, presence of ketosis)
→ R/O IGT
→ R/O hyperglycemia secondary to prescription medications (diuretics, glucocorticosteroids)
→ Following diagnosis, consider the following (although doubtful) as contributing factors:
- Cushing's syndrome
- acromegaly
- pheochromcytoma
- glucagonoma
- acute severe stress (Foster 1980)

PLAN

DIAGNOSTIC TESTS

→ Screen individuals with one or more risk factors or symptomatic patients with fasting glucose (see **Table 10D.1**).
→ If random blood sugar or FBS is within normal limits but still have high index of suspicion for diabetes, order oral glucose tolerance test.
→ If FBS is > 115 mg/dl order the following:
- creatinine.
- thyroid function tests.
- cholesterol.
- LDL.
- HDL.
→ Obtain urine:
- ketones.
- glucose.
→ EKG.
→ If patient is symptomatic, order the following:
- WBC count.
- serum ketones.
- bicarbonate.
- pH.
- potassium.
- sodium.

TREATMENT/MANAGEMENT

→ If there is no acute illness present, the patient is asymptomatic, and blood glucose is less than 300 mg/dl:
- if patient is obese, refer to a registered dietitian for diet recommendations or advise patient to follow the ADA weight-reduction diet.
- if not obese, refer for ADA diet.
  - The amount of carbohydrate should be 55 percent to 60 percent of total caloric intake.
  - The amount of daily protein should be 0.8 g/kg body weight.
  - Fat intake should be less than 30 percent of total caloric intake.
  - Total cholesterol should be less than 300 mg/day.
  - Total caloric intake is calculated to achieve and maintain ideal body weight (ADA 1991-1992).
  - Alcohol is advised in moderation only.
    - May inhibit liver production of glucose during the fasted state and increase the hypoglycemia effect of oral medication and insulin (Heins and Beeke 1992).

–Limit intake to 1 to 2 drinks 1 to 2 times per week (ADA 1991-1992).
- ▪ prescribe exercise program.
  - • Consult with physician regarding ordering treadmill (ADA recommends stress EKG in patients older than 35 years) (ADA 1991-1992).
  - • Recommend warm-up exercises for 5 to 10 minutes followed by aerobic exercise (50 percent to 70 percent of patient's maximum oxygen uptake) 3 times per week or more for 20 to 45 minutes each; cool-down period for 5 to 10 minutes (ADA 1991-1992).
→ If little change in blood glucose results with diet and exercise after trial period, start on oral agents (see **Table 10D.5, Biochemical Indices of Metabolic Control: Top Limits**, and **Table 10D.6, Sulfonylurea Comparison**).
- ▪ Counsel women of childbearing age that they should use birth control measures if on oral agent.
  - • If planning to get pregnant, switch to insulin and attempt normal $HgbA_{1C}$ before conception. Refer to perinatologist for pre-conception counseling.
→ If little change in blood glucose results with diet, exercise, or maximum-dose oral agents, discontinue oral agents and start on insulin. If unable to maintain blood glucose below 200 mg/dl during the day, initiate insulin therapy (Karam 1993).
- ▪ Total daily dose of insulin is calculated as 0.3 units/kg/day-0.5 units/kg/day.
- ▪ There are many different insulin regimens (see also **Table 10D.3**):
  - • BID injection: before breakfast and before dinner with split mixed dose of short-acting (regular) and intermediate acting (NPH) in a ratio 2:1.
  - • TID injection: split mixed dose before breakfast; regular before dinner and NPH at bedtime.

- • QID injection: regular before each meal and NPH at bedtime (Hollander et al. 1990).
- ▪ Adjust insulin dose, depending on SBGM results.
- ▪ Prescribe glucagon kit (per physician consultation).
- ▪ Advise on lifestyle changes.
→ SBGM (See "Patient Education" section).
- ▪ SBGM up to the provider's discretion, but may be useful for the patient to see the results.
- ▪ Two types of SBGM: visual method or machine; visual less expensive but more risk of user error.
  - • Older people may have more visual problems.
- ▪ Recommend SBGM using machine for all Type II patients on insulin.
- ▪ SBGM is useful for Type II patients on oral agents to monitor hypoglycemia more closely.
- ▪ If patient is on diet alone, SBGM is up to the provider and patient's discretion. It may be an educational tool and motivating force for the patient to see the results of the diet and exercise program.

CONSULTATION

→ Physician consultation for initiation and adjustment of oral agents or insulin.
→ Physician referral for hospital management if DKA or HHNKC is suspected.
→ Referral to a nutritionist may be necessary for counseling/adjustment to ADA diet.
→ Refer for ophthalmological examination upon diagnosis and then at least annually.
→ Refer to appropriate specialist when indicated (i.e., cardiologist, neurologist, nephrologist, ophthalmologist, podiatrist, perinatologist).

PATIENT EDUCATION

→ SBGM.
- ▪ Instruct on use of meter, including check strip, cleaning, and memory. Choose a meter that is easy to use, has fewer steps, and is reliable (e.g., One Touch II by Lifescan).

Table 10D.5. BIOCHEMICAL INDICES OF METABOLIC CONTROL: TOP LIMITS

	Normal	Acceptable	Fair	Poor
Fasting plasma glucose	115 mg/dl	150 mg/dl	200 mg/dl	>200 mg/dl
Postprandial plasma glucose	140 mg/dl	175 mg/dl	235 mg/dl	>235 mg/dl
Glycosylated hemoglobin	6%	8%	10%	10%

Source: Reprinted with permission from Haire-Joshu, D. 1992. *Management of diabetes mellitus*, p. 631. St. Louis: C.V. Mosby.

Table 10D.6. SULFONYLUREA COMPARISON

Drug	Total Daily Dose	No. of Doses Per Day	Considerations
Acetohexamide (Dymelor)	250 mg-1500 mg	1-2	Renally excreted metabolite may have greater activity than parent compound; adjust dose for renal failure.
Chlorpropamide (Diabinese)	100 mg-500 mg	1	Highest incidence of side effects; longest duration; adjust dose in presence of renal failure.
Glipizide (Glucotrol)	2.5 mg-40 mg	1-2	Metabolized to inactive metabolites that are excreted renally.
Glyburide (Diabeta, Micronase)	1.25 mg-20 mg	1-2	Metabolized to less active forms; 50 percent excreted renally, 50 percent via feces.
Tolbutamide (Orinase)	500 mg-3000 mg	2-3	Shortest-acting; metabolites inactive.
Tolazamide (Tolinase)	100 mg-1000 mg	1-2	Converted to inactive metabolites.

Source: Reprinted with permission from White, J., and Campbell, K. 1992. Pharmacologic therapies in the management of diabetes mellitus. In *Management of diabetes mellitus*, ed. D. Haire-Joshu, p. 145. St. Louis: C.V. Mosby.

- Advise patient to bring meter to all appointments. Recheck technique each visit.
- Instruct on use of finger-sticking device and lancets.
  - Choose any finger.
    - Use sides of fingers and tips (avoid finger pads) and rotate sites.
  - Wash hands with soap and warm water
    - Avoid using alcohol (unless in dirty environment) as it toughens skin.
  - Hang hand at side for 30 to 60 seconds to obtain blood sample more easily.
- Instruct on how to record blood glucose results in record book (see **Appendix 10C.1, How to Obtain Patient-Education Handouts**, p. 10-31).
  - Advise patient to bring record book to all appointments.

→ Instruct on urine testing for ketones.
- Advise testing for ketones when blood glucose over 240 mg/dl or when patient is ill.
- Advise patient to call if ketones are moderate or large.
- Advise patient to drink extra water if ketones are small.

→ Instruct on insulin administration.
- Instruction regarding insulin to include types, source, dose onset, peak, and duration (see **Table 10D.2**).
- Instruct on technique for drawing, measuring, and injecting insulin (see **Appendix 10C.1**, p. 10-31 for information on how to obtain patient handout on drawing and injecting insulin).
  - Do not aspirate before injecting.
- Instruct patient on sites rotation (see **Appendix 10C.1**, p. 10-31).

- Abdomen has best absorption, followed by arms, thighs, buttocks.
- Stay in same region, same time of day.
- Avoid injections in exercising muscle.
- Change site by one inch each time.
- Do not use same site more than once every three to four weeks.
- Advise patient to re-use needles if she has good personal hygiene, no acute illness or ongoing problems with infection, and is physically capable of safely recapping a syringe. Needles may be re-used until they become dull or bent (ADA 1991-1992).
  - If needle is re-used, recap after each use (ADA 1991-1992).
- Use needle clipper device to dispose of needle. Discard syringe and lancets in a hard plastic or needle container
  - Check local county policy for syringe take-back program.
- Advise on insulin storage.
  - Keep bottles currently in use at room temperature, out of sunlight for up to one month, then discard. If stored, store in door of refrigerator and discard bottle after three months.

→ Review symptoms, causes, treatment, and prevention of hypoglycemia with patient and family (see **Table 10D.4**).
- Advise patient to obtain medical alert bracelet.
- If patient is on insulin, review glucagon kit with patient and family members.
- Advise patient to call provider if blood sugar falls below 60 mg/dl daily or weekly.

→ Review symptoms, causes, treatment, and prevention of hyperglycemia, including DKA.

→ Teach patient about proper sick day management (e.g., colds, flu, infection):
- explain HHNKC causes, treatment, and prevention.
- explain that illness, stress, infection may raise blood sugar.
- advise patient never to stop taking insulin unless advised by provider or patient experiences severe hypoglycemia.
- advise patient to check blood sugar and urine ketones every four hours.
- advise patient to call if blood sugar remains over 300 mg/dl, if ketones are moderate or large, vomiting or persistent diarrhea occur, or patient has trouble breathing (may be sign of DKA).
- advise patient to drink extra liquids (such as water, diet soda, and tea) ½-¾ cup every ½ hour to one hour.
- advise patient to weigh herself daily and if more than five-pound loss, to call her provider.
- advise patient to check her temperature and call if temperature is greater than 101°F (38.3°C).

→ Advise patient to have ophthalmological examination yearly.

→ Instruct on foot care (see **Appendix 10C.2, Patient-Education Handout: Foot Care,** p. 10-32).

→ Recommend dental examination every six months.

→ Review local community resources.

→ Emphasize importance of following prescribed meal plan to improve blood sugar control.
- Encourage patient to check blood sugars one to two hours after meals to assess the effects of different foods on blood sugar levels.

→ Instruct patient regarding effects of smoking, alcohol, and drugs on diabetes. Counsel on lifestyle modification techniques when indicated.

→ Provide education for family on all aspects of diabetes care.

FOLLOW-UP
→ Number of visits depends on blood glucose control, change in treatment regimen, presence of complications.

→ May need to contact patient weekly to check on SBGM results.

→ See patient within several weeks to one month if major changes are made.

→ See patient on insulin every three to six months if in good control; other patients twice a year.

→ The interim history should include:
- frequency, causes, and severity of hypoglycemia or hyperglycemia,
- results of regular glucose monitoring,
- adjustments by the patient of the therapeutic regimen,
- problems with adherence,
- symptoms suggesting development of the complications of diabetes,
- psychosocial status,
- other medical illnesses, and
- current medications.

→ Physical examination should include:
- yearly physical examination.
- check weight, blood pressure, and feet every visit.
- yearly eye examination by an ophthalmologist.

→ Diagnostic tests:
- HgbA$_{1C}$ twice a year; possibly quarterly if on insulin.
- cholesterol, HDL, triglycerides yearly.
- urinalysis yearly; after five years of diabetes, obtain microalbuminuria (Haire-Joshu 1992).

→ Patient education.
- Review SBGM results.
- Teach patients to trouble-shoot machine/testing equipment.
- Teach signs of chronic complications.
- Review diet.
- Review exercise program—compliance, roadblocks to compliance.
- Review foot care.
- Review causes, symptoms, treatment, and prevention of hyperglycemia.
- Review psychological adjustment (CDC 1991a).
- Review habits: smoking, alcohol, drugs.
- See "Treatment/Management" section.

→ Document in progress notes and problem list.

10-E
Bibliography

American Diabetes Association. 1991. Standards of medical care for patients with diabetes mellitus. *Diabetes Care* 14(2):10–13.

———. 1991–1992. Clinical practice recommendations. *Diabetes Care* 15(2):474.

Antony, A.C. 1991. Megaloblastic anemia. In *Hematology: Basic principles and practice*, eds. R. Hoffman, E. Benz, S.J. Shattil, B. Furie, and H. Cohen, pp. 392–416. New York: Churchill Livingstone.

Baker, W.F. 1993. The clinical evaluation of the patient with anemia. In *Hematology: Clinical and laboratory practice*, ed. R.L. Bick, pp. 203–230. St Louis: C.V. Mosby.

Berliner, N., and Duffy, T.P. 1991. The approach to the patient with anemia. In *Hematology: Basic principles and practice*, eds. R. Hoffman, E. Benz, S.J. Shattil, B. Furie, and H. Cohen, pp. 302–310. New York: Churchill Livingstone.

Beulter, E. 1988. Common anemias. *Journal of the American Medical Association* 259:2433–2437.

Boots Pharmaceuticals. 1991. *Thyroid disease: Hypothyroidism and hyperthyroidism.* Lincolnshire, IL: Boots Pharmaceuticals.

Brittenham, G.M. 1991. Disorders of iron metabolism: Iron deficiency and overload. In *Hematology: Basic principles and practice*, eds. R. Hoffman, E. Benz, S.J. Shattil, B. Furie, and H. Cohen, pp. 327–345. New York: Churchill Livingstone.

Bunn, H.F. 1991. Pathophysiology of the anemias. In *Harrison's principles of internal medicine*, eds. J. Wilson, E. Braunwald, K. Isselbacher, R. Petersdorf, J. Martin, A. Fauci, and R. Root, vol. 1, 12th ed., pp. 1489–1493. New York: McGraw-Hill.

Bushnell, F. 1992. A guide to primary care of iron-deficiency anemia. *The Nurse Practitioner* 17(11):68–74.

Carmel, R. 1993. The clinical aspects of megaloblastic anemia. In *Hematology: Clinical and laboratory practice*, ed. R.L. Bick, pp. 437–450. St Louis: C.V. Mosby.

Centers for Disease Control. 1991a. *Take charge of your diabetes: A guide for patients.* Atlanta: National Center for Chronic Disease Prevention and Health Promotion.

———. 1991b. *The prevention and treatment of complications of diabetes mellitus, a guide for primary care practitioners.* Atlanta: National Center for Chronic Disease Prevention and Health Promotion.

Colbum, M. 1995. Patient handout: Foot care. Walnut Creek, CA: Kaiser Permanente Medical Center. (1425 South Main Street).

Damon, L. 1992a. Anemias of chronic disease in the aged: Diagnosis and treatment. *Geriatrics* 47(4):47–57.

———. 1992b. New concepts in evaluation and treatment of anemia. *Primary care medicine: Principles and practice*, pp. 251–270. San Francisco: University of California, San Francisco, Division of General Internal Medicine.

Desnick, R.J., and Anderson, K.E. 1991. Heme biosynthesis and its disorders: The porphyrias and sideroblastic anemias. In *Hematology: Basic principles and practice*, eds. R. Hoffman, E. Benz, S.J. Shattil, B. Furie, and H. Cohen, pp. 350–364. New York: Churchill Livingstone.

Diabetes Control and Complications Trial Research Group. 1993. The effect of intensive treatment of diabetes on the development and progression of long-term complications in insulin-dependent diabetes mellitus. *The New England Journal of Medicine* 329:977–986.

Djulbegovic, B., Hadley, T., and Pasic, R. 1989. The new algorithm for diagnosis of anemia. *Postgraduate Medicine* 85:119–130.

Eisenbarth, G.S., and Kahn, C.R. 1990. Etiology and pathogenesis of diabetes mellitus. In *Principles and practice of endocrinology and metabolism,* ed. K.L. Becker, pp. 1074–1084. Philadelphia: J.B. Lippincott.

Esposito, N. 1992 Thalassemia: Simple screening for hereditary anemia. *The Nurse Practitioner* 17(2):50–61.

Foster, D.W. 1980. Diabetes mellitus. In *Harrison's principles of internal medicine,* ed. T.R. Harrison, pp. 1741–1755. New York: McGraw-Hill.

Goroll, A.H., May, L.A., and Mulley, A.G. 1995. *Primary care medicine: Office evaluation and management of the adult patient,* 3rd ed. Philadelphia: J.B. Lippincott.

Groop, L.C. 1992. Sulfonylureas in NIDDM. *Diabetes Care* 15(6):737–754.

Groop, L.C., Groop, P.H., and Stenman, S. 1990. Combined insulin-sulfonylurea therapy in treatment of NIDDM. *Diabetes Care* 13(Suppl. 3):47–52.

Haire-Joshu, D., ed. 1992. *Management of diabetes mellitus.* St Louis: C.V. Mosby.

Halstead, J.A., and Halstead, C.A. 1981. *The laboratory in clinical medicine: Interpretation and application,* 2nd ed, pp. 457–467. Philadelphia: W.B. Saunders.

Heins, J.M., and Beeke, C.A. 1992. Nutritional management of diabetes mellitus. In *Management of diabetes mellitus,* ed. D. Haire-Joshu, pp. 21–73. St. Louis: C.V. Mosby.

Herbert, V. 1988. Anemias. In *Clinical Nutrition,* 2nd ed., ed. D. Paige, p. 593. St Louis: C.V. Mosby.

Hollander, P., Castle, G., Joynes, J.O., and Nelson, J. 1990. *Intensified insulin management for you.* Minneapolis: DCI Publishing.

Kaplan, M.E. 1988. Hemolytic disorders: Introduction. In *Cecil's textbook of medicine,* eds. J.B. Wyngaarden, L.H. Smith, and J.C. Bennett, pp. 855–856. Philadelphia: W.B. Saunders.

Karam, J.H. 1993. Diabetic mellitus and hypoglycemia. In *Current medical diagnoses and treatment,* ed. L.M. Tierney, pp. 912–948. Norwalk, CT: Appleton & Lange.

Kee, J.L. 1990. *Handbook of laboratory and diagnostic tests with nursing implications.* Norwalk, CT: Appleton & Lange.

Linker, C.A. 1992. Blood. In *Current medical diagnosis and treatment,* eds. S.A. Schroeder, L.A. Tierney Jr., S.J. McPhee, M.A. Papadakis, and M.A. Krupp, pp. 387–437. Norwalk, CT: Appleton & Lange.

Marge, S., and University of California at Berkeley Wellness Letter, eds. 1992. *The wellness encyclopedia of food and nutrition: How to buy, store and prepare every variety of fresh food.* New York: Rebus.

McPhee, S.J., and Hughes, E.F. 1991. Anemia. In *Current practice of emergency medicine,* ed. M.L. Callaham, pp. 777–783. Philadelphia: B.C. Decker.

Meek, J.C. 1990. Tests of thyroid function: Update in the diagnosis and management of thyroid disease. *Comprehensive Therapy* 16(7):20–27.

Metzger, B.E., ed. 1991. Proceedings of the Third International Workshop Conference on Gestational Diabetes Mellitus. *Diabetes* 40(Suppl. 2):1–201.

Meyers, F.J., Welborn, J.L., and Lewis, J.P. 1988. Improved approach to patients with normocytic anemia. *American Family Physician* 38:191–195.

Mohler, E. 1992. Iron deficiency and anemia of chronic disease: Clues to differentiating these conditions. *Postgraduate Medicine* 92(4):123–126.

Peters, A.L., and Davidson, M.B. 1991. Insulin plus sulfonylurea agent for treating type II diabetes. *Annals of Internal Medicine* 115:45–53.

Ratner, R.E. 1992. Overview of diabetes mellitus. In *Management of diabetes mellitus,* ed. D. Haire-Joshu, pp. 3–20. St. Louis: C.V. Mosby.

Ross, D.S. 1991a. Evaluation of the thyroid nodule. *The Journal of Nuclear Medicine* 32(11):2181–2192.

———. 1991b. Subclinical hypothyroidism. In *Werner and Ingbar's the thyroid: A fundamental and clinical text,* eds. L.E. Braverman and R.D. Utiger, 6th ed., pp. 1256–1262. Philadelphia: J.B. Lippincott.

Schectman, J.M., and Pawlson, G. 1990. The cost-effectiveness of three thyroid function testing strategies for suspicion of hypothyroidism in a primary care setting. *Journal of General Internal Medicine* 5(1):8–15.

Schuman, C.R. 1988. Diabetes mellitus: Definition, classification and diagnosis. In *Diabetes mellitus,* eds. J.A. Galloway, J. Potvin, and C.R. Schuman, 9th ed., pp. 2–13. Indianapolis: Eli Lilly and Co.

Schwartz E., Berkman, E.M., and Silberstein, L.E. 1991. The autoimmune hemolytic anemias. In *Hematology: Basic principles and practice,* eds. R. Hoffman, E. Benz, S.J. Shattil, B. Furie, and H. Cohen, pp. 422–437. New York: Churchill Livingstone.

Schwartz, E., and Benz, E.J. 1991. Thalassemia. In *Hematology: Basic principles and practice,* eds. R. Hoffman, E. Benz, S.J. Shattil, B. Furie, and H. Cohen, pp. 368–390. New York: Churchill Livingstone.

Sobel, D.S., and Ferguson, T. 1985. *The people's book of medical tests.* New York: Summit Books.

Star, W.L. 1990. Gestational diabetes. In *Ambulatory obstetrics: Protocols for nurse practitioners/nurse-midwives,* 2nd ed., eds. W.L. Star, M.T. Shannon, L.N. Sammons, and Y. Gutierrez. San Francisco: University of California, San Francisco.

Tattersall, R.B., and Pyke, D.A. 1972. Diabetes in identical twins. *Lancet* 2:1120–1125.

U.S. Department of Agriculture. 1975. *Nutritive value of American foods in common units: Handbook 456.* Washington, DC: U.S. Government Printing Office.

Wallerstein, R.O. 1987. Laboratory evaluation of anemia. *Western Journal of Medicine* 146:443–451.

Wartofsky, L., and Ingbar, S.H. 1991. Diseases of the thyroid. In *Harrison's principles of internal medicine,* eds. J.D. Wilson, E. Braunwald, K.J. Isselbacher, R.G. Petersdorf, J.B. Martin, A.S. Fauci, and R.K. Root, 12th ed., vol. 2, pp. 1692–1712. New York: McGraw-Hill.

Waterbury, L. 1991. Anemia. In *Principles of ambulatory medicine,* eds. L.R. Barker, J.R. Burton, and P.D. Zieve, 3rd ed., pp. 549–562. Baltimore: Williams and Wilkins.

Wheby, M.S. 1987. Anemia: Classification, mechanisms, diagnosis and physiologic effects. In *Leavell and Throup's fundamentals of clinical hematology,* pp. 163–183. Philadelphia: W.B. Saunders.

White, J.R., and Campbell, R.K. 1992. Pharmacologic therapies in the management of diabetes mellitus. In *Management of diabetes mellitus,* ed. D. Haire-Joshu, pp. 249–308. St. Louis: C.V. Mosby.

White, N.H., and Henry, D.N. 1992. Special issues in diabetes management. In *Management of diabetes mellitus,* ed. D. Haire-Joshu, pp. 249–309. St. Louis: C.V. Mosby.

Woolf, P.D. 1990. Thyroiditis. In *Thyroid disease: Endocrinology, surgery, nuclear medicine, and radiotherapy,* ed. S. Falk, pp. 307–321. New York: Raven Press.

SECTION 11

Infectious Diseases

11-A

Chronic Fatigue Syndrome

Chronic fatigue syndrome (CFS) or *chronic fatigue immune dysfunction syndrome* (CFIDS) is characterized by a constellation of signs and symptoms dominated by a disabling fatigue of unknown origin. The illness usually affects adults in their 20s or early 30s, with a higher incidence noted in women compared to men (3:1 ratio) (Gorensek 1991). Although the illness is often thought to be relatively new, similar syndromes have been described in the literature for over two centuries (Gorensek 1991; *San Francisco Epidemiologic Bulletin* 1992).

Initially, CFS was thought to occur as a result of some type of chronic viral infection—e.g., Epstein-Barr virus (EBV), human-T-lymphotrophic viruses I and II (HTLV-I, HTLV-II). However, a causal relationship has not been clearly established (Gorensek 1991; Levine et al. 1992). A recent study by Buchwald et al. (1992) suggests a possible link between CFS and human herpes virus type 6 (HHV-6), resulting in an immune-mediated chronic inflammation of the central nervous system.

Other proposed theoretical causes include immune dysfunction (Lloyd et al. 1989), psychiatric disorders (e.g., somatization disorder, depression) (Abbey and Garfinkel 1991), muscle dysfunction (Lloyd, Gandenia, and Hales 1991), and possibly endocrine dysfunction (Demitrak et al. 1991), all of which have conflicting results reported in the literature. Thus far, there is no evidence that CFS is transmitted through close household or intimate contact.

Diagnosing CFS is difficult because general fatigue is one of the most frequently reported problems in primary care settings, with an estimated prevalence as high as 25 percent (Schroeder and McPhee 1993). Additionally, fatigue is a subjective symptom which is difficult to quantify and qualify.

Although general fatigue is a hallmark symptom of CFS, other symptoms and signs also must be present to make the diagnosis of CFS. To clarify the criteria essential for a diagnosis of CFS, the Centers for Disease Control and Prevention (CDC) has developed a working case definition as a guideline for practitioners and researchers (see **Table 11A.1, CDC Working Case Definition of Chronic Fatigue Syndrome/Chronic Fatigue Immune Dysfunction Syndrome**). This definition requires the presence of a specific number of major and minor criteria in order to meet the CDC definition of CFS (Holmes et al. 1988; *San Francisco Epidemiologic Bulletin* 1992; Schluederberg et al. 1992).

DATABASE

SUBJECTIVE

→ Symptoms may include:
- fatigue:
  - recent onset of persistent or relapsing debilitating fatigue or easy fatigability that does not resolve after bed rest in a person without a previous history of similar symptoms.
  - the patient's activities of daily living (ADL) are reduced by ≥50 percent below their ADL level prior to the onset of fatigue for at least six months.
  - prolonged (≥24 hours) generalized fatigue after exercise that the patient had been able to tolerate prior to the onset of symptoms.
- mild fever (oral temperature between 37.5°C to 38.6°C/99.5°F to 101.4°F) which may be recurrent.

Table 11A.1.   CDC WORKING CASE DEFINITION OF CHRONIC FATIGUE SYNDROME/CHRONIC FATIGUE IMMUNE DYSFUNCTION SYNDROME

In order for a person to be diagnosed with chronic fatigue syndrome/chronic fatigue immune dysfunction syndrome, specific criteria must be met. These include two major criteria and the following minor criteria, which include at least six of the eleven symptom criteria.

Major Criteria
1. New onset of persistent or relapsing debilitating fatigue or easy fatigability—in a person without a previous history of similar symptoms—that does not resolve with bed rest and that is severe enough to reduce or impair average daily activity below 50 percent of the patient's premorbid activity level for at least six months.
2. Clinical conditions that may produce symptoms similar to CFS/CFIDS must be excluded by a thorough evaluation (including history, physical examination, and laboratory data). These other clinical conditions include:
   - Malignancy.
   - Autoimmune disease.
   - Localized infection (e.g., occult abscess).
   - Chronic or subacute bacterial disease (e.g., endocarditis, tuberculosis, Lyme disease).
   - Fungal disease (e.g., coccidiomycosis, histoplasmosis).
   - Parasitic disease (e.g., giardiasis, amebiasis, toxoplasmosis).
   - Human immunodeficiency virus (HIV)-related disease.
   - Chronic psychiatric disease, either newly diagnosed by history or chronic use of major tranquilizers, lithium, or antidepressive medications.
   - Chronic inflammatory disease (e.g., chronic hepatitis).
   - Neuromuscular disease (e.g., multiple sclerosis).
   - Endocrine disease (e.g. diabetes mellitus, hypothyroidism).
   - Drug dependency or abuse.
   - Side effects of a chronic medication or toxic agent (e.g., chemical solvent, pesticide, heavy metal).
   - Other known or defined chronic pulmonary, cardiac, gastrointestinal, hepatic, renal, or hematologic disease.

Minor Criteria
1. *Symptom Criteria:* Six or more of the following symptoms *and* two or more of the physical criteria, *or* at least eight of the following symptoms (without the minimum number of physical criteria) must be fulfilled if a diagnosis of CFS/CFIDS is to be made. The symptom(s) must have started at or following the time of onset of the fatigue and must have persisted or recurred over a period of six months (although individual symptoms may or may not have occurred simultaneously). The following symptoms are those included in the symptom criteria for CFS/CFIDS:
   - Chills or a low-grade fever (i.e., an oral temperature between 37.5°C to 38.6°C if measured by the patients). **Note:** Oral temperatures of 38.6°C are less indicative of CFS/CFIDS, and evaluation for other causes of illness should be considered.
   - Sore throat.
   - Painful lymph nodes—anterior or posterior cervical or axillary distribution.
   - Unexplained generalized muscle weakness.
   - Myalgia.
   - Prolonged (≥24 hours) generalized fatigue after levels of exercise that would have been easily tolerated in the patient's premorbid state.
   - Generalized headaches (different in type, severity, and/or pattern from headaches the patient experienced in the premorbid state).
   - Migratory arthralgia without joint swelling or redness.
   - One or more of the following neuropsychological complaints—photophobia, transient visual scotomata, forgetfulness, excessive irritability, confusion, inability to concentrate, difficulty thinking, depression.
   - Sleep disturbance (insomnia or hypersomnia).
   - Patient describes the main symptom complex as initially developing over a few hours to a few days. **Note:** This is not a true symptom, but may be considered equivalent to the above symptoms in meeting the case definition requirement.
2. *Physical Exam Criteria:* A health care provider must document the presence of the physical criteria on at least two occasions a minimum of one month apart.
   - Low-grade temperature—oral temperature between 37.5°C to 38.6°C, or a rectal temperature between 37.8°C to 38.8°C.
   - Pharyngitis (non-exudative).
   - Enlarged, palpable, or tender anterior or posterior cervical or axillary lymph nodes. **Note:** Lymph nodes greater than 2 cm diameter suggest other causes of adenopathy and further evaluation is warranted.

Source: Adapted with permission from Holmes, G.P. 1988. Chronic fatigue syndrome: A working case definition. *Annals of Internal Medicine* 108(3):387-389; Chronic fatigue syndrome/chronic fatigue immune dysfunction syndrome. 1992. *San Francisco Epidemiologic Bulletin* 8(9):33-37.

- chills.
- sore throat.
- enlarged, tender anterior or posterior cervical or axillary nodes.
- myalgia.
- muscle weakness.
- migratory joint pain without edema or erythema of joints.
- headaches—generalized and different from headaches experienced by patient prior to onset of fatigue.

- insomnia or hypersomnia (excessive sleeping).
- neuropsychiatric symptoms including forgetfulness, irritability, confusion, problems with concentration or thinking clearly, depression, transient scotomata, and photophobia.

→ Symptoms reportedly develop within a few hours to a few days.

→ Patient denies a history of other conditions which may produce similar symptoms (e.g., malignancy, infection, autoimmune disorders, chronic diseases, neuromuscular disease, fungal or parasitic diseases, psychiatric disease, allergies, substance abuse, or drug side effects).

OBJECTIVE

→ Patient may appear depressed, anxious, or with normal affect.

→ Patient may present with:
  ▪ low-grade temperature elevation:
    • oral temperature of 37.6°C to 38.6°C/99.6°F to 101.4°F, rectal temperature of 37.8°C to 38.8°C/100.0°F to 101.8°F.
  ▪ erythema of pharynx without exudate.
  ▪ enlarged and/or tender anterior or posterior cervical and/or axillary nodes. Lymph nodes >2 cm in diameter require further evaluation to rule out other pathology.

→ Patient may demonstrate tenderness in multiple trigger points (joints). (Holmes et al. 1988; Gorensek 1991; *San Francisco Epidemiologic Bulletin* 1992).

ASSESSMENT

→ Chronic fatigue syndrome (chronic fatigue immune dysfunction syndrome)

→ R/O anemia

→ R/O chronic infections (e.g., hepatitis, tuberculosis)

→ R/O fibromylagia

→ R/O endocrine disease (e.g., thyroid dysfunction, diabetes mellitus)

→ R/O autoimmune disease

→ R/O renal disease

→ R/O malignancy

→ R/O human immunodeficiency virus (HIV) infection

→ R/O psychiatric disease

→ R/O neuromuscular disease

PLAN

DIAGNOSTIC TESTS

→ The following tests should be considered routinely in the evaluation of a patient with CFS to rule out other causes for the symptomatology:
  ▪ complete blood count (CBC) with differential, indices, and platelet count—within normal limits (WNL) in patients with CFS.

▪ urinalysis—WNL.
▪ PPD—negative.
▪ chemistry panel (electrolytes, liver function, BUN, creatinine, calcium, and fasting glucose)—WNL.
▪ sedimentation rate frequently <5 mm/hr.
▪ thyroid function tests—WNL.
▪ anti-nuclear antibodies—may demonstrate a low level positive result.
▪ syphilis tests (VDRL or RPR)—nonreactive.

→ The following additional tests should be considered to rule out other causes of symptomatology based on the patient's history and physical examination:
  ▪ anti-thyroid antibodies—may demonstrate a low-level positive result.
  ▪ lyme disease serology—negative.
  ▪ hepatitis serologies—negative.
  ▪ HIV antibody—negative.
    NOTE: HIV antibody testing may need to be repeated at 3 and 6 months after initial test is done if patient reports a recent history of activities associated with an increased risk of HIV transmission (see **Human Immunodeficiency Virus [HIV]** Protocol).
  ▪ chest x-ray—WNL.
  ▪ skin testing for anergy (e.g., *Candida*, mumps, and/or tetanus)—may not demonstrate a reaction to antigens.
  ▪ lymph node biopsy as indicated—WNL.
  ▪ serologies and cultures as indicated—WNL/ negative.
  ▪ cosyntropin (Cortrosyn) stimulation test (to rule out adrenal insufficiency)—WNL.
  ▪ magnetic resonance imaging (MRI) (to rule out demyelinating disease)—WNL.
  ▪ stool for ova and parasites—WNL.
  ▪ fecal occult blood—negative.
  ▪ quantitative immunoglobulins—WNL.
  ▪ lumbar puncture—WNL.
  ▪ evaluation for myasthenia gravis (e.g., acetylcholine receptor antibody test, electrophysiological tests)—WNL.

TREATMENT/MANAGEMENT

→ Multiple therapeutic interventions have been attempted in the treatment of CFS, but few have been studied adequately to demonstrate proven efficacy.
  ▪ Nevertheless, clinicians managing the care of patients with CFS do attempt to treat some CFS symptoms with treatments proven effective in

other diseases to help diminish some of the debilitating effects of CFS.

NOTE: Several patients with CFS appear to have increased sensitivity to several drugs, and, therefore, medications are often initiated at ¼ to ½ usual adult doses (*San Francisco Epidemiologic Bulletin* 1992).

→ Because sleep disturbances can contribute to an increase in other symptoms associated with CFS, attempts to relieve these sleep disorders are important and should include non-pharmacological recommendations such as establishing a consistent bedtime, and avoidance of caffeine and other stimulants in the late afternoon or evening, comfortable room temperature (usually a cool environment is beneficial), and avoidance of late snacks and daytime naps.

■ When medication is indicated, prescribing clonazepam (Klonopin®) 0.25 mg to 2.0 mg p.o. at bedtime or cyclobenzaprine (Flexeril®) 10 mg to 20 mg p.o. at bedtime may be helpful).

NOTE: Warn the patient about possible side effects associated with these medications (e.g., the habit-forming potential of clonazepam). Consult *Physicians' Desk Reference* (*PDR*) for additional information.

→ Pain associated with myalgias, arthralgias, and neuralgias can be quite severe and can require pharmacological interventions with nonsteroidal anti-inflammatory drugs (NSAIDs) including:

■ naproxen (Naprosyn®) 250 mg to 500 mg p.o. BID.

■ naproxen sodium (Anaprox®) 275 mg to 550 mg p.o. BID.

■ ibuprofen (Advil®, Motrin®) 400 mg p.o. TID–QID.

NOTE: Warn patients about potential side effects (e.g., gastritis, gastrointestinal bleeding, hepatotoxicity) and drug interactions. Consult *PDR* for additional information.

→ Muscle relaxants—cyclobenzaprine (Flexeril®) 10 mg p.o. TID may be helpful.

→ Headaches can be treated with NSAIDs (see above) or dichloralphenazone (Midrin®) 2 tablets p.o. STAT and 1 tablet p.o. every day up to 5 tablets/24 hrs (*San Francisco Epidemiologic Bulletin* 1992).

→ Fatigue and lethargy often are debilitating and may require evaluation and education about proper nutrition, rest, and daily exercise within the physical capabilities of the patient.

■ If medication is needed, a low-dose, non-sedating antidepressant, such as fluoxetine (Prozac®) 5 mg p.o. every day, may be initiated if there are no contraindications to its use (*San Francisco Epidemiologic Bulletin* 1992).

→ Depression may require therapeutic interventions—including individual or group counseling—which are often common with other types of chronic diseases.

■ If antidepressant medication is indicated, the dosages should be prescribed in ¼ to ½ the usual adult dose because of CFS patients' sensitivity to drugs.

• If antidepressants are to be used, their initiation should be under the supervision of a physician managing the patient's psychiatric care.

→ Other therapies tried in CFS patients with some reported relief of symptoms, despite their lack of proven efficacy or adequate clinical trials, include:

■ vitamin and mineral therapy consisting of one or all of the following:

• multivitamin with additional magnesium and zinc (e.g., Optivites®) 4 to 6 tablets every day.

• magnesium sulfate 1 gm every week for 6 weeks.

• high-dose Vitamin B_{12} injections with a maximum dose of 300 mg twice a week. (Patient also must be taking multivitamin supplement.)

■ antiviral therapy with acyclovir (Zovirax®) has been used without demonstrated efficacy in controlled trials.

• However, other antiviral medications are being investigated (including intravenous ampligen—an immune-modulating antiviral drug currently being investigated by the Food and Drug Administration [FDA]) (*San Francisco Epidemiologic Bulletin* 1992).

■ immunoglobulin therapy with 2 cc to 4 cc/week (based on weight) or 5 gm/week for 6 to 12 weeks given intravenously or intramuscularly (*San Francisco Epidemiologic Bulletin* 1992).

• Although conflicting results have been reported from double-blind studies investigating this therapy in CFS patients (Lloyd et al. 1990; Strauss 1990), some patients have shown improvement after 3 months of immunoglobulin therapy (Lloyd et al. 1990).

▪ kutapressin (a porcine liver extract) has reportedly helped relieve symptoms in some CFS patients who received a series of intramuscular injections over a period of several weeks.
  • The exact mechanism of action is unknown.

→ Documented evidence of other specific pathology (e.g., thyroid dysfunction, anemia) should be treated as indicated.
NOTE: Although a patient may have CFS, other illnesses also can occur in CFS patients and will warrant appropriate evaluation and treatment.

CONSULTATION

→ Consultation with a physician as indicated, but is warranted if underlying pathology is evident during work-up (e.g., malignancy, psychiatric disorder, thyroid disease).

→ As needed for prescription(s).

PATIENT EDUCATION

→ Educate the patient about CFS, including theoretical causes, diagnostic work-up required to document CFS, chronicity of illness, therapeutic options, prognosis, and community resources available including:
▪ The CFS Association
  Community Health Services
  P.O. Box 220398
  Charlotte, NC 28222-0398
  (704) 362-2343.

▪ The CFS Society
  Box 230108
  Portland, OR 97223
  (503) 684-5261.
▪ The National CFS Association
  919 Scott Avenue
  Kansas City, KS 66105
  (913) 321-2278.
▪ Information pamphlet:
  Centers for Disease Control and Prevention
  Department of Health and Human Services
  Public Health Service, CDC
  Atlanta, GA 30333
  (404) 332-4555 (Hotline).

→ If other pathology is evident (e.g., anemia, thyroid disease), educate the patient about these specific problems, their causes, treatment options, prognosis, and follow-up as indicated.

→ Educate patient's family about CFS, especially emphasizing the noncontagious nature of the disease.

FOLLOW-UP

→ Follow-up visits with patient will vary and depend upon the patient's symptoms, success of chosen therapies, and/or need for additional consultation for evaluation of possible problems (e.g., psychiatric evaluations and/or therapy).

→ Document in progress notes and problem list.

Maureen T. Shannon, C.N.M., F.N.P., M.S.

11-B

Diarrhea—Infectious

Infectious diarrhea is an increase in the frequency, fluidity, and volume of stools as a result of exposure to a pathogen (Berquist 1990). In the United States, 25 million individuals experience enteric infections annually (Cohen 1988). Usually such infections are self-limited and resolve without serious sequelae.

However, complications are reported in association with infectious diarrhea including severe dehydration, bacteremia/sepsis, hypoglycemia, hypokalemia, hemorrhagic colitis, and disseminated intravascular coagulation (DIC). There are 10,000 deaths attributed to enteric infections each year, with the majority of these reported in young children (Cohen 1988). Although a substantial amount of information exists regarding infectious diarrhea in children, limited data are available on this condition in adults.

Certain variables have been noted to increase an individual's risk of experiencing infectious diarrhea including the individual's age, immune functioning, type(s) of exposure, and geographic regions where the individual lives or which she has visited. Transmission of the infectious pathogen occurs through fecal-oral spread (person to person) or through exposure to contaminated food or water. Once transmitted, the pathogen can affect the gastrointestinal (GI) tract by directly invading epithelial cells (e.g., *Shigella*) or through the secretion of an enterotoxin (e.g., *Staphylococcus*).

Several types of pathogens can cause infectious diarrhea with varying incubation periods and symptoms (see **Table 11B.1, Infectious Diarrhea, Selected Organisms**). Viral pathogens are the most common cause of infectious diarrhea in the United States, including rotavirus, Norwalk-like viruses, and enteric adenoviruses. These infections often are associated with upper respiratory symptoms, and the epidemics have a seasonal pattern (Fairchild and Blackblow 1988).

Bacterial pathogens commonly associated with infectious diarrhea include *Escherichia coli* (*E. coli*), *Staphylococcus aureus* (*S. aureus*), *Salmonella* species (*S. paratyphi*, *S. typhi*), *Shigella* species (*S. sonnei*, *S. flexneri*, *S. dysenteriae*), and *Campylobacter jejuni*. Bacterial infectious diarrhea is most frequently associated with ingestion of contaminated food or water. Often there is a clustering of individuals reporting similar symptoms, and such epidemiological information contributes to the diagnosis.

In the United States, parasitic organisms are the least common cause of infectious diarrhea behind viral or bacterial organisms. *Giardia lamblia* (*G. lamblia*), *Cryptosporidium*, and *Entamoeba histolytica* (*E. histolytica*) are the most frequently reported parasitic organisms, often causing mild clinical presentations in immunocompetent individuals.

DATABASE

SUBJECTIVE

→ Risk factors. The patient may be:
- elderly.
- day care center attendee.
- parent of a child with a history of diarrhea.
- engaged in laboratory work involving exposure to pathogens.
- have a history of:
  - recent foreign travel to a country in a region with an increased likelihood of exposure to pathogens (e.g., Africa, Latin America, Middle East, Asia).

Table 11B.1. INFECTIOUS DIARRHEA (SELECTED ORGANISMS)

Bacterial Organisms	Incubation Period	Vomiting	Diarrhea	Fever	Transmission	Susceptible Individuals	Clinical Features
Escherichia coli (some strains)	24-72 hours	±	−	−	Food-borne and water-borne routes	Individuals who ingest contaminated food or water	Usually abrupt onset of diarrhea; vomiting rare. A serious infection in neonates. In adults, a cause of "traveler's diarrhea," usually self-limited, resolving in 1-3 days. Use diphenoxylate with atropine but no antimicrobials unless patient has an ↑ risk of complications.
Salmonella spp	8-40 hours	±	+	+	Food-borne; rarely fecal-oral route. ↑ during summer/fall months	↑ in very young (<20 years) and very old (>70 years)	Gradual or abrupt onset of diarrhea and low-grade fever. No antimicrobials unless systemic dissemination is suspected. Stool cultures are positive. Prolonged carriage is frequent.
Shigella spp (mild cases)	24-72 hours	±	+	+	Food-borne; fecal-oral route. ↑ during summer/fall months	Individuals who ingest contaminated foods	Abrupt onset of diarrhea, often with blood and pus in stools, cramps, tenesmus, and lethargy. Stool cultures are positive. Often mild and self-limited. In severe cases, give trimethoprim-sulfamethoxazole, ampicillin, or chloramphenicol. Do not give opiates. Restore fluids.
Staphylococcus	1-8 hours, rarely up to 18 hours	+	+	−	Fecal-oral route, food-borne outbreaks (animal protein)	Individuals who ingest contaminated foods	Abrupt onset, intense vomiting for up to 24 hours, regular recovery in 24-48 hours. Occurs in persons eating the same food. No treatment usually necessary except to restore fluids and electrolytes.
Campylobacter jejuni	2-10 days	±	+	+	Food-borne and water-borne routes. ↑ during warmer months in temperate climates	↑ in children and young adults. Can cause traveler's diarrhea.	Fever, diarrhea; polymorphonuclear leukocytes (PMNs) and fresh blood in stool, especially in children. Usually self-limited. Stool cultures are positive. Erythromycin in severe cases. Usual recovery in 5-8 days.
Vibrio cholerae (mild cases)	6-96 hours	+	+	−	Food-borne or use of contaminated water in food preparation	Ingestion of contaminated food	Abrupt onset of diarrhea in persons consuming the same food, especially if ingestion of crabs and other seafood. Recovery is usually complete in 1-3 days. Food and stool cultures are positive.
Vibrio cholerae (mild cases)	24-72 hours	+	+	−	Water-borne route	Ingestion of contaminated water and/or foods prepared using contaminated water	Abrupt onset of liquid diarrhea in endemic area. Needs prompt replacement of fluids and electrolytes I.V. or orally. Tetracyclines shorten excretion of vibrios. Stool cultures positive.

Continued

- immunosuppression.
- exposure via intimate contact with a partner with infectious diarrhea.
- exposure to a recent food-borne or water-borne outbreak.
→ Symptoms may include:

■ abrupt onset of one or more of the following symptoms ranging from mild to severe intensity (see **Table 11B.1**):
- fever.
- malaise.
- headache.
- anorexia.
- nausea.

Table 11B.1. INFECTIOUS DIARRHEA (SELECTED ORGANISMS)(CONTINUED)

Viral Organisms	Incubation Period	Vomiting	Diarrhea	Fever	Transmission	Susceptible Individuals	Clinical Features
Norwalk-like	24-48 hours	+	+	+	Unknown. Probably fecal-oral route, community food-borne or water-borne spread. Winter outbreaks common.	Adults and school-age children; family- and community-wide epidemics often occur.	Abrupt onset of vomiting and/or diarrhea, anorexia, nausea, abdominal cramping, malaise, headache, and myalgia. Stools are loose and watery without mucus, blood, or fecal leukocytes. Illness is usually mild and self-limited, lasting 2-5 days. Stool cultures are positive.
Rotavirus	24-72 hours	+	+	+	Probably fecal-oral, possible fecal-respiratory. Usually occurs during cooler months in temperate climates.	Infants and very young children. Can cause traveler's diarrhea in adults; diarrhea in parents of infected children, immuno-compromised patients, and elderly.	Abrupt onset of fever (often low-grade) and vomiting, followed by profuse, watery diarrhea. Milder symptoms in adults including upper respiratory infection symptoms. Illness can last up to 8 days. Stool cultures are positive.

Parasitic Organisms

Parasitic Organisms	Incubation Period	Vomiting	Diarrhea	Fever	Transmission	Susceptible Individuals	Clinical Features
Giardia lamblia	5-25 days	−	+	−	Person-to-person through hand-to-mouth transfer of cysts from feces	↑ in children (especially in day care); ↑ in mountain communities with contaminated water	Usually asymptomatic; can cause chronic diarrhea, steatorrhea, abdominal cramps, bloating, weight loss, fatigue. Stools often pale, loose, greasy. Identification of trophozoites in feces (string test). Metronidzole, quinacrine, or furazolidone can be used to treat patients.
Entamoeba histolytica	8 days up to 4 weeks	+	+	±	Person-to-person, fecal-oral routes	↑ in foreign travelers, homosexual men, immigrants	Asymptomatic to severe colitis symptoms. Usually mild to moderate recurrent diarrhea, abdominal cramps, intermittent constipation, mucus in stools. Severe symptoms include semiformed to liquid blood-streaked stools. May have extra-intestinal infection (e.g., liver). Evidence of trophozoites or cysts in stools in 90% of serial stool specimens.
Cryptosporidium	1-12 days	+	+	±	Person-to-person, fecal-oral, animal-to-person, water-borne.	↑ incidence of symptomatic infection in immune-deficient patients	Asymptomatic to profuse, watery diarrhea; may have anorexia, nausea, vomiting, malaise, fever. Symptoms are intermittent but usually resolve within 30 days in immune-competent patients; can continue in patients with advanced immunodeficiency. Presence of oocysts in fecal smear is diagnostic.

Source: Adapted with permission from Jacobs, R.A. 1993. General problems in infectious diseases. In *Current medical diagnosis and treatment*, 32d ed., 999-1000, eds. L.M. Tierney, Jr., S.J. McPhee, M.A. Papadakis, and S.A. Schroeder. Norwalk, CT: Appleton & Lange. Copyright 1993 by Appleton & Lange.

- vomiting.
- abdominal cramping or pain that is often located in the right lower quadrant (RLQ) or periumbilical region.
- increased flatulence that may be foul-smelling.
- increased frequency of defecation.
- consistency of stools watery, mucoid, slimy, or bloody (**Note:** *Salmonella* and *Shigella* infections are associated with bloody, mucoid stools.).
- foul-smelling stools.
- fecal urgency.
- rectal tenesmus.
- weight loss.
- lightheadedness, vertigo, syncope in patients with significant dehydration.
- upper respiratory infection (URI) symptoms if the diarrhea is associated with viral pathogen (e.g., rotavirus) (Fairchild and Blackblow 1988).

OBJECTIVE

→ Physical examination of the patient may be unremarkable or reveal any of the following findings:

- vital signs may be WNL or may demonstrate an elevated temperature and decreased weight.
- postural changes in the patient's pulse and blood pressure will be evident with significant dehydration.
- tissue turgor will be poor if the patient is significantly dehydrated.
- examination of the mouth may reveal dry buccal mucosa with significant dehydration.
- abdominal examination:
  - auscultation may reveal hyperactive bowel sounds.
  - percussion may demonstrate increased resonance.
  - palpation may reveal tenderness, guarding, and rebound.
- rectal examination will be WNL, or anal erythema and edema may be evident.

ASSESSMENT

→ Infectious diarrhea (viral, bacterial, parasitic)
→ R/O dehydration
→ R/O hemorrhagic colitis
→ R/O bacteremia/sepsis
→ R/O acute abdomen (e.g., appendicitis)
→ R/O functional bowel disease (e.g., diverticulosis)

→ R/O drug toxicity (e.g., *Clostridium difficile*)
→ R/O pelvic inflammatory disease
→ R/O inflammatory bowel disease
→ R/O other causes of diarrhea

PLAN

DIAGNOSTIC TESTS

→ Because diagnostic testing for infectious diarrhea pathogens can be costly—with results often not available until after the patient's symptoms have resolved—diagnostic tests are not routinely ordered in patients with mild symptoms (e.g., no fever, abdominal pain, bloody stools, mucous in stools, significant dehydration, and no exposure to unusual organisms [e.g., cholera]) (Bergquist 1990).

→ In patients exhibiting moderate to severe symptoms or who have fever (≥ 38.8°C/101.8°F), bloody stools, or dehydration, the following tests can be ordered in consultation with a physician (Berquist 1990; Brownlee, Jr. 1990; Thorne 1988):

- microscopic examination of fecal smears can be done in an office setting at minimum cost to the patient and can help determine the need for additional testing. The following tests can be done:
  - *methylene blue stain:*
    - obtain a small fecal specimen with blood and mucous (if possible), mix with 2 drops of methylene blue stain, and place a coverslip over the specimen.
    - evidence of increased polymorphonuclear cells suggests an invasive inflammatory process of the colon (e.g., *Shigella, Salmonella, Campylobacter* infections or ulcerative colitis) (Johnson and Ericcson 1990).
  - *gram stain:*
    - standard gram staining of a fecal smear may reveal an etiological organism such as *S. aureus* and may demonstrate increased leukocytes (Berquist 1990).
  - *Guaiac.*
    - Standard guaiac testing will be positive if there is blood in the fecal specimen.
- stool culture and sensitivity should be considered when a patient has evidence of leukocytes on microscopic evaluation of the fecal smear.

- Collection of stool specimens on 3 alternate days will increase the likelihood of identification of a pathogen.
- In many laboratories, clinicians must specifically request that evaluations for particular pathogens are performed (e.g., *Campylobacter*).
- Positive results are diagnostic of an etiological pathogen.
- Sensitivities may be helpful in identifying a resistant organism and in determining the most effective therapeutic agent.
- Negative results do not eliminate the possibility of a particular pathogen, since it is often difficult to obtain adequate stool specimens in some patients.
  NOTE: One suggested way to obtain stool specimens is to have the patient place a sheet of plastic wrap under the toilet seat and pass the feces onto the plastic. The patient can then transfer the feces to the specimen cup. Advise the patient to avoid urine or water touching the specimen (Ware and Jones 1991).
- specimens for ova and parasite determination also can be sent as indicated by the patient's history.
  - Collection of a stool specimen on 3 alternate days usually is necessary to obtain adequate sampling.
  - Because microscopic evaluation of such specimens requires experience on the part of the examiner, clinicians should send specimens for such tests to qualified laboratories.
- cultures of food suspected to be contaminated with a pathogen (e.g., *S. aureus*) (Berquist 1990).
- CBC may demonstrate leukocytosis with increased bands (i.e., left shift).
- paired sera can be obtained and sent for hemagglutination titer with a rise in titer, specific to the pathogen suggestive of infection (Berquist 1990).
- proctoscopy or sigmoidoscopy may be necessary in patients with bloody or mucoid diarrhea (usually ordered by the physician consultant).
- the string test (Entero Test) can be done to identify parasites of the upper intestines (e.g., *G. lamblia*) but should be ordered by the physician consultant.

TREATMENT/MANAGEMENT

→ In the majority of patients, infectious diarrhea is a self-limited illness that usually resolves within 2 to 5 days (see **Table 11B.1**).
- Symptomatic treatment for infectious diarrhea includes:
  - avoidance of food for at least 24 hours or until the diarrhea substantially decreases or stops.
  - once food intake resumes, begin with easily digestible foods such as toast, crackers, rice, broth-based soups, and decaffeinated tea.
    –Avoid foods high in fat and protein (e.g., meat, eggs), as well as raw fruits and vegetables, until the symptoms are resolving.
    –Milk and milk products should not be resumed until after the acute phase of the illness, because many patients develop a transient lactase deficiency which could aggravate the diarrhea (Johnson and Ericcson 1990).
- Replacement of fluids and electrolytes is essential and should begin early in the illness with:
  - hourly ingestion of 8 ounces of fruit juice (apple or orange juice) mixed with a pinch of table salt and a teaspoon of honey or sugar
                OR
  - decaffeinated, nondiet soda drinks that have lost their carbonation (leave bottle of soda uncapped for several hours to eliminate carbonation).
  - an 8-ounce glass of water with ¼ teaspoon of baking soda should also be ingested.
- Use of over-the-counter (OTC) replacement fluids—may be initiated with one of the following (DiJohn and Levine 1988):
  - pedialyte RS® solution which has a higher concentration of sodium and chloride than other solutions (for replacement therapy if moderate to severe diarrhea with or without vomiting).
  - pedialyte® or Lytren® solutions.
  - infalyte® which is available in powder form.
→ Antidiarrheal medications should be avoided if inflammatory bowel disease or parasitic infections (e.g., patients with high fever, bloody or mucoid diarrhea) are suspected because of an increased risk of toxic megacolon.
- In patients where these conditions are not suspected, the use of the following medications can be initiated:

- bismuth subsalicylate (Pepto Bismol®) 30 ml or 2 tablets p.o. up to 8 doses per day.
  NOTE: Side effects include black stools and tongue. Also, patients should be advised that this drug contains salicylates and the concomitant use of aspirin should be avoided (Johnson and Ericcson 1990).
- loperamide (Imodium®) 4 mg p.o. initially, then 2 mg after each unformed stool (maximum dose 16 mg per day).
  NOTE: Discontinue use in patients with an increase in symptoms, if patient develops blood or mucous in her stool, or if no improvement after 48 hours.
- diphenoxylate and atropine (Lomotil®) 5 mg p.o. initially then 2.5 mg to 5.0 mg p.o. after each unformed stool (maximum 8 tablets a day).
  NOTE: Patients can develop drug dependence using this agent. Other side effects include central nervous system (CNS) depression, headaches, confusion, intestinal obstruction, nausea, vomiting, and pancreatitis. Atropine effects include possible increased intraocular pressure, urinary retention, tachycardia, flushing, and dry skin and mucous membranes. Contraindications for use include obstructive jaundice and pseudomembraneous colitis (Ellsworth et al. 1991).

→ Antimicrobial therapy in suspected or documented infectious diarrhea is controversial, because most episodes are self-limited and resolve without complications.
  ■ Antimicrobial therapy is indicated in patients with a history of immunosuppression (e.g., HIV infection), bacteremia, typhoid fever, enteric fever, or metastatic infection (Bartlett 1991).
  ■ If antimicrobial therapy is being considered, consultation with a physician is indicated.
  ■ The following antimicrobial agents can be prescribed depending upon the patient's status and the results of diagnostic tests:
    • ampicillin (Principen®) 500 mg p.o. QID for 5 days (will cover *Salmonella*, and entero-invasive and enterohemorrhagic strains of *E. coli*).
    • trimethoprim (TMP)/sulfamethoxazole (SMX) (Septra DS®, Bactrim®) 160 mg/800 mg p.o. BID for 5 days (will cover *Shigella* and entero-invasive and enterohemorrhagic strains of *E. coli*).

- erythromycin (E-Mycin®, Ery Tab®) 500 mg p.o. QID for 5 days (will cover *C. jejuni*).
- ciprofloxacin (Cipro®) 500 mg p.o. BID for 5 days (will cover some strains of *E. coli*); 500 mg p.o. BID for 7 days (will cover *C. jejuni*); 500 mg p.o. QID for 14 days (will cover *S. typhi* typhoid fever).
- quinacrine (Atabrine®) 100 mg p.o. TID for 5 days (will cover *G. lamblia*).
- metronidazole (Flagyl®) 750 mg p.o. TID for 5 to 7 days followed by diloxanide furoate 500 mg p.o. TID for 10 days (will cover *E. histolytica*).

→ Antimicrobial therapy has had a documented efficacy in the treatment of traveler's diarrhea; however, currently it is not recommended for prophylaxis or for routine use in mild cases, because the illness is usually self-limited in most individuals.
  ■ However, patients with moderate symptoms or patients with an increased risk of severe symptoms or complications (e.g., immuno-suppressed patients) should initiate empiric therapy with one of the following (Wolfe 1990):
    • TMP/SMX 160 mg/800 mg (Septra DS®, Bactrim®) 1 tablet p.o. BID for 3 days plus loperamide (Imodium®) 4 mg p.o. initially followed by 2 mg p.o. after each unformed stool (maximum dose 16 mg p.o. per day).
      NOTE: The combination of these drugs has demonstrated better efficacy than the use of either drug alone (Ericcson et al. 1990).
    • TMP/SMX 160 mg/800 mg (Septra DS®, Bactrim®) 1 tablet p.o. BID for 5 days.
    • doxycycline (Vibramycin®) 100 mg BID p.o. for 5 days.
    • ciprofloxacin (Cipro®) 500 mg p.o. BID for 5 days.
    • norfloxacin (Noroxin®) 400 mg p.o. BID for 5 days.

CONSULTATION

→ Consultation with a physician is indicated in any patient:
  ■ with severe symptoms (e.g., dehydration, high fever, or bloody or mucoid stools).
  ■ with symptoms that persist longer than 48 hours.
  ■ with conditions placing her at an increased risk of bacteremia/sepsis (e.g., elderly, immunocompromised patients).

- if abdominal or rectal pain is reported (Brownlee, Jr. 1990).
→ As needed for prescription(s).

___

PATIENT EDUCATION

→ Educate the patient about the cause of diarrhea, clinical course, plan of care, possible complications, possible side effects of medications, preventive measures (e.g., handwashing, proper food preparation), and the indicated follow-up.

→ If perianal discomfort is reported, review symptomatic relief measures including sitz baths three times a day, witch hazel solution or pads to clean perineal area, and use of soft tissue or absorbent cotton to dry perineal area.

→ Educate the patient about ways to prevent further exposure and/or transmission of enteric pathogens through the proper handling and cooking of food, use of pasteurized milk, and handwashing with soap prior to and after handling food (CDC 1993c).

→ Educate the patient who is planning to travel to an area where there is an increased risk of exposure to enteric pathogens associated with traveler's diarrhea (e.g., Africa, Latin America, Middle East, Asia) regarding ways to reduce exposure including:
  - avoiding ingesting raw vegetables, unpeeled fruits, ice or untreated water, and foods that are served uncooked or cold.
  - disinfecting water by boiling for at least five minutes, treating water chemically with commercially available disinfectants, or using a mixture of five-percent chlorine bleach, two drops (0.1 ml) in a liter of water, and allowing 30 minutes at room temperature before using (Tellier and Keystone 1992).
  - avoiding purchasing and ingesting food from street vendors.

- using drugs when symptoms first begin:
  - mild diarrhea (< three loose stools a day without fever, pus, or blood)—patient can initiate therapy with loperamide (Imodium®) or bismuth subsalicylate (Pepto Bismol®) as described in "Treatment/Management" section.
  - moderate diarrhea—antimicrobial therapy can be started with regimens described in "Treatment/Management" section.
  - severe or persistent diarrhea with dehydration, fever, blood, and/or mucous in stools—patient should seek medical evaluation (Bartlett 1991).

→ Educate patients planning foreign travel about preventive immunizations that are recommended (e.g., *S. typhi* vaccination to prevent typhoid fever) prior to travel.
  - Advice about preventive measures, possible therapeutic regimens, and recommended immunizations for international travelers can be obtained by calling the Centers for Disease Control and Prevention at (404) 332-4559.

___

FOLLOW-UP

→ See "Consultation" section.

→ Any patient experiencing persistent or worsening symptoms, or possible side effects associated with therapeutic interventions should return as soon as possible for evaluation.

→ Many of the pathogens causing infectious diarrhea (e.g., *Salmonella, Shigella*) are state-mandated reportable diseases and require a morbidity report to be filed with the department of public health. Contact the local department of public health for a complete list of pathogens that require morbidity reports be filed.

→ Document in progress notes and problem list.

11-C

Hepatitis—Viral

Viral hepatitis is a systemic infection that primarily affects the liver. The most common causes of viral hepatitis are the:

→ hepatitis A virus (HAV)

→ hepatitis B virus (HBV)

→ hepatitis delta virus (HDV)

→ three different viruses associated with non-A, non-B hepatitis (NANB): hepatitis C virus (HCV), hepatitis E virus (HEV), and possibly another parenterally transmitted NANB type of hepatitis. The less common causes of viral hepatitis include Epstein-Barr virus, cytomegalovirus, herpes simplex virus, Ebola fever virus, Lassa fever virus, Marburg virus, rubella virus, yellow fever virus, and HIV infection (Padilla and Schiff 1991).

Hepatitis A Virus (HAV)

Also known as *infectious hepatitis*, hepatitis A has an incubation period of 15 to 45 days and is transmitted by fecal-oral routes, commonly with contamination of food or drinking water. Transmission occurs rarely through contaminated needles. Blood and stool are infectious during the incubation period and through the first week of illness when peak transaminase levels are achieved.

The disease is more common in young children who often have mild or subclinical cases. Adults commonly present with jaundice. Hepatitis A does not cause a chronic state but one percent of cases may progress to fulminant hepatitis.

Hepatitis B Virus (HBV)

Also known as *serum hepatitis*, Hepatitis B has an incubation period varying from 45 to 180 days and is transmitted through a break in the skin, via mucous membranes, or through parenteral or perinatal exposure. Approximately ten percent of adults contracting Hepatitis B will become chronic carriers defined by abnormal aminotransferase levels and histopathological findings that persist longer than six months. Approximately 25 percent to 30 percent of chronic carriers will progress to cirrhosis with an increased risk for hepatocellular carcinoma (Padilla and Schiff 1991).

There are two subclasses of chronic hepatitis: *chronic persistent hepatitis* (CPH) and *chronic active hepatitis* (CAH). The distinction between these is determined through liver biopsy and is characterized by the extent of liver involvement, with CAH extending beyond the portal area and having a poorer prognosis.

Hepatitis D Virus (HDV)

Hepatitis D, *delta hepatitis*, can cause infection only in the presence of Hepatitis B virus. It is most commonly transmitted through parenteral routes (intravenous drug use and multiple transfusions). It occurs as a co-infection (acute HDV simultaneous with acute HBV) or as a superinfection (acute HDV superimposed on a Hepatitis B carrier). Acute delta hepatitis is self-limiting. Approximately five percent of patients with delta co-infection develop chronic infection. Approximately 80 percent of patients with superinfection develop chronic hepatitis. Approximately 75 percent of patients with chronic delta hepatitis develop cirrhosis.

NON-A, NON-B HEPATITIS

Hepatitis C Virus (HCV)

Hepatitis C has an incubation period varying from 45 to 180 days. It is primarily transmitted thought the parenteral route (blood transfusion and intravenous drug use) and is the primary cause of post-transfusion non-A, non-B hepatitis (95 percent). Acute HCV infections are usually mild. Approximately 50 percent of patients with HCV will develop chronic hepatitis and approximately 20 percent of those will develop cirrhosis. Hepatitis C is also a frequent cause of community-acquired (sporadic) hepatitis. Anti-HCV cannot be detected until six to eight weeks after onset of clinical hepatitis, which makes testing undesirable for diagnosis of acute HCV infection.

Hepatitis E Virus

Hepatitis E has an incubation period of two to nine weeks and is transmitted by the fecal-oral route. It is one of the primary causes of viral hepatitis in developing countries. In the United States, the only cases that have been reported were acquired in endemic countries. It does not cause chronic liver disease but one percent to two percent of cases are fatal. In pregnancy, case fatality can be as high as 20 percent. No serological test has been developed (Padilla and Schiff 1991).

The third NANB virus is thought to account for some cases of non-C, post-transfusion hepatitis known as non-A, non-B, non-C (NANBNC) hepatitis.

DATABASE

SUBJECTIVE

→ Symptoms are extremely variable from asymptomatic to fulminating disease.

→ General symptoms in the prodromal phase may include:
- abrupt or insidious onset.
- malaise, fatigue.
- myalgia, arthralgia.
- upper respiratory symptoms (nasal discharge, pharyngitis).
- headache.
- photophobia.
- anorexia.
- nausea, vomiting.
- diarrhea or constipation.
- fever rarely over 39.5°C/103.1°F.
- altered taste and smell with distaste for smoking.

→ General symptoms in the icteric phase may include:
- jaundice usually appearing five to ten days after symptom onset when prodromal symptoms begin to diminish.
  - Patient may never experience jaundice.
  - Prodromal symptoms may intensify with onset of jaundice followed by symptom improvement.
- right upper quadrant/epigastric pain aggravated by jarring or exertion.
- dark urine, clay-colored stools present with jaundice.

→ General symptoms in the convalescent phase may include:
- disappearance of jaundice.
- return of appetite.
- resolving abdominal pain.

→ Acute illness subsides after two to three weeks and is gone by six to eight weeks.

Hepatitis A

→ Risk factors include:
- recent foreign travel.
- exposure to individual with hepatitis.
- child in day care center.
- residency or employment in institutions for mentally handicapped.
- intravenous drug use.

→ Forty percent of individuals have no identifiable risk factor (Hallam and Kerlin 1991).

→ Patient may be asymptomatic or have symptoms as listed above under general symptoms.

Hepatitis B

→ Risk factors include those who are (Hallam and Kerlin 1991):
- health workers exposed to blood or blood products.
- hemodialysis staff and patients.
- intravenous drug users.
- recipients of blood products or multiple transfusions.
- homosexual men.
- persons with multiple sexual partners.
- prisoners, employees, and patients in institutions for mentally handicapped.
- sexual and household contacts of HBsAG carriers.
- travelers to endemic areas planning extended stays or intimate contact with locals.

- neonate of HBsAG mothers who have not received routine immunization.
→ Symptoms may include those listed previously under "General Symptoms."
→ Thirty to 40 percent experience icteric phase.
→ Five to ten percent of cases may be complicated by urticaria, skin rashes, and joint pains.
→ May present with cholestatic illness with pruritus lasting longer than one month.
→ Fulminant hepatitis is a complication most commonly associated with Hepatitis B, with symptoms of liver failure, encephalopathy, ascites, and coagulopathy.
→ Symptoms of chronic persistent hepatitis vary from asymptomatic to various degrees of fatigue, malaise, and anorexia.
→ Symptoms of chronic active hepatitis include jaundice (20 percent) and amenorrhea.

Hepatitis D

→ Risk factors are the same as for Hepatitis B.
→ Prodromal symptoms may include those listed previously under "General Symptoms."
→ With co-infection, a single episode of acute hepatitis may occur or a biphasic illness characterized by two sets of symptoms may present.
→ Approximately three percent of patients with co-infection will develop fulminant hepatitis (see Hepatitis B symptoms).
→ Superinfection is characterized by symptoms of acute hepatitis (see Hepatitis B symptoms) in a previously asymptomatic carrier.

Hepatitis C

→ Patients at risk include:
- those who require blood or blood products.
- intravenous drug users.
- hemodialysis patients.
- homosexual men.
- female contacts of intravenous drug users.
- those who have heterosexual contact with individuals with Hepatitis C.
→ Symptoms may include those listed previously under "General Symptoms."
→ Only approximately 25 percent develop jaundice.

Hepatitis E

→ Risk factors include exposure to endemic areas.
→ Symptoms may include those listed previously under "General Symptoms."

OBJECTIVE

→ Patient may present with:
- hepatomegaly, tenderness.
- splenomegaly.
- jaundice, icteric conjunctiva.
- palatial petechiae.
- enlarged lymph nodes, especially epitrochlear and cervical.
- arthralgia with or without arthritis.
- white blood cell (WBC) count normal to low.
- elevated aspartate aminotransferase (AST, SGOT) and alanine aminotransferase (ALT, SGPT).
- elevated bilirubin and alkaline phosphatase.
- mild proteinuria.
- bilirubinuria preceding onset of jaundice.
- prolonged prothrombin time (PT) in severe hepatitis.

Hepatitis A

→ Physical findings same as those listed just previously.
→ Aminotransferase elevations (in the hundreds) may precede or coincide with onset of prodromal symptoms.
→ Bilirubin elevation is five to ten times normal.
→ Labs usually normal after nine weeks.

Hepatitis B

→ Physical findings same as above.
→ Five to ten percent may present with urticaria, maculopapular rash, fever, polyarthritis, and arthralgia.
→ Patient may present with cholestatic illness with marked jaundice and elevation of serum alkaline phosphatase and cholesterol.
→ Fulminant hepatitis is more commonly associated with Hepatitis B, presenting with signs of liver failure, encephalopathy, ascites, and coagulopathy.
→ Aminotransferase elevation is in hundreds to thousands depending on disease severity.
→ Labs usually normal by 16 weeks.
→ Clinical signs for chronic persistent hepatitis are usually absent. Intermittent or persistent aminotransferase elevation two to three times normal.

→ Signs for chronic active hepatitis include:
  - multiple spider nevi.
  - acne.
  - hirsutism.
  - multiple system involvement (lungs, bowels, kidneys, joints).
  - Coombs-positive hemolytic anemia.
  - absent Hepatitis B markers.

Hepatitis D

→ Physical findings, signs same as those listed just previously.

→ With co-infection, a single episode of acute hepatitis may occur or a biphasic illness characterized by two sets of signs and aminotransferase peaks may occur.

→ Super-infection is characterized by signs of acute hepatitis and elevated aminotransferase level in a previously asymptomatic carrier (see Hepatitis B signs).

→ Approximately three percent of patients will develop fulminant hepatitis (see Hepatitis B signs).

Hepatitis C

→ Physical findings same as above though usually milder.

→ Peak transferase level lower than in HBV or HAV infection evident.

→ ALT levels may fluctuate, especially in chronic Hepatitis C, but also may be monophasic or plateau-like.

→ Labs usually normal by 16 weeks.

Hepatitis E

→ Physical findings same as Hepatitis C.

ASSESSMENT

→ Viral hepatitis
  - Hepatitis A
  - Hepatitis B
  - Hepatitis D
  - Hepatitis C
  - Hepatitis E
→ R/O infectious mononucleosis
→ R/O cytomegalovirus
→ R/O HSV infection
→ R/O drug-induced liver disease
→ R/O influenza

→ R/O upper respiratory tract infection
→ R/O biliary tract disease

PLAN

DIAGNOSTIC TESTS

→ At diagnosis (positive serological marker; see **Figures 11C.1 through 11C.5**) and at 2 and 12 weeks obtain:
  - ALT and AST.
  - CBC.
  - PT.
  - bilirubin.
  - albumin/globulin.
  - urinalysis.

Hepatitis A

→ See **Figure 11C.1, Serological Diagnosis: Acute Hepatitis A.**
  - IgM antibody to HAV (anti-HAV) will develop early in acute infection and persist for 6 to 12 months.
  - IgG anti-HAV will indicate previous exposure to HAV, non-infectivity and immunity to recurring HAV infection.

→ ALT will peak at onset of clinical disease and return to normal after three months.

Hepatitis B

→ See **Figure 11C.2, Serological Diagnosis: Acute Hepatitis B.**
  - Hepatitis B surface antigen (HBsAG) indicates infection or chronic hepatitis.
  - IgM anti-HBc indicates acute infection (high titer).
  - IgG antibody to HBcAG (anti-HBc) indicates chronic disease if HBsAG positive or prior exposure if HBsAG negative.
  - Antibody to HBsAG (anti-HBs) indicates immunity.
    • There is a "window period" between the time that HBsAG is cleared and anti-HBs appears. Infectivity has been demonstrated during this period.
  - HBeAG indicates acute infectious state. Denotes a more highly replicative chronic infection, associated with increased infectivity and liver injury.
  - Antibody to HBeAG (anti-HBe) indicates convalescence or ongoing infection.

→ ALT will peak at onset of clinical disease and return to normal after 4 to 5 months.

Figure 11C.1. SEROLOGICAL DIAGNOSIS: ACUTE HEPATITIS A

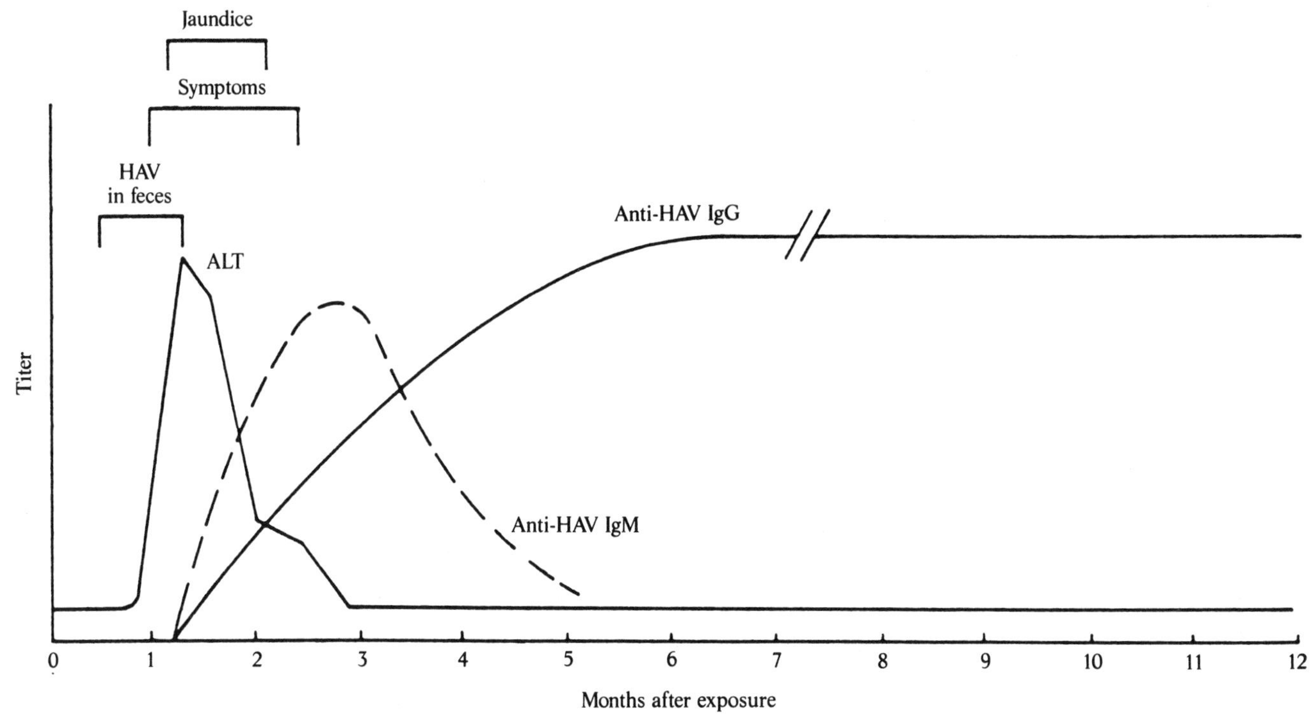

SOURCE: Reprinted with permission from Clarke, D.D., and Kao, H. 1983. Meaningful markers for hepatitis Dx and Px. *Contemporary Ob/Gyn Special Issue* 21:31-50.

→ See **Figure 11C.3, Serological Course of the Chronic HBsAG Carrier.**

■ HBsAG for longer than 6 months.

→ Liver biopsy is indicated for diagnosis of chronic hepatitis to distinguish between chronic persistent and chronic active hepatitis.

Hepatitis D

→ See **Figure 11C.4, Serological Diagnosis: Hepatitis D Co-Infection.**

■ Antibody to HDV (anti-HDV) along with Hepatitis B markers: HBsAG and IgM anti-HBc.

■ Rising titers of anti-HDV indicate acute infection.

■ Sustained high titer of anti-HDV indicates chronic Hepatitis D infection. A single or biphasic aminotransferase peak may occur.

→ See **Figure 11C.5, Serological Diagnosis, Hepatitis D Super-Infection.**

■ HBsAG and anti-HDV in absence of IgM anti-HBc.

■ Elevated aminotrasferase level in previous asymptomatic carrier.

Hepatitis C

→ Antibody to HCV (anti-HCV) is positive in 95 percent of patients with post-transfusion hepatitis and in 50 percent with sporadic infection.

→ Presence of anti-HCV in serum can be detected as early as 6 to 8 weeks or as late as 9 to 10 months after onset of clinical manifestations (Aach 1992; Knauer 1993).

→ Anti-HCV not applicable to diagnosis of acute Hepatitis C infection.

→ Recovery or chronic carrier state cannot be determined.

→ ALT may be fluctuating, especially in chronic hepatitis, but may be monophasic or plateau-like.

Hepatitis E

→ No serological testing available.

→ Diagnosis by clinical setting and detection of IgG anti-HAV indicating resolved past infection to Hepatitis A, which may clinically resemble Hepatitis E.

Figure 11C.2. SEROLOGICAL DIAGNOSIS: ACUTE HEPATITIS B

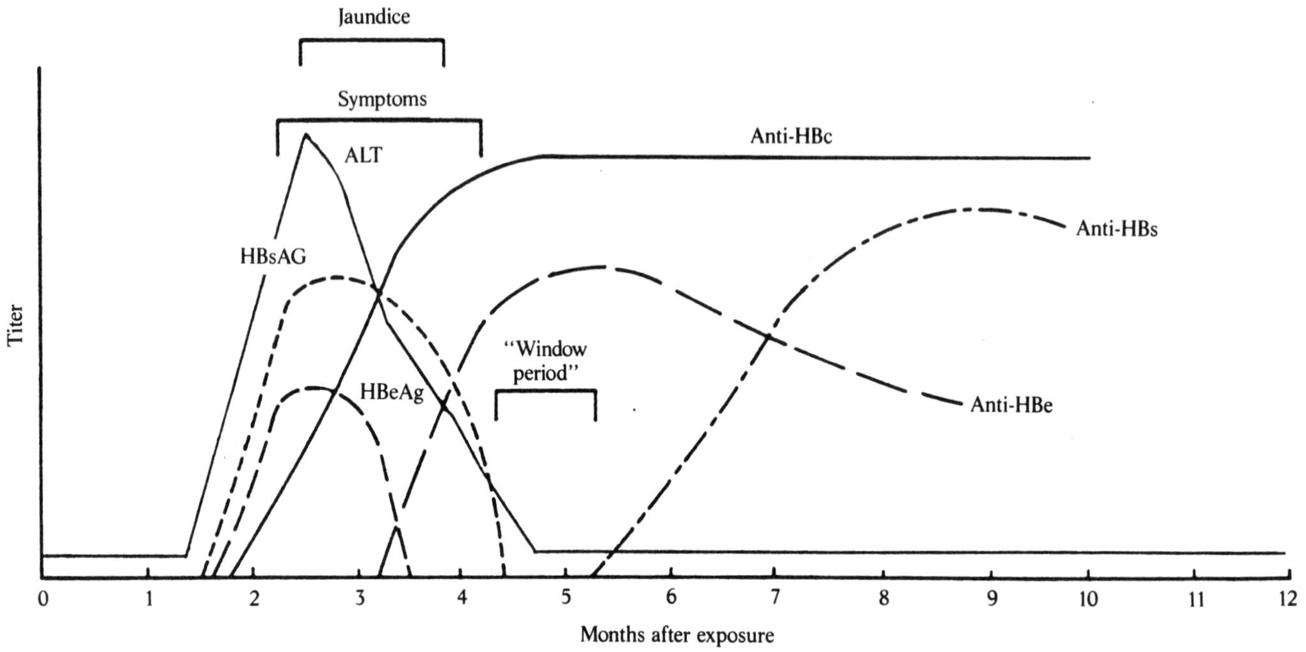

SOURCE: Adapted with permission from Clarke, D.D., and Kao, H. 1983. Meaningful markers for hepatitis Dx and Px. *Contemporary Ob/Gyn Special Issue* 21:31-50.

TREATMENT/MANAGEMENT

→ Supportive therapy is the mainstay of treatment with acute viral hepatitis.

→ Adequate nutrition should be encouraged with small, frequent meals.

→ Bed rest has not been proven to alter disease course.

→ Physical activity should be encouraged as tolerated.

→ Hepatotoxic agents should be eliminated—e.g., medications and alcohol. Oral contraceptives do not have to be discontinued (Dienstag 1995).

→ Nausea and vomiting can be controlled with nonphenothiazine antiemetics.

→ Pruritus can be controlled with cholestyramine.

Hepatitis A

→ Disease is self-limiting. Supportive measures are recommended.

→ Once jaundice is present, fecal shedding has ceased but hygiene precautions are highly recommended. See "Patient Education" section.

→ Pre-exposure prophylaxis recommended when traveling to endemic areas of Asia, Africa, and India where hygiene standards are not strictly controlled.
  ▪ Immunoglobulin 0.02 ml/kg I.M. within 2 weeks of arrival for stay less than 2 months.
  ▪ If staying longer than 2 months, recommended dosage is immunoglobulin 5 ml/kg I.M. every 5 months (Knauer 1993).

→ Post-exposure prophylaxis recommended to household or personal contacts, day care staff or attendees, residents and staff in prisons or institutions for mentally handicapped.
  ▪ 8 percent effective in preventing symptomatic hepatitis if given within 2 weeks of exposure (Hallam and Kerlin 1991).
  ▪ immunoglobulin 0.02 ml/kg I.M. (Knauer 1993).

Hepatitis B

→ There is no specific treatment for acute or chronic infection. Several studies are underway looking at interferon alfa-2b (Kools 1992).

→ Liver transplantation has been effective treatment for patients with end-stage liver disease.

Figure 11C.3.   SEROLOGICAL COURSE OF THE CHRONIC HBsAG CARRIER

SOURCE: Reprinted with permission from Clarke, D.D., and Kao, H. 1983. Meaningful markers for hepatitis Dx and Px. *Contemporary Ob/Gyn Special Issue* 21:31-50.

→ Immunoprophylaxis is recommended for all individuals at risk for infection. See Hepatitis B risk factors in "Subjective" section.

- Recipients must have a negative HBsAG and HBcAb before immunization.
- The Immunization Practices Advisory Committee (ACIP) of the U.S. Department of Health and Human Services recommends routine vaccination of all infants (CDC 1991d). See *PDR* for newborn and pediatric dosages.
- Hepatitis B recombinant vaccine (Recombivax HB®) 10 µg I.M. in deltoid at 0, 1, and 6 months,

OR

- Hepatitis B recombinant vaccine (Engerix-B®) 20 µg I.M. in deltoid at 0, 1, and 6 months (Shapiro and Margolis 1992).
- Three doses of vaccine induce protective antibody levels in 90% of adult recipients and confer protection from HBV infection in essentially all vaccine responders (Alter and Margolis 1990).

→ Post-exposure prophylaxis is recommended after a needlestick or transmucosal inoculation.

- Blood should be drawn from the donor and recipient and analyzed for HBV markers.
- Also consider HCV- and HIV-antibody status if the donor is at risk for these viruses.
- After the blood is drawn, give to the recipient Hepatitis B immunoglobulin (H-BIG®, Hep-B-Gammagee®, HyperHep®) 0.06 ml/kg I.M. within 7 days of exposure and again at 30 days (Knauer 1993).

→ If the donor is negative for HBsAG and recipient negative for HBsAG and anti-HBs, begin immunization with Hepatitis B recombinant vaccine (Recombivax HB®).

- 10 µg I.M. within 7-14 days of exposure and at 1 and 6 months (Ergun and Miskovitz 1990).

→ Immunocompromised and hemodialysis patients and the aged are considered poor responders to vaccine. It has been recommended that if these individuals are again exposed to Hepatitis B they receive post-exposure Hepatitis B immuno-globulin (Hallam and Kerlin 1991).

Figure 11C.4. SEROLOGICAL DIAGNOSIS: HEPATITIS D CO-INFECTION

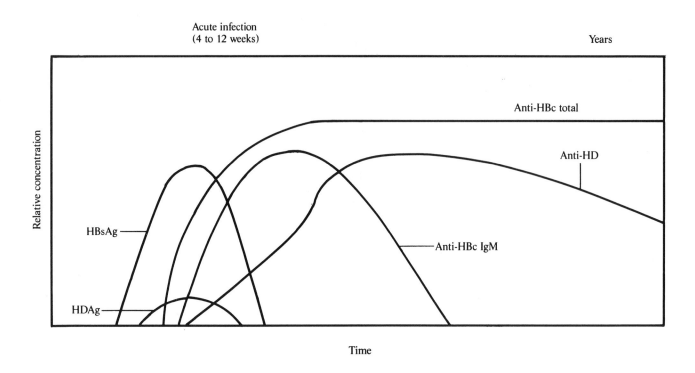

SOURCE: Reprinted with permission from Stremmel, W., Schwarzendrobe, J., Niederau, C., and Strohmeyer, G. 1991. Epidemiology, clinical course, and treatment of chronic viral hepatitis. *Hepatogastroenterology* 38(1):22-28.

Hepatitis D

→ There is no effective treatment for Hepatitis D.

→ Immunophrophylaxis would be the same as for Hepatitis B.

Hepatitis C

→ There is no effective treatment for acute Hepatitis C.

→ Interferon alfa-2b has been approved for treatment of chronic Hepatitis C.

→ No immunoprophylaxis is available.

Hepatitis E

→ No effective treatment is available.

→ No immunoprophylaxis is available.

CONSULTATION

→ Referral to a physician is warranted for patients:
- who are elderly.
- who are immunocompromised.
- who have difficult-to-manage underlying chronic disorders.

- with severe symptoms and with inadequate caloric and fluid intake.
- whose symptoms are worsening.
- who have clinical manifestations of fulminant disease.

→ Physician referral is warranted in patients with chronic hepatitis to determine specific diagnosis.
- Patients with chronic persistent hepatitis may be followed in consultation with the physician.
- Patients with chronic active hepatitis should be managed by a physician.

→ As needed for prescription(s).

PATIENT EDUCATION

→ The following recommendations are general guidelines that may be appropriate to all types of hepatitis.

→ Teach patient and family risk factors, pathophysiology, management plan, state of infectivity, and prophylaxis availability of hepatitis vaccines.

→ Advise patient regarding transmission precautions until period of infectivity has passed.

Figure 11C.5.   SEROLOGICAL DIAGNOSIS: HEPATITIS D SUPER-INFECTION

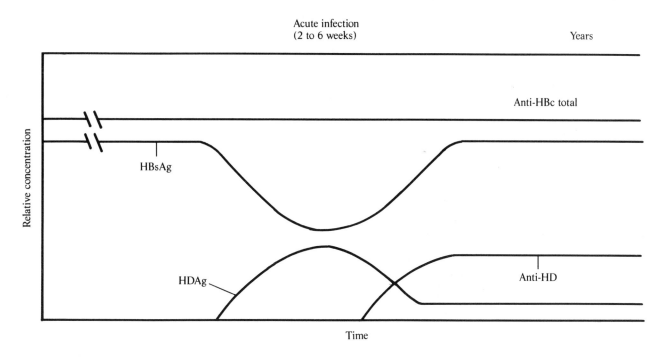

SOURCE: Reprinted with permission from Stremmel, W., Schwarzendrobe, J., Niederau, C., and Strohmeyer, G. 1991. Epidemiology, clinical course, and treatment of chronic viral hepatitis. *Hepatogastroenterology* 38(1):22-28.

→ Patients with carrier or chronic state should be advised to continue transmission precautions.

→ Teach patient good personal hygiene:
  ▪ wash hands with soap after using the bathroom.
  ▪ dispose of tampons, peripads, and bandages in plastic bags.
  ▪ use separate drinking cups, utensils, razors, toothbrushes, manicure sets.

→ Advise patient not to prepare or serve food to others.

→ Advise patient that intimate contact (sharing of bodily fluids) should be avoided.

→ Advise patient that male sex partner(s) should use condoms.

→ Advise thorough hand washing for those who come in contact with utensils, bedding, or clothing.

→ Educate intravenous drug users to clean their needles properly with bleach: Discuss availability of new needles through needle exchange services.

→ Teach health care workers to dispose of blood and blood products properly and not to recap needles. (Special waste containers should be available.)

→ Advise patient to encourage exposed contacts to consult their provider as soon as possible for prophylaxis and/or immunization if appropriate.

→ Advise patient regarding a nutritious diet (see **General Nutrition Guidelines**).

→ Advise patient regarding measures to reduce nausea including consumption of small frequent meals, carbohydrates.

→ Advise patient about regular physical activity as tolerated and to avoid becoming over-tired.

→ Teach patient to omit hepatotoxic agents—e.g, drugs and alcohol.

→ Advise patient to inform all health care providers regarding hepatitis infection.

FOLLOW-UP

→ Recommendation is for patient evaluation at two weeks after diagnosis and in three months for repeat laboratory studies.
  ▪ Patients who are more than mildly symptomatic may need to be evaluated more often.

→ Patients with persistent symptoms or laboratory abnormalities beyond 12 weeks should be monitored every four weeks with:
- ALT and AST.
- bilirubin.
- PT.
- albumin/globulin.
- serological marker for virus type.

→ Referral to a physician is recommended for persistent symptoms or abnormal laboratory values lasting longer than six months.

→ Patients with chronic hepatitis should be followed by a physician.
- In particular, patients with chronic active hepatitis should be followed closely.

→ A public health nurse referral may assist the family with preventive care and teaching in the home.

→ Referral to drug treatment program is recommended for patient using drugs.

→ Document in progress notes and problem list.

Maureen T. Shannon, C.N.M., F.N.P., M.S.

11-D

Human Immunodeficiency Virus (HIV)

Human immunodeficiency virus (HIV) infection is a complex infectious disease caused by a retrovirus and resulting in chronic immune dysfunction involving multiple organs and systems of the body. The majority of individuals infected with HIV will eventually develop *acquired immunodeficiency syndrome* (AIDS), a condition considered to represent end-stage HIV disease and with a significantly high mortality rate (CDC 1994).

As of June 1994, over 401,749 individuals in the United States had been diagnosed with AIDS, with 13 percent of those cases reported in women (CDC 1994). AIDS is the number one cause of death for African American women of reproductive age in New York, and the fifth leading cause of death for women of reproductive age nationally (Chu, Buehler, and Berkelman 1990).

An estimated one million individuals in the United States are HIV-positive (CDC 1993a): the majority of these are asymptomatic. Approximately 100,000 are women, 80,000 of whom are estimated to be of reproductive age (Minkoff 1991).

An in-depth presentation of the complex pathogenesis of HIV is beyond the scope of this protocol. However, a brief summary of the clinical progression of individual infected with HIV will be provided.

When a person becomes infected with HIV, the virus must seek out and attach to CD4 receptor sites located on the surface of cells in the human body. Once the virus has attached to these cells, it can enter the host cell and begin to replicate after encoding its genetic message onto the host cell's DNA. To accomplish this process the virus must utilize an enzyme called reverse transcriptase.

The human body contains a number of CD4 receptor sites including *T-lymphocytes* (specifically *T-helper*

cells [CD4 lymphocyte cells]) and *macrophages.* When HIV replicates within a CD4 lymphocyte cell, the host cell is eventually destroyed in the process of viral replication. However, macrophages are not destroyed during the process of viral replication and remain capable of further production of the virus when stimulated. In addition, a recent report has documented evidence of viral activity in lymphoid tissue during periods of clinical latency when minimal viral activity is demonstrated in the peripheral blood (Pantaleo et al. 1993).

The exact mechanism that triggers viral replication resulting in clinical symptomatology after a long latency period in HIV-infected persons is still unknown. However, since viral replication in CD4 lymphocytes results in cell destruction, the CD4 lymphocyte count is presently the major laboratory marker used to evaluate HIV disease progression. The average count in normal non-infected individuals is at least 800 cells/mm³. During the first year of infection after seroconversion there is an average decline of 200 to 300 cells/mm³, with a subsequent yearly decline of approximately 50 to 80 cells/mm³ (see **Figure 11D.1, Natural History of HIV Infection Based on CD4 Cell Counts** and **Table 11D.1, Natural History of HIV Infection**) (Bartlett 1992).

Knowledge of an individual's CD4 count is useful in staging HIV disease and developing a plan of care. Certain therapeutic interventions (e.g., antiretroviral therapy) are indicated at various stages of HIV disease in both symptomatic and asymptomatic patients.

Furthermore, patients with CD4 counts less than 200 cells/mm³ are at significantly higher risk of developing several major opportunistic infections (OIs) including *Pneumocystis carinii* pneumonia (PCP), toxoplasmosis encephalitis, cryptococcal meningitis, esophageal

Figure 11D.1. NATURAL HISTORY OF HIV INFECTION BASED ON CD4 CELL COUNTS*

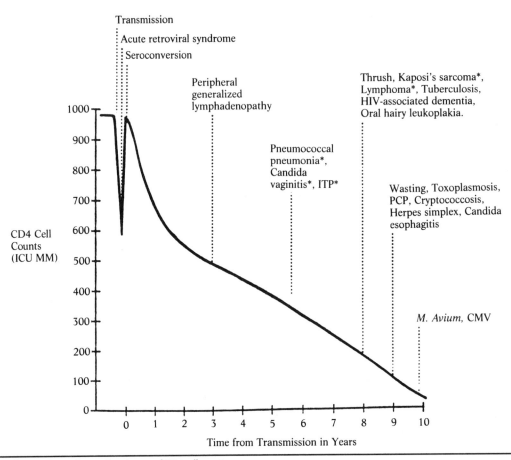

*Indicates conditions that are observed over a broad range of CD4 cell counts.

Decline in CD4 cell count based on sequential tests in 318 seroconverters in the MAC study (JID 165:352, 1992). Approximate time of complications relevative to CD4 cell count is based on experience of MACS with 888 AIDS-defining diagnoses (A. Munoz, personal communication) and multiple published reports.

Source: Reprinted with permission from Bartlett, J.G. 1992. *1992-1993 recommendations for the medical care of persons with HIV infection*, 2nd. ed., p. 19. Baltimore: Critical Care America. Copyright 1992 by the Johns Hopkins Medical Institutions.

candidiasis, and disseminated *Mycobacterium avium intracellulare* (MAI).

The clinical manifestations of HIV infection vary depending upon the level of immune deficiency that the person is experiencing (see **Table 11D.2, Major Diagnostic Considerations by Organ System**). Initially, a person infected with HIV may experience an acute retroviral syndrome that usually occurs two to four weeks after infection. A period of latency follows and may last as long as ten years. During this time, the HIV-infected person remains relatively asymptomatic, although the development of persistent generalized lymphadenopathy, anemia, leukopenia, and thrombocytopenia may be observed.

As the person's immune functioning continues to decline, clinical manifestations associated with minor OI (e.g., oral candidiasis, hairy leukoplakia) and AIDS-defining conditions are observed (see **Table 11D.3, AIDS**

Case Surveillance Definition for Adults, U.S. Centers for Disease Control and Prevention).

As HIV infection progresses in women, an increased incidence of certain gynecological complications also are noted including recurrent, recalcitrant vaginal candidiasis which usually precedes the development of oral candidiasis (Carpenter et al. 1991; Imam et al. 1990; Rhoads et al. 1987); cervical dysplasia with an estimated eight- to eleven-fold increase compared to noninfected women (Maiman et al. 1990; Marte et al. 1992); and pelvic inflammatory disease (PID) (Bartlett 1992; Carpenter et al. 1991). As a result of the observed gynecological complications associated with HIV infection in women, the Centers for Disease Control and Prevention (CDC) added invasive cervical carcinoma to the list of AIDS-defining conditions in January 1993 (CDC 1992b; *San Francisco Epidemiologic Bulletin* 1993).

Table 11D.1. NATURAL HISTORY OF HIV INFECTION*

Time from Transmission (average)	Observation	CD4 Cell Count
0	Viral transmission	Normal: 1000 ± 500/cu mm
2-4 weeks	Self-limited infectious mononucleosis-like illness with fever, adenopathy, splenomegaly, morbilliform rash, leukopenia with atypical lymphocytes; may present with aseptic meningitis	Transient decrease
6-12 weeks	Seroconversion (rarely requires ≥ 3 months for seroconversion)	Normal
0-8 years	Asymptomatic HIV infection ± peripheral generalized lymphadenopathy (PGL)	Gradual reduction with average decrease of 50/cu mm-80/cu mm/yr
4-8 years	AIDS-related complex (ARC) or early symptomatic HIV infection; thrush, oral hairy leukoplakia, ITP, constitutional symptoms—fever, weight loss, fatigue; bacterial infections	50/cu mm-300/cu mm
6-10 years	AIDS*; most common late complications are AIDS-defining diagnoses (in order by frequency as initial AIDS-defining diagnosis): *P. carinii*, wasting syndrome, Candida esophagitis, Kaposi's sarcoma, HIV-associated dementia, disseminated *M. avium*, lymphoma, cryptococcal meningitis	< 200/cu mm (mean count with most AIDS-defining opportunistic infections is 50/cu mm-100/cu mm)
8-12 months after AIDS-defining diagnosis*	Death	< 50/cu mm

*Natural history indicates course of HIV infection in absence of antiretroviral treatment. The AIDS-defining diagnosis utilizes the CDC criteria of 1987-1992 (MMWR. 1987). 36:36.

Source: Reprinted with permission from Bartlett, J.G. 1992. *1992-1993 recommendations for the medical care of persons with HIV infection*, 2nd ed., p. 21. Baltimore: Critical Care America. Copyright 1992 by the Johns Hopkins Medical Institutions.

An in-depth presentation of the plan of care for an HIV-positive woman throughout the course of this disease is beyond the scope of this protocol. However, the therapeutic options available to a woman during the asymptomatic phase of the disease, as well as therapeutic interventions for common minor OIs, are presented with the understanding that current management strategies for HIV infection are changing continually. The rapid evolution of therapies and clinical trials available to HIV-positive women requires that practitioners constantly update their knowledge regarding this disease, utilize infectious disease and/or HIV specialists as consultants, and make appropriate referrals so that HIV-positive women receive timely and effective therapy.

DATABASE

SUBJECTIVE

→ Risk factors may include:
- history of injection drug use (IDU), needle-sharing behavior.
- history of sexual contact with a person with an increased risk of HIV infection including:
  - history of injection drug use.
  - history of bisexuality.
- having symptoms of or diagnosed with HIV infection or AIDS.
- hemophilia.
- lived in an area where HIV infection is endemic.
- receiving a blood transfusion, blood products, or tissue between mid-1970s to June 1985.
- sexual partner(s) at risk for HIV infection.
- transfusion, blood product, or tissue recipient between mid-1970s to June 1985.
- lived in an area where HIV infection is endemic (e.g., Central Africa).
- has child(ren) diagnosed with HIV infection or AIDS.
- had an unscreened artificial insemination.
- had occupational exposure to human blood or body fluids.
- has clinical signs/symptoms associated with HIV infection.

→ Other factors that may be associated with HIV risk:
- drug use (e.g., alcohol, crack).
- exchanging sex for money, drugs, food, shelter.
- history of sexually transmitted diseases (STDs).
- multiple sexual partners.

Table 11D.2. MAJOR DIAGNOSTIC CONSIDERATIONS BY ORGAN SYSTEM

Conditions	CD4 > 300/cu mm	CD4 < 200/cu mm
LYMPHADENOPATHY	PGL* (syphilis, lymphoma, KS, TB)**	PGL (CMV*, TB*, KS*, MA*)
EYE (FUNDI) Exudate + hemorrhage Cotton wool spots	HIV retinopathy	CMV retinitis HIV retinopathy
ORAL White patches Ulcers Red-purple nodular lesions Esophagus (dysphagia)	Thrush, OHL HSV,* aphthous ulcers KS	Thrush, OHL HSV, aphthous ulcers, (CMV) KS *Candida* (HSV, CMV, aphthous ulcers)
ABDOMEN Diarrhea Hepatomegaly Splenomegaly	*Salmonella, C. difficile, Campylobacter, Shigella* Hepatitis (usually HBV or HCV)	*Cryptosporidia*, bacterial agents, *Microsporidia*, MA, CMV, AIDS enteropathy, small bowel overgrowth, (histoplasmosis, isospora, blue-green algae) Hepatitis, CMV, MA, lymphoma, HIV, fatty liver 2° malnutrition Lymphoma, MA, histoplasmosis, HIV
SKIN Purple-black nodular lesions Vesicles Maculopapular lesions Plaques, scaling lesions Umbilicated papules Petechiae, purpura Nodules	KS (bacillary angiomatosis, prurigo nodularis) H. simplex, H. zoster Adverse drug reaction, syphilis Seborrhea (psoriasis, eczema) Molluscum ITP*	KS (bacillary angiomatosis, prurigo nodularis) H. simplex, H. zoster Adverse drug reaction, syphilis Seborrhea (psoriasis, eczema) Molluscum (*cryptococcus*) ITP *Cryptococcus*, histoplasmosis
LUNGS Pneumonia Cavity nodules	S. pneumoniae, H. influenzae, TB TB (*S. aureus* with I.V. drug users)	PCP (TB, MA, KS, CMV, cryptococcus, bacterial infection, lymphoid interstitial pneumonia) TB (*cryptococcus, nocardia*, KS, lymphoma, MA, *M. kansasii*, atypical PCP, *rhodococcus*)
NEUROLOGICAL Aseptic meningitis Chronic meningitis Dementia	Neurosyphilis, viral Tuberculosis, fungal meningitis Trauma, tumor, depression, hypothyroid	Cryptococcal meningitis *Cryptococcus* or tuberculosis HIV-associated dementia
CONSTITUTIONAL (FUO,* weight loss, etc.)	Lymphoma, TB	MA, CMV, histoplasmosis, HIV cryptococcosis, PCP, lymphoma

*CMV = Cytomegalovirus, PCP = Pneumocystis *carinii* pneumonia, MA = *Mycobacterium avium*, TB = Tuberculosis, OHL = Oral hairy leukoplakia, PGL = Peripheral generalized lymphadenopathy, HSV = Herpes simplex virus, KS = Kaposi's sarcoma, ITP = Idiopathic thrombocytopenia, FUO = Fever of unknown origin.

**Conditions in parentheses indicate less likely diagnosis.

Source: Reprinted with permission from Bartlett, J.G. 1992. *1992-1993 recommendations for the medical care of persons with HIV infection*, 2nd ed., p. 8. Baltimore: Critical Care America. Copyright 1992 by the Johns Hopkins Medical Institutions.

■ sexual partner with a history of incarceration.
NOTE: Heterosexual transmission is now the leading mechanism for the acquisition of HIV by women in the United States (CDC 1993b). Therefore, women with a history of unprotected sexual contact with a partner of unknown HIV status should be considered at risk.

→ Symptoms may include:

Acute HIV Retroviral Syndrome
■ fever.
■ sweats.
■ rigors.
■ malaise.
■ sore throat.
■ gastrointestinal symptoms including anorexia, nausea, vomiting, and diarrhea.
■ generalized rash.
■ enlarged lymph nodes.
■ headaches.

Table 11D.3.   AIDS CASE SURVEILLANCE DEFINITION FOR ADULTS, U.S. CENTERS FOR DISEASE CONTROL AND PREVENTION

Without laboratory evidence of HIV infection:
1. Candidiasis of the esophagus, trachea, bronchi, or lungs.
2. Cryptococcosis, extrapulmonary.
3. Cryptosporidiosis with diarrhea persisting >1 month.
4. Cytomegalovirus disease of an organ other than liver, spleen, or lymph nodes.
5. Herpes simplex virus infection causing a mucocutaneous ulcer that persists longer than 1 month, or bronchitis, pneumonitis, or esophagitis for any duration.
6. Kaposi's sarcoma affecting a patient <60 years of age.
7. Lymphoma of the brain (primary) affecting a patient <60 years of age.
8. *Mycobacterium avium* complex or *M. kansasii* disease, disseminated (at a site other than or in addition to lungs, skin, or cervical or hilar lymph nodes).
9. *Pneumocystis carinii* pneumonia.
10. Progressive multifocal leukoencephalopathy.
11. Toxoplasmosis of the brain.

With laboratory evidence for HIV infection:
1. Recurrent pneumonia.
2. Coccidioidomycosis, disseminated (at a site other than or in addition to lungs or cervical or hilar lymph nodes).
3. HIV encephalopathy (also called HIV dementia or substance encephalitis due to HIV).
4. Histoplasmosis, disseminated (at a site other than or in addition to lungs or cervical or hilar lymph nodes).
5. Isosporiasis with diarrhea persisting >1 month.
6. Kaposi's sarcoma at any age.
7. Lymphoma of the brain (primary) at any age.
8. Other non-Hodgkin's lymphoma of B-cell or unknown immunologic phenotype.
9. Any mycobacterial disease caused by mycobacteria other than *M. tuberculosis*, disseminated (at a site other than or in addition to lungs, skin, or cervical or hilar lymph nodes).
10. Disease caused by *M. tuberculosis*.
11. Salmonella (nontyphoid) septicemia, recurrent.
12. HIV wasting syndrome (emaciation, "slim disease").
13. Invasive cervical carcinoma.
14. CD_4+ lymphocyte count less than or equal to 200/mm^3, or a CD_4+ lymphocyte percentage less than or equal to 14%.

Source: Reprinted with permission from Centers for Disease Control. 1992b. 1993 Revised classification system for HIV infection and expanded surveillance case definition for AIDS among adolescents and adults. *Morbidity and Mortality Weekly Report* 41(RR-17):1-19; Cohn, J.A. 1993. Human immunodeficiency virus and AIDS. *Journal of Nurse Midwifery* 38(2):70.

- photophobia.
- altered mental status.

Progressive HIV Infection
- HIV-infected individuals may remain asymptomatic for up to ten years after seroconversion.
- generalized manifestations may be reported including:
  - enlarged lymph nodes.
  - fatigue.
  - night sweats.
  - intermittent low-grade fever.
  - weight loss.
- dermatological manifestations may be reported including:
  - dry skin (generalized).
  - erythematous, scaly skin of scalp, eyebrows, nasolabial folds, trunk, groin (may indicate seborrheic dermatitis).
  - grouped vesicles of lips, genitalia, or perianal region that are usually painful and recurrent (may indicate HSV infection).
  - painful eruption of blisters in a wide distribution (dermatomal pattern) usually unilateral and occurring on the trunk, head, or neck (may indicate herpes zoster).
  - scaly patches with areas of central clearing (may indicate tinea infection).
  - thick, crumbling of fingernails or toenails (may indicate tinea infection).
  - thick, erythematous, red plaques with well-defined margins; intermittently pruritic; usually reported at site of trauma (may indicate psoriasis).
  - erythematous papular, pustular lesions at hair follicles of the face and/or trunk; may be tender and/or pruritic (may indicate folliculitis).
  - oval nodules that become reddish-purple in color; 1 cm to 2 cm; reported on face, truck, legs, and hard palate of oral cavity (may indicate Kaposi's sarcoma [KS], rarely reported in HIV-infected women).
  - petechiae (may indicate thrombocytopenia).

- ophthalmic manifestations may be reported including:
  - abrupt onset of small floating spots in field of vision.
  - intermittent or persistent blurred vision.
  - intermittent flashes of light.
  - photophobia.
  - loss of vision.
- oral manifestations may be reported including:
  - "canker sores" of tongue and buccal mucosa.
  - grouped vesicles or ulcers of lips or buccal mucosa (may indicate HSV infection).
  - white patches on buccal mucosa and/or tongue that may or may not scrape off (may indicate oral candidiasis or hairy leukoplakia).
  - erythema, edema, bleeding of gums (may indicate gingivitis).
  - nodules that are reddish-purple in color; usually reported on hard palate (may indicate KS).
- respiratory manifestations may be reported including:
  - dyspnea.
    - –May be mild to severe depending upon underlying condition.
  - shortness of breath.
    - –May be mild to severe.
  - a persistent dry, hacking cough (often noted in *Pneumocystis carinii* pneumonia).
  - abrupt onset of productive cough with minimal to copious amounts of purulent mucous (see **Pneumonia** Protocol).
- gastrointestinal manifestations may be reported including:
  - chronic, intermittent diarrhea with or without bloating.
  - odynophagia.
  - dysphagia.
  - jaundice.
  - hemetemesis, melena (rare).
- neurological manifestations may be reported including:
  - memory lapses, mental confusion, inability to think clearly.
  - frequent or persistent headaches with or without fever.
  - dysesthesia of extremities.
  - problems with coordination or balance.
- gynecological manifestations may be reported including:
  - erythema and/or pruritis of vulvovaginal and/ or perianal areas.

- vaginal discharge that is indicative of candidiasis, trichomonas, bacterial vaginosis, chlamydia, or gonorrhea (see specific **Vaginitis** and **Sexually Transmitted Diseases** protocols).
- recurrent, painful blister(s) or ulcer(s) in vulvovaginal and/or perianal regions (indicative of HSV).
- verruciform lesions of the vulvovaginal, perineal, or anal regions that may be recurrent (indicative of condyloma).
- a history of or documented evidence of rapid development of cervical intraepithelial neoplasia (CIN).

OBJECTIVE
→ The physical examination may be WNL or demonstrate significant pathological findings depending upon the immune status of the patient and any concomitant conditions that may be present.
- General examination may reveal a thin, wasted body type.
- Vital signs are usually WNL but will change depending upon any underlying illness (e.g., bacterial pneumonia) that may coexist.
- Examination of the skin may reveal evidence of the following conditions:
  - xerosis.
  - seborrheic dermatitis.
  - folliculitis.
  - psoriasis.
  - tinea infection.
  - herpes simplex or zoster.
  - molluscum contagiousum (see specific protocols for descriptions of these conditions).
  - flat or elevated reddish-purple nodule(s) or plaques varying in size from 1 cm to 2 cm may be observed (KS, rare in women).
- Examination of the eyes may reveal:
  - cotton wool patches with or without evidence of hemorrhage (finding is not necessarily associated with a specific disease) (Shin and Avers 1988).
  - dry, granular, white retinal opacification with hemorrhage (evidence of retinopathy).
  - bright red subconjunctival hemorrhage (may indicate KS).
  - visual field defects, optic atrophy, pupillary abnormalities, cranial nerve palsies (may indicate neuro-opthalmic signs of intracranial disease or other conditions).
- Examination of the oropharynx may reveal:

- erythema, edema, hypertrophy of gingiva (gingivitis).
- smooth, erythematous patches of the hard or soft palate, buccal mucosa, or dorsum of the tongue (atrophic candidiasis).
- raised white patches on tongue or buccal mucosa that scrape off with tongue blade. Patches may be on an erythematous base (candidiasis).
- white or whitish-gray raised, irregularly shaped lesions with vertical folds or corrugations of the lateral (often posterior, inferior) tongue that do not scrape off (hairy leukoplakia).
- small erythematous, eroded, or fissured lesions at corners of mouth (angular chelitis).
- reddish-purple-blue-colored flat or elevated single or multiple lesions of the mouth (may indicate KS).
- small vesicular or ulcerated painful lesions of the lips, palate, or gingiva (may indicate HSV infection).
- single or multiple verruciform lesions that may be cauliflower-like or flat (may indicate human papillomavirus infection [HPV]).
- Examination of the lungs will reveal findings consistent with any concomitant disease (see **Respiratory/Otorhinolaryngological Disorders** Protocol).
  NOTE: Pulmonary problems in HIV-positive patients (e.g., PCP, bacterial pneumonia) often present with subtle physical examination findings such as:
  - tachypnea.
  - rales.
- Cardiac examination is usually WNL. If significant disease (e.g., endocarditis in injection drug use patients, cardiomyopathy) coexists, the following symptoms may be evident:
  - increased pulse rate.
  - murmur.
  - S$_3$ gallop.
- Abdominal examination may reveal enlarged
  - liver.
  - spleen.
- Palpation of the patient's lymph nodes may reveal:
  - enlarged, soft, mobile lymph nodes of the occiput, anterior, and posterior cervical chains, axilla, epitrochlear region, inguinal, femoral, and popliteal regions with or without tenderness.
- single or multiple hard, enlarged node(s) (may indicate lymphoma).
- Neurological examination may reveal:
  - a flat affect.
  - diminished recent memory.
  - decreased fine and gross motor movements.
  - decreased proprioception.
  - abnormal, symmetrical or asymmetrical deep tendon reflexes.
  - paraparesis.
  - ataxia.
- Musculoskeletal examination may reveal decreased muscle:
  - tone.
  - strength.
- Pelvic examination may reveal physical findings consistent with:
  - vaginitis.
  - cervicitis.
  - condyloma acuminata.
  - molluscum contagiousum.
  - HSV infection.
  - other sexually transmitted diseases (STDs).
  - vulvar/vaginal/cervical intraepithelial neoplasia (see specific protocols for descriptions of physical findings).

ASSESSMENT

→ HIV infection

→ R/O HIV infection

→ R/O AIDS

→ R/O minor OIs (e.g., oral candidiasis)

→ R/O immune dysfunction from other causes (e.g., neoplasms, autoimmune disorders)

→ R/O STDs

→ R/O psychological disorders associated with chronic disease (e.g., depression)

→ Assess factors associated with increased risk of HIV infection

PLAN

DIAGNOSTIC TESTS

→ Verification of the HIV status of a new patient presenting for HIV-specific care is essential (either through obtaining a copy of previous test results or by repeat testing of the patient) prior to the initiation of any plan of care, particularly pharmacological interventions.

- See "Patient Education" section for information regarding informed consent and disclosure of HIV test results.
→ The following tests may be ordered to document the HIV status of a patient:
  - HIV-antibody tests will usually demonstrate a positive result 6 to 12 weeks after infection with the virus.
    • However, in some individuals, it may take as long as 6 months to demonstrate detectable antibodies after infection with the virus.
    • The following tests can be performed:
      –the enzyme-linked immunosorbent assay (ELISA) test is a very sensitive but less specific antibody test used as an initial screening for the presence of HIV antibodies.
        ▸ If the initial test is positive, the test is usually repeated on the same specimen.
        ▸ If the repeat ELISA test is positive, a confirmatory antibody test is done on the same specimen (e.g., Western Blot, immunofluorescence assay [IFA]).
      –IFA can be done to confirm the initial ELISA testing and involves a process whereby a fluorescein label is attached to HIV antibodies present in a specimen. This specimen is then evaluated under an ultraviolet microscope for the presence of bright spots of fluorescence indicating a positive test.
        ▸ This test can be used to confirm positive ELISA results.
      –Western Blot is a confirmatory test that involves direct evaluation of the specimen for the presence of antibodies to specific HIV proteins.
        ▸ It is a very sensitive and specific antibody test with strict guidelines used for the interpretation of findings and is the preferred test for confirmation of positive ELISA results.
        ▸ A fully reactive Western Blot test confirms HIV-seropositive ELISA results.
        NOTE: When both the ELISA and Western Blot test results are positive, the sensitivity and specificity are each greater than 99 percent (Bartlett 1992; Grady and Vogel 1993). In patients with indeterminant test results, repeat testing should be performed at an interval appropriate to the last known HIV exposure (i.e., 6 to 12 weeks after last exposure).
  - HIV antigen (p24) is a measurement of the presence of HIV core protein in a specimen.
    • When HIV replication is active, there is an increased concentration of this antigen in the patient's blood; however, during latency periods, p24 antigen may be undetectable. Therefore, this test may be negative in an infected patient and should not be used to determine HIV serostatus in the general population.
    • In some clinical settings this test is done to monitor HIV disease-progression response to therapeutic interventions, or to detect early HIV infection (e.g., during the acute HIV retroviral syndrome) (Grady and Vogel 1993).
  - HIV cultures can be performed on a number of body fluids and tissues and may be positive depending upon the concentration of the virus in the specimen.
    • HIV cultures are expensive, the virus is difficult to grow, and meticulous laboratory procedures are essential to ensure accurate results.
    • Erratic results can occur due to a number of factors (e.g., contamination of a specimen, low concentration of virus in the specimen). For these reasons, this process is not commonly used to determine HIV status in adult populations (Cohn 1993).
  - polymerase chain reaction (PCR) is a technique that amplifies the DNA of cells from a specimen to determine the presence of HIV in the cell.
    • It is very sensitive and specific with results available within a few days. However, this test is expensive and requires an experienced laboratory staff with meticulous technique to perform the test.
    • False positive results are possible since any trace of a DNA sequencing pattern similar to HIV may be interpreted as positive (Grady and Vogel 1993).
→ CBC, differential, and platelet count should be obtained and may be WNL or reveal the following (Bartlett 1992):
  - leukopenia.
  - lymphocytopenia.
  - decreased red blood cells (RBCs), hematocrit (Hct), or hemoglobin (Hgb).
  - increased MCV to l05 fl to 110 fl in patients taking zidovudine (ZDV, AZT).

- thrombocytopenia.
→ Complete T-lymphocyte count should be ordered and may reveal (Bartlett 1992):
  - decreased T-helper cell (CD4) count (normal count is more than 800 cells/mm³).
  - increased T-suppressor cell (CD8) count.
  - inversion of T-helper to T-suppressor ratio (normal ratio 2:1).
    NOTE: There is considerable intra-laboratory and inter-laboratory variation in T-lymphocyte count results. Ideally, tests should be done at the same laboratory after being obtained at approximately the same time of day as a means of attaining some consistency in values. Furthermore, T-lymphocyte counts should be obtained 2 to 3 weeks after recovering from any complication or illness, since intercurrent illness and complications can affect baseline levels (Bartlett 1992).
→ A chemistry panel should be performed and may be WNL or reveal the following in the presence of concomitant disease(s):
  - elevated ALT, AST (in presence of hepatitis).
  - elevated alkaline phosphatase (in presence of liver disease).
  - elevated lactate dehydrogenase (LDH) (may be evidence of PCP if CD4 count is lower than 200).
  - decreased serum cholesterol (may be depleted because of chronic disease state with wasting).
→ A syphilis serology (e.g., VDRL or RPR) should be obtained.
→ Hepatitis screening should be done and include Hepatitis C-antibody testing in patients at risk for this infection (see **Hepatitis—Viral** Protocol).
→ Toxoplasmosis serology (IgG) should be done to determine the patient's serostatus. This is helpful to have documented should the patient develop symptoms of encephalitis and a diagnosis of toxoplasmosis is being considered (Bartlett 1992).
→ G6PD level should be obtained since patients with a deficiency of this enzyme will develop a hemolytic anemia when placed on some of the medications frequently used during the course of HIV disease (e.g., dapsone, sulfonamides, primaquine) (Cosby and Stringari 1991).
→ Tuberculin skin testing should be done using a purified protein derivative (PPD) and two controls (candida and mumps or tetanus).

- Induration of ≥5 mm or greater at the site of the PPD is considered to be a positive tuberculin skin test.
- A negative PPD test is valid only in patients where one of the control skin tests demonstrates a reaction.
- If the patient does not have a reaction to any skin test, she is considered to be anergic, and a chest x-ray should be done to eliminate the possibility of active tuberculosis infection.
→ Cervical cytology should be performed on any patient who has not had one performed during the past 6 to 12 months.
  - Guidelines regarding the frequency of Pap smears in HIV-positive women vary. However, the following schedules have been proposed:
    - upon entry to care, women with early HIV infection without a history of any abnormal cervical cytology should have two Pap smears obtained 6 months apart.
      - If both results are benign, then annual Pap smear testing can be done (CDC 1990; Caschetta 1992; El-Sadr et al. 1994).
    - women should have a repeat PAP smear if there is no evidence of endocervical cells on their smears, or after treatment of any cervical lesion or underlying inflammation (El-Sadr et al. 1994).
    - women without a history of abnormal cervical cytology who have symptomatic disease or a CD4 count of less than 500 should have Pap smear testing every 6 months (ACOG 1992; El-Sadr et al. 1994; Minkoff and Dehovitz 1991).
    - women with *any* abnormality noted on cervical cytology (including atypical squamous cells of undetermined significance) or who have a history of untreated squamous intraepithelial lesions (SILs) should be referred for colposcopy with repeat evaluation(s) and Pap smears per recommendation of the colposcopist (ACOG 1992; El-Sadr et al. 1994; Minkoff and Dehovitz 1991).
    - women should have appropriate cervical cultures to rule out the presence of STDs (e.g., chlamydia, gonorrhea, HSV) as indicated.
    - a wet mount of vaginal secretions should be done to evaluate for the possibility of vaginal/cervical pathogens requiring treatment (e.g., candidiasis, trichomonas, bacterial vaginosis).

→ Pregnancy testing should be considered in women of reproductive age when the possibility of conception is reported or suspected, especially prior to the initiation of systemic medications with known or unknown adverse fetal effects.

→ The following tests are ordered to monitor HIV disease progression by some authorities (Bartlett 1992; Hernandez 1990):
- beta$_2$ microglobulin level—may be WNL or elevated.
- sedimentation rate—may be WNL or elevated.
- p24 antigen level—may be undetectable or increased.

→ Routine follow-up tests of an HIV-positive patient should be done based upon the patient's HIV disease progression and therapeutic interventions that are involved in the patient's plan of care.
- The following regimen for repeat laboratory testing has been recommended (Bartlett 1992; El-Sadr et al. 1994):
  - CD4 cell counts:
    - ≥600/mm^3: repeat every 3 to 6 months.
    - 200-600/mm^3: repeat every 3 to 4 months.
    - <500/mm^3: repeat 1 to 2 weeks after obtaining initial value <500/mm^3 (to determine whether or not to offer antiretroviral therapy).
    - <200/mm^3: repeat 1 week after obtaining initial value (to determine whether or not to initiate PCP prophylaxis and zidovudine [ZDV], if the patient has not already started antiretroviral therapy).
    - <200/mm^3: repeat testing determined by the need to monitor effectiveness of therapeutic interventions, eligibility for various prophylactic interventions, and possibility of clinical trial enrollment.
  - CBC should be repeated as clinically indicated.
    - A patient beginning ZDV therapy should have a CBC done prior to initiation of ZDV and monthly for 3 months after initiating ZDV therapy.
      - ► If these results are normal, a CBC should be done every 3 months unless there is evidence of hematological side effects (Sande and Volberding 1994).
  - chemistry panel should be repeated as indicated.
    - A patient taking ZDV should have a repeat chemistry panel every 3 to 6 months to monitor transaminase values.

- VDRL or RPR should be repeated annually or more frequently as indicated (Cosby and Stringari 1991).
- chlamydia and gonorrhea cultures and vaginal/cervical wet mounts should be repeated annually, or more frequently as indicated, in sexually active individuals.
- PPD and control skin tests should be done annually unless otherwise indicated (see **Tuberculosis** Protocol).
- Pap smear testing.

TREATMENT/MANAGEMENT

→ The plan of care for an HIV-positive woman is based on her stage of HIV disease.

→ As HIV disease progresses to advanced immune dysfunction (CD4 < 200/mm^3), the risk of developing a major OI or other condition associated with an AIDS diagnosis increases significantly, and prophylactic administration of a number of pharmacological agents may be indicated.
- The management of patients who have progressed to this stage of HIV infection and/or who have a major OI or other AIDS-defining condition is beyond the scope of this protocol.

→ The following therapeutic interventions are those commonly recommended for HIV-positive women who are *asymptomatic* and less advanced in their disease progression.
- An HIV-positive patient should be given the following immunizations after obtaining informed consent (CDC 1991c):
  - pneumococcal vaccination 0.5 ml I.M. (see **Pneumonia** Protocol for additional information).
  - hepatitis B vaccination if at risk for Hepatitis B infection.
    - The series consists of three 0.5 ml I.M. injections given at appropriate time intervals (see **Hepatitis—Viral** Protocol for additional information).
  - influenza vaccination annually prior to the influenza season (see **Influenza** Protocol).

NOTE: See Table 11D.4, Recommendations for Routine Vaccination of HIV-Infected Persons, United States, for current CDC recommendations for immunizations of HIV-positive adults.
- Antiretroviral therapy should be offered to an asymptomatic patient with a CD4 count <500/mm^3 documented by results from the

Table 11D.4. RECOMMENDATIONS FOR ROUTINE VACCINATION OF HIV-INFECTED PERSONS*, UNITED STATES

Vaccine/toxoid +	HIV Infection	
	Known asymptomatic	Symptomatic
DTP/Td	Yes	Yes
OPV	No	No
eIPV$	Yes	Yes
MMR	Yes	Yes#
HbCV**	Yes	Yes
Pneumococcal	Yes	Yes
Influenza	Yes#	Yes

*Appropriate for human immunodeficiency virus (HIV)-infected children and adults.

+The vaccine/toxoid abbreviations are defined as follows: DTP = Diphtheria and tetanus toxoids and pertussis vaccine, adsorbed (pediatric); Td = Tetanus and diphtheria toxoids, adsorbed (for adult use); OPV = Oral poliovirus vaccine; eIPV = Enhanced-potency inactivated poliovirus vaccine; MMR = Measles, mumps, and rubella vaccine; HbCV—*Hemophilus influenzae* type B conjugate vaccine; and Pneumococcal—Pneumococcal polysaccharide vaccine.

$For adults older than 18 years of age, use only if indicated.

#Should be considered.

**May be considered for HIV-infected adults.

Source: Reprinted from Centers for Disease Control. 1991c. Update on adult immunization: Recommendations of the Immunization Practices Advisory Committee. *Morbidity and Mortality Weekly Report* 40(RR-12):59.

same laboratory from specimens drawn at least 1 to 2 weeks apart.

■ Initiation of antiretroviral therapy is recommended for any patient with symptomatic disease, or who is asymptomatic but has a CD4 count <200 documented by results from the same laboratory from specimens drawn 1 to 2 weeks apart (Goldschmidt and Dong 1994; Sande et al. 1993).

• The recommended first-choice therapeutic agent is:
  –zidovudine (Retrovir®) 100 mg p.o. 5 times a day or 200 mg TID.
  –zidovudine (Retrovir®) 100 mg p.o. TID can be prescribed to patients with a CD4 count >200/mm^3 demonstrating an intolerance to the drug, but this dose is the lowest dose recommended since any dose less than 300 mg a day has been shown to be less therapeutic (Bartlett 1992).

NOTE: Hematological side effects associated with this drug include bone marrow suppression with the development of anemia and granulocytopenia. Interruption or permanent discontinuation of therapy is indicated in patients with severe anemia (Hgb<8 g/dl) and/or an absolute neutrophil count (ANC) <750/cu (Bartlett 1992). Myopathy (with elevation of creatinine

phosphokinase [CPK]) has been reported in patients with long-term use (Goldschmidt and Dong 1994). Therefore, a baseline CPK level should be drawn when ZDV therapy is initiated. Two potentially fatal, albeit rare, side effects reported with ZDV use include lactic acidosis and severe hepatomegaly with steatosis observed in 6 patients. Five of the 6 affected patients were mildly to moderately obese women. The relationship between these conditions and ZDV is unknown at this time, and caution is advised when considering ZDV therapy for a patient with a history of liver disease or hepatomegaly. Appropriate monitoring of transaminase levels is recommended (Burroughs Wellcome Company, personal communication, June 1, 1993).

■ A patient demonstrating intolerance to ZDV or a diminished response to ZDV (based on laboratory and clinical evidence) may begin therapy with alternative antiretroviral therapeutic agents after consultation with a physician.

• Currently there are two medications approved for use in such patients (Bartlett 1992; Cosby and Stringari 1991; Goldschmidt and Dong 1994; Sanford et al. 1994):

• ddC (Dideoxycytidine®, Hivid®) 0.375 mg - 0.75 mg p.o. TID
  NOTE: Side effects associated with ddC include painful peripheral neuropathy (reversible), mucocutaneous eruptions, pancreatitis (rare), and seizures.

• ddI (Dideoxyinosine®, Videx®) may be prescribed in combination with ZDV or used as a single agent. The dose is based upon the patient's weight as follows:
  –>75 kg—300 mg tablet or 375 mg buffered powder p.o. BID.
  –50-74 kg—200 mg tablet or 250 mg buffered powder p.o. BID.
  –35-49 kg—125 mg tablet or 167 mg buffered powder p.o. BID.
  NOTE: Pancreatitis, peripheral neuropathy, hepatic failure, and cardiomyopathy have all been reported in association with ddI use. Patients should be advised to avoid alcohol use. Concurrent use of other pancreatic toxins (e.g., systemic pentamidine) should be avoided (Goldsmith and Dong 1994).

• Other antiretroviral agents (e.g., d4T [Stavudine®, Zerit®], nevirapine) are being studied and may be available to a patient through her enrollment in a clinical trial (see

"Patient Education" section for information on clinical trials).

- PCP primary prophylaxis should be initiated in a patient with a CD4 count <200/mm³ or <20 percent of total lymphocytes documented by two test results done at the same laboratory 1 to 2 weeks apart (Bartlett 1992).
  - Recommendations for such treatment involve systemic medications since extrapulmonary PCP has been documented in patients undergoing aerosolized pentamidine therapy for PCP prophylaxis (Goldschmidt and Dong 1994).
  - The following therapeutic agents can be initiated if there is no contraindication for their use (Goldschmidt and Dong 1994):
    - —trimethoprim (TMP)/sulfamethoxazole (SMX) 160 mg/800 mg (Septra DS®, Bactrim®) 1 tablet p.o. 3 times a week.
    - —TMP/SMX 160 mg/800 mg (Septra DS®, Bactrim®) 1 tablet p.o. every day.
    - —dapsone 50 mg-100 mg p.o. every day.
    - —dapsone 100 mg p.o. twice a week.
- Patients with CD4 counts <200/mm³ with contraindications to systemic agents for primary PCP prophylaxis should begin aerosolized pentamidine treatments if there are no contraindications to such therapy (e.g., pulmonary disease).
  - The following regimen is recommended:
    - —aerosolized pentamidine 300 mg every 4 weeks or 150 mg every 2 weeks delivered by Respirgard II® or Ultra Vent® Nebulizers.
- A patient with evidence of oral candidiasis and no clinical evidence of esophagitis (e.g., dysphagia, odynophagia, retrosternal pain when swallowing) should be treated with one of the following (Goldschmidt and Dong 1994):
  - clotrimazole oral troches (Mycelex®)—1 troche 5 times a day for 1 to 2 weeks (advise the patient to suck, not swallow, the troche until it completely dissolves).
  - nystatin (Mycostatin®) 500,000 units (5 ml)—swish and swallow 5 times a day for 1 to 2 weeks.
    NOTE: Nystatin is reported to be less effective than clotrimazole, ketoconazole, or fluconazole in the treatment of oral candidiasis (Goldschmidt and Dong 1994).
  - ketoconazole (Nizoral®) 200 mg to 400 mg p.o. every day for 1 to 2 weeks or fluconazole (Diflucan®) 100 mg to 200 mg p.o. for 1 to 2 weeks can be prescribed in recurrent or resistant cases of oral candidiasis.

NOTE: Ketoconazole requires gastric acid for absorption. Advise the patient to take this medication with orange juice. Because hepatotoxicity is a possible complication of ketoconazole use, this drug should not be used unless other therapies have been unsuccessful. Appropriate monitoring of a patient's liver function tests (LFTs) is indicated with ketoconazole use.

- A patient with evidence of vaginitis, cervicitis, or other STDs should be treated as indicated (see **Vaginitis, Sexually Transmitted Diseases** protocols).
- A patient with a positive tuberculin skin test should be treated according to current CDC recommendations (see **Tuberculosis** Protocol).
- A patient with evidence of gingivitis and/or other dental disease should be referred for a dental examination and appropriate treatment.
  - The following agents can be used (Goldschmidt and Dong 1994):
    - —hydrogen peroxide—gargle for 30 seconds BID indefinitely.
    - —chlorhexidine gluconate (Peridex®) oral rinse—15 ml swished in mouth for 30 seconds BID indefinitely.
    NOTE: Peridex® can cause staining of teeth.
- A patient with any abnormality noted on cervical cytology should be evaluated and treated as indicated by an experienced colposcopist.

CONSULTATION

→ Physician consultation is indicated regarding the plan of care for any patient suspected of being HIV-positive or with documented evidence of HIV-seropositive status with or without symptomatic disease.

→ Physician consultation is warranted in any HIV-positive patient with evidence of a major OI or AIDS-defining condition, lack of response to therapeutic interventions, serious side effects or suspected toxicity to a medication, or who is being considered for maintenance therapy (e.g., ketoconazole for candidiasis) or prophylactic therapy (e.g., Septra DS® for PCP prophylaxis).

→ In clinical settings where physician consultation is limited or unavailable, current information regarding management of HIV disease is available through the HIV Telephone Consultation Service of the Community Provider AIDS Training

Project. The telephone consultation service number is 800-933-3413.

→ Psychological or psychiatric consultation is indicated in patients with evidence of moderate to severe psychiatric symptoms (e.g., anxiety, depression) or who may be exhibiting neuro-psychiatric manifestations of HIV (e.g., HIV dementia).

→ As needed for prescription(s).

PATIENT EDUCATION

→ Educate the patient about HIV infection including the clinical course (especially the chronicity of the disease), indicated diagnostic tests, therapeutic options available, modes of transmission, prevention of further exposure to HIV and other STDs in sexually active women (see Table **13A.2, Safer Sex Guidelines**, p. 13-9), symptoms of complications requiring immediate evaluation, and indicated follow-up.
  ■ A number of patient education materials are available through the CDC National AIDS Hotline, 800-342-AIDS.

→ Discuss with patient any referrals that are recommended and the importance of keeping such appointments.

→ Discuss with the patient the need for testing of individuals who may have had exposure through sexual contact or needle-sharing activities. If a woman has children, assess the possible need for testing of her children based upon the woman's history of exposure, date of first positive test result, and ages of her children.

→ A patient who is continuing to inject drugs should be educated about the adverse effects on her health, the need to consider drug treatment, and the importance of avoiding sharing needles to prevent transmission of HIV and other infectious diseases (e.g., Hepatitis B and Hepatitis C).

→ Prior to obtaining a patient's medical records, discuss with her the need for confirmation of her HIV status and how this can be obtained.
  ■ In many locations, a special consent for disclosure of HIV test results must be signed by the patient in addition to standard medical record release forms.
  ■ Furthermore, informed consent of a patient (in some states this is written consent) regarding HIV testing is required prior to obtaining such tests.

  ■ Disclosure of HIV test results should involve only the patient and the provider or counselor who obtained the test.
  ■ Ideally, the patient should return to the provider or counselor to receive her results in person and to receive follow-up counseling regarding implication(s) of the results (including repeat testing in at-risk patients with ongoing high-risk behaviors).

→ Advise the patient regarding any potential short-term or long-term side effects associated with medications and when immediate evaluation may be indicated.

→ Advise the patient that she should not donate blood products or consent to organ donation.

→ Advise the patient not to share personal hygiene implements that could be contaminated with blood (e.g., toothbrush, razors).

→ Teach the patient ways to reduce the risk of becoming infected with toxoplasmosis—including properly cooking meat and, if the patient has a cat, recommending that another household member change the litter box.
  ■ If the patient lives alone and must change the litter box, she should wear a mask and use disposable gloves during the task and thoroughly wash her hands once done.

→ Educate reproductive-age women who are sexually active and who want to postpone childbearing about the need to combine effective STD and contraceptive methods.
  ■ Currently there are limited data available regarding the various contraceptive methods and the impact on HIV disease and/or transmission.
  ■ Most methods are acceptable if combined with effective STD prevention strategies.
    • Intrauterine devices are not recommended because of the risk of uterine infections associated with their use (Minkoff 1991; Rompalo, Anderson, and Quinn 1992).

→ An HIV-positive woman considering pregnancy should be referred to an obstetrician or perinatologist experienced in the care of HIV-positive pregnant women for an in-depth presentation of current information.
  ■ It is imperative to present current information regarding the effects of pregnancy on HIV disease progression, the effects of HIV infection on pregnancy outcome, perinatal transmission rates, interventions that reduce perinatal

transmission rates (e.g., use of ZDV during antepartum, intrapartum, and neonatal periods), therapeutic interventions for the woman during pregnancy, care of an HIV-positive infant, and clinical trials available to the woman and her infant.

→ Advise the woman regarding the need to disclose her HIV status to other medical providers so that appropriate therapy for any illness or condition can be prescribed.

→ Educate the patient about community resources available to her for psychosocial support (e.g., HIV-specific women's groups, legal counseling, financial aid).

→ Educate the patient about clinical trials that may be available to her.
  ▪ For information about NIH- and FDA-approved efficacy trials call the AIDS Clinical Trials Information Service at 800-TRIALS-A (800-874-2572).

FOLLOW-UP

→ See "Consultation" section.

→ Recommend follow-up evaluation of the asymptomatic HIV-positive woman with a CD4 count greater than $600/mm^3$ is every six months for an HIV-specific evaluation (including laboratory tests).
  ▪ See "Diagnostic Tests" section for recommendations for additional follow-up tests and evaluations.

→ A patient with any symptoms of a possible complication or side effect(s) of a medication should return for evaluation as soon as possible.

→ An AIDS diagnosis is a reportable condition with notification of the local public health department mandated by law. Contact the local public health department for the appropriate forms and the procedure(s) to follow.

→ Document in progress notes and problem list (as appropriate and without breaching patient confidentiality).

Maureen T. Shannon, C.N.M., F.N.P., M.S.

11-E

Lyme Disease

Lyme disease is a tick-borne systemic illness that can affect the skin, heart, joints, and nervous system, resulting in clinical manifestations that may persist for years. The disease was identified in 1977 in Lyme, Connecticut, because of a cluster of children in the area who were initially thought to have juvenile rheumatoid arthritis (RA).

Investigation into clusters of patients with similar symptoms revealed physical findings implicating an arthropod-borne infectious disease. It was not until 1982 that the organism responsible for the illness was identified. At that time, a previously unrecognized spirochete, now called *Borrelia burgdorferi*, was isolated and later recovered from patients with Lyme disease in the United States and patients with similar disorders in Europe (Buchstein and Gardner 1991; Steere 1989).

Since the identification of Lyme disease and the pathogen responsible for it, 43 states have reported cases. Among these states, nine (New York, New Jersey, Connecticut, Massachusetts, Rhode Island, Pennsylvania, Wisconsin, Minnesota, and California) have reported more than 90 percent of cases (Buchstein and Gardner 1991; Rahn and Malawista 1991; Steere 1989).

Ixodes ticks are the vectors of Lyme disease, with various types responsible for transmission of the spirochete in different regions of the United States and Europe. In the United States, the eastern deer tick, *Ixodes dammini*, is the vector in the Northeast and Midwest; the western black-legged tick, *Ixodes pacificus*, is the vector along the West Coast; and the black-legged tick, *Ixodes scapularis* is the vector responsible for transmission in the Southeast.

Infection rates among *Ixodes* ticks vary among sites, and knowledge of these rates can be beneficial when assessing the possibility of Lyme disease in a patient presenting with a tick bite. In Connecticut, infection among *I. dammini* ticks has been reported to be between 10 percent to 35 percent; in some areas of New York (e.g., Shelter Island) the infection rate is over 50 percent; and along the West Coast the infection rate for *I. pacificus* ticks is between one percent to three percent.

The major hosts for vectors are the white-footed mouse, during the larval and nymph stages, and the white-tailed deer during the tick's adult life. However, ticks have been found in several other types of wild animals and birds. Although clinical Lyme disease has been observed in domestic animals (e.g., dogs, cattle, horses), pet ownership has not demonstrated any increased risk of infection (Buchstein and Gardner 1991).

The incidence of Lyme disease has a temporal pattern, with the majority of cases reported during summer months, followed by spring and autumn months, respectively. This temporal pattern of reported cases is directly related to the two-year life cycle of the tick. During each stage of the life cycle (e.g., larval, nymph, and adult stages) the tick must feed once. The feeding times for the tick vary according to its stage of development, with larvae feeding once between July and September, nymphs feeding during May to July, and adults feeding during autumn (Steere 1989). It is during these feedings that the tick acquires the spirochete from an infected host and may transmit the spirochete to uninfected hosts.

In vitro and animal studies have demonstrated that for the spirochete to be transmitted effectively from the infected tick to a host, the tick must remain attached for at least 24 hours. Because larvae and nymphs are small and do not produce pain when biting a host—thereby remaining unnoticed—the highest incidence of transmission and reported cases of Lyme disease is noted during the months that the immature ticks, particularly nymphs, are feeding (e.g., spring through summer).

Asymptomatic infection is reportedly common, although the long-term sequelae associated with asymptomatic infection is unknown (Buchstein and Gardner 1991). However, in many instances, once a person has been bitten by an infected tick, a broad spectrum of clinical manifestations reflecting multisystem involvement can occur.

As is common with other types of spirochetal diseases (e.g., syphilis), the complex, protean nature of this illness has required the classification of the disease process into various stages as a means of establishing guidelines for therapeutic interventions for each stage of Lyme disease (see **Table 11E.1, Lyme Disease National Surveillance Case Definition**). Development of the characteristic skin lesion associated with Lyme disease—erythema chronica migrans—at the site of the tick's attachment, usually develops in 70 percent of persons two to 30 days after the tick bite (Buchstein and Gardner 1991; Kantor 1994; Steere 1989) and is classified as *stage 1 disease*. Regional lymphadenopathy also occurs in stage 1 disease.

Stage 2 disease reflects the hematological and lymphatic spread of the spirochete, resulting in disseminated infection with clinical manifestations ranging from mild to severe multisystem problems. These include musculoskeletal, dermatological, neurological, cardiac, lymphatic, ocular, gastrointestinal, genitourinary, and constitutional symptoms. Stage 2 disease usually occurs within a few days to weeks after inoculation of the spirochete.

Stage 3 disease indicates late, persistent infection with a range of symptoms developing months to several years after the initial stage of the infection. The most common symptoms reported during this stage involve musculoskeletal problems (e.g., arthritis), neurological problems (e.g., chronic encephalomyelitis, chronic axonal polyradiculopathy), ocular problems (e.g., keratitis), dermatological problems (e.g., acrodermatitis chronica atro-

---

Table 11E.1. LYME DISEASE NATIONAL SURVEILLANCE CASE DEFINITION*

Lyme disease is a systemic, tick-borne disease with protean manifestations, including dermatological, rheumatological, neurological, and cardiac abnormalities. The best clinical marker for the disease is the initial skin lesion, erythema migrans, that occurs in 60 percent to 80 percent of patients.

Case definition for the national surveillance of Lyme disease:
1. A person with erythema migrans, *or*
2. A person with at least one late manifestation and laboratory confirmation of infection.

General definitions:
1. Erythema migrans: For purposes of surveillance, erythema migrans is a skin lesion that typically begins as a red macule or papule and expands over a period of days or weeks to form a large, round lesion, often with partial central clearing. To be considered to be erythema migrans, a solitary lesion must measure at least 5 cm. Secondary lesions may also occur. Annular erythematous lesions developing within several hours of a tick bite represent hypersensitivity reactions and do not qualify as erythema migrans. In most patients, the expanding erythema migrans lesion is accompanied by other acute symptoms, particularly fatigue, fever, headache, mildly stiff neck, arthralgias, and myalgias. These symptoms are typically intermittent. The diagnosis of erythema migrans must be made by a physician. Laboratory confirmation is recommended for patients with no known exposure.
2. Late manifestations: These manifestations include any of the following *when an alternate explanation is not found:*
   a. Musculoskeletal system: Recurrent, brief attacks (lasting weeks or months) of objective joint swelling in one or a few joints sometimes followed by chronic arthritis in one or a few joints. Manifestations that are not considered to be criteria for diagnosis include chronic progressive arthritis that is not preceded by brief attacks and chronic symmetric polyarthritis. Additionally, arthralgias, myalgias, or fibromyalgia syndromes alone are not accepted as criteria for musculoskeletal involvement.
   b. Nervous system: Lymphocytic meningitis, cranial neuritis, particularly facial palsy (may be bilateral), radiculoneuropathy, or, rarely, encephalomyelitis alone or in combination. Encephalomyelitis must be confirmed with evidence of antibody production against *Borrelia burgdorferi* in the cerebrospinal fluid, shown by a higher titer of antibody in the cerebrospinal fluid than in the serum. Headache, fatigue, paresthesias, or mildly stiff neck alone are not accepted as criteria for neurological involvement.
   c. Cardiovascular system: Acute-onset, high-grade (second- or third-degree) atrioventricular conduction defects that resolve in days to weeks and are sometimes associated with myocarditis. Palpitations, bradycardia, bundle-branch block, or myocarditis alone are not accepted as criteria for cardiovascular involvement.
3. Exposure: Exposure is defined as having been in wooded, brushy, or grassy areas (potential tick habitats) in an endemic county not more than 30 days before the onset of erythema migrans. A history of tick bite is not required.
4. Endemic county: A county in which at least two definite cases have been previously acquired or in which a tick vector has been shown to be infected with *B. burgdorferi*.
5. Laboratory confirmation: Laboratory confirmation of infection with *B. burgdorferi* is established when a laboratory isolates the spirochete from tissue or body fluid, detects diagnostic levels of immunoglobulin M or immunoglobulin G antibodies to the spirochete in the serum or the cerebrospinal fluid, or detects an important change in antibody levels in paired acute and convalescent serum samples. States may determine the criteria for laboratory confirmation and diagnostic levels of antibody. Syphilis and other known biological causes of false positive serological test results should be excluded when laboratory confirmation is based on serological testing alone.

*This epidemiological case definition is intended for surveillance purposes only.

Source: Reprinted with permission from Rahn, D.W., and Malawista, S.E. 1991. Lyme disease: Recommendations for diagnosis and treatment. *Annals of Internal Medicine* 114(6):473.

phicans), and generalized fatigue (Buchstein and Gardner 1991; Kantor 1994; Logigian, Kaplan, and Steere 1990; Rahn and Malawista 1991; Steere 1989).

Although very rare, congenital infection associated with adverse fetal/neonatal outcomes (e.g., congenital cardiac malformations, encephalitis) has been reported in women who had experienced Lyme borreliosis during pregnancy (Markowitz et al. 1986; Schlesinger et al. 1985; Weber et al. 1988). Despite the extensive morbidity associated with Lyme disease, there is a very low mortality rate observed.

DATABASE

SUBJECTIVE

→ Patients may be asymptomatic or report one or more of the symptoms as follows.

Stage 1 Disease

→ Symptoms usually occur two to 30 days after the tick bite and include:
- development of erythema migrans lesion:
  - an erythematous (color ranging from pink to violaceous), annular plaque with a central area of clearing at the site of the tick bite (most commonly noted in the axilla, thigh, or groin).
  - usually the lesion begins two to 20 days after inoculation and resolves in three to four weeks.
  - it is observed in 50 percent to 70 percent of patients and is pathognomonic of Lyme disease.
  - atypical presentations include vesicular, pruritic, or scaling lesions with indurated centers (Buchstein and Gardner 1991).
- fever.
- chills.
- malaise.
- myalgia.

Stage 2 Disease

→ Symptoms may develop within days to weeks after the tick bite.

→ Constitutional symptoms include:
- severe fatigue.
- severe malaise.

→ Dermatological manifestations include:
- secondary annular lesions similar to the initial lesion but smaller in size.
- malar rash.
- diffuse erythema or urticaria.
- lymphocytoma:

- a small, erythematous plaque or nodule that develops on the nipple in adults and on the ear in children.
  - Very rare, occurring in only one percent of patients.
  - Primarily seen in European populations.

→ Neurological manifestations including:
- headache (often intermittent).
- stiff neck (usually mild).
- Bell's palsy symptoms—pain, paralysis of face in cranial nerve VII or X distribution.
- pain along spinal nerve distribution (radiculoneuritis).

→ Musculoskeletal manifestations include:
- migratory pain in joints, tendons, muscles, bursae, or bones.
- swollen, red joints (usually episodes are transient and brief).

→ Lymphatic system manifestations including:
- regional and/or generalized lymphadenopathy.
- splenomegaly.

→ Cardiac manifestations including:
- shortness of breath and dyspnea on exertion in patients with myocarditis, pericarditis, or severe heart block.
- pleural pain—pericardial or substernal chest pain which may radiate to the neck, shoulders, back, or epigastrium.

→ Ocular manifestations include:
- conjunctival erythema and discharge.
- visual disturbances if severe ocular disease (e.g., in cases of iritis, retinal hemorrhage or detachment, panophthalmitis).

→ Gastrointestinal manifestations include:
- mild and/or recurrent signs and symptoms of hepatitis (see **Hepatitis—Viral** Protocol).

→ Respiratory manifestations include:
- sore throat.
- nonproductive cough.
- signs and symptoms of respiratory distress in cases of adult respiratory distress syndrome (very rare).

Stage 3 Disease

→ Symptoms may appear months to several years after a tick bite.
- Constitutional manifestations including chronic fatigue.
- Dermatological manifestations including:
  - development of acrodermatitis chronica.

- atrophicans lesions characterized by the gradual swelling and bluish-red to violaceous discoloration of a distal extremity.
  –Later the lesions become atrophic and sclerotic.
- Musculoskeletal manifestations including:
  - swollen, erythematous, warm, painful joints (usually the knee) noted chronically or intermittently.
- Neurological manifestations including:
  - headache—mild to severe, episodic without associated auras.
  - hypersomnia.
  - problems with memory or thinking clearly.
  - tingling, burning, shooting pains in the extremities or trunk.
  - pain in the cervical, thoracic, or lumbosacral area of the spine.
  - progressive stiffness, weakness of the extremities.
  - urinary frequency, urgency, and incontinence.

OBJECTIVE

→ Patient may exhibit one or more of the following physical findings depending upon the stage of Lyme disease:

Stage 1 Disease
- temperature may be slightly elevated.
- erythema migrans lesion may be observed at site of tick bite (see "Subjective" section for description).
- palpable enlarged lymph node(s) in area of tick bite.

Stage 2 Disease
- vital signs may reflect an irregular heart rate (if heart block) and increased respiratory rate (if myocarditis, pericarditis, or pancarditis).
- dermatological physical findings may be present and include:
  - small, discrete, erythematous annular plaque-like lesions (similar to erythema migrans lesion) on body.
  - small reddish nodule or plaque on nipple (lymphocytoma).
  - erythematous eruption over cheekbones.
  - diffuse erythema.
→ Neurological physical findings may be present and include:
  - nuchal rigidity.
  - diminished or absent facial movement in the distribution of cranial nerves VII and X.

- diminished sensation to light touch or pinprick in affected areas.
- hyperreflexia.
- unsteady or uneven gait.
- subtle evidence of memory problems.
→ Musculoskeletal physical findings may be present and include:
  - muscle weakness.
  - erythematous, edematous joints which are tender to palpation.
→ Cardiac physical findings may be present and include:
  - irregular heart rate with the apical pulse rate greater than peripheral pulses (in atrio-ventricular nodal heart block).
  - tachycardia.
  - gallop rhythm (in myocarditis).
  - pericardial friction rub (in pericarditis).
→ Ocular physical findings may be present and consistent with conjunctivitis, keratitis, iritis, or panophthalmitis (see **Opthalmalogical Disorders** Protocol).
→ Gastrointestinal physical findings may be present and consistent with hepatitis (see **Hepatitis—Viral** Protocol).
→ Respiratory physical findings may be present and include:
  - tachypnea (if myocarditis, pericarditis, or pancarditis).
  - auscultation of lungs usually WNL but may reveal crackles at the bases if congestive heart failure associated with severe myocarditis.

Stage 3 Disease
→ Vital signs will be WNL.
→ Dermatological physical findings may include:
  - evidence of acrodermatitis chronica atrophicans:
    - edematous, doughy, bluish-red to violaceous colored extremities; or atrophic, sclerotic lesions of the extremities.
→ Musculoskeletal physical findings may include:
  - muscular weakness in affected extremities.
  - edematous, erythematous, tender joints (usually knee joints).
  - evidence of subluxations inferior to lesions of acrodermatitis chronica atrophicans.
→ Neurological physical findings may include:
  - evidence of memory impairment upon neurological evaluation.

- evidence of depression upon psychiatric evaluation.
- diminished sensation to light touch or pinprick.
- hyporeflexia or hyperreflexia with ankle clonus and Babinski signs.
- mild weakness of the extremities.
- unsteady or uneven gait.

→ Ocular physical findings may be present and consistent with evidence of keratitis (see **Keratitis** Protocol).

ASSESSMENT

→ Lyme disease (Stage 1, 2, or 3)

→ R/O chronic fatigue syndrome

→ R/O fibromyalgia

→ R/O other spirochetal diseases (e.g., syphilis, Rocky Mountain spotted fever)

→ R/O neurological disease (e.g., multiple sclerosis)

→ R/O autoimmune disease

→ R/O cardiac disease

→ R/O other infectious disease (e.g., HIV infection)

PLAN

DIAGNOSTIC TESTS

→ The diagnosis of Lyme disease is made *primarily* on clinical manifestations and secondarily on the basis of laboratory data.

- Demonstration of the spirochete by culture or direct visualization is difficult except when biopsy of skin lesions is performed.
- Therefore, the most practical approach to laboratory confirmation is through the utilization of antibody titers.
- However, the lack of standardization among laboratories, the ablation of antibody titers in patients who receive antibiotic therapy early in the disease, and the incidence of both false positive and false negative results makes confirmation of the diagnosis difficult in some situations (Buchstein and Gardner 1991; Dattwyler et al. 1988; Rahn and Malawista 1991; Steere 1989).

→ Serology tests:
- serum antibody titers:
  • IgM antibody against 41kd antigen (a protein present on all strains of the pathogen) begins to rise between 2 to 4 weeks after the initial infection but has cross reactivity with other spirochetal antigens (e.g., syphilis, Rocky Mountain spotted fever, autoimmune disease).
  • IgM antibody peaks and then begins to decline at between 6 to 8 weeks after initial infection. IgM antibody to lower molecular weight antigens (surface proteins) begins to increase in some patients later in the disease process (Buchstein and Gardner 1991; Steere 1989).
  • IgG antibody titer increase gradually occurs weeks to months after initial infection.
- cerebrospinal fluid antibody titers:
  • positive IgM and/or IgG antibody titers are strong evidence of spirochetal infection of the central nervous system (Logigian, Kaplan, and Steere 1990; Rahn and Malawista 1991).
- immunoblot testing (e.g., Western Blot):
  • positive immunoblot testing after an equivocal or suspected false positive result may be indicative of disease; a positive result may not be demonstrated until several months after initial infection (Rahn and Malawista 1991).
- polymerase chain reaction (PCR):
  • currently under investigation for use in identification of spirochetal DNA in patient tissue and fluids, as well as in ticks; not available for clinical use at this time (Rahn and Malawista 1991).

→ Other tests (e.g., electrophysiological, electrocardiogram) may be indicated depending upon systemic manifestations of the disease and should be ordered in consultation with a physician.

TREATMENT/MANAGEMENT

→ Essential to the treatment of the patient is the removal of the tick if still present. (It is important to remember that these ticks are immature and, therefore, smaller than adult ticks.)

- The best means of doing this is by mechanical removal of the head of the tick (i.e., using tweezers) (see "Patient Education" section).
- If removal of the tick occurs within 24 hours after attachment, the likelihood of spirochete transmission is significantly reduced.

→ Antibiotic therapy for the treatment of Lyme disease is based on clinical manifestations and includes the use of oral and/or parenteral antibiotics.

- If parenteral therapy is indicated, the patient should be referred to a physician.

- The following are recommended regimens for the treatment of Lyme disease at various stages (Rahn and Malawista 1991; Steere 1989):
  - early disease (e.g., erythema migrans) without systemic involvement:
    - doxycycline (Vibramycin®) 100 mg p.o. BID for 10 to 21 days
      OR
    - amoxicillin 500 mg p.o. TID for 10 to 21 days
      OR
    - erythromycin (E-Mycin®, Ery Tab®) 250 mg p.o. QID for 10 to 21 days (less effective than doxycycline or amoxicillin).
  - cardiac disease:
  - first-degree heart block (PR interval <0.3 sec):
    - doxycycline (Vibramycin®) 100 mg p.o. BID for 14 to 21 days
      OR
    - amoxicillin 500 mg p.o. TID for 14 to 21 days.
  - high-degree heart block and/or other cardiac disease:
    - ceftriaxone (Rocephin®) 2 g I.V. every day for 14 days
      OR
    - penicillin G 20 mu I.V. every 4 hours for 14 days.
- Neurological disease:
  - Bell's palsy without evidence of other neurological disease (e.g., meningitis)—oral antibiotic therapy with doxycycline or amoxicillin as listed above under early disease.
  - general neurological disease:
    - parenteral antibiotic therapy with ceftriaxone or penicillin G as listed above.
    - alternative therapy if allergy to ceftriaxone (Rocephin®) or penicillin includes doxycycline (Vibramycin®) 100 mg p.o. BID for 30 days
      OR
    - chloramphenicol (Chloromycetin®) 250 mg I.V. QID for 14 days.
- Lyme arthritis (intermittent or chronic):
  - doxycycline (Vibramycin®) 100 mg p.o. BID for 30 days
    OR
  - amoxicillin 500 mg p.o. TID for 30 days
    OR
  - ceftriaxone (Rocephin®) 2 g I.V. every day for 14 days
    OR

- penicillin G 20 mu I.V. every 4 hours for 14 days.
- Pregnant women:
  - asymptomatic seropositive—no treatment indicated.
  - early, localized infection—amoxicillin 500 mg p.o. for 21 days.
  - disseminated early disease or any manifestation of late disease—penicillin G 20 mu I.V. every day for 14 to 21 days.
  NOTE: Jarisch-Herxheimer reaction can occur in patients receiving antibiotic therapy for Lyme disease (see **Syphilis** Protocol for a description of this reaction).
→ The use of prophylactic antibiotics for the treatment of deer-tick bites without evidence of Lyme disease (e.g., erythema migrans) currently is not recommended (Rahn and Malawista 1991; Shapiro et al. 1992).
→ Symptomatic treatment may be indicated and include the use of analgesics (i.e., NSAIDs) and bed rest at various stages of the disease. The use of corticosteroids is not recommended in the treatment of Lyme disease.

CONSULTATION

→ Consultation with a physician is indicated in all cases of suspected disseminated or late-stage Lyme disease, in pregnant women with evidence of Lyme disease, or in any patient with symptoms indicating the need for hospitalization.

→ As needed for prescription(s).

PATIENT EDUCATION

→ Educate the patient about Lyme disease including its cause, clinical course, possible complications, treatment options, and indicated follow-up.

→ If the patient is pregnant, discuss possible perinatal complications, but reassure her these are rare.

→ Instruct the patient in ways to reduce exposure to ticks including:
- avoiding tick habitats (e.g., tall grass, bushes, forests) during seasons when tick activity is at its peak.
- wearing clothing that reduces tick exposure (e.g., tightly woven, light-colored, long-sleeved shirts and long pants tucked into socks; hats; closed shoes).

■ use of tick repellent as indicated (advise patient to use as directed and to wash off the repellent as soon as possible after outdoor activity).
  • Clothing pesticide (e.g., permethrin) may be used on trouser legs and socks.
  • If the patient has outdoor pet(s), advise inspecting the pet(s) frequently for ticks and use anti-tick collars and baths as indicated.

→ Educate the patient about the importance of checking for and removing ticks immediately once they are discovered as a means of reducing transmission of spirochetes.

■ Instruct the patient in the proper removal of ticks (e.g., grasping the head of the tick, not the body, with a tweezer and exerting steady upward pressure to remove it).
■ Advise the patient not to attempt to burn or suffocate the tick prior to removal. Once the tick is removed, instruct the patient to cleanse the area with soap and water.

FOLLOW-UP

→ See "Consultation" section.
→ Document in progress notes and problem list.

11-F

Measles (Rubeola)

Measles (rubeola) is an acute systemic illness caused by one of the paramyxoviruses. It usually occurs in pre-school-age children, but outbreaks in adolescent and adult populations have been documented. From 1989 to 1991, a major increase in measles cases was reported in the United States (American Academy of Pediatrics 1994b; CDC 1992a).

Although measles infection most often is associated with a lack of or incomplete immunization, a small percentage of cases has been reported in patients with apparently adequate immunization histories (CDC 1992a). An atypical measles syndrome has been reported in adults and adolescents who received inactivated measles vaccine or live measles vaccine before one year of age. These individuals develop a hypersensitivity rather than protective immunity to measles and, when infected by the measles virus, experience a severe systemic illness that can be fatal (Shandera and Gill 1994).

Measles is transmitted by direct exposure to infectious droplets or, less frequently, by airborne spread, and is contagious three to five days prior to the eruption of the acute exanthem (American Academy of Pediatrics 1994b). Patients remain contagious for four days after the appearance of the exanthem; however, immunocompromised patients may remain contagious for the duration of the illness due to prolonged viral excretion in respiratory droplets (American Academy of Pediatrics 1994b). The incubation period is eight to 12 days from exposure to the onset of prodromal symptoms.

Complications associated with measles infection include cervical adenitis, otitis media, pneumonia, encephalitis (0.1 percent to 0.2 percent incidence) and death (0.2 percent in children in the United States) (CDC 1992a; American Academy of Pediatrics 1994b;

Shandera and Gill 1994). Highest complication rates are reported in children younger than five years of age, but complications have been noted in adolescents and adults as well (CDC 1992a).

In immunosuppressed individuals, measles infection can result in an acute encephalitis which may progress from seizures and neurological deficits to stupor and death (Shandera 1993). An extremely rare complication of measles infection is sub-acute sclerosing panencephalitis (SSPE). SSPE is a progressive, degenerative central nervous system disease resulting from persistent measles virus infection. SSPE is characterized by intellectual and behavioral deterioration and convulsions (American Academy of Pediatrics 1994b; Shandera and Gill 1994). SSPE usually develops several years after the initial measles infection and is not contagious (American Academy of Pediatrics 1994b).

DATABASE

SUBJECTIVE

→ Prodrome symptoms may include:
- fever (often 40°C/104°F or higher).
- cough (non-productive, persistent).
- coryza (rhinorrhea, nasal congestion, sneezing, pharyngitis).
- eye discharge, erythema.
- photosensitivity.

→ Symptoms may include:
- Koplik's spots (pathognomonic of measles):
  - tiny, white, crystal-like lesions on the buccal mucosa, inner conjunctiva, or vagina occurring approximately two days before the rash and remaining for one to four days.

- eruption of confluent erythematous irregular maculopapular rash beginning on the face and extending to the trunk and then the extremities; develops three to four days after onset of prodrome symptoms.
- with atypical measles, patients reporting a high fever, arthalgias, headache, abdominal pain, a rash without Koplik's spots, and a history of measles vaccination.

OBJECTIVE

Classic Measles

→ Patients may present with:
- elevated temperature (may be 40°C/104°F or higher).
- erythematous conjunctiva with or without discharge.
- pharyngeal edema.
- tonsillar exudate (usually yellow).
- white coating on dorsum of tongue with erythema of margins and tip.
- Koplik's spots on buccal mucosa, inner conjunctival folds.
- generalized lymphadenopathy.
- erythematous, irregular maculopapular rash with distinctive eruptive pattern:
  - first day, rash begins on face; second day, facial eruption begins to coalesce and eruption begins on trunk; third day, facial rash fades, trunk eruption coalesces, and rash begins on extremities.
  - after the third day, rash continues to fade, reversing the pattern in which it appeared, with slight desquamation often observed (Shandera and Gill 1994).
- after rash subsides, hyperpigmentation observed in severe cases or in fair-skinned patients.

Atypical Measles (Shandera and Gill 1994)

→ Patient may present with:
- elevated temperature.
- maculopapular, hemorrhagic rash:
  - may be confluent.
  - usually starts with extremities and progresses to trunk.
- absence of Koplik's spots.
- tenderness to abdominal palpation may be present.
- decreased breath sounds (if coexistent pleural effusion).

ASSESSMENT

→ Measles (rubeola)
→ R/O typical measles
→ R/O rubella
→ R/O mononucleosis
→ R/O scarlet fever (Group A beta-hemolytic streptococcus)
→ R/O drug reaction

PLAN

DIAGNOSTIC TESTS

→ CBC with differential—leukopenia may be present.
→ Urinalysis—proteinuria is present.
→ Immunoglobulin testing (acute and convalescent serum antibody titers):
- acute sera should be obtained after appearance of the rash with the convalescent titer obtained 2 to 4 weeks later.
  - Usually a fourfold increase in titer is observed.
- a single specimen can be obtained and sent for the presence of measles-specific IgM antibody, but the specimen must not be taken during the first 2 days of the rash or 30 to 60 days after the onset of the rash.
  - If specimens are obtained during these times, a false negative IgM result will occur.
→ SSPE—high titers of measles antibody may be demonstrated in cerebrospinal fluid and serum.
→ Presence of measles in tissue culture is diagnostic; however, viral isolation usually is not available and is technically difficult to perform (American Academy of Pediatrics 1994b).
→ Chest x-ray may reveal evidence of pneumonia or pleural effusion in patients with these complications.

TREATMENT/MANAGEMENT

→ Respiratory isolation of the patient for 4 days after the onset of the rash will reduce transmission to other susceptible individuals.
- Immunocompromised patients should maintain respiratory isolation for the duration of the illness (American Academy of Pediatrics 1994b).
→ Bed rest, increased fluids, and acetaminophen as needed should be recommended for relief of fever.

→ No antiviral medication is available for treatment of measles infection.

→ Initiate appropriate antibiotic therapy for specific secondary bacterial infections (e.g., otitis media, pneumonia).

→ Treatment of neurological complications (e.g., encephalitis, SSPE) requires hospitalization and is managed by the consulting physician.

→ If susceptible individuals have known exposure to measles, administration of the live-virus vaccine within 72 hours of exposure can provide protection.

- Obtain informed consent prior to immunization administration.

- If susceptible individuals report an exposure beyond 72 hours but within 6 days of contact, administration of immunoglobulin 0.25 mg/kg can help prevent clinical illness.

    • Active immunization with live measles-virus vaccine is recommended 3 months later (American Academy of Pediatrics 1994b). **NOTE:** If susceptible individuals have not received immunizations for mumps or rubella, consider vaccination with measles, mumps, and rubella live vaccine (MMR) (0.5 ml) unless contraindicated (i.e., pregnant women, women who are considering pregnancy within 3 months after vaccination). Live measles vaccine should not be given to patients with significant immunocompromise. MMR may be given to HIV-infected patients (see **Human Immunodeficiency Virus [HIV]** Protocol). Mumps vaccine is contraindicated in patients with a history of anaphylaxis to eggs or neomycin.

CONSULTATION

→ Indicated for patients suspected of having atypical measles infection and/or patients with possible serious complications (e.g., pneumonia, encephalitis).

→ As needed for prescription(s).

PATIENT EDUCATION

→ Discuss the communicability, symptomatic treatment, need for isolation (when appropriate), and possible complications of measles infection. Advise the patient to call or return to the office if signs/symptoms of complications develop.

→ Educate the patient about the possible need for immunizing family members and/or close contacts.

- Determination of susceptible close contacts and appropriate interventions could reduce infection and/or clinical illness.

FOLLOW-UP

→ At three months, immunize with live measles-virus vaccine those susceptible patients who received gamma globulin administration after exposure to measles.

→ If confirmation of measles diagnosis is desired, patients with suspected measles should have a measles-specific IgM antibody test drawn between three days and 30 to 60 days after the onset of the rash.

→ Document in progress notes and problem list.

11-G

Mononucleosis

Infectious mononucleosis is an acute infectious disease caused by the Epstein-Barr virus (EBV), a herpes virus. Cytomegalovirus (CMV) infection also can cause a similar infectious mononucleosis and is most commonly observed in adolescents and young adults between the ages of 10 years and 35 years.

Although the mode of transmission is not fully understood, it usually requires close contact with a person shedding the virus, probably through infectious oropharyngeal secretions. Transmission through blood transfusions has been reported but occurs rarely (American Academy of Pediatrics 1994a). A person with infectious mononucleosis can have viral shedding for several months after the acute clinical phase of the disease. The incubation period is estimated to be five to 50 days (American Academy of Pediatrics 1994a; Shandera and Gill 1994).

The clinical manifestations of infectious mononucleosis are extremely variable, ranging from asymptomatic infection to severe infection which can result in death. Recovery from the acute infection may take three weeks to two months. Complication rates range between 2.5 percent to 5 percent in some populations (Cheeseman 1988) and include splenic rupture, hemolytic anemia, immune thrombocytopenia, cardiac complications (e.g., heart block, pericarditis), pneumonia, encephalitis, meningitis, and Guillain-Barré syndrome.

A syndrome called chronic active mononucleosis also has been reported. It is characterized by persistent or recurrent fatigue, fever, headache, hepatitis, pharyngitis, and depression. A patient with this syndrome must have experienced these symptoms for at least one year and have a previous history of infectious mononucleosis and an absence of other underlying causes of chronic infection (Anderson and Ernberg 1988; Shandera 1993).

DATABASE

SUBJECTIVE

→ Patient may be asymptomatic or may report one or more of the following:
- fever.
- pharyngitis.
- malaise.
- headache.
- nausea.
- vomiting.
- anorexia.
- myalgia.
- lymphadenopathy.
- jaundice.

→ If myocardial involvement, the patient may report chest pain or dyspnea.

→ In CNS involvement, the patient may report photophobia, stiff neck, or neuritis.

OBJECTIVE

→ Physical examination may reveal one or more of the following:
- elevated temperature.
- palpable lymph nodes, particularly in the posterior cervical chain.
- erythematous posterior pharynx/tonsils with or without exudate.
- palatal petechiae.
- palpebral edema.
- maculopapular or petechial rash (noted in 15 percent of patients with mononucleosis; also noted in more than 90 percent of patients with

mononucleosis who have taken ampicillin during
the infection).
- jaundice (if hepatitis).
- hepatosplenomegaly.
- nuchal rigidity, photosensitivity in patients with
CNS involvement.

ASSESSMENT

→ Acute infectious mononucleosis

→ R/O acute pharyngitis

→ R/O CMV infection

→ R/O acute hepatitis

→ R/O thrombocytopenia

→ R/O rubella

→ R/O toxoplasmosis

→ R/O hemolytic anemia

→ R/O pneumonia

→ R/O encephalitis, meningitis

→ R/O myocarditis

→ R/O influenza

→ R/O other viral syndromes

PLAN

DIAGNOSTIC TESTS

→ CBC:
  - decreased hematocrit if anti-i antibodies.
    present.
→ Differential:
  - decreased granulocytes, increased leukocytes
    secondary to increased lymphocytes with many
    atypical lymphocytes noted.
→ Platelet count:
  - decreased if associated thrombocytopenia.
→ Monospot test:
  - usually becomes positive by the fourth week
    after clinical manifestations.
→ Heterophile antibody test:
  - usually becomes positive by the fourth week
    after clinical manifestations.
  - if heterophile antibody test is negative, consider
    testing for other viral pathogens (e.g.,
    cytomegalovirus).
→ Serum EBV antibody testing (American Academy
  of Pediatrics 1994a):
  - antibody to viral capsid antigen IgG (Anti-VCA
    IgG) titers rise rapidly early after onset of
    infection and remain elevated for long periods.

Because of this, paired sera for anti-VCA IgG
may not be helpful in determining acute
mononucleosis infection.
- a rise in antibody against VCA IgM is observed
  during acute illness.
- a rise in antibody titer against early antigen
  indicates recent infection.
- antibody against EBV nuclear antigen is not
  detected until 3 to 4 weeks after the onset of
  infection and excludes recent infection when
  present.
→ Liver function tests (e.g., ALT, AST) will be
  elevated when hepatitis is present.
→ Cerebrospinal fluid will demonstrate increased
  pressure, abnormal lymphocytes, and protein if
  there is CNS involvement.
→ Electrocardiogram may demonstrate abnormal T-
  waves and prolonged PR intervals if there is
  myocardial involvement.

TREATMENT/MANAGEMENT

→ Symptomatic treatment of infectious mononucleosis includes rest and the use of analgesics
  and antipyretics (e.g., acetaminophen, NSAIDs)
  as needed for the relief of fever, myalgia, and
  pharyngitis.
  - Warm saline gargles (i.e., 1 tsp. salt in 8 oz.
    warm water) TID-QID may further relieve
    pharyngitis symptoms.
→ Corticosteroid therapy can be initiated in severely
  ill patients with enlarged lymphoid tissue
  (possibly causing airway obstruction), severe
  thrombocytopenia, or autoimmune hemolytic
  anemia.
  - Consultation with a physician is indicated in
    such cases.
→ Isolation of patients with mononucleosis is not
  necessary.

CONSULTATION

→ Physician consultation and management is
  indicated in patients with severe complications
  associated with mononucleosis (e.g., severe
  thrombocytopenia, myocardial involvement, CNS
  involvement).
→ As needed for prescription(s).

PATIENT EDUCATION

→ Educate the patient about infectious
  mononucleosis including the cause, clinical
  course, treatment, possible method of

transmission and infectivity, and possible complications. Reassure the patient that isolation is not necessary.

→ Advise the patient not to donate blood for several months after infection because of the possibility of transmission via blood transfusions.

FOLLOW-UP

→ In complicated cases, follow-up is on recommendation of the consulting physician.

→ Document in progress notes and problem list.

Maureen T. Shannon, C.N.M., F.N.P., M.S.

11-H

Mumps

Mumps, an infectious disease caused by a paramyxovirus, results in inflammation of the salivary glands. With the introduction of live mumps vaccine in 1977, reported cases have declined steadily in the United States. In recent years, however, reported mumps cases have increased nationally. Although the majority of mumps infections occur in children ages five years to 14 years, risk has increased for adolescents 15 years old and older due to lack of immunization (CDC 1989a, 1989b).

Mumps is transmitted through infected respiratory droplets and has a usual incubation period of 14 to 21 days, although some cases have occurred in individuals exposed 12 to 25 days prior to symptoms. Patients are most infectious one to two days prior to and five to nine days after parotid gland swelling (American Academy of Pediatrics 1994c). Although most persons with mumps experience painful salivary gland inflammation, 30 percent may have a subclinical infection. Both acute and subclinical mumps infections provide lifelong immunity.

Mumps is usually a self-limited disease resolving within seven to nine days. However, mumps infection may result in serious complications including meningoencephalitis (up to 5 per 1,000 mumps cases), deafness (0.5 to 5.0 per 1,000 mumps cases), pancreatitis, oophoritis, and orchitis (20 percent to 30 percent of mumps cases in postpubertal males) (CDC 1989b; Shandera and Gill 1994). The encephalitis case fatality rate is reportedly 1.4 percent (CDC 1989b).

Overall mortality rates associated with mumps infection are low; however, approximately 50 percent of mumps-associated deaths have been reported in persons 20 years of age or older (CDC 1984). Although mumps infection during pregnancy has not been associated with an increased rate of congenital malformations, there is an increased rate of spontaneous abortions (as high as 27 percent) reported in women who are infected with mumps during the first trimester (CDC 1989b).

DATABASE

SUBJECTIVE

→ Patient may report:
- lack of immunization to mumps.
- exposure to a person with mumps infection.

→ Symptoms may include:
- fever (may be high if associated with meningitis).
- malaise.
- painful swelling of one or both salivary glands.
- headache, lethargy, stiff neck (if associated meningitis).
- nausea, vomiting, upper abdominal pain (if associated pancreatitis) (American Academy of Pediatrics 1994c; CDC 1989b; Shandera and Gill 1994).

OBJECTIVE

→ Patient may present with:
- elevated temperature (may be high if associated with meningitis or pancreatitis).
- tender, enlarged parotid gland(s) (70 percent of mumps infection).
- enlarged, tender submaxillary and sublingual lymph glands.
- erythema, edema of Stensen's duct.
- meningitis/encephalitis-associated symptoms— nuchal rigidity, positive Kernig sign, positive Brudzinski sign, confusion.

- Meningeal signs have been reported in up to 15 percent of mumps cases (CDC 1989b).
  - pancreatitis-associated symptoms:
    - upper abdomen tender to palpation usually without guarding, rebound, or rigidity; abdomen may be distended.
  - oophoritis-associated symptoms:
    - lower abdominal/pelvic pain, ovarian enlargement.
  - diminished hearing if eighth cranial nerve damage (American Academy of Pediatrics 1994c; Shandera and Gill 1994).

ASSESSMENT

- → Mumps
- → R/O parotitis from other causes (e.g., bacteria, other viruses, drug reaction)
- → R/O cervical adenitis
- → R/O parotid gland calculi
- → R/O meningitis/encephalitis
- → R/O oophoritis
- → R/O eighth cranial nerve neuritis (deafness rare)
- → R/O pancreatitis

PLAN

DIAGNOSTIC TESTS

- → CBC with differential:
  - lymphocytosis is present.
- → Serum amylase:
  - often is elevated even without pancreatitis.
- → Culture of saliva and cerebrospinal fluid samples:
  - will demonstrate mumps virus.
- → Paired sera complement:
  - fixation testing will demonstrate a fourfold increase in mumps antibody titers.
- → Cerebrospinal fluid:
  - lymphocytic pleocytosis (glucose level normal to low) is present with meningitis.
- → Audiometry tests may demonstrate decreased hearing (American Academy of Pediatrics 1994c; Fischbach 1988; Shandera and Gill 1994).

TREATMENT/MANAGEMENT

- → Treatment of patients with mumps infection depends on symptoms.
  - Bed rest is advised during the febrile phase.
  - Acetaminophen with or without codeine may be necessary for analgesia.

- Alkaline mouthwashes may reduce some discomfort.
- Adequate hydration (i.e., force fluids) should be recommended.
- → Isolation of patient until parotid gland swelling subsides is necessary to reduce possible transmission.
- → Hospitalization is indicated in patients with serious sequelae (e.g., meningitis/encephalitis, severe pancreatitis).
- → Mumps immune globulin has been proven to be ineffective in the treatment of susceptible patients exposed to mumps and is no longer available for use (CDC 1989b).
- → Live mumps vaccine given to susceptible persons exposed to mumps infection has not been effective in preventing illness.
  - However, future protection from mumps infection in such individuals can result from immunization at this time.
  - No increased risk of reactions or complications has been associated with live mumps vaccination when administered to a patient during the incubation phase of the infection or to a person already immune to mumps (CDC 1989b; American Academy of Pediatrics 1994c).
  - If susceptible individuals have not received immunizations for measles or rubella, consider vaccination with MMR 0.5 ml unless contradicted.
    - MMR should not be given to a pregnant woman or a woman who is considering becoming pregnant within 3 months of vaccination.
    NOTE: Mumps vaccine is contraindicated in persons with a history of anaphylaxis reaction to eggs or neomycin, an immunodeficiency disease, or those who are receiving immuno-suppressive therapy or large doses of corti-costeroids, antimetabolites, radiation, or alkylating agents (American Academy of Pediatrics 1994c). Patients with HIV infection may receive MMR vaccination (see **Human Immunodeficiency Virus [HIV]** Protocol).

CONSULTATION

- → Physician consultation is warranted for patients suspected of having serious complications (e.g., meningitis, encephalitis, pancreatitis).
- → As needed for prescription(s).

PATIENT EDUCATION

→ Educate the patient about the course of the illness, symptomatic relief measures, symptoms of complications, and the need for isolation until parotid gland swelling resolves.

→ Educate the patient about the need for future immunization with measles-rubella vaccine if the patient was born after 1957 and cannot document vaccination against or actual infection with measles or rubella (CDC 1991a).

FOLLOW-UP

→ See "Consultation" section.

→ Follow-up evaluation is not necessary in uncomplicated mumps infection.

→ Document in progress notes and problem list.

11-I

Rubella

Rubella infection is a systemic illness caused by a toga-virus transmitted by inhalation of infectious nasopharyngeal secretions. The period of communicability is from a few days prior to until seven days after the onset of the rash (American Academy of Pediatrics 1994d). The incubation period is from 14 to 21 days. Generally, rubella is a mild infection and may be asymptomatic or subclinical in 25 percent to 50 percent of patients (American Academy of Pediatrics 1994d).

Encephalitis and thrombocytopenia are complications associated with rubella infection and are observed more frequently in adolescents and adults than in school-age children. Encephalitis (one in 5,000 to 6,000 cases) usually occurs one to six days after the development of the rash and is associated with a 20 percent mortality rate (Shandera and Gill 1994; Wharton, Cochi, and Williams 1990).

The greatest morbidity and mortality rates associated with rubella result from exposure during pregnancy. Rubella infection occurring during pregnancy is associated with spontaneous abortion, stillbirth, or congenital rubella in the neonate. Congenital rubella syndrome (CRS) is a constellation of abnormalities including ophthalmic anomalies (e.g., glaucoma, cataracts, chorioretinitis), cardiac anomalies (e.g., atrial or ventricular septal defects, patent ductus arteriosus), neurological problems (e.g., mental retardation, microcephaly), sensorineural deafness, and other complications such as growth retardation, thrombocytopenia, and jaundice (American Academy of Pediatrics 1994d; Shandera and Gill 1994).

The risk of CRS is highest during the first 20 weeks of pregnancy. Occurrence rates of 50 percent, 75 percent, and 10 percent have been reported during the first, second, and third months, respectively (ACOG 1981). During the second and third trimesters the risk of CRS is reportedly one percent (ACOG 1981).

Although rubella immunization has dramatically reduced the incidence of both postnatal rubella infection and CRS in the United States, a fivefold increased incidence was reported in 1988, with over 50 percent of cases occurring among individuals 15 years of age and older (CDC 1991b). Furthermore, eleven cases of CRS were reported in 1990 (CDC 1991b). An estimated six percent to 11 percent of young adults in the United States remain susceptible to rubella (CDC 1991b).

DATABASE

SUBJECTIVE

→ Patient may be asymptomatic or report any of the following symptoms:
- history of exposure to a person with rubella infection during past three weeks.
- prodromal symptoms (usually seven days prior to rash eruption), including:
  - low-grade fever.
  - headache.
  - malaise.
  - anorexia.
  - sore throat.
  - mild conjunctivitis.
  - rhinitis.
  - nonproductive cough.
  - suboccipital, postauricular, and/or cervical lymph node enlargement.
- eruption of a fine rash beginning on the face and neck and progressing to the trunk and

extremities within two to three days after the facial rash appears. Patient may report rapid disappearance of the rash (within one day after eruption is evident) (Shandera 1993; Wharton, Cochi, and Williams 1990).

▪ joint pain in 25 percent of adults which may continue for one week or longer (Shandera and Gill 1994).

OBJECTIVE

→ Patient may present with:
  ▪ temperature slightly elevated, but usually WNL.
  ▪ fine, pink, discrete maculopapular rash on face, neck, trunk, and/or extremities.
  ▪ postauricular, occipital, and/or cervical lymphadenopathy.
  ▪ erythema of the palate and posterior pharynx (Shandera and Gill 1994).
  ▪ evidence of tender, edematous joints in a symmetrical pattern (Hellman 1994).

ASSESSMENT

→ Rubella infection

→ R/O measles (rubeola)

→ R/O atypical measles

→ R/O infectious mononucleosis

→ R/O drug reaction

→ R/O enterovirus infection

PLAN

DIAGNOSTIC TESTS

→ Diagnostic tests usually are done only if confirmation of rubella diagnosis is indicated (e.g., in pregnant women).
  ▪ Consider a urine or serum pregnancy test in any woman of reproductive age presenting with suspected rubella and a history of no contraception and/or unprotected coitus (unless she has just completed her menses).

→ Culture for rubella virus can be done with specimens obtained from throat swabs, blood, urine, and cerebrospinal fluid (as clinically indicated) and will be positive.

→ Acute and convalescent serum specimens can be obtained and sent for rubella virus hemagglutination inhibition (HI) testing (see **Figure 11I.1, Immune Response in Acute Rubella Infection**).

▪ If a patient has a recent infection, a fourfold or higher increase in HI titer will be reported (American Academy of Pediatrics 1994d).

→ Recently, more sensitive tests for rubella have been made available and include fluorescent immunoassays, latex agglutination tests, passive hemagglutination tests, enzyme immunoassay tests, and hemolysis-in-gel tests.
  ▪ These tests have demonstrated positive results in patients who did not demonstrate immunity using the HI tests.
  ▪ It is advisable to consult the laboratory that will be performing diagnostic tests for rubella to determine which tests it is able to perform and what the sensitivity is for each available test.

→ Presence of rubella-specific IgM antibody (serum testing) indicates recent acute infection.

→ CBC—may demonstrate leukopenia in early infection.

→ Platelet count may be decreased if thrombocytopenia is present.

→ Tests for rheumatoid factor will be negative in patients with rubella-associated arthritis.

TREATMENT/MANAGEMENT

→ Supportive treatment consists of bed rest while febrile, analgesics for arthritis/arthralgia, and antipyretics (e.g., acetaminophen) as needed.

→ Isolation of the patient from susceptible individuals is indicated until 1 week after the initial eruption of the rash. **NOTE:** It is estimated that 10 percent to 20 percent of postpubertal populations in the United States lack evidence of rubella immunity and are susceptible to infection if exposed.

CONSULTATION

→ Patients with suspected encephalitis should be referred to a physician for further evaluation and treatment as indicated.

→ Pregnant women with suspected rubella infection should be referred to an obstetrician/perinatologist for further evaluation, counseling, and follow-up.

PATIENT EDUCATION

→ Educate the patient about rubella infection, duration of symptoms, infectivity, possible complications, and symptomatic treatment options.

Figure 11I.1. IMMUNE RESPONSE IN ACUTE RUBELLA INFECTION

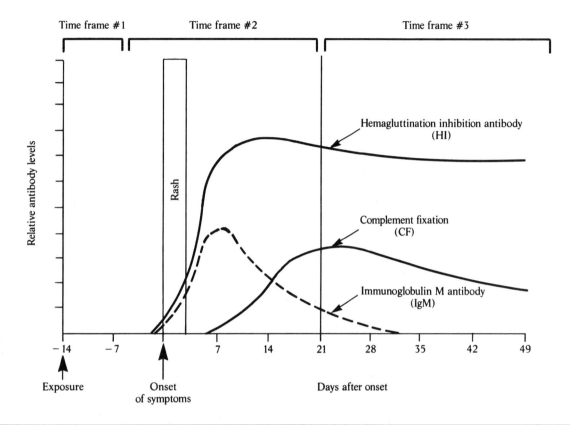

Source: Reprinted with permission from Mann, J.M., Preblud, S.R., Hoffman, R.E., Brandling-Bennett, A.D., Hinman, A.R., and Herrmann, K.L. 1981. Assessing risks of rubella infection during pregnancy. A standardized approach. *Journal of the American Medical Association* 245(16):1651.

→ Educate the patient about the need to avoid contact with susceptible individuals until one week after initial eruption of the rash.

→ If patient is pregnant, discuss perinatal risks associated with acute rubella infection.

→ In postpubertal patients without documented evidence of rubella vaccination or rubella immunity, immunization with rubella vaccine (0.5 ml) or in combination with measles (MR) vaccine or MMR vaccine should be considered.

- Rubella vaccine is contraindicated in pregnant women due to the theoretical risk of congenital rubella.

- Non-pregnant women of childbearing age who receive rubella vaccine should be advised not to become pregnant until three months after the immunization.

- Rubella vaccine is a live virus vaccine and is contraindicated in patients with immuno-deficiency diseases, who are receiving immunosuppressive therapy, or who are receiving large doses of corticosteroids, antimetabolites, radiation, or ankylating agents (American Academy of Pediatrics 1994d).

- Patients with HIV infection may receive an MMR (see **Human Immunodeficiency Virus [HIV]** Protocol).

FOLLOW-UP

→ See "Consultation" section.

→ Document in progress notes and problem list.

11-J

Varicella Zoster Virus

Varicella zoster virus is a human herpes virus responsible for two distinct illnesses: *primary varicella zoster virus* infection (chickenpox) and reactivation of *latent varicella zoster virus* (herpes zoster or shingles). Because these illnesses have different clinical manifestations and treatments, each is presented individually.

Primary Varicella Zoster Virus Infection (Chickenpox)

Approximately three million cases of primary varicella zoster virus infection (chickenpox) are reported each year in the United States (Straus et al. 1988). The majority of cases occur in children less than ten years of age (American Academy of Pediatrics 1994e). However, infection in adolescents and adults is of concern since approximately five percent to ten percent of healthy adults in the United States are susceptible to chickenpox (Hardy and Gershon 1990).

Chickenpox is highly contagious. It is spread by direct contact with varicella lesions or by inhalation of infectious respiratory droplets. The incubation period is usually 14 to 16 days, but the range is between nine and 21 days. Shorter incubation periods have been reported in immunocompromised patients and longer incubation periods (up to 28 days) have been noted in patients who receive varicella zoster immune globulin (VZIG) (American Academy of Pediatrics 1994e). Patients are contagious from one to two days prior to the onset of varicella lesions and remain infectious until all lesions have crusted (Straus et al. 1988). The duration of varicella from prodrome to disappearance of all lesions is usually less than two weeks.

Although rare, asymptomatic primary infection has been reported. An episode of varicella usually provides lifelong immunity against subsequent outbreaks, although reinfections have been reported (Straus et al. 1988).

Except for neonatal cases of varicella zoster infection, chickenpox in adults is associated with higher morbidity and mortality rates than in children (Hardy and Gershon 1990). Varicella-related viral pneumonia is responsible for the majority of hospitalizations and deaths in adults (Hardy and Gershon 1990; Straus et al. 1988). Other complications associated with varicella include bacterial superinfection of lesions, encephalitis, Reye's syndrome (rare in adults), hepatitis, thrombocytopenia, arthritis, conjunctivitis, carditis, nephritis, and neurological disorders such as transverse myelitis, aseptic meningitis, and Guillain-Barré syndrome (Straus et al. 1988).

Varicella during pregnancy is associated with a number of maternal, fetal, and neonatal complications. Pregnant women with varicella are at an increased risk for varicella-related pneumonia. If varicella occurs during the first or second trimester, there is a one percent to ten percent chance of fetal malformations including limb atrophy, growth retardation, chorioretinitis, cataracts, scarring of the skin, deafness, and cortical atrophy (American Academy of Pediatrics 1994d; Shandera and Gill 1994; Straus et al. 1988).

Maternal varicella occurring between five days prior to and two days after delivery is associated with severe neonatal varicella, which has an associated case fatality rate of up to 30 percent (American Academy of Pediatrics 1994d). Both in utero varicella and neonatal varicella can result in herpes zoster during infancy (Straus et al. 1988).

DATABASE

SUBJECTIVE

→ The patient may report one or more of the following:

■ exposure to chickenpox or suspected chickenpox during past three weeks.

■ prodromal symptoms of fever, headache, myalgia, arthralgia, or anorexia (may occur 24 hours prior to eruption of the rash) (Shandera 1993; Straus et al. 1988).

■ pruritic rash with discrete lesions ranging from macular to papular to vesicular to crusted.

■ centripetal (extremities to trunk) distribution of rash.

■ if varicella pneumonia is present, the patient may report the development of fever, dry cough, dyspnea, and possibly pleuritic chest pain and/ or hemoptysis approximately one to six days after the eruption of the rash (Straus et al. 1988).

■ if encephalitis is present, the patient may report seizures, altered sensorium, headache, and/or ataxia (Shandera and Gill 1994; Straus et al. 1988).

■ if severe thrombocytopenia is present, the patient may report unexplained bruising.

OBJECTIVE

→ Temperature may be elevated.

→ Patient presents with evidence of macular, papular, vesicular, and crusted lesions on body, including scalp and mucous membranes. Various types of lesions are present simultaneously.

→ If pneumonia coexists, physical findings may be minimal and include an increased respiratory rate and presence of crackles when auscultating lungs.

→ If encephalitis coexists, the patient may demonstrate ataxia, nystagmus, and nuchal rigidity.

→ If thrombocytopenia coexists, the patient may demonstrate petechiae and ecchymosis.

ASSESSMENT

→ Primary varicella zoster virus infection (chickenpox)

→ R/O disseminated zoster

→ R/O disseminated HSV infection

→ R/O eczema vaccinia

→ R/O generalized vaccinia

→ R/O atypical measles

→ R/O rickettsial pox

→ R/O thrombocytopenia

→ R/O other vesicular eruptions (e.g., poison oak)

PLAN

DIAGNOSTIC TESTS

→ Diagnosis is usually made on clinical findings but adjunctive laboratory tests may be ordered if a definitive diagnosis is indicated.

→ CBC may reveal leukopenia.

→ Platelet count will be decreased if thrombocytopenia exists.

→ Cultures of vesicular fluid or lesion scrapings will be positive.

■ Several days are needed to obtain results.

→ Skin biopsy or cytological smears (e.g., Tzanck smear) are positive in 50 percent to 60 percent of varicella cases but do not indicate whether lesions are due to varicella zoster or herpes simplex infections (Straus et al. 1988).

→ Fluorescent antibody to membrane antigen (FAMA) test of smear obtained from lesion will be positive. Although considered to be highly sensitive and specific, this test is used as a research tool because of the cost and technical elements.

→ Enzyme-linked immunosorbent assay (ELISA) tests are very sensitive (86 percent to 97 percent) and specific (82 percent to 89 percent) antibody tests that can be used to determine which individuals are susceptible to varicella zoster virus and which have had the infection in the past (Hardy and Gershon 1990).

→ Complement-fixation test of a varicella patient's serum will be positive. Complement-fixation tests are not useful in determining immune status because antibody levels diminish with time (Hardy and Gershon 1990; Straus et al. 1988).

→ Chest x-ray of patient suspected of having pneumonia may reveal a "patchy or diffuse bilateral nodular infiltrate with prominent peribronchial distribution" (Straus et al. 1988, 225).

TREATMENT/MANAGEMENT

→ Isolation of patient is recommended until primary crusts have disappeared. Lesions should be kept clean.

→ Bed rest should be maintained while the patient is febrile.

- Acetaminophen should be used for analgesia and fever because the use of aspirin has been associated with an increased risk of Reye's syndrome.

→ Topical therapy for relief of pruritus may include the application of calamine lotion to lesions and/or colloidal oatmeal baths as needed.

- If necessary, systemic antihistamines such as diphenhydramine (Benadryl®) 25 mg capsule p.o. once every 4 to 6 hours can be recommended.
  - Advise patients taking antihistamines about the possible side effects (e.g., drowsiness) and the need to avoid activities which require concentration (e.g., driving).

→ If secondary bacterial infection of the lesions occurs, topical antibiotic creams such as mupirocin 2 percent (Bactroban®) ointment can be applied TID–QID.

- If extensive bacterial infection is evident, consider prescribing antistaphylococcal oral antibiotics such as dicloxacillin (Dynapen®) 250 mg p.o. QID for 10 days.

→ In immunocompromised patients, antiviral therapy (acyclovir 30 mg/kg/day in 3 divided doses intravenously for 7 days) should be initiated as soon as possible to decrease the risk of serious sequelae.

- Antiviral therapy also is indicated in immunocompetent patients with severe varicella-associated complications (e.g., pneumonitis) (Shandera and Gill 1994).

→ VZIG 125 units/10 kg body weight (up to a total dose of 625 units) I.M. should be given to susceptible persons at *high risk* of developing progressive varicella (See **Table 11J.1, Types of Exposure to Varicella or Zoster for which VZIG Is Indicated** and **Table 11J.2, Candidates for VZIG, Provided Significant Exposure Has Occurred**).

- VZIG must be administered within 96 hours of exposure to varicella to be effective. The duration of the protective effect of VZIG is unknown.
- If an individual continues to be exposed to a patient with varicella, a second injection should be administered 3 weeks after the initial dose.
- Because asymptomatic varicella is known to occur, laboratory tests for varicella immune status in high-risk susceptible individuals can

Table 11J.1. TYPES OF EXPOSURE TO VARICELLA OR ZOSTER FOR WHICH VZIG IS INDICATED*†

1. Household: Residing in the same household.
2. Playmate: Face-to-face‡ indoor play.
3. Hospital:
   Varicella:
   a) In same 2-person to 4-person bedroom, or adjacent beds in large ward,
   b) Face-to-face‡ contact with an infectious staff member or patient, *or*
   c) Visit by a person deemed contagious.
   Zoster: Intimate contact (e.g., touching or hugging) with a person deemed contagious.
4. Newborn infant: Onset of varicella in the mother 5 days or less before delivery or within 48 hours after delivery. VZIG is not indicated if the mother has zoster.

*Patients should meet criteria of both significant exposure and candidacy for receiving VZIG, as given in Table 11J.2.

†VZIG should be administered within 96 hours (preferably sooner) after exposure.

‡Experts differ in the duration of face-to-face contact that warrants the administration of VZIG. However, the contact should be nontransient. Some experts suggest a contact of 5 or more minutes as constituting significant exposure for this purpose; others define close contact as more than 1 hour.

Source: Reprinted with permission from American Academy of Pediatrics. 1994e. *Report of the Committee on Infectious Diseases*, 23rd ed., p. 514. Elk Grove Village, IL: the Author.

Table 11J.2. CANDIDATES FOR VZIG, PROVIDED SIGNIFICANT EXPOSURE* HAS OCCURRED

1. Immunocompromised children without history of chickenpox.†
2. Susceptible, pregnant women.
3. Newborn infant of a mother who had onset of chickenpox within 5 days before delivery or within 48 hours after delivery.
4. Hospitalized premature infant (≥ 28 weeks gestation) whose mother has no history of chickenpox.
5. Hospitalized premature infant (<28 weeks gestation or ≤1,000 grams), regardless of maternal history.

*See Table 11J.1.

†Immunocompromised adolescents and adults are likely to be immune, but, if susceptible, they should also receive VZIG.

Source: Reprinted with permission from American Academy of Pediatrics. 1994e. *Report of the Committee on Infectious Diseases*, 23rd ed., p. 515. Elk Grove Village, IL: the Author.

be done prior to administration of VZIG if performing such tests will not delay VZIG administration beyond 96 hours after exposure. **NOTE:** VZIG is not recommended for low-risk susceptible individuals.

CONSULTATION

→ As indicated, especially in patients with an increased risk of serious sequelae (e.g., pregnant women, immunosuppressed patients) or patients with clinical evidence of severe disease (e.g.,

pneumonia, encephalitis) requiring hospitalization.
→ As needed for prescription(s).

PATIENT EDUCATION

→ Educate the patient about varicella including transmission, infectivity, clinical course, treatment(s), signs and symptoms of possible complications, and when further evaluation may be needed.
→ Assess the possible need to administer VZIG to any high-risk susceptible person in close contact with the patient.
→ If hospitalization is indicated (e.g., in case of pneumonia), the physician responsible for the patient's care should discuss this decision, as well as indicated treatment(s), with the patient.
→ If the patient is pregnant, discuss the possible perinatal risks associated with varicella infection.

FOLLOW-UP

→ Follow-up visits will be based on the clinical presentation or determined by the managing physician.
→ Document in progress notes and problem list.

Herpes Zoster (Shingles)

Herpes zoster (shingles) is a reactivation of latent varicella zoster virus infection, reportedly experienced by 10 percent to 20 percent of the population (Straus et al. 1988). Generally, it is thought to result from decline in cell-mediated immunity usually associated with advanced aging, immunosuppression, and certain malignancies, although herpes zoster can occur in otherwise healthy persons. The characteristic eruption of cutaneous herpes zoster is a painful vesicular → pustular → crusted confluent rash along single or multiple dermatomes. The rash usually resolves in 14 to 21 days. The patient usually reports a history of chickenpox.

The most frequent complication associated with herpes zoster is postherpetic neuralgia (pain which lasts more than one month after zoster). This complication is increasingly more prevalent in older patients. Postherpatic neuralgia usually resolves within two months in 50 percent of patients and within one year after the onset of pain in 70 percent to 80 percent of patients (Straus et al. 1988).

Other severe complications include cutaneous scarring, cellulitis, encephalitis, myelitis, motor neuropathies (in five percent of herpes zoster patients, usually transient), Guillain-Barré syndrome, cerebrovasculopathy (usually associated with ophthalmic zoster and with a mortality rate of 25 percent), ocular inflammation (e.g., optic neuritis, keratitis, conjunctivitis, optic atrophy, second-degree glaucoma) and vasculopathy (e.g., thrombosis), pneumonitis, enterocolitis, myocarditis, pancreatitis, and esophagitis.

The Ramsay Hunt syndrome is a complication noted in some patients with cutaneous lesions in the external auditory canal, facial palsy, vertigo, and tinnitus. It is associated with diminished hearing (Shandera and Gill 1994; Straus et al. 1988). The more severe complications are more commonly associated with disseminated herpes zoster or immunosuppressed patients.

DATABASE

SUBJECTIVE

→ Patient may report one or more of the following:
- a history of chickenpox, immunosuppression, previous herpes zoster episode.
- prodromal symptoms of fever, headache, dysesthesia(s), malaise one to four days prior to eruption of lesions.
- eruption of painful vesicles in a dermatome pattern.
- evolution of blisters into pustules three to four days after initial eruption, with crusting usually occurring seven to ten days after initial eruption.
- symptoms specific to nerve involvement (e.g., facial weakness if trigeminal involvement, peripheral motor weakness if motor neuropathies coexist).
- symptoms associated with complications (e.g., headache, stiff neck, problems with coordination if encephalitis/meningoencephalitis coexist).
- dyspnea, if pneumonitis coexists.
- symptoms of visual disturbances and pain, if ocular complications coexist.

OBJECTIVE

→ Vital signs usually WNL unless complications such as encephalitis, pneumonitis coexist.
- If such complications occur, there may be an elevated temperature, heart rate, and respiratory rate.
→ Examination of skin will reveal vesicular → pustular → crusted grouped lesions, usually along a single dermatome (most often thoracic and lumbar nerve root distributions; trigeminal and cervical distribution is less common). Evidence of

eruption on the tip of the nose indicates involvement of the ophthalmic division.

→ In disseminated herpes zoster, there will be evidence of 20 lesions or more outside the primary and adjacent dermatome(s), usually appearing 4 to 11 days after eruption of the lesions in the primary dermatome (Straus et al. 1988).
  ▪ This finding occurs in up to 26 percent of patients (usually immunosuppressed patients) and is associated with ocular, visceral, or neurological involvement in 50 percent of patients with dissemination (Straus et al. 1988).

→ If coexistent pneumonia, pulmonary symptoms, including increased respiratory rate and crackles, will be evident.

→ If encephalitis or meningoencephalitis coexists, examination may reveal associated symptoms of nuchal rigidity, nystagmus, and evidence of ataxia.

→ If there are coexistent motor neuropathies, examination may reveal evidence of abnormalities in area of nerve distribution (e.g., facial palsy if trigeminal nerve involvement).

→ If there is coexistent ocular involvement, examination may reveal evidence of abnormalities suggestive of pathology specific to site (e.g., conjunctivitis, keratitis). See specific **Ophthalmological Disorders** Protocol for physical findings and treatment.

→ If there is coexistent Ramsay Hunt syndrome, examination may reveal evidence of lesion in external auditory canal and the tympanic membrane, with facial palsy and diminished hearing.

ASSESSMENT

→ Herpes zoster (shingles)
→ R/O disseminated herpes zoster
→ R/O zosteriform HSV infection
→ R/O cellulitis
→ R/O encephalitis/meningoencephalitis
→ R/O pneumonia
→ R/O herpes zoster-associated neuropathies
→ R/O herpes zoster ocular complications
→ R/O immunosuppression
→ R/O other vesicular eruptions

PLAN

DIAGNOSTIC TESTS

→ The classic dermatome eruption characterizing herpes zoster is usually sufficient to diagnose this condition. However, the following tests may be ordered as indicated:
  ▪ culture of vesicular fluid may be indicated to rule out zosteriform herpes simplex virus infection and confirm varicella zoster virus infection.
  ▪ chest x-ray may be ordered if pneumonia is suspected. The presence of interstitial infiltrates will confirm the diagnosis.
  ▪ Lumbar puncture may be performed in patients suspected of having encephalitis/meningoencephalitis, although laboratory confirmation of this condition is difficult primarily because varicella virus is rarely recovered from CSF.
    • Additionally, up to 40 percent of all patients with herpes zoster have increased spinal fluid cell counts and/or elevated CSF protein concentrations.
    • However, elevation of antibody titers to varicella viral membrane antigens are observed in the CSF of patients with encephalitis but not evident in patients with uncomplicated herpes zoster (Straus et al. 1988).

→ See "Diagnostics Tests" under "Primary Varicella Zoster Infection."

→ If disseminated herpes zoster or severe complications of herpes zoster occurs in a patient without a history of immunosuppression, consider diagnostic tests (as indicated) to identify possible cause(s) of immunosuppression (e.g., HIV antibody testing, evaluation for possible malignancy).

TREATMENT/MANAGEMENT

→ Isolation of the patient from varicella-susceptible individuals in the household (or hospital) is indicated whenever possible.

→ Because virus can be recovered from vesicular fluid, precautions should be taken by any varicella-susceptible individuals who may be caring for a patient with herpes zoster (e.g., use gloves when in contact with lesions).

→ Symptomatic treatment of discomfort associated with herpes zoster includes acetaminophen or more potent prescription medications as indicated.

→ To reduce the likelihood of secondary bacterial infection, the lesions should be kept clean through gentle cleansing and drying of involved areas. If secondary bacterial infection occurs, initiation of antibiotic therapy specifically effective against staphylococci and streptococci is indicated (e.g., amoxicillin and clavulanic acid [Augmentin®] 500 mg p.o. TID for 7-10 days.).

→ Antiviral therapy for herpes zoster infection is based on the immune status of the patient and the severity of the illness (e.g., dermatomal versus disseminated herpes zoster, presence of pneumonia or encephalitis, ophthalmic complications).

■ To be effective, acyclovir should be started within 4 days of symptom onset or while lesions are still forming.

■ The following antiviral treatment recommendations have been made (Bartlett 1991; Bartlett 1992; Shandera and Gill 1994; Straus et al. 1988):

• dermatomal herpes zoster:
  –immunocompetent patient: Acyclovir (Zovirax®) 800 mg p.o. 5 times a day for 7 to 10 days.
  –immunosuppressed patient: Acyclovir (Zovirax®) 30 mg/kg/day I.V. for at least 7 days

OR

800 mg p.o. 5 times a day for at least 7 days.

• ophthalmic zoster:
  –immunocompetent patient: Same acyclovir dose and route as for dermatomal zoster; however, ophthamology consultation is warranted.
  –immunosuppressed patient: Acyclovir (Zovirax®) 30 mg/kg to 36 mg/kg/day I.V. for at least 7 days. Ophthalmology consultation is warranted.

• disseminated herpes zoster, herpes zoster pneumonia, visceral and neurological complications:
  –immunocompetent and immunosuppressed patient: Acyclovir (Zovirax®) 30 mg/kg to 36 mg/kg/day I.V. for at least 7 days; or vidarabine (Vira-A®) 10 mg/kg/day I.V. for 5 to 7 days (alternative treatment for disseminated herpes zoster, or visceral or neurological complications).

NOTE: Patients with severe disease or complications should be hospitalized with antiviral treatment determined by the physician responsible for the patient's care.

–steroid therapy has been reported to decrease postherpetic neuralgia in some patients. However, steroid use remains controversial. If initiated, the following is recommended: prednisone (Deltasone®) 40 mg p.o. every day tapered over the next 10 to 14 days (Bartlett 1991; Shandera and Gill 1994).

CONSULTATION

→ Physician consultation is warranted in patients with severe disease (e.g., disseminated herpes zoster), zoster-associated complications, or immunosuppression.

→ As needed for prescription(s).

PATIENT EDUCATION

→ Educate the patient about the cause of herpes zoster, its duration, possible complications, treatment options including any side effects of treatment, and possibility of recurrence (approximately 10 percent to 20 percent) (Straus et al. 1988).

→ Educate the patient about the infectivity of the vesicular fluid and the need to have varicella-susceptible individuals (e.g., household members) avoid contact with the lesions until they crust over.

→ If there is evidence of disseminated herpes zoster or complications, educate the patient about the possible need for further evaluation to rule out underlying immunosuppressive conditions (e.g., HIV infection, malignancy).

→ Educate the patient to avoid direct sun exposure to affected area(s) to prevent hyperpigmentation of skin.

FOLLOW-UP

→ Patients hospitalized and managed by a physician should return for follow-up as recommended by the physician.

→ In uncomplicated, dermatomal herpes zoster, the patient should return for evaluation if any complications (including postherpatic neuralgia) develop.

→ Document in progress notes and problem list.

11-K

Bibliography

Aach, R.D. 1992. The emerging clinical significance of hepatitis C. *Hospital Practice* 27(5a):19–22.

Abbey, S.E., and Garfinkel, P.E. 1991. Chronic fatigue syndrome and depression: Cause, effect, or covariate. *Review of Infectious Diseases* 13(Suppl):S73–S83.

Alter, M.J., and Margolis, H.S. 1990. The emergence of hepatitis B as a sexually transmitted disease. *Medical Clinics of North America* 74(6):1529–1541.

American Academy of Pediatrics. 1994a. *Report of the Committee on Infectious Diseases*, 23rd ed., pp. 273–275. Elk Grove Village, IL: the Author.

———. 1994b. *Report of the Committee on Infectious Diseases*, 23rd ed., pp. 308–323. Elk Grove Village, IL: the Author.

———. 1994c. *Report of the Committee on Infectious Diseases*. 23rd ed., pp. 329–333. Elk Grove Village, IL: the Author.

———. 1994d. *Report of the Committee on Infectious Diseases*, 23rd ed., pp. 406–412. Elk Grove Village, IL: the Author.

———. 1994e. *Report of the Committee on Infectious Diseases*. 23rd ed., pp. 510–517. Elk Grove Village, IL: the Author.

American College of Obstetricians and Gynecologists. 1981. Rubella: A clinical update, ACOG Technical Bulletin 62. Washington, DC: the Author.

———. 1992. Human immunodeficiency virus infections. *ACOG Technical Bulletin* 165. Washington, DC: the Author.

Anderson, J., and Ernberg, I. 1988. Management of Epstein-Barr virus infections. *American Journal of Medicine* 85(Suppl 2A):107–115.

Bartlett, J.G. 1991. *1991–1992 pocketbook of infectious disease therapy*, 3rd ed. Baltimore: Williams & Wilkins.

———. 1992. *1992–1993 recommendations for the medical care of persons with HIV infection*, 2d ed. Baltimore: Critical Care America.

Berquist, E.J. 1990. The office evaluation of infectious diarrhea. *Primary Care* 17(4):853–866.

Brownlee, H.J. Jr., 1990. Family practitioner's guide to patient self-treatment of acute diarrhea. *The American Journal of Medicine* 88(Suppl. 6A):27S–29S.

Buchstein, S.R., and Gardner, P. 1991. Lyme disease. *Infectious Disease Clinics of North America* 5(1):103–116.

Buchwald, D., Cheney, P.R., Peterson, D.L., Henry, B., Wormsley, S.B., Geiger, A., and Ablashi, D.V. 1992. A chronic illness characterized by fatigue, neurologic, and immunologic disorders and active human herpes virus type 6 infection. *Annals of Internal Medicine* 116(2):103–113.

Carpenter, C.C.J., Mayer, K.H., Stein, M.D., Leibman, B.D., Fisher, A., and Fiore, T.C. 1991. Human immunodeficiency virus infection in North American women: Experience with 200 cases and a review of the literature. *Medicine* 70(5):307–325.

Caschetta, M.B. 1992. A review of reports on women and HIV. *Treatment Issues* 6(10):2–6.

Centers for Disease Control. 1984. *Mumps surveillance, January 1977–December 1982*. Atlanta: U.S. Department of Health and Human Services, Public Health Service.

———. 1989a. Mumps—United States, 1985–1988. *Morbidity and Mortality Weekly Report* 38(7):101–105.

————. 1989b. Mumps prevention. *Morbidity and Mortality Weekly Report* 38(22):388–400.

————. 1990. Risk for cervical disease in HIV-infected women—New York City. *Morbidity and Mortality Weekly Report* 38:846–849.

————. 1991a. Recommendations of the Immunization Practices Advisory Committee (ACIP). *Morbidity and Mortality Weekly Report* 40(RR–12):22–23, 60.

————. 1991b. Update on adult immunization recommendations of the Immunization Practices Advisory Committee (ACIP). *Morbidity and Mortality Weekly Report* 40(RR–12):24–26.

————. 1991c. Update on adult immunization recommendations of the Immunization Practices Advisory Committee. *Morbidity and Mortality Weekly Report* 40(RR-12):59.

————. 1991d. Hepatitis B virus: A comprehensive strategy for eliminating transmission in the United States through universal childhood vaccination. *Morbidity and Mortality Weekly Report* 40 (RR-13):1–25.

————. 1992a. Measles surveillance—United States, 1991. *Morbidity and Mortality Weekly Report* 41(SS-6):1–12.

————. 1992b. 1993 Revised classification system for HIV infection and expanded surveillance case definition for AIDS among adolescents and adults. *Morbidity and Mortality Weekly Report* 41(RR-17):1–19.

————. 1993a. CDC HIV programs to undergo review. *HIV/AIDS Prevention* 4(1):1–12.

————. 1993b. Update: Acquired immunodeficiency syndrome—United States, 1992. *Morbidity and Mortality Weekly Report* 42:547–557.

————. 1993c. Preliminary report: Foodborne outbreak of *Escherichia coli* 0157:H7 infections from hamburgers—western United States, 1993. *Morbidity and Mortality Weekly Report* 42(4):85–86.

————. 1994a, June. *HIV/AIDS surveillance*, pp. 1–27. Atlanta: U.S. Department of Health and Human Services, Public Health Service.

Cheeseman, S.H. 1988. Infectious mononucleosis. *Seminars in Hematology* 25(3):261–268.

Chu, S.Y., Buehler, J.W., and Berkelman, R.L. 1990. Impact of the human immunodeficiency virus epidemic on mortality in women of reproductive age, United States. *Journal of the American Medical Association* 264(2):225–229.

Clarke, D.D., and Koa, H. 1983. Meaningful markers for hepatitis Dx and Px. *Contemporary Ob/Gyn* 21(Special Issue):31–50.

Cohen, M.L. 1988. The epidemiology of diarrheal disease in the United States. *Infectious Disease Clinics of North America* 2(30):557–570.

Cohn, J.A. 1993. Human immunodeficiency virus and AIDS. *Journal of Nurse Midwifery* 38(2):65–85.

Cosby, C.D., and Stringari, S.E. 1991. Primary care for the HIV-seropositive adult: Nurse practitioners prepare for the challenge of the 1990s. *Nurse Practitioner Forum* 2(2):116–125.

Dattwyler, R.J., Volkman, D.J., Luft, B.J., Halperin, J.J., Thoman, J., and Golightly, M.G. 1988. Seronegative Lyme disease. *New England Journal of Medicine* 319(22):1441–1446.

Demitrak, M.A., Dale, J.K., Straus, S.E., Lave, L., Listwak, S.F., Kruesi, M.J., Chrousos, G.P., and VanGold, P.W. 1991. Evidence for impaired activation of the hypothalamic pituitary adrenal axis in patients with chronic fatigue syndrome. *Journal of Clinical Endocrinology and Metabolism* 73(6):1224–1234.

Dienstag, J.L. 1995. Management of hepatitis. In *Primary care medicine*, eds. A.H. Goroll, L.A. May, and A.G. Gulley, pp. 399–407. Philadelphia: J.B. Lippincott.

DiJohn, D., and Levine, M.M. 1988. Treatment of diarrhea. *Infectious Disease Clinics of North America* 2(3):719–745.

Ellsworth, A.J., Bray, R.F., Bray, B.S., and Geyman, J.P. 1991. *The family practice drug handbook*. St. Louis: Mosby Year Book.

El-Sadr, W., Oleske, J.M., Agins, B.D., Bauman, K., Brosgart, C., et al. 1994. Evaluation and management of early HIV infection. Clinical practice guideline No. 7, AHCPR Publication No. 94-0572. Rockville, MD: Agency for Health Care Policy and Research, Public Health Service, U.S. Department of Health and Human Services.

Ergun, G.A., and Miskovitz, P.F. 1990. Viral hepatitis. *Postgraduate Medicine* 88(5):69–76.

Ericcson, C.D., DuPont, H.L., Mathewson, J.J., West, M.S., Johnson, P.C., and Bitsura, J.A. 1990. Treatment of traveler's diarrhea with sulfamethoxazole and trimethoprim and loperamide. *Journal of the American Medical Association* 263(2):257–261.

Fairchild, P.G., and Blackblow, N.R. 1988. Viral diarrhea. *Infectious Disease Clinics of North America* 2(3):677–685.

Fischbach, F. 1988. *A manual of laboratory diagnostic tests*, 3rd ed., pp. 309–310. Philadelphia: J.B. Lippincott.

Fischl, M.A. 1994. Treatment of HIV infection. In *The medical management of AIDS*, 4th ed., eds. M.A. Sande and P.A. Volberding, pp. 141–160. Philadelpia: W.B. Saunders.

Friedman, L.S. 1987. Management of cirrhosis and chronic liver failure. In *Primary care medicine*, eds. A.H. Goroll, L.A. May, and A.G. Gulley, pp. 355–358. Philadelphia: J.B. Lippincott.

Goldschmidt, R.H., and Dong, B.J. 1994. Current report—HIV. Treatment of AIDS and HIV-related conditions—1994. *Journal of the American Board of Family Practice* 7(2):155–178.

Gorensek, M.J. 1991. Chronic fatigue and depression in the ambulatory patient. *Primary Care* 18(2):397–419.

Grady, C., and Vogel, S. 1993. Laboratory methods for diagnosing and monitoring HIV infection. *Journal of the Association of Nurses in AIDS Care* 4(2):11–21.

Hallam, A., and Kerlin, P. 1991. Viral hepatitis A to E: An update. *Australian Family Physician* 20(6):760–770.

Hardy, I.R.B., and Gershon, A.A. 1990. Prospects for use of a varicella vaccine in adults. *Infectious Disease Clinics of North America* 4(1):159–173.

Hellman, D.B. 1994. Arthritis and musculoskeletal disorders. In *Current medical diagnosis and treatment*, eds. L.M. Tierney, Jr., S.J. McPhee, and M.A. Papadakis, 33rd ed., pp. 664–710. Norwalk, CT: Appleton & Lange.

Hernandez, S.R. 1990. Laboratory testing and management of HIV-infected patients. In *The AIDS knowledge base*, eds. P.T. Cohen, M.A. Sande, and P.A. Volberding, pp. 1–11. Waltham, MA: The Medical Publishing Group.

Holmes, G.P., Kaplan, J.E., Gantz, N.M., Kamaroff, A.L., Schonberger, L.B., Straus, S.E., Jones, J.F., Dubois, R.E., Cunningham-Rundles, C., Pahwa, S., Tosato, G., Zegans, L.S., Purtilo, D.T., Brown, N., Schooley, R.J., and Brus, I. 1988. Chronic fatigue syndrome: A working case definition. *Annals of Internal Medicine* 108(3):387–389.

Imam, N., Carpenter, C.C.J., Mayer, K.H., Fisher, A., Stein, M., and Danforth, S.B. 1990. Hierarchical pattern of mucosal candida infections in HIV-seropositive women. *The American Journal of Medicine* 89:142–146.

Jacobs, R.A. 1993. General problems in infectious diseases. In *Current medical diagnosis and treatment*, eds. L.M. Tierney, Jr., S.J. McPhee, M.A. Papadakis, and S.A. Schroeder, 32d ed., pp. 999–1000. Norwalk, CT: Appleton & Lange.

Johnson, P.C., and Ericcson, C.D. 1990. Acute diarrhea in developed countries. A rationale for self-treatment. *The American Journal of Medicine* 88(Suppl. 6A):5S–9S.

Kantor, K.S. 1994. Disarming Lyme disease. *Scientific American* 271(3):34–39.

Knauer, C.M. 1993. Liver, biliary tract and pancreas. In *Current medical diagnosis and treatment*, eds. L.M. Tierney, S.J. McPhee, M.A. Papadakis, and S.A. Schroeder, pp. 503–537. Norwalk, CT: Appleton & Lange.

Kools, A.M. 1992. Hepatitis A, B, C, D, E. *Postgraduate Medicine* 91(3):109–114.

Levine, P.H., Jacobson, S., Pocinki, A.G., Cheney, P., Peterson, D., Connelly, R.R., Weil, R., Robinson, S.M., Ablashi, D.V., Salahuddin, S.Z., Pearson, G.R., and Hoover, R. 1992. Clinical epidemiologic and virologic studies in four clusters of the chronic fatigue syndrome. *Archives of Internal Medicine* 152:1611–1616.

Lloyd, A.R., Gardenia, S.C., and Hales, P. 1991. Muscle performance, voluntary activation, twitch properties, and perceived effort in normal subjects and patients with chronic fatigue syndrome. *Brain* 114:85–98.

Lloyd, A.R., Hickie, I., Wakefield, D., Boughton, D.R., and Dwyer, J.M. 1990. A double-blind placebo-controlled trial of intravenous immunoglobulin therapy in patients with chronic fatigue syndrome. *American Journal of Medicine* 89:561–568.

Lloyd, A.R., Wakefield, D., Boughton, C.R., and Dwyer, J.M. 1989. Immunological abnormalities in the chronic fatigue syndrome. *Medical Journal of Australia* 151:122–124.

Logigian, E.L., Kaplan, R.F., and Steere, A.C. 1990. Chronic neurologic manifestations of Lyme disease. *New England Journal of Medicine* 323(21):1438–1444.

Maiman, M., Fruchter, R.G., Serur, E., Remy, J.C., Feuer, G., and Boyce, J. 1990. Human immunodeficiency virus infection and cervical neoplasia. *Gynecologic Oncology* 38:377–382.

Mann, J.M., Preblud, S.R., Hoffman, R.E., Brandling-Bennett, A.D., Hinman, A.R., and Herrmann, K.L. 1981. Assessing risks of rubella infection during pregnancy. A standardized approach. *Journal of the American Medical Association* 245(16):1647–1652.

Markowitz, L.E., Steere, A.C., Benach, J.L., Slade, J.D., and Broome, C.V. 1986. Lyme disease during pregnancy. *Journal of the American Medical Association* 255:3394–3396.

Marte, C., Cohen, M., Fruchter, R., and Kelly, P. 1992. Pap test and STD findings in HIV-positive women at ambulatory care sites. *American Journal of Obstetrics and Gynecology* 166(4):1232–1237.

Minkoff, H.L. 1991. Gynecologic care of HIV-infected women. *Contemporary Ob/Gyn* 35(9):46–60.

Minkoff, H., and Dehovitz, J.A. 1991. HIV infection in women. *AIDS Clinical Care* 3(5):33–35.

Padilla, V.M., and Schiff, E.R. 1991. Current topics in viral hepatitis. *Comprehensive Therapy* 17(9):7–12.

Pantaleo, G., Graziosi, C., Demarest, J.F., Butini, L., Montroni, M., Fox, C.H., Orenstein, J.M., Kotler, D.P., and Fauci, A.S. 1993. HIV infection is active and progressive in lymphoid tissue during the clinically latent stage of disease. *Nature* 362(6418):355–358.

Podolsky, D.K., and Isselbacher, K.J. 1991. Cirrhosis of the liver. In *Principles of internal medicine*, eds. J.D. Wilson, E. Braunmald, K. Isselbacher, R.G. Petersdorf, J.B. Martin, A.S. Fauci, and R.K. Root, 12th ed., pp. 1340–1350. New York: McGraw-Hill.

Rahn, D.W., and Malawista, S.E. 1991. Lyme disease: Recommendations for diagnosis and treatment. *Annals of Internal Medicine* 114(6):472–481.

Rhoads, J.L., Wright, C., Redfield, R.R., and Burke, D. S. 1987. Chronic vaginal candidiasis in women with human immunodeficiency virus infection. *Journal of the American Medical Association* 257(22):3105–3107.

Rompalo, A.M., Anderson, J.R., and Quinn, T.C. 1992. Reproductive tract infections and their management in women infected with the human immunodeficiency virus. *Infectious Diseases in Clinical Practice* 1(5):277–286.

Saag, M.S. 1994. AIDS testing now and in the future. In *The medical management of AIDS*, eds. M.A. Sande and P.A. Volberding, 4th ed., pp. 65–88. Philadelphia: W.B. Saunders.

Sande, M.A., Carpenter, C.C., Cobbs, C.G., Holmes, K.K., and Sanford, J.P. 1993. Antiretroviral therapy for adult HIV-infected patients. *Journal of the American Medical Association* 270:2583–2589.

Sanford, J.P., Sande, M.A., Gilbert, D.N., and Gerberding, J.L. 1994. *The Sanford guide to HIV/AIDS therapy*. Dallas: Antimicrobial Therapy, Inc.

San Francisco Epidemiologic Bulletin. 1992. Chronic fatigue syndrome/chronic fatigue immune dysfunction syndrome 8(9):33–37.

———. 1993. 1993 Revision of the HIV infection classification system and the AIDS surveillance definition. 9(1):1–6.

Schlesinger, P.A., Duray, P.H., Burke, B.A., Steere, A.C., and Stillman, M.T. 1985. Maternal-fetal transmission of the Lyme disease spirochete, *Borrelia burgdorferi*. *Annals of Internal Medicine* 103:67–69.

Schluederberg, A., Straus, S.E., Peterson, P., Blumenthal, S., Komaroff, A.L., Spring, S.B., Landay, A., and Buchwald, D. 1992. Chronic fatigue syndrome research. Definition and medical outcome assessment. *Annals of Internal Medicine* 117(4):325–331.

Schroeder, S.A., and McPhee, S.J. 1993. General approach to the patient: Health maintenance and disease prevention; principles of diagnostic test selection and use; common symptoms. In *Current medical diagnosis and treatment*, eds. L.M. Tierney, Jr., S.J. McPhee, M.A.

Papadakis, and S. A. Schroeder, 32d ed., pp. 1–20. Norwalk, CT: Appleton & Lange.

Shandera, W., and Gill, E.P. 1994. Infectious diseases: Viral and rickettsial. In *Current medical diagnosis and treatment*, eds. L.M. Tierney, Jr., S.J. McPhee, and M.A. Papadakis. 33rd ed., pp. 1098–1128. Norwalk, CT: Appleton & Lange.

Shapiro, C.N., and Margolis, H.S. 1992. Impact of hepatitis B virus infection on women and children. *Infectious Disease Clinics of North America* 6(1):75–98.

Shapiro, E.D., Gerber, M.A., Holabird, N.B., Berg, A.T., Feder, H.M., Bell, G.L., Rys, P.N., and Persing, D.H. 1992. A controlled trial of antimicrobial prophylaxis for Lyme disease after deer tick bites. *New England Journal of Medicine* 327(25):1769–1773.

Shin, D.M., and Avers, J. 1988. *AIDS/HIV reference guide for medical professionals*, 3d ed. Los Angeles: Regents of the University of California.

Steere, A.C. 1989. Lyme disease. *New England Journal of Medicine* 321(9):586–596.

Straus, S.E., Ostrave, J.M., Inchauspe G., Felser, J.M., Freifeld, A., Croen, K.D., and Sawyer, M.H. 1988. Varicella zoster virus infections. Biology, natural history, treatment, and prevention. *Annals of Internal Medicine* 108(2):221–237.

Stremmel, W., Schwarzendrobe, J., Niederau, C., and Strohmeyer, G. 1991. Epidemiology, clinical course, and treatment of chronic viral hepatitis. *Hepatogastroenterology* 38(1):22–28.

Tellier, R., and Keystone, J.S. 1992. Prevention of traveler's diarrhea. *Infectious Disease Clinics of North America* 6(2):333–354.

Thorne, G.M. 1988. Diagnosis of infectious diarrheal diseases. *Infectious Disease Clinics of North America* 2(3):747–774.

Ware, B.R., and Jones, J.E. 1991. The office diagnosis of common intestinal parasitic diseases. *Primary Care* 18(1):185–193.

Weber, K., Bratzke, H.J., Neubert, U., Wilske, B., and Duray, P.H. 1988. *Borrelia burgdorferi* in a newborn despite oral penicillin for Lyme borreliosis during pregnancy. *Pediatric Infectious Disease* 7:286–289.

Wharton, M., Cochi, S.L., and Williams, W.W. 1990. Measles, mumps, and rubella vaccines. *Infectious Disease Clinics of North America* 4(1):47–59.

Wolfe, M.S. 1990. Acute diarrhea associated with travel. *The American Journal of Medicine* 88(Suppl. 6A):34S–37S.

SECTION 12

Genitourinary Disorders

(Each section contains its own Bibliography)

12-A

Abnormal Uterine Bleeding

Abnormal uterine bleeding is defined as a significant variation from one's usual menstrual pattern. *Menses* are considered abnormal if they occur more often than every 21 days, persist longer than seven days, and/or if total blood loss is greater than 80 ml (Engel and Moison 1991). Abnormal uterine bleeding can be classified under two major etiological categories: organic (25 percent of cases) and dysfunctional (nonorganic, 75 percent of cases) (Field 1988; Long and Gast 1990; Murata 1989). See **Table 12A.1, Classification of Abnormal Uterine Bleeding**. Organic causes include local (genital) factors, gross endocrinopathies, systemic disease, and iatrogenic factors (Benjamin and Seltzer 1987).

Genital tract factors are among the most common causes of organic bleeding. Normal ovulatory function is generally not disturbed in these cases (Field 1988). Gross endocrinopathies cause abnormal bleeding by indirectly interfering with gonadotropin-releasing hormone (GnRH), follicle-stimulating hormone (FSH), or luteinizing hormone (LH), and/or estrogen/progesterone function (Benjamin and Seltzer 1987). Systemic disease can cause abnormal uterine bleeding via deficiencies in hormone metabolism, conjugation, or clearance, or, in the case of blood dyscrasias, by defects in specific clotting factors (Benjamin and Seltzer 1987).

Blood dyscrasias usually accompany ovulatory cycles and account for about 20 percent of cases of heavy bleeding among adolescent females. Iatrogenic factors mainly include drugs and medications which may cause abnormal bleeding by their direct uterine effects or effects on the clotting abilities of menstrual blood (Long and Gast 1990).

Dysfunctional uterine bleeding (DUB) is a diagnosis of exclusion when organic causes of abnormal

bleeding have been ruled out. Ninety percent of DUB is due to *anovulation*. Anovulation results from disturbances of the feedback signals of the hypothalamic-pituitary-ovarian (HPO) axis and/or from within the ovary itself (March 1991; Speroff, Glass, and Kase 1989, 1994). Approximately 50 percent of women with DUB are in the 40- to 50-year-old age group; 20 percent are adolescents (March 1991).

Anovulatory uterine bleeding patterns depend upon the duration and intensity of endometrial estrogen stimulation and on the response of the endometrium to specific hormonal stimuli (ACOG 1989). Classic anovulatory bleeding involves constant estrogen stimulation with resultant endometrial overgrowth and eventual breakdown, occurring over a variable period of time. Sporadic and uncoordinated loss of the endometrial lining occurs, resulting in varying presentations of uterine bleeding such as *menorrhagia, amenorrhea, oligomenorrhea*, or *polymenorrhea* (Field 1988; Long and Gast 1990). In many cases the cycle interval is prolonged, and bleeding is heavy. All anovulatory patterns have one common denominator—the absence of progesterone influence on the endometrium (ACOG 1989).

Prolonged exposure to unopposed estrogen may lead to *endometrial hyperplasia*. One type of hyperplasia, adenomatous hyperplasia, increases the risk for atypical cellular changes of the endometrium. Atypical hyperplasia is a precursor of endometrial adenocarcinoma. In most cases of DUB, however, morphology of the endometrium is normal (ACOG 1989).

Ovulatory cycles are present in 10 percent of cases of DUB and are mostly encountered in the adult reproductive age group (Field 1988). Ovulatory DUB is defined as abnormal uterine bleeding superimposed on

Table 12A.1.   CLASSIFICATION OF ABNORMAL UTERINE BLEEDING

Organic Causes 25%	Dysfunctional Causes 15%.
Local Pelvic Factors Leiomyomas Polyps Endometriosis Uterine neoplasm Pelvic inflammatory disease Ovarian tumors Pregnancy-related events Intrauterine device Foreign body Other genital lesions: anatomical, benign masses, inflammatory, infection, sexually transmitted disease	**Anovulatory** HPO axis disturbances **Ovulatory** Persistent corpus luteum Luteal phase deficiency Decreased estrogen at midcycle Increased endometrial fibrinolysins

Gross Endocrinopathy
Hypothalamic disorders
   psychogenic
   polycystic ovary syndrome
   organic diseases
Pituitary diseases
   hyperprolactinemia
   acromegaly
Thyroid dysfunction
Diabetes mellitus
Adrenal diseases
   congenital adrenal hyperplasia
   Cushing's syndrome
   Addison's disease
   tumors	

Systemic Disease
Blood dyscrasias
   idiopathic thrombocytopenia purpura
   Von Willebrand's disease
   other hematological disorders: leukemia; lupus; factor II, V, VII,
      XI, and prothrombin deficiencies
Increased endometrial fibrinolysins
Hepatic diseases
Renal disease
Obesity	

Iatrogenic Factors Anticoagulants Hormones Digitalis Aspirin Major tranquilizers Chemotherapeutic agents	
Extragenital Factors Urinary tract Gastrointestinal tract	

Source: Adapted from Benjamin, F., and Seltzer, V.L. 1987. Excessive menstrual bleeding, menorrhagia, and dysfunctional uterine bleeding. In *Gynecology principles and practice*, eds. Z. Rosenwaks, F. Benjamin, and M.L. Stone. New York: Macmillan.

regular cyclic menstruation (Gomel, Munro, and Rowe 1990). It may manifest a variety of bleeding patterns due to several different pathophysiological mechanisms.

Menorrhagia is one of the most commonly encountered abnormal ovulatory bleeding patterns. It may affect 15 percent to 20 percent of otherwise healthy women (Long and Gast 1990; Zacur and Morales 1990). In the absence of disease, a locally enhanced fibrinolysis and shift in prostaglandin synthesis toward platelet ag-

gregation inhibition and vasodilatation promotion may result in "essential" menorrhagia (van Eijkeren et al. 1992).

When progesterone production is prolonged, as with a persistent *corpus luteum* (Halban's disease), "irregular shedding" may occur, with drawn out, heavy, but regular bleeding (Field 1988). Premenstrual or postmenstrual spotting is due to disordered corpus luteum regression or an irregular follicular response, respectively. Midcycle spotting/bleeding may result from a temporary decrease of estrogen during this time. *Luteal phase deficiency* (LFD), also known as corpus luteum insufficiency, occurs when insufficient progesterone is produced post-ovulation. Variations in cycle length, duration/amount of flow, and postmenstrual spotting, as well as infertility or recurrent pregnancy loss, may be encountered with LFD (Field 1988).

Abnormal uterine bleeding (due to organic causes) and dysfunctional uterine bleeding may coexist or seem to overlap, and the terms often are used interchangeably.

DATABASE

SUBJECTIVE

→ A patient with abnormal bleeding may present with any of the following bleeding patterns (Connell 1989; Field 1988; Gomel, Munro, and Rowe 1990; Johnson 1991; March 1991; Shulman 1990; Speroff, Glass, and Kase 1994):

■ menorrhagia: Prolonged and/or excessive (>80 ml) uterine bleeding occurring at regular intervals (also known as hypermenorrhea).
  • Etiologies may include polyps, myomas, adenomyosis, infection, intrauterine device (IUD), systemic diseases, thyroid disease, endocrinopathies, HPO axis disturbances, polycystic ovarian disease, obesity, ovarian neoplasms, endometrial hyperplasia, carcinoma, blood dyscrasias, and arteriovenous malformation of uterine wall (rare).

■ metrorrhagia: Uterine bleeding occurring between normal menses (intermenstrual bleeding), variable in amount.
  • Etiologies may include oral contraceptives, IUD, endogenous or endogenous unopposed estrogen, thyroid dysfunction, coagulopathies, pregnancy complications, benign or malignant genital lesions, trauma or foreign bodies, cervical eversion or dysplasia, infection, polyps, myomas, malignancy, functional ovarian cysts, ovarian tumors, endometriosis, physiological decrease of estrogen at midcycle, luteal phase defect.

■ menometrorrhagia: Prolonged uterine bleeding occurring at irregular intervals. (See etiologies listed previously.)

■ postmenopausal bleeding: Uterine bleeding occurring less than one year after the last menstrual period in a woman with ovarian

failure. (Some clinicians use six months as a cutoff.)
  • Etiologies may include atrophy, hyperplasia, or malignancy of the endometrium; polyps; atrophic vaginitis; urethral caruncle; hormone replacement therapy; trauma; infection; and vulvar lesions.

■ polymenorrhea: Cycle intervals of less than 21 days. The proliferative phase may be less than 10 days or the secretory phase less than 14 days.
  • Etiologies may include immature HPO axis; systemic, endocrine, or metabolic disorders; or psychogenic causes.

■ oligomenorrhea: Cycle intervals ranging from 35 days to six months.
  • Etiologies may include oral contraceptives, HPO axis dysfunction, systemic diseases, endocrinopathies, and drug abuse.

■ hypomenorrhea: Abnormally small amount of menstrual bleeding.
  • Etiologies may include Asherman's syndrome, Cushing's syndrome, ovarian failure, congenital obstruction of the outflow tract, or oral contraceptives.

■ amenorrhea: Absence of menstrual bleeding for six months or more than three of the previous cycle intervals.
  • Disorders of any of the following compartments may be the cause: outflow tract, ovary, anterior pituitary, or CNS (hypothalamus) (Speroff, Glass, and Kase 1989).

→ Specific symptoms associated with genital infection: pregnancy; thyroid, liver, renal, or adrenal disease; diabetes; and/or infertility may exist. It is beyond the scope of this protocol to list the specific symptoms associated with all of these entities. (Refer to other protocols.)

→ History of the patient with abnormal/dysfunctional bleeding requires systematic consideration of the many possible etiologies, which may include, but not be limited to:

■ menstrual cycle and obstetrical/gynecological history:
  • last normal menstrual period.
  • previous normal menstrual periods (ideally the last three).
  • usual cycle interval, duration of flow, presence of clots.
  • onset/change in menstrual cycle characteristics.

- number of pads/tampons per day during normal and abnormal bleeding episodes, and degree of saturation.
- aggravating factors associated with abnormal bleeding (e.g., exercise, trauma, intercourse, douching).
- associated physical symptoms/molimina:
  - bloating.
  - cramping.
  - irritability.
  - breast tenderness.
  - mittelschmerz.
  - abnormal vaginal discharge, odor, or itching.
  - abdominal/pelvic pain.
  - urinary frequency, urgency, dysuria.
  - fever.
  - chills.
  - nausea.
  - vomiting.
  - diarrhea or constipation.
- age at menarche/menopause.
- gravidy.
- parity.
- number of abortions (spontaneous or induced).
- Pap smear history.
- previous episodes of abnormal bleeding and/ or diagnosis of other gynecological disorders, and how they were managed.
- history of sexually transmitted diseases (STDs).
- gynecological surgery.
- last delivery.
- complications of pregnancy.
- current breast-feeding status.
■ sexual history:
  - sexual preference, number of partners, sex practices, date of last coitus, sexual partner history.
■ contraceptive history:
  - type/use of oral contraceptives; use of Norplant® or Depo-Provera®; use of condoms, spermicides, diaphragm, or cervical cap; IUD use (time of insertion, complications); sterilization (patient and partner); desire for future fertility.
■ medical history:
  - including general health, present/past major medical disorders and how managed (systemic, endocrine, metabolic, etc.), including:
    - trauma.
    - bleeding tendencies.

- childhood illnesses.
- hospitalizations.
- surgeries.
- medications.
- habits: tobacco, drugs, alcohol, exercise.
- nutritional status.
- environmental/occupational hazards.
- review of systems: weight, hair, or appetite changes; petechiae; bruising; hot flushes; hot/cold sensitivity; fatigability; weakness; headaches; galactorrhea; vaginal dryness; recent illness; and any other symptoms of systemic, endocrine, or metabolic disease, and/or genitourinary or gastrointestinal disorders.
■ social history:
  - education/occupation, marital/partner/social support status, psychosocial stressors, anxiety level, life satisfaction, etc.
■ family history:
  - bleeding disorders, endometriosis, ovarian/ endometrial cancer.

OBJECTIVE

→ Ideally, a thorough physical examination should be performed. Important components to assess may include, but are not limited to (Clark-Coller 1991; Shulman 1990):
■ vital signs:
  - blood pressure, pulse, postural vital signs as indicated.
■ general:
  - height, weight, skin pallor, stature, habitus, posture, motor activity, gait, dress, grooming, personal hygiene, manner, mood, affect, developmental stage of secondary sex characteristics, stigmata of systemic or endocrine disease.
■ hair:
  - texture, loss of axillary/pubic hair, hirsutism.
■ eyes, ears:
  - stare, lid lag, exophthalmos, visual field defects, auditory acuity, fundoscopic changes.
■ neck:
  - thyroid masses/enlargement, lymph nodes, "buffalo hump."
■ skin:
  - dry, moist, warm, cold, rough, petechiae, ecchymoses, acne, facial plethora, palmar erythema, nail bed color.
■ deep tendon reflexes.
■ extremities:
  - edema, wasting.

- heart/lungs:
  - general assessment.
- breasts:
  - striae, masses, tenderness, galactorrhea.
- abdomen:
  - striae, organomegaly, masses, tenderness, inguinal nodes, pulses.
- pelvis:
  - complete assessment of mons pubis, vulva, vagina, cervix, uterus, adnexa and rectum, noting any abnormalities.
    - –assess for pubic hair distribution, clitoral hypertrophy, visible bleeding sites, vaginal or cervical lesions, evidence of trauma/foreign body, atrophy, polyps, abnormal discharge, Chadwick's/Hegar's signs, presence of uterine enlargement/tenderness, adnexal fullness/tenderness, rectal or cul-de-sac masses/fullness/nodularity, nodularity of sacrospinous ligaments, fixation of pelvic organs.
    - –if patient is wearing perineal pad or tampon assess the degree of bleeding.

ASSESSMENT

→ Abnormal uterine bleeding (organic causes)

→ Dysfunctional uterine bleeding, may be anovulatory or ovulatory

→ R/O pregnancy in reproductive-age woman

PLAN

DIAGNOSTIC TESTS

→ Menstrual calendars should be utilized to establish an abnormal bleeding pattern when the history is unclear.

→ Methods for direct measurement of menstrual blood loss are generally unavailable.
  - Determination of number of tampons/pads is an unreliable means for assessing the amount of blood loss.

→ Ordering of laboratory tests should be individualized based on the patient's age, clinical presentation, and consideration of the differential diagnoses.
  - May consult with physician to determine necessary laboratory work.

→ Disorders of pregnancy should be considered in all cases of abnormal bleeding (unless patient is clearly postmenopausal), thus qualitative or quantitative serum HCG tests should be ordered.

→ Additional lab tests may include, but are not limited to:
  - complete blood count (CBC).
  - ferritin (or other tests of iron status).
  - reticulocyte count.
  - erythrocyte sedimentation rate (ESR).
  - coagulation profile, including prothrombin time (PT), partial thromboplastin time (PTT), bleeding time, and platelet count.
  - prolactin.
  - thyroid function tests (TSH, T_3, T_4, FTI).
  - serum androgens (testosterone, dehydroepiandrosterone sulfate [DHEA-S]).
  - midluteal progesterone, FSH, LH, and renal/hepatic function tests (creatinine, blood urea nitrogen (BUN), serum transaminases).
  - adrenal function testing (serum cortisol, 17-hydroxyprogesterone).
  - fasting blood sugar (FBS) (Long and Gast 1990; Nesse 1991).

→ Pap smear and endocervical cultures for *Neisseria gonorrhoeae* and *Chlamydia trachomatis* are suggested.

→ Wet mounts may be performed as indicated.

→ Biopsy of any suspicious vulvar, vaginal, or cervical lesion. Refer to/consult with a physician.

→ Basal body temperature (BBT) recordings and cervical mucus charting may differentiate between ovulatory and anovulatory cycles.

→ Pelvic ultrasound (preferably with transvaginal probe) may be used for diagnosis of early pregnancy disorders or intrauterine/intrapelvic disease (e.g., myomata, ovarian masses) and measurement of endometrial thickness (Herbst et al. 1992; Long and Gast 1990).

→ Endometrial biopsy (EMB) is indicated in women over age 35 years since malignancy potential is increased in this age group.
  - Endometrial biopsy also may be done in younger women with persistent abnormal bleeding associated with longstanding anovulation (ACOG 1989).
  - Young teenagers with anovulatory cycles generally do not require biopsy.
  - Consult with a physician.

→ Computerized tomographic (CT) scan and magnetic resonance imaging (MRI) are used in staging/follow-up of gynecological malignancies, and also can be used for high-resolution viewing of intramyometrial structures (Long and Gast 1990).

→ Hysteroscopy often is used to rule out an endometrial polyp, submucous myoma, hyperplasia, or an atrophic endometrium (Rueda et al. 1991).
- Biopsies may be done under direct visualization.
  - This technique may better identify both isolated and generalized uterine pathologies missed by blind biopsy or curettage (Long and Gast 1990).
- Refer to a physician.

→ Hysterosalpingogram (HSG) may be used as an adjunctive tool in identifying space-occupying lesions within the uterus (Long and Gast 1990).
- This test should not be performed when patient is bleeding and only if the pregnancy test is negative (March 1991).
- Refer to a physician.

→ Dilatation and curettage (D and C) is used in emergency situations, such as when heavy bleeding is associated with profound anemia, when there is evidence of hyperplasia on EMB, or when the EMB is insufficient to exclude malignancy, and when abnormal bleeding persists despite medical management (March 1991; Nesse 1991).
- Refer to a physician.

TREATMENT/MANAGEMENT

→ There is no single approach to use with all patients. The primary goals are to normalize the bleeding and seek underlying causes (ACOG 1989). Pregnancy should always be ruled out.

Acute, hemorrhagic bleeding

→ Patient should be hospitalized and *managed by a physician*.
- Full discussion of inpatient therapy is beyond the scope of this protocol.

→ Conjugated estrogens (Premarin®) in 25 mg doses I.V. every 4 hours until bleeding stops (up to 3 doses), followed by oral conjugated estrogen 2.5 mg-3.75 mg/day for 21 days.
- During the last 7-10 days of the estrogen regimen, add a progestational agent (e.g., medroxyprogesterone acetate [Provera®]) 10 mg p.o. (ACOG 1989; Connell 1989; Speroff, Glass, and Kase 1989, 1994).
- Alternatively, a combined oral contraceptive may be given for 21 days following intravenous therapy (Field 1988; Speroff, Glass, and Kase 1994).
  - Patient may be maintained on oral contraceptive if pregnancy is not desired.

→ If bleeding has not stopped in 12 to 24 hours, a D and C usually is performed (Speroff, Glass, and Kase 1989). D and C may be considered initially on the basis of age, evidence of hypovolemia, and/or severe anemia (March 1991).

Acute, heavy bleeding

→ Combined low-dose monophasic estrogen-progestin oral contraceptive: 1 pill 2-4 times/day for 5-7 days (Speroff, Glass, and Kase 1989, 1994). (An antiemetic may be needed with QID dosing.)
- Bleeding usually stops in 12-24 hours.
- If bleeding does not stop, consider other pathologies (e.g., polyps, incomplete abortion, neoplasia) (Speroff, Glass, and Kase 1989, 1994).
- Warn patient to expect a heavy, crampy flow 2-4 days after last pill.
- On day 5 of flow, begin a low-dose combined oral contraceptive, 1 pill/day for 21 days. After 1 week off, begin oral contraceptive again and repeat this process for 3-6 months (Field 1988; Speroff, Glass, and Kase 1989, 1994).
- Oral contraceptives may be continued indefinitely if the patient needs a form of birth control and is doing well with the pill.
- Alternatively, the pill may be discontinued after 3 months to assess the woman's bleeding pattern.
- If menses does not resume, a progestin regimen may be employed after ruling out pregnancy (see following discussion on "Chronic anovulatory bleeding") (Speroff, Glass, and Kase 1989, 1994).

→ Alternatively, acute bleeding may be controlled with oral estrogen. Regimens include:
- 1.25 mg conjugated estrogen p.o. for 7-10 days (Speroff, Glass, and Kase 1994).
- 2.0 mg estradiol p.o. for 7-10 days (Speroff, Glass, and Kase 1994).
- 1.25 mg conjugated estrogen
  OR
  2.0 mg estradiol p.o. every 4 hours for 24 hours, followed by the single daily dose for 7-10 days. This regimen is designed for more moderately heavy bleeding (Speroff, Glass, and Kase 1994).
  NOTE: All of the above must be followed by progestin therapy and a withdrawal bleed (Speroff, Glass, and Kase 1994). Patient may thereafter be managed with low-dose oral contraceptives. WARNING: Any high-dose

estrogen therapy (i.e., more than one oral contraceptive/day and multiple doses of oral or intravenous estrogen/24 hours) has a theoretical risk of precipitating a thrombotic event (Speroff, Glass, and Kase 1994). Physician consultation should be sought and the patient's risk factors considered in the decision making process.

→ Postmenopausal acute heavy bleeding is best managed by D and C in the hospital (Connell 1989).

Chronic anovulatory bleeding (oligomenorrhea, amenorrhea with terminal menorrhagia, polymenorrhea)

→ Rule out uterine pathology with EMB, hysteroscopy, HSG, D and C, etc., especially in women over age 35 years and in any patient who has frequent, heavy, or prolonged bleeding (Field 1988).
  ▪ An EMB should be performed prior to hormonal therapy in women who are anovulatory for extended periods of time (ACOG 1989).

→ Medroxyprogesterone acetate (Provera®) 10 mg/day p.o. for 10 days/month may be prescribed.
  ▪ Withdrawal bleeding will occur 2-7 days after the last pill of each cycle.
  ▪ If irregular bleeding is not ameliorated by progestin therapy, re-evaluate for uterine pathology or other causes of abnormal bleeding (March 1991; Speroff, Glass, and Kase 1989, 1994).

→ Progesterone in oil 250 mg I.M. may be given to control bleeding.
  ▪ Withdrawal flow will ensue 10-14 days later.
  ▪ Progesterone in oil 50 mg-100 mg I.M. may be given at 4-week intervals instead of oral progestin medication (ACOG 1989).
  ▪ Long-acting depo-medroxyprogesterone acetate (Depo-Provera®) 150 mg I.M. every 3 months may also be used to inhibit ovarian function and create an atrophic endometrium (ACOG 1989).
  ▪ Consult with a physician.

→ Sexually active women desiring hormonal contraception may be best managed with low-dose oral contraceptives on a monthly basis.

→ Perimenopausal patients may require conjugated estrogen (Premarin®) 0.625 mg-1.25 mg p.o. daily with medroxyprogesterone acetate (Provera®) 10 mg p.o. on days 1-12, after endometrial pathology has been ruled out (March 1991).

  ▪ Alternatively, patients in the 40- to 50-years age group may be treated with low-dose combined oral contraceptives provided they do not have risk factors of smoking, diabetes, hypertension, obesity, and/or hypercholesterolemia (ACOG 1989). Consult with physician.

→ Observation alone may suffice, provided bleeding is not heavy/frequent or patient does not develop amenorrhea.
  ▪ Recommend menstrual calendar.

Metrorrhagia

→ Attempt to ascertain the cause of bleeding through history and physical examination.

→ Order appropriate laboratory tests as indicated, including pregnancy test, CBC, ESR, midluteal phase serum progesterone, Pap smear, endocervical cultures, and others.

→ An EMB, hysteroscopy, HSG, D and C, etc., may be used as indicated.
  ▪ Consult with a physician.

→ Observation alone may suffice if no organic pathology is identified (Field 1988).
  ▪ Recommend menstrual calendar.
  ▪ Basal body temperature and mucus charting also may be recommended to document ovulation.

→ Identified organic pathology should be treated appropriately. Consult with a physician as indicated.

→ Premenstrual spotting: medroxyprogesterone acetate (Provera®) 10 mg/day p.o. for 7-12 days beginning on day 15 of the menstrual cycle may be prescribed if patient desires therapy and is not attempting pregnancy, and organic pathology has been ruled out (Field 1988; Gomel, Munro, and Rowe 1990).

→ Midcycle spotting: conjugated estrogen (Premarin®) 1.25 mg-2.5 mg/day p.o. or ethinyl estradiol 10 mg-20 mg/day p.o. from 1-3 days before to 2-4 days after ovulation may be used if patient desires therapy, is not attempting pregnancy, and organic pathology has been ruled out (Field 1988; Gomel, Munro, and Rowe 1990).

→ Postmenstrual spotting: Prostaglandin synthetase inhibitors (see following discussion) (Field 1988).

→ Oral contraceptives also may be used for premenstrual/postmenstrual, or midcycle spotting/bleeding (Field 1988), provided organic pathology has been ruled out and patient is not interested in achieving pregnancy.

Menorrhagia

→ Patients with chronic ovulatory menorrhagia should have intrauterine pathology ruled out. The goal of long-term therapy is to reduce blood loss (March 1991).

→ Prostaglandin synthetase inhibitors (nonsteroidal anti-inflammatory drugs [NSAIDs]). Regimens include:
  ▪ mefenamic acid (Ponstel®) 500 mg p.o. TID for 3 days during menstrual bleeding.
  ▪ ibuprofen (Motrin®, Advil®, or Nuprin®) 400 mg-600 mg TID for 3 days during menstrual bleeding.
  ▪ naproxen (Naprosyn®) 500 mg p.o. initially, then 250 mg p.o. TID for 3-5 days during menstrual bleeding (Field 1988; Herbst et al. 1992; Long and Gast 1990).
  ▪ **NOTE:** These agents are contraindicated in patients with an ulcer or bronchospastic lung disease (Rueda et al. 1991); NSAIDs also may reduce bleeding in IUD wearers and possibly in women with myomas (ACOG 1989).

→ Danazol (Danocrine®) 200 mg-400 mg/day p.o. for 12 weeks results in endometrial atrophy and has been used in cases of excessive uterine bleeding (March 1991).
  ▪ Consult with a physician.

→ Combined low-dose oral contraceptives (March 1991).

→ Prolonged progestin use—i.e., medroxyprogesterone acetate (Provera®) 10 mg/day p.o. for 10 days each month (March 1991).
  ▪ Sexually active women not desiring pregnancy may be best managed with combined low-dose oral contraceptives.

→ Long-acting depo-medroxyprogesterone acetate (Depo-Provera®) 150 mg I.M. every 3 months also may be used to inhibit ovarian function and create an atrophic endometrium (ACOG 1989; Gomel, Munro, and Rowe 1990).

→ Progestasert® IUD may be of short-term benefit (Field 1988).

→ GnRH-agonist therapy leads to a suppression of gonadotropins and lowering of estradiol to the menopausal range; thus menstruation is arrested (Rueda et al. 1991).
  ▪ Bone loss is a concern with this therapy.
  ▪ Consult with a physician.

→ Antifibrinolytic agents—e.g., *E*-amino-caproic acid (EACA) and tranexamic acid (AMCA) have been used to reduce menorrhagia. Side effects are common, however, and these drugs have been associated with thromboembolic events, thus their use is limited (Long and Gast 1990).

→ Ergot derivatives are not recommended (March 1991).

→ Aspirin does not diminish blood loss and may even increase loss (van Eijkeren 1992).

→ Endometrial ablation via the Nd:Yag laser, resectoscope, or roller ball are newer surgical techniques to control excessive uterine bleeding (Ke and Taylor 1991).
  ▪ These techniques are performed by an experienced physician under general or regional anesthesia.
  ▪ Best results are obtained when the endometrium has been suppressed with danocrine, GnRH-agonist, or medroxyprogesterone acetate for 4 to 6 weeks prior to surgery (Long and Gast 1990; Rueda et al. 1991).

→ Hysterectomy is the last resort in the treatment of menorrhagia.

Additional considerations

→ Iron replacement therapy should be prescribed when anemia is present. (See **Anemia** Protocol.)

→ Identified underlying endocrine dysfunction, coagulation disorders, systemic illness, or behavioral alterations should be treated appropriately. (See appropriate **Genitourinary Disorders, Hematological/Endocrine Disorders,** and **Behavioral Disorders** protocols.) Refer patient to appropriate health care provider as indicated.

→ Ovulation induction is indicated for anovulatory patients desiring pregnancy. (See **Infertility** Protocol.)

→ Patients with recurrent pregnancy loss should be referred to a gynecologist or infertility specialist.

CONSULTATION

→ Consultation with a physician is recommended for all cases of abnormal bleeding and for endometrial biopsy and/or other genital biopsies as necessary.

→ Refer to gynecologist as indicated by clinical presentation.
  ▪ Patients with acute, heavy bleeding should be managed by a physician.

→ Patients with identified endocrine or systemic pathologies, coagulation disorders, or underlying conditions should be referred to a specialist.

→ As needed for prescription(s).

PATIENT EDUCATION

→ Thoroughly explain identified etiologies of abnormal bleeding. Specific recommendations for care will depend upon the identified pathology/ disorder.
  ■ Patient-education handouts are a helpful adjunct to teaching.

→ Discuss planned hormonal therapy, and include patient in the decision making. Ascertain the woman's/couple's desire for pregnancy.

→ Encourage compliance with prescribed medication and follow-up visits. Discuss side effects of medication prescribed, and alert patient to the anticipated withdrawal bleeding episodes.

→ Advise a menstrual calendar and encourage patient to bring it with her to all office visits.
  ■ A BBT and cervical mucus chart also may be suggested.

→ Ask the patient to keep track of pad/tampon use and degree of saturation, if indicated, to aid in establishing amount of blood loss, although this information can provide only a crude estimate.

→ Provide psychological support to the woman experiencing infertility or recurrent pregnancy loss. Refer patient to a mental health professional as indicated.

→ Address issues of weight loss/gain, proper nutrition, exercise, and stress management.

FOLLOW-UP

→ Patients with acute bleeding should return for re-evaluation if bleeding does not subside after administration of medication.

→ Return visit schedules will vary depending upon the pathology identified and the therapy provided.
  ■ Patient should be evaluated initially at regular intervals (e.g., three to six months) or as necessary.
  ■ Carefully assess growth of myomas if identified. (See **Pelvic Masses** Protocol.)

→ Annual visits should include thorough reassessment of the patient's gynecological and medical history and a thorough physical examination.

→ Follow up on all lab work ordered. Review abnormal labs with physician as indicated.

→ Refer patient to the appropriate health care provider when endocrine or systemic pathology has been identified.

→ Document in progress notes and problem list.

Bibliography

American College of Obstetricians and Gynecologists. 1989. *Dysfunctional uterine bleeding.* Technical Bulletin. Washington, DC: the Author.

Benjamin, F., and Seltzer, V. L. 1987. Excessive menstrual bleeding, menorrhagia, and dysfunctional uterine bleeding. In *Gynecology principles and practice*, eds. Z. Rosenwaks, F. Benjamin, and M.L. Stone. New York: Macmillan.

Clark-Coller, T. 1991. Dysfunctional uterine bleeding and amenorrhea. *Journal of Nurse-Midwifery* 36(1):49–62.

Connell, A. 1989. Abnormal uterine bleeding. *Nurse Practitioner* 14(4):40–57.

Engel, T., and Moison, S. 1991. Abnormal uterine bleeding. In *Ob/Gyn secrets*, eds. H.L. Frederickson and L. Wilkins-Haug, pp. 18–20. St. Louis: Mosby Year Book.

Field, C. S. 1988. Dysfunctional uterine bleeding. *Primary Care* 15(3):561–575.

Frederickson, H.L., and Wilkins-Haug, L.W., eds. 1991. *Ob/Gyn secrets.* St. Louis: Mosby Year Book.

Gomel, V., Munro, M.G., and Rowe, T.C. 1990. *Gynecology. A practical approach.* Baltimore: Williams & Wilkins.

Herbst, A.L., Mishell, D.R., Stenchever, M.A., and Droegemueller, W. 1992. *Comprehensive gynecology*, 2d ed. St. Louis: Mosby Year Book.

Johnson, C.A. 1991. Making sense of dysfunctional uterine bleeding. *American Family Physician* 44(1):149–157.

Ke, R.W., and Taylor, P.J. 1991. Endometrial ablation to control excessive uterine bleeding. *Human Reproduction* 6(4):574–580.

Lichtman, R., and Papera, S. 1990. *Gynecology. Well-woman care.* Norwalk, CT: Appleton & Lange.

Long, C.A., and Gast, M.J. 1990. Menorrhagia. *Obstetrics and Gynecology Clinics of North America* 17(2):343–359.

March, C.M. 1991. Dysfunctional uterine bleeding. In *Infertility, contraception, and reproductive endocrinology*, 3rd ed., eds. D.R. Mishell, V. Davajan, and R.A. Lobo, pp. 488–502. Boston: Blackwell Scientific Publications.

Murata, J.M. 1989. Abnormal genital bleeding and secondary amenorrhea. Common gynecological problems. *Journal of Obstetric, Gynecologic, and Neonatal Nursing* 19(1):26–36.

Nesse, R. E. 1991. Managing abnormal vaginal bleeding. *Postgraduate Medicine* 89(1):205–214.

Nilsson, L., and Rybo, G. 1971. Treatment of menorrhagia. *American Journal of Obstetrics and Gynecology* 110:713.

Rueda, R., Falcone, T., Hemmings, R., and Tulandi, T. 1991. Dysfunctional uterine bleeding: A reappraisal. *Current Problems in Obstetrics, Gynecology, and Infertility* 14(3):71–96.

Shulman, J.F. 1990. Bleeding disorders. In *Gynecology: Well-woman care*, eds., R. Lichtman and D. Papera. Norwalk, CT: Appleton & Lange.

Speroff, L., Glass, R.H., and Kase, N.G. 1989. *Clinical gynecologic endocrinology and infertility*, 4th ed. Baltimore: Williams & Wilkins.

———. 1994. *Clinical gynecologic endocrinology and infertility*, 5th ed. Baltimore: Williams & Wilkins.

Van Eijkeren, M.A., Christiaens, G.C.M.L., Scholten, P.C., and Sixma, J.J. 1992. Menorrhagia. Current drug treatment concepts. *Drugs* 43(2):201–209.

Zacur, H.A., and Morales, A. 1990. Menstrual disorders and their management. *Current Opinion in Obstetrics and Gynecology* 2(3):405–411.

Lynn N. Hanson, N.P., M.S.

12-B

Abnormal Cervical Cytology

Several classification systems for *cervical cytology* are in use today. Recently, the Bethesda System was developed in an attempt to standardize and clarify cytopathological reports (Lundberg 1989). The Bethesda System provides detailed descriptive information and recommendations for follow-up on abnormal findings. The format of the report includes three components:

- a statement on the adequacy of the specimen.
- a general categorization (within normal limits or other).
- a descriptive diagnosis.

The descriptive diagnosis component may report the following:

- infection.
- reactive and reparative changes.
- epithelial cell abnormalities.
- nonepithelial malignant neoplasm.
- hormonal evaluation (vaginal smears only).

Cytological abnormalities representing the spectrum from atypia, to premalignancy, to squamous cell carcinoma are reported under the category "epithelial cell abnormalities." Atypia of undetermined signficance may represent an early lesion with progressive potential and should be accompanied by a recommendation for further evaluation. This diagnosis is distinguished from inflammatory atypia which may resolve after antibiotic or other therapy.

Two new terms have been introduced to describe premalignant lesions: *low-grade squamous intraepithelial lesion* (LGSIL), and *high-grade squamous intraepithelial lesion* (HGSIL). The LGSIL encompasses changes associated with human papillomavirus (koilocytosis) and mild dysplasia (cervical intraepithelial neoplasia 1). The HGSIL includes abnormalities previously graded as moderate to severe dysplasia and carcinoma-in-situ (cervical intraepithelial neoplasia 2-3). (See **Table 12B.1, The Bethesda System for Reporting Cervical/Vaginal Cytological Diagnoses**).

Likely many factors contribute to the etiology of squamous cell carcinoma of the cervix, but a dominant agent, the *human papillomavirus* (HPV) is usually present (Richart 1987). This virus is sexually transmitted and is known to cause venereal warts (*Condylomata acuminata*). Over 60 distinct genotypes of HPV have been identified to date, of which certain types have a greater oncogenic potential than others. HPV is associated with malignant transformation in the vagina, vulva, anus, and the cervix (Spitzer, Krumholz, and Seltzer 1989).

Because of the high prevalence of HPV, the sexually active female population should have a Pap smear (cervical cytology) at least annually. Cervical cytology screening is the first step in detection of cervical abnormalities. Proper technique is essential to reduce false-negative sampling errors (see **Table 12B.2, Obtaining a Cytological Sample**). The DNA hybridization techniques which detect and type the papillomavirus are also available, but their clinical application has not been universally defined as yet. (See **Human Papillomavirus** Protocol.)

Colposcopy and *directed biopsy* are methods for evaluating patients with abnormal cytology. Clinicians with specialized training may perform colposcopic examinations and therapeutic procedures in certain settings. While it is not the intent of this protocol to serve as a guide for colposcopy, aspects of the colposcopic examination and therapeutic options will be mentioned to

Table 12B.1. THE BETHESDA SYSTEM FOR REPORTING CERVICAL/VAGINAL CYTOLOGICAL DIAGNOSES

Format of the Report:
  a. A statement on Adequacy of the Specimen for Evaluation
  b. A General Categorization which may be used to assist with clerical triage (optional)
  c. The Descriptive Diagnoses

Adequacy of the Specimen
Satisfactory for evaluation
Satisfactory for evaluation but limited by . . . (specify reason)
Unsatisfactory for evaluation . . . (specify reason)

General Categorization (Optional)
Within normal limits
Benign cellular changes: see Descriptive Diagnoses
Epithelial cell abnormality: see Descriptive Diagnoses

Descriptive Diagnoses
Benign cellular changes
  Infection
    Trichomonas vaginalis
    Fungal organisms morphologically consistent with *Candida* spp
    Predominance of coccobacilli consistent with shift in vaginal flora
    Bacteria morphologically consistent with *Actinomyces* spp.
    Cellular changes associated with herpes simplex virus
  Other

Reactive changes
  Reactive cellular changes associated with:
    Inflammation (includes typical repair)
    Atrophy with inflammation ("atrophic vaginitis")
    Radiation
    Intrauterine contraceptive device (IUD)
  Other

Descriptive Diagnoses (continued)
Epithelial Cell Abnormalities
  Squamous Cell
    Atypical squamous cells of undetermined significance: qualify*
    Low-grade squamous intraepithelial lesion encompassing:
      HPV[†]
      Mild dysplasia/CIN 1
    High-grade squamous intraepithelial lesion encompassing:
      Moderate and severe dysplasia
      CIS/CIN 2 and CIN 3
  Squamous cell carcinoma
Glandular Cell
  Endometrial cells, cytologically benign, in a postmenopausal woman
  Atypical glandular cells of undetermined significance: qualify*
  Endocervical adenocarcinoma
  Endometrial adenocarcinoma
  Extrauterine adenocarcinoma
  Adenocarcinoma, not otherwise specified (NOS)
Other malignant neoplasms: specify
Hormonal evaluation (applied to vaginal smears only)
  Hormonal pattern compatible with age and history
  Hormonal pattern incompatible with age and history: specify
  Hormonal evaluation not possible due to: specify

---

*Atypical squamous or glandular cells of undetermined significance should be further qualified as to whether a reactive or a premalignant/malignant process is favored.

[†]Cellular changes of human papillomavirus (HPV)—previously termed koilocytosis atypia or condylamatous atypia—are included in the category of low-grade squamous intraepithelial lesion.

Source: Reprinted with permission from American College of Obstetricians and Gynecologists. Technical Bulletin, August 1993. No. 183, p. 3. *Cervical cytology: Evaluation and management of abnormalities.* Washington, DC: the Author.

---

assist reader comprehension. Clinicians who perform colposcopy should refer to site-specific protocols.

Colposcopy and directed biopsy allow the clinician to rule out the presence of invasive carcinoma and to select the best method of treatment by determining the location and extent of pre-invasive lesions. Three-percent to five-percent acetic acid is applied to the tissue surfaces in question, and these are then viewed under magnification with the colposcope. The location of the squamocolumnar junction is noted; it may appear on the cervical portio or may be located in the endocervical canal. The squamocolumnar junction is an area where abnormalities are likely to arise, and its location will influence treatment decisions.

Atypical lesions may be represented by acetowhite epithelium (leukoplakia without magnification), punctuation, mosaic structures, and/or abnormal blood vessels. Directed biopsy of these lesions allows for histological confirmation of colposcopic findings. An endocervical curettage usually is performed to determine if abnormal tissue is present in the endocervical canal. Col-

poscopic evaluation of the vaginal and vulvar surfaces is often indicated to assess for multifocal genital tract lesions. (See **Human Papillomavirus** Protocol.)

After histological, cytological, and colposcopic findings are compared and evaluated, treatment decisions may be made. Treatment may include local destructive methods such as cryotherapy, laser ablation, chemical ablation (with 5-fluorouracil in cream), excisional biopsy, loop electrosurgical excision procedure (LEEP), and conization (laser or cold knife). In some settings, LGSIL is followed with expectant management—i.e., with colposcopy and Pap smears at three- to six-month intervals. Treatment is initiated if the lesion progresses to HGSIL, or if the patient desires therapy.

DATABASE

SUBJECTIVE

→ Risk factors may include:
  ▪ history of HPV infection.
  ▪ multiple sexual partners.

Table 12B.2.   OBTAINING A CYTOLOGICAL SAMPLE

An endocervical brush and plastic spatula are the ideal materials for obtaining a cervical sample. A single slide for both ectocervical and endocervical sampling may be used. Vaginal pool sampling has a high false negative rate and should be avoided. The following steps are recommended in sampling the cervix:

■ A speculum moistened with water and not lubricant (which may contaminate the specimen) should be inserted into the vagina. Bimanual examination should be performed after the cytological smear is obtained.

■ Excessive amounts of cervical or vaginal discharge should be gently removed with a cotton swab, with care taken to avoid scraping the cervical epithelium. Cervical cultures should be performed after the cytological sampling.

■ Cytological sampling should be avoided during times of heavy menstrual bleeding. If bleeding is minimal, the sample may be taken and will usually be adequate for evaluation.

■ The ectocervix should be sampled first by scraping the entire cervical portio with a plastic spatula.

■ The endocervical canal is sampled by inserting the brush gently until resistance is met, then turning the brush only one-quarter turn to prevent excessive bleeding. When both samples have been obtained, they should rapidly be applied to the slide in a uniform fashion and be fixed (ideally within 4 seconds).

■ Spray fixatives should be held at least 10 inches from the side to prevent distortion of the cells (ACOG 1993).

Copyright © L. Hanson 1995.

■ early age at first intercourse.
■ sexual partner with HPV or history of HPV exposure.
■ drug, alcohol, and/or tobacco use.
■ poor health habits, including infrequent Pap smears.
■ immunosuppressive disease or therapy.

→ Symptoms may include:
■ vaginal discharge, odor, intermenstrual or postcoital bleeding (sometimes seen with cervical malignancy).
■ weight loss, fatigue (late signs of cervical carcinoma).

→ History to include:
■ age and age at first intercourse.
■ number of sexual partners.
■ birth control method, use of barrier method.
■ history of HPV or other sexually transmitted infections in self or partner(s).
■ date of last Pap smear and result.
■ prior abnormal Pap smear.
■ history of diethylstilbestrol (DES) exposure in utero.
■ history of drug, alcohol, or tobacco abuse.

■ history of medical conditions (including HIV status) or therapies which alter the function of the immune system.

OBJECTIVE

NOTE: Colposcopic evaluation and directed biopsy should be performed only by clinicians with special training. Aspects of this examination have been italicized to emphasize this distinction.

→ External genitalia may exhibit erythema, discharge, or gross lesions (including condylomata, leukoplakia); acetowhite lesions with or without vessels may be present after application of 3-percent to 5-percent acetic acid, suggesting a subclinical HPV infection or vulvar intraepithelial neoplasia. (Data indicate that some acetowhite lesions represent a benign, non-HPV entity) (Bergeron et al. 1990).

→ Speculum examination may reveal discharge, erythema of cervix and/or vagina, and gross lesions including condylomata and leukoplakia. Cervical carcinoma may present as an ulceration, a raised friable lesion, necrosis, or it may appear as normal cervical tissue. Classic DES changes may be noted (cervical sulcus, collar).

→ Wet smear may indicate fungal, bacterial, or trichomonal infection.

→ Cervical cultures may indicate chlamydia, gonorrhea, herpes, or other infections.

→ *Colposcopic examination (after application of 3-percent to 5-percent acetic acid) may reveal acetowhite lesions of the vulva, vagina, and cervix with or without the presence of abnormal vessels (punctations, mosaicism, atypical vessels). Location of squamocolumnar junction should be identified.*

→ Non-staining cervical and vaginal tissue may be observed after application of an iodine solution (Schiller test).

→ Bimanual examination may reveal a hard, enlarged, and fixed cervix (in late cervical carcinoma).

→ See **Human Papillomavirus** Protocol.

ASSESSMENT

→ Cytology diagnosis
→ R/O condylomata acuminata
→ R/O vaginitis/cervicitis
→ R/O concomitant STDs

→ *Assess presence of colposcopic vulvar, vaginal, and/or cervical lesion(s), including location, extent, and characteristics of lesion(s)*

→ *Assess location of squamocolumnar junction*

PLAN

DIAGNOSTIC TESTS

→ Pap smear may be repeated.

→ Wet mounts as indicated to assess for vaginitis.

→ Appropriate genital cultures to rule out STDs.

→ *Cervical, vaginal, and/or vulvar biopsies as indicated.*

→ See "Objective" section.

TREATMENT/MANAGEMENT

→ Benign, inflammation.
  ▪ No action, or evaluate/treat if symptomatic.

→ Benign, no endocervical cells.
  ▪ Repeat, especially if history of abnormal Pap smear or HPV.

→ Inflammatory atypia.
  ▪ Evaluate (including wet smear, cervical cultures) and treat.
  ▪ If no identifiable cause, may use broad-spectrum antibiotic such as doxycycline.
  ▪ In the postmenopausal client, inflammatory atypia may result from atrophy.
    • If not contraindicated, treat with topical or oral estrogen for 2 to 3 months. (See **Perimenopausal Symptoms and Hormone Therapy** Protocol.)
  ▪ Repeat Pap smear in 2 to 3 months.
    • If abnormality persists, refer for or *perform colposcopy.*

→ Atypical squamous cells.
  ▪ Repeat pap smear in 2 to 3 months.
    • If condition persists refer for or *perform colposcopy.*
  ▪ If follow-up Pap smear benign, repeat in 6 to 12 months.

→ Atypical endocervical cells.
  ▪ Refer for or *perform colposcopy and endocervical curettage.*

→ LGSIL.
  ▪ Refer for or *perform colposcopy; expectant management or treatment of biopsy-proven lesions if within scope of practice,* or refer for treatment.

→ HGSIL.
  ▪ Refer for or *perform colposcopy.*
  ▪ Refer to physician as indicated by site-specific policy for definitive therapy if biopsy-proven HGSIL.

→ Malignant cells.
  ▪ Refer to physician for evaluation and definitive therapy.

CONSULTATION

→ As indicated by cytology and clinical findings.

→ Referral to physician as indicated for colposcopy and/or definitive therapy. See "Treatment/ Management" section.

→ Depending on site-specific policy, referral to physician for colposcopy may be required if client has HGSIL on cervical cytology.

→ Depending on site-specific policy, referral to physician for colposcopy may be required if client is pregnant and has abnormal cytology.

→ Referral to physician is mandatory if cytology or clinical findings indicate malignancy.

PATIENT EDUCATION

→ Discuss the concept that cervical cancer and its precursors are related to infection by a sexually transmitted agent (i.e., HPV).
  ▪ Advise regarding sexual transmission of HPV and methods to prevent spread and reinfection.
  ▪ See **Table 13A.2, Safer Sex Guidelines,** p. 13-9 and **Table 12I.1, Recommendations for Individuals to Prevent STD/PID,** p. 12-96.

→ Discuss the possible premalignant nature of cervical intraepithelial neoplasia and the need for close and continuous follow-up.

→ Discuss the emotional effect of an abnormal cytological finding on the client's self-esteem, body image, and sexuality.
  ▪ Refer for counseling when indicated.

→ Discuss possible relationship of cigarette smoking as a co-carcinogen. (See **Human Papillomavirus** Protocol.)

FOLLOW-UP

NOTE: Site-specific practices for follow-up will vary.

→ Client with condylomata, treated.
  ▪ Pap smear every six to 12 months.

→ Client with atypia that reverts to normal with or without treatment for inflammation.
  ▪ Annual Pap smear.

→ Client treated for LGSIL/HGSIL.

- Pap smear every three months for one year (colposcopy, endocervical curettage on first visit), then every six months.

→ Client treated for cervical carcinoma.
- Pap smear every three months for two years, then every six months.

→ In some settings, partner(s) of clients with abnormal cytology will be referred for evaluation. This is controversial. (See **Human Papillomavirus** Protocol.)

→ Document in progress notes and problem list.

Bibliography

American College of Obstetricians and Gynecologists. 1993. *Cervical cytology: Evaluation and management of abnormalities.* Technical Bulletin No. 183, 1–7. Washington, DC: the Author.

Bergeron, C., Ferenczy, A., Richart, R.M., and Guralnick, M. 1990. Micropapillomatosis labialis appears unrelated to human papillomavirus. *Obstetrics and Gynecology* 76(2):281–286.

Coppelson, M., Pixley, E., and Reid, B. 1986. *Colposcopy*, 3rd ed. Springfield, IL: Charles C. Thomas.

Herbst, A.L., Jones III, H., Reid, R., and Richart R. 1993. Interpreting the new Bethesda classification system. *Contemporary Ob/Gyn* 38(8):86–107.

Lundberg, G.D. 1989. The 1988 Bethesda system for reporting cervical/vaginal cytological diagnoses. *Journal of the American Medical Association* 262(7):931–934.

Nelson, J.H., Averette, H.E., and Richart, R.M. 1984. Dysplasia, carcinoma in situ, and early invasive cervical carcinoma. *Ca-A Cancer Journal for Clinicians* 34(6):306–327.

Richart, R.M. 1987. Causes and management of cervical intraepithelial neoplasia. *Cancer* 60(8):1951–1959.

Spitzer, M., Krumholz, B.A., and Seltzer, V.L. 1989. The multicentric nature of disease related to human papillomavirus infection of the female lower genital tract. *Obstetrics and Gynecology* 73(3):303–307.

12-C

Amenorrhea—Secondary

Secondary amenorrhea is defined as the absence of menses for a length of time equivalent to three previous cycle intervals or a total of six months without menstrual bleeding (Speroff, Glass, and Kase 1989, 1994). Once pregnancy has been eliminated as a cause of missed menses, the approach to evaluation of the amenorrheic patient can be broken down into four "compartments" where pathology may be encountered (Speroff, Glass, and Kase 1989, 1994).

Compartment 1: Disorders of the Uterus

Destruction of the endometrium as a result of curettage, uterine surgery, or infection may result in uterine scarification or synechiae formation. This condition, known as *Asherman's syndrome*, may partially or completely obliterate the endometrial cavity or the internal cervical os, or combinations of both these areas. Extensive uterine scarring may be associated with such complications as reproductive failure, premature labor, placenta accreta/previa, and postpartum hemorrhage (Richart 1987; Speroff, Glass, and Kase 1989, 1994).

Tuberculosis and schistosomiasis are other rare conditions of the uterus that can cause *granulomatous endometritis* leading to fibrosis of the endometrium (Gomel, Munro, and Rowe 1990). Intrauterine devices (IUDs) and severe pelvic infection also may cause Asherman's syndrome.

Compartment 2: Disorders of the Ovary

Ovarian failure is a fairly common reason for secondary amenorrhea. This condition normally presents at the time of menopause, which occurs, on average, at age 50 years

to 51 years. *Premature ovarian failure* (POF) is defined as a failure of ovarian estrogen production occurring in a hypergonadotrophic state developing at any age between menarche and 35 years (Davajan and Kletzky 1991).

While in most cases the etiology of POF is unknown, autoimmune disease is widely believed to play a role. Autoimmune thyroid disease is the most common concomitant disorder. Other rare conditions associated with POF include myasthenia gravis, rheumatoid arthritis (RA), idiopathic thrombocytopenia purpura (ITP), vitiligo, and autoimmune hemolytic anemia (Speroff, Glass, and Kase 1989, 1994). Other conditions that may cause follicle destruction and ovarian failure are mumps, radiation to the ovary, and/or chemotherapeutic agents (Gomel, Munro, and Rowe 1990).

In rare instances, POF patients have reduced or absent gonadotropin receptors on the follicles with follicular development to the antrum stage only; this is known as the *resistant* or *insensitive ovary syndrome* (or the Savage syndrome). These women, for the most part, should be considered sterile and receive hormone replacement therapy (Davajan and Kletzky 1991; Speroff, Glass, and Kase 1989).

Ovaries of patients with POF do not secrete enough estrogen to maintain a negative feedback on the hypothalamus; thus, gonadotropins are elevated into the postmenopausal range (Davajan and Kletzky 1991). Women under age 25 years with POF should have a karyotype performed to establish the presence of a silent Y chromosome, which is associated with the potential for malignant change within the gonads (25 percent incidence) (ACOG 1989; Davajan and Kletzky 1991; Speroff, Glass, and Kase 1989).

Androgen-secreting tumors of the ovary, such as Sertoli-Leydig cell tumors and granulosa-theca cell tumors also are rare, but cause rapidly progressing symptoms of androgen excess and associated secondary amenorrhea (Lobo 1991a).

Compartment 3: Disorders of the Anterior Pituitary

Non-neoplastic lesions and pituitary tumors are the two main problems encountered at this level. Non-neoplastic lesions may occur as a result of Sheehan's syndrome (infarction of the pituitary after postpartum hemorrhage/hypotension), radiation, surgery, or trauma to the pituitary gland (Gomel, Munro, and Rowe 1990). Other masses of the pituitary may include gummas, tuberculomas, and fat deposits. Suspicion of a pituitary tumor may be increased if the patient has signs of acromegaly or Cushing's disease, with excessive secretion of growth hormone and adrenocorticotropic hormone (ACTH), respectively. Malignant tumors of the pituitary are quite rare (Speroff, Glass, and Kase 1989, 1994).

The most common tumor of the pituitary is a prolactin-secreting adenoma. As many as one-third of patients with secondary amenorrhea will have a pituitary adenoma (Speroff, Glass, and Kase 1989, 1994). If less than 1 cm in diameter, the tumor is referred to as a *microadenoma*; tumors larger than 1 cm are termed *macroadenomas* (Speroff, Glass, and Kase 1989).

About one-third of women with hyperprolactinemia have galactorrhea. One-third of galactorrheic women will have normal menstrual cycles (Speroff, Glass, and Kase 1994). An associated complication of elevated prolactin levels may be *hypoestrogenism*, with its attendant risk of osteoporosis (Zacur and Seibel 1989). Serum FSH and LH levels are low or normal, and estradiol levels may be quite low (<40 pg/ml) in hyperprolactinemic, hypoestrogenic patients (Davajan and Kletzky 1991).

Hyperprolactinemia may occur with no evidence of a pituitary tumor on CT scan or MRI. Patients may have a tumor too small to visualize (nanoadenoma) or generalized pituitary hyperplasia. Alterations in central dopamine metabolism can occur, most commonly as a result of drugs such as phenothiazines. Idiopathic hyperprolactinemia may be a result of hypothalamic dysfunction rather than a pituitary disorder (see following section). (See also "Diagnostic Tests" section for additional causes of hyperprolactinemia.)

The empty sella syndrome is another (mostly benign) entity that may be associated with galactorrhea and normal or elevated prolactins. This condition is characterized by herniation of the subarachnoid membrane into the sella turcica through a congenital defect in the sellar diaphragm (Kletzky and Davajan 1991; Speroff, Glass, and Kase 1989). Compression of the pituitary gland with resultant hyperprolactinemia or galactorrhea may ensue; a prolactin-secreting adenoma also may coexist (Speroff, Glass, and Kase 1989).

An indirect pituitary effect causing amenorrhea is hypothyroidism. Primary hypothyroidism (usually Hashimoto's thyroiditis) is responsible for about three percent to five percent of cases of galactorrhea/hyperprolactinemia (Kletzky and Davajan 1991). When thyroxine (T$_4$) production is low, the hypothalamus releases increased amounts of thyrotropin-releasing hormone (TRH), which in turn stimulates the release of thyroid-stimulating hormone (TSH) from the pituitary gland. The TRH also may act directly on the pituitary to cause prolactin release.

Compartment 4: Disorders of the Central Nervous System (Hypothalamus)

Hypothalamic dysfunction (or failure) is one of the most common causes of amenorrhea and usually is diagnosed when pituitary lesions are excluded (Speroff, Glass, and Kase 1989). Hypothalamic dysfunction may be idiopathic or can be caused by weight loss, anorexia nervosa, stress, exercise, or drugs (e.g., phenothiazines and other psychotropic drugs, contraceptives, antihypertensives, and narcotics).

The exact pathophysiological mechanisms are not completely clear. Abnormal patterns of GnRH pulsatility are present, most likely due to a neurotransmitter alteration or a hypothalamic derangement (Davajan and Kletzky 1991). The FSH and LH levels will be in the normal or low-normal range. Estradiol levels will depend upon the degree of hypothalamic suppression and, in some cases, may be quite low (e.g., exercise-induced amenorrhea, anorexia nervosa). Since osteoporosis is a concern in amenorrheic women with low estradiol levels, these patients may require hormone therapy if the hypothalamic dysfunction is long-standing. Rare hypothalamic lesions associated with amenorrhea may include craniopharyngioma, tuberculous granuloma, sarcoidosis, and meningoencephalitis sequelae (Davajan and Kletzky 1991).

Polycystic ovary syndrome (PCO) or *hyperandrogenic chronic anovulation* (HCA) is a multilevel abnormality characterized by chronic anovulation and hyperandrogenism. No single factor is responsible for the abnormalities associated with this syndrome, and there is debate whether the disorder is primarily a hypothalamic-pituitary disturbance or an ovarian-adrenal abnormality (Lobo 1991b).

It is postulated that the hypothalamus of PCO patients is vulnerable to alterations in feedback control and/or to stress events. Evidence exists that either the amplitude or the frequency of GnRH pulses is increased in PCO, with significant elevations in LH release from the anterior pituitary, consequent ovarian stromal and thecal hypertrophy, and increased ovarian androgen production (i.e., testosterone and androstenedione) (Gomel, Munro, and Rowe 1990). In addition, hyperandrogenism is associated with hyperinsulinemia and insulin resistance; with insulin stimulating ovarian androgen production (Lobo 1991b).

Androgen excess causes decreased sex-hormone-binding globulin (SHBG) from the liver, and an increase in free estradiol and serum estrone, which, in turn, diminishes release of FSH from the pituitary (Gomel, Munro, and Rowe 1990). The LH:FSH ratio in women with PCO is greater than in normally cycling women. Lowered FSH results in reduced FSH-induced aromatase activity in the granulosa cells of ovarian follicles with resultant inability of thecal and stromal androgens to be converted (by aromatase) to estrogen (Gomel, Munro, and Rowe 1990). Androgens, thus, are released into the systemic circulation.

Typical polycystic ovaries demonstrate a thickened capsule, subcortical cysts, and increased stromal density (Lobo 1991b). The role of the adrenal gland in PCO is controversial. Dehydroepiandrosterone sulfate (DHEA-S), an adrenal androgen, is elevated in a majority of patients.

The chronic anovulatory state of PCO patients with the unopposed estrogen effect on the endometrium may lead to benign hyperplasia or atypical hyperplasia, a precursor to endometrial cancer. Abnormal lipoprotein levels also may exist in PCO, placing these patients at risk for coronary artery disease (CAD) (Lobo 1991b). Besides amenorrhea, features associated with PCO may include acne, obesity, hirsutism, and infertility.

Additional Causes of Secondary Amenorrhea/Anovulation

These may include hyperthyroidism, virilizing adrenal tumors, Cushing's disease, adult-onset congenital adrenal hyperplasia (CAH), exposure to environmental/occupational hazards, pseudocyesis, high fever, and lactation (Clark-Coller 1991).

DATABASE

SUBJECTIVE

→ Patient will typically present with hypomenorrhea, oligomenorrhea, or amenorrhea, at times with terminal menorrhagia, depending upon the pathology involved.
  ▪ Symptoms associated with amenorrhea are variable and depend upon the compartment affected.
  ▪ A number of systems may be affected as described previously.
→ Stress, exercise, malnutrition, and obesity are common associated factors.
→ Certain medications, listed previously, may be involved.
→ History of the patient with amenorrhea requires systematic consideration of the many possible etiologies, including but not limited to:
  ▪ menstrual cycle and obstetrical/gynecological history:
    • age at menarche/menopause.
    • gravidity.
    • parity.
    • number/date of abortions (spontaneous/induced).
    • last normal menstrual period.
    • previous normal menstrual periods (ideally, the last three).
    • usual cycle interval, duration, and amount of flow, and onset/change in menstrual cycle characteristics.
    • molimina (bloating, cramping).
    • irritability, breast tenderness, mittelschmerz, etc.
    • associated physical symptoms (abnormal vaginal discharge, odor, itching; abdominal/pelvic pain; dyspareunia; urinary frequency, urgency, or dysuria; fever; chills; nausea; vomiting; diarrhea; constipation; etc.).
    • Pap smear history.
    • diagnosis of other gynecological disorders, and how managed.
    • STD history.
    • gynecological surgery.
    • last delivery.
    • complications of pregnancy or delivery.
    • current breast-feeding status.
  ▪ sexual history:
    • sexual preference, number of partners, sex practices (e.g., nipple stimulation), date of last coitus, sexual partner history.

- contraceptive history:
  - use/type of oral or other hormonal contraceptives; use of condoms, spermicides, diaphragm, cervical cap; use of intrauterine device (IUD), including date of insertion, complications; sterilization (patient and partner); desire for future fertility.
- medical history:
  - general health, present and past major medical disorders and how managed (systemic, endocrine, metabolic, etc.).
- childhood illnesses, particularly mumps.
- environmental/occupational hazards.
- hospitalizations.
- surgeries.
- trauma:
  - particularly chest wall trauma; chronic chest wall irritation.
- radiation exposure.
- medications.
- habits—tobacco, drugs, alcohol, exercise.
- nutritional status—dieting, anorexia, bulimia.
- review of systems:
  - weight, hair, appetite changes.
  - bruisability.
  - hot flushes.
  - night sweats.
  - hot/cold sensitivity.
  - fatigability.
  - muscle wasting.
  - weakness.
  - increased lanugo hair.
  - headaches.
  - visual changes (especially visual field).
  - galactorrhea.
  - defeminizing signs (loss of female body *Androgen* contour, decrease in breast size).
  - signs of virilization (temporal baldness, hirsutism, deepening of voice, clitoromegaly).
  - vaginal dryness.
  - decreased cervical mucus.
  - libido changes.
  - mental status changes.
  - recent illness.
  - and any other symptoms of systemic, endocrine, metabolic disease.
- psychosocial history:
  - education/occupation, marital/partner status, social support, environmental/psychologic stressors, anxiety level, life satisfaction, etc.
- family history:
  - amenorrhea, PCO, infertility, genetic problems.

OBJECTIVE

→ Pay attention to the stigmata of thyroid disease, adrenal disease, signs of virilization, and pregnancy.

→ Ideally, a thorough physical examination should be performed. Important components to assess may include (but are not limited to) (Clark-Coller 1991; Lichtman and Papera 1990):

- vital signs:
  - blood pressure, pulse.
- general:
  - height, weight, stature, habitus, posture, motor activity, gait, dress, grooming, personal hygiene, manner, mood, affect, developmental stage of secondary sex characteristics, stigmata of systemic or endocrine disease.
- hair:
  - texture, loss of axillary/pubic hair, hirsutism.
- eyes:
  - stare, lid lag, exophthalmus, visual field defects, fundoscopic changes.
- ears:
  - auditory acuity.
- neck:
  - thyroid masses/enlargement, lymph nodes, "buffalo hump."
- skin:
  - dry, moist, warm, cold, rough, acne, facial plethora, palmar erythema.
- deep tendon reflexes.
- extremities:
  - edema, wasting.
- heart/lungs:
  - general assessment.
- breasts:
  - striae, masses, tenderness, galactorrhea; Tanner stage.
- abdomen:
  - striae, organomegaly, masses, tenderness, inguinal nodes, pulses.
- pelvis:
  - complete assessment of mons pubis, vulva, vagina, cervix, uterus, adnexa, and rectum, noting any abnormalities and all pertinent findings.
    - Pay attention to any virilizing signs (e.g., clitoromegaly) or indications of pregnancy (e.g., Chadwick's/Hegar's signs, enlarged uterus).
- other:

- calculation of body mass index (BMI). Normal is 20 to 25. BMI = weight [kg]/height squared [m²] (Eden 1991).
- milky secretions of breast may be examined microscopically for evidence of fat.
- formal visual field testing by an ophthalmologist may be indicated when patient has headaches/visual changes, which could be evidence of a pituitary macroadenoma (>10 mm) or suprasellar extension of a pituitary lesion (ACOG 1989; Speroff, Glass, and Kase 1989; Zacur and Seibel 1989).

ASSESSMENT

→ Amenorrhea—secondary

→ R/O pregnancy

→ Attempt to establish etiological diagnosis within Compartments 1 to 4

PLAN

DIAGNOSTIC TESTS

See **Figure 12C.1, Algorithm for Amenorrhea.** (**NOTE:** The diagnostic protocol may vary according to the case presentation, site-specific procedures, and consultation with the physician.)

→ Elaboration on certain specifics of algorithm.

- *Progestin challenge:* Purpose is to assess endogenous estrogen level and outflow tract competence (ACOG 1989; Davajan and Kletzky 1991; Gomel, Munro, and Rowe 1990; Speroff, Glass, and Kase 1989, 1994).
  - Medroxyprogesterone acetate (Provera®) 5 mg-10 mg p.o./day for 5 to 10 days

    OR

    30 mg p.o./day for 3 days

    OR
  - Progesterone in oil 100 mg-200 mg I.M.

  NOTE: It is suggested that if withdrawal bleeding does not occur after oral progestin (absorption may be variable), I.M. progesterone should be tried (Davajan and Kletzky 1991).
- *Withdrawal bleeding:* Patient may bleed within 2 to 14 days.
  - "Bleeding in any amount beyond a few spots is considered a positive withdrawal response." (Speroff, Glass, and Kase 1994, 406).
  - Only a few spots implies marginal levels of endogenous estrogen. Patient should be

followed closely and re-evaluated periodically (Speroff, Glass, and Kase 1994).

- *Prolactin:* Draw between 8:00 a.m. and 12:00 noon.
  - Prolactin levels may be increased by many factors: food ingestion, major stress, suckling, breast/pelvic examinations, coitus, certain drugs (e.g., sedatives, tranquilizers, antihypertensives, narcotics, oral contraceptives), epilepsy, surgery, migraines, chronic chest wall irritation or chest trauma, herpes zoster, and pregnancy.
  - Repeat sampling is suggested if results are ambiguous or elevated.
  - Normal values will vary depending upon laboratory (DeVane 1989; Kletzky and Davajan 1991).
- *Estrogen and progestin cycle:* Purpose is to challenge Compartment 1 capacity with exogenous estrogen. Administer conjugated estrogen (Premarin®) 1.25 mg/day p.o. for 21-25 days and medroxyprogesterone acetate (Provera®) 5mg-10 mg/day p.o. on the last 5-10 days.
  - A second course may be used if no withdrawal bleeding occurs after the first cycle (ACOG 1989; Speroff, Glass, and Kase 1994).
  - As noted, this step may be omitted in a patient with normal genitalia and no history of uterine curettage (Speroff, Glass, and Kase 1994).
- *Gonadotropin assay:* Purpose is to determine cause of estrogen deficiency as either a follicular (Compartment 2) or a CNS-pituitary (Compartment 3-4) defect (Speroff, Glass, and Kase 1994).

→ Additional considerations.

- Simple evaluation of ovulation may be undertaken by the patient with BBT charting, observation of cervical mucus changes, and attention to secondary fertility signs such as mittelschmerz, menstrual molimina, etc.
  - LH kits may be used when achievement of pregnancy is desired.
  - See **Infertility** Protocol.
- Additional laboratory tests may include but are not limited to: CBC, ESR, FBS, T₃, T₄, free thyroxine index (FTI), thyroid antibodies, antinuclear antibody (ANA), rheumatoid factor (RF), total serum protein, albumin/globulin ratio, calcium, phosphorus, random cortisol,

Figure 12C.1. ALGORITHM FOR AMENORRHEA

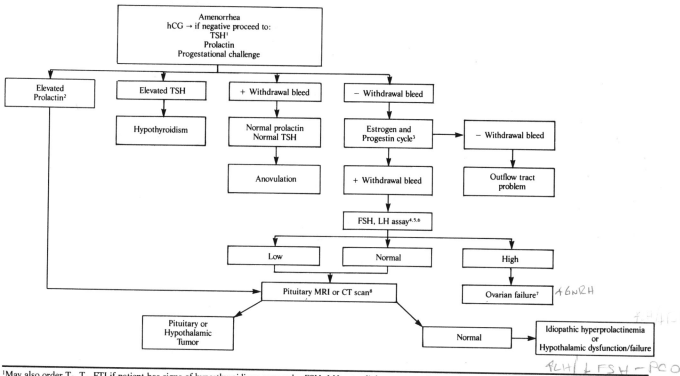

[1]May also order T_3, T_4, FTI if patient has signs of hyperthyroidism; may order FSH, LH, estradiol at outset or later as shown.

[2]Cut-off levels vary. Consult with physician.

[3]May be omitted in patient with normal pelvic exam and no history of curettage.

[4]Wait 2 weeks to assay if exogenous estrogen was used.

[5]May order estradiol.

[6]If LH:FSH ratio ≥ 3:1 or LH > 25 mIU consider PCO; may order testosterone, DHEA-S.

[7]If under age 35 years, may order the following to rule out autoimmune disease: thyroid antibodies, cortisol, calcium, phosphorus, CBC, sedimentation rate, total protein, albumin/globulin ratio, rheumatoid factor, antinuclear antibody. If under age 25 years, order a karyotype. Consult with a physician.

[8]Coned-down view of sella turcica may be substituted if cost is a factor. However if coned-down view is abnormal, prolactin > 60 ng-100 ng/ml, or the patient has a history of visual problems or headaches, proceed to MRI or CT.

Source: Adapted with permission from Speroff, L., Glass, R.H., and Kase, N.G. 1989. *Clinical gynecologic endocrinology and infertility*, 4th ed. Baltimore: Williams & Wilkins.

Additional sources: Davajan, V., and Kletzky, O.A. 1991. Secondary amenorrhea without galactorrhea or androgen excess. In *Infertility, contraception, and reproductive endocrinology*, 3rd ed., eds. D.R. Mishell, V. Davajan, and R.A. Lobo, pp. 372-395. Boston: Blackwell Scientific Publications; Kletzky, O.A., and Davajan, V. 1991. Hyperprolactinemia: Diagnosis and treatment. In *Infertility, contraception, and reproductive endocrinology*, 3rd ed., eds. D.R. Mishell, V. Davajan, and R.A. Lobo, pp. 396-421. Boston: Blackwell Scientific Publications.

estradiol, testosterone, DHEA-S (ACOG 1989; Davajan and Kletzky 1991). See algorithm. **NOTE:** Many of these tests are expensive. Consultation with a physician is recommended prior to ordering.

- Ultrasound imaging or MRI of the ovaries has been used by some clinicians to assist in diagnosis of PCO (Loy and Seibel 1988).
- Consult with a physician and refer patient to an endocrinologist if there is suspicion of:
  - a virilizing tumor (rapid progression of virilizing signs).
  - Cushing's syndrome (signs include hypertension, acne, hirsutism, plethoric appearance, centripetal obesity, abdominal striae, "buffalo hump," muscle wasting, thin skin, lanugo hair, etc.)

    OR

  - adult-onset CAH (clinical presentation identical to that of PCO patient). Patients with these signs will require specialized tests to make the diagnoses—e.g., serum testosterone, androstenedione, DHEA, DHEA-S, CT, or MRI; dexamethasone-suppression test, serum 17-hydroxyprogesterone level (17-OHP); ACTH stimulation test, human leukocyte antigen (HLA) typing (Eden 1991; Lobo 1991a).
    –See **Hirsutism** Protocol.
- Some clinicians will attempt to differentiate between hypothalamic and pituitary etiologies of hyperprolactinemia by the use of TRH stimulation or insulin tolerance testing.
  - This is within the purview of physician practice.

TREATMENT/MANAGEMENT

→ Diagnostic work-up will attempt to establish etiology.

→ Ongoing treatment/management will be determined by the location of the identified pathology of amenorrhea and the fertility goals of the patient.

Compartment 1

→ Asherman's syndrome.

- Refer to physician. Therapy will vary according to physician responsible for patient's care.
- Patient is usually evaluated with hysteroscopy, or hysterosalpingography. Synechiae/adhesions can be treated with hysteroscopic lysis.
- After the procedures, antibiotics may be given, and an IUD or pediatric Foley catheter may be placed, followed by 2 months of high stimulatory doses of estrogen, e.g., conjugated estrogen (Premarin®) 2.5 mg/day p.o. 3 weeks out of 4, with medroxyprogesterone acetate (Provera®) 10 mg/day p.o. during the third week. Antiprostaglandin medications may be given if cramping is present (ACOG 1989; Richart 1987; Speroff, Glass, and Kase 1994).

Compartment 2

→ Premature ovarian failure.

- If patient is under age 35 years, consider autoimmune disease as a cause.
  - Refer to specialist.
  - In consultation with physician, order selected blood tests for autoimmune disease.
  - See diagnostic algorithm, **Figure 12C.1.**
- If patient is under age 25 years, order a karyotype and refer to physician if abnormal.
- Hormone therapy should be given to prevent osteoporosis and cardiovascular disease in patients with POF.
  - See **Perimenopausal Symptoms and Hormone Therapy** Protocol.
- Contraception is advisable for women with POF while on hormone therapy if pregnancy is not desired (a very remote possibility). These patients may be recipients of oocyte donation and embryo transfer (ACOG 1989).

→ Suspected androgen-producing ovarian (or adrenal) tumors.

- Patient will present with rapidly progressing signs of androgen excess.
  - Refer to endocrinologist.
  - May order serum testosterone, DHEA, and DHEA-S levels.
  - Vaginal ultrasonography, CT, or MRI may be considered.
  - See **Hirsutism** Protocol.

Compartment 3

→ Galactorrhea/hyperprolactinemia/pituitary adenomas.

- Patient usually is referred to a physician if care is anticipated to be long-term or when treating pituitary adenomas. In some settings, the primary care provider may co-manage patient in close consultation with the specialist.
  - Goals of therapy include elimination of galactorrhea, establishment of regular menstrual cycles and/or normal estrogen secretion, treatment of prolactin-secreting tumors, correction of hypothyroidism, and/or

induction of ovulation (Kletzky and Davajan 1991).

- In most women, hyperprolactinemia (with or without microadenoma) has a benign clinical course (Kletzky and Davajan 1991).
  - –Management includes observation, drug therapy, surgery, and radiation.

■ When imaging studies indicate a pituitary abnormality, tumors other than a prolactinoma should also be ruled out.
- Consult with a physician regarding appropriate tests (e.g., growth hormone level, cortisol, LH and FSH measurements) (Zacur and Seibel 1989).

■ Observation may be all that is indicated for galactorrheic menstruating women with normal or idiopathic prolactin elevation and for some women with microadenomas.
- Order yearly prolactin levels and MRI or CT scan periodically.
- Consult with physician.

■ For idiopathic hyperprolactinemia with associated oligomenorrhea/amenorrhea in euestrogenic women:
- medroxyprogesterone acetate (Provera®) 5 mg-10 mg/day p.o. for at least 12 days every 1-2 months to induce regular bleeding; consult with physician.
- oral contraceptives may be an option for cycle control; consult with physician.

■ For hyperprolactinemia with associated low serum estradiol (<30 pg/ml) without evidence of pituitary adenoma:
- oral contraceptives.
- cyclic estrogen/progestin (see **Perimenopausal Symptoms and Hormone Therapy** Protocol for hormone regimens).
- bromocriptine (Parlodel®).
- consult with physician.

■ For hyperprolactinemia-associated dysfunctions (e.g., amenorrhea with or without galactorrhea/infertility, and prolactin-secreting micro-macroadenomas), bromocriptine (Parlodel®) may be employed.
- Patient should be managed by a physician.

■ Transsphenoidal resection of pituitary adenomas may be employed in certain cases (e.g., failure to comply or poor compliance with medical therapy).

■ Radiation may arrest the growth of a pituitary adenoma, but it is not recommended over bromocriptine (Kletzky and Davajan 1991).

■ For associated infertility, ovulation induction with clomiphene citrate (Clomid®) may be attempted in euestrogenic women without evidence of a pituitary adenoma (Kletzky and Davajan 1991).
- Refer patient to a physician. (Periovulatory transient increases in prolactin require no therapy unless associated with infertility.)

■ Visual field testing by an ophthalmologist to assess optic nerve compression may be indicated when the patient has visual symptoms/headaches, evidence of a macroadenoma, or suprasellar extension of the prolactinoma (ACOG 1989; Speroff, Glass, and Kase 1989; Zacur and Seibel 1989).

■ Bone mass determination via single or dual photon densitometry, or CT scan should be considered in individuals with hyperprolactinemia who have evidence of hypoestrogenism (i.e., serum estradiol <30 pg/ml) (Zacur and Seibel 1989). Calcium supplementation and hormone therapy in the absence of a pituitary adenoma is advisable in hyperprolactinemic, hypoestrogenic women (ACOG 1989).
- See **Perimenopausal Symptoms and Hormone Therapy** Protocol and **General Nutrition Guidelines.**

■ Conception may occur in sexually active women who are hyperprolactinemic. Birth control methods should be employed if the patient does not desire pregnancy.

■ When primary hypothyroidism is established as the cause of hyperprolactinemia, thyroxine replacement therapy is indicated (Kletzky and Davajan 1991).
- See **Thyroid Disorders** Protocol.
- Refer patient to a physician as indicated.

■ If galactorrhea develops while patient is on a prescribed medication, stop the drug if possible, and measure serum prolactin 1 month later if galactorrhea persists (Kletzky and Davajan 1991).
- If unable to stop the medication, assess prolactin:
  - –if <50 ng/ml, no further work-up necessary, measure prolactin yearly.
  - –if >50 ng/ml, proceed with pituitary evaluation—i.e., coned down view of sella turica, MRI, or CT scan (Kletzky and Davajan 1991).
- Consult with a physician.

→ Empty sella syndrome.

■ MRI or CT will establish definitive diagnosis.
  • Advise patient that prognosis usually is benign and endocrine abnormalities are unlikely.
  • May follow with yearly prolactin levels.
  • Consult with a physician.
→ Other pituitary lesions.
  ■ Patients with radiographic evidence of a large pituitary lesion (e.g., macroadenoma) or a history suggestive of Sheehan's syndrome should have an insulin-tolerance test to determine pituitary growth hormone, prolactin, and ACTH reserve (Davajan and Kletzky 1991; Kletzky and Davajan 1991).
    • Refer patient to a physician.
→ See **Galactorrhea** Protocol.

Compartment 4

→ Hypothalamic dysfunction/failure.
  ■ Attempt to ameliorate the underlying cause of hypothalamic dysfunction or failure.
  ■ Basic to caring for these patients is nutritional counseling and discussion regarding exercise patterns, weight loss, and stress management techniques.
    • Refer to nutritionist as indicated.
    • Refer to psychiatrist or other mental health provider and physician as indicated for patients with anorexia nervosa or bulimia, especially in severe cases.
  ■ Patients with hypothalamic dysfunction should have uterine bleeding induced at least every 60 days with progestins (e.g., medroxyprogesterone acetate [Provera®] 5 mg-10 mg/day p.o. for at least 12 days).
    • If withdrawal bleeding fails to occur, pituitary gland imaging is in order (Davajan and Kletzky 1991).
    • Alternately, a cyclic oral contraceptive may be used if patient needs a form of birth control.
  ■ In cases of hypothalamic-pituitary failure (i.e., estradiol <30 ng/ml), hormone therapy is indicated for the hypoestrogenic state.
    • Cyclic estrogen/progestin or oral contraceptives may be used.
    • A diet that provides 1000 mg-1500 mg/day of calcium is suggested (Speroff, Glass, and Kase 1994).
    • See **Perimenopausal Symptoms and Hormone Therapy** Protocol and **General Nutrition Guidelines.**

■ Hyperprolactinemic patients with hypothalamic dysfunction/failure should have pituitary imaging to rule out a tumor. Prolactins should be reassessed yearly if no tumor is found; pituitary imaging studies (CT or MRI) may also be ordered periodically for follow-up. Consult with a physician (Davajan and Kletzky 1991).
  • See "Compartment 3," "Treatment/ Management" section.
■ Bone mineral density assessment of the spine and hip is suggested in patients who have been amenorrheic for longer than 2 years (Smith and Zook 1986).
■ Amenorrhea following the discontinuance of oral contraceptives should be evaluated if the patient has not resumed normal menstruation after 6 months, if galactorrhea is present, or if the patient is very anxious or desires pregnancy (Davajan and Kletzky 1991).
  • Proceed as detailed in "Diagnostic Tests" section.
  • Advise the patient to use an alternate method of contraception if pregnancy is not desired.
■ Patients with associated infertility should be referred for ovulation induction.

→ Polycystic ovary syndrome (PCO).
  ■ The goal in anovulatory PCO patients is to prevent endometrial hyperplasia and atypia that may result from unopposed estrogen stimulation. In cases of long-standing anovulation/amenorrhea, endometrial biopsy may be performed.
    • Consult with/refer to a physician.
  ■ Patients with PCO should be treated with intermittent progestins—e.g., medroxyprogesterone acetate (Provera®) 5 mg-10 mg/day p.o. for at least 12 days every 1-2 months.
  ■ Alternately cyclic oral contraceptives may be used, provided risk factors are not significant (ACOG 1989; Davajan and Kletzky 1991; Speroff, Glass, and Kase 1989, 1994).
    –Androgenic oral contraceptives, such as levonorgestrel products, should be avoided.
    –Estrogenic oral contraceptives also are used in management of the hirsute patient with PCO. See **Hirsutism** Protocol.
  ■ Besides amenorrhea, problems of PCO patients may include hirsutism, obesity, acne, infertility, and dysfunctional uterine bleeding.
    • Therapy should be individualized.
    • See specific protocols.

- Baseline testosterone and DHEA-S levels may be ordered in PCO patients.
→ Craniopharyngioma.
  - Refer to physician for surgery.

CONSULTATION

→ Consultation with a physician:
  - is suggested for all patients with amenorrhea.
  - may be indicated to determine necessary diagnostic tests.
→ Patients with Asherman's syndrome, endocrinopathies, autoimmune disorders, pituitary or hypothalamic lesions, galactorrhea, infertility, or severe anorexia nervosa or bulimia should be referred to a specialist (e.g., gynecologist, endocrinologist or reproductive endocrinologist, rheumatologist, psychiatrist) for medical management. Depending upon the policies of the practice setting, certain patients may be co-managed with the physician.
→ As needed for endometrial biopsy in cases of PCO with long-standing amenorrhea.
→ As needed for prescription(s).

PATIENT EDUCATION

→ Specific patient education will depend upon the etiology of the amenorrhea. Discussion regarding diagnostic tests and procedures should be as detailed as possible in terms the patient will understand.
  - Patient-education materials are a useful adjunct to teaching.
→ When patient is referred to a specialist, the physician should detail the specific diagnostic and therapeutic modalities.
  - Co-managed patients should be cared for with a comprehensive plan in mind.
  - The primary care provider should complement and supplement the specialist's care and ensure the patient's goals and objectives of health care are taken into consideration.
→ Reassurance is indicated for patients with obvious causes of amenorrhea.
  - For example, a woman with "post-pill" amenorrhea should be told there is no long-term effect on fertility and that normal menstrual cycles should resume within six months without therapy.

→ Patients with POF need psychological support if loss of fertility is a major issue.
  - They should be directed to the appropriate sources if interested in pursuing pregnancy via oocyte donation or embryo transfer. Discuss the need for contraception if on hormone therapy, though the possibility of conception is rare.
→ Discussion regarding healthy eating patterns should be undertaken as indicated.
  - Explain that reduced food intake and underweight status interfere with ovarian function and may lead to amenorrhea.
  - Women with anorexia nervosa or bulimia usually require counseling about the disorder.
  - See **Eating Disorders** Protocol.
→ If obesity is a concern, the patient may benefit from joining a weight loss program. Weight loss improves the insulin-resistant state in obesity and may ameliorate gonadotropin/sex steroid secretion leading to better regulation of menstrual cycles and improved fertility (Loy and Seibel 1988). In addition, PCO patients may be at increased risk for lipoprotein abnormalities; thus, counseling regarding low fat/low cholesterol diet is important.
  - See **General Nutrition Guidelines.**
→ Address the potential for hyperplastic endometrial change in PCO patients with chronic anovulation. Also discuss the importance of periodic progestins or combined oral contraceptives.
→ A change in lifestyle (e.g., moderation of exercise and weight gain) will be appropriate for some amenorrheic athletes.
  - Reduction in exercise plus an optimal diet is often enough to restore a normal menstrual cycle (Genazzani et al. 1991).
→ Address the concerns regarding hypoestrogenism, stress fractures, and osteoporosis in amenorrheic athletes.
  - Adequate calcium and hormone therapy is indicated for athletes when amenorrhea is long-standing.
    • Patients should understand that they will have withdrawal bleeding while on hormone therapy. However, on discontinuing, amenorrhea is likely to recur.
  - Women declining hormonal therapy should be encouraged to have bone density evaluation if their estradiol levels are low.

→ When infertility is a problem, ovulation induction often is indicated. Discuss with patient the need for referral to an infertility specialist.

→ With affected patients, discuss the small risk (5 percent) of a pituitary microadenoma progressing to a macroadenoma.

→ Despite amenorrhea, spontaneous ovulation may occur. Discuss contraceptive options.

FOLLOW-UP

→ Follow-up of amenorrheic patients will vary and is dependent upon the identified underlying condition. Establish a plan of care with a consultant as indicated.

→ See "Treatment/Management" section.

→ Document in progress list and problem notes.

Bibliography

American College of Obstetricians and Gynecologists. 1989. *Amenorrhea.* Technical Bulletin No. 128. Washington, DC: the Author.

Baker, E.R., Stumpf, P., and Lloyd, T.A. 1986. Menstrual irregularity and athletic injury. *Contemporary Ob/Gyn* 28:45–50.

Barnea, E.R., and Tal, J. 1991. Stress-related reproductive failure. *Journal of In Vitro Fertilization and Embryo Transfer* 8(1):15–23.

Barnes, R., and Rosenfield, R.L. 1989. The polycystic ovary syndrome: Pathogenesis and treatment. *Annals of Internal Medicine* 110(5):386–399.

Blackwell, R.E. 1989. How to manage the hyperprolactinemic patient. *Contemporary Ob/Gyn* 34(3):109–118.

Bronson, F.H., and Manning, J.M. 1991. The energetic regulation of ovulation: A realistic role for body fat. *Biology of Reproduction* 44:945–950.

Clark-Coller, T. 1991. Dysfunctional uterine bleeding and amenorrhea. *Journal of Nurse-Midwifery* 36(1):49–62.

Cullins, V.E., and Huggins, G.R. 1990. Disorders leading to amenorrhea. *Contemporary Ob/Gyn* 35(9):67–82.

Davajan, V., and Kletzky, O.A. 1991. Secondary amenorrhea without galactorrhea or androgen excess. In *Infertility, contraception, and reproductive endocrinology*, 3rd ed., eds. D.R. Mishell, V. Davajan, and R.A. Lobo, pp. 372–395. Boston: Blackwell Scientific Publications.

De Cree, C., Vermeulen, A., and Ostyn, M. 1991. Are high-performance young women athletes doomed to become low-performance old wives? *The Journal of Sports Medicine and Physical Fitness* 31(1):108–114.

DeVane, G.W. 1989. Prolactin measurement: What is normal? *Contemporary Ob/Gyn* 34(3):99–104.

Eden, J.A. 1991. The hazards of amenorrhea. *The Medical Journal of Australia* 154:536–542.

Genazzani, A.R., Petraglia, F., De Ramundo, B.M., Genazzini, A.D., Amato, F., Algeri, I., Galassi, M.C., Botticelli, G., and Bidzinska, B. 1991. Neuroendocrine correlates of stress-related amenorrhea. *Annals of the New York Academy of Sciences* 626:125–129.

Gomel, V., Munro, M.G., and Rowe, T.C. 1990. *Gynecology: A practical approach.* Baltimore: Williams & Wilkins.

Gindoff, P.R., and Jewelewicz, R. 1987. Polycystic ovarian disease. *Obstetrics and Gynecology Clinics of North America* 14(4):931–953.

Kletzky, O.A., and Davajan, V. 1991. Hyperprolactinemia: Diagnosis and treatment. In *Infertility, contraception, and reproductive endocrinology*, 3rd ed., eds. D.R. Mishell, V. Davajan, and R.A. Lobo, pp. 396–421. Boston: Blackwell Scientific Publications.

Kustin, J., and Rebar, R.W. 1989. Addressing concerns of amenorrheic athletes. *Contemporary Ob/Gyn* 28:35–43.

Lichtman, R., and Papera, S. 1990. *Gynecology: Well-woman care.* Norwalk, CT: Appleton & Lange.

Lobo, R.A. 1991a. Androgen excess. In *Infertility, contraception, and reproductive endocrinology*, 3rd ed., eds. D.R. Mishell, V. Davajan, and R.A. Lobo, pp. 422–446. Boston: Blackwell Scientific Publications.

———. 1991b. The syndrome of hyperandrogenic chronic anovulation. In *Infertility, contraception, and reproductive endocrinology*, 3rd ed., eds. D.R. Mishell, V. Davajan, and R.A. Lobo, pp. 447–487. Boston: Blackwell Scientific Publications.

Loy, R., and Seibel, M. 1988. Evaluation and therapy of polycystic ovarian syndrome. *Endocrinology and Metabolism Clinics of North America* 17(4):785–813.

Mauvais-Jarvis, P., and Bricaire, C. 1989. Pathophysiology of polycystic ovary syndrome. *Journal of Steroid Biochemistry* 33(4B):791–794.

Prough, S.G., and Aksel, S. 1987. Overweight, endocrine function, and infertility. *Contemporary Ob/Gyn* 30(4):63–79.

Richart, R. 1987. Managing Asherman's syndrome hysteroscopically. *Contemporary Ob/Gyn* 30(2):147–150.

Salisbury, J., and Mitchell, J.E. 1991. Bone mineral density and anorexia nervosa in women. *American Journal of Psychiatry* 148(6):768–774.

Smith, E.L., and Zook, S.K. 1986. Exercise can reduce bone loss. *Contemporary Ob/Gyn* 28:53–61.

Speroff, L., Glass, R.H., and Kase, N.G. 1989. *Clinical gynecologic endocrinology and infertility*, 4th ed. Baltimore: Williams & Wilkins.

———. 1994. *Clinical gynecologic endocrinology and infertility*, 5th ed. Baltimore: Williams & Wilkins.

Warren, M.P. 1991. Exercise in women. *Clinics in Sports Medicine* 10(1):131–139.

Zacur, H.A., and Seibel, M.M. 1989. Steps in diagnosing prolactin-related disorders. *Contemporary Ob/Gyn* 34(3):84–96.

Joan R. Murphy, R.N., C., M.S., N.P., C.N.S.

12-D

Dysmenorrhea

Dysmenorrhea is synonymous with painful menstruation or menstrual cramps. Characteristically, dysmenorrhea causes a painful cramping sensation in the lower abdomen, often accompanied by systemic symptoms such as gastrointestinal upset, low backache, headache, syncope, and fatigue (Dawood 1985; Treybig 1989).

Dysmenorrhea is one of the most frequently encountered gynecological disorders. In the United States over half of the women of childbearing age experience some degree of painful menstruation (Treybig 1989). Approximately 10 percent of these women have dysmenorrhea severe enough to render them incapacitated for one to three days each month, resulting in increased absenteeism and economic loss. Decreased productivity and disruption of family and personal life are also common (Dawood 1985, 1990).

Dysmenorrhea is classified as either *primary* or *secondary*. Specific clinical features differentiate one type from the other (Dawood 1990). Primary dysmenorrhea occurs in the absence of pelvic pathology, whereas secondary dysmenorrhea occurs as a result of some underlying organic pelvic disease such as endometriosis, adenomyosis, pelvic inflammatory disease (PID), fibroids, cervical stenosis, or müllerian duct malformations (Dawood 1985, 1990; Droegemueller et al. 1987; Treybig 1989). Endometriosis is the most common cause of secondary dysmenorrhea but may be mistaken for primary dysmenorrhea (Treybig 1989).

The pain experienced with primary dysmenorrhea is characteristically suprapubic, spasmodic, and colicky in nature, and usually starts at or soon after menarche (six to 12 months), when ovulatory cycles are established (Dawood 1985, 1990; Hoffman 1988; Treybig 1989). Menstrual pain usually lasts 48 to 72 hours

and can begin as early as a few hours before or just after the onset of bleeding. It is most severe during the first or second day of menses. Systemic symptoms occur in approximately 50 percent of patients. Physical examination will be within normal limits in patients experiencing primary dysmenorrhea (Dawood 1985, 1990).

Primary dysmenorrhea is thought to be due to excessive production and release of prostaglandins, resulting in increased uterine contractions and vasospasm of uterine arterioles. Consequently, tissue ischemia occurs, causing painful cramping (Dawood 1985, 1990; Treybig 1989). (See **Figure 12D.1, Postulated Mechanism of Pain in Primary Dysmenorrhea**.)

Systemic symptoms associated with primary dysmenorrhea are due to entry of prostaglandins into the circulation (Treybig 1989). Women with primary dysmenorrhea produce eight to 13 times more prostaglandins than nondysmenorrhic women and produce prostaglandins seven times faster. The increased pain experienced during the first 48 to 72 hours of menstruation correlates well with the increased production and release of prostaglandins that occur during this time period (Dawood 1985).

Primary dysmenorrhea occurs mainly in women in their teens and early 20s. The rate tends to decrease with age, especially after age 35 years. Unmarried women experience primary dysmenorrhea more frequently than married women do. Pregnancy and vaginal delivery do not resolve it. Occupation and physical condition also do not affect the frequency of primary dysmenorrhea (Dawood 1985, 1990). The severity of primary dysmenorrhea is associated with duration of menstrual flow, cigarette smoking, and early menarche (Droegemueller et al. 1987; Sundell, Milsom, and Andersch 1990). Dys-

Figure 12D.1.   POSTULATED MECHANISM OF PAIN IN PRIMARY DYSMENORRHEA

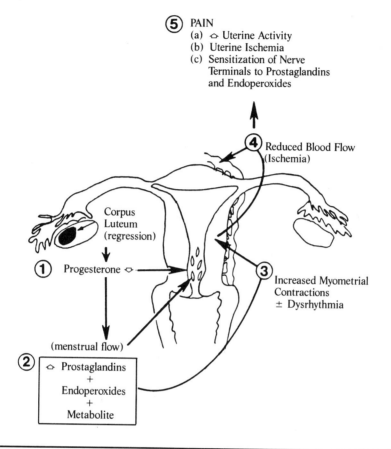

Source: Reprinted with permission from Dawood, Y.M. 1985. Dysmenorrhea. *The Journal of Reproductive Medicine* 30(3): 160.

menorrhea also is increased among mothers and sisters of women with painful menses (Droegemueller et al. 1987).

Secondary dysmenorrhea should be considered when there is a history of recurrent PID, irregular menstrual cycles, menorrhagia, IUD use, or infertility (Dawood 1990). With secondary dysmenorrhea, the pelvic examination may reveal physical clues about the cause of the pain.

Cervical stenosis may cause secondary dysmenorrhea due to impediment of the menstrual flow through the cervical canal and subsequent increased intrauterine pressure. A history of scant menstrual flow and severe cramping throughout the menstrual period should alert the clinician to the possibility of cervical stenosis (Droegemueller et al. 1987).

Endometriosis should be considered if dysmenorrhea becomes more severe as menses progresses. Pelvic infections or PID can cause pelvic adhesions which may be aggravated at the time of menses (Droegemueller

et al. 1987). Adenomyosis is more common during the fourth and fifth decades of life.

DATABASE

SUBJECTIVE

Primary dysmenorrhea

→ Onset is usually one to two years after menarche.

→ Patient describes cramping as:
  ■ suprapubic.
  ■ sharp/colicky.
  ■ possibly radiating to inner thighs, groin, sacrum; beginning within hours of onset of menses.
  ■ diminishing within 24 to 48 hours.

→ Associated symptoms may include:
  ■ nausea.
  ■ diarrhea.
  ■ headache.
  ■ bloating.

- breast tenderness.
- flushing.
- anxiety.
- palpitations.
→ Risk factors may include:
  - single.
  - delayed childbearing.
  - overweight.
  - smoking.
  - positive family history.
  - higher socioeconomic status.
  - retroflexed uterus.

Secondary dysmenorrhea

→ Onset of dysmenorrhea is in adulthood with a possible history of previous pain-free menstrual cycles.

→ Pain may be described as dull in character, starting earlier and lasting longer than cramping associated with primary dysmenorrhea or may be similar to pain experienced with primary dysmenorrhea.

→ The patient may complain of pelvic pain throughout the menstrual cycle.

→ Pain may occur during ovulation and with intercourse.

→ Pain increases with age.

→ There are no associated visceral symptoms.

→ Patient may have a history of PID, irregular menstrual cycles, menorrhagia, IUD use, infertility.

Primary and secondary dysmenorrhea

→ History to include:
  - description of usual menstrual pattern.
  - age at menarche.
  - description of menstrual pain.
    - Including onset, character, duration, severity, and timing during the menstrual cycle, and age when first started.
  - history of analgesic use, palliative measures, efficacy of treatment.
  - associated symptoms.
  - thorough obstetrical and gynecological history (may help to differentiate between primary and secondary dysmenorrhea) (Treybig 1989).

OBJECTIVE

Primary dysmenorrhea

→ Pelvic and abdominal examination usually within normal limits (WNL).

Secondary dysmenorrhea

→ May find pelvic pathology on pelvic or abdominal examination, sonogram, laparoscopy, hystero-salpingogram, or hysteroscopy.

ASSESSMENT

→ Dysmenorrhea (primary or secondary)

→ R/O possible causes of secondary dysmenorrhea:
  - endometriosis
  - PID
  - fibroids
  - adenomyosis
  - cervical stenosis
  - congenital müllerian duct malformations
  - presence of an IUD
  - chronic pelvic pain
  - ovarian cysts/tumors
  - intrauterine adhesions (Asherman's syndrome)

PLAN

DIAGNOSTIC TESTS

Primary dysmenorrhea

→ None specific.

Secondary dysmenorrhea

→ Tests may include:
  - sonogram.
  - laparoscopy.
  - hysteroscopy.
  - hysterosalpingogram.
  - laboratory tests as indicated. These may include: CBC, RPR, pregnancy test, cervical cultures for *N. gonorrhoeae* and *C. trachomatis*, Pap smear.

TREATMENT/MANAGEMENT

Primary dysmenorrhea

→ Pharmacological agents useful in treatment may include (see **Figure 12D.2, Management of Primary Dysmenorrhea**):
  - oral contraceptives.
    - Drug of choice if patient also desires birth control pills as method of contraception (Dawood 1985).
    - Combination oral contraception with low estrogen to progesterone ratio reported as most effective (Treybig 1989).
    - Mechanism:
      - decreased menstrual fluid volume secondary to suppression of endometrial growth.

Figure 12D.2. MANAGEMENT OF PRIMARY DYSMENORRHEA

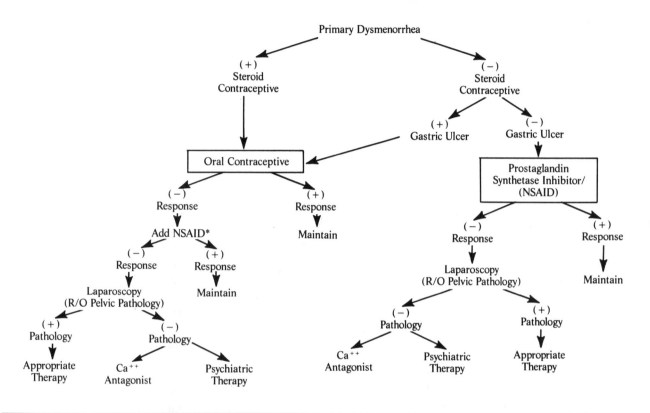

Outline of management of primary dysmenorrhea. "+" indicates 1) subject wishes to have or has; 2) positive or favorable response; or 3) present. "–" indicates 1) subject does not wish to have or does not have; 2) negative or poor response; or 3) absent.

*Except with gastric ulcer

NOTE: Adapted with permission from Dawood, Y.M. 1990. Dysmenorrhea. *Clinical Obstetrics and Gynecology* 33(1):174.

–suppression of ovulation, resulting in low levels of prostaglandins.
- Effective in 90 percent or more of cases.
- A trial of oral contraceptives for 3 to 4 months is reasonable to evaluate effectiveness.
  –If no relief, an NSAID may be added, unless there is a history of peptic ulcer disease or gastritis (Dawood 1985, 1990; Treybig 1989).
- NSAIDs, also known as prostaglandin synthetase inhibitors.
  - Mechanism:
    –inhibits prostaglandin synthesis and release in endometrial tissue, which results in suppression of menstrual fluid prostaglandins.
    –also has direct analgesic properties (Dawood 1985, 1990).
    –75 percent to 90 percent effective (Treybig 1989).

- Advantages over oral contraceptives:
  –taken only for 2 to 3 days of the menstrual cycle.
  –does not suppress the pituitary-gonadal axis.
  –oral-contraceptive-related metabolic effects are not present (Dawood 1984, 1985, 1990).
- Should start taking NSAID as soon as menstrual pain begins or at the onset of menstruation.
  –Should not administer prior to this time as risk of NSAID use in early pregnancy is not known.
- Options—4 major groups of NSAIDs and dosages shown to be effective in the treatment of dysmenorrhea (see **Table 12D.1, Prostaglandin Synthetase Inhibitors Shown to Be Effective in Treatment of Primary Dysmenorrhea**):
  –indole-acetic acid derivatives (indomethacin [Indocin®]).

Table 12D.1. PROSTAGLANDIN SYNTHETASE INHIBITORS SHOWN TO BE EFFECTIVE IN TREATMENT OF PRIMARY DYSMENORRHEA

Nonsteroidal Anti-Inflammatory Drug Group	Examples	Dose
Indole-acetic acid derivative	Indomethacin	25 mg every 4-8 hrs.
Fenamate	Mefenamic acid	500 mg initially then 250 mg every 6 hrs.
Arylpropionic acids	Ibuprofen Naproxen Naproxen sodium Ketoprofen	400 mg every 4 hrs. 500 mg initially then 250 mg every 6-8 hrs. 550 mg initially then 275 mg every 6-8 hrs. 25-50 mg every 6-8 hrs.
Oxicam	Piroxicam	20 mg/day

Source: Adapted with permission from Dawood, Y.M. 1990. Dysmenorrhea. *Clinical Obstetrics and Gynecology* 33(1):175.

–fenamates (mefenamic acid [Ponstel®]).
–arylpropionic acids (ibuprofen [Motrin®], naproxen [Naprosyn®], naproxen sodium [Anaprox®], and ketoprofen [Orudis®]).
–oxicams (piroxicam [Feldene®]).
NOTE: Drug of choice is either an arylproprionic acid derivative or a fenamate (Dawood 1985).
• Treatment.
  –Continue NSAID treatment through the first 48 to 72 hours of menstrual flow rather than on an as needed basis. Rationale:
    ▸ corrects the biochemical derangement caused by excessive production and release of prostaglandins (Dawood 1990).
    ▸ maximal prostaglandin release is during the first 48 hours of the menstrual flow (Dawood 1990).
• If dysmenorrhea persists during the first few hours after the NSAID is taken, increase the starting dose by 50 percent or double at the onset of the next cycle, while keeping the maintenance dose essentially the same.
  –If this fails to relieve the dysmenorrhea, try an NSAID from a different group (Dawood 1985).
• A trial of up to 6 months should be adequate to determine effectiveness of treatment (Dawood 1990).
• Contraindications to NSAIDs:
  –gastrointestinal ulcers, hypersensitivity to ASA or similar agents (Dawood 1985).
• Side effects of NSAIDs:
  –uncommon due to the intermittent use of these drugs, with the exception of gastro-intestinal (GI) disturbances (Dawood 1988).
  –GI side effects can be reduced if NSAID is taken with food or an antacid. See

Physicians' Desk Reference (*PDR*). **NOTE:** Toxic effects of NSAIDs may include nephrotoxicity, hepatotoxicity, and platelet dysfunction/blood dyscrasias.
→ Non-drug therapies:
  ▪ exercise:
    • suppresses prostaglandin release.
    • releases beta endorphins which decrease pain perception.
    • shunts blood away from the uterus (Treybig 1989).
  ▪ dietary changes:
    • decreased salt intake and increased consumption of foods that are natural diuretics to decrease water retention.
    • vitamin E:
      –Mild prostaglandin inhibitor, improves circulation to the uterus secondary to its ability to reduce arteriolar spasm (Treybig 1989).
  ▪ sexual activity:
    • Sexual excitement and orgasm may decrease dysmenorrhea secondary to uterine arteriolar vasodilation (Treybig 1989).
  ▪ pregnancy:
    • reduces the number of adrenergic nerves which only partially regenerate after delivery. This may result in a decrease or absence of pain (Treybig 1989).
  ▪ application of local heat (heating pad, hot water bottle):
    • increases blood flow and decreases muscle spasm (Treybig 1989).
  ▪ transcutaneous electrical nerve stimulation (TENS):
    • may be useful for:

–patients who have contraindications or experienced side effects with oral contraceptives or NSAIDs.
   –patients who do not get adequate pain relief from NSAIDs.
 • may not be widely available or affordable.
 • mechanism:
   –inhibits propagation of pain-related impulses ("gate-control" theory).
   –increases the release of endorphins, with subsequent pain relief (Dawood 1990; Dawood and Ramos 1990).

Secondary dysmenorrhea

→ Specific therapy should be aimed at correcting the underlying cause of the condition. See protocols for **Pelvic Pain—Acute, Pelvic Pain—Chronic, Endometriosis, Pelvic Masses, Pelvic Inflammatory Disease,** and **Abnormal Uterine Bleeding.**

→ Stress relief/hypnosis/psychotherapy may be helpful.

→ Referral to a support group may be indicated.

→ Record keeping.
  ▪ Patient should keep a diary of symptomatology and BBT for the first 2 to 4 months of treatment.
    • Useful for assessing the characteristics of the pain, associated symptoms, and efficacy of treatment (Treybig 1989).

CONSULTATION

→ For evaluation of possible causes of secondary dysmenorrhea, if suspected.

→ As needed for prescription(s).

PATIENT EDUCATION

→ Explain the process of menstruation and etiology of dysmenorrhea. Patients with primary dysmenorrhea should be reassured that their condition is not caused by pelvic pathology.

→ Review daily living modifications.

→ Instruct patient in use of oral contraceptives and NSAIDs if used in treatment.

→ Discuss diary keeping.

→ Encourage regular exercise and proper nutrition.

→ Encourage follow-up visits as outlined.

FOLLOW-UP

→ Re-evaluation in one month recommended to assess treatment efficacy.

→ Document in progress notes and problem list.

Bibliography

Dawood, Y.M. 1984. Ibuprofen and dysmenorrhea. *The American Journal of Medicine* 77:87–94.

———. 1985. Dysmenorrhea. *The Journal of Reproductive Medicine* 30(3):154–167.

———. 1988. Nonsteroidal anti-inflammatory drugs and changing attitudes toward dysmenorrhea. *The American Journal of Medicine* 84(Suppl. 5A):23–29.

———. 1990. Dysmenorrhea. *Clinical Obstetrics and Gynecology* 33(1):168–178.

Dawood, Y.M., and Ramos, J. 1990. Transcutaneous electrical nerve stimulation (TENS) for the treatment of primary dysmenorrhea: A randomized crossover comparison with placebo TENS and ibuprofen. *Obstetrics and Gynecology* 75:656–660.

Droegemueller, W., Herbst, A.L., Mishell, D.R., and Stenchever, M.A. 1987. Dysmenorrhea and premenstrual syndrome. In *Comprehensive gynecology*, pp. 941–952. St. Louis: C.V. Mosby.

Hoffman, P. G. 1988. Primary dysmenorrhea and the premenstrual syndrome. In *Office gynecology*, 3d ed., ed. R.H. Glass, pp. 209–229. Baltimore: Williams & Wilkins.

Pernoll, M.L., and Benson, R.C. 1987. Complications of menstruation, abnormal uterine bleeding. In *Current obstetric and gynecologic diagnosis and treatment*, pp. 613–614. Norwalk, CT: Appleton & Lange.

Sullivan, N. 1990. Dysmenorrhea. In *Gynecology: Well-woman care*, eds. R. Lichtman and S. Papera, pp. 345–353. Norwalk, CT: Appleton & Lange.

Sundell, G., Milsom, J., and Andersch, B. 1990. Factors influencing the prevalence and severity of dysmenorrhea in young women. *British Journal of Obstetrics and Gynecology* 97:588–594.

Treybig, M. 1989. Primary dysmenorrhea or endometriosis? *Nurse Practitioner* 14(5):8–18.

Women's Primary Care Program. Dysmenorrhea/Premenstrual Syndrome. Spring 1989. Lecture presented at the University of California, San Francisco, School of Nursing.

Maureen Shannon C.N.M., F.N.P., M.S.

12-E

Ectopic Pregnancy

Ectopic pregnancy is a pregnancy that occurs outside normal implantation sites within the uterine cavity. The fallopian tubes are the most frequent sites for implantation of an ectopic pregnancy. The ampulla, isthmus, infundibulum, and fimbria of the fallopian tubes are involved in 55 percent, 25 percent, and 17 percent of ectopic pregnancies, respectively (Sanfilippo and Woodworth 1992). Other extrauterine sites for implantation include cervical (0.1 percent of ectopic pregnancies), ovarian (0.5 percent), and abdominal sites (0.03 percent) (Sanfilippo and Woodworth 1992). In addition, heterotopic pregnancies (simultaneous intrauterine and extrauterine pregnancy) have been noted in one out of 2,600 pregnancies (Sanfilippo and Woodworth 1992).

A significant increased incidence of ectopic pregnancies has been noted since the 1970s. In 1989, over 88,000 ectopic pregnancies were reported in the United States, with an incidence rate of 16.1 per 1,000 reported pregnancies and an annual cost of $1.1 billion (Washington and Katz 1993). The highest rates of ectopic pregnancies are reported in nonwhite women 35 years of age and older and women between the ages of 15 years to 24 years (Doyle, DeCherney, and Diamond 1991; Gale, Stovall, and Muram 1990). Multiple factors have been implicated in this increased incidence, including an increase in STDs, assisted reproduction (e.g., ovulation induction, in vitro fertilization, gamete intrafallopian transfer [GIFT]), and earlier diagnosis of ectopic pregnancies due to improved technology and provider awareness (Doyle, DeCherney, and Diamond 1991).

Ectopic pregnancy is the second leading cause of maternal death in the United States. The case fatality rate for black women is three times higher than that for white women (Doyle, DeCherney, and Diamond 1991;

Sanfilippo and Woodworth 1992). Most maternal deaths are attributed to a delay in diagnosis, either because patients failed to seek evaluations and treatment or providers failed to diagnose and treat the condition in a timely manner. However, the mortality rate associated with ectopic pregnancy has had a sevenfold decline since 1970. This is presumably because of earlier detection and intervention as a result of improved technology, a higher index of suspicion on the part of clinicians, and more conservative treatment options currently available (Sanfilippo and Woodworth 1992).

A number of pathophysiological mechanisms have been cited as probable causes of ectopic pregnancies. *Tubal ectopic pregnancies* are a result of inhibition or prevention of normal tubal transport of an embryo because of damage to the mucosal lining of the fimbria and/or fallopian tube. The etiology of such damage may be secondary to infection (e.g., PID), inflammation (e.g., chronic salpingitis, tubal diverticula), tubal/uterine surgery, and DES exposure (Doyle, DeCherney, and Diamond 1991).

Other possible causes of ectopic pregnancies include ovum defects (e.g., premature or delayed ovulation, postmature ovum), hormonal dysfunction (e.g., hyperestrogenism), mechanical interference with implantation (e.g., IUDs), sterilization failure (e.g., tubal ligation with subsequent conception), and assisted reproduction technologies (e.g., GIFT) (Doyle, DeCherney, and Diamond 1991; Guirgis and Craft 1991).

Complications associated with an ectopic pregnancy can be severe and life threatening. They are related to the length of gestation, site of implantation, any delay or failure to diagnose the condition, and method of treatment chosen. The most emergent complication is excessive blood loss due to tubal rupture or development of a pelvic hematocele. Such blood loss may result in anemia, the need for transfusions, and, rarely, the development of disseminated intravascular coagulopathy (DIC) or death. Regardless of the therapeutic intervention chosen in the management of a patient with an ectopic pregnancy, careful monitoring for any evidence of acute or chronic blood loss is essential.

An increased incidence of repeated ectopic pregnancy is another complication reported in the literature. Recurrence rates between four percent to seven percent have been documented. Women with a history of predisposing conditions involving tubal damage are more likely to have repeated ectopic pregnancies (Russell and Rodgers 1991). In addition, the type of therapeutic intervention chosen can have an impact on recurrence rates. The incidence of repeat ectopic pregnancies is less with conservative treatments (e.g., expectant management, medical management, conservative surgical procedures), compared to more extensive surgical procedures and procedures involving more manipulation of the fallopian tube(s) (e.g., "milking" the tube to remove the products of conception [POCs]) (Russell and Rodgers 1991; Sanfilippo and Woodworth 1992).

Persistent ectopic pregnancy can occur when retained trophoblastic tissue continues to proliferate at the site of implantation (Sanfilippo and Woodworth 1992). This complication has been reported in conjunction with conservative therapeutic interventions, and the rate may be as high as 20 percent following conservative surgical procedures (Seifer, Diamond, and DeCherney 1991). Persistent ectopic pregnancy can result in hemorrhage, continued tubal destruction, and, rarely, the development of choriocarcinoma (Seifer, Diamond, and DeCherney 1991). Clinicians should consider this possible complication in any patient with persistent elevation of serum human chorionic gonadotropin (hCG) levels after therapy for an ectopic pregnancy (Sanfilippo and Woodworth 1992).

DATABASE

SUBJECTIVE

→ Risk factors may include:
■ patient reporting a history of one or more of the following (Doyle, DeCherney, and Diamond 1991; Sanfilippo and Woodworth 1992; Stock 1988):
• prior ectopic pregnancy.
• episode of PID.
• tubal or uterine surgery.
• infertility.
• current or past use of an IUD.

• factors associated with uterine or tubal anatomic abnormalities (e.g., DES exposure, salpingitis, isthmica nodosa).
• induced superovulation (e.g., Clomid® or Pergonal®).
• assisted reproduction (e.g., GIFT, in vitro fertilization).
• prior therapeutic abortion with complications (i.e., endometritis, retained POCs).
NOTE: Although several risk factors associated with ectopic pregnancy have been reported in the literature, in one report as many as 42 percent of women with ectopic pregnancies did not have an identifiable risk factor (Stock 1988).

→ Symptoms may include one of more of the following:
■ abdominal pain, which is reported by more than 90 percent of women experiencing an ectopic pregnancy.
• Pain may range in intensity and character from a mild, dull, cramp-like sensation to a severe, sharp pain.
• Women experiencing acute blood loss associated with tubal rupture usually report the sudden onset of severe lower quadrant abdominal pain that may be intermittent and associated with backache, dizziness, and fainting.
• Women experiencing chronic blood loss from "minor" tubal ruptures may report less severe abdominal symptoms.
■ amenorrhea.
■ abnormal vaginal bleeding, which may vary from slight intermenstrual spotting to profuse vaginal bleeding.
■ associated symptoms of pregnancy (e.g., nausea, vomiting, breast tenderness/enlargement) may or may not be reported depending upon the gestation of the pregnancy (i.e., after eight weeks gestation the patient may not notice any associated symptoms).
■ if significant blood loss, lightheadedness, vertigo, and/or syncopal episodes.
■ shoulder pain, which may be reported by patients experiencing hemorrhage as blood pools under the diaphragm.
■ in addition to abdominal pain, a patient with an abdominal pregnancy may report persistent nausea and vomiting, general malaise, painful fetal movements, fetal movements high in the abdominal cavity, and decreased fetal movements (Martin and McCaul 1990;

Osguthorpe and Keating 1988; Sanfilippo and Woodworth 1992).

OBJECTIVE

→ Physical examination may reveal one or more of the following findings:

- vital signs WNL or demonstrate changes associated with significant blood loss (e.g., decreased blood pressure, rapid/thready pulse, rapid respirations, orthostatic changes).
- patient may appear in no distress, or loss of consciousness may be evident.
- skin pallor may be observed in patients with significant blood loss.
- upon abdominal examination:
  - decreased bowel sounds may be noted if a mild paralytic ileus has occurred (may be noted in patients with chronic abdominal blood loss).
  - if hemoperitoneum present, tenderness to palpation with or without rebound, guarding.
  - Cullen's sign (bluish discoloration of the umbilical area) may be noted and is associated with hemoperitoneum.
  - if abdominal pregnancy present, uterine size less than dates, a distinct mass may be observed outside the uterus, fetal parts may be easily palpated, and fetal activity may be noted high within the abdomen (Martin and McCaul 1990; Osguthorpe and Keating 1988).
- upon pelvic examination:
  - speculum may reveal varying amounts of blood (minimal to profuse) at the introitus, in the vaginal vault, and/or coming from the cervical os.
  - bimanual may be WNL if the pregnancy is in an early stage of gestation or reveal an adnexal mass that is with or without tenderness to palpation.
    - There may be a doughy sensation when the pouch of Douglas is palpated (posterior vaginal wall) due to the accumulation of blood in this area secondary to a hemoperitoneum.

ASSESSMENT

→ Ectopic pregnancy (tubal, cervical, ovarian, abdominal)

→ R/O appendicitis

→ R/O spontaneous abortion

→ R/O gestational trophoblastic neoplasia

→ R/O ruptured corpus luteum cyst

→ R/O ruptured ovarian follicle

→ R/O intrauterine gestation earlier than suggested by menstrual dates

→ R/O intrauterine pregnancy with corpus luteum cyst

→ R/O PID

→ R/O urinary calculi

PLAN

DIAGNOSTIC TESTS

→ Most ectopic pregnancies are diagnosed through a number of tests and procedures ordered depending on the patient's status (i.e., stable versus in shock) as well as the point in gestation when the patient presents for an evaluation.

- Since a patient with a suspected ectopic pregnancy is at risk for significant morbidity and mortality due to hemorrhage, physician management of such patients is warranted and any diagnostic tests should be ordered in consultation with the physician.
- CBC may reveal decreased RBC count, Hgb, and Hct consistent with acute or chronic blood loss, as well as a mild leukocytosis.
- Pregnancy tests.
- Quantitative serum beta-human chorionic gonadotropin (B-hCG) radioimmunoassay.
  - Currently, this is considered the "gold standard" pregnancy test for the evaluation of patients with a possible ectopic pregnancy.
    - A positive result can be obtained 7 to 10 days after conception and is highly sensitive (99 percent).
    - However, results of the test are usually not available for 24 hours.
    - In normal early intrauterine pregnancies, a doubling of this hormone level is expected every 2 days.
    - Although abnormal results do not confirm the existence of an ectopic pregnancy, they may assist the clinician in formulating a plan of care when ectopic pregnancy is suspected.
    - Serial testing can be done to determine if a normal or abnormal pregnancy is occurring.

NOTE: Usually, B-hCG levels are reported in international units/liter (IU/L) using a standard international reference preparation to determine the hormone level. Initially, the Second International Standard (2nd IS) was used to quantify hCG levels. However, this preparation was found to contain large amounts of the alpha subunit of hCG, which can cross-react with other gonadotropic hormones (e.g., luteinizing hormone). The First International Standard (1st IS) is a purified, homogeneous preparation that provides a more accurate B-hCG level and is the preferred preparation for quantifying hCG levels. Conversion of 2nd IS values to 1st IS values can be calculated by multiplying the 2nd IS value by 1.7 (Sanfilippo and Woodworth 1992). It is important to know which reference range has been used, especially if the patient has had previous levels drawn at a different clinical site. For consistency and accuracy of results, the patient should have all further serial B-hCG specimens performed at the same laboratory.

- B-hCG levels that demonstrate less than 66 percent increase over 48 hours are associated with ectopic pregnancies or a spontaneous abortion of intrauterine pregnancies in 85 percent of patients.
- In abdominal pregnancies, the B-hCG may be abnormally elevated for the stage of gestation.
- Discriminatory zone of B-hCG: B-hCG levels can be used in conjunction with ultrasonography to determine the presence of an early ectopic pregnancy (especially at a gestational stage [i.e., less than 10 weeks gestation] when tubal rupture is less likely to occur).
  –Discriminatory zones of B-hCG levels are the levels at which an intrauterine gestational sac should be reliably visualized by ultrasound.
  –When the B-hCG is between 6000 to 6500 IU/L (International Reference Preparation), an intrauterine gestational sac should be seen by transabdominal ultrasound in more than 90 percent of pregnant patients (Ory 1992).
  –When an ultrasound is done using a vaginal transducer, the discriminatory zone for B-hCG is reportedly in the range of 1200 to 1500 IU/L (International Reference Preparation) (Ory 1992).
    ‣ At these levels, if an intrauterine gestational sac is not visualized the pregnancy may not be viable or it may be an ectopic implantation.
    ‣ However, the visualization of an intrauterine gestational sac does not absolutely eliminate the possibility of an

ectopic pregnancy since heterotopic pregnancy, although rare, can occur (Sanfilippo and Woodworth 1992).
NOTE: Individual institutions should establish their specific discriminatory zone ranges based upon the quality of ultrasonography available within their institution, the B-hCG radioim-munoassay techniques utilized, and the reference standard that is used to quantify the B-hCG level. Clinicians must be knowledgeable regarding the discriminatory zones currently used in their institutions in order to evaluate the patient properly.

- Urine hCG tests: Several rapid, ultrasensitive monoclonal antibody urine tests are available to assess B-hCG levels (Tandem Icon II®, First Response®).
  –These tests can reliably detect pregnancy 7 to 10 days after conception and can offer rapid screening of women for ectopic pregnancy; however, additional testing with serum B-hCG and ultrasonography may also be indicated.
  –The reported false negative rate of rapid urine hCG tests is 1 percent.
- Serum progesterone levels.
- Low levels of progesterone have been associated with abnormal pregnancies, including spontaneous abortions and ectopic pregnancies (Sanfilippo and Woodworth 1992).
- A single serum progesterone level does not confirm the existence of an ectopic pregnancy; however, a low level can alert the clinician to the possibility of a potentially abnormal pregnancy requiring further evaluation and testing.
- The results from this test usually can be obtained the day the specimen is drawn.
- Ultrasonography (sonogram).
- Both transabdominal and transvaginal ultrasonography can be used in the evaluation of a patient suspected of having an ectopic pregnancy, either by ruling out the presence of an intrauterine pregnancy or demonstrating the presence of a gestational sac outside the uterus.
- The accuracy of ultrasound results in determining an ectopic pregnancy is based on the stage of gestation of the pregnancy, the implantation site, the type of ultrasound being performed, and the capabilities of the sonographer.

- Abdominal ultrasound (de Crespigny 1987; Ory 1992; Sanfilippo and Woodworth 1992).
  - –Absence of an intrauterine gestational sac 6 weeks from the patient's last menstrual period or absence of a fetal pole 7 weeks from the last menstrual period may indicate an ectopic pregnancy, especially if serum *B*-hCG levels are between 6000 to 6500 IU/L.
  - –The presence of a gestational sac and fetal pole does not eliminate the possibility of an ectopic pregnancy in all patients since heterotopic pregnancy can occur.
  - –Evidence of a gestational sac or fetus outside of the uterine cavity (e.g., interstitial portion of the fallopian tube, abdomen, ovary) would confirm the diagnosis of an ectopic pregnancy at these sites.
  - –The presence of an intrauterine gestational sac-like structure (i.e., "pseudogestation sac") may be observed with an ectopic pregnancy and can be confused with an intrauterine gestational sac.

NOTE: A pseudogestation sac can result from accumulation of blood in the uterine cavity, the development of the decidual lining without a trophoblastic rim, or the development of a thick proliferative endometrium (de Crespigny 1987).

- Transvaginal ultrasound.
  - –The use of transvaginal ultrasound in the evaluation of ectopic pregnancy has been documented in several studies and is reportedly more accurate than abdominal ultrasound in locating early-gestation ectopic pregnancies and determining the size of the gestational sac.
    - ▸ Evidence of extrauterine fetal cardiac pulsations indicates an ectopic pregnancy.
    - ▸ Visualization of a sac-like adnexal ring is indicative of an ectopic pregnancy.
    - ▸ Visualization of echogenic fluid may indicate an ectopic pregnancy. This finding also correlates with a hemoperitoneum in many patients.
    - ▸ Evidence of fluid in the cul-de-sac may indicate an ectopic pregnancy.
- Culdocentesis can be performed.
  - Aspiration of nonclotted blood indicates intraperitoneal bleeding and an ectopic pregnancy in patients with signs and symptoms associated with this condition.
  - Absence of fluid from the cul-de-sac does not eliminate the possibility of an ectopic pregnancy.

- If the patient has had a recent therapeutic abortion, the pathology report on the POCs may be able to confirm an intrauterine pregnancy, in which case the likelihood of a simultaneous ectopic pregnancy is remote (Hatcher et al. 1990).
- Laparoscopy often is performed when confirmation and further intervention is indicated.
  - This procedure can locate the site of an extrauterine pregnancy, assess bleeding, and, if indicated, accomplish removal of the ectopic conceptus in some patients.

TREATMENT/MANAGEMENT

→ The care of the patient suspected of having an ectopic pregnancy should be by a physician qualified to manage this condition.
  - Therapeutic options and interventions are determined by the physician based on the patient's status, symptoms, site of implantation, stage of gestation, and the patient's desire to maintain fertility.
  - The decision making regarding the various treatment options is beyond the scope of this protocol. However, a brief presentation of these therapeutic interventions will be presented in this section.

→ Expectant management.
  - Spontaneous resolution of extrauterine pregnancies has been reported in the literature (Doyle, DeCherney, and Diamond 1991). Based upon these observations, expectant management of patients with ectopic pregnancies has been studied (Fernandez et al. 1991a; Fernandez et al. 1991b; Ory 1992; Pansky et al. 1991).
    - Results from these studies indicate that close observation without the use of medical or surgical interventions can be offered to a very select group of patients with ectopic pregnancies. The criteria used for inclusion in such a plan of care varied among studies but generally required the following:
      - –an initial serum *B*-hCG level ≤ 2000 IU/L.
      - –a consistent decline in hCG level.
      - –no symptoms reported by the patient.
      - –no evidence of tubal rupture or bleeding (by ultrasound and/or laparoscopy), and
      - –patient compliance with required serial testing and follow-up visits.
        - ▸ possible complications associated with this plan include late tubal rupture,

hemorrhage, and persistent ectopic pregnancy.
  ‣ tubal patency and return of reproductive performance in patients involved in expectant management strategies have been higher than what has been observed in patients undergoing surgical interventions (Fernandez et al. 1991b; Pansky et al. 1991).

→ Medical interventions.
  ▪ The use of pharmacological agents in the treatment of ectopic pregnancies has been studied. The various success rates depend upon the type of agent used, the method of administration (i.e., systemic versus local injection), patient tolerance of the agent, stage of gestation of the pregnancy, and size of the gestational sac.
    • Highest efficacy rates are reported in patients who receive methotrexate (either systemically or locally) (Ory 1991; Ory 1992; Pansky et al. 1991; Stovall, Ling, and Buster 1990; Stovall, Ling, and Gray 1991; Stovall et al. 1991).
    • However, other agents such as systemic RU 486 (mifepristone) and local injections of prostaglandins, actinomycin D, and potassium chloride have been studied with varying efficacy rates noted (Ory 1991; Pansky et al. 1991; Vejtorp, Vejerslev, and Ruge 1989).
    • Complications associated with this plan of care include possible adverse effects of the pharmacological agent(s), tubal rupture, bleeding, and persistent ectopic pregnancy.
    • Tubal patency and reproductive performance were reportedly higher in eligible women receiving medical treatment compared to women undergoing surgical interventions (Fernandez et al. 1991a; Stovall, Ling, and Buster 1990).
  ▪ Women who are Rh negative and antibody-screen (Du) negative should be given Rh immune globulin (RhIG) at the following recommended doses:
    • 50 µg of RhIG (Micro RhoGam®) I.M. should be given if the ectopic gestation is < 13 weeks.
    • 300 µg of RhIG (RhoGam®) I.M. should be given if the gestation is > 13 weeks (ACOG 1990).
→ Surgical interventions.
  ▪ Various surgical interventions are used in the management of ectopic pregnancies.

▪ Decisions regarding which surgical procedure is indicated are based upon the status of the patient, threat or evidence of rupture, bleeding, size of the gestational sac, accessibility of the ectopic pregnancy, desire of the patient to maintain fertility, skill of the surgeon, and availability of various operative instruments (i.e., laparoscopic instruments).
▪ The following are surgical procedures that may be performed:
  • laparoscopy with removal of the POC and/or oviduct.
  • linear salpingostomy.
  • segmental resection of the fallopian tube.
  • salpingectomy.
  • laparotomy.
  • hysteroscopy (Nager and Murphy 1991; Ory 1992; Osguthorpe and Keating 1988; Sanfilippo and Woodworth 1992).
▪ The more conservative surgical interventions are less life-threatening and have a higher likelihood of maintaining tubal patency than more extensive procedures.
▪ Complications associated with the surgical procedures include hemorrhage, infection, anesthesia complications, persistent ectopic pregnancy (primarily associated with conservative surgical procedures), decreased tubal patency, decreased reproductive performance, and death.

CONSULTATION

→ Consultation with a physician is warranted for any patient suspected of having an ectopic pregnancy.
  ▪ The evaluation and management of the woman should be by the consulting physician.

→ Consultation with a psychologist or psychiatrist may be indicated in patients and their partners who are experiencing prolonged, severe depression associated with pregnancy loss.
  ▪ This may be especially important for women or couples who have had assisted reproduction procedures (e.g., GIFT, in vitro fertilization) and are facing the loss of a desired pregnancy and the possibility of further reduction in fertility as a result of this condition.
  ▪ In addition, the threat of loss of the woman's life may precipitate a psychological crisis, for the woman and/or her partner, requiring crisis intervention.

PATIENT EDUCATION

→ Education of the patient with a suspected or documented ectopic pregnancy should include information about the condition, diagnostic tests that will be ordered, treatment options, possible complications associated with the condition and treatment(s), and indicated follow-up.
  ▪ Ideally, such discussions should occur between the patient and the physician responsible for her care.
  ▪ In situations where the patient's condition is unstable, a discussion about the plan of care should occur between the physician, the patient, and a patient's relative or partner whenever possible.

→ Women undergoing outpatient therapy (e.g., expectant or medical management) should be educated about the possibility of sudden rupture of an ectopic pregnancy and the rapid blood loss associated with this condition.
  ▪ A thorough review of signs and symptoms that occur should be undertaken.
  ▪ The patient should be advised not to operate motor vehicles or be involved in similar activities that require concentration because of the possibility of syncopal episodes that can occur with tubal rupture and significant blood loss.
  ▪ The patient should have a plan for immediate access to medical treatment if any signs and/or symptoms associated with tubal rupture and hemorrhage develop (e.g., someone should be immediately available to drive her to the hospital).

→ Referral of the patient and her partner to community resources that provide support as they work through the loss of a pregnancy may be necessary.

→ Education of all sexually active women of reproductive age regarding ways to prevent STDs will help prevent and eventually decrease the incidence of ectopic pregnancies (especially tubal pregnancies).

→ If a woman with risk factors is contemplating pregnancy, she should be educated about the possibility of an ectopic pregnancy and the need to obtain an evaluation as soon as possible after conception so that her pregnancy can be carefully monitored for evidence of extrauterine implantation.

→ After a woman has completed therapy for an ectopic pregnancy, she should be counseled about the need to postpone conception for three months to allow complete recovery of the ectopic implantation site (Ory 1992).
  ▪ Contraception should be provided after a discussion of available methods.

FOLLOW-UP

→ Follow-up evaluation of the patient with an ectopic pregnancy is by the physician responsible for her care.

→ Serum *B*-hCG levels should be monitored in a woman with an ectopic pregnancy to determine resolution of the condition.
  ▪ The frequency of testing is based upon the gestation of the pregnancy and the type of treatment the woman is undergoing.
  ▪ Testing should be recommended by the physician managing the woman's care.
  ▪ A consistent decline in *B*-hCG levels should be observed (Ory 1992). A level that plateaus or increases warrants further evaluation and possibly a change in therapy.

→ Women being treated for an ectopic pregnancy without evidence of immunity to rubella should be considered for rubella immunization during the follow-up period.
  ▪ Thorough counseling regarding the need to postpone conception until at least three months after immunization, as well as provision of an effective contraceptive method during this period, is essential.
  ▪ Document in progress notes and problem list.

Bibliography

American College of Obstetricians and Gynecologists. 1990. *Prevention of D isoimmunization.* ACOG Technical Bulletin 147. Washington, DC: the Author.

De Crespigny, L.C. 1987. The value of ultrasound in ectopic pregnancy. *Clinical Obstetrics and Gynecology* 30(1):136–147.

Doyle, M.B., DeCherney, A.H., and Diamond, M.P. 1991. Epidemiology and etiology of ectopic pregnancy. *Obstetrics and Gynecology Clinics of North America* 18(1):1–17.

Fernandez, H., Lelaidier, C., Thouvenez, V., and Frydman, R. 1991a. The use of a pretherapeutic, predictive score to determine inclusion criteria for the nonsurgical treatment of ectopic pregnancy. *Human Reproduction* 6(7):995–998.

Fernandez, H., Lelaidier, C., Baton, C., Bourget, P., and Frydman, R. 1991b. Return of reproductive performance after expectant management and local treatment for ectopic pregnancy. *Human Reproduction* 6(10):1474–1477.

Gale, C.L., Stovall, T.G., and Muram, D. 1990. Tubal pregnancy in adolescence. *Journal of Adolescent Health Care* 11(6):485–489.

Guirgis, R.R., and Craft, I.L. 1991. Ectopic pregnancy resulting from gamete intrafallopian transfer and in vitro fertilization: Role of ultrasonography in diagnosis and treatment. *The Journal of Reproductive Medicine* 36(11):793–796.

Hatcher, R.A., Stewart, F., Trussell, J., Kowal, D., Guest, F., Stewart, G.K., and Cates, W. 1990. *Contraceptive technology 1990–1992*, 15th ed., pp. 431–444. New York: Irvington Publishers.

Margolis, A.J., and Greenwood, S. 1993. Ectopic pregnancy. In *Current medical diagnosis and treatment,* 32d ed., eds. L. M. Tierney, Jr., S.J., McPhee, M.A. Papadakis, and S.A. Schroeder, pp. 598–599. Norwalk, CT.: Appleton & Lange.

Martin, J.N., and McCaul, J.F. 1990. Emergent management of abdominal pregnancy. *Clinical Obstetrics and Gynecology* 33(3):438–447.

Nager, C.W., and Murphy, A.A. 1991. Ectopic pregnancy. *Clinical Obstetrics and Gynecology* 34(2):403–411.

Ory, S.J. 1991. Chemotherapy for ectopic pregnancy. *Obstetrics and Gynecology Clinics of North America* 18(1):123–134.

———. 1992. New options for diagnosis and treatment of ectopic pregnancy. *Journal of the American Medical Association* 267(4):534–537.

Osguthorpe, N.C., and Keating, C.E. 1988. Ectopic pregnancy. Surgical intervention and perioperative nursing care. *AORN Journal* 48(2):254–267.

Pansky, M., Golan, A., Budovsky, I., and Caspi, E. 1991. Nonsurgical management of tubal pregnancy: Necessity in view of the changing clinical appearance. *American Journal of Obstetrics and Gynecology* 164(3):888–895.

Russell, J.B., and Rodgers, M.S. 1991. Repeated ectopic pregnancy. *Obstetrics and Gynecology Clinics of North America* 18(1):145–152.

Sanfilippo, J.S., and Woodworth, S.H. 1992. Ectopic pregnancy. *TeLinde's Operative Gynecology Updates* 1(4):1–14.

Seifer, D.B., Diamond, M.P., and DeCherney, A.H. 1991. Persistent ectopic pregnancy. *Obstetrics and Gynecology Clinics of North America* 18(1):153–159.

Stock, R.J. 1988. The changing spectrum of tubal eccyesis. *Obstetrics and Gynecology* 71:885–888.

Stovall, T.G., Ling, F.W., and Buster, J.E. 1990. Reproductive performance after methotrexate treatment of ectopic pregnancy. *American Journal of Obstetrics and Gynecology* 162(6):1620–1624.

Stovall, T.G., Ling, F.W., and Gray, L.A. 1991. Single-dose methotrexate for treatment of ectopic pregnancy. *Obstetrics and Gynecology* 77(5):754–757.

Stovall, T.G., Ling, F.W., Gray, L.A., Carson, S.A., and Buster, J.E. 1991. Methotrexate treatment of unruptured ectopic pregnancy: A report of 100 cases. *Obstetrics and Gynecology* 77(5):749–753.

Vejtorp, M., Vejerslev, L.O., and Ruge, S. 1989. Local prostaglandin treatment of ectopic pregnancy. *Human Reproduction* 4(4):464–467.

Washington, A.E., and Katz, A. 1993. Ectopic pregnancy in the United States: Economic consequences and payment source trends. *Obstetrics and Gynecology* 81(2):287–292.

12-F

Endometriosis

Endometriosis is defined as the presence of endometrium in ectopic sites. Although the actual prevalence is unknown, endometriosis is suspected to affect two percent to 15 percent of reproductive age women. It is also believed to affect 20 percent to 40 percent of infertile women (Mahmood and Templeton 1990). Endometriosis usually occurs in the pelvis with the most common sites being the ovaries (55 percent), the posterior and uterosacral ligaments (35 percent and 28 percent, respectively), and the anterior and posterior cul-de-sacs (35 percent and 34 percent, respectively) (Gerbie and Merrill 1988). It also has been found in virtually every organ, as well as in males being treated for prostatic cancer with long-term estrogen therapy.

Even though endometriosis was described in the 1800s and has been studied extensively, confusion still exists surrounding its etiology, pathogenesis, natural history, and relationship to infertility diagnosis and management. Etiological theories include celomic metaplasia, embryonic cell rests, and retrograde menstruation.

The theory of celomic metaplasia refers to the ability of the peritoneal mesothelium to undergo metaplasia and produce ectopic endometrium. Although much has been written about this theory, little evidence supports it (Metzger and Haney 1989).

The embryonic cell rest theory is based on the assumption that cells of müllerian origin may develop into functioning endometrium. To date, there have been no reports of such cell rests (Metzger and Haney 1989).

The clinical pattern of endometriosis suggests that most cases are due to menstrual effluent that has passed out of the fallopian tubes. There is evidence that the endometrial cells present in the effluent can be transplanted to areas outside the pelvis via vascular, lymphatic,

and iatrogenic routes of dissemination (Metzger and Haney 1989). Thus, this theory could explain the presence of endometrial implants in the pelvis as well as in other parts of the body, but it does not explain the cases of endometriosis occurring in men. Moreover, retrograde menstruation appears to be a universal phenomenon, although only a small percentage of women develop endometriosis.

Although endometriosis may regress spontaneously, most cases appear to be progressive (Mahmood and Templeton 1990). The pathophysiological changes, including bleeding from the lesions and the development of endometrial cysts, adhesions, and adverse anatomical alterations, often are responsible for the symptoms of endometriosis. Evidence suggests that ovarian steroid hormones are not necessary for the initiation of the process but do play a role in maintaining the implants, since endometriosis is found almost solely in menstruating women (Gerbie and Merrill 1988).

Prostaglandins and autoimmune factors also are suspected in the pathophysiology, but their role is unclear. Other factors may include genetics, race, menstrual factors (earlier menarche, longer flow, shorter cycles, and dysmenorrhea), delayed childbearing, outflow obstruction, the hormonal milieu, smoking, exercise, and immunological factors (Metzger and Haney 1989; Shaw 1991).

Although endometriosis is considered a benign condition, 105 cases of malignant neoplasms arising from endometriosis have been reported since 1925 (Heaps, Nieberg, and Berek 1990). Endometriosis also may be related to an increased rate of spontaneous abortion, but more research is needed to explore this relationship (Lichtman and Smith 1990).

Endometriosis is very common in women who are infertile, but the exact nature of this relationship is unclear. In moderate or severe cases of endometriosis, anatomical defects (e.g., pelvic adhesions, ovarian capsular scarring) may interfere with ovulation, ovum pick-up, or embryo transport. In the absence of an anatomical alteration, however, there is no clear explanation for the infertility. Factors under consideration include ovulatory dysfunction, hormonal abnormalities, autoimmunity, a hostile pelvic environment, and spontaneous abortions. The possibility exists that delayed childbearing or infertility may actually predispose a woman towards endometriosis and not vice versa (Mahmood and Templeton 1990).

A definitive diagnosis can be made only by visualization of the implants in the pelvis, usually via laparoscopy. In addition to the classical implants (powder-burn, blue-black, chocolate ovarian masses, etc.), endometriosis may be associated with many other types of lesions (e.g., red lesions, white lesions, vesicular lesions). It is strongly recommended that any suspicious lesion be biopsied for histological confirmation. To complicate diagnosis further, electron microscopy has demonstrated the presence of microscopic lesions in a visually normal peritoneum (Barlow 1991, Shaw 1991). It is not known whether the variety of lesions represents different stages in progression or a different pathogenesis.

Since so many aspects of this condition are poorly understood, a wide variety of therapeutic regimens exists, including ablative surgery with surgical castration, expectant management, conservative surgical therapy, medical therapy, and superovulation therapies such as in vitro fertilization and gamete intrafallopian tube transfer (GIFT) when infertility is an issue.

DATABASE

SUBJECTIVE

→ Symptoms:
- although endometriosis is associated with the classic triad of increasing dysmenorrhea, pelvic pain, and dyspareunia, some women present with a wide spectrum of symptoms, while others have none.
  - The severity of symptoms does not correlate with the extent of the disease, but may correlate with the site. (See **Table 12F.1, Symptoms of Endometriosis in Relation to Site of Endometriotic Implants.**)

→ Risk factors include:

Table 12F.1. SYMPTOMS OF ENDOMETRIOSIS IN RELATION TO SITE OF ENDOMETRIOTIC IMPLANTS

Reproductive tract
Dysmenorrhea (50 percent)
Dyspareunia/pain (20 percent)
Infertility (25 percent)
Abnormal bleeding (up to 5 percent)

Gastrointestinal tract
Cyclical tenesmus/rectal bleeding
Diarrhea
Colonic obstruction

Urinary tract
Cyclical hematuria/pain
Ureteral obstruction

Lung
Cyclical hemoptysis

Source: Adapted with permission from Shaw, R.W. 1991. Endometriosis: The next ten years. *British Journal of Clinical Practice* 72(Suppl.):61.

- women of Japanese descent.
- menstrual history of early menarche, short cycles, long flow.
- history of infertility.
- history of outflow obstruction.
- family history, primarily in first-degree relatives.

→ Exercise is thought to have a *protective* effect.

→ A complete health history should be obtained with particular attention to current and historical description of symptomatology.

OBJECTIVE

→ A complete abdominal and pelvic examination should be performed. A rectal examination should be included to assess nodularity appropriately.

→ Physical examination may reveal:
- tender uterosacral nodularity.
- retroversion of the uterus.
- adnexal masses.
- diffuse focal tenderness (especially in the cul-de-sac or the posterior surface of the lower uterine segment or cervix).
- limited pelvic mobility.

→ Most often in the absence of nodularity or an adnexal mass, the pelvic examination is WNL. **NOTE:** The American Fertility Society (AFS) Classification of Endometriosis has been used as a descriptive tool to document the extent of disease after laparoscopic evaluation of the pelvis. (See **Figure 12F.1, The American Fertility Society Revised Classification of Endometriosis.**) Pain symptomatology and reproductive prognosis do not

Figure 12F.1.   THE AMERICAN FERTILITY SOCIETY REVISED CLASSIFICATION OF ENDOMETRIOSIS

Patient's Name _____ Date _____

Stage I   (Minimal)   —1-5

Stage II   (Mild)   —6-15   Laparoscopy _____ Laparotomy _____ Photography _____

Stage III (Moderate) —16-40   Recommended Treatment _____

Stage IV (Severe)   —> 40   _____

Total _____   Prognosis _____

	ENDOMETRIOSIS	< 1 cm	1-3 cm	> 3 cm
PERITONEUM	Superficial	1	2	4
	Deep	2	4	6
OVARY	R Superficial	1	2	4
	Deep	4	16	20
	L Superficial	1	2	4
	Deep	4	16	20
	POSTERIOR CUL-DE-SAC OBLITERATION	Partial		Complete
		4		40
	ADHESIONS	< 1/3 Enclosure	1/3-2/3 Enclosure	> 2/3 Enclosure
OVARY	R Filmy	1	2	4
	Dense	4	8	16
	L Filmy	1	2	4
	Dense	4	8	16
TUBE	R Filmy	1	2	4
	Dense	4*	8*	16
	L Filmy	1	2	4
	Dense	4*	8*	16

*If the fimbriated end of the fallopian tube is completely enclosed, change the point assignment to 16.

Additional Endometriosis: _____   Associated Pathology: _____

_____   _____

_____   _____

_____   _____

To Be Used with Normal Tubes and/or Ovaries

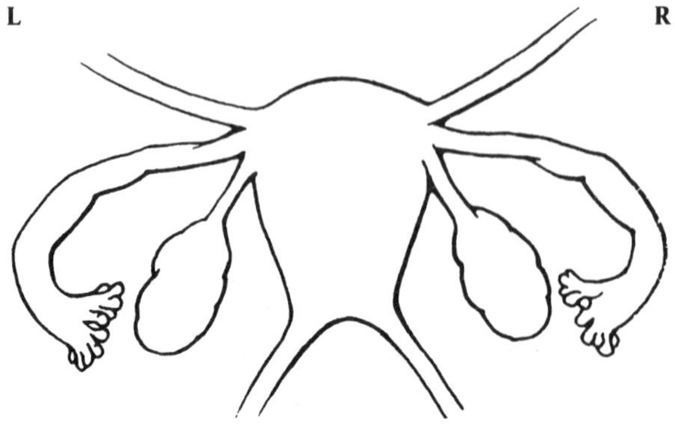

To be Used with Abnormal Tubes and/or Ovaries

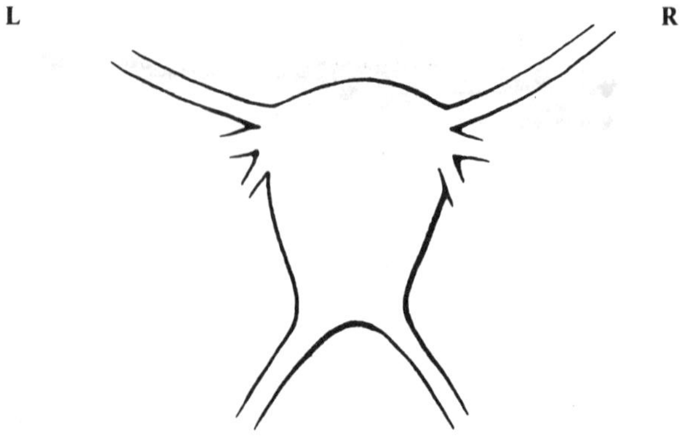

Source: Reprinted with permission from the American Fertility Society. 1985. *Revised classification of endometriosis*. Birmingham, AL: the Author.

Women's Primary Health Care: Protocols for Practice

EXAMPLES AND GUIDELINES

STAGE I (MINIMAL)

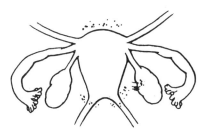

PERITONEUM
　Superficial Endo　–　1-3 cm　– 2
R. OVARY
　Superficial Endo　–　< 1 cm　– 1
　Filmy Adhesions　–　< 1/3　– 1
　　　TOTAL POINTS　　　4

STAGE II (MILD)

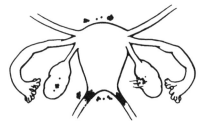

PERITONEUM
　Deep Endo　　　–　> 3 cm　– 6
R. OVARY
　Superficial Endo　–　< 1 cm　– 1
　Filmy Adhesions　–　< 1/3　– 1
L. OVARY
　Superficial Endo　–　< 1 cm　– 1
　　　TOTAL POINTS　　　9

STAGE III (MODERATE)

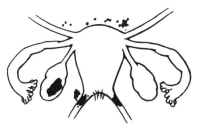

PERITONEUM
　Deep Endo　　　–　> 3 cm　– 6
CUL-DE-SAC
　Partial Obliteration　　　　– 4
L. OVARY
　Deep Endo　　　–　1-3 cm　– 16
　　　TOTAL POINTS　　　26

STAGE III (MODERATE)

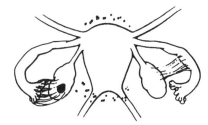

PERITONEUM
　Superficial Endo　–　> 3 cm　– 4
R. TUBE
　Filmy Adhesions　–　< 1/3　– 1
R. OVARY
　Filmy Adhesions　–　< 1/3　– 1
L. TUBE
　Dense Adhesions　–　< 1/3　– 16*
L. OVARY
　Deep Endo　　　–　< 1 cm　– 4
　Dense Adhesions　–　< 1/3　– 4
　　　TOTAL POINTS　　　30

STAGE IV (SEVERE)

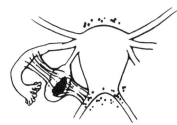

PERITONEUM
　Superficial Endo　–　> 3 cm　– 4
L. OVARY
　Deep Endo　　　–　1-3 cm　– 32**
　Dense Adhesions　–　< 1/3　– 8**
L. TUBE
　Dense Adhesions　–　< 1/3　– 8**
　　　TOTAL POINTS　　　52

　*Point asignment changed to 16
　**Point assignment doubled

STAGE IV (SEVERE)

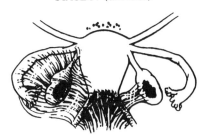

PERITONEUM
　Deep Endo　　　–　> 3 cm　– 6
CUL-DE-SAC
　Complete Obliteration　　　– 40
R. OVARY
　Deep Endo　　　–　1-3 cm　– 16
　Dense Adhesions　–　< 1/3　– 4
L. TUBE
　Dense Adhesions　–　> 2/3　– 16
L. OVARY
　Deep Endo　　　–　1-3 cm　– 16
　Dense Adhesions　–　> 2/3　– 16
　　　TOTAL POINTS　　　114

　Determination of the stage or degree of endometrial involvement is based on a weighted point system. Distribution of points has been arbitrarily determined and may require further revision or refinement as knowledge of the disease increases.

　To ensure complete evaluation, inspection of the pelvis in a clockwise or counterclockwise fashion is encouraged. Number, size, and location of endometrial implants, plaques, endometriomas, and/or adhesions are noted. For example, five separate 0.5 cm superficial implants on the peritoneum (2.5 cm total) would be assigned 2 points. (The surface of the uterus should be considered peritoneum.) The severity of the endometriosis or adhesions should be assigned the highest score only for peritoneum, ovary, tube, or cul-de-sac. For example, a 4 cm superficial and a 2 cm deep implant of the peritoneum should be given a score of 6 (not 8). A 4 cm deep endometrioma of the ovary associated with more than 3 cm of superficial disease should be scored 20 (not 24).

　In those patients with only one adnexa, points applied to disease of the remaining tube and ovary should be multiplied by two.** Points assigned may be circled and totaled. Aggregation of points indicates stage of disease (minimal, mild, moderate, or severe).

　The presence of endometriosis of the bowel, urinary tract, fallopian tube, vagina, cervix, skin, etc., should be documented under "additional endometriosis." Other pathology such as tubal occlusion, leiomyomata, uterine anomaly, etc., should be documented under "associated pathology." All pathology should be depicted as specifically as possible on the sketch of pelvic organs, and means of observation (laparoscopy or laparotomy) should be noted.

necessarily correlate with the amount or degree of visible endometriosis (Candiani et al. 1991).

ASSESSMENT

→ R/O endometriosis

→ R/O dysmenorrhea

→ R/O PID

→ R/O uterine fibroids

→ R/O ovarian cysts

→ R/O appendicitis

→ R/O inflammatory bowel disease or obstruction

→ R/O neoplasm

→ R/O urinary tract infection (UTI)

→ R/O ectopic pregnancy

→ R/O ruptured endometrioma (a rare occurrence that may lead to generalized peritonitis) (Lichtman and Smith 1990)

→ See **Abnormal Uterine Bleeding, Abdominal Pain, Pelvic Pain—Acute, Pelvic Pain—Chronic, Infertility, Sexual Dysfunction, Dysmenorrhea, Pelvic Masses,** and **Ectopic Pregnancy** protocols

PLAN

DIAGNOSTIC TESTS

→ Definitive diagnosis is made by direct visualization of the pelvis via laparoscopy.

→ Appropriate tests to rule out other conditions may include: pregnancy test, cultures for gonorrhea/ chlamydia, urine culture and sensitivity, pelvic ultrasound, and CBC. (See protocols listed previously.)

TREATMENT/MANAGEMENT

→ Treatment should be individualized and based on the following:
  ▪ the desire for pregnancy.
  ▪ age.
  ▪ duration of infertility.
  ▪ extent of the disease.
  ▪ associated pelvic pathology.
  ▪ the severity of symptoms.
  ▪ the wishes of the patient.

→ Expectant management.
  ▪ Expectant management is appropriate for women with mild or moderate endometriosis presenting with infertility.
  ▪ If used in conjunction with the correction of other infertility factors, expectant management

has been shown to produce pregnancy rates similar to those achieved with drug therapy or conservative surgery.

→ Conservative surgery.
  ▪ Various procedures can be done with laparoscopic cautery or laser surgery. Conservative surgery is indicated:
    • to confirm the diagnosis.
    • when an anatomical alteration (e.g., adhesions) is interfering with conception.
    • for chocolate cysts of the ovary.
    • when medical therapy fails to result in conception or the relief of symptoms.

→ Complete surgery.
  ▪ Total hysterectomy and bilateral salpingo-oophorectomy is an option when all other medical and surgical interventions have failed and the woman no longer wishes to maintain reproductive function.

→ Induction of pseudopregnancy.
  ▪ This treatment approach is used to eliminate cyclical changes and bleeding resulting in the reabsorption of endometrial implants.
  ▪ Low-dose combination oral contraceptives or progestational therapy is used for 6 to 9 months. Medications used:
    • any combination oral contraceptives with 30 μg-35 μg of ethinyl estradiol: 1 tablet p.o. every day; increase to 2 tablets if break-through bleeding occurs.
    • medroxyprogesterone acetate (MPA) (Provera®): 30 mg-100 mg p.o. every day.
    • gestrione (not currently available in United States): dosages range from 1.25 mg p.o. 2 times per week to 2.5 mg 3 times per week (Saltiel and Garabedian-Ruffalo 1991).
  ▪ Symptoms are improved in 60 percent to 94 percent of patients, pregnancy rates range from 43 percent to 55 percent, recurrence rates are about 5 percent to 10 percent annually (Saltiel and Garabedian-Ruffalo 1991).

→ Induction of pseudomenopause.
  ▪ Danazol (Danocrine®) once was considered the medical treatment of choice for endometriosis, but now GnRH agonists are becoming more popular (see following discussion).
    • Variable success rates for danazol have been achieved in the alleviation of symptoms, pregnancy rates, and recurrence rates.
    • Usual dose of danazol is 400 mg-800 mg p.o. per day (titrated until menses ceases) for 6 to 9 months.

- Side effects of danazol include hirsutism, weight gain, acne, and an adverse effect on lipoproteins.
- GnRH agonists result in a drastic reduction of gonadotropins from the pituitary and as a result, serum estradiol levels plunge to those of women who have undergone oophorectomy. Medications used:
  - nafarelin (Synarel®) (first drug in this class to be FDA-approved for endometriosis): usual dose is 1 spray (200 μg) intranasally BID.
  - leuprolide acetate (Lupron®): recommended dosage is a single 3.75 mg I.M. injection once a month (every 28-33 days), not to exceed 6 months.
  - side effects of these medications are consistent with hypoestrogenism, including hot flashes, dyspareunia, vaginal dryness, decreased libido, and adverse effects on bone metabolism.
    - Nasal stinging may occur with Synarel®.
    - Research is continuing on GnRH agonists with the concurrent use of a progestin to determine if bone loss can be decreased.

CONSULTATION

→ Physician consultation should be considered in all suspected cases and is required in cases where more conservative measures do not provide relief of symptoms (e.g., dysmenorrhea, dysparuenia, abnormal bleeding) or if conception cannot be achieved.

→ Consultation with psychological services may be required for women experiencing dyspareunia, infertility, or debilitating pain.

PATIENT EDUCATION

→ Discuss proposed etiological theories regarding endometriosis.

→ Provide patient education regarding risks/benefits of surgical and drug therapies and include patient in decision making. Drug regimens vary considerably in cost, and patients should be informed of the expense involved.

→ Advise patients that the natural history of endometriosis is unknown and that response to treatments may be unpredictable (Candiani et al. 1991).

→ Inform patients of alternative/supplemental forms of symptom management including the use of herbal teas, prostaglandin inhibitors, hot water

bottles, massage, Vitamin E supplements (see **Dysmenorrhea** Protocol).
- Advise patients to contact the National Endometriosis Association at 800-992-ENDO for additional information.

→ Encourage exercise, especially for clients receiving danazol therapy, since exercise has been shown to decrease side effects.

→ Since endometriosis tends to be a chronic condition, refer patient to an endometriosis support group for help.
- Advise patient to contact the National Endometriosis Association at telephone number provided previously.

→ See additional appropriate protocols for further patient education.

FOLLOW-UP

→ Since the condition tends to progress, women should be encouraged to obtain follow-up care. This will be tailored to the individual case.

→ For patients already diagnosed and undergoing management, evaluate the effectiveness of treatment regimens and monitor for side effects of drug therapy.

→ Monitor for occurrences in sites outside of pelvis.
- Symptoms often cyclical. See **Table 12F.1**.

→ Ongoing psychological support is an important component of care.

→ Document in progress notes and problem list.

Bibliography

American Fertility Society. 1985. *Revised classification of endometriosis.* Birmingham, AL: the Author.

Barlow, D.H. 1991. What is endometriosis in the 1990s? *British Journal of Clinical Practice* 72(Suppl.):1–7.

Candiani, G.B., Vercellini, P., Fedele, L., Colombo, A., and Candiani, M. 1991. Mild endometriosis and infertility: A critical review of epidemiologic data, diagnostic pitfalls, and classification limits. *Obstetrical and Gynecological Survey* 46(6):374–378.

Gerbie, A.B., and Merrill, J.A. 1988. Pathology of endometriosis. *Clinical Obstetrics and Gynecology* 31(4):779–786.

Heaps, J.M., Neiberg, R.K., and Berek, J.S. 1990. Malignant neoplasms arising in endometriosis. *Obstetrics and Gynecology* 75(6):1023–1028.

Lichtman, R., and Smith, S.M. 1990. Multiorgan disorders. In *Gynecology: Well-woman care*, eds. R.

Lichtman and S. Papera, p. 323. Norwalk, CT: Appleton & Lange.

Mahmood, T.A., and Templeton, A. 1990. Pathophysiology of mild endometriosis: Review of literature. *Human Reproduction* 5(7):765–784.

Metzger, D.A., and Haney, E.F. 1989. Etiology of endometriosis. *Obstetrics and Gynecology Clinics of North America* 16(1):1–14.

Saltiel, E., and Garabedian-Ruffalo, S.M. 1991. Pharmacologic management of endometriosis. *Clinical Pharmacy* 10(7):518–531.

Shaw, R.W. 1991. Endometriosis: The next ten years. *British Journal of Clinical Practice* 72(Suppl.):59–63.

12-G

Hirsutism

Hirsutism is defined as cosmetically or objectively excessive growth of bodily hair. It should not be confused with *hypertrichosis*, which implies any generalized increase in relatively fine (vellus) body hair, usually on the forehead, forearms, or lower legs (Hatch et al. 1981; Lobo 1991).

In women, the excessive amount of hair may appear where hair normally grows or where coarse body hair usually is absent—on the cheeks; above the upper lip; on the chin, chest, or intermammary region; on the inner thighs, or along the midline lower back entering the intergluteal area; or as a male escutcheon (ACOG 1987; Lobo 1991).

This excessive hair growth generally occurs in response to an abnormally increased level of circulating androgens. Other symptoms which may coexist include acne, oligomenorrhea, amenorrhea, and frank virilization. More pronounced androgenization may be manifested by virilization. Associated symptoms include temporal balding, deepening of the voice, increased muscle mass, enlargement of the clitoris, and loss of female secondary sex characteristics including decreased breast size and loss of female body contour (ACOG 1987; Lobo 1991).

Ethnicity, race, other genetic factors, and age greatly influence the characteristics and distribution of body hair. For instance, Asians, Native Americans, light-skinned whites, and some blacks have less hair; women of Mediterranean descent commonly have coarse hair on the upper lip, arms, and legs. Elderly women may have increased facial hair but diminished pubic/axillary hair (Lobo 1991; Nestler 1989). Cultural and societal attitudes affect individual perception regarding body hair. It is estimated that as many as 30 percent of white females may have symptoms of hirsutism (Breckwoldt, Zahradnik, and Wieacker 1989).

Two types of body hair occur: *vellus* hair (short, fine, nonpigmented hair) and *terminal* hair (long, coarse, pigmented hair). The latter is responsive to circulating reproductive hormones. Increased androgen levels associated with puberty cause the pilosebaceous units (PSU) on the axilla, pubis, back, face, chest, abdomen, and extremities to differentiate into an androgen-sensitive end-unit, either a terminal hair follicle or a sebaceous follicle (Ehrmann and Rosenfield 1990). Local conversion of testosterone to its 5-alpha reduced product, dihydrotestosterone (DHT), is necessary for normal growth of androgen-dependent hair (Leshin 1987).

A basic endocrinology review helps understand the pathophysiology of hirsutism. The androgens are secreted by both the ovary and adrenal gland in response to pituitary-derived trophic hormones LH and adrenocorticotropic hormone (ACTH). The main androgenic hormones are testosterone, DHEA, DHEA-S, and androstenedione.

Testosterone comes from three sources: ovary, adrenal, and peripheral conversion (in liver, skin, fat). In women, approximately 50 percent of testosterone comes from peripheral conversion of androstenedione, and 50 percent is secreted by the adrenal gland and ovary in equal amounts (Speroff, Glass, and Kase 1989, 1994). Biological activity of testosterone is mediated largely by its 5-alpha reduced product, DHT (Ehrmann and Rosenfield 1991). DHEA-S is derived largely from the adrenal gland, and 90 percent of DHEA is adrenal in origin (Speroff, Glass, and Kase 1989, 1994).

In the circulation, androgens are present in either the free or bound (conjugated) form. The bioavailability of androgens is determined by the degree of binding to sex hormone-binding globulin (SHBG)

(Breckwoldt, Zahradnik, and Wieacker 1989). Estrogens and hyperthyroidism increase SHBG; androgens, glucocorticoids, hyperinsulinemia, and obesity decrease SHBG concentration (Ehrmann and Rosenfield 1990; Lobo 1991). The etiology of hirsutism can be attributed to abnormalities that result from increased androgen production, altered peripheral androgen metabolism, and decreased androgen binding (ACOG 1987; Lobo 1991).

Increased Androgen Production

Excessive hair growth occurs in response to an increase in circulating androgens and may be associated with abnormal gonadal/sexual development, exogenous or iatrogenic factors, polycystic ovarian disease (PCO), stromal hyperthecosis, androgen-producing tumors of the ovaries or adrenals, Cushing's syndrome, or adult-onset congenital adrenal hyperplasia (CAH) (Ehrmann and Rosenfield 1990; Leshin 1987; Lobo 1991). Hirsutism caused by an adrenal enzyme defect (such as CAH) usually is more severe and begins typically at puberty (Speroff, Glass, and Kase 1994). Twenty-one-hydroxylase deficiency accounts for more than 90 percent of cases of CAH (Barnes 1991).

Rapidly progressing virilization suggests the presence of an androgen-producing tumor. Exogenous/iatrogenic causes may include medications such as anabolic steroids, synthetic progestins (e.g., 19-nortestosterone oral contraceptives), testosterone creams, danazol, deladumone, minoxidil, diazoxide, phenytoin, corticosteroids, penicillamine, and cyclosporine (ACOG 1987; Lobo 1991; Nestler 1989).

Altered Peripheral Androgen Metabolism

Altered peripheral androgen metabolism is thought to be the actual cause of what is termed *idiopathic hirsutism*, a condition which occurs in association with normal menstrual cycles and normal serum testosterone and DHEA-S levels (Lobo 1991). Idiopathic hirsutism (also known as *constitutional* or *familial hirsutism*) is due to altered androgen activity at the PSU due to increased 5-alpha reductase activity (ACOG 1987; Lobo 1991). Together with PCO, idiopathic hirsutism accounts for more than 90 percent of all instances of hirsutism. Certain ethnic groups, especially people of Mediterranean descent, are affected more often.

Decreased Androgen Binding

Decreased androgen binding is associated with relative estrogen deficiency and usually is seen during meno-

pause. Estrogen deficiency, with its resultant diminution of SHBG, may increase free testosterone and lead to increased hair growth (ACOG 1987).

HAIR-AN

A recently described syndrome associated with hirsutism is called HAIR-AN: hyperandrogenism, insulin resistance, and acanthosis nigricans (Nestler 1989). This syndrome is an inherited defect of insulin receptor action.

In-depth discussion of all the etiologies associated with hirsutism is beyond the scope of this protocol. The reader is directed to the "Bibliography" for additional information.

DATABASE

SUBJECTIVE

→ Patient may have:
  ▪ increased hair growth.
  ▪ progressive virilization (rapid progression of symptoms of androgen excess).
  ▪ menstrual irregularities:
    • oligomenorrhea or amenorrhea.
    • menorrhagia.
    • menometrorrhagia.
  ▪ pelvic pain, pressure.
  ▪ increased abdominal girth.
  ▪ weight gain, obesity.
  ▪ infertility.
  ▪ symptoms/signs associated with Cushing's syndrome (Lobo 1991):
    • centripetal obesity.
    • abdominal striae.
    • supraclavicular and dorsal neck fat pads.
    • muscle wasting.
    • weakness.
    • thin skin.
    • bruisability.
    • fine (vellus) hair on face, back, and extremities.
    • amenorrhea.
    • symptoms of diabetes.
    • hypertension.
    • psychosis.
  ▪ signs/symptoms of thyroid disease (see **Thyroid Disorders** Protocol).
→ History should include:
  ▪ ethnicity.
  ▪ age of onset and rate of progression of hirsutism.
  ▪ history of menstrual abnormalities.

- increased libido, clitoromegaly, and other signs of masculinization.
- environmental factors.
- drug use history.
- pregnancy symptoms.
- signs/symptoms associated with Cushing's syndrome (hypertension, truncal obesity, acne, facial plethora, ecchymosis, petechiae, striae, proximal muscle weakness, etc.).
- psychosocial impact of hirsutism, emotional response to hair growth, etc. (Leshin 1987; Speroff, Glass, and Kase 1994).

OBJECTIVE

→ Ideally, a complete physical examination is performed. Specific features may include:
- hypertension.
- short stature.
- excessive hair growth present on the face, chest, breasts, abdomen, lower back, arms, or legs.
- acne, oily skin.
- excessive vellus hair growth.
- frontal/temporal baldness, deepening of voice, increased muscle mass.
- features associated with Cushing's syndrome. (See "Subjective" section.)
- galactorrhea.
- palpable abdominal/pelvic masses.
- clitoromegaly (clitoral index 100 mm² or clitoral shaft diameter >1 cm). **NOTE:** The clitoral index is obtained by multiplying the vertical and horizontal dimensions of the clitoris; normal size is ≤35 mm² (Nestler 1989).
- findings associated with the HAIR-AN syndrome may include velvety, hyperpigmented, thickened verrucous skin changes around the neck, axilla, intertriginous areas, vulva and under the breasts.

→ A hirsutism scoring scale by Ferriman and Gallwey (1961) has been utilized to quantify the degree of hirsutism. See **Figure 12G.1, Hirsutism Scoring**. A total score of ≥8 signifies hirsutism; however, it is important to interpret the findings in relation to the ethnic background of the patient.

ASSESSMENT

→ Hirsutism

→ R/O nonspecific sources: exogenous/iatrogenic factors; abnormal/gonadal sexual development

→ R/O peripheral sources: idiopathic hirsutism

→ R/O ovarian causes: PCO, stromal hyperthecosis, ovarian tumors

→ R/O adrenal sources: adrenal tumors, Cushing's syndrome, adult-onset CAH (Lobo 1991)

→ R/O HAIR-AN syndrome

→ R/O hypertrichosis

→ Assess contribution of age, ethnic, racial, and genetic factors

→ Assess psychosocial factors

PLAN

DIAGNOSTIC TESTS

→ The 3 lab tests that follow are best obtained in the follicular phase of the menstrual cycle or just after a withdrawal bleed (Azziz 1992). **NOTE:** Confer with a physician regarding diagnostic tests. Check with the laboratory for regional normal values.
- Serum total testosterone: normal range = 20-80 ng/dl (Speroff, Glass, and Kase 1994). Values >200 ng/dl require further investigation for an androgen-producing tumor. Refer to a physician.
- Serum DHEA-S: upper limit of normal = 350 μg/dl in most labs. A value >700 μg/dl is a marker for abnormal adrenal function (Speroff, Glass, and Kase 1994). Refer to a physician.
- 17-hydroxyprogesterone (17-OHP): baseline level = <200 ng/dl. Levels from 200ng/dl-800 ng/dl require ACTH testing. Levels >800 ng/dl are diagnostic of 21-hydroxylase deficiency (CAH) (Speroff, Glass, and Kase 1994). Refer to a physician.

→ Patients presenting with rapid virilization, an abdominal/pelvic mass, and/or very high levels of testosterone or DHEA-S should be evaluated for an adrenal/ovarian tumor.
- Tests may include ultrasound, CT scan, MRI, and ovarian/adrenal vein catheterization.
- Refer to a physician.

→ Evaluation of suspected Cushing's syndrome may include an overnight dexamethasone suppression test: 1 mg of dexamethasone orally at bedtime with plasma cortisol measurement at 8:00 A.M. the following day; plasma cortisol <5 μg/dl rules out Cushing's; a level >5 μg/dl suggests need for further testing with 24-hour urinary-free cortisol and plasma ACTH measurements (Lobo 1991; Lobo and Kletzky 1991; Speroff, Glass, and Kase 1994).
- Refer to a physician.

Figure 12G.1. HIRSUTISM SCORING

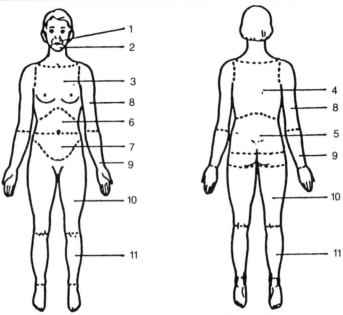

(Grade 0 at all sites indicates absence of terminal hair.)

Site	Grade	Definition
1. Upper Lip	1 2 3 4	A few hairs at outer margin. A small moustache at outer margin. A moustache extending halfway from outer margin. A moustache extending to mid-line.
2. Chin	1 2 3 & 4	A few scattered hairs. Scattered hairs with small concentrations. Complete cover, light and heavy.
3. Chest	1 2 3 4	Circumareolar hairs. With mid-line hair in addition. Fusion of these areas, with three-quarter cover. Complete cover.
4. Upper back	1 2 3 & 4	A few scattered hairs. Rather more, still scattered. Complete cover, light and heavy.
5. Lower back	1 2 3 4	A sacral tuft of hair. With some lateral extension. Three-quarter cover. Complete cover.
6. Upper abdomen	1 2 3 & 4	A few mid-line hairs. Rather more, still mid-line. Half and full cover.
7. Lower abdomen	1 2 3 4	A few mid-line hairs. A mid-line streak of hair. A mid-line band of hair. An inverted V-shaped growth.
8. Arm	1 2 3 & 4	Sparse growth affecting not more than a quarter of the limb surface. More than this; cover still incomplete. Complete cover, light and heavy.
9. Forearm	1, 2, 3, 4	Complete cover of dorsal surface; 2 grades of light and 2 of heavy growth.
10. Thigh	1, 2, 3, 4	As for arm.
11. Leg	1, 2, 3, 4	As for arm.

NOTE: Scores in each area are added. Total score of ≥ 8 indicates hirsutism.

Source: Reprinted with permission from Ferriman, D., and Gallwey, J.D. 1961. Clinical assessment of a body hair growth in women. *Journal of Clinical Endocrinology and Metabolism* 21:1440.

→ Evaluation of suspected CAH may include early-morning (8:00 A.M.) serum 17-OHP and an ACTH stimulation test.

- Consult with a physician.

- It has been suggested that high-risk ethnic groups be screened when the index of suspicion is high. This includes Ashkenazi Jews, Hispanics, and women of central European descent (Lobo 1991).

→ Additional lab tests/procedures will depend upon the clinical presentation and may include (but are not limited to): LH, FSH, prolactin, estradiol, thyroid function tests, endometrial biopsy, and a 3-hour oral glucose-tolerance test measuring insulin and glucose.

TREATMENT/MANAGEMENT

→ The wishes of the patient play an important part in treatment strategies. Reassurance may be all that is indicated. Discuss treatment approaches with a physician.

→ When possible, drugs which cause hirsutism should be discontinued.

→ Medical treatment of hirsutism is aimed at ovarian suppression, adrenal suppression, and/or peripheral inhibition of androgens (Falcone et al. 1993).

- Options include:
  - combined low-dose oral contraceptives—inhibit ovarian and adrenal androgen production and are the drug of choice for patients with nonneoplastic hyperandrogenic disorders.
    - Theoretically best are formulations with desogestrel, gestodene, and norgestimate. These are associated with greater increases in SHBG and decreases in free testosterone (Speroff, Glass, and Kase 1994).
    - Six months of treatment usually are necessary before results are obtained. Adjunctive treatment with electrolysis may be used after this time.
    - Oral contraceptive use may be continued for 1 to 2 years, at which time therapy may be stopped to reevaluate the patient (Falcone et al. 1993; Lobo 1991; Speroff, Glass, and Kase 1994).
  - oral or depo forms of medroxyprogesterone acetate (Provera® or Depo-Provera®)—may be used when oral contraceptives are contraindicated.

    - Doses are 20 mg-40 mg p.o. every day
        OR
      150 mg I.M. every 3 months (Lobo 1991; Speroff, Glass, and Kase 1994).
  - spironolactone (Aldactone®):
    - an aldosterone antagonist and antiandrogen, inhibits testosterone synthesis, increases testosterone conversion to estradiol, and inhibits a 5-alpha reductase activity.
    - it may be tried when an oral contraceptive is unacceptable or ineffective.
    - the dose is 200 mg/day p.o. After some time, dose may be lowered to a maintenance dose of 25 mg-50 mg/day p.o.; maximal effect is demonstrated only after 6 months (Speroff, Glass, and Kase 1994). See *PDR* for side effects.
    - ideally, spironolactone should be used in combination with an oral contraceptive, which provides for a better clinical effect as well as a means of adequate contraception (Falcone et al. 1993; Lobo 1991; Speroff, Glass, and Kase 1994).
  - flutamide (Eulexin®), an antiandrogen, blocks androgen receptors.
    - The dose is 250 mg p.o. BID-TID.
    - Ideally, it should be used in combination with an oral contraceptive (Falcone et al. 1993). **NOTE:** Antiandrogens may cause feminization of a male fetus. Adequate contraception—ideally with oral contraceptives—should be employed.
  - cyproterone acetate (may not be currently available in United States):
    - potent progestational agent, inhibits gonadotropin secretion and blocks androgen action by binding to androgen receptor (Speroff, Glass, and Kase 1994). Consult with physician.
    - dose is 100 mg p.o. daily on days 5-14, combined with 30 μg-50 μg of ethinyl estradiol on days 5-25 (this regimen is termed the "reversed sequential regimen") (Speroff, Glass, and Kase 1994). Improvement is seen by third month of treatment.
    - cyproterone is available in many parts of the world as an oral contraceptive "Diane" (2 mg cyproterone acetate and 50 μg ethinyl estradiol) *or* "Dianette" (2 mg cyproterone acetate and 35 μg ethinyl estradiol) (Speroff, Glass, and Kase 1994).

–side effects of treatment include fatigue, edema, loss of libido, weight gain, mastalgia (Speroff, Glass, and Kase 1994).

• GnRH agonists—markedly suppress gonadotropin secretion, ovarian androgen and estrogen (Azziz 1992):

–leuprolide acetate (Lupron®) 0.5 mg-1.0 mg/ day S.C. injection

OR

3.75 mg-7.5 mg monthly I.M. injection.

–goserelin acetate (Zoladex®) 3.6 mg implant.

–nafarelin (Synerel®) intranasal spray 400 mc/g-800 mc/g per dose BID.

–GnRH agonists and oral contraceptives used in combination prevent hypoestrogenic side effects (e.g., osteoporosis) (Azziz 1992; Lobo 1991).

–monitoring testosterone levels is advised (Speroff, Glass, and Kase 1994).

–relatively complicated expensive treatment; reserved for severe cases of ovarian hyperandrogenism (Speroff, Glass, and Kase 1994).

• ketoconazole (Nizoral®) blocks adrenal/ ovarian steroidogenesis by inhibiting cytochrome P_{450}-dependent enzyme pathways and decreases testosterone, androstenedione, and DHEA-S. The dose is 400 mg-1000 mg/ day (Falcone et al. 1993; Lobo 1991).

NOTE: Last resort. Hepatotoxic. See *PDR*. Requires frequent monitoring of liver function.

• corticosteroids are reserved for patients with marked adrenal hyperandrogenism (e.g., CAH) to suppress adrenal androgen production:

–dexamethasone (Decadron®) 0.25 mg-0.5 mg p.o. at bedtime (Falcone et al. 1993; Speroff, Glass, and Kase 1994).

–prednisone 2.5 mg-7.5 mg p.o. every day or every other day (Lobo 1991; Speroff, Glass, and Kase 1994).

▪ Other agents tried: cimetidine 300 mg QID (disappointing clinical response); progesterone skin cream (frequent application required, concentrated action at point of application) (Speroff, Glass, and Kase 1994).

→ Patients with suspected Cushing's syndrome, CAH, stromal hyperthecosis, androgen-producing tumors of the ovaries or adrenals, or HAIR-AN syndrome should be managed by a physician.

→ Physical methods for hirsutism management include:

▪ bleaching: commercial products are available.

▪ shaving: one of oldest methods of hair depilation.

• Will not increase rate/coarseness of subsequent hair growth.

▪ plucking (tweezing):

• may cause postepilation pustule or scar.

▪ waxing: certain hair length necessary.

• Use with caution to prevent thermal burns.

• May be done professionally.

▪ chemical depilatory agents: mild topical corticosteroid or skin moisturizer may be applied after use to prevent irritant contact dermatitis. (See **Table 12TB1, Potency Ranking of Topical Corticosteroids**, p. 12-228.)

▪ hair-removing gloves of fine sandpaper or pumice stone.

▪ electrolysis/thermolysis or a combination: professional method of permanent hair removal.

• At least 6 months of systemic therapy for underlying causes of hirsutism must be used prior to treatment with electrolysis.

• Keloids and postinflammatory hypopigmentation/hyperpigmentation may occur after treatment (Wagner 1990).

NOTE: These methods, except for electrolysis/ thermolysis, are temporary measures.

→ If oligomenorrhea, amenorrhea, or dysfunctional bleeding is a problem, cyclic progestins or oral contraceptives may be used. (See **Amenorrhea— Secondary** and **Abnormal Uterine Bleeding** protocols.)

→ If infertility is an issue, ovulation induction may be indicated. (Refer to **Infertility** Protocol.)

→ Nutritional aspects of obesity should be addressed. Refer to nutritionist as indicated.

▪ Patient may be referred to a weight loss program.

▪ Encourage a regular exercise program. (See **General Nutrition Guidelines**.)

CONSULTATION

→ Consultation with a physician is recommended in all cases of hirsutism.

→ Scope of practice regarding evaluation/ management of hirsute women will vary depending on policies of the setting.

→ Evaluation and management of patients with suspected Cushing's syndrome, CAH, stromal hyperthecosis, androgen-producing tumors of the ovaries or adrenals, or HAIR-AN syndrome should be undertaken by a physician, ideally an endocrinologist or reproductive endocrinologist.

PATIENT EDUCATION

→ Discussion should include the etiologies of hirsutism, usual treatment/management modalities, physical methods of depilation, and permanent methods of hair removal.

→ When patient is on a systemic drug, review side effects. Consult *PDR*.
- With antiandrogens (e.g., spironolactone, flutamide), alert patient to the possibility of feminization of a male fetus if pregnancy should occur.
  • Adequate contraception is therefore advisable.

→ Be sure the patient understands that diminution of the hirsute condition may not occur until after six months of drug therapy because of the physiology of hair growth.
- Temporary methods of depilation may be used during this time, but electrolysis should not be used until after six months of hormonal suppression.
- The best response to treatment occurs in a woman who has had a short duration of hirsutism.

→ The usual response to treatment is initial reduction of new hair followed by thinning/ softening of existing terminal hair and less frequent need for depilation (Leshin 1987).

→ Psychosocial implications of hirsutism may be a factor for some women. Ensure patient has some form of social support and utilize appropriate referral sources as indicated.

FOLLOW-UP

→ Patients should be encouraged to continue treatment for one to two years.
- Clinical response and patient desires will dictate when therapy should be discontinued.
- It is reasonable to stop therapy after one to two years to reevaluate the patient's condition. In some cases, hirsutism will not recur and in others therapy will need to be reinstituted.

→ Follow-up appointments will depend upon medical management.
- The patient may be seen at three- to six-month intervals or more often as indicated.

→ Serial photographs of the hirsute patient's response to therapy may be helpful to both the clinician and patient.

→ Failure of drug therapy in suppressing hair growth after six to 12 months should arouse suspicion of adrenal disease or an ovarian tumor (Speroff, Glass, and Kase 1989).

→ Ongoing psychological support of the hirsute woman is important.

→ Document in progress notes and problem list.

Bibliography

American College of Obstetricians and Gynecologists. 1987. *Evaluation and treatment of hirsute women.* Technical Bulletin. Washington, DC: the Author.

Azziz, R. 1992. Treating hirsutism with GnRH agonists. *Contemporary Ob/Gyn* 37(6):33–48.

Barnes, R.B. 1991. Adrenal dysfunction and hirsutism. *Clinical Obstetrics and Gynecology* 34(4):827–834.

Breckwoldt, M., Zahradnik, H.P., and Wieacker, P. 1989. Hirsutism: Its pathogenesis. *Human Reproduction* 4(6):601–604.

Ehrmann, D.A., and Rosenfield, R.L. 1990. An endocrinologic approach to the patient with hirsutism. *Journal of Clinical Endocrinology and Metabolism* 71(1):1–4.

Erkkola, R., and Ruutiainen, K. 1990. Hirsutism: Definitions and etiology. *Annals of Medicine* 22:99–103.

Falcone, T., Bourque, J., Granger, L., Hemmings, R., and Miron, P. 1993. Polycystic ovarian syndrome. *Current Problems in Obstetrics, Gynecology and Fertility* 16(2):65–95.

Ferriman, D., and Gallwey, T.J. 1961. Clinical assessment of a body hair growth in women. *Journal of Clinical Endocrinology and Metabolism* 21:1440.

Hatch, R., Rosenfield, R.L., Kim, M.H., and Tredway, D. 1981. Hirsutism: Implications, etiology, and management. *American Journal of Obstetrics and Gynecology* 140(7):815–830.

Kessel, B., and Liu, J. 1991. Clinical and laboratory evaluation of hirsutism. *Clinical Obstetrics and Gynecology* 34(4):805–816.

Leshin, M. 1987. Southwestern internal medicine conference: Hirsutism. *American Journal of the Medical Sciences* 294(5):369–383.

Lobo, R.A. 1991. Androgen excess. In *Infertility, contraception, and reproductive endocrinology*, 3rd ed., eds. D.R. Mishell, V. Davajan, and R.A. Lobo, pp. 422–446. Boston: Blackwell Scientific Publications.

Lobo, R.A., and Kletzky, O.A. 1991. Dynamics of hormone testing. In *Infertility, contraception, and reproductive endocrinology*, 3rd ed., eds. D.R. Mishell, V. Davajan, and R.A. Lobo, pp. 518–534. Boston: Blackwell Scientific Publications.

Nestler, J.E. 1989, August. Evaluation and treatment of the hirsute woman. *Virginia Medical*: 310–315.

Speroff, L., Glass, R.H., and Kase, N. G. 1989. *Clinical gynecologic endocrinology and infertility*, 4th ed. Baltimore: Williams & Wilkins.

Speroff, L., Glass, R.H., and Kase, N.G. 1994. *Clinical gynecologic endocrinology and infertility*, 5th ed., pp. 483-513. Baltimore: Williams & Wilkins.

Wagner, R.F. 1990. Physical methods for the management of hirsutism. *Cutis* 25:319–326.

12-H

Infertility

Infertility is defined as the inability or diminished ability to produce offspring (Bernstein and Mattox 1982). Statistically, approximately 25 percent of women under the age of 35 years conceive in the first cycle of unprotected intercourse, 60 percent within six months, 80 percent in nine months, and 85 percent within one year.

Infertility is a shared concern for a couple. The problems of infertility are distributed equally between the male and female. Approximately 35 percent of problems are with the male partner, and 35 percent are with the female partner. Twenty-five percent of infertility problems are due to combined male/female factors, and approximately 3.5 percent are of undetermined etiology. Limiting the evaluation to one member of a couple would be incomplete and may result in a delay of diagnosis and treatment.

Generally, the diagnosis of infertility is not made unless the couple has been sexually active for one year without the use of contraception. Exceptions to this one-year period should include advanced maternal age (35 years or older), irregular or absent menses, previously diagnosed infertility problems, history of genital infections, DES exposure in utero (for either the male or female), or abnormal development of sexual organs.

The goal of the primary provider is to provide the couple with an accurate diagnosis, information, and treatment resulting in a positive outcome for the couple—ideally, a pregnancy, or, at least, a decision to pursue alternative avenues or to accept no further treatment.

Infertility represents a very real loss to the couple. Loss of self-esteem, of feminine and masculine identities, of mutual marital goals unfulfilled, and, especially, of the unconceived child, are keenly felt by the couple, particularly with the onset of menses. The media, fertile friends, and overbearing family members add to the feelings of loss and frustration. The infertility evaluation can be very trying for the couple due to the cost, loss of privacy, and invasiveness of testing. The primary provider should recognize that infertility represents a life crisis for couples, and be aware of the intensity and variety of emotional responses that couples may manifest. Counseling may be indicated.

Upon completion of the infertility evaluation, the couple will fall into one or more of the following categories:
- male-factor infertility.
- pelvic-factor infertility.
- endocrine-factor infertility.
- immunological infertility.
- unexplained infertility.
- age-related infertility.

The primary provider should then focus treatment of the couple to minimize or remedy the infertility factor(s).

Male-factor Infertility

The male partner is recognized as a contributor to infertility in approximately 30 percent to 40 percent of infertile couples (Berkowitz 1986). To be classified as fertile, a man should be able to produce sperm capable of fertilizing a human oocyte (Grunfeld 1989). Although therapy for treatment of male-factor infertility is limited, early evaluation of the male is important.

Findings of complete male infertility are made with at least two abnormal semen analyses (see **Table 12H.1, Normal Semen Analysis**). Findings may include but are not limited to:

Table 12H.1. NORMAL SEMEN ANALYSIS

Volume	—	2 ml-6 ml
Viscosity	—	liquefaction in 1 hour
Count	—	20 million/ml or more
Morphology	—	at least 60 percent normal morphology and viability
Motility	—	at least 50 percent with forward progression
pH	—	7-8

Source: Reprinted with permission from Speroff, L., Glass, R.H., and Kase, N. 1989. *Clinical gynecologic endocrinology and infertility.* Baltimore: Williams & Wilkins, p. 568.

Anatomic defects of the penis, testicles, or excretory ducts (e.g., varicocele)

Varicoceles result from dilation of the spermatic vein, and can cause oligospermia in a variety of ways, including elevation of scrotal temperatures, reflux of adrenal hormones into the spermatic vein, and stagnation of blood (Marsman 1987).

Antisperm antibodies

Autoimmunity to sperm can result in decreased fertility. Assays such as the immunobead test and mixed agglutination reaction look for sperm-bound antibodies. Evaluation of female serum or cervical mucus for antibodies using immunobead techniques also is necessary.

Sperm penetration disorders

For several years, a mixed gamete penetration assay has been utilized by Overstreet (Overstreet et al. 1980). This test is performed to evaluate the spermatozoa's ability to penetrate the zona pellucida of the human egg. The most commonly used test for predicting the fertilizing capacity of the human sperm is the sperm penetration assay (SPA). The test is performed by coincubation of prepared human sperm with fresh human eggs retrieved from hysterectomy specimens or with denuded hamster eggs. Further investigation is needed to show that the test is an absolute predictor of infertility (Grunfeld 1989).

Infections of the genital tract

Infection can play a role in infertility. Epididymal or prostatic infections with *Neisseria gonorrhoeae, Chlamydia trachomatis,* or gram-negative organisms can cause ductal obstruction or orchitis (Grunfeld 1989).

Treatment of other organisms such as mycoplasma and ureaplasma involves more controversy. Rehewy et al. (1978) did not find improvement in the pregnancy rate with eradication of the organism, while Toth et al. (1983) found a substantially higher pregnancy rate in the organism-free groups. The value of treating mycoplasma still needs to be determined.

Low semen volume

Low semen volume may be due to retrograde ejaculation, ductal obstruction, or male accessory glands.

Abnormal liquification

Semen liquification usually occurs 20 to 30 minutes after ejaculation. Semen that does not undergo normal liquification and is associated with a poor postcoital test, may be a factor in infertility.

Low sperm count (concentration)

Low sperm count may be due to illness or temperature variations.

Decreased motility

Decreased sperm motility may be related to trauma, infection, or exposure.

Decreased normal morphology

Decreased normal morphology may be a consequence of toxic exposure or neoplasm.

Intrauterine insemination is the treatment of choice for many of the diagnoses associated with male-factor infertility (see **Appendix 12H.1, Indications for Intrauterine Insemination**, p. 12-72).

Pelvic-factor Infertility

Pelvic-factor infertility includes Asherman's syndrome, cervical factor, endometriosis, and tubal disease or obstruction.

Asherman's syndrome

With this disorder, ovulation may occur normally but there is no lush endometrial lining on which the embryo can implant. This syndrome results from scarring and damage secondary to a traumatic D and C (Toaff and Ballas 1978). Patients may present with amenorrhea, because there is no uterine lining to shed. However, regular bleeding has been documented in women presenting with Asherman's syndrome (Reid et al. 1992). Diagnosis is confirmed by either hysterosalpingogram (HSG) or hysteroscopy.

Cervical factor

Approximately 10 percent to 15 percent of women with infertility problems will have poor sperm transport mechanism as the etiology. The causes may include, but are not limited to, cervical stenosis, poor quality or quantity of cervical mucus, and varicosities of the endocervical canal. As seen through the colposcope, the endocervical canal will have a poorly developed columnar epithelium with prominent superficial varicosities, which may respond to cryosurgery or laser cautery. Postcoital testing is done to assess for cervical factor infertility.

Endometriosis

Endometriosis is the presence of endometrial tissue on the peritoneal cavity, fallopian tubes, ovaries, bladder, and bowel. It is theorized that there is a reflux of endometrial tissue during menses, enabling the tissue to "implant" on to the pelvic organs. These implantations are called endometriomas, and may continue to "leak" endometrial tissue to the surrounding pelvic organs.

In the general population, there is a seven percent to eight percent incidence of endometriosis, while in the infertile population the incidence may be as high as 10 percent to 50 percent. Symptoms may include dysmenorrhea, dyspareunia, and chronic pelvic pain. The diagnosis of endometriosis can be made only after direct visualization by laparoscopy or during pelvic surgery. The condition is then classified depending on the extent of the disease, utilizing the system set forth by the American Fertility Society which stages the disease from Stage I to Stage IV based on a numerical scoring system (see **Figure 12F.1**, pp. 12-46 and 12-47). Classification of the disease is necessary to determine the best treatment modality.

The underlying mechanism causing infertility in women with increased amounts of endometriosis is scarring and adhesion formation following the inflammatory process of the disease. These adhesions can interfere with tubal-ovarian interaction, preventing fertilization. However, in patients with minimal endometriosis, the causative factor is not as clear. Theories include altered smooth muscle contractility of the fallopian tube secondary to increased prostaglandin production by the disease, uterine irritability, or altered ovarian steroidogeneses also due to increased prostaglandin production (Older 1983). (See **Endometriosis** Protocol.)

Tubal disease/Obstruction

Tubal disease and/or obstruction can be the result of adhesion formation from previous pelvic surgery, trauma (e.g., from an IUD), or disease such as PID or endometriosis. Tubal patency also may be damaged due to a previous ectopic pregnancy, or surgically altered as in the case of an elective tubal ligation for sterilization.

Adhesion formation secondary to PID is usually the result of a previous infection or multiple infections, with *N. gonorrhoeae* and *C. trachomatis* being the causative agents. An inflammatory response follows sexual transmission of the agent, and patients with fulminant PID will often present with high fever, severe pelvic pain, and mucopurulent vaginal discharge. These patients are treated with antibiotics, though damage to the fallopian

tubes may have already occurred by the time the patient receives treatment.

Patients may also contract an STD with ensuing PID and damage to the fallopian tubes without experiencing any symptoms. Therefore, it is important to do chlamydia and gonorrhea cultures at the first visit. Pelvic inflammatory disease may also result from a septic abortion or IUD use. Patients with a history of Dalkon Shield use should be evaluated early in the infertility work-up for tubal integrity. (See also **Pelvic Inflammatory Disease** and **Sexually Transmitted Diseases** protocols.)

Endocrine Infertility

Primary amenorrhea

Women presenting with primary amenorrhea (no spontaneous uterine bleeding by age 17 years) must be evaluated for chromosomal abnormalities, congenital absence of the uterus, or androgen-insensitivity syndrome. Management of primary amenorrhea is beyond the scope of this protocol.

Hypothalamic factors

Hypothalamic dysfunction/failure may result from stress, excessive exercise (e.g., long-distance running or ballet) and/or severe weight loss resulting from eating disorders (anorexia/bulimia). All these conditions have an effect on estrogen production and the pulsatility of GnRH (Thatcher 1989). Ovulatory cycles generally resume when stress is reduced and there is a return to normal weight and exercise patterns, though this may be delayed for up to a year.

A vast number of milder, even subclinical forms of hypothalamic dysfunction may also result in anovulation. The ovulatory disorder may be treated relatively easily, while the underlying etiology of the disturbance may be more difficult to treat.

Pituitary factors

Increased circulating prolactin (PRL) is recognized as a common cause of amenorrhea, anovulation, and other defects of the hypothalamic-pituitary-ovarian (HPO) axis. Women with hyperprolactinemia may present with galactorrhea, polymenorrhea, oligomenorrhea, amenorrhea, decreased libido, and infertility. Hyperprolactinemia may be due to hypothyroidism, or secondary to medications such as antihistamines, tranquilizers, antidepressants, antihypertensives, antiemetics, or oral contraceptives.

The most common cause of hyperprolactinemia is a prolactin-secreting adenoma (prolactinoma). Hyperprolactinemia also has been found in association with luteal-phase deficiency due to defective folliculogenesis and inhibition of progesterone secretion caused by higher concentrations of PRL (100 ng/ml) (Jones 1989). Chronic anovulation may be due to hyperprolactinemia in 38 percent of women (Jones 1989). It appears that increased PRL secretion inhibits hypothalamic GnRH release, resulting in decreased circulating LH and FSH.

Sheehan's syndrome is pituitary failure resulting from a disturbance to the pituitary circulation immediately following childbirth. In this rare condition, the pituitary shuts down LH and FSH production; consequently the follicles do not develop.

Thyroid factors

Disorders affecting thyroid function are common in women of reproductive age. Menorrhagia, anovulation, oligomenorrhea, and amenorrhea may be associated with hypofunction and hyperfunction of the thyroid. (See **Thyroid Disorders** Protocol). Hypothyroidism has been found to be a causative factor in infertility due to hyperprolactinemia. There are myriad clinical presentations of abnormal thyroid function; therefore, a high level of suspicion is advisable.

Adrenal factors

Dysfunction of the adrenal glands or ovaries can result in increased androgen levels, which in turn result in abnormal estrogen levels that interfere with FSH and LH feedback systems (as in PCO). The three principal androgens in women are testosterone, androstenedione, and DHEA. Hyperandrogenism describes an elevation of the circulating level of testosterone, DHEA-S, and/or androstenedione.

The pathophysiological consequences of hyperandrogenism in women may include virilization, hirsutism, acne, diminished breast size, dysfunctional uterine bleeding, and anovulation (Marut 1989). (See **Hirsutism** Protocol). Androgen-secreting tumors of the ovary or adrenals are rare but should always be ruled out when androgen levels are high (DHEA-S ≥ 9 ng/ml).

Androgen secretion (either of adrenal or ovarian origin) serves as a precursor of the extraglandular production of estrogen. This conversion occurs in adipose tissue and the brain. Obesity, with its inherent increase in adipose tissue, is frequently associated with hyperandrogenism (Marut 1989). A consequence of chronically elevated, acyclic estrogen levels will include an exaggerated pulsatile LH level. The failure of elevation of FSH levels in association with the rise in LH can result in an alteration of the sensitive feedback system necessary for ovulation (as in PCO). The association of hyperprolactinemia with hyperandrogenism may also result from the chronically elevated estrogen levels.

Polycystic ovary syndrome

PCO is the most common cause of ovarian dysfunction. An excess of ovarian androgen production results in chronic anovulation. Decreased FSH stimulation results in impaired follicle development, and the increased androgen production causes elevated LH, which interferes with GnRH. Often patients with PCO have ovaries that are encapsulated in a tough, fibrous covering, hindering the release of a mature ovum from the follicle. The end result is an ovary that contains multiple cysts in various stages of development and difficulty for any one follicle in achieving dominance (Marut 1989). Patients with PCO often present with amenorrhea, obesity, hirsutism and acne. Lab data reveal an elevated LH to FSH ratio (at least 2:1), and increased testosterone (more than 70 ng/dl) and DHEA-S levels.

Premature ovarian failure

In this condition, oocytes are "used up" prior to the age of 40 years. Patients with this condition will present with amenorrhea and, possibly, menopausal symptoms. Clinically, early follicular FSH and LH levels are greater than 50 mIU/ml on more than one occasion. Irradiation for Hodgkin's disease may cause this condition, though the cause is usually unclear.

Luteinized unruptured follicle (LUF)

In patients with this syndrome, ovulation may appear to have occurred according to hormonal laboratory data, but the ovum is not released from the follicular cavity. This may be caused by inadequate follicular development, premature LH surge, or progesterone release, and is difficult to diagnose consistently. Diagnosis is by visualization of the ovary using ultrasound or laparoscopy. The syndrome may occur normally in all women intermittently.

Immunological Infertility

Controversy exists about the relationship between positive sperm antibodies and infertility. Serum IgG, IgM, and IgA have been evaluated by modifications of the direct and indirect Coombs assay, and some correlation with infertility has been established. Also, immunoglobulins have been detected on the surface of sperm with use of an immunobead test. (See "Antisperm antibodies" subsection under "Male-factor infertility.") Antibodies against the sperm surface become harmful due to phagocytosis and complement-mediated cytotoxicity (Serafini and Batzofin 1989). Postcoital testing in immunologically affected couples usually reveals no cervical spermatazoa in a woman whose partner is known to have sperm, in contrast to what was previously thought to be absence of sperm motility.

Unexplained Infertility

Ten percent to fifteen percent of infertile couples who have a thorough evaluation will be "diagnosed" with unexplained or idiopathic infertility. Infertility evaluation and treatment is not an exact science, and it is possible that the cause of couples' infertility is still unknown.

Age-related Infertility

A measurable decline in fertility is associated with aging in the female (i.e., 35 years of age and older). This is especially significant when considering assisted reproductive technology procedures. In over 3,000 in vitro fertilization (IVF) cycles performed in 1991 in the United States, no woman beyond age 42 years conceived and delivered an infant using IVF (personal communication, S. Feigenbaum 1993). Women over age 39 years experience more luteal-phase abnormalities, and the rate of miscarriage is 50 percent or higher in women 44 years and older.

Other Factors

Repeated pregnancy loss

Two categories of patients who have experienced repeated pregnancy loss include those with:
- three or more *consecutive* pregnancy losses at any gestational age, and
- an unexplained second trimester loss and any number of subsequent pregnancy losses at any gestational age.

The risk of another miscarriage after three consecutive losses is 30 percent to 45 percent (Speroff, Glass, and Kase 1994).

Luteal-phase deficiencies

The luteal-phase defect or inadequate luteal phase is believed to be caused by insufficient FSH and/or LH release and stimulation causing suboptimal corpus luteum development. This results in inadequate progesterone production. Consequently, the endometrial lining develops inadequately and implantation of the fertilized ovum is unsuccessful. This defect also may be caused by a lack of cellular receptors for progesterone in the endometrium (Serafini and Batzofin 1989).

A short luteal phase is when the time interval between the LH peak and the onset of menses is less than 10 days due to insufficient duration of progesterone pro-

duction. The short luteal phase is confirmed by BBT readings during at least two to three cycles.

The inadequate luteal phase is a histological diagnosis whereby the endometrial biopsy shows a lag of two or more days in two different menstrual cycles (Witten and Martin 1985). Normally fertile women may, on occasion, have an out-of-phase endometrial biopsy. Daily luteal-phase progesterone levels in women with luteal-phase defect are generally lower than in normal women, though the difference may be minimal.

DATABASE

SUBJECTIVE

→ A review of health history should include:
- age of both members of the couple.
- approximate date couple stopped using contraception.
- history and outcome of any previous pregnancies involving both partners:
  - couples with a history of three or more spontaneous pregnancy losses should be referred for further evaluation, including genetic karyotyping.
- length and regularity of menstrual cycle, magnitude of flow, age at menarche.
- symptoms, treatment of dysmenorrhea or dyspareunia.
- history, treatment of abnormal bleeding.
- symptoms of ovulation—e.g., breast tenderness, acne, mittelschmerz, mood changes, spotting, changes in libido, increased mid-cycle vaginal discharge.
- frequency of coitus, use of lubricants, perception of couple with respect to whether or not ejaculation is completed in vagina.
- religious practices that may relate to intercourse or fertility.
- duration of amenorrhea, if any:
  - presence of physical or emotional stress, weight fluctuation or medication taken prior to cessation of menses.
- presence or history of galactorrhea.
- history of STD, PID; treatment and/or sequellae.
- previous pelvic or other surgery; complications if any.
- review of any previous infertility evaluation and treatment.
- pertinent medical history suggestive of endocrine disorder.
- history of serious medical illnesses.
- DES exposure.

- history of IUD use; sequellae, if any.
- history of oral contraceptive use.
- social history:
  - use of alcohol, prescription, OTC drugs (e.g., laxatives or antihistamines), recreational drugs; smoking history.
- eating habits:
  - any habits suggestive of eating disorders.
- exercise history/habits.
- family history with attention to endocrine, genetic, or reproductive abnormalities.
- history of exposure to radiation or toxic chemicals.
- use of saunas or hot tubs.

→ Investigation of a woman with repeated pregnancy loss should include:
- review of systems with attention to systemic diseases including diabetes, collagen vascular disorders, thyroid dysfunction, history of thromboembolic events (e.g., stroke, deep vein thrombosis [DVT], pulmonary emboli).
- description of work environment with attention to possible toxic exposures.
- prior surgical history, including whether previous losses were associated with curettage.
- prior obstetrical history with attention to possible curettage for retained products.
- family history of inborn errors of metabolism (e.g., Tay Sachs disease, chromosomal anomalies, stillborns, early infant deaths, pregnancy loss).
- medication history.
- DES exposure.
- social history including smoking, alcohol consumption, use of illicit drugs.

OBJECTIVE

→ A comprehensive physical examination should be conducted, with special attention to:
- vital signs.
- height, weight:
  - assess desirable body weight (see **General Nutrition Guidelines**).
- signs of hyperandrogenism: acne, oily skin, hirsutism, etc.
- thyroid examination:
  - assess for masses.
  - note if patient has any signs of hypothyroidism or hyperthyroidism (see **Thyroid Disorders Protocol**).
- abdominal examination:
  - assess for scars, masses, tenderness.

- breast examination:
  - assess for galactorrhea.
- pelvic, rectal examination—assess for:
  - normal hair distribution.
  - signs of clitoromegaly.
  - signs of vaginal/cervical infection.
  - cervical mucus relative to time of menstrual cycle.
  - uterine or adnexal abnormalities.
  - nodularity of the uterosacral ligaments or cul-de-sac.
  - rectal masses.
- see **Hirsutism** Protocol.

ASSESSMENT

→ Infertility: primary or secondary
→ R/O male-factor infertility
→ R/O pelvic-factor infertility
→ R/O endocrine infertility
→ R/O immunological infertility
→ R/O unexplained infertility
→ R/O age-related infertility
→ R/O repeated pregnancy loss
→ R/O luteal-phase infertility

PLAN

DIAGNOSTIC TESTS

→ Tests should proceed from simpler, less invasive to more complicated and invasive.

→ Routine laboratory tests (values may vary by laboratory) may include:
- rubella titer.
- VDRL or RPR.
- LH and FSH (day 2 to 3 of cycle).
  - FSH and LH <10 mIUml (hypothalamic-pituitary dysfunction or failure).
  - FSH and LH as high as 75 mIU/ml (ovarian dysfunction).
  - FSH > 50 mIU/ml in the follicular phase during 2 separate cycles (premature ovarian failure).
  - High LH with low or normal FSH (ratio of LH:FSH 3:1 or higher) (PCO).
    NOTE: While a 3:1 or higher ratio is typical of PCO, this condition should not be ruled out if ratio is less than 3:1.
- prolactin (early to mid-morning; no breast stimulation 24 hours prior to test (normal = 4 to 20 ng/ml).

- TSH (normal = 0.2-3.2 μIU/ml).
- Pap smear, gonorrhea, chlamydia cultures.
- mycoplasma culture.
  NOTE: *T. mycoplasma*, now referred to as *Ureaplasma urealyticum*, has been reported as a possible factor in cases of infertility with unknown etiology. This is controversial; studies comparing colonization in fertile and infertile populations are plagued by conflicting results and poor controls (Grunfeld 1989).
- testosterone (normal = < 70 ng/dl total).
- DHEA-S (normal = 15-17 years, 35-535 μg/dl; 18-30 years, 29-781 μg/dl; 31-50 years, 12-379 μg/dl).

→ Specific infertility tests and procedures.
  - The primary care provider can order tests, interpret results in consultation with a physician, and provide couples with information regarding tests and procedures. *Tests listed here should be done in order suggested.*
  - BBT charting.
    • Two to three cycles of BBT monitoring sufficient for purpose of suggesting that ovulation has occurred.
    • BBT readings also used for guiding woman about:
      −when to start testing using LH predictor kits.
      −scheduling of postcoital testing.
      −timing of intrauterine insemination (IUI).
    • See **Fertility Awareness** Protocol for details of BBT charting.
  - Urine LH predictor kits.
    • LH surge ovulation predictor kits (e.g., Ovuquick®) detect the normal preovulatory surge of LH and translate the surge as an abrupt color change over colorless readings seen prior to surge.
    • LH kits available over the counter:
      −used daily by the woman, starting 2 to 3 days prior to expected ovulation until an obvious color change is seen, signaling that ovulation will occur in next 24 to 36 hours.
    • LH kit readings now used routinely by primary providers for optimal timing of postcoital testing and IUI, as well as timing of coitus during peak ovulation.
    • LH kit *predicts* ovulation, whereas ovulatory readings are *retrospective* from BBT readings.
    • If woman's history strongly suggests anovulation, kits should not be used because of their cost.

    • LH kit readings should not be used as a diagnostic tool without confirmation by laboratory and clinical data.
  - Mid-luteal phase serum progesterone.
    • Should be obtained 7 days after presumed ovulation as determined by LH predictor kit.
    • Normal = 10-15 ng/ml as an indirect indicator of ovulation; higher values expected in clomiphene citrate (CC) cycle.
    • False positive result possible if sample obtained too early or too late in luteal phase due to normal pulsatile variations of serum progesterone.
  - Sonography/serum estradiol.
    • Pre-ovulatory sonography highly useful for evaluating adequate follicular development.
    • Sector scanner with high resolution easily used in practice setting; vaginal transducer provides sonographer improved image of ovarian follicles.
    • Potential ovulation defined as follicles measuring ≥ 16 mm to 18 mm.
    • Serum estradiol (E2) drawn at the time follicles measure ≥ 16 mm to 18 mm should show a level of 400 pg/ml (site-specific values vary).
  - Examination of semen.
    • Semen analysis should be obtained early in the infertility evaluation.
    • Values for the same individual will fluctuate over time; one abnormal result not sufficient to make a diagnosis.
    • At least 2 to 3 abnormal semen analyses done over 2 to 3 months necessary before classifying male-factor infertility.
    • In the event of abnormal findings, referral to a urologist specializing in male-factor infertility should be instituted as necessary.
    • See **Table 12H.1,** for normal semen analysis parameters, and **Appendix 12H.2, Collection of Sample for Semen Analysis**, p. 12-73, for description regarding sample collection.
  - Immune tests.
    • Immunobead test.
      −Looks for the presence of sperm-bound antibodies by binding a marker substance coated with antibodies directed against human immunoglobin to sperm.
    • Only the immunobead test can localize site of antibody binding on the sperm.
    • Binding to the sperm detected easily with microscopic examination for presence of latex particles bound to sperm.

Table 12H.2. INTERPRETATION OF POST-COITAL TEST

Parameter	Poor	Fair-Good	Excellent
Amount of mucus	none	scant-dribble	cascade
Spinnbarkeit	none	slight-moderate (uninterrupted mucus thread may be drawn approx. ¼ to ½ of the distance between external os and vulva	pronounced
Ferning	none-amorphous	linear-partial	complete
Cervix	closed, pale pink	partially open, mucosa pink	gaping-mucosa hyperaemic
Number of Sperm	none	at least 5 motile/HPF	> 5 motile/HPF
Forward motility	no motility	1 + to 2 +	3 +
WBCs present	many	occasional	none

Copyright © L. Weseman 1995

• Binding requires motile sperm for detection; test is useless when motility or sperm count very low.

▪ SPA.
  • Evaluates spermatazoa's ability to penetrate zona pellucida of human egg.
  • Fresh human eggs retrieved from hysterectomy specimens ideal, if available; denuded hamster eggs, if not.
  • Penetration rates correlated with fertile male populations; infertile populations identified by a penetration rate of 15 percent or less.

▪ Postcoital testing.
  • Postcoital (or Sims-Huhner's) test evaluates sperm survival in cervical mucus.
  • Performed just prior to ovulation as determined by color change on LH predictor (See **Appendix 12H.3, Instructions for Postcoital Test**, p. 12-74. In the event of an abnormal result (See **Table 12H.2, Interpretation of Post-Coital Test**), test should be repeated every 2 days until BBT rises to ensure that test was performed at time of maximum estrogen stimulation.

▪ Endometrial biopsy.
  • May be performed by a physician or primary provider following on-site training.
  • Done to confirm ovulation or to diagnose luteal-phase defect.
  • Specimen obtained several days prior to expected onset of menses (between cycle days 24 to 26 in a 28- to 30-day cycle).
  • Results should reveal histological evidence that endometrium appears as expected for the stated postovulatory day on which the biopsy was taken.
  • A single abnormal result is common and not indicative of pathology unless confirmed by a second biopsy.

▪ HSG.
  • Should generally precede diagnostic laparoscopy and hysteroscopy.
  • Performed by a physician, findings interpreted by radiologist and gynecologist.
  • Involves injection of water or oil-based dye into uterine cavity to evaluate fallopian tubal patency and uterine abnormalities.
  • Done under fluoroscopy shortly after menses in the follicular phase prior to anticipated ovulation.
  • Studies have reported an improved pregnancy rate following the HSG with the use of an oil-based dye, indicating that there may be some therapeutic value to HSG.

▪ Laparoscopy.
  • Performed by a physician at end of infertility evaluation unless there is a history of major pelvic pathology.
  • Performed under general anesthesia during follicular phase of cycle to prevent possible disruption of early pregnancy.
  • HSG is commonly performed again during laparoscopy to evaluate tubal patency by directly observing dye spill from fimbriated ends of fallopian tube.

▪ Hysteroscopy.
  • Usually done at the time of laparoscopy.
  • Involves direct visualization of uterine cavity for adhesions, tumors, or anomalies such as endometrial and endocervical polyps and fibroids.

→ Tests, procedures for women with repeated pregnancy loss.
  ▪ Maternal and paternal karyotype.

- Karyotype of abortus material may also be appropriate with advance arrangement with genetics laboratory.
- LH, FSH cycle day 1 to 3.
- TSH.
- Prolactin.
- Antinuclear antibody (ANA).
- PTT, platelets.
- Lupus anticoagulant.
- Anticardiolipin antibody.
- Mid-luteal serum progesterone.
- Chlamydia, gonorrhea culture.
- Mycoplasm culture (or empiric treatment of couple with doxycycline 100 mg twice a day for 10 days).
- Endometrial biopsy 7 days postovulation and prior to onset of menses.
- Study of uterine cavity with sonography, hysterosalpingogram, and hysteroscopy.

TREATMENT/MANAGEMENT

→ Diagnostic evaluation as outlined above.

→ Specific therapy based on patient's history and findings of diagnostic evaluation.

Male-factor infertility

→ Treatment of male-factor infertility focuses on intrauterine insemination. (See **Appendix 12H.1,** p. 12-72, and **Appendix 12H.4, Timing of Intrauterine Insemination,** p. 12-75.)

→ Additional male infertility problems and treatment may include:
- varicocele—surgical repair (varicocelectomy):
  - rate of improved fertility following surgery is variable.
- pyospermia—empiric therapy:
  - 5 weeks of doxycycline 100 mg twice daily for male partner (prostate poorly vascularized, seminiferous tubules sheltered by blood-testes barrier).
  - 10-14 days of doxycycline 100 mg twice daily for female partner (to coincide with last 2 weeks of male's therapy).
- antisperm antibodies—intrauterine insemination (IUI) (see **Appendix 12H.1,** p. 12-72):
  - if unsuccessful after 6 cycles of IUI, may progress to IVF (see **Appendix 12H.5, Assisted Reproductive Technology,** p. 12-76).
  - steroid therapy may be considered, though there is concern regarding reactions to glucocorticoids.
    - poor semen analysis with poor sperm

penetration assay results—donor sperm or IVF—micromanipulation.
- infections of the genital tract:
  - antibiotic therapy for the couple.
  - repeat semen analysis after 1 month; if leukospermia (> 8 white blood cells per high-power field) persists, semen should be cultured.
    –Refer to urologist.
- low semen volume:
  - refer to urologist for complete evaluation.
  - use multiple ejaculates for IUI.
- abnormal liquification:
  - refer to urologist for evaluation of prostate and seminal vesicles.
- low sperm count:
  - if persistent or azospermic, refer to urologist for complete evaluation.
- decreased motility:
  - refer to urologist.
- decreased normal morphology:
  - refer to urologist.

Pelvic-factor infertility

→ Asherman's syndrome:
- lysis of adhesions by hysteroscopy (performed by a physician).
- hormone administration may be utilized after surgical intervention to prevent reoccurrence of scarring.
  - Regimen: Premarin® 1.25 mg for 6 weeks, plus Provera® 10 mg for 12 days during last 2 weeks of Premarin®.

→ Cervical-factor infertility.
- IUI now treatment of choice. (See **Appendix 12H.1,** p. 12-72 for indications for IUI, and **Appendix 12H.4,** p. 12-75 for timing of IUI.)
- Refer for assisted reproductive technology as necessary. (See **Appendix 12H.5,** p. 12-76.)

→ Endometriosis.
- See **Endometriosis** Protocol.
- Consider referral for assisted reproductive technology in the event medical and surgical therapy do not produce positive outcome.

→ Tubal disease/obstruction.
- Refer to a physician adept at microsurgical technique.
- Operative laparoscopy more cost-effective than laparotomy.
  - Involves atraumatic instrumentation, tissue handling, various methods of adhesion prevention.

- Prognosis for pregnancy following surgery for bilateral tubal disease very poor. If, after 18 months no pregnancy ensues following extensive surgery and woman is less than 37 years old, repeat procedure is considered. If woman reaches her 37th birthday, refer for assisted reproductive technology. (See **Appendix 12H.5**, p. 12-76.)
  - Tubal ligation reversal.
- Reconstructive surgery.
- Ability to reverse sterilization procedures determined by amount of tubal damage incurred at time of sterilization procedure, length of remaining tubes for reanastomosis, type of surgical technique used.

Endocrine infertility

→ Primary amenorrhea.
  - Refer to endocrinologist.
  - Hypothalamic factors.
    - Refer for treatment of eating disorder as necessary (see **Eating Disorders** Protocol).
    - Return to ovulatory status may require a change in exercise habits.
      –Counsel or refer as necessary.
    - Ovulation induction by administration of CC. (See **Clomiphene Citrate** Protocol.)
    - May require ovulation induction by "super-ovulation therapy" (e.g., Pergonal®).
      –Refer as necessary.
    - Refer for assisted reproductive technology as necessary if woman fails to conceive with ovulation induction therapy.
    - See also **Amenorrhea—Secondary** Protocol.
  - Pituitary factors.
    - Prolactin level greater than 100 ng/ml highly suggestive of pituitary-secreting adenoma.
      –Refer woman for MRI and treatment by endocrinologist.
    - Administration of bromocriptine mesylate (Parlodel®) 2.5 mg-7.5 mg per day to normalize prolactin level (See **Clomiphene Citrate** Protocol.).
      –Consult with physician.
    - Administration of Parlodel® and CC. (See **Clomiphene Citrate** Protocol).
    - In the event of hyperprolactinemia due to hypothyroidism, begin thyroid hormone replacement. (See **Thyroid Disorders** Protocol.)
    - See **Amenorrhea—Secondary** Protocol.
  - Sheehan's syndrome.

- Refer to a reproductive endocrinologist for treatment.
- Hypothyroidism.
  - See **Thyroid Disorders** Protocol.
  - Maintain TSH in normal range by administration of Synthroid® 0.1 mg to 0.15 mg per day (site policies may vary).
    –Consult with physician.
  - Refer to endocrinologist for treatment of other thyroid disorders.
- Adrenal factors.
  - Androgen-secreting tumors of the ovary or adrenals are rare; should be ruled out when androgen levels are high.
  - Women with abnormal levels should be referred to an endocrinologist.
  - See **Hirsutism** Protocol.
  - Abnormal (low) testosterone level.
    –Treat with dexamethasone 0.5 mg at bedtime to decrease nighttime ACTH production (a low testosterone reflects low ovarian output, so these women may respond poorly to ovulation induction therapy without addition of dexamethasone).
    –Consult with physician.
- Polycystic ovary syndrome (PCO).
  - Referral to a safe, structured weight loss program recommended for the obese PCO woman, though the parameters for success with weight loss and return to normal ovulatory status are hard to measure.
  - Induce ovulation by administration of CC. (See **Clomiphene Citrate** Protocol.)
  - If woman fails to conceive after 3 to 6 ovulatory cycles on CC therapy, refer for more aggressive therapy.
    –Administration of urinary menotropins (e.g., Pergonal®, Metrodin®).
  - Refer for assisted reproductive technology if not responsive to CC or Pergonal® and age is appropriate.
  - See **Amenorrhea—Secondary** Protocol.
- Premature ovarian failure.
  - Refer for assisted reproductive technology.
    –Donor oocytes or use of the GnRH pump to attempt to induce ovulation—success limited.
  - Estrogen replacement for protection of bones and cardiovascular system.
    –Therapy will be patient- and site-specific.
    –See also **Perimenopausal Symptoms and Hormone Therapy** Protocol.

- Refer couple with premature ovarian failure for crisis counseling as this diagnosis is naturally quite devastating.
- Counsel couples to consider options of adoption, surrogacy (check state laws pertaining to surrogacy), and child-free living.
- See **Amenorrhea—Secondary** Protocol.
■ Luteinized unruptured follicle (LUF).
- Administer human chorionic gonadotropin for injection (Profasi®).
  – Acts like LH surge to induce ovulation which should occur 24 to 36 hours after the injection.
  – Consult with physician.
  – Couple is instructed to have intercourse on day of injection and every other day thereafter until follicle rupture as evidenced by ultrasound.
  – See section in **Clomiphene Citrate** Protocol for description of ultrasound evidence of ovulation.
- Clomiphene citrate therapy and Profasi® or Pergonal® therapy and Profasi® also are used as a treatment for LUF in some practices.

Immunological infertility

→ Suppressive therapy with the use of steroid therapy has had limited success.

→ Use IUI to attempt to bypass immobilizing antibodies secreted in cervical mucus.

→ Refer for assisted reproductive technology if no pregnancy after 6 IUI cycles or sooner depending on woman's age.

→ Counsel couple to consider options of adoption, surrogacy, child-free living.

Unexplained infertility

→ Treat couple empirically for mycoplasma.
  ■ Doxycycline 100 mg twice a day for a minimum of 10 days. (Site-specific policies will vary.)

→ Ovulation induction alone (see **Clomiphene Citrate** Protocol) or CC combined with ultrasound monitoring and IUI for 6 ovulatory cycles.
  ■ If unsuccessful refer for Pergonal®/IUI therapy.

→ Refer for assisted reproductive technology as appropriate.

→ Counsel couple, keep them actively involved in decision making, help them to "let go" when all avenues of therapy have been exhausted, and encourage them to explore adoption, surrogacy, and child-free living.

Age-related infertility

→ Counsel couples that empiric therapy over age 43 years is not efficacious or cost-effective.
  ■ Counsel regarding donor oocytes, adoption, surrogacy, or child-free living.

→ In the event of age-related luteal-phase abnormalities, treatment includes CC therapy with support of the luteal phase by administration of progesterone vaginal suppositories (25 mg-50 mg every 12 hours) until positive pregnancy test.
  ■ At that time, intramuscular injections (12.5 mg progesterone in oil) are given daily until the tenth week of pregnancy.
  ■ Consult with a physician.

Repeated pregnancy loss (Treatment depends on causative factor.)

→ Müllerian anomalies or fibroids impinging on uterine cavity.
  ■ Refer to a physician for appropriate surgery (e.g., hysteroscopic resection of uterine septum).

→ Karyotypic abnormalities.
  ■ Refer for genetic counseling; possible referral for assisted reproductive technology with donor gametes.

→ Intrauterine synechiae.
  ■ Refer for appropriate surgery.

→ Age 44 years or older.
  ■ Spontaneous abortion rate is over 50 percent; treatment generally is not successful.

→ DES exposure.
  ■ No specific treatment.
  ■ Refer for colposcopic examination.
  ■ Counsel regarding risk of pathology secondary to DES exposure to cervix.
  ■ Counsel to consider adoption, surrogacy, child-free living.

→ Prior history of thrombosis/embolic events or with abnormality in bleeding times and positive anticardiolipin autoantibodies.
  ■ Administer low-dose aspirin, 60 mg-80 mg per day (one "baby aspirin").
  ■ Consult with a physician.
  ■ Immediately refer to a perinatologist upon documentation of pregnancy by appropriately rising hCG titers, as these pregnancies are at high risk for sudden fetal loss.

→ Isolated abnormal immune tests of low titer (e.g., ANA 1:80 or low positive IgG anticardiolipin antibody).

- Administer aspirin, 60 mg-80 mg per day (empiric).
- Refer to a perinatologist upon documentation of pregnancy viability.

→ Unexplained early losses for women with well-documented luteal-phase deficiency.
- Luteal-phase support or CC and luteal-phase support with progesterone.
- Illicit drug use, smoking, or chronic alcohol use.
- Advise appropriate counseling.

Luteal-phase defect

→ Administration of progesterone vaginal suppositories 25 mg-50 mg twice daily or progesterone in oil 12.5 mg I.M. every day in the luteal phase until onset of menses, or, in the event of a pregnancy, continue until early in the second trimester at which time it is presumed that placental production of progesterone is adequate.
- Consult with a physician.

→ Clomiphene citrate and Profasi® 10,000 I.M. (see **Clomiphene Citrate** Protocol).
- Consult with a physician.
- Measure serum progesterone level 7 days following administration of Profasi® (15-30 ng/ml normal in CC-enhanced cycle).
- Refer to BBT charting to monitor length of luteal phase and assess efficacy of treatment.

Counseling

→ Provide initital counseling done at intake with ongoing discussion to evaluate emotional needs.

→ Evaluate couple's coping skills and whether additional couseling is needed.

→ Infertility counseling is based on brief psychotherapy or a crisis-intervention model.
- In some cases, the infertility experience triggers responses that are linked to past losses, unresolved grief, or poor self-esteem (Mahlstedt 1985).
- Several important features should be kept in mind when counseling the couple:
  - couples need information about their medical situation and options to give them a sense of control.
  - they need to identify feelings that have resulted directly from the infertility.
  - they may need help restoring self-esteem.
  - they need to discuss and explore the feelings of loss and guilt before resolution is possible.
  - they may need help with decision making in terms of treatment modalities.

→ Refer to physician for consultation regarding any abnormal clinical findings, and for discussion of treatment modalities.

→ Refer to specific specialists as indicated (e.g., reproductive endocrinologist, urologist, counselor).

→ Refer to support groups/counseling (e.g., RESOLVE peer-support group).

→ Hold ongoing discussion with infertility team to ensure that woman's treatment continues to be up-to-date.

→ As needed for prescription(s).

PATIENT EDUCATION

→ Provide information regarding basic anatomy and physiology, with emphasis on normal menstrual cycle, ovulation, frequency, timing of and positions for intercourse.

→ Advise against use of lubricants and douches. Explain effects of drugs, heat, excessive alcohol consumption on spermatogenesis. See **Fertility Awareness** Protocol.

→ Hold comprehensive discussion with couple to describe infertility evaluation, risks, expected overall cost, time involved, and expectations of couple.

→ Refer to office manager or accountant to discuss insurance reimbursement and costs of individual tests.

→ Discuss laparoscopy/hysteroscopy:
- classified as same-day surgery; post-operative patients may resume normal activities in one to three days.
- common after-effects may include generalized stiffness, sore throat, shoulder pain (referred pain secondary to carbon dioxide application to abdomen for insertion and visualization with a laparoscope), and bloating of the abdomen, as well as abdominal wall tenderness.

FOLLOW-UP

→ Careful interpretation and explanation of all laboratory data or clinical findings is necessary. Institute necessary treatment modalities.

→ Specific treatment follow-up should assess management plan, assess for possible side effects of drug therapies and changes in physical status, or test for pregnancy following any treatment regimen.

→ Patient may need assurance that infertility evaluation is progressing in a thorough, timely manner; that tests are done properly; assistance with scheduling of tests or treatments.

→ Ongoing consultation with infertility team, regarding patient's clinical data, treatment modalities, emotional status, is necessary.

→ Offer patient pertinent referrals to specialists in the event of unusual findings.

→ Ongoing assessment of couple's emotional status and pertinent counseling is recommended. Refer to counselor experienced with infertility crisis.
  ▪ Have a variety of specialists on referral list from varying religious backgrounds.
  ▪ Give couple access to referrals for adoption resources.

→ Referral to endometriosis support group in the area.
  ▪ The Endometriosis Foundation has many regional chapters and publishes a newsletter (P.O. Box 92187, Milwaukee, WI 53202).

→ Referral to RESOLVE infertility peer-support group.

→ Document in progress notes and problem list.

Bibliography

Berkowitz, G.S. 1986. Epidemiology of infertility and early pregnancy wastage. *Reproductive failure.* London: Churchill Livingstone.

Bernstein, J., and Mattox, J.H. 1982. An overview of infertility. *Journal of Obstetric, Gynecologic and Neonatal Nursing* 11(5):309–314.

Grunfeld, L. 1989. Workup for male infertility. *Journal of Reproductive Medicine* 34(2):143–149.

Henzl, M. 1989. Role of nafarelin in the management of endometriosis. *Journal of Reproductive Medicine* 34(12):1021–1024.

Jones, E. 1989. Hyperprolactinemia and female infertility. *Journal of Reproductive Medicine* 34(2):117–125.

Mahlstedt, P.P. 1985. The psychological component of infertility. *Fertility and Sterility* 43(3):335–346.

Marsman, J.W.P. 1987. Clinical versus subclinical variococeles: Venographic findings and improvement of fertility after embolization. *Radiology* 155(3):635–638.

Marut, E.L. 1989. Polycystic ovary syndrome. *Journal of Reproductive Medicine* 34(1):104–107.

Mazor, M., and Simons, H. 1983. Infertility: Medical, emotional, and social considerations. New York: Human Sciences Press.

Older, J. 1983. *Endometriosis.* New York: Scribner.

Ollivier, S., Lesser, C., and Bell, K. 1984. Providing infertility care. *Journal of Obstetric, Gynecologic and Neonatal Nursing.* March-April:415.

Overstreet, J.W., Yanagimachi, R., Katz, D.F., Hayashi, K., and Hanson, F.W. 1980. Penetration of human spermatozoa into the human zona pellucida and the zona-free hamster egg: A study of fertile donors and infertile patients. *Fertility and Sterility* 33(5):534–542.

Rehewy, M.S.E., Thomas, A.J., Hafez, E.S.E., Brown, W.J., Mughissi, K.S., and Jaszczak, S. 1978. Ureaplasma urealyticum (T-mycoplasm) in seminal plasma and spermatazoa from infertile and fertile volunteers. *European Journal of Obstetrics and Gynecologic Reproductive Biology* 8(5):247–251.

Reid, P.C., Thurrell, W., Smith, J.H., Kennedy, A., and Sharp F. 1992. YAG laser endometrial ablation: Histological aspects of uterine healing. *International Journal of Gynecological Pathology* 11(3):174–179.

Serafini, P., and Batzofin, J. 1989. Diagnosis of female infertility: A comprehensive approach. *Journal of Reproductive Medicine* 34(1):29–37.

Speroff, L., Glass, R.H., and Kase, N. 1989. *Clinical gynecologic endocrinology and infertility*, 4th ed. Baltimore: Williams & Wilkins.

———. 1994. *Clinical gynecologic endocrinology and infertility*, 5th ed. Baltimore: Williams & Wilkins.

Thatcher, S. 1989. Anovulatory infertility causes and cures. *Journal of Reproductive Medicine* 34(1):17–24.

Toaff, R., and Ballas, S. 1978. Traumatic hypomenorrhea-amenorrhea (Asherman's syndrome). *Fertility and Sterility* 30(4):379–387.

Toth, A., Lesser, M.L., Brooke, A., Brooks, M.A., and Labriola, D. 1983. Subsequent pregnancies among 161 couples treated for T-mycoplasma genital tract infection. *New England Journal of Medicine* 308(9):505–507.

Witten, B.I., and Martin, S.A. 1985. The endometrial biopsy as a guide to the management of luteal phase defect. *Fertility and Sterility* 44(4):460–465.

APPENDIX 12H.1

Indications for Intrauterine Insemination

Indications for simple sperm wash without swim-up

- coital dysfunction
- retrograde ejaculation
- cervical mucus abnormalities
- anatomical defects of genital organs

Indications for IUI with swim-up and various column techniques

- antisperm antibodies (male and female)
- donor insemination
- low semen volume (collect and combine multiple ejaculates over 1-4 hour period)
- oligoasthenospermia
- seminal fluid liquefaction defect
- teratospermia
- vasectomy reversal
- unexplained infertility
- in conjunction with ovulation induction

APPENDIX 12H.2

Collection of Sample for Semen Analysis

- Abstinence prior to specimen collection should be two to five days.

- Specimen obtained by masturbation into a clear container (usually provided by laboratory).

- Couple advised not to use lubrication (spermicidal).

- Milex sheath (condom which is nontoxic to sperm) may be used if religious practices prohibit masturbation.

- Deliver specimen to laboratory within 1-2 hours from time of collection.

- Specimen to be kept warm in transit (next to body usually adequate).

APPENDIX 12H.3

Instructions for Post-Coital Test

- Couple to observe normal interval of abstinence prior to test to reflect accurate picture.

- Test performed in office of primary provider on the morning following an obvious color change on LH predictor kit, or one to three days prior to expected rise in BBT.

- Intercourse to take place morning of office visit, test to be performed within 2 hours to 2½ hours after coitus, as maximum number of sperm present in cervical canal at this time.

- No lubricants or douches to be used during or after intercourse.

APPENDIX 12H.4

Timing of Intrauterine Insemination

Natural cycles | Inseminate day following color change on LH surge kit

Ovulation-induced cycles | Inseminate 2 days after Profasi® injection

If frozen sperm used | Inseminate day of color change on LH surge and day after color change (better results with 2 inseminations for frozen sperm). Wash all frozen sperm first before IUI.

APPENDIX 12H.5

Assisted Reproductive Technology

Type		Indications
In-vitro fertilization	IVF	Tubal disease, unexplained infertility, male-factor infertility, endometriosis, immunological infertility, DES exposure, cervical-factor infertility, possibly resistant anovulation
Gamete intrafallopian transfer	GIFT	Unexplained infertility, male-factor infertility, mild endometriosis, possibly immunological infertility, DES exposure, cervical-factor infertility, possibly resistant anovulation
Zygote intrafallopian transfer	ZIFT	Unexplained infertility
Tubal embryo transfer	TET	IVF failure when poor sperm is involved
Peritoneal oocyte and sperm transfer	POST	Unexplained infertility
Subzonal insertion of sperm by microinjection	SUZI	Male-factor infertility
Intracytoplasmic sperm injection	ICSI	Male-factor infertility

Lori M. Weseman, R.N., M.S., N.P.

12-HA INFERTILITY
Clomiphene Citrate

As many as 30 percent to 40 percent of women with infertility have some form of ovulatory dysfunction secondary to a variety of endocrine factors. Clomiphene citrate (CC) is first-line pharmacological therapy for induction of ovulation in women with evidence of endogenous estrogen production. Clomiphene citrate is a non-steroidal agent with estrogenic and anti-estrogenic properties, and supports events that occur in normal ovulatory cycles. GnRH secretion occurs first under the influence of CC, causing increased pulse frequency of LH and FSH. Simply put, because the body is tricked into thinking that there is a lack of estrogen, an increased production of FSH and LH ensues.

Recently, CC has been combined with bromocriptine mesylate (Parlodel®) in patients with galactorrhea and/or hyperprolactinemia. Patients with increased prolactin secretion (prolactin-secreting adenomas should be ruled out) and a positive progesterone withdrawal bleed may be treated with Parlodel® or a combination of CC and Parlodel® to decrease prolactin concentration and allow ovulation to occur. Parlodel® is a dopamine receptor agonist and is used in women with idiopathic hyperprolactinemia when anovulation is the causative factor (Jones 1989).

The exact mechanism of prolactin-induced anovulation is unclear; evidence suggests that prolactinemic inhibition of normal ovulation occurs at the level of the hypothalamus. A disturbance in amplitude and frequency of LH pulsations occurs in women with hyperprolactinemia (Jones 1989). Clinically, patients with hyperprolactinemia may present with galactorrhea, menstrual dysfunction, hirsutism, diminished libido, or unexplained infertility.

Hyperprolactinemia also has been found in association with a shortened luteal phase and deficient luteal function due to effects on ovarian steroidogenesis and folliculogenesis. Higher concentrations (100 ng/ml) of prolactin appear to inhibit progesterone secretion (Check, Wu, and Adelson 1989). Certain metabolic disturbances—in particular, hypothyroidism—also may be associated with hyperprolactinemia. Treatment of the causative disorder may result in a return to normal prolactin level; however CC and Parlodel® therapy is an effective treatment option for many infertile women.

Among women treated with CC, ovulation is achieved in an average of 75 percent to 80 percent of well-selected patients, with a pregnancy rate of 35 percent to 40 percent. Patients with hypothalamic-pituitary failure do not respond to CC therapy. Pregnancy occurs at a higher rate in the first three ovulatory cycles, with as high as 85 percent in the first three cycles, dropping to seven percent in the fourth cycle, and to approximately five percent occuring at six cycles or more (Hammond, Halme, and Talbert 1983). Clearly, extending CC therapy beyond three to six ovulatory cycles is not as effective and may place considerable stress on the couple.

DATABASE

SUBJECTIVE

→ Review of health history to include:
- age of both members of the couple.
- approximate date couple stopped using contraception.
- history and outcome of any previous pregnancies for both partners; length of time to conceive for previous pregnancies.

- length and regularity of menstrual cycle, magnitude of flow, age at menarche.
- symptoms, treatment of dysmenorrhea or dyspareunia.
- history of abnormal bleeding; treatment.
- symptoms of ovulation—i.e., breast tenderness, acne, mittelschmerz, mood changes, spotting, changes in libido, increased mid-cycle vaginal discharge.
- frequency of coitus, use of lubricants, perception of couple with respect to whether or not ejaculation is completed in vagina.
- religious practices that may relate to intercourse or fertility.
- duration of amenorrhea, if any.
  • Presence of physical or emotional stress, weight fluctuation, or medication taken prior to cessation of menses.
- presence or history of galactorrhea.
- history of STDs, PID; treatment and/or sequellae.
- previous pelvic or other surgery; complications, if any.
- review of any previous infertility evaluation and treatment.
- pertinent medical history suggestive of endocrine disorder.
- history of serious medical illnesses.
- DES exposure.
- history of IUD use; sequellae if any.
- history of oral contraceptive use.
- social history:
  • use of alcohol, prescription, or OTC drugs (e.g., laxatives, antihistamines), or recreational drugs; smoking history.
- eating habits:
  • any habits suggestive of eating disorder.
- exercise history/habits.
- family history with attention to endocrine, genetic, or reproductive abnormalities.
- history of exposure to radiation or toxic chemicals.
- use of saunas or hot tubs.

OBJECTIVE
See **Infertility** Protocol.

ASSESSMENT

→ Ovulatory dysfunction requiring ovulation induction by administration of clomiphene citrate
→ R/O endocrine infertility

- R/O hypothalamic-pituitary dysfunction/failure
- R/O PCO
- R/O androgen abnormalities
→ R/O unexplained infertility
→ R/O luteal-phase infertility

PLAN

DIAGNOSTIC TESTS
→ Normal values will vary by laboratory.
→ Rubella titer is indicated.
→ VDRL or RPR is indicated.
→ Chlamydia and gonorrhea cultures are recommended.
→ Laboratory tests to evaluate dysovulation are directed at evaluation of the hypothalamic-pituitary-ovarian axis.
  - Fasting prolactin (no breast stimulation 48 hours prior to test).
  - FSH—day 2 to 3 of cycle.
  - LH—day 2 to 3 of cycle.
    • FSH and LH <10 mIU/ml (hypothalamic-pituitary dysfunction or failure).
    • FSH and LH as high as 75 mIU/ml (ovarian dysfunction).
    • FSH > 50 mIU/ml in the follicular phase during 2 separate cycles (premature ovarian failure).
    • High LH with low or normal FSH (ratio of LH:FSH 3:1 or higher) PCO.
    NOTE: While a 3:1 or higher ratio is typical of PCO, it should not be ruled out if ratio less than 3:1.
  - Mid-luteal phase progesterone.
  - TSH.
  - DHEA-S.
  - Testosterone.
    • Clinical signs of excess androgen include hirsutism and acne.
    • An elevated DHEA-S indicates over-active adrenal contribution to circulating androgens.
    • Highly elevated testosterone levels may be indicative of an androgen-secreting neoplasm in the ovary.
    • In presence of high normal values, especially of DHEA-S, patients may respond poorly to CC without addition of dexamethasone 0.5 mg at bedtime to decrease nighttime ACTH production.
  - 2 to 3 months of BBT readings helpful for assessment of the woman's menstrual cycle; not

necessary for women with infrequent, spontaneous menses.
  • Refer to **Fertility Awareness** Protocol for discussion of BBT charting.
- LH predictor kits recommended for use in women with regular menses.
- Consider endometrial biopsy in women with longstanding (longer than 3 months) amenorrhea to rule out hyperplasia; otherwise not necessary as a pre-CC evaluatory test.
- Progesterone withdrawal/challenge:
  • rule out pregnancy by beta-hCG assay prior to challenge.
  • progesterone administered orally (Provera® 10 mg daily for 5 to 7 days) or I.M. (progesterone in oil 100 mg-150 mg—1 dose) to determine existence of endogenous estrogen production. (Site-specific policies may vary.) Use 10 mg for 12 days for patients with longstanding amenorrhea to achieve full conversion of endometrium.
  • optimal candidates for CC therapy are those who have a withdrawal bleed following progesterone administration.
    –Bleeding is evidence of intact hypothalamic-pituitary-ovarian (HPO) axis.
  • those who do not respond may have premature ovarian failure or hypothalamic-pituitary failure and will not respond to CC. These patients should be referred for assisted reproductive technology (ART) (See **Appendix 12H.5,** p. 12-76) and/or counseling.
  • semen analysis is necessary prior to CC administration to rule out male-factor infertility. Refer to **Appendix 12H.2,** p. 12-73.

TREATMENT/MANAGEMENT

→ Contraindications to CC therapy include:
- primary pituitary or ovarian failure.
- thyroid or adrenal disease (these conditions may be treated first, followed by CC administration if still necessary).
- abnormal uterine bleeding of undetermined origin.
- liver disease or dysfunction (check liver function tests before initiating CC in women with a positive history).
- ovarian enlargement or ovarian cysts (larger than 6 cm).
- pregnancy.

→ Dosage/administration of CC (Clomid®, Serophene®).
- Recommended initial dose is 50 mg/day p.o. for 5 consecutive days beginning cycle day 5.
- If ovulation not achieved at 50 mg dose, increase dose in steps by 50-mg increments each month.
- Dosage is the same when treating patients with luteal-phase defects or unexplained infertility (Refer to **Infertility** Protocol).
  NOTE: CC acts negatively on cervical mucus, especially at doses of 150 mg-200 mg. Treat with Premarin® 0.625 mg/day p.o. for one week after the last CC pill to improve quality of cervical mucus. IUI is also an option in patients with compromised cervical mucus. (Refer to **Infertility** Protocol for discussion of IUI).
- Once ovulation is achieved, continue CC therapy at effective dose until woman conceives or until termination of treatment.
  • Prognosis is poor if conception does not occur after 6 months of well-timed intercourse/IUI.
- Ovulation is anticipated approximately 5 to 10 days after stopping CC treatment.
- CC cycles can be longer than spontaneous cycles; 30 to 33 day cycles not unusual.
- Intercourse recommended every other day from day 15 until a rise on BBT chart occurs.
- LH predictor kit recommended starting day of rise on BBT chart or within 24 hours of rise.
- Menstruation expected 14 days after ovulation.
- Rule out pregnancy if spontaneous menstruation does not occur, especially if temperature on BBT chart remains elevated.
- If regular CC protocol fails and all other infertility factors have been ruled out or are being managed, may use extended CC protocol, though it is controversial.
  • Use 250 mg CC for 8 days plus 10,000 units human chorionic gonadotropin for injection (Profasi®) 6 days later.
  • Most clinicians now recommend urinary menotropins (e.g., Pergonal®) for CC therapy failure.
- If the history suggests oligo-ovulation as the sole cause of infertility, treat with CC for 3 cycles.
  • If no response, do further work-up.
  • See **Infertility** Protocol.
→ Pergonal®
- Pergonal® is a purified preparation of gonadotropins, extracted from the urine of

postmenopausal women, and consisting of FSH and LH. It is administered by I.M. injection.
- Pergonal® acts directly on the ovaries to stimulate growth of follicles; bypasses the hypothalamic-pituitary axis.
- Ovarian function must be present to ensure that follicles are capable of being stimulated by FSH and LH.
- Pergonal® does not trigger ovulation.
  • Profasi® must be administered after Pergonal® to mimic the endogenous LH surge, thus stimulating ovulation.
- Pergonal® and Profasi® given in a sequential manner are indicated for the induction of ovulation:
  • as first-line therapy for anovulatory infertile women with low to normal levels of FSH and LH.
  • as second-line therapy in women who fail to ovulate or conceive after optimal doses of CC. **NOTE:** Induction of ovulation with Pergonal® requires advanced training of health care providers as well as constant monitoring and follow-up. The primary provider should refer the woman requiring Pergonal® therapy to a clinician experienced in super-ovulation therapy.
→ CC and bromocriptine:
- CC has been combined with bromocriptine (Parlodel®) in patients with evidence of increased prolactin secretion.
  • Women with increased prolactin.
    –First-line therapy is Parlodel®. Add CC if Parlodel® does not restore ovulatory function.
  • Women without increased prolactin and no evidence of galactorrhea.
    –Addition of Parlodel® to CC therapy is controversial; efficacy is not established.
  • Women with increased prolactin and galactorrhea.
    –Treat with Parlodel®.
- dosage—administered orally in divided doses:
  • 2.5 mg-7.5 mg p.o. daily to normalize prolactin levels. CC therapy remains as discussed.
  • women with luteal-phase defects on CC and Parlodel® therapy may require progesterone vaginal suppositories (25 mg) 2 times daily.
- discontinue CC and Parlodel® when pregnancy confirmed.
- side effects:

- nausea, vomiting, dizziness, syncope.
- give small, divided doses with meals or at bedtime, gradually increasing dosage to therapeutic dosage, to ameliorate side effects.
- can also insert intravaginally to avoid side effects, especially nausea.
→ Complications associated with CC therapy:
- ovarian hyperstimulation/enlargement (occurs rarely).
  • Ovaries significantly enlarged, tender, and fragile with hyperstimulation.
  • Pelvic examinations, transvaginal sonogram contraindicated if this is suspected.
  • CC therapy should be discontinued for 1 to 2 cycles if symptoms do not abate spontaneously.
- rupture of ovarian cyst.
  • Ovarian hyperstimulation followed by rupture of ovarian cysts can cause internal bleeding, low blood pressure, and severe dizziness, necessitating hospitalization and/or surgery.
    –Patients complaining of pelvic pain after receiving CC should be evaluated carefully.
  • If enlargement (> 6 cm) of the ovary occurs, CC is to be discontinued until ovaries return to pretreatment size. Dosage should be reduced for the next cycle.
  • Cyst size < 6 cm rarely ruptures. It is safe to continue under these conditions.
- congenital malformations/spontaneous abortion.
  • Several large, long-term studies have shown that rates of congenital malformations and spontaneous abortions in CC pregnancies are not greater than in spontaneous pregnancies (Scialli 1986).
- multiple gestation.
  • Most commonly twins—occurs in 3 percent to 5 percent of CC pregnancies.
  • Less than 1 percent results in triplets or more.
  • Starting CC on cycle day 3 instead of day 5 recruits more follicles and is associated with higher multiple gestation rate.
→ Monitoring ovulation during CC:
- BBT charts.
  • Ovulation is presumed if BBT rises by 1°F.
- home LH kits.
  • Used by patient to pinpoint ovulation, timing of coitus, postcoital test, or IUI.
- postcoital test.
  • Anti-estrogenic properties of CC may cause cervical mucus to become thick, tenacious, and cellular, impairing sperm transport and survival.

- Postcoital test at mid-cycle can be used to assess for antiestrogenic effects.
- IUI in conjunction with CC therapy should be considered in the event that cervical mucus quality is compromised.
- May also treat with Premarin® 0.625 mg p.o. for 1 week after last CC pill.
▪ serum estradiol levels.
- Preovulatory estradiol levels should measure above 200-300 pg/ml.
▪ ultrasound.
- Using vaginal transducer, ultrasound should be performed starting around day 10, then every other day until the dominant follicle measures 14 mm, then daily until it measures 16 mm to 18 mm (follicle grows 1 mm to 3 mm/day).
- Profasi® is administered when there is no response to maximum dose or there is a short luteal phase. Timing of administration of Profasi® is calculated with the use of ultrasound measurements.
- Ultrasound evidence of ovulation (presumptive) includes:
  - disappearance of dominant follicle with or without fluid in the cul-de-sac.
  - cystic change in dominant follicle with crenated border.
  - "filling in" of dominant follicle (appears "cob-webby").
  - collapse of follicle (emergence of corpus luteum).
▪ endometrial biopsy.
- Obtained 2 days prior to expected menstruation.
- Results should indicate a proper secretory endometrium (not more than 2 days out of phase).
- Serum beta-hCG prior to the biopsy should be drawn to rule out pregnancy, though patients can be reassured that risk of the biopsy interrupting an early pregnancy is extremely low.
▪ mid-luteal progesterone.
- Progesterone level should be drawn around 7 days after expected ovulation to determine whether ovulation has occurred and what the potential is for a normal luteal phase.
- Normal = 15-30 ng/ml in a CC-enhanced cycle.
- Support of the luteal phase with administration of progesterone suppositories (25 mg-50 mg every 12 hours) or I.M. progesterone (12.5 mg progesterone in oil I.M. daily) is suggested by many infertility practitioners.

CONSULTATION

→ Physician consultation is recommended regarding laboratory data, clinical findings, and correct administration of ovulation induction therapy.
→ Referral to specialist is indicated in the event of unusual laboratory data or clinical findings (e.g., abnormal androgen levels, ovarian failure).
→ Referral to physician for second-line therapy (i.e., Pergonal®) is recommended in the event of failure of patient to achieve ovulation or pregnancy on CC therapy or for IUI in the event that cervical mucus is found to be compromised with CC therapy.
→ Ongoing discussion with infertility care team is recommended to ensure that patient's care continues to be up-to-date and effective.
→ Referral for counseling and treatment of eating disorders or to a weight loss program, as necessary.
→ As needed for prescription(s).

PATIENT EDUCATION

→ Discussion and explanation should include:
  ▪ normal reproductive cycle.
  ▪ factors contributing to patient's specific dysovulation diagnosis (e.g., excessive exercise, PCO).
  ▪ recommended treatment regimen; action of CC; realistic chances for ovulation and conception.
    - Ovulation occurs in 75 percent to 80 percent of well-selected patients with pregnancy rate of 10 percent.
  ▪ correct medication administration—amount, days of the cycle, duration of the therapy (five days).
  ▪ when ovulation is expected, when intercourse should take place; possible physical signs of ovulation, though many patients experience no symptoms (Reassure patient).
  ▪ thorough description of potential side effects, especially those which should be reported to the office immediately (e.g., visual disturbance or abdominal or pelvic pain).
    - Side effects may include, but are not limited to:
      - vasomotor flushes.
      - insomnia.
      - bloating.

–breast tenderness.

–fatigue.

–mild mood alterations—lability, irritability, or depression.

–nausea.

–dizziness, headaches.

–abdominal or pelvic pain, mild to severe.

  ▸ Contact provider or return to office.

–visual disturbances—blurring, spots, flashes of light (Talbert 1983).

  ▸ Contact provider or return to office.

• Less frequent side effects may include:

–abnormal uterine bleeding.

–increased urination.

–urticaria and allergic dermatitis.

–weight gain.

–reversible hair loss.

▪ monitoring techniques, timing of tests (e.g., BBT instruction, home LH kits, biopsies, ultrasonography, postcoital testing, blood tests).

▪ additional treatment options in the event that patient does not achieve ovulation or pregnancy with CC therapy.

→ Reassure patient that side effects generally resolve spontaneously with discontinuation of CC.

→ Patient also needs to be aware of any adverse reactions to CC therapy (discussed previously in this protocol).

→ Offer educational handouts listing correct administration of medication, schedule of tests, side effects, and when to call the office.

FOLLOW-UP

→ Rule out pregnancy if no menses after CC cycle; refer for prenatal care as needed.

→ Interpret laboratory data and clinical findings pertaining to documentation of ovulation.

▪ If ovulation has occurred, instruct woman to continue at same dose next cycle.

▪ If no evidence of ovulation, increase dose by 50 mg.

→ Advise woman to return to office in the event of moderate to severe pain.

▪ Discontinue CC until ovaries are normal size and non-tender.

▪ Refer to physician as necessary.

→ Hold ongoing discussion with woman regarding CC therapy, dose changes, side effects, emotional status. Telephone follow-up is often adequate.

→ Hold ongoing discussion with physician/infertility team regarding ovulation status, medication changes, patient's condition.

→ Refer as necessary for second-line therapy (i.e., Pergonal®, Metradin®) or IUI; carefully explain to couple.

→ Encourage woman to take a one- to two-month break from treatment if she appears overwhelmed.

→ Refer to specialist in the event that the woman has a medical problem beyond scope of the primary provider.

→ Refer to counselor/support group as necessary.

→ Document in progress notes and problem list.

Bibliography

Check, J., Wu, C., and Adelson, H. 1989. Bromocriptine versus progesterone therapy for infertility related to luteal-phase defects in hyperprolactinemic patients. *International Journal of Fertility* 34(3):209–214.

Hammond, M.G., Halme, J.K., and Talbert, L.M. 1983. Factors affecting the pregnancy rate in clomiphene citrate induction of ovulation. *Obstetrics and Gynecology* 62(2):196–202.

Jones, E. 1989. Hyperprolactinemia and female infertility. *Journal of Reproductive Medicine* 34(2):117–125.

Scialli, A.R. 1986. The reproductive toxicity of ovulation induction. *Fertility and Sterility* 45(3):315–323.

Talbert, L.M. 1983. Clomiphene citrate induction of ovulation. *Fertility and Sterility* 39(6):742–743.

12-HB INFERTILITY
Fertility Awareness

Fertility awareness (FA) and *natural family planning* (NFP) methods are defined as techniques used to plan or avoid pregnancy through observation of naturally occurring signs and symptoms of fertility during the menstrual cycle. Natural family planning is not a method of contraception: rather, the phrase refers to the timing of intercourse in relation to the identified fertile phase of the menstrual cycle in order to achieve or prevent a pregnancy (Spieler and Thomas 1989). The reasons for using natural methods to control fertility vary from discontent with available contraceptives to fear of contraceptive side effects, religious and cultural reasons, and the desire to plan a pregnancy (Barbato and Bertolotti 1988).

Fertility awareness education may be a useful initial step in the care of the client presenting with infertility. Education and information help the client develop realistic expectations regarding the treatment process. Encouraging couples to attend fertility awareness classes together is a way to stress the concept of mutual fertility, and both partners can acquire the vocabulary to discuss sexuality, infertility, and fertility treatment options. This will decrease any stress or discomfort associated with these topics (McCusker 1982).

It has been estimated that 74 percent of couples with normal fertility achieve pregnancy within the first three cycles when they know their fertile days, and some couples with unexplained infertility will achieve pregnancy after investigation is completed through simple explanations, reassurance, and time (Klaus 1983; McCusker 1982).

Natural methods of family planning are grouped under the term natural family planning but actually include five separate methods: the basal body temperature method, the cervical mucus or ovulation method, the symptothermal method, and the fertility awareness

method. The fifth, the calendar rhythm method, although the most widely practiced natural method, is not considered to be as scientific or reliable as the other methods (Spieler and Thomas 1989).

Each method has its own specific rules. Calendar rhythm uses the average length of a woman's cycle to calculate her fertile period, at which time intercourse should occur to achieve pregnancy (Johnson and Reich 1986). Newer NFP techniques teach women to observe bodily changes that signal ovulation on a daily basis and are therefore more sophisticated and effective. The ovulation method relies on observation of changes in the consistency and appearance of cervical mucus to signal the fertile period and implies abstinence during this time.

The basal body temperature (BBT) method relies on temperature observation alone, and is based on the fact that the BBT rises in response to progesterone production following ovulation, thus serving as an indicator that ovulation has occurred. The symptothermal method utilizes both cervical mucus observation to predict ovulation and BBT to indicate the occurrence of ovulation. The symptothermal method may incorporate other fertility signs and symptoms such as breast tenderness, abdominal pain, spotting, mood changes, and heightened libido.

The fertility awareness method combines the use of barrier methods of contraception and observation of fertility signs. During the identified fertile phase of the menstrual cycle, a barrier method, such as a condom or diaphragm, would be utilized to prevent pregnancy (Johnson and Reich 1986; Kass-Annese and Hammond 1992). Technological refinements that allow more accurate prediction of ovulation may make NFP appealing to more women and couples by assisting in the timing of intercourse for achieving pregnancy and by decreasing required days of abstinence when attempting to avoid pregnancy (Flynn 1989; Robertson 1987; Zinamen 1988).

Considerable advances have been made in the field of home testing for fertility. The luteinizing hormone (LH) surge that immediately precedes ovulation has been used as a reference marker for timing ovulation. Dipstick immunoassay kits for detecting the LH surge in urine are available commercially and are useful in assisting couples to time intercourse when planning a pregnancy (France 1988). Digital and electronic thermometers are useful as they provide a reliable reading and reduce the recording time from five minutes to 45 seconds (Flynn 1989; France 1988; Zinamen 1988).

DATABASE

SUBJECTIVE

→ Obtain complete medical history with particular attention to menstrual cycle and fertility. See **Infertility** Protocol.
→ Women who have a greater chance of achieving pregnancy using fertility awareness include those who:
  ▪ have regular ovulatory cycles.
  ▪ are low risk for acquisition of STDs.
  ▪ are not lactating.
  ▪ are motivated to learn and use a natural method.
  ▪ have no medical conditions associated with infertility.
  ▪ have a male partner who has no medical condition associated with infertility (see **Infertility** Protocol).

OBJECTIVE

→ Primary fertility signs are the clinical indicators, or signs and symptoms, of the fertile period.
  ▪ These indicators reflect the underlying changes in estrogen and progesterone throughout the menstrual cycle and are observed and recorded by a woman using NFP (see **Figure 12HB.1, Sample Chart #1: Charting**).
→ Basal body temperature demonstrates a biphasic pattern during the menstrual cycle due to the thermogenic properties of progesterone.
  ▪ A shift of approximately 0.2°C-0.4°C (0.4°F-0.8°F) occurs after ovulation over a 24- to 48-hour period.
    • This shift is preceded by a dip, or nadir, in approximately 30 percent of cycles.

  ▪ A sustained rise in BBT generally is accepted as indicative of ovulation (Gross 1989).
→ Cervical mucus is secreted by the columnar epithelial cells of the cervix and also is regulated by estrogen and progesterone. As estrogen increases in response to follicular growth, mucus secretion begins and a moist vaginal secretion is observed.
  ▪ The mucus may be thick, pasty, yellow, or white but gradually increases in volume and becomes clear and watery.
    • The last day of watery mucus is described as the "peak day" which has been shown to be closely correlated with the LH peak.
    • After ovulation, under the influence of progesterone, the mucus becomes thick and sticky or dries up altogether (Gross 1989).
    • Penetration of sperm through the cervical mucus is maximal when viscoelasticity is minimal, which occurs just prior to ovulation. Sperm penetration begins to drop immediately after the peak in LH secretion (Katz 1991).
→ Other fertility signs can be observed along with BBT and mucus but should not be used alone to determine the fertile and infertile phases of the menstrual cycle.
  ▪ The changes in the cervical os follow a pattern similar to the changes in cervical mucus.
    • After menses, the cervix is easily reached by inserting fingers into the vagina and feels firm and closed.
    • As estrogen increases, the cervix softens and rises higher in the vagina and the os dilates.
    • After ovulation, the os closes and returns to a lower position in the vagina.
→ Additional signs and symptoms that occur and are associated with ovulation include mittelschmerz (intermenstrual pain), vaginal spotting or bleeding, backache, vulvar swelling, breast tenderness, skin and hair changes, and mood changes (Gross 1989; Kass-Annese and Hammond 1992).

ASSESSMENT

→ Use of fertility awareness or natural family planning methods to achieve or prevent pregnancy
→ Preovulatory infertile phase (Phase I)
→ Fertile phase (Phase II)
→ Postovulatory infertile phase (Phase III)
→ R/O anovulation

Figure 12HB.1. SAMPLE CHART # 1: CHARTING

CYCLE HISTORY:
Shortest **26**
Longest **29**
Last Cycle **29**
NAME _____

Month **August**   Year **1994**   Cycle Number **7**

Usual Time of Day: **7:00 AM**

Basal Body Temperature (scale 96.9 – 99.1)

99.1
99.0
98.0
97.0
96.9

Cycle Day: 1 2 3 4 5 6 7 8 9 10 11 12 13 14 15 16 17 18 19 20 21 22 23 24 25 26 27 28 29 30 31 32 33 34 35 36 37 38 39 40

Date

Day

Intercourse: ✓✓✓ (days 4,5,6) ✓ (day 19) ✓ (day 22) ✓✓ (days 24,25)

Mucus: * * * * D D D ? D M M M (M)(M)(M)(M) M M M D D D D D D D D *

Cervix: ° ° ° • •

Notes:

Mucus Description / Sensation:
- Dry
- woke @ 8:00am
- sticky, tacky, "paste"
- slippery, wet
- "egg white", sticky
- Dry
- bleeding

Disturbances, Schedule Changes, etc.:
- cramping
- cramping

MUCUS SYMBOLS:

*	S	D	M	(M)	(X)
Menses	Spotting	Dry day — No mucus (and dry vaginal sensation)	Sticky, pasty, crumbly mucus (and dry vaginal sensation)	Slippery, stretchy, wet mucus (and wet vaginal sensation)	Last day of very wet, slippery, stretchy mucus (and wet vaginal sensation)

CERVIX SYMBOLS: • • ° ○ ° • •

Source: Reprinted with permission from Kass-Annese, B., and Hammond, K. F. 1992. *Fertility awareness manual—an instructional guide for clients.* San Francisco: James Bowman.

→ R/O pregnancy

→ R/O premature ovarian failure

→ R/O menopause

PLAN

DIAGNOSTIC TESTS

→ Fertility assay kits utilizing detection of the LH surge in urine can be used to predict ovulation and plan the timing of intercourse.

→ See "Objective" section for discussion of primary and secondary fertility signs used in assessment of ovulation.

TREATMENT/MANAGEMENT

→ Determine if client is using fertility awareness or natural family planning methods to achieve or prevent pregnancy.

→ See "Patient Education" section for discussion regarding BBT and cervical mucus observations.

→ Recommend that couples abstain from intercourse for one cycle, or at least until the end of the fertile phase, so that the woman can become familiar with observing and charting her mucus pattern.

  ▪ Women who are familiar with observing and charting mucus patterns are prepared to use this information to assist in achieving pregnancy if desired.

  ▪ The effectiveness of NFP methods relies on a woman's daily observation and charting her fertility signs.

Basic natural family planning rules (see **Figure 12HB.2, Sample Chart #2: Natural Family Planning, Basic Rules**).

→ Counsel patient to abstain from intercourse during menstrual bleeding so as not to miss observation of cervical mucus.

→ Dry Days Rule.

  ▪ Intercourse can occur on the evening of any "dry" day when attempting to prevent pregnancy. (A dry day is when no mucus is observed and there is a dry vaginal sensation.)

  ▪ If semen is present in the vagina, it may take up to 24 hours to observe mucus again.

→ Early Mucus Rule.

  ▪ The fertile phase (Phase II) begins when any type of mucus appears or there is a wet vaginal sensation. When attempting to achieve pregnancy, intercourse should occur after mucus appears.

→ Peak Day Rule.

  ▪ The postovulatory infertile phase (Phase III) begins on the evening of the fourth day after the "peak" day.

  ▪ The "peak" day is the last day of wet, lubricative, or stretchy mucus or a wet vaginal sensation.

→ Thermal Shift Rule.

  ▪ The postovulatory infertile phase (Phase III) begins on the evening of the third day in a row that the BBT is above the coverline.

  ▪ The "coverline" is drawn 0.1°F above the highest of the first 10 temperatures of the menstrual cycle.

  ▪ The BBT may remain high during menses as a result of progesterone from the previous cycle. Disregard any abnormally high temperatures when drawing the coverline.

→ Phase III begins when both Peak Day Rule and the Thermal Shift Rule have been observed and applied (Kass-Annese and Hammond 1992, 20).

Optional natural family planning rules (for experienced users for avoiding pregnancy—see **Figure 12HB.3, Sample Chart #3: Natural Family Planning, Optional Rules**).

→ First 5 Days Rule.

  ▪ The first 5 days of the cycle are safe for unprotected intercourse if the Peak Day Rule and the Thermal Shift Rule were both observed in the previous cycle.

→ Modified Peak Day Rule.

  ▪ The postovulatory infertile phase (Phase III) begins on the evening of the third day after the peak day if the Thermal Shift Rule has been completed.

→ Cervix Open Rule.

  ▪ The postovulatory infertile phase (Phase III) begins on the evening of the fourth day after the cervix is the highest, softest, and most open. (This rule is used only to confirm the Peak Day or Thermal Shift Rules.)

→ 21 Day Rule.

  ▪ The preovulatory infertile phase (Phase I) is determined by subtracting 21 days from the number of days in the previous cycle if it was a normal cycle and there was a thermal shift (Kass-Annese and Hammond 1992).

Figure 12HB.2. SAMPLE CHART # 2: NATURAL FAMILY PLANNING, BASIC RULES

CYCLE HISTORY:

Usual Time of Day: 7:00 AM

Shortest 26
Longest 29

Last Cycle 29

NAME _____

Month August   Year 1994   Cycle Number 7

Basal Body Temperature

| | 99.1 | 99.0 | ... | 98.0 | ... | 97.0 | 96.9 |

Cycle Day: 1 2 3 4 5 6 7 8 9 10 11 12 13 14 15 16 17 18 19 20 21 22 23 24 25 26 27 28 29 30 31 32 33 34 35 36 37 38 39 40

Date

Day

Intercourse: ABSTAIN ✓✓✓

Mucus: * * * * D D D ? D M M M M M M M M M M D D D D D D D *

Cervix: P 1 2 3 4

Notes:

DRY DAY RULE

EARLY MUCUS RULE

PEAK DAY RULE

Mucus Description

Sensation

Disturbances, Schedule Changes, etc.

MUCUS SYMBOLS:

*	S	D	M	Ⓜ	⊗
Menses	Spotting	Dry day No mucus (and dry vaginal sensation)	Sticky, pasty crumbly mucus (and dry vaginal sensation)	Slippery, stretchy, wet mucus (and wet vaginal sensation)	Last day of very wet, slippery, stretchy mucus (and wet vaginal sensation)

CERVIX SYMBOLS: ●● ○ ○ ○ ●●

Source: Reprinted with permission from Kass-Annese, B., and Hammond, K. F. 1992. *Fertility awareness manual—an instructional guide for clients.* San Francisco: James Bowman.

Figure 12HB.3. SAMPLE CHART # 3: NATURAL FAMILY PLANNING, OPTIONAL RULES

CYCLE HISTORY:

Shortest _26_
Longest _29_

Last Cycle _29_

NAME ____ *previous cycle had a thermal shift and peak a*

Month _August_   Year _1994_   Cycle Number _7_

Usual Time of Day
7:00 AM

Basal Body Temperature

(temperature grid from 99.1 down to 96.9 with charted BBT readings)

Cycle Day	1	2	3	4	5	6	7	8	9	10	11	12	13	14	15	16	17	18	19	20	21	22	23	24	25	26	27	28	29	30	31	32	33	34	35	36	37	38	39	40

Date

Day

Intercourse: P 1 2 3 4

Mucus: * * * * D D D D D M M M (M)(M)(M)⊗ M M M D D D D D D D *

Cervix: (cervix symbols)

Notes: FIRST VERY LAST   C 1 2 3 4 R
FFDR FIRST
DR DAY RULE
TWENTY-ONE DAY RULE

CERVIX OPEN RULE

MODIFIED DAY RULE

Mucus Description

Sensation

Disturbances, Schedule Changes, etc.

MUCUS SYMBOLS:	*	S	D	M	(M)	⊗
	Menses	Spotting	Dry day No mucus (and dry vaginal sensation)	Sticky, pasty crumbly mucus (and dry vaginal sensation)	Slippery, stretchy, wet mucus (and wet vaginal sensation)	Last day of very wet, slippery, stretchy mucus (and wet vaginal sensation)

CERVIX SYMBOLS: ●● ○ ○ ○ ●●

Source: Reprinted with permission from Kass-Annese, B., and Hammond, K. F. 1992. *Fertility awareness manual—an instructional guide for clients.* San Francisco: James Bowman.

CONSULTATION

→ Clients who plan to use NFP to plan or prevent pregnancy should be referred to an NFP class taught by a trained instructor.

→ Clients whose charts show an abnormal bleeding pattern, short luteal phase, monophasic BBT pattern, or other abnormalities should be evaluated further to rule out pregnancy, anovulation, menopause, infertility, or other menstrual irregularities in consultation with a physician.

PATIENT EDUCATION

→ Teach the client her fertility signs during routine examination.

→ Reinforce need for formal instruction by a trained NFP instructor if client desires to use NFP for achieving or preventing pregnancy.

→ Advise client that effectiveness of natural methods depends on consistency in observation and charting of fertility signs.

→ Teach patient to obtain BBT as follows:
- should be taken after three hours of sleep.
- should be taken every day at the same time prior to activity, eating, drinking, or smoking.
- may be taken orally, rectally, or vaginally but same route must be used throughout the cycle.
- should be taken with a BBT thermometer, either glass or digital.
- a glass thermometer should be shaken down the night before and will hold the temperature until this is done.
- for an accurate reading, a glass thermometer must be kept in place for five minutes and a digital thermometer for 30 to 60 seconds.
- if a BBT reading on a glass thermometer is between two lines, record the lower temperature so as not to assume a rise.
- an alternative method of measuring BBT is to obtain first morning urine in a styrofoam cup, place a glass thermometer into the cup, and read the temperature when it is convenient.
- basal body temperature can be affected by stress, fever, travel, alcohol use, use of an electric blanket, and oversleeping, and these disturbances should be noted on the chart when they occur.

→ Teach client to check cervical mucus as follows:
- cervical mucus should be checked several times daily after menstrual bleeding stops and the most "fertile" observation of that day should be noted on the chart.
- vaginal sensations (wet or dry) should be noted as they may precede the observation of mucus.
- cervical mucus can be checked externally or internally.
- to check externally, wipe a piece of clean, white toilet paper across the vaginal opening and note the presence, quality, and consistency of mucus that appears on the paper.
- to check internally, insert two clean fingers into the vagina, gently press the fingers against the cervix, withdraw the fingers, and note quality and consistency of mucus between fingers.
- Kegel's exercises may help to push mucus closer to the vaginal opening for observation.
- mucus should not be checked when sexually aroused as vaginal lubrication may interfere with mucus observation.
- mucus observation can be affected by stress, illness, medications (antibiotics, antihistamines, vaginal spermicides, creams, and suppositories), douching, or the presence of semen.
- it takes 24 hours to clear the vagina; mucus observation may be unreliable during this time.

FOLLOW-UP

→ Advise client to return to clinic or NFP instructor to review or interpret charts as needed.

→ Document in progress notes and problem list.

Bibliography

Barbato, M., and Bertolotti, G. 1988. Natural methods for fertility control: A prospective study-first part. *International Journal of Fertility* (Suppl.):48–51.

Flynn, A.M. 1989. Natural family planning and the new technologies. *International Journal of Gynecology and Obstetrics* (Suppl.):123–127.

France, J.T. 1988. The development of fertility assay kits: An overview. *International Journal of Fertility* (Suppl.):5–10.

Gross, B.A. 1989. Clinical indicators of the fertile period. *International Journal of Gynecology and Obstetrics* (Suppl.):45–51.

Johnson, J.H., and Reich, J. 1986. The new politics of natural family planning. *Family Planning Perspectives* 18(6):277–282.

Kass-Annese, B., and Hammond, K.F. 1992. *Fertility awareness manual—An instructional guide for clients.* San Francisco: James Bowman.

Katz, D.F. 1991. Human cervical mucus: Research update. *American Journal of Obstetrics and Gynecology* 165(6):1984–1986.

Klaus, H. 1983. The role of the clinician in natural family planning. *Journal of American College Health* 32:114–120.

McCusker, M.P. 1982. The subfertile couple. *Journal of Obstetric, Gynecologic, and Neonatal Nursing* 11(3):157–162.

Queenan, J.T., and Moghissi, K.S. 1991. Natural family planning: Looking ahead. *American Journal of Obstetrics and Gynecology* 165(16):1979–1980.

Rice, F.J., Lanctot, C.A., and Garcia-Devesa, C. 1981. Effectiveness of the sympto-thermal method of natural family planning: An international study. *International Journal of Fertility* 26(3):22–230.

Robertson, E.M., ed. 1987. Psychology as a vital technology in natural family planning. *Contraceptive Technology Update* 8(7):85–87.

Spieler, J., and Thomas, S. 1989. Demographic aspects of natural family planning. *International Journal of Gynecology and Obstetrics* (Suppl.):133–144.

Trussell, J., and Grummer-Strawn, L. 1991. Further analysis of contraceptive failure of the ovulation method. *American Journal of Obstetrics and Gynecology* 165(6):2054–2059.

Zinamen, M.J. 1988. Why you should know about natural family planning. *Contemporary Ob/Gyn Special Issue* 69–86.

Winifred L. Star, R.N., C., N.P., M.S.

12-1

Pelvic Inflammatory Disease

By definition, the ascent of microorganisms from the lower to the upper genital tract is the cause of *pelvic inflammatory disease* (PID) (Peterson, Galaid, and Cates 1990). PID is a polymicrobial infection that encompasses endometritis, salpingitis, parametritis, oophoritis, pelvic peritonitis, tubo-ovarian abscess (TOA), or perihepatitis (Fitz-Hugh-Curtis [FHC] syndrome) (Paavonen 1990). In the United States, 1 million women are treated each year for PID, with staggering costs reaching $4.2 billion in 1990 (CDC 1991a).

Two major groups of microorganisms are responsible for the disease. One group includes sexually transmitted agents—predominantly *Neisseria gonorrhoeae* and *Chlamydia trachomatis*. The second group includes a wide variety of anaerobic and aerobic (facultative) organisms of the lower genital tract—*Escherichia coli, Hemophilus influenzae, Bacteroides, Gardnerella vaginalis, Peptococcus, Peptostreptococcus, Staphylococcus, Actinomyces*, and genital mycoplasmas. Distribution of etiological agents recovered from the upper genital tract in women with PID show 25 percent to 50 percent to be *N. gonorrhoeae*, 10 percent to 43 percent to be *C. trachomatis*, and 25 percent to 84 percent consisting of nongonococcal, nonchlamydial bacteria (Sweet 1991).

Infection of the upper genital tract may be precipitated by surgery, gynecological procedures, or extension of infection from the gastrointestinal (GI) tract, and may follow pregnancy or miscarriage/abortion (Keith, Berger, and Lopez-Zeno 1986). Bacterial vaginosis also has been suggested as an antecedent lower genital tract infection that may lead to acute PID (CDC 1991a; Eschenbach et al. 1988).

Theories regarding the mechanisms for transport of bacteria to the upper genital tract include vector transmission via sperm (or trichomonads), canalicular spread, passive transport of particulate matter, uterine contractions, movement by menstrual reflux or an intrauterine device (IUD) string, and hematogenous or lymphatic spread (Cates, Rolfs, and Aral 1990; Keith, Berger, and Lopez-Zeno 1986; Shafer and Sweet 1989). *N. gonorrhoeae* and *C. trachomatis* may pave the way for some cases of PID that are ultimately caused by secondary invasion with endogenous organisms (Cates, Rolfs, and Aral 1990; Keith, Berger, and Lopez-Zeno 1986; Westrom and Mardh 1990). STD pathogens more often are isolated from women with milder, short-standing infection, whereas endogenous organisms are associated with more advanced disease (Westrom and Mardh 1990). Male sexual contacts of women with PID have infection rates for gonorrhea and chlamydia up to 41 percent and 53 percent, respectively (CDC 1991a).

Because of the wide variation in signs and symptoms of PID among women, clinical diagnosis is difficult and imprecise. A broad clinical spectrum exists with acute, silent, and atypical PID; the PID residual syndrome (chronic PID); and postpartum/postabortal PID (CDC 1991a). Mild symptoms and vague, subtle signs are not easily recognized as PID and many cases go undiagnosed (CDC 1991a). Recently, there has been increasing evidence of an epidemic of silent asymptomatic infection; however, the magnitude of this problem has yet to be defined (Cates, Rolfs, and Aral 1990; Westrom and Mardh 1990). HIV-infected women with PID may be more clinically ill and refractory to medical management (CDC 1991a).

Perihepatitis, also known as FHC syndrome, is an extrapelvic manifestation of the dissemination of PID. Both *N. gonorrhoeae* and *C. trachomatis* are causative agents. Progression of the condition causes "violin-string" adhesions between the abdominal wall and liver. Incidence is 15 percent to 30 percent of all cases of PID.

Sequelae of PID are significant and include recurrent infection, ectopic pregnancy, involuntary infertility, pelvic adhesions, TOA, premature hysterectomy, chronic pelvic pain, and psychological depression. Delay in diagnosis and treatment probably contributes to inflammatory sequelae in the upper reproductive tract (CDC 1993).

After only one episode of PID, ectopic pregnancy risk increases sevenfold. Twelve percent of women are infertile after a single episode, 25 percent after two episodes, and over 50 percent after three or more episodes of PID (CDC 1991a). Thus, prevention of PID is of paramount importance. Health care providers can play a major role by maintaining up-to-date knowledge, providing appropriate preventive services—including medical management and risk-reduction counseling—and promoting sex partner evaluation (CDC 1991a).

DATABASE

SUBJECTIVE

→ Risk factors include:
- sexually active teenager (one-fifth of total cases; three times more likely to have PID diagnosis than 25-year to 29-year-old [CDC 1991a]).
- young age at first intercourse.
- high frequency of sexual intercourse.
- new/multiple sexual partners (especially within previous 30 days).
- partner with penile discharge/urethral symptoms/STD.
- STDs.
- previous PID.
- bacterial vaginosis.
- menses (within seven days of onset for STD-related PID).
- cervical ectopy (eversion).
- uterine instrumentation.
- pelvic surgery.
- bowel inflammation.
- tubercle infection.
- impairment of local/systemic defense mechanisms: congenital/acquired immunodeficiency syndromes, systemic diseases, immunosuppressive drugs, local defense mechanisms (iatrogenic injuries, immature local immune system).
- douching.
- alcohol and illicit drug use.

- IUD use (primarily in first few months after insertion; may not be STD-related).
- no/nonbarrier method of contraception.
- oral contraception (enhances cervical ectopy and increases *C. trachomatis* risk; symptomatic PID risk lowered).
- nonwhite race.
- lower socioeconomic status.
- never married; divorced, or separated.
- urban residence.
- smoking.
- behavioral factors: risk-taking, poor health-seeking behaviors (i.e., poor motivation/compliance with diagnosis/treatment/follow-up).

→ Symptoms may include:
- asymptomatic.
- bilateral lower abdominal or pelvic pain, most common symptom.
  - Pain is subacute at onset, usually within first week of menstrual cycle, non-radiating, with unspecific character, and unrelieved by position change.
- increase or change in vaginal discharge.
- dysuria, frequency, urgency.
- dyspareunia.
- dysmenorrhea.
- irregular bleeding: menorrhagia, menometrorrhagia, oligomenorrhea amenorrhea, post-coital bleeding.
- rectal symptoms: frequent stools, passage of mucus, tenesmus.
- fever, chills, malaise, nausea, vomiting in severe cases.
- right upper quadrant pain with FHC syndrome.
- complaints associated with silent or atypical infection.
  - May consist only of metrorrhagia, abnormal vaginal discharge, or urinary tract symptoms.

→ History:
- menstrual cycle history.
- contraceptive history.
- description of symptoms.
  - Onset, duration, quality/quantity, frequency, course, aggravating/relieving factors, associated symptoms.
- previous history of same/similar problem.
- STD history (including dates, treatment).
- sensitive questioning regarding recent sexual activity (including date of last exposure, sex practices, sites of exposure, number of partners

in past one to two months, use of condoms/spermicides).
- sex partner history.
- general health, including acute/chronic illness.
- surgical history.
- medications.
- allergies.
- habits.
- history of laboratory tests for syphilis, Hepatitis B, HIV.
- review of systems (CDC 1991b).

OBJECTIVE

NOTE: Traditional clinical criteria used in assessment/diagnosis of PID can be insensitive and nonspecific. A "low threshold" for diagnosis is recommended (CDC 1991a). See following discussion of "Diagnostic Tests, Diagnostic Criteria."

→ Patient may appear ill, distressed in severe cases.

→ Physical examination may reveal the following:
- vital signs:
  - fever present in <50 percent of cases (>38°C or >100.4°F).
  - assess for orthostatic changes in blood pressure and pulse as indicated.
- abdominal examination:
  - decreased bowel sounds, tenderness, rebound tenderness/guarding may be present.
  - right upper quadrant tenderness may be present in FHC syndrome.
- pelvic examination:
  - vagina: profuse, abnormal discharge may be present.
  - cervix: mucopurulent discharge may be present.
    - See details in "Diagnostic Tests" section of **Chlamydia Trachomatis** Protocol.
    - cervical motion tenderness (CMT) common.
    - cervical friability and/or erythema/edema in zone of ectopy may be present.
  - uterus: usually tender; assess size, shape, consistency, mobility.
  - adnexa: usually tender bilaterally; fullness or masses may be present.
  - recto/vaginal: may be tender; fullness/masses in cul-de-sac may be palpable.

NOTE: Pay attention to mucopurulent discharge and/or subtle signs of uterine/adnexal tenderness. Silent or atypical PID or subclinical endometritis may be present. Acute disease is more often associated with *N. gonorrhoeae* while silent disease is

thought to be due to *C. trachomatis* (Hemsell 1988).

→ gram stain of endocervical mucus may reveal ≥10-30 WBCs/oil immersion field and/or gram negative intracellular diplococci (gonorrhea).

→ wet mounts of vaginal discharge may reveal clue cells/amines indicative of bacterial vaginosis, or an increased number of WBCs associated with mucopurulent cervicitis and PID.
- Motile trichomonads and increased WBCs may be present with concomitant trichomoniasis.

→ endocervical cultures (or other direct tests) for *N. gonorrhoeae* and/or *C. trachomatis* may be positive.

→ WBC count may be >10,000/mm³ (two-thirds of cases).

→ ESR may be >15 mm/hour (three-fourths of cases).

→ C-reactive protein may be >2 mg/dl.

→ serological chlamydia antibodies may be present and are indicative of either past or present infection (have been found in 20 percent to 40 percent of women with a history of PID [CDC 1991a]).

→ serum levels of CA-125 are elevated in 25 percent to 35 percent of patients with PID.

ASSESSMENT

→ Pelvic inflammatory disease

→ R/O chlamydia and/or gonorrhea

→ R/O ectopic/intrauterine pregnancy

→ R/O appendicitis

→ R/O tubo-ovarian abscess

→ R/O FHC syndrome

→ R/O other causes of acute lower abdominal pain: dysmenorrhea, endometriosis, mittelschmerz, ovarian cyst, hemorrhagic ovarian cyst, ovarian torsion, ovarian tumor, polycystic ovaries, leiomyomata, threatened abortion, pelvic congestion, pelvic adhesions, constipation, gastroenteritis, diverticulitis, irritable bowel syndrome, inflammatory bowel disease, cystitis, pyelonephritis, kidney stone (Hemsell 1988; Shafer and Sweet 1989).

PLAN

DIAGNOSTIC TESTS

→ See previous "Objective" section.
- Clinical diagnosis of PID is imprecise. No single historical, physical, or lab finding is both sensitive and specific for diagnosis (CDC 1993).

→ Health care providers should maintain a low threshold of diagnosis for PID (CDC 1993).

→ Minimum diagnostic criteria:
- lower abdominal tenderness.
- adnexal tenderness.
- cervical motion tenderness (CDC 1991a, 1991b; CDC 1993; *San Francisco Epidemiologic Bulletin* 1992).
  NOTE: All three are necessary for diagnosis.

→ Additional diagnostic criteria (used to increase specificity of diagnosis):
- routine:
  - oral temperature >38.3°C (>101°F).
  - WBC count >10,000 mm³.
  - abnormal cervical or vaginal discharge.
  - mucopurulent cervicitis.
  - elevated ESR.
  - endocervical smear (gram stain) positive for gram-negative intracellular diplococci.
  - elevated C-reactive protein.
  - laboratory documentation of cervical infection with *N. gonorrhoeae* or *C. trachomatis*.
- Elaborate:
  - histopathological evidence of endometritis on endometrial biopsy.
  - purulent material in the peritoneal cavity obtained by culdocentesis or laparoscopy.
  - TOA on ultrasound or radiological test.
  - laparoscopic abnormalities consistent with PID (CDC 1991a, 1991b; CDC 1993; *San Francisco Epidemiologic Bulletin* 1992).

→ Additional considerations:
- endocervical cultures or antigen detection tests for *C. trachomatis* and endocervical cultures for *N. gonorrhoeae* should be performed.
- quantitative beta hCG as indicated to rule out ectopic pregnancy.
- serological HIV testing should be offered.
- endometrial biopsy may be performed to assess for presence of plasma cells indicative of endometritis, but not recommended if there is strong suspicion of PID. Consult with physician.
- culdocentesis may be performed to provide culture material and to assist in ruling out ectopic pregnancy or hemorrhagic ovarian cyst.

- ultrasound can aid in diagnosis and follow-up of TOA, identify dilated tubes suggestive of pyo-salpinx or hydrosalpinx, and identify fluid in the cul-de-sac (Paavonen 1990). A CT scan may on occasion be used to assess TOA (Soper 1991).
- laparoscopy (considered by many to be the "gold standard" for diagnosis as it provides direct evidence of inflamed fallopian tubes and allows culturing of specific intrapelvic site) may be considered when appendicitis cannot be ruled out, when PID diagnosis is questionable, and when the patient does not respond to conventional therapy (Morgan 1991).
  - Grading of the severity of salpingitis can be made via laparoscopy:
    - *mild*—tubes freely movable, erythema/ edema, purulent fimbrial exudate.
    - *moderate*—gross purulent material, more marked edema/erythema, tubes may not be freely movable.
    - *severe*—abscess, pyosalpinx, or inflammatory complex present (Jacobson and Westrom 1969).
- laparotomy is indicated in more severe cases (e.g., generalized peritonitis with sepsis due to ruptured TOA or severe PID with TOA refractory to medical management [Soper 1991]).
- additional tests may include (but are not limited to): Pap smear, VDRL or RPR, urinalysis, urine culture and sensitivities, liver enzymes, total bilirubin, alkaline phosphatase, amylase, Hepatitis B screen.

TREATMENT/MANAGEMENT

→ The goals of therapy are to preserve fertility, prevent ectopic pregnancy, and reduce long-term sequelae (Sweet 1991). Thus, it is important to attempt to make an accurate diagnosis and treat promptly.
- Subtle signs of uterine tenderness should be considered as possible atypical PID or subclinical endometritis.
- The three minimum criteria for pelvic inflammation, as detailed above, should be used to initiate empiric treatment in the absence of other established causes (CDC 1993).
- Therapy should not be withheld in a woman who fails to meet the criteria outlined above if PID is suspected (CDC 1991a; *San Francisco Epidemiologic Bulletin* 1992).

→ Ideally, patients with PID should be hospitalized, but this is not always practical. Hospitalization should be considered in the following instances:
- uncertain diagnosis.
- surgical emergencies such as ectopic pregnancy and appendicitis cannot be excluded.
- patient is an adolescent, is pregnant, has coexistent HIV infection, has nausea, is vomiting, or is severely ill.
- suspicion of pelvic abscess.
- patient is unable to follow, tolerate, or has failed to respond to an outpatient regimen.
- clinical follow-up in 72 hours is uncertain (CDC 1989; *San Francisco Epidemiologic Bulletin* 1992).
  - Discussion of inpatient therapy is beyond the scope of this protocol. Refer to 1993 CDC citation in bibliography.
- Choice of treatment regimen may be influenced by cost issues, patient acceptability, and regional differences in bacterial resistance (Peterson, Galaid, and Zenilman 1990).
  - Antimicrobial options should be broad-spectrum to include coverage for *N. gonorrhoeae, C trachomatis*, gram-negative bacteria, streptococci, and anaerobes (CDC 1993; *San Francisco Epidemiologic Bulletin* 1992).

→ Outpatient treatment:
- regimen A:
  - cefoxitin (Mefoxin®) 2 grams I.M., plus probenecid (Benemid®) 1 gram p.o. in a single dose concurrently,
                OR
    ceftriaxone (Rocephin®) 250 mg I.M. (or other parenteral third-generation cephalosporin—e.g., ceftizoxime [Cefizox®] or cefotaxime [Claforan®])
                PLUS
  - doxycycline (Vibramycin®) 100 mg p.o. BID for 14 days (CDC 1993).
- regimen B (broader coverage but more expensive):
  - ofloxacin (Floxin®) 400 mg p.o. BID for 14 days
                PLUS
  - clindamycin (Cleocin®) 450 mg p.o. QID for 14 days,
                OR
    metronidazole (Flagyl®) 500 mg BID for 14 days (CDC 1993).

NOTE: Refer to *PDR* regarding contraindications and adverse reactions of above medications.

→ Additional considerations:
- patients with FHC syndrome may be treated with the same antibiotic regimens as for PID (Soper 1991).
- IUD wearers should have the device removed soon after antimicrobial therapy has been initiated (CDC 1989).
  - Discuss alternative options for contraception.
- surgical intervention (laparoscopy or laparotomy) is indicated when medical management fails. A TOA that fails to respond to antibiotics or ruptures also will require surgery (laparoscopic drainage or drainage by culdocentesis) (Paavonen 1990).
- pregnant women with PID (or suspicion thereof) should be hospitalized and treated with parenteral antibiotics (CDC 1993).

→ Partner therapy:
- Evaluation and treatment of sexual partners is imperative.
  - Partners should be treated empirically with regimens effective against *N. gonorrhoeae* and *C. trachomatis* (CDC 1989, 1991a, 1993).
  - Provide referrals to provider/facility that offers appropriate STD care as indicated.

CONSULTATION

→ Consultation is recommended in all cases of PID. Co-management with a physician is appropriate for patients undergoing outpatient therapy. Cases of severe PID should be referred to a physician for management.

→ Referral to a physician is indicated when considering invasive diagnostic procedures (e.g., endometrial biopsy, culdocentesis) and for surgery.

→ When alternate diagnoses are suspected (e.g., ectopic pregnancy, appendicitis), refer patient to a physician.

→ If patient fails to respond to outpatient therapy, refer to a physician for further management.

PATIENT EDUCATION

→ Discuss the etiology, course, treatment, follow-up, and potential sequelae of PID and the importance of partner treatment.
- Patient-education materials are a helpful adjunct to teaching.
  - Written materials may be obtained from:

Information Services
Center for Prevention Services
Centers for Disease Control and Prevention,
EO6
Atlanta, Georgia 30333
(404) 639-1819

→ Advise patient to finish full course of medication and return for follow-up. Advise abstinence from intercourse until both patient and partner complete the prescribed medication.

→ Advise pelvic rest, adequate sleep/hydration/ nutrition. Analgesics may be taken (e.g., acetaminophen) as needed.

■ If symptoms worsen or recur, patient should return for reevaluation promptly.

→ Additional recommendations for all patients (especially teenagers) include: maintenance of healthy sexual behaviors, appropriate health-seeking behaviors, and use of barrier methods of contraception and spermicides. See **Table 12I.1, Recommendations for Individuals to Prevent STD/PID**, and **Table 13A.2, Safer Sex Guidelines**, p. 13-9.

→ Routine screening for STDs in high-risk groups and settings is advisable. These include adolescents; high-prevalence groups such as women with multiple partners, prostitutes, illicit drug users, individuals trading sex for drugs; facilities where high STD levels occur such as jails, emergency rooms (CDC 1991a).

→ Allow patient to ventilate her feelings of surprise, shame, fear, anger regarding diagnosis of an STD as indicated. Psychological support may be important for the patient in gaining control over her sexual situation and to enable her to prevent future STDs.

FOLLOW-UP

→ Patient should return for reassessment within 72 hours.

■ Criteria for clinical improvement include: defervescence, reduction in abdominal tenderness (direct or rebound), and reduction in uterine, adnexal, and cervical motion tenderness (CDC 1993).

■ Patients who do not respond to therapy (or worsen) within 72 hours should be hospitalized (CDC 1989). Physician consultation mandatory.

■ Symptoms that persist two to 14 days after outpatient treatment should arouse suspicion for an alternate diagnosis (e.g., appendicitis, endometriosis, ruptured ovarian cyst, adnexal

Table 12I.1. RECOMMENDATIONS FOR INDIVIDUALS TO PREVENT STD/PID

General preventive measures	Specific recommendations
Maintain healthy sexual behavior	Postpone initiation of sexual intercourse until at least 2 to 3 years after menarche.
	Limit number of sex partners.
	Avoid casual sex and sex with high-risk partners.
	Ask potential sex partners about STDs and inspect their genitals for lesions/discharge.
	Avoid sex with infected partners.
	Abstain from sex if STD symptoms appear.
Use barrier methods of contraception	Use condoms, diaphragms, and/or vaginal spermicides for STD protection and use consistently and correctly throughout all sex.
Adopt healthy medical-care-seeking behaviors	Seek medical evaluation promptly after having unprotected sex with someone who is suspected of having an STD.
	Seek medical care immediately when genital lesions/discharge appear.
	Seek routine check-ups for STDs if not in mutually monogamous relationship, even if there are no symptoms.
Comply with management instructions	Take all medications as directed, regardless of symptoms.
	Return for follow-up evaluation as instructed.
	Abstain from sex until symptoms resolve and treatment is completed.
Ensure partner evaluation	Notify all sex partners when diagnosed with an STD. Tell them to seek evaluation and treatment. If preferred, assist health care provider in identifying partner.

Adapted from Centers for Disease Control. 1991. Pelvic inflammatory disease: Guidelines for prevention and management. *Morbidity and Mortality Weekly Report* 40(RR-5):1-25.

torsion); laparoscopy may be considered in such cases (Morgan 1991).

• Alternative/additional antibiotic therapy also should be considered (CDC 1991a).

→ Follow-up cervical cultures should be performed seven to 10 days after completing therapy. Rescreening for both *C. trachomatis* and *N. gonorrhoeae* also may be performed four to six weeks after completing therapy (CDC 1993).

→ History on follow-up of ambulatory patients should include symptom status, medication compliance, drug reaction/side effects, partner therapy, sexual exposure, and use of condoms.

→ Follow up on all laboratory tests ordered. Treat all concomitant STDs and other identified conditions.

→ Negative HIV tests may be repeated in three to six months. Continue to encourage safer sex.

→ HIV-positive results should be conveyed in person and by a provider who has received training in the complexities of test disclosure.
  ▪ HIV-positive persons should be referred to the appropriate provider/agency for early intervention services.
  ▪ HIV-infected women with PID may be at increased risk for a complicated clinical course and should be followed closely.
→ Hepatitis B antigen-positive individuals should have liver function tests and receive counseling regarding the implications of their positive status and need for immunoprophylaxis of sex partners and household members.
  ▪ See **Hepatitis—Viral** Protocol.
→ In March, 1989, PID became a reportable communicable disease in California. A strict surveillance definition has been developed to determine which cases require reporting.
  ▪ Only those cases meeting the following criteria need to be reported (*San Francisco Epidemiologic Bulletin* 1992):
    • major criteria:
      –history of lower abdominal pain and presence of lower abdominal tenderness.
      –bilateral adnexal tenderness.
      –cervical motion tenderness.
      –absence of other causes of pelvic inflammation.
    • supporting criteria:
      –oral temperature >38°C (100.4°F).
      –gram stain of endocervical discharge revealing gram-negative intracellular diplococci.
      –gram stain of endocervical discharge revealing a minimum of 10 WBCs/oil immersion.
      –presence of a pelvic mass on examination.
      –gonococcal or chlamydial infection of the cervix.
  NOTE: Probable PID requires all four major criteria and any one of the supporting criteria; possible PID requires two of the four major criteria (*San Francisco Epidemiologic Bulletin* 1992).
→ Gonorrhea is a reportable disease in all states and chlamydia increasingly is reported (CDC 1991a). Providers should check with their local public health authorities regarding reporting criteria for STDs.
→ Document in problem list and progress notes.

Bibliography

Anderson, J.R., and Wilson, M. 1990. Caring for teenagers with salpingitis. *Contemporary Ob/Gyn* 35(8):103–111.

Cates, W., Rolfs, R.T., and Aral, S.O. 1990. Sexually transmitted diseases, pelvic inflammatory disease, and infertility: An epidemiologic update. *Epidemiologic Reviews* 12:199–220.

Centers for Disease Control. 1989. 1989 sexually transmitted disease treatment guidelines. *Morbidity and Mortality Weekly Report* 38(S-8).

———. 1991a. Pelvic inflammatory disease: Guidelines for prevention and management. *Morbidity and Mortality Weekly Report* 40(RR-5):1–25.

———. 1991b. *Sexually transmitted diseases. Clinical practice guidelines.* Atlanta: the Author.

———. 1993. 1993 sexually transmitted disease treatment guidelines. *Morbidity and Mortality Weekly Report* 42(RR-14):75–81.

Cunha, B.A., 1990. Treatment of pelvic inflammatory disease. *Clinical Pharmacy* 9:275–285.

Eschenbach, D.A., Hillier, S., Critchlow, C., Stevens, C., DeRouen, T., and Holmes, K.K. 1988. Diagnosis and clinical manifestations of bacterial vaginosis. *American Journal of Obstetrics and Gynecology* 158(4):819–827.

Forrest, K.A., Washington, A.E., Daling, J.R., Sweet, R.L. 1989. Vaginal douching as a possible risk factor for pelvic inflammatory disease. *Journal of the National Medical Association* 81(2):159–165.

Hemsell, D.L. 1988. Acute pelvic inflammatory disease. Etiologic and therapeutic considerations. *The Journal of Reproductive Medicine* 33(1):119–123.

Jacobson, L., and Westrom, L. 1969. Objectivized diagnosis of acute pelvic inflammatory disease: Diagnostic and prognostic value of routine laparoscopy. *American Journal of Obstetrics and Gynecology* 105:1088–1098.

Keith, L.G., Berger, G.S., and Lopez-Zeno, J. 1986. New concepts on the causation of pelvic inflammatory disease. *Current Problems in Obstetrics, Gynecology and Infertility* 9(1):7–77.

Morgan, R.J. 1991. Clinical aspects of pelvic inflammatory disease. *AFP Practical Therapeutics* 43(5):1725–1732.

Paavonen, J. 1990. Pelvic inflammatory disease. *Seminars in Dermatology* 9(2):126–132.

Peterson, H.B., Galaid, E.I., and Cates, W. 1990. Pelvic inflammatory disease. *Medical Clinics of North America* 74(6):1603–1615.

Peterson, H.B., Galaid, E.I., and Zenilman, J.M. 1990. Pelvic inflammatory disease: Review of treatment options. *Reviews of Infectious Diseases* 12(Suppl. 6):S656–S664.

Peterson, H.B., Walker, C.K., Kahn, J.G., Washington, A.E., Eschenbach, D.A., and Faro, S. 1991. Pelvic inflammatory disease: Key treatment issues and options. *Journal of the American Medical Association* 266(18):2605–2611.

Rice, P.A., and Schacter, J. 1991. Pathogenesis of pelvic inflammatory disease: What are the questions? *Journal of the American Medical Association* 266(18):2587–2593.

San Francisco Epdemiologic Bulletin. 1992. San Francisco: Department of Public Health, Bureau of Epidemiology and Disease Control.

Shafer, M., and Sweet, R.L. 1989. Pelvic inflammatory disease in adolescent females. *Pediatric Clinics of North America* 36(3):513–533.

Soper, D.E. 1991. Surgical considerations in the diagnosis and treatment of pelvic inflammatory disease. *Surgical Clinics of North America* 71(5):947–963.

Sweet, R.L. 1991. Acute salpingitis treatment—an update. *Contemporary Ob/Gyn* 36(12):43–52.

Washington, A.E., Cates, W., and Wasserheit, J.N. 1991. Preventing pelvic inflammatory disease. *Journal of the American Medical Association* 266(18):2574–2580.

Washington, A.E., Aral, S.O., Wolner-Hanssen, P., Grimes, D.A., and Holmes, K.K. 1991. Assessing risk for pelvic inflammatory disease and its sequelae. *Journal of the American Medical Association* 266(18):2581–2586.

Wasserheit, J.N. 1987. Pelvic inflammatory disease and infertility. *Maryland Medical Journal* 36(1):58–63.

Westrom, L., and Mardh, P.-A. 1990. Acute pelvic inflammatory disease. In *Sexually transmitted diseases*, 2d ed., eds, K.K. Holmes, P.-A. Mardh, P.F. Sparling, P.J. Wiesner, W. Cates, Jr., S.M. Lemon, and W.E. Stamm, pp. 593–613. New York: McGraw-Hill.

Wolner-Hanssen, P., Kiviat, N.B., and Holmes, K.K. 1990. Atypical pelvic inflammatory disease: Subacute, chronic, or subclinical upper genital tract infection in women. In *Sexually transmitted diseases.* 2d ed., eds. K.K. Holmes, P.-A. Mardh, P.F. Sparling, P.J. Wiesner, W. Cates, Jr., S.M. Lemon, and W.E. Stamm, pp. 615–620. New York: McGraw-Hill.

12-J

Pelvic Masses

Patients with *pelvic masses* may present with various symptoms and signs or may be completely asymptomatic. The etiologies of pelvic masses are quite varied and may stem from the genital tract, GI tract, or urinary tract. See **Table 12J.1, Pelvic Masses—Differential Diagnoses.** Management of pelvic masses depends, to a large extent, on the age of the patient, size and nature of the mass, and symptoms involved. Common types of pelvic masses by age group will be highlighted.

During adolescence, imperforate hymen, vaginal agenesis, or a vaginal septum may give rise to a hematocolpos or hematometrium with secondary pelvic or abdominal masses. The majority of adnexal masses in this age group are functional ovarian cysts. Benign cystic teratoma is the most common neoplastic entity. Solid adnexal tumors, although rare in adolescence, are usually dysgerminomas or malignant teratomas. Paraovarian and paratubal cysts and extragenital masses need to be considered as well (Herbst et al. 1992).

Masses seen in women during the reproductive years develop from the uterus, cervix, adnexa, and other organ systems. Findings include ectopic pregnancy, trophoblastic disease, myomas, and a variety of adnexal masses including functional ovarian cysts, benign cystic teratomas, endometriomas, and cancer. A pelvic kidney is one of the more common extragenital tumors in this age group.

In the perimenopause and menopause, endometrial adenocarcinoma, sarcoma, and mixed uterine tumors are more common. The chance of malignancy associated with an adnexal mass increases during this time. Ovarian endometriomas, especially in women on hormone replacement, also should be considered. Extragenital masses are quite common, including diverticulitis, and bowel, kidney,

musculoskeletal and lymphatic system tumors. Sex-cord stromal tumors may occur at any age but are found predominantly during menopause.

The pelvic masses detailed in this section are representative of some of the more commonly encountered gynecological pathologies in women's primary care.

Fibroids and Adenomyosis

Leiomyomata uteri, commonly known as *fibroids*, are estrogen-sensitive, essentially benign muscle cell tumors of the uterus. They are the most frequently encountered tumors of the pelvis, with the highest incidence in a woman's fifth decade of life. Etiology is unknown, but it is estimated that myomas occur in about ten percent of whites and 30 percent of blacks over the age of 35 years. This prevalence increases to 30 percent and 50 percent, respectively, by age 50 years (DiSaia and Creasman 1989; Lichtman and Papera 1990).

After menopause, fibroids generally regress secondarily to reduced estrogen stores. Myomas are classified into subgroups according to their anatomic location. (See following "Objective" section.) Complications arising from fibroids may include degeneration, infarction, infection, infertility, pregnancy complications, and sarcomatous change (0.3 percent to 0.7 percent) (Herbst et al. 1992).

Adenomyosis is a result of aberrant growth of endometrial glands and stroma from the basalis layer of the endometrium into the myometrium. The stimulus for this benign invasion is unknown; estimated incidence is ten percent to 20 percent (Gomel, Munro, and Rowe 1990). The diagnosis commonly is made incidentally by the pathologist at hysterectomy or autopsy. The signifi-

Table 12J.1. PELVIC MASSES—DIFFERENTIAL DIAGNOSES

Vaginal

Developmental anomalies
–imperforate hymen
–vaginal septum
Relaxation
–cystocele
–rectocele
–enterocele

Foreign body
Bartholin's/Gartner's duct cyst
Neoplasm
–sarcoma botryoides
–vaginal cancer
–benign lesions

Cervical

Nabothian cyst
Fibroid

Ectopic
Carcinoma

Uterine

Pregnancy
–cornual
–cervical
Displacement
–retro
–lateral
Fibroids
Adenomyosis
Round ligament tumors
Malignancies
–endometrial adenocarcinoma
–adenosquamous carcinoma
–sarcoma

Rare tumors
–hemangiopericytoma
Congenital anomalies
–defects in Müllerian fusion
–associated urinary tract
 anomalies
Hematometra/Pyometra
–transverse vaginal septum
–vaginal atresia
–cervical stenosis
–cervical cancer

Tubal

Mesonephric duct remnants
–paraovarian cyst
–hydatid of Morgagni
Ectopic
Acute salpingitis
–pyosalpinx
–tubo-ovarian abscess
Chronic salpingitis
–hydrosalpinx
Tuberculosis

Other chronic granulomas
Benign neoplasms
–fibroids/fibromas
–teratomas
–rare lipomas, hemangiomas,
 adenoid tumors
–salpingitis isthmica nodosa
Tubal carcinoma

Ovarian

Epithelial stromal tumors
–serous
–mucinous
–endometroid
–clear cell
–Brenner
–mixed
–undifferentiated carcinoma
–unclassified
Germ cell tumors
–dysgerminoma
–endodermal sinus tumor
–embryonal carcinoma
–polyembryoma
–choriocarcinoma
–teratoma
–mixed forms
Sex-cord stromal tumors
–granulosa-stromal
–androblastomas:Sertoli-
 Leydig
–gynadroblastoma
–unclassified

Lipid (lipoid) cell tumors
Gonadoblastoma
–pure
–mixed
Soft tissue tumors
Unclassified tumors
Secondary (metastatic) tumors
Tumor-like conditions
–pregnancy luteoma
–hyperplasia of ovarian
 stroma, hyperthecosis
–massive edema
–follicle cyst
–corpus luteum cyst
–polycystic ovaries
–luteinized follicle cysts and/
 or corpora lutea
–endometriosis
–surface-epithelial inclusion
 cysts
–simple cysts
–paraovarian cysts
–inflammatory lesions

Extragenital

Endometriosis
Inflammatory
–appendicitis
–diverticulitis
–perirectal abscess
Hematocele
Ascites
Urological
–bladder
–urachal cysts
–pelvic kidney
–transplant
–tumor
Gastrointestinal
–inflammatory
–tumor
–stool/gas

Retroperitoneal
–teratoma
–meningomyelocele
–presacral chordoma
–lymphocyst
–lymphoma
–sarcoma group
Abdominal wall lesions
–hematoma
–muscle tumor
–abscess
–lipoma
–scar implants
Foreign body

Source: Adapted from Serov, S.F., and Sculley, R.E. 1973. Histological typing of ovarian tumors. International histological typing of tumors, 9. Geneva: World Health Organization; Gates, E. 1990. Pelvic masses—Lecture notes. University of California, San Francisco.

cance of adenomyosis is its similarity to leiomyomata, with uterine enlargement and symptoms which may mimic fibroids. Other pelvic pathology such as myomas, endometriosis, endometrial hyperplasia, or cancer may coexist (Herbst et al. 1992).

Ovarian Masses

The finding of an enlarged ovary may be indicative of a non-neoplastic functional cyst or the presence of a benign or malignant cystic or solid neoplasm. A wide range of types and patterns of ovarian tumors exist due to the complexity of ovarian embryology (Margolis and Greenwood 1993) (see **Table 12J.1**). Within each category of

ovarian tumor, a designation is made regarding its nature as benign, of low malignant or borderline malignant potential, or malignant (Lichtman and Papera 1990).

Treatment of ovarian masses depends on the etiology and age of the patient. In the premenarchal and postmenopausal female, ovarian masses must be considered highly suspect for malignancy and promptly investigated (DiSaia and Creasman 1989). Most pelvic masses occur during the reproductive years, with both benign and malignant lesions presenting; the majority, however, are benign. Some of the more common ovarian neoplasms are discussed in this protocol.

Among the most frequently encountered ovarian masses are *functional cysts*. A *follicular cyst* may form if the dominant follicle fails to ovulate or when other follicles fail to undergo normal atresia (Neinstein 1991). Estrogen may be produced by the cyst and cause menstrual irregularity. Normally, these cysts resolve in one to two months.

Corpus luteum cysts are less common. They occur after ovulation when limited spontaneous bleeding fills the central cavity of the corpus luteum with blood. Subsequently, the blood is resorbed, and a cystic space remains. If bleeding is excessive, the corpus luteum may rupture and precipitate a surgical emergency. Corpus luteum cysts are more likely than follicular cysts to produce menstrual irregularities. Smaller corpus luteum cysts often resolve spontaneously.

Other physiological ovarian cysts, known as *theca lutein cysts,* may be associated with hydatidiform mole, choriocarcinoma, or chorioadenoma destruens (Griffiths and Berkowitz 1986). These regress after removal of the trophoblastic tissue. *Simple cysts* frequently occur in postmenopause.

Benign cystic teratomas (dermoids) are unique germ cell tumors that contain among other features teeth, hair, and sebaceous glands. They are the most common ovarian neoplasms in women under age 30 years, comprising 20 percent to 25 percent of all ovarian neoplasms and 33 percent of all benign tumors (excluding follicular and corpus luteum cysts).

Complications of dermoids include torsion, rupture, infection, and hemorrhage; malignant transformation occurs in one percent to two percent, usually in women over 40 years of age. An association with thyrotoxicosis, carcinoid syndrome, and autoimmune hemolytic anemia may occur with dermoid cysts (Herbst et al. 1992). *Serous and mucinous cystadenomas* are other common benign lesions that may also have a malignant variety (DiSaia and Creasman 1989).

Fibromas are the most common benign solid tumors of the ovary, usually occurring in women in their late 40s. They constitute about five percent of all benign ovarian neoplasms and 20 percent of all solid tumors of the ovary. Their potential toward malignancy is less than one percent (Herbst et al. 1992). *Endometriosis* of the ovary is another very common cause of ovarian enlargement. See **Endometriosis** Protocol for further discussion.

Torsion of the ovary (or tube and ovary) is an uncommon but important cause of pelvic pain associated with a pelvic mass. Most torsions occur with benign ovarian masses of 8 cm to 12 cm. Pregnancy and enlarged ovaries due to ovulation induction are predisposing factors. The relative risk of torsion also is increased with dermoids, paraovarian cysts, solid benign tumors, and serous cysts. Most often the right ovary is involved; in ten percent of cases the contralateral adnexa may torse at a future time (Herbst et al. 1992). TOA is discussed in the **Pelvic Inflammatory Disease** Protocol.

Sex-cord stromal tumors account for about six percent of ovarian neoplasms and the majority of hormonally active tumors. Some of these tumors will produce hirsutism and other signs of masculinization (Herbst et al. 1992).

The risk of malignancy in an ovarian tumor is 33 percent in a woman over age 45 years, and less than one in 15 for women 20 years to 45 years of age. More than half of ovarian cancers are found in women over age 50 years. Ovarian cancer is the leading cause of death from gynecological cancer. Unfortunately, this type of cancer does not often cause symptoms until metastasis has occurred. The lower reproductive tract, the GI tract, and the breast are the most frequent sites of origin of tumors metastatic to the ovary (Herbst et al. 1992).

DATABASE

SUBJECTIVE

Fibroids and adenomyosis

→ The majority of women with fibroids are asymptomatic.

→ Symptoms of fibroids may include:
  ▪ abnormal bleeding (30 percent of women):
    • menorrhagia, hypermenorrhea, metrorrhagia; severity of bleeding and other symptoms depend upon location, size, and number of fibroids.
  ▪ pelvic pressure, pelvic pain/dull ache/heaviness, dysmenorrhea, urinary urgency/frequency/incontinence, constipation, or other lower GI or rectal symptoms.
  ▪ increased abdominal girth without appreciable weight change.
  ▪ infertility, spontaneous abortion.
  ▪ dyspnea.
  ▪ symptoms of anemia (see **Anemia** Protocol).
  ▪ severe, acute pelvic pain may be associated with sudden degeneration or torsion of fibroid.

→ Features of adenomyosis may include:
  ▪ woman usually multiparous; onset between ages 35 years to 50 years.
  ▪ secondary dysmenorrhea.
  ▪ menorrhagia, hypermenorrhea, polymenorrhea, or premenstrual spotting.
  ▪ dyspareunia occasionally—deep, midline pelvis.
  ▪ uterine tenderness before and during menstruation.
  ▪ increasing symptom severity in untreated cases.

- fifty percent of cases with associated leiomyomas.
→ Inquire regarding previous diagnosis of fibroids/adenomyosis, prior uterine size, diagnostic modalities, associated symptoms, and treatment regimens.

Ovarian masses

→ Most ovarian neoplasms are asymptomatic unless rupture or torsion occurs, in which case sudden severe unilateral lower abdominal and pelvic pain, intraperitoneal hemorrhage, and signs of shock may ensue. Internal bleeding from a corpus luteum cyst may follow coitus, trauma, exercise, or a pelvic examination.

→ Symptoms are usually not specific to the type of tumor. Complaints may include:
- mild lower abdominal or pelvic discomfort, ache, pain, pressure, heaviness, or unilateral cramping.
  - Pain may be referred to the iliac or inguinal area; inner, upper thigh; or vulva.
- dyspareunia.
- increased abdominal girth; a mass or ascites.
- in some cases, specific symptoms may be dependent upon the size, location, and type or tumor.

→ Additional symptoms may include:
- irregularity of the menstrual cycle—e.g., delayed flow, irregular/intermittent spotting or menorrhagia; oligomenorrhea, amenorrhea.
- urinary frequency/obstruction/incontinence.
- anorexia, nausea, vomiting, eructation, flatulence, constipation, or other alteration in bowel habits.
- edema/varicosities of lower extremities.
- dyspnea.
- symptoms/signs of feminization or masculinization.
- signs of Cushing's syndrome or hyperthyroidism.

→ Moderate anorexia, nausea, vague abdominal or pelvic discomfort, abdominal enlargement or distention, increased flatulence or bloating, and/or indigestion should arouse suspicion for ovarian cancer.

→ Colicky pain, melena, altered bowel habits, or diminution of stool caliber is associated with sigmoid cancer.

→ Postulated risk factors for ovarian cancer include: asbestos, talc, intake of animal fat, nulliparity, family history of ovarian cancer, early menarche, late menopause, history of ovarian dysfunction, genetic disorders, Peutz-Jeghers syndrome, Jewish lineage, and a history of breast, endometrial, or colorectal cancer (Lichtman and Papera 1990).

→ History should include thorough evaluation of the menstrual cycle characteristics, last normal and previous normal menstrual periods, signs/symptoms of pregnancy, questioning regarding nature of pain and other associated symptoms as above, sexual/contraceptive history, medical history, medication history, family history of gynecological cancer.

OBJECTIVE

Fibroids and adenomyosis

→ Thorough abdominal, pelvic, and rectovaginal examinations should be performed.
- Patient should void prior to examination.

→ Typical findings related to fibroids include a firm, irregular, mobile, nontender enlarged uterus; the adnexa may be difficult to palpate secondary to the enlarged or laterally displaced uterus.
- Description of uterine size is generally in gestational weeks; e.g., ten-week size.

→ A normal retroverted uterus may mimic a posterior wall myoma projecting into the cul-de-sac; a pedunculated fibroid may be confused with an ovarian tumor.

→ Degenerating myomas may result in the uterus becoming softer and more cystic.

→ Uterine fixation or tenderness may indicate infection or endometriosis.

→ A menopausal woman's fibroids should demonstrate regression in size.
- An enlarging uterus after menopause should arouse suspicion for sarcomatous degeneration or possibly an ovarian neoplasm.

→ In adenomyosis, the uterus is diffusely enlarged, globular with a finely nodular surface, possibly tender; usually it is two to three times normal size but often not greater than 14-week size unless there are concomitant fibroids.

→ Anatomical location of fibroids may include:
- *interstitial* (intermural): most common; within the uterine wall, rounded shape.
- *submucosal*: protruding into uterine cavity; five percent to ten percent of all myomas; associated with bleeding problems, infertility, spontaneous abortion; growth may lead to pedunculation.

- *subserosal* (subperitoneal): bulging through outer uterine wall; unlikely related to infertility unless obstructing fallopian tubes.
- *interligamentous*: within broad ligament.
- *pedunculated*: myoma with thin pedicle attached to base of uterus; unlikely related to infertility unless obstructing fallopian tubes; difficult to distinguish from ovarian masses.
- *parasitic*: extruding from uterus with accessory blood supply; may grow laterally into broad ligament and produce hydroureter; difficult to distinguish from ovarian masses.
- *cervical*: three percent to eight percent of myomas; most small, asymptomatic; may become pedunculated and protrude through external os leading to ulceration/infection. (Herbst et al. 1992; Lichtman and Papera 1990).

Ovarian masses

→ All patients must void prior to examination.

→ Vital signs as indicated.
  - Temperature may be elevated and hypotension/tachycardia present in cases of rupture.

→ Complete abdominal examination, including inspection, auscultation, percussion, and palpation, and a complete pelvic examination are mandatory. Rectovaginal examination is mandatory to fully palpate the surface of a mass in the posterior cul-de-sac and/or nodularity of the uterosacral ligaments.
  - Note location of the mass with respect to the uterus and its mobility, adherence, consistency, contour, size, and bilaterality.
  NOTE: Pelvic examinations should be performed gingerly so rupture is not caused inadvertently.

→ Abdominal rigidity with local/rebound tenderness may be present if rupture of an ovarian cyst or TOA has occurred.

→ Dullness over the mass, tympany in the flanks, and no tone difference with position change is characteristic of a cyst. Shifting dullness in the flanks is characteristic of ascites.

→ Lower abdominal veins may be distended in the presence of large ovarian cysts.

→ The majority of ovarian neoplasms are lateral or posterior to the uterus (an exception is the dermoid, which is anterior to the broad ligament).

→ A smooth, regular surface, softness/flaccidity, and mobility suggest a benign cyst; a uniformly firm or tensely fluctuant mass suggests a benign

neoplasm; an irregular/nodular surface is more indicative of malignancy.

→ Fixation suggests endometriosis, an inflammatory process, adhesions, or malignancy.

→ Firm cul-de-sac nodules or uterosacral ligamentous nodularity in association with an ovarian mass strongly suggests endometriosis or metastatic carcinoma.

→ A palpable ovary in a postmenopausal female suggests the possibility of malignancy. Bilateral ovarian findings in any age group also may be indicative of malignancy.

→ Follicular cysts may be from a few millimeters to 15 cm (average 2.5 cm to 3 cm), solitary or multiple; corpus luteum cysts range from 3 cm to 10 cm in diameter (average 4 cm).

→ Dermoids range from a few millimeters to 25 cm; the majority are less than 10 cm. They may be single or multiple and may occur bilaterally in ten percent to 15 percent of cases.

→ Fibromas range in size from small nodules to 50-pound tumors with an average diameter of 6 cm; the majority are unilateral.
  - Ascites and hydrothorax may occur with fibromas or other ovarian tumors (Meigs' syndrome).
  - The effusion must be tapped by a physician for cytological evaluation.

→ Manifestations of hormone-producing tumors also should be evaluated.

ASSESSMENT

→ Uterine mass
  - R/O uterine fibroid(s) (also known as myoma(s), leiomyoma(s), fibromyoma(s))
    • R/O leiomyosarcoma
    • R/O endometrial carcinoma
  - R/O adenomyosis
    • R/O endometriosis
    • R/O multiple leiomyomas
    • R/O salpingitis isthmica nodosa
    • R/O idiopathic uterine hypertrophy of multiparity (fibrosis uteri)
    • R/O pelvic congestion syndrome
  - R/O ovarian/bowel tumors
  - R/O pregnancy
  - R/O anemia
  - R/O uterine/urinary tract infection
  - R/O endometrial hyperplasia/cancer

→ Ovarian mass

- R/O benign versus malignant lesion
- R/O ectopic/intrauterine pregnancy
- R/O rupture/torsion
- R/O pyosalpinx, hydrosalpinx, TOA
- R/O appendicitis
- R/O conditions mimicking ovarian neoplasms: pedunculated fibroid, low-lying, distended cecum, redundant sigmoid colon, appendiceal abscess, impacted feces, carcinoma of the sigmoid colon, diverticulitis, hematoma of rectus muscle, urachal cyst, retroperitoneal neoplasm/ abscess, pelvic kidney

PLAN

DIAGNOSTIC TESTS

Fibroids and adenomyosis

→ Presumptive diagnosis usually made on abdominal and bimanual pelvic examination.

→ Pelvic ultrasound may be ordered for confirmation, baseline assessment, and clinical follow-up of fibroid size progression.
- A sonogram also is indicated in cases where symptoms are suggestive of fibroids but none are palpable.
- Ultrasonography also will be useful to distinguish fibroids from the most common misdiagnosis of ovarian neoplasm and in identifying adenomyotic implants in the myometrium.

→ Although quite costly, MRI has been used to assess number, size, and location of fibroids, to distinguish other pathological disease states, and to evaluate fibroid size progression and response to therapy.

→ Abdominal x-ray may be less commonly used to identify concentric uterine calcifications. Generally it is not clinically useful to rule out fibroids; however, fibroids may be diagnosed incidentally by x-ray when ordered for other reasons.

→ Hysteroscopy may be used to demonstrate filling of small myometrial cavities, but is indicated only in rare cases to direct management.

→ Definitive diagnosis can be made only by histopathology of the lesion obtained via laparoscopy or laparotomy, though these procedures are not generally performed unless indicated for management (see "Treatment/ Management" section).

→ Endometrial hyperplasia should be ruled out with endometrial biopsy if a woman has associated abnormal bleeding or adenomyosis.

→ Additional tests may include (but are not limited to): Pap smear, pregnancy test, CBC, urinalysis, urine culture and sensitivities, ESR, endocervical cultures, hysteroscopy, hysterosalpingogram (HSG), and intravenous pyelogram (IVP).

Ovarian masses

→ Preliminary diagnosis usually is made on bimanual pelvic examination.

→ If the bowel is filled with fecal material and the examination is difficult or inconclusive, a cathartic or enema may be prescribed. Re-examination should be performed after the patient's bowel has been evacuated.

→ Abdominal or transvaginal ultrasound, CT scanning, and MRI are the techniques used in the evaluation and diagnosis of ovarian neoplasms.

→ X-ray evaluation may identify calcified lesions— e.g., teeth of a dermoid cyst.

→ Culdocentesis performed by a physician is used in acute cases when intraperitoneal bleeding or hemorrhage is suspected.

→ Pap smears may pick up transmigrating ovarian carcinoma cells.

→ Paracentesis is indicated for evaluation of ascitic fluid.

→ Laparoscopy may be indicated for diagnostic evaluation when the source of the mass is unclear. Definitive diagnosis of tumor type is made by histological diagnosis when surgery is indicated.

→ Endoscopy is indicated if there has been GI bleeding or with suggestion of rectosigmoid disease. An upper GI series also may be indicated.

→ Additional tests may include (but are not limited to): CBC; ESR; specific ovarian tumor markers: beta-hCG, CA-125, alpha-fetoprotein (AFP), carcinoembryonic antigen (CEA), placental alkaline phosphatase (PLAP), lactic dehydrogenase (LDH), fibrin split products, lipid-associated sialic acid in plasma (LSA), urinary gonadotropin fragments (UGF), neuron-specific enolase (NSE), TA-4, NB/70K, TAG 72, and/or CA 15-3; testosterone; DHEAS; urinalysis; urine culture and sensitivities; electrolytes; blood coagulation studies; renal function studies; liver chemistries; chest x-ray; EKG; IVP; contrast study of the colon. Consult with physician regarding ordering of specific tests.

→ See protocols on **Endometriosis, Ectopic Pregnancy, Amenorrhea—Secondary** (for polycystic ovary disease), and **Pelvic Inflammatory Disease** (for TOA) for additional diagnostic tests.

TREATMENT/MANAGEMENT

Fibroids and adenomyosis

→ Conservative management is all that is required in an asymptomatic woman. Re-examination after confirmation of fibroids (or suspicion of adenomyosis) is done initially in 3 months and usually every 6 months thereafter (more often as indicated).

→ Indications for definitive treatment of myomas include abnormal bleeding, pain, urinary tract or bowel disorders, infertility problems, recurrent spontaneous abortion, rapidly enlarging fibroids, anemia.

→ More aggressive treatment modalities are tailored to the individual patient based on severity of symptoms and plans for childbearing.
  ▪ Surgical options include removal via the resectoscope during hysteroscopy, laparoscopic removal techniques, myomectomy, and hysterectomy.
    • Indications for hysterectomy may include:
      –large multiple fibroids.
      –a symptomatic woman who has completed her childbearing.
      –cases of intractable bleeding or rapidly enlarging fibroids.
      –a uterus >12 weeks gestational size.
      –concomitant pelvic pathology such as endometriosis and adhesions.

→ GnRH agonists may be employed to induce a hypogonadotrophic, hypogonadal state.
  ▪ These costly agents may be used preoperatively to reduce the size of the fibroids/uterus, in cases of severe anemia, in the perimenopause to avoid surgery, or when medical conditions preclude surgery.
    • Reduction may be 30 percent to 50 percent in 3 to 6 months, but after therapy, uterine fibroids usually return to pretreatment size.
  ▪ Side effects of GnRH therapy are varied and may include: hot flushes, vaginal dryness, weight gain, amenorrhea, loss of bone density, decreased libido/breast size, depression, fatigue,

headaches, insomnia, arthralgias/myalgias, and adverse effects on lipid metabolism.
    • To counter some of these effects, "add-back" estrogen/progestin therapy may be used.
  ▪ Fibroid size reduction during therapy must be monitored via ultrasound or MRI.
  ▪ No change should arouse suspicion for leiomyosarcoma.
  ▪ Specific protocols for GnRH therapy have been developed. (See references Friedman and Barbieri 1988 and Anderson 1992a.) Patient generally is managed by a physician.
  ▪ Depo-medroxyprogesterone acetate (Depo-Provera®) also has been used as a medical treatment. Consult with a physician.
  ▪ Iron-deficiency anemia must be treated. See **Anemia** Protocol.
  ▪ Medical treatment for adenomyosis is largely ineffective. Oral contraceptives or prostaglandin synthetase inhibitors may be tried. Hysterectomy is the definitive therapy and is indicated in certain cases. Malignancy should be ruled out with endometrial biopsy prior to surgery (Herbst et al. 1992).

Ovarian masses

→ Goals of management include: establishment that the mass is ovarian in origin, distinguishing between physiological cysts and neoplastic cysts/tumors, and determination of the benign or malignant nature of the mass (Lichtman and Papera 1990).

→ In consultation with physician, set up appropriate diagnostic testing.

→ Patients in whom ruptured cysts/masses are suspected require prompt intervention and immediate referral to an emergency facility.

→ When an ovarian malignancy is suspected, immediate referral to a physician is warranted.
  ▪ Further management will be undertaken by the physician.
  ▪ Details of management of cancer patients are beyond the scope of this protocol.

→ Indications for surgical intervention include: presence of an adnexal mass after menopause, solid mass at any age, cystic mass >8 cm or cystic mass from 5 cm-8 cm persisting for more than 8 weeks in a reproductive-age woman (Herbst et al. 1992).

→ Functional ovarian cysts may be treated conservatively and usually resolve within 4 to 8 weeks.

- If <8 cm, perform a pelvic examination every 3 to 4 weeks. Oral contraceptives for 4 to 8 weeks may be employed to prevent ovulation.
- Cysts >8 cm or those which persist through 2 menstrual cycles require surgery (Herbst et al. 1992; Griffiths and Berkowitz 1986).

→ Corpus luteum cysts may be managed expectantly, provided there is no active intraperitoneal bleeding.

→ Treatment of benign cystic teratomas is surgical.
- Treatment of suspected malignancy is laparotomy, usually including total hysterectomy and bilateral salpingoophorectomy.

→ Unilocular cystic masses <5 cm in a postmenopausal woman are usually benign.
- In some settings, these patients may be conservatively managed with utilization of serial transvaginal ultrasound, possibly in conjunction with CA-125 levels.
- Pelvic washings obtained via laparoscope also may be sent for cytological evaluation.
- These patients generally are managed by a physician.
- See protocols on **Endometriosis, Ectopic Pregnancy, Amenorrhea—Secondary** (for polycystic ovary disease), and **Pelvic Inflammatory Disease** (for TOA) for additional management.

CONSULTATION

→ Suggested for all pelvic masses.

→ For a rapidly enlarging uterus or if a malignancy in the pelvis is suspected, refer patient to a physician.

→ Diagnostic procedures performed by the physician may include culdocentesis, paracentesis, and laparoscopy.

→ For endometrial biopsy, consultation with a physician prior to the procedure is suggsted.

→ For medical management with GnRH agonists or Depo-Provera®, generally the patient is managed by a physician.
- This depends, however, on the practice setting.

→ Patients with severe anemia, infertility, or recurrent pregnancy losses should be referred to a physician.

→ For all surgical candidates, refer to a physician.

→ Patients with suspected rupture/torsion or TOA require emergency intervention.

PATIENT EDUCATION

→ Discuss the nature of uterine fibroids, or adenomyosis if this is suspected.
- Informative patient-education pamphlets with good illustrations are a useful adjunct to teaching.
  • The American College of Obstetricians and Gynecologists (ACOG) has a useful pamphlet on fibroids.
- Reassurance regarding the benign nature of fibroids is important.
- Alert the patient to the signs and symptoms of an enlarging uterus.
- Discuss the need for regular follow-up and the various treatment options for fibroids and/or adenomyosis.
  • Adenomyosis, unfortunately, has no satisfactory form of medical management; hysterectomy generally is the definitive therapy.

→ Ascertain the patient's desire regarding contraception and childbearing and discuss appropriate contraception.
- Oral contraceptives are options provided the patient is followed carefully to assess potential fibroid growth from the hormones.
- Intrauterine devices are not advisable.
- Diaphragm may be used if it does not exacerbate symptoms.

→ Women with infertility or recurrent pregnancy losses require psychological support throughout the investigation. Refer to an infertility specialist as indicated.

→ When a suspected ovarian mass is encountered, discuss the physical findings with the patient and outline possible treatment options. Definitive management in many cases will be by physician, who should fully discuss the treatment approaches with the patient. Benign ovarian tumors have an excellent prognosis.

→ If ovarian malignancy is suspected, try not to alarm the patient. This is a difficult position for the clinician. Utilize appropriate resources and refer to a physician promptly.
- Suggest a support person accompany the patient to the doctor's appointment.
- Set up appropriate diagnostic tests in consultation with the physician and ensure the patient understands the importance of follow-up. These patients also are at risk of developing

breast and endometrial cancer (Herbst et al. 1992).

FOLLOW-UP

→ After initial discovery of fibroids, uterine re-assessment should be in three months and every six months thereafter, more often as indicated.

→ Utilization of pelvic ultrasound or MRI may be indicated in difficult cases to follow myoma progression, determine response to medical therapy, or as an adjunct to routine, intermittent assessment of the pelvis.

→ Monitoring for worsening of dysmenorrhea is warranted for a patient with adenomyosis who has been placed on oral contraceptives.

→ Follow-up of ovarian masses will be dependent upon the case presentation and in many cases will be handled by the physician.

→ Cystic ovarian masses <8 cm may be followed by the primary care provider.
  ▪ The patient should have a pelvic examination every three to four weeks.
  ▪ Cysts that persist for more than two menstrual cycles require surgery. Refer patient to a physician.

→ Supportive care for the cancer patient and her family is paramount to the recovery process.
  ▪ Prognosis for ovarian cancer is dependent upon cell type, stage, and grade.
  ▪ Body image and sexuality issues need to be addressed.
  ▪ Patients will be closely followed by a gynecological oncologist and possibly an oncological clinical nurse specialist as available.

→ Ensure that ovarian cancer patients follow the American Cancer Society Guidelines for mammography. See **Breast Disorders** Protocols.

→ Document in progress notes regarding pelvic masses should include onset, nature of the mass, progression, rapidity/stability of growth, timing/results of monitoring modalities, and definitive therapy as indicated. Update the problem list periodically.

Bibliography

Anderson, F. 1992a. Treating uterine fibroids with GnRH agonists. *Contemporary Ob/Gyn* 37(7):62–75.

Anderson, F. 1992b. How GnRH agonists facilitate fibroid surgery. *Contemporary Ob/Gyn* 37(8):55–67.

Anderson, R.E., Serafini, P.C., Paulson, R.J., Sauer, M.V., and Marrs, R.P. 1990. Detection and management of pathological, non-palpable, cystic adnexal masses. *Human Reproduction* 5(3):279–281.

DiSaia, P.J., and Creasman, W.T. 1989. *Clinical gynecologic oncology*, 3d ed. St. Louis: C.V. Mosby.

Entman, S.S. 1988. Uterine leiomyoma and adenomyosis. In *Novak's textbook of gynecology*, eds. H.W. Jones, A.C. Wentz, and L.S. Burnett. Baltimore: Williams & Wilkins.

Fleischer, A.C. 1991. Transabdominal and transvaginal sonography of ovarian masses. *Clinical Obstetrics and Gynecology* 34(2):433–442.

Friedman, A.J., and Barbieri, R.L. 1988. Leuprolide acetate: Applications in gynecology. *Current Problems in Obstetrics, Gynecology, and Infertility* 11:205.

Gates, E. 1990. *Pelvic Masses.* Lecture Notes. University of California, San Francisco.

Goldstein, S.R., Subramanyam, B., Snyder, J.R., Beller, U., Raghavendra, N., and Beckman, E.M. 1989. The postmenopausal cystic adnexal mass: The potential role of ultrasound in conservative management. *Obstetrics and Gynecology* 73(1):8–10.

Gomel, V., Munro, M.G., and Rowe, T.C. 1990. *Gynecology. A practical approach.* Baltimore: Williams & Wilkins.

Griffiths, C.T., and Berkowitz, R. 1986. The ovary. In *Gynecology: Principles and practice*, ed. R.W. Kistner, pp. 289–377. Chicago: Year Book Medical Publishers.

Herbst, A.L., Mishell, D.R., Stenchever, M.A., and Droegemueller, W. 1992. *Comprehensive gynecology*, 2d ed. St. Louis: Mosby Year Book.

Kistner, R.W. 1986. *Gynecology: Principles and practice*, 4th ed. Chicago: Year Book Medical Publishers.

Lichtman, R., and Papera, S. 1990. *Gynecology. Well-woman care.* Norwalk, CT: Appleton & Lange.

Margolis, A.J., and Greenwood, S. 1993. Gynecology and obstetrics. In *Current medical diagnosis and treatment*, eds. L.M. Tierney, Jr., S.J. McPhee, M.A. Papadakis, and S.A, Schroeder. Norwalk, CT: Appleton & Lange.

Neinstein, L.S. 1991. *Adolescent health care. A practical guide*, 2d ed. Baltimore: Urban & Schwarzenberg.

Olt, G., Berchuck, A., and Bast, R.C. 1990. The role of tumor markers in gynecologic oncology. *Obstetrical and Gynecological Survey* 45(9):570–576.

Schwartz, P.E. 1991. Ovarian masses: Serologic markers. *Clinical Obstetrics and Gynecology* 34(2):423–432.

Schriock, E.D. 1989. GnRH agonists. *Clinical Obstetrics and Gynecology* 32(3):550–563.

Scoutt, L.M., and McCarthy, S.M. 1991. Imaging of ovarian masses: Magnetic resonance imaging. *Clinical Obstetrics and Gynecology* 34(2):443–451.

Silva, P.D., and Sloane, K.A. 1992. Uterine leiomyomata: An overview. *The Female Patient* 17:49–56.

Underwood, P.B. 1983. Adnexal masses in teenagers. *Contemporary Ob/Gyn* 21(1):177–190.

World Health Organization (WHO). As cited in Serov, S.F., and Scully, R.E. 1973. Histological typing of ovarian tumors. *International histological typing of ovarian tumors* 9. Geneva: WHO.

12-K

Pelvic Pain—Acute

Acute pelvic pain may be a manifestation of a pathologic condition stemming from the genital, GI, or urinary tracts; the vascular or musculoskeletal systems; or the integument; or it may be of metabolic origin. In most instances, acute pelvic pain is new in onset and not previously experienced by the patient. The management goal for acute, severe pain is timely diagnosis and treatment, with referral to a physician in cases requiring hospitalization or surgery. See **Table 12K.1, Differential Diagnosis of Acute Pelvic Pain**. Quality and duration of the pain, associated symptoms, and specific physical examination findings form the basis of the differential diagnosis.

DATABASE

SUBJECTIVE

→ Obtain a comprehensive menstrual, sexual, contraceptive, medical, surgical, medication, psychosocial, and habits history.

→ Obtain a complete description of the pain, including onset, location and radiation, character, intensity, duration, aggravating and relieving factors, relationship to menstrual cycle and coitus, and associated symptoms.

→ Following are characteristics of common pathologies of pelvic pain:
  ▪ onset:
    • sudden onset suggests a mechanical cause such as ovarian torsion; ruptured ectopic pregnancy, tuboovarian or diverticular abscess, or ovarian cyst; degenerating myoma; hemorrhage into peritoneum; blockage of a ureter; bowel perforation; or ischemic infarction of a pelvic structure.

Table 12K.1. DIFFERENTIAL DIAGNOSIS OF ACUTE PELVIC PAIN

Genital Tract Causes	Non-Genital Tract Causes
Pregnancy related –Abortion –Ectopic pregnancy	**Urinary Tract** –Acute infection: cystitis, pyelonephritis –Renal calculus
Other causes *Ovary* –Rupture/torsion of cyst –Bleeding corpus luteum cyst –Mittelschmerz –Endometrioma –Tuboovarian abscess –Ovarian hyperstimulation	**Gastrointestinal** –Appendicitis –Inflammatory bowel disease –Mesenteric adenitis –Bowel perforation/obstruction –Meckel's diverticulitis
Fallopian Tubes –Torsion –Poststerilization stump torsion –Acute salpingitis –Tuboovarian abscess –Endometrial implants	**Vascular** –Mesenteric disease –Aortic aneurysm **Integument** –Rectus hematoma –Herpes zoster
Uterus –Degeneration/torsion of fibroid –Dysmenorrhea –Retrograde menstruation –Endometritis –Pyometra –Adenomyosis	**Metabolic** –Porphyria –Sickle cell crisis **Psychosomatic**

Source: Reprinted with permission from Taylor, P.J., and Gomel, V. 1987. *Current Problems in Obstetrics, Gynecology and Fertility* 10(9):404.

• insidious onset suggests an inflammatory condition.
▪ location: See **Table 7A.1, Common Anatomical Pain Sites for Specific Disease States**, p. 7-4.
▪ character:
  • crampy, intermittent, colicky pain is characteristic of contractions of hollow

muscular viscus, e.g., uterus—dysmenorrhea, threatened abortion; fallopian tube—ectopic pregnancy; ureter—stone; bowel—obstruction.

- dull, aching pain which radiates to the lower back or thighs is often associated with endometritis, salpingitis, or urinary tract infection.
- constant, steadily increasing pain is suggestive of increasing distension of hollow viscus or peritoneal irritation from blood, pus, or other fluid.

▪ duration:

- severe pain lasting for more than four hours is indicative of a condition that requires consideration for surgical evaluation or concentrated medical management (e.g., ruptured ovarian cyst, ruptured ectopic pregnancy, infarcted adnexal structure, or perforated viscus).
- in inflammatory conditions or acute appendicitis, pain may be present for a longer period (after insidious onset).

▪ relationship to menstrual cycle:

- during menstruation may indicate dysmenorrhea.
- at midcycle may indicate mittelschmerz (ovulatory pain).
- after delayed menses, rule out pregnancy event.

▪ radiation:

- kidney stone: Pain radiates down involved flank and into pelvis.
- appendicitis: Pain is initially periumbilical, then shifts to right lower quadrant in several hours.
- musculoskeletal: If lower back is affected, pain may radiate down one or both legs.
- dysmenorrhea and endometriosis: Pain may radiate to lower back or down legs (associated rectal pain in endometriosis may be referred or secondary to perirectal lesions).

▪ associated symptoms:

- fever, chills, malaise, and associated symptoms are indicative of infection from any source.
- lightheadedness, dizziness, fainting, shouldertip pain may be associated with intraperitoneal bleeding.
- genital tract source: Amenorrhea, menorrhagia, metrorrhagia, or other abnormal vaginal bleeding; leukorrhea; dyspareunia.
- urinary tract source: Urinary urgency, frequency, dysuria, hematuria, or flank pain.

- GI source: Nausea, vomiting, diarrhea, constipation, hematochezia, or melena. GI or urinary tract may be secondarily involved in inflammatory processes from the genital tract (Gomel, Munro, and Rowe 1990).

→ See "Subjective" sections of the following protocols: **Abdominal Pain** and other associated **Gastrointestinal Disorders** Protocols; **Pelvic Pain—Chronic, Ectopic Pregnancy, Pelvic Masses, Urinary Tract Infection, Interstitial Cystitis, Pelvic Inflammatory Disease, Vaginitis, Sexually Transmitted Diseases, Abnormal Uterine Bleeding,** and **Musculoskeletal Disorders.**

OBJECTIVE

→ Assess vital signs in patients with acute pelvic pain. Fever may be present in inflammatory and infectious states. Orthostatic changes in pulse and blood pressure may be indicative of intraperitoneal bleeding.

→ Perform a complete abdominal, pelvic, and rectovaginal examination.

▪ The abdominal examination should include:

- inspection for presence of distension, visible peristalsis, scarring, masses.
- auscultation for altered bowel sounds.
- percussion to delineate masses, free air.
- palpation for hepatosplenomegaly, guarding, rebound tenderness, site of maximal tenderness, masses, costovertebral angle (CVA) tenderness. See **Table 7A.2, Abdominal Palpation,** p. 7-7.

▪ The pelvic examination should include:

- inspection of external genitalia for lesions, discharge, bleeding.
- speculum examination to inspect for vaginal or cervical lesions, discharge, bleeding.
- bimanual examination to assess for cervical motion tenderness (CMT); palpation for uterine size, shape, consistency, mobility, tenderness; and adnexal palpation for masses, tenderness, fullness, fixation.

▪ The rectovaginal examination should include:

- assessment of masses, tenderness, nodularity in the cul-de-sac or rectum and the presence or absence and consistency of stool.
- fecal occult blood testing as indicated.

→ Objective findings associated with an acute abdomen due to rupture (e.g., of ectopic pregnancy, TOA, appendix) may include the following:

- fever, signs of shock.
- peritoneal signs.
- extreme cervical motion and pelvic tenderness.
- pelvic mass.
- adnexal induration or fixation.
- positive pregnancy test; decreased Hgb/Hct; leukocytosis; increased ESR.
- if performed, pelvic ultrasound showing a complex adnexal mass, and possibly culdocentesis revealing nonclotting blood or pus.

  NOTE: Patients with an acute abdomen should be referred immediately for emergency care.

→ Objective findings associated with inflammatory/infectious gynecological conditions may include the following:
  - fever.
  - abnormal vaginal discharge or bleeding.
  - CMT and uterine/adnexal tenderness.
  - adnexal mass.
  - increased WBCs revealed by wet mounts.
  - leukocytosis with immature polymorphonuclear leukocytes revealed by CBC.
  - elevated ESR.
  - endocervical cultures positive for *N. gonorrhoeae* and/or *C. trachomatis*.

→ Objective findings associated with urological disorders (depending on the etiology) may include the following:
  - restlessness, fever, associated vomiting.
  - CVA tenderness, suprapubic tenderness.
  - gross hematuria.
  - urinalysis significant for bacteria, white blood cells, red blood cells, casts.
  - leukocytosis with increased polymorphonuclear leukocytes revealed by CBC.
  - stone and dilated ureter determined by diagnostic ultrasound or intravenous pyelogram (IVP).

→ GI disorders manifest with acute abdominal pain and a multiplicity of associated symptoms and physical examination findings. See **Abdominal Pain** Protocol.

→ Musculoskeletal disorders present typically after injury or exercise and may be confused with pain originating from the urinary tract. See specific **Musculoskeletal Disorders** Protocols.

→ See "Objective" sections of specific associated protocols.

ASSESSMENT

→ Pelvic pain—acute

→ See **Table 12K.1**.

PLAN

DIAGNOSTIC TESTS

→ Initial diagnostic tests should be prioritized for patients with acute, severe pain warranting immediate referral. Tests may include beta-hCG, CBC, urinalysis, urine culture and sensitivities, endocervical cultures for *N. gonorrhoeae* and *C. trachomatis*, pelvic ultrasound, flat and upright x-rays of the abdomen (including diaphragm), culdocentesis, diagnostic laparoscopy.

→ Laboratory evaluation of stable patients depends upon diagnostic considerations and may include (but is not limited to) sensitive pregnancy test, CBC, ESR, urinalysis, urine culture and sensitivities, endocervical cultures, Pap smear, wet mounts, gram stain, liver enzymes, total bilirubin, alkaline phosphatase, amylase, electrolytes, stool examination, pelvic ultrasound, flat and upright x-rays of the abdomen, IVP, CT scan, diagnostic laparoscopy.

→ See "Diagnostic Tests" sections of specific associated protocols.

TREATMENT/MANAGEMENT

→ Patients with evidence of peritoneal irritation, rupture, or obstruction should be referred to an emergency facility immediately.

→ Consult with physician to establish appropriate diagnostic tests and plan a management approach as indicated.

→ Specific treatment/management will depend upon the underlying identified problem (see specific protocols).

→ When the diagnosis is uncertain, repeated histories and physical examinations may unfold new data and allow for appropriate diagnosis, referral, and treatment.

CONSULTATION

→ Consultation is suggested for all patients with acute pelvic pain.

→ Patients with acute, severe pain should be referred to a physician immediately.

→ Referral to a mental health provider is warranted when psychosomatic pain is suspected or in the presence of depression, neurosis, or hysteria.

PATIENT EDUCATION

→ Patient education will depend upon underlying disorder. Refer to appropriate protocols.

→ Encourage compliance with therapeutic regimens and follow-up care.

FOLLOW-UP

→ Follow-up will depend on patient presentation, diagnosis, and treatment/management modalities

→ When the diagnosis is uncertain, reassessment is indicated. Pain diary, menstrual calendar, and perimenstrual symptoms calendar may aid in clarifying the diagnosis.

→ Document significant pelvic pathology in problem list. Thorough progress notes are important.

Bibliography

American College of Obstetricians and Gynecologist 1989. *Chronic Pelvic Pain*, Technical Bulletin No. 12(Washington, DC: the Author.

Andrews, M.C. 1987. Pelvic pain. In *Gynecology princ ples and practice*. New York: Macmillan.

Beard, R.W., Reginald, P.W., and Wadsworth, J. 198 Clinical features of women with chronic lower abdor inal pain and pelvic congestion. *British Journal of O stetrics and Gynaecology* 95:153–161.

Burnett, L.S. 1988. Gynecologic causes of the acute a domen. *Surgical Clinics of North America* 68(2):38! 398.

Faro, S., and Maccato, M. 1990. Pelvic pain and infe tions. *Obstetrics and Gynecology Clinics of Nor America* 17(2):441–455.

Gaul, J.N. 1988. Evaluation of chronic pelvic pain. *Mi nesota Medicine* 71:546–548.

Gomel, V., Munro, M.G., and Rowe, T. 1990. *Gynecol-ogy: A practical approach*. Baltimore: Williams & Wilkins.

Herbst, A.L., Mishell, D.R., Stenchever, M.A., and Droegemueller, W. 1992. *Comprehensive gynecology*, 2d ed. St. Louis: Mosby Year Book.

Kresch, A.J. 1992. Kresh pain analysis and mapping. Palo Alto, CA: Fertility and Gynecology Center of Northern California.

Muse, K.N. 1990. Cyclic pelvic pain. *Obstetrics and Gynecology Clinics of North America* 17(2):427–439.

Quan, M. 1987. Chronic pelvic pain. *The Journal of Family Practice* 25(3):283–288.

Rapkin, A.J., and Reading, A.E. 1991. Chronic pelvic pain. *Current Problems in Obstetrics, Gynecology and Fertility* 14(4):99–137.

Reiter, R.C. 1990a. A profile of women with chronic pelvic pain. *Clinical Obstetrics and Gynecology* 33(1): 130–136.

———. 1990b. Occult somatic pathology in women with chronic pelvic pain. *Clinical Obstetrics and Gynecology* 33(1):154–160.

Roseff, S.J., and Murphy, A.A. 1990. Laparoscopy in the diagnosis and therapy of chronic pelvic pain. *Clinical Obstetrics and Gynecology* 33(1):137–144.

Slocumb, J.C. 1990a. Chronic somatic, myofacial, and neurogenic abdominal pelvic pain. *Clinical Obstetrics and Gynecology* 33(1):145–153.

———. 1990b. Operative management of chronic abdominal pelvic pain. *Clinical Obstetrics and Gynecology* 33(1):196–204.

Stovall, T.G., Ling, F. 1991. Relieving chronic pelvic pain through surgery. *Contemporary Ob/Gyn* 36(4):11–22.

Wood, D.P., Wiesner, M.G., and Reiter, R.C. 1990. Psychogenic chronic pelvic pain: Diagnosis and management. *Clinical Obstetrics and Gynecology* 33(1):179–195.

Taylor, P.J., and Gomel, V. 1987. Pelvic pain. *Current Problems in Obstetrics, Gynecology and Fertility* 10(9): 393–437.

12-L

Pelvic Pain—Chronic

Chronic pelvic pain (CPP) is defined as pain, localized to the pelvic area, that has persisted for more than six months (Quan 1987; Rapkin and Reading 1991). It has also been defined as "noncyclic pain of at least six months duration refractive to previous treatment and without an obvious pathologic source on examination." (Gaul 1988, 546). Sources of chronic pelvic pain may be of gynecological, GI, urological, neurological, or musculoskeletal origin. See **Table 12L.1, Causes of Chronic Pelvic Pain**. The most common findings at laparoscopy in CPP patients are endometriosis or adhesions, or the syndrome may lack obvious pathology (Roseff and Murphy 1990).

Pelvalgia is the term used to refer to cases of CPP with no obvious somatic pathology. Pelvalgia may occur 14 percent to 76 percent of the time (Quan 1987; Reiter 1990a). The psychogenic theory is the most popular theory regarding the pathogenesis of this type of CPP. It suggests that CPP is a manifestation of an underlying psychiatric disturbance (e.g., hysteria, depression, anxiety, or hypochondriasis).

Other theories advocate an organic basis for pelvalgia, suggesting it is due to syndromes such as pelvic congestion syndrome—a disorder of the pelvic autonomic system with smooth muscle spasm and venous congestion of the ovaries, uterus, and vulva, triggered by emotional stress or occurring in a psychologically predisposed woman—or pelvic myofascial syndrome—trigger points of pain, or hyperirritable spots, within taut bands of skeletal muscle or in abdominal/vaginal/sacral muscle fascial areas, the pathophysiology of which is unclear (Quan 1987; Rapkin and Reading 1991; Slocumb 1990a). Additional research is needed to sort out the contribution of these factors to CPP.

Pain is a multidimensional phenomenon with neurophysiological and psychosocial components. It is theorized that pain behavior in CPP patients becomes linked to environmental consequences, which sets the stage for operant learning. When reinforcement of pain behavior by favorable outcomes occurs (i.e., sympathy from significant others), the pain behavior may continue despite lessening or discontinuation of the initiating pain stimulus (Quan 1987).

CPP can be one of the most frustrating and time-consuming matters in women's primary care, presenting a major clinical challenge. The significance of CPP is the long-standing suffering and disability associated with it. Thus, the approach to the CPP patient must incorporate a meticulous history, thorough psychosocial assessment, careful physical examination, and concerted effort at treatment. A review of the mechanisms of pain perception is beyond the scope of this protocol. (See "Bibliography" for further reading.)

DATABASE

SUBJECTIVE

NOTE: Good patient/clinician rapport is important in obtaining a comprehensive history regarding somatic and sensitive psychosocial matters; compassionate, but non-codependent, behavior toward the CPP patient should be displayed.

→ Complete history will include:
- characteristics of the pain:
  - onset, quality or character, quantity, location and radiation, timing.
  - aggravating and relieving factors.

Table 12L.1. CAUSES OF CHRONIC PELVIC PAIN

Gynecological	Neurological
Noncyclical	Nerve entrapment syndrome
Adhesions	Neuroma
Endometriosis	
Salpingo-oophoritis	**Musculoskeletal**
Ovarian remnant syndrome	Low back pain syndrome
Pelvic congestion syndrome	Congenital anomalies
Ovarian neoplasms	Scoliosis/kyphosis
Pelvic relaxation	Spondylolysis
	Spondylolisthesis
Cyclical	Spinal injuries
Primary dysmenorrhea	Inflammation
Secondary dysmenorrhea	Tumors
–Imperforate hymen	Osteoporosis
–Transverse vaginal septum	Degenerative changes
–Cervical stenosis	Coccydynia
–Uterine anomalies	
–Intrauterine synechiae	**Myofascial Syndrome**
–Endometrial polyps	
–Uterine leiomyoma	**Systemic**
–Adenomyosis	Acute intermittent porphyria
–Pelvic congestion syndrome	Abdominal migraine
–Endometriosis	Systemic lupus erythematosus
	Lymphoma
Atypical cyclical	Neurofibromatosis
Endometriosis	
Adenomyosis	**No Obvious Organic Pathology**
Ovarian remnant syndrome	
Chronic functional ovarian	
cysts	
Gastrointestinal	
Irritable bowel syndrome	
Ulcerative colitis	
Crohn's disease	
Carcinoma	
Infectious diarrhea	
Recurrent partial small bowel	
obstruction	
Diverticulitis	
Hernia	
Abdominal angina	
Recurrent appendiceal colic	
Genitourinary	
Recurrent/relapsing	
cystourethritis	
Urethral syndrome	
Interstitial cystitis	
Urethral diverticuli/polyps	
Carcinoma of bladder	
Ureteral obstruction	
Pelvic kidney	

Source: Adapted with permission from Rapkin, A.J., and Reading, A.E. 1991.
Chronic pelvic pain. *Current Problems in Obstetrics, Gynecology and Fertility*
14(4):110.

- effect of menstrual cycle, exercise, work, stress, coitus, orgasm.
- associated symptoms:
  - sleep disturbance; appetite changes; fatigue, headache, or other constitutional symptoms.

- depressed mood, anxiety, hypochondriasis, loss of interest in social activities, reduced physical/sexual activity.
- abnormal bleeding, discharge, dyspareunia, dysmenorrhea.
- constipation, diarrhea, flatulence, tenesmus, hematochezia, changes in caliber of stool.
- dysuria, urgency, frequency, suprapubic pain.
- low back pain, sciatica, difficulty walking, other musculoskeletal symptoms.
- complete past medical, surgical, obstetrical/ gynecological, sexual and contraceptive history; injuries; hospitalizations; medications; chemical dependency; prior pain evaluations and their outcomes.
- historical questions specific to pathologies in **Table 12L.1.**
- psychosocial history:
  - marital/partner status, children, employment status.
  - history of physical, sexual, emotional abuse; suicide attempts.
  - impact of the pain on lifestyle and interpersonal relationships; attitudes and behavior of significant other regarding patient's pain.
  - stressors; coping mechanisms; leisure activities.
  - symptoms of depression, anxiety, etc.
  - patient's understanding of the cause of the pain.
- family history:
  - significant gynecological problems or psychological disorders.
    - It may be necessary to interview family members (with patient's consent) regarding their perceptions of the problem and how they are coping with it.

→ The overall profile of a woman with pelvalgia has been shown to include the following characteristics (ACOG 1989; Quan 1987):
- parous woman.
- onset of pain is between ages 20 years and 40 years (mean age 30.4 years), usually following obstetric delivery.
- average duration of pain is 2.5 ± 1.9 years (range 0.5 years to 12.5 years).
- character of pain is dull ache in pelvic area, aggravated premenstrually and with deep penetration during intercourse; pain is out of proportion to reality.

- associated symptoms are likely to include abdominal pain, nausea, dizziness, weakness, shortness of breath, difficulty walking, dysmenorrhea, and depression (Wood, Wiesner, and Reiter 1990). Often physiological functions such as menses, ovulation, bladder fullness, intercourse and orgasm exacerbate the pain (Slocumb 1990a).
- incomplete pain relief with most previous treatments.
- impaired function at home/work; altered family roles.

→ A few specific causes of CPP that are not covered elsewhere in this book are treated in the following discussions.

- Symptoms associated with pelvic congestion syndrome may include bilateral lower pelvic pain aggravated with menses, nervous tension, chronic fatigue, breast tenderness, spastic colon, and PMS symptoms (Rapkin and Reading 1991).
- Nerve entrapment syndrome may occur months to years after Pfannensteil incision.
  - Pain is sudden, stabbing, and colicky along lateral edge of rectus muscle and may be elicited by exercise.
    - May be associated with burning pain radiating horizontally or diagonally toward linea alba and along flank/sacroiliac areas.
    - May be exacerbated by full bladder, nausea, menses, bloating.
  - Bedrest relieves the pain (Rapkin and Reading 1991).
- Myofascial pelvic pain is typically aggravated by activity in the deeper visceral structures that share the same dermatome innervation.
  - Associated symptoms include dysmenorrhea, irritable bowel/bladder symptoms; aggravating factors are menses, bladder/rectal fullness, intercourse, cervical motion.
  - Associated autonomic phenomena may include tearing, visual disturbances, dizziness, tinnitus (Rapkin and Reading 1991; Slocumb 1990a).

→ Psychological profiles of women with CPP (both with and without surgically documented pathology), using the Minnesota Multiphasic Personality Inventory (MMPI), have included the following characteristics:

- hypochondriasis, hysteria, depression, neuroses, and borderline personality disorder.

- other instruments used in psychological evaluation have shown higher prevalences of substance abuse, sexual dysfunction, somatization, history of childhood/adult sexual abuse, suicidal ideation, anxiety, family dysfunction, dependency.
- women with pelvalgia are more prone to a history of sexual abuse, difficulty with close relationships, somatic overconcern, strong dependency needs, feelings of inadequacy or dissatisfaction with the female role, emotional insecurity and immaturity, impulsiveness, unusual thought processes, internalization of stress/hostility (Wood, Weisner, and Reiter 1990).

→ Evidence of an association between pelvalgia and post-traumatic stress disorder (PTSD) is accumulating.

- Symptoms of PTSD may include fear, anxiety, guilt, depression, sleep disturbances, sexual difficulties, compulsive repetition, reenactment of the stressful event, ego constriction, disturbed expressions of anger (Wood, Weisner, and Reiter 1990).

→ See "Subjective" sections of the following protocols: **Endometriosis, Pelvic Pain—Acute, Abdominal Pain** and other specific **Gastrointestinal Disorders** Protocols, **Pelvic Inflammatory Disease, Dysmenorrhea, Pelvic Masses, Perimenstrual Symptoms and Premenstrual Syndrome, Sexual Assault, Sexual Dysfunction, Urinary Tract Infection, Vulvodynia, Low Back Pain—Acute, Low Back Pain—Chronic,** and selected **Behavioral Disorders** Protocols.

OBJECTIVE

NOTE: Because of the multiple tissue layers between the abdominal and vaginal fingers, the physical examination of CPP patients may be misleading about the specific area of tenderness during palpation. In general, there is poor correlation between the pelvic examination findings and existence of pelvic pathology in CPP patients (Quan 1987).

→ A complete physical examination should be performed with specific attention to the abdominal, back, pelvic, and rectovaginal areas, *noting carefully* any abnormal findings.

- Palpation of these areas should attempt to reproduce the patient's pain.
- Abdominal examination should include tension of the abdominal muscles (by straight leg raising

or lifting head and shoulders) to differentiate abdominal wall and visceral sources of pain (Carnett's test).

- Abdominal wall pain is augmented while visceral pain is diminished by these maneuvers.

- CPP patients may have normal pelvic examinations or palpable abnormalities reflective of the underlying disorder—e.g., uterosacral nodularities consistent with endometriosis, uterine nonmobility indicative of pelvic adhesions, or a pelvic mass.

- Commonly, CPP patients have generalized tenderness on pelvic examination or sharp pain elicited by stretching the uterosacral ligaments by lifting the uterus forward, but often no other palpable abnormalities.

→ Objective findings of a few specific causes of CPP that are not covered elsewhere in this book are treated in the following discussion.

- Pelvic congestion patients may have tenderness/bulkiness over the uterine fundus/cervix and enlarged cystic ovaries.

- The examiner can localize pain in patients with nerve entrapment syndrome with the fingertip to the maximal point of tenderness at the rectus margin, inferior and anterior to the iliac spine; with the abdomen tensed, single-finger pressure by the examiner on the outer side of the muscle will exacerbate the pain (Rapkin and Reading 1991).

- With myofascial pain, finger point palpation of trigger points in the abdominal wall and paracervical and sacral regions will evoke acute local and referred pain (to arm, head, down back); patient may jump, muscle may twitch.

→ See "Objective" sections of the protocols mentioned previously.

ASSESSMENT

→ Pelvic pain—chronic. See differential diagnoses in **Table 12L.1**.

→ R/O acute causes of pelvic pain. See **Table 12K.1, Differential Diagnosis of Acute Pelvic Pain**, p. 12-109.

PLAN

DIAGNOSTIC TESTS

→ Basic general laboratory tests may include CBC; ESR; VDRL or RPR, urinalysis, urine culture and sensitivities; endocervical cultures for *N.*

gonorrhoeae and *C. trachomatis*; wet mounts; Pap smear; stool guaiac; stool culture if diarrhea present.

→ Pelvic ultrasound may be performed if there is suggestion of a mass, if the pelvic examination is indeterminate as to the cause of pain, or if the examination is technically difficult.

→ Diagnostic laparoscopy is the most valuable test and considered mandatory for comprehensive evaluation of the CPP patient (Roseff and Murphy 1990).

→ Additional tests may include fiber-optic or radiographic imaging if signs and symptoms are indicative of potential pathology in a specific organ system—e.g., upper GI series (UGI), barium enema, sigmoidoscopy, cystoscopy, intravenous pyelogram (IVP), hysteroscopy, hysterosalpingogram (HSG), MRI of the spine.

- These tests are ordered in consultation with a physician.

→ Tentative diagnosis of nerve entrapment can be confirmed by nerve block injections of local anesthetic into the abdominal wall.

- Performed by a physician.

→ Trigger point injections for evaluation (and treatment) of myofascial pain have been used.

- Performed by a physician.

→ Diagnostic modalities for pelvic congestion syndrome have included fluoroscopic venography and intravenous dihydroergotamine (DHE) injection (Rapkin and Reading 1991; Reiter 1990b).

→ Psychological testing should be a *routinely applied* evaluation tool.

- No special skills are necessary to administer the MMPI; however, the clinician may prefer that it be administered by a clinical psychologist.

- Other commonly used instruments include the SCL-90, the Zung Self-Rating Depression and Anxiety Scale, the National Institutes of Health Diagnostic Interview Schedule, the Melzack-McGill Pain Questionnaire, and the Middlesex Hospital Questionnaire (Quan 1987; Wood, Weisner, and Reiter 1990).

TREATMENT/MANAGEMENT

→ It is important to establish a firm diagnosis and separate out the relative contributions of physical disease and psychological factors. A multidisciplinary approach with multiple patient visits is required.

- Care of the CPP patient may be beyond the scope of an individual clinician's practice; thus, early referrals are in order.
- It is reasonable to perform a thorough history and physical examination and initiate basic laboratory work.

→ A logical approach to management has been suggested by Rapkin and Reading (1991). Site-specific procedures will, of course, vary. Consultation with a physician is essential to a coordinated approach to management. See also Wood, Weisner, and Reiter (1990).

- Visit 1:
  - obtain thorough history as outlined in "Subjective" section of this protocol.
  - perform a complete physical examination.
  - order laboratory tests as indicated by history and physical examination findings.
  - initiate daily symptom calendar:
    - patient to note onset, location, quality, intensity of pain; aggravating and relieving factors; associated symptoms; interference of pain with daily activities; medications taken.
    - diary to be maintained for 2 months. See **Figure 12L.1, Daily Symptom Calendar** for an example of calendar.
  - request patient's prior medical records.
  - treat any identified acute condition(s).
  NOTE: See also pain questionnaire, and pain descriptor and mapping forms, **Figures 12L.2, 12L.3,** and **12L.4.**
- Visit 2 (2 weeks later):
  - continue/update psychosocial and sexual history.
  - review with patient results of laboratory work, prior records, and pain diary.
  - repeat abdominal, back, and pelvic examination with particular attention to abdominal, lumbosacral, and vaginal trigger points. Trigger points may be treated with local anesthetic.
    - Refer to physician.
  - treat any identified subacute condition(s).
  - initiate psychological evaluation. Patient should be referred to a psychologist, preferably one who is well versed in all aspects of CPP.
  - consult with or refer patient to other specialists as indicated by suspected or confirmed somatic pathology, e.g., gynecologist, urologist, gastroenterologist, orthopedist, neurologist.

- Visit 3 (1 to 2 weeks later):
  - review symptom diary.
  - diagnostic laparoscopy may be indicated at this time. Therapy of endometriosis and adhesions may be performed through the laparoscope.
    - Refer to physician.
  - initiate physical therapy referral for patient with persistent trigger point pain.
  - discuss case with psychologist.
- Visit 4 (1 to 2 weeks later):
  - if somatic pathology has been ruled out, proceed with nonsurgical, multidisciplinary pain management modalities. These may include relaxation techniques, hypnosis, biofeedback, guided imagery, stress management, cognitive-behavioral approaches, sexual therapy, couples therapy.
    - Refer patient to specialists in these areas.
  - patient may be referred to a multidisciplinary pain management center. Health insurance coverage and cost factors are issues to explore.

→ Additional considerations in the treatment/ management of CPP patients are as follows:
- long-term narcotic use has no place in the management of CPP patients; when required, narcotics are used as interim therapy.
  - Non-narcotics (e.g., NSAIDs, salicylates, acetaminophen) may be used continuously.
  - Patient needs to understand that these medications are not a panacea and are used to ameliorate, not eliminate, pain. Dosage may be reduced over time (ACOG 1989).
  - Antidepressants may also be necessary. Consult with or refer patient to psychiatrist for medication management.
- hysterectomy, presacral neurectomy, and uterosacral nerve ablation have limited application in CPP patients. These modalities are generally reserved for patients with intractable, severely disabling pain.
- a discussion of the treatment of a few specific causes of CPP that are not presented elsewhere in this book follows.
  - Nerve entrapment: Anesthetic nerve block; surgical removal of involved nerves.
    - Refer to physician.
  - Myofascial pain: Hyperstimulation analgesia (e.g., cold spray), local anesthetic/steroid injection, transcutaneous electrical nerve stimulation (TENS) units, acupuncture.
    - Refer to specialist.

Figure 12L.1. DAILY SYMPTOM CALENDAR

Day of cycle	1	2	3	4	5	6	7	8	9	10	11	12	13	14	15	16	17	18	19	20	21	22	23	24	25	26	27	28	29	30	31
Date																															
Menses																															
Medications																															
Cramps-pelvic																															
Cramps-other																															
Backache																															
Pelvic pain-left																															
Pelvic pain-right																															
Pelvic pain-low middle																															
Pelvic pain-other																															
Painful bowel movement																															
a. before																															
b. during																															
c. after																															
Painful sexual intercourse																															
a. during																															
b. after																															
Urinary problems																															
a. pain																															
b. urgency																															
c. frequency																															
General aches/pains																															
Feeling the blues																															
Feeling depressed																															

Menses:

X = Menses

S = Spotting

For medications, list the initials and medications used:

_____ = _____

_____ = _____

_____

Grading of pain and/or symptoms:

1 = Mild, but does not interfere with activities.

5 = Moderate and interferes with activities but not disabling.

10 = Severe and disabling, unable to function.

Note: To be given to patient after initial assessment. Patient to maintain for two months.

• Pelvic congestion syndrome: Reassurance, psychotherapy, hormonal suppression (e.g., medroxyprogesterone acetate [Provera®] 30 mg/day for 3 months) (Rapkin and Reading 1991).

▪ see protocols in other sections of this book for treatment of specific disease states.

CONSULTATION

→ Indicated for all patients with chronic pain. Consultation with a physician is essential to a coordinated approach to management.

→ Patients may be co-managed by physician, psychologist, psychiatrist, and other specialists.

PATIENT EDUCATION

→ It is essential that the patient understand the etiology of CPP and the basic pathways of pain expression.

▪ When no obvious pathology can be identified, CPP patients are often resistant to the suggestion that their pain may be of nonorganic origin.

▪ These patients will need a lot of support and encouragement to follow through with psychological assessment and must understand this is a *requisite part* of a thorough evaluation.

▪ It is important, however, not to attribute CPP to psychological causes until the presence of organic pathology has been ruled out.

→ CPP patients often have unrealistic expectations regarding therapy and eradication of their pain.

Figure 12L.2. PAIN QUESTIONNAIRE (FORM A)

Date: _____   Name: _____

By: _____   Age: _____ G: _____ P: _____

LMP: _____   Cycle day: _____

1. Pain Location. List each different location and number it.	2. Date first noticed	3. Pain Description. Adjectives that *patients use* to describe typical pain. List cycle days it occurs.	4. Pain Intensity. Rate each pain separately. (1 – 10)*		
Pain Location	**Onset**	**Description and Cycle days**	**Worst**	**Avg**	**Least**

5. Overall interference of pain with life (1 – 10) _____

Work	School	Social activities	Child care relationships	Sports and exercise	Sex	Other: _____
_____	_____	_____	_____	_____	_____	_____

*1 - Mild: but does not interfere with activities.
 5 - Moderate: present interferes with activities but not disabling.
10 - Severe: disabling. Unable to function.

NOTE: Designed to be used by interviewer (not patient) during initial visit. See Fig. 12L.3 for list of pain descriptors.

Source: Adapted with permission from Kresch, A.J. 1992. *Kresch pain analysis and mapping.* Palo Alto, CA: The Fertility and Gynecology Center of Northern California.

Figure 12L.3.   PAIN DESCRIPTORS (FORM B)

Some of the words below may describe your present pain. Refer to Figure 12L.2 (Form A) for your pain locations. Circle only those words that best describe the pain in each of these locations and write that location number next to the word here. Leave out any category that is not suitable.

1 Flickering Quivering Pulsing Throbbing Beating Pounding	2 Jumping Flashing Shooting	3 Pricking Boring Drilling Stabbing	4 Sharp Cutting Lacerating
5 Pincing Pressing Gnawing Cramping Crushing	6 Tugging Pulling Wrenching Searing	7 Hot Burning Scalding Stinging	8 Tingling Itchy Smarting
9 Dull Sore Hurting Aching Heavy	10 Tender Taut Rasping Splitting	11 Tiring Exhausting	12 Sickening Suffocating
13 Fearful Frightful Terrifying	14 Punishing Grueling Cruel Vicious Killing	15 Wretched Blinding Miserable	16 Annoying Troublesome Miserable Intense Unbearable
17 Spreading Radiating Penetrating Piercing	18 Tight Numb Drawing Squeezing Tearing	19 Cool Cold Freezing	20 Nagging Nauseating Agonizing Dreadful Torturing

Source: Adapted with permission from Kresch, A.J. 1992. *Kresch pain analysis and mapping.* Palo Alto, CA: The Fertility and Gynecology Center of Northern California.

The clinician must outline a realistic approach to care and ensure that the patient understands limitations.

- Goals include maximizing functioning and minimizing suffering and disability (Rapkin and Reading 1991).
- Codependent behavior on the part of the provider should be avoided.

→ All consultants should agree on an approach to managing the patient's treatment and should dialogue regularly on the patient's progress. Patient should be made aware that this communication exists.

→ When a benign treatable condition has been identified, the patient should be reassured. Treatment approaches should be detailed by the physician responsible for the definitive care.

→ Drug dependency issues should be addressed. The patient should understand that long-term narcotic use has no place in management.

FOLLOW-UP

→ As noted, CPP patients should be seen at regular intervals. Family members should be included as indicated. Focusing on topics other than the pain component is valuable for the patient's self-esteem.

→ It is recommended that any clinician caring for CPP patients become familiar with the current literature on the subject, since it is a multifaceted phenomenon.

→ Document in progress notes and problem list.

Figure 12L.4. PAIN MAP (FORM C)

Instructions:
Put highest intensity in each square that is applicable.
May use color codes for different pains.

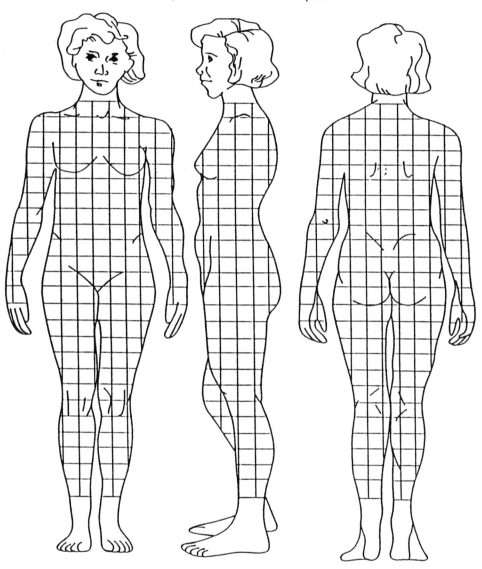

Pain intensity scale
 1—Mild: but does not interfere with activities
 5—Moderate: present and interferes with activities but not disabling
10—Severe: disabling. Unable to function.

NOTE: Patient may use this form to map out the intensity level of her pain. For use during interview.

Source: Adapted with permission from Kresch, A.J. 1992. *Kresch pain analysis and mapping.* Palo Alto, CA: Fertility and Gynecology Center of Northern California.

Bibliography

American College of Obstetricians and Gynecologists. 1989. *Chronic Pelvic Pain*, Technical Bulletin No. 129. Washington, DC: the Author.

Andrews, M.C. 1987. Pelvic pain. In *Gynecology principles and practice*. New York: Macmillan.

Beard, R.W., Reginald, P.W., and Wadsworth, J. 1988. Clinical features of women with chronic lower abdominal pain and pelvic congestion. *British Journal of Obstetrics and Gynaecology* 95:153–161.

Burnett, L.S. 1988. Gynecologic causes of the acute abdomen. *Surgical Clinics of North America* 68(2):385–398.

Faro, S., and Maccato, M. 1990. Pelvic pain and infections. *Obstetrics and Gynecology Clinics of North America* 17(2):441–455.

Gaul, J.N. 1988. Evaluation of chronic pelvic pain. *Minnesota Medicine* 71:546–548.

Gomel, V., Munro, M.G., and Rowe, T. 1990. *Gynecology: A practical approach*. Baltimore: Williams & Wilkins.

Herbst, A.L., Mishell, D.R., Stenchever, M.A., and Droegemueller, W. 1992. *Comprehensive gynecology*, 2d ed. St. Louis: Mosby Year Book.

Kresch, A.J. 1992. *Kresh pain analysis and mapping*. Palo Alto, CA: Fertility and Gynecology Center of Northern California.

Muse, K.N. 1990. Cyclic pelvic pain. *Obstetrics and Gynecology Clinics of North America* 17(2):427–439.

Quan, M. 1987. Chronic pelvic pain. *The Journal of Family Practice* 25(3):283–288.

Rapkin, A.J., and Reading, A.E. 1991. Chronic pelvic pain. *Current Problems in Obstetrics, Gynecology and Fertility* 14(4):99–137.

Reiter, R.C. 1990a. A profile of women with chronic pelvic pain. *Clinical Obstetrics and Gynecology* 33(1):130–136.

———. 1990b. Occult somatic pathology in women with chronic pelvic pain. *Clinical Obstetrics and Gynecology* 33(1):154–160.

Roseff, S.J., and Murphy, A.A. 1990. Laparoscopy in the diagnosis and therapy of chronic pelvic pain. *Clinical Obstetrics and Gynecology* 33(1):137–144.

Slocumb, J.C. 1990a. Chronic somatic, myofacial, and neurogenic abdominal pelvic pain. *Clinical Obstetrics and Gynecology* 33(1):145–153.

———. 1990b. Operative management of chronic abdominal pelvic pain. *Clinical Obstetrics and Gynecology* 33(1):196–204.

Stovall, T.G., Ling, F. 1991. Relieving chronic pelvic pain through surgery. *Contemporary Ob/Gyn* 36(4):11–22.

Wood, D.P., Wiesner, M.G., and Reiter, R.C. 1990. Psychogenic chronic pelvic pain: Diagnosis and management. *Clinical Obstetrics and Gynecology* 33(1):179–195.

Taylor, P.J., and Gomel, V. 1987. Pelvic pain. *Current Problems in Obstetrics, Gynecology and Fertility* 10(9):393–437.

12-M

Perimenopausal Symptoms and Hormone Therapy

Overview of menopause

Menopause, the cessation of menstruation and the end of reproductive potential in women, occurs at an average age of 50 years (Treloar 1974). Menopause is not an abrupt event but is preceded by a five- to six-year transition in hormonal and menstrual functioning (Treloar 1982). While the age of menarche has slowly decreased over generations, the age of menopause has remained stable for hundreds of years.

The First International Congress on Menopause in 1976 and the World Health Organization (WHO) in 1981 recommended standard definitions of the stages of menopause. These definitions, while imprecise, provide general clinical guidelines. *Menopause* is defined as the permanent cessation of menstruation due to loss of ovarian follicular activity and is clinically defined as 12 months of amenorrhea. *Perimenopause* is a variable period of years on either side of menopause during which characteristic symptoms and signs of ovarian involution are present. *Premenopause* is a poorly defined period prior to perimenopause, and *postmenopause* is the entire span of life following last menses (WHO 1981). Menopause is considered premature when it occurs before age 40 years and is referred to as premature ovarian failure.

Induced menopause is defined as the removal of both ovaries before the onset of menopause. When menopause is induced, the closure of menstrual life occurs precipitously and symptoms will vary depending on the age of the woman (Voda and George 1986). Induced menopause in a young woman may result in severe somatic and affective changes not present in an older woman whose body has begun to adapt to a changing internal environment. In addition, women who have had a surgically induced menopause appear to be more at risk for serious health problems than do women who experience natural menopause (Cobb 1989; Office of Technology Assessment [OTA] 1992; Voda and Eliasson 1983).

Recent evidence suggests that bilateral oophorectomy increases risk for coronary artery disease and osteoporosis (Chakravarti et al. 1977; Johannson et al. 1975). Some studies have suggested that women who have had this procedure have greater loss of bone density and higher incidence of osteoporotic fractures than do women of equivalent age with intact ovaries (OTA 1992).

Despite increased attention to midlife women and their health, research on menopause has been dominated by a biomedical disease model suggesting that hormonal changes alone are responsible for perimenopausal symptoms and disease. Research that demonstrates alterations in sensitivity in the neuroendocrine systems of the brain and peripheral glands supports an alternative model to the disease model of menopause etiology (Dyrenfurth 1982; Henrik 1982; Voda 1992).

Decline in hypothalamic-pituitary-ovarian (HPO) sensitivity to follicle-stimulating hormone (FSH) and leutenizing hormone (LH) occurs after menopause because of anatomical ovarian changes. Changes in negative and positive feedback action by ovarian steroids create an increased threshold to estrogen feedback, which produces incomplete inhibition of pituitary secretion when combined with reduced estrogen. Constant high levels of FSH and LH overstimulate a still functional ovary, leading to a decline in ovarian activity.

Hormone Therapy

While hormone therapy (HT) (estrogen and progesterone combined) can be an effective regimen for treating osteoporosis or alleviating severe perimenopausal symptoms in women experiencing surgical or premature menopause, the risks and dangers of HT have been seriously underestimated and under-reported. There has been increased media attention on the preventive effects of estrogen and progesterone on diseases related to menopause. Although some scientific reports were claiming that taking estrogen would protect older women from heart disease and heart attacks, the FDA Fertility and Maternal Health Drugs Advisory Committee did not recommend adding prevention of cardiovascular disease to the existing benefits of conjugated estrogens.

Until the Postmenopausal Estrogen Progestogen Intervention (PEPI) study—the first randomized, prospective experiment, begun in 1991, to evaluate the effects of HT on lipids, blood pressure, and bone density—there had been no randomized clinical trials of estrogen therapy (ET) or HT to establish "gold standards" for determining the validity and side effect potential of pharmaceutical therapies. Furthermore, case-control studies of white, middle-class women have been used to predict risks and benefits to the total population of perimenopausal women.

Hormone Therapy: Risks and Controversies

Most of the existing research on the risks and benefits of HT is based on ET only. As a result of the discovery that endometrial cancer is associated with ET, progestins were added to the ET regimen. However, because of the short duration of many studies and the use of statistical formulas to calculate risk, how the addition of exogenous steroids will affect women's health remains unclear.

Osteoporosis

Estrogen plays an important role in bone manufacture and reduces bone demineralization. After menopause, bone demineralization occurs more rapidly than bone resorption, resulting in accelerated bone loss for several years postmenopause (Riggs et al. 1982). While all postmenopausal women have declining levels of estrogen, only five percent to ten percent are diagnosed with vertebral fractures (Riggs 1987). Osteoporotic hip fractures occur in 30 percent of Caucasian women by 90 years of age. Clinical research data have shown that:

→ ET taken within five to six years of menopause effectively protects against incidence of bone fracture, reducing its likelihood by more than 50 percent (Hutchinson, Polansky, and Feinstein 1979; Weiss et al. 1980).

→ Any interruption in ET results in return to pretreatment bone loss rate (Lindsay et al. 1978).

→ Daily ET (≥0.625 mg conjugated estrogen) retards bone loss as long as drug is taken (Christiansen, Christiansen, and Transbol 1981).

→ Fracture rates in women with osteoporosis are reduced most effectively by a combination of calcium, fluoride, and ET.

→ ET has little or no effect on bone fracture risk in obese women, but its greatest beneficial effect is in thin women smokers (Williams et al. 1982).

→ Estrogen does not increase bone mass, and newer nonhormonal regimens are being tested that increase both bone density and bone mass, which is the optimal therapy for osteoporosis.

Cancer

Clinical studies support that overstimulation of a target tissue by hormones is likely to play an important role in causing cancers, particularly those of the breast and reproductive tract (Henderson 1989). Current risk assessments, however, can only speculate about level of risk for developing cancer; they cannot predict actual risk.

Endometrial cancer

In the mid-1970s, studies found that ET alone increased the incidence of uterine cancer from five-fold to 14-fold (Mack et al. 1976; Smith et al. 1975; Ziel and Finkel 1975).

→ Relative risk was linked to dosage and duration of ET.

→ Adding progestins to ET was found to reduce the risk.

Breast cancer

Endogenous estrogens have been found to play an important role in breast cancer (Kelsey and Berkowitz 1988). While some studies have found little or no connection between breast cancer and ET (Kaufman et al. 1984; Wingo et al. 1987), the FDA Fertility and Maternal Health Drugs Advisory Committee found an increased risk of breast cancer in postmenopausal women treated with ET (FDA 1990). Selected studies of breast cancer risk with HT have shown:

→ Long duration of ET use (six to 15 years) appears to increase the risk of breast cancer by 30 percent to 80 percent. Risk applies to natural and surgical menopause (Brinton, Hoover, and Fraumeni 1986;

Colditz, Stampfer, and Willett 1990; Daling 1990; FDA 1991; Hoover et al. 1976; Ross et al. 1980).

→ HT does not protect against breast cancer and may increase the risk (Bergkvist et al. 1989; Ewertz 1988; Hulka 1990).

→ Breast cancer risk is highest in women who use higher ET doses (≥1.25 mg) and increases 2.7 times after ten years with ET doses greater than 0.625 mg/day (Hoover et al. 1976). Lower doses of shorter duration (<0.625 mg/day) may not pose a "substantially increased risk" of breast cancer (Steinberg et al. 1991).

→ While breast cancer incidence increases with duration of ET use, mortality remains stable. One study demonstrates that ET may stimulate the growth of slow-growing, low-grade, less aggressive tumors (OTA 1992). Furthermore, when ET is withdrawn, breast cancer survival is better than among women who have never used ET (Colditz, Stampfer, and Willett 1990).

→ In summary, the OTA *Report on Menopause and Hormone Therapy* recommends "a cautious interpretation of the best available data is that estrogen therapy is associated with an increase in the risk of breast cancer. This increased risk is on the order of 30 percent to 80 percent and appears to be no larger than a doubling of the risk" (OTA 1992, 42).

Cardiovascular disease (CVD)

The fact that postmenopausal women suffer more heart attacks and strokes than younger women has caused speculation that declining estrogen levels may be a causative factor. According to the recent OTA review of menopausal hormones, "only randomized, controlled clinical trials can demonstrate conclusively that oral estrogen use reduces the incidence of cardiovascular disease" (OTA 1992, 27). Studies on the effects of hormones and CVD have indicated:

→ Postmenopausal ET decreases low-density lipoprotein (LDL) cholesterol and increases high-density lipoprotein (HDL) cholesterol (Bain et al. 1981; Krauss et al. 1979), which protects against atherosclerosis (Longcope et al. 1990).

→ The relative risk of ischemic heart disease (IHD) in ET-treated versus untreated women shows beneficial risk ratio (RR) = 0.4 (Ross et al. 1980).

→ Though no evidence exists that ET *actually* reduces myocardial infarction (MI) incidence in

older women, several studies suggest a reduction of MI in women on ET (Bain et al. 1981).

→ Women with early bilateral oophorectomy are at increased risk for CVD compared with women with intact ovaries (Bush et al. 1983; Stampfer and Colditz 1991).

→ Addition of progestins to decrease endometrial cancer may neutralize CVD benefit (Notelovitz 1982) because of stimulation of hyperinsulinemia/hyperglycemia, which increases atherogenic effect (Stout 1987). Addition of progestin to ET reduced HDL levels by as much as 31 percent (Bush and Miller 1987). Furthermore, no experimental study has demonstrated that ET/HT is *preventive* for CVD.

→ Preliminary results from the PEPI trial reveal statistically significant improvement in lipid metabolism (↑ HDL, ↓ LDL) in women taking ET and HT (especially conjugated equine estrogen [CEE]/micronized progesterone) compared to placebo control group. While final results will not be complete until 1997-1998, preliminary results show no difference in the incidence of new CVD or new breast or endometrial cancers (The Writing Group for the PEPI trial 1995).

→ Heart disease in women can be reduced by 90 percent through exercise, weight loss, reduction in fat intake, smoking cessation, and hypertension treatment.

Coagulation and thrombosis

Ovarian hormones produce several effects on the vascular system, but determining net effect is difficult.

→ Estrogen reduces endothelial prostacyclin production (Elam et al. 1980); progestins may increase or decrease prostacyclin activity (Makila et al. 1982; Rongaglioni et al. 1979).

→ Platelet aggregation is unchanged by estrogens; thromboembolism is not increased in postmenopausal women receiving ET.

→ Clotting factors are elevated by synthetic estrogens and are dose-related.

Liver/Gall bladder

→ ET in creams or skin patches bypass liver metabolism but quickly induce high serum levels; no known risks have been evaluated (Chetkowski et al. 1986; Martin et al. 1979).

→ One hundred thirty-one out of 100,000 cases of gallbladder disease are due to ET (Honore 1980).

→ Effect of ET on gall bladder disease persists after discontinuation (Petitti, Sidney, and Perlman 1988).

Neurological effects

→ ET may potentiate headaches and migraines; dose reduction reduces headache symptoms by 58 percent (Kudrow 1975).

→ Migraine headaches are a relative contraindication to ET.

For most women, menopause is accomplished with minimal discomfort and little need for pharmacologic intervention. Many women want more control over decision making regarding their health rather than a prescription for hormones. They are asking for assistance from health professionals in sorting out the myths of menopause from the facts. They want to be active participants in decisions about health care and treatment and are interested in the full range of options for managing symptoms, preventing disease, and maintaining their health into old age.

DATABASE

SUBJECTIVE

→ Symptomatology of the perimenopausal transition is highly variable regardless of ethnicity or culture, with some women reporting few or no symptoms and others reporting extreme distress and discomfort. Symptoms may include:
  - vasomotor symptoms: Hot flashes (flushes) (vary in frequency/intensity; may continue for a few months to years), night sweats, dizziness, nausea, lightheadedness, palpitations, nervousness.
  - oligomenorrhea, polymenorrhea.
  - menorrhagia, metrorrhagia, hypermenorrhea, hypomenorrhea, menometrorrhagia.
  - sudden amenorrhea.
  - genitourinary symptoms: Vaginal dryness, itching, or discharge; urinary urgency, frequency, dysuria, or stress incontinence; dyspareunia.
  - negative affect symptoms: Depression, irritability, emotional lability, tension, heightened stress response.
  - physical discomfort: Headaches; insomnia, sleep disruption, fatigue (secondary to nocturnal hot flashes); breast tenderness; musculoskeletal aching; appetite changes; constipation.
  - cognitive changes: Decreased concentration, forgetfulness.

  - sexual changes: Decreased libido, diminished arousal.
  - symptom severity declines in one to five years (except for vaginal atrophy).
  - symptoms may be more severe and longer in women who undergo surgical menopause.

→ Gynecological history should include:
  - status of uterus, ovaries.
  - history of fibroids, cancer, abnormal cervical cytology.
  - menstrual cycle changes.
  - abnormal bleeding patterns.
  - change in sexual desire, orgasmic potential, lubrication; dyspareunia.
  - need for contraception.

→ Complete medical history should include:
  - major medical illness: Cardiovascular, breast, liver, gall bladder disease; cancer; diabetes; hypertension; obesity; arthritis.
  - mental health history.
  - medications including current and previous hormone use.
  - habits: Smoking, drugs, alcohol, exercise, nutrition.

→ Psychosocial history should include:
  - living situation.
  - social support.
  - economic stability.
  - life event changes.
  - coping/stress management skills.

→ Complete family history should include:
  - cardiovascular disease.
  - breast, uterine, ovarian cancer.
  - hypercholesterolemia.
  - osteoporosis.

→ Osteoporosis risk factors:
  - premature or surgically induced menopause.
  - smoking.
  - poor nutrition.
  - light- or yellow-skinned race.
  - small stature, low weight.
  - history of eating disorder, hyperthyroidism, hyperparathyroidism, gastric/small bowel resection.
  - family history of osteoporosis, stress fractures.
  - excessive alcohol intake.
  - long-term use of corticosteroids.
  - inactivity.

→ Cardiovascular risk factors:
  - recent MI, cerebral vascular accident (CVA), transient ischemic attack (TIA).

- acute thrombosis or emboli.
- established IHD or hypertension.
- family history of early-onset coronary artery disease, hypercholesterolemia.

OBJECTIVE

→ Physical examination (Barger 1988):

- mental/sensory status, affect: Assess for signs of anxiety, depression; cognitive function loss; sensory loss.
- height, weight, vital signs: Compare with previous findings, if available.
- general: Assess for increased facial hair, increased/decreased skin pigmentation, changes in body contour (kyphosis).
- head, eyes, ears, nose, throat: Assess for masses, lesions; funduscopic examination and visual acuity as indicated.
- neck: Assess for lymphadenopathy.
- thyroid: Assess for thyromegaly, masses.
- heart and lungs: Assess for signs of cardiorespiratory disease.
- extremities: Assess for edema, varicosities.
- breasts: Assess for masses, skin/nipple changes, lymphadenpopathy, galactorrhea, atrophy of breast tissue.
- abdomen: Assess for organomegaly, masses, scars, tenderness.
- complete pelvic examination:
  - external genitalia/urethra: Assess for thinning/fusing of labia majora/minora, introital shrinkage (kraurosis), urethral ectopy.
  - vagina: Assess vault (may be shortened); assess for paleness/erythema of vaginal epithelium, atrophy of vaginal mucosa, vaginal dryness, loss of rugosity, petechial hemorrhages, lesions, signs of infection, cystocele, rectocele; assess muscle tone.
  - cervix: Assess color, texture, patency of os (may become stenotic); portio may no longer protrude into vagina.
  - uterus: Assess uterine size, shape, consistency, mobility, tenderness (uterus decreases in size after menopause).
  - adnexa: Assess for pelvic masses, tenderness (ovaries should be nonpalpable in a post-menopausal woman).
- rectal examination: Assess for masses; stool for occult blood may be performed.

→ Additional objective findings:

- wet mount may reveal:
  - increased number of parabasal cells/WBCs (see **Atrophic Vaginitis** Protocol).
  - other pathogens may be identified with concomitant infection, e.g., *C. albicans, T. vaginalis*, clue cells). See specific protocols.
  - decreased lactobacilli.
- vaginal pH increased.
- cytological evaluation (Pap smear) may reveal atypia associated with atrophic changes of the cervix.
- cholesterol/triglycerides rise postmenopausally (rapidly in oophorectomized women); HDL cholesterol decreases.

→ See "Diagnostic Tests" section.

ASSESSMENT

→ Menopause (natural or surgically induced)

→ R/O premature ovarian failure

→ R/O perimenopausal symptoms

→ R/O osteoporosis

→ R/O cardiovascular disease

→ R/O mental health problems

→ R/O abnormal uterine bleeding

→ R/O pregnancy

→ R/O urinary tract/vaginal infection

PLAN

DIAGNOSTIC TESTS

→ Self-assessment: Self-evaluation of symptoms, stress, and daily activities will be a helpful first step in the evaluation of the perimenopausal patient.

- Prospective charting for 1 to 2 menstrual cycles (or 1 to 2 months if cycle is irregular) may be undertaken by the patient using a symptom checklist or calendar method.
- Method should include a severity rating scale and allow for women to record positive symptom experiences. See **Perimenstrual Symptoms and Premenstrual Syndrome** Protocol for an example of one type of calendar.

→ Perimenopausal history: Evaluate patient's complete medical history and risk factors (see "Subjective" section).

→ Additional diagnostic studies as indicated, considering age, risk status, or symptoms:

- cytological evaluation of cervix (Pap smear): Perform yearly.
  NOTE: Perform careful sampling since transition zone may recede high up into endocervical canal. Atypical (nondysplastic) changes may be noted in the presence of an atrophic cervix.
- vaginal sampling for maturation index reflecting state of estrogen activity (out of vogue in many settings).
- wet mounts of vaginal secretions as indicated to assess the relative ratio of parabasal to superficial epithelial cells and/or to assess for the presence of vaginal infection.
- mammography: recommended schedule (every 2 years age 40 years to 50 years; annually after age 50 years).
- CBC or Hgb/Hct.
- urinalysis.
- stool for occult blood.
- fasting blood glucose if family history of diabetes.
- lipid profile: Total cholesterol, triglycerides, HDL, LDL; see **Hypercholesterolemia** Protocol for specifics.
- liver function tests.
- FSH level (results depending on laboratory):
  - premenopausal range: 1-30 mIU/ml.
  - perimenopausal range: 30-200 mIU/ml.
  - postmenopausal range: 100-200 mIU/ml; ≥50 mIU/ml considered postmenopausal.
- estradiol levels: Indicate extraovarian sources or absorption of estrogen in ET. Serum estradiol levels of 184pmol-220 pmol/l (50 pg/ml-60 pg/ml) ensure protection against bone loss (Ruggiero 1992).
- bone densitometry: Dual photon absorptiometry of spine, femur, radius in selected cases (i.e., in cases where patient is considering HT for osteoporosis prevention but requires more data to assist in decision making).
- endometrial biopsy (EMB) as indicated for:
  - abnormal bleeding.
  - women in higher risk categories for endometrial changes, including obesity, diabetes, dysfunctional uterine bleeding, anovulation, infertility, high alcohol intake, hepatic disease, hypothyroidism (Speroff, Glass, and Kase 1989).
  NOTE: Consult with physician regarding need for EMB based on the patient's history, risk factors, and clinical presentation.

TREATMENT/MANAGEMENT

→ The primary care provider is likely to have contact with women in the perimenopausal transition who are seeking help for bothersome symptoms, seeking information about menopause and the need for HT as well as overall, ongoing health care.
  - For women to make personal and informed decisions about perimenopausal symptom management and disease prevention strategies, certain issues must be addressed:
    - education and information about the natural course of menopause.
    - discussion of accurate knowledge and myths of menopause.
    - balance between potential risks and benefits of various treatment regimens.
    - personal values and choices about midlife health and perimenopausal transition.
→ The approach to management of the perimenopausal woman must be individualized according to each specific case. Currently, there are only 3 medical indications for hormone therapy: menopausal discomforts, surgical menopause, and osteoporosis prevention.

Hormonal therapy
(See **Tables 12M.1** and **12M.2, Hormone Therapy: Select Preparations, Advantages, Disadvantages** and **Hormone Therapy: Typical Prescribing Regimens**, respectively.)

→ Estrogens:
  - indicated for treatment of menopausal symptoms and prevention of osteoporosis.
  - FDA-approved indications for estrogen include hot flashes; vaginal dryness; itching and thinning of the vaginal wall; and urinary incontinence, urgency, dysuria unrelated to infection.
  - ET is recommended for women younger than 45 years following oophorectomy or hysterectomy.
  - FDA has recommended that women at high risk for osteoporosis take ET (see "Risk Factors" in "Subjective" section of this protocol).

→ Androgens (treatment using progesterone or testosterone):
  - progestins are added to ET to decrease the risk of endometrial cancer and to reduce osteoporosis risk in women unable to use ET; progestin preparations do not have FDA approval for treatment of menopausal symptoms, although current standard practice is to

Table 12M.1.   HORMONE THERAPY: SELECT PREPARATIONS, ADVANTAGES, DISADVANTAGES

<u>Estrogen Preparations</u>

Conjugated estrogens (CE):	33% equine estrogens, 60% estrone sulfate
Brand name	*Premarin*®
Dose available	oral—0.3 mg, 0.625 mg, 0.9 mg, 1.25 mg, 2.5 mg; vaginal—0.625 mg/g
Advantages	most clinical data available favorable lipid patterns Estrone (E1): Estradiol (E2) ratio >1 available in oral, vaginal, parenteral routes
Disadvantages	first-pass effect in liver dose duration = 24 hrs overstimulation of endometrium
Esterified estrogens (EstE):	85% equine estrogens, 15% estrone sulfate
Brand name	*Estratab*®
Dose available	0.3 mg, 0.625 mg, 1.25 mg, 2.5 mg (0.625 mg EstE = 0.625 mg CE)*
Advantages	favorable lipid patterns
Disadvantages	little clinical data unavailable in vaginal, parenteral routes others—same as for CE
Estropipate (EP):	Estrone sulfate with piperazine from pregnant mare urine
Brand name	*Ogen*®
Dose available	oral—0.625 mg, 1.25 mg, 2.5 mg, 5.0 mg vaginal—1.5 mg/g (0.625 mg EP = 0.625 mg CE)*
Advantages	favorable lipid patterns oral and vaginal preparations
Disadvantages	more expensive than CE (almost twice the cost) others—same as for CE
17-Beta Estradiol (E2):	Micronized E2
Brand names	*Estrace*®, *Estraderm*®, *Delestrogen*®, *Depo-estradiol*®
Dose available	*Estrace*®: oral—1 mg, 2 m; vaginal—0.01% (0.1 mg/g) *- vag drying* (1 mg = 0.625 mg CE)* *Estraderm*® (transdermal patch): 0.05 mg or 0.1 mg, applied 2×/week (0.05 mg = 0.625 mg CE)*
Advantages	favorable lipid pattern vaginal cream without fragrance; alternative to oral route for local symptom relief transdermal route avoids first-pass effect in liver
Disadvantages	little clinical data not FDA-approved for osteoporosis prevention

*Equivalency based on inhibition of bone resorption (Brenner and Mishell 1991; Gambrell 1994; Genant et al. 1990; Harris et al. 1991; Lobo 1987; Speroff, Glass, and Kase 1994).

Continued

prescribe progestin with ET for endometrial protection. Current labeled indications for progestins include secondary amenorrhea, abnormal uterine bleeding related to hormonal imbalance (fibroids, cancer), and endometriosis.

■ testosterone is added to ET to control extreme vasomotor instability not controlled by ET alone, increase energy level and feelings of well-being, and increase sexual desire and orgasmic capacity (Sherwin 1985); testosterone combined with ET does not have FDA approval.

→ Contraindications to the use of hormone therapy will change with results from prospective clinical trials. Existing contraindications to the use of estrogens, progestins, and testosterone include:

■ absolute contraindications (*PDR* 1993):
  • known or suspected pregnancy.
  • known or suspected breast cancer.

Table 12M.1. HORMONE THERAPY: SELECT PREPARATIONS, ADVANTAGES, DISADVANTAGES (CONTINUED)

Progestins and Testosterone Preparations

Medroxyprogesterone (MPA)   most frequently used progestin for combined hormone therapy

Brand names	*Provera®, Amen®*
Dose available	2.5 mg, 5 mg, 10 mg
Advantages	reduces HDL cholesterol less than other progestins, positive effects on bone mineralization
Disadvantages	uterine cramping, bloating, depression, breast tenderness

Norethindrone (NET)   used when control of bleeding unsatisfactory with MPA

Brand names	*Micronor®, Nor-Q D®*
Dose available	Micronor® & Nor-Q D®—0.35 mg (NET 0.7 mg-1.05 mg = 10 mg MPA)**
Advantages	positive effects on bone mineralization; may be associated with fewer side effects than MPA; may offer better control of breakthrough bleeding
Disadvantages	adverse lipid effect compared with MPA

Norgestrel (NG)

Brand name	*Ovrette®*
Dose available	0.075 mg (0.150 mg = 10 mg MPA)**
Advantages	more potent progestin than MPA and NET; may offer better control of breakthrough bleeding; may be associated with fewer side effects than MPA
Disadvantages	nausea, depression, weight gain, breast tenderness; adverse lipid effect compared with MPA

Progesterone (P)   micronized form administered in oral, vaginal, sublingual routes

Dose available	100 mg micronized (capsulized by pharmacist) (200 mg-300 mg = 10 mg MPA)**‡
Advantages	positive effects on bone mineralization; may be associated with fewer side effects than MPA
Disadvantages	few controlled studies; available only from selected pharmacies†

Depomedroxyprogesterone acetate

Brand name	Depo-Provera®
Dose available	100 mg/ml, 5 ml; 400 mg/ml, 2.5 ml (dose weight-dependent)
Advantages	infrequent administration (50 mg-200 mg I.M. every 3 mos.); substitute for estrogen for relief of hot flushes; decreases urinary calcium excretion
Disadvantages	bleeding, weight gain, depressive symptoms

Methyltestosterone (MT)

Brand names	*Oreton®, Metandren®*
Doses available	1.25 mg, 2.5 mg, 5 mg; 75 mg pellet sq
Advantages	with ET, helps control hot flashes; increased sexual desire and orgasmic capacity
Disadvantages	hirsutism, weight gain; few controlled studies; difficult to obtain

Estrogen/Testosterone combination

Brand names/Doses	*Estratest®:* EstE 1.25 mg + MT 2.5 mg *Estratest® HS:* EstE 0.625 mg + MT 1.25 mg *Premarin® + MT:* CE 0.625 mg + MT 5 mg CE 1.25 mg + MT 10 mg *Estrapel®:* 25 mg estradiol in testosterone pellet (investigational)
Advantages	see MT
Disadvantages	high dose of HT in combination with estrogen; most women require ≤2.5 mg; ↑ intolerance and side effects at higher doses.

**Equivalency (approximate) based on endometrial protection if used for at least 12 days each month (Gambrell 1994; Moyer et al. 1993; Whitehead et al. 1987).

†See **Perimenstrual Symptoms and Premenstrual Syndrome** Protocol.

‡Equivalencies still being investigated.

Table 12M.2 HORMONE THERAPY: TYPICAL PRESCRIBING REGIMENS

Cyclical/Continuous Estrogen Therapy (ET)
–Oral estrogen (0.625 mg CE or equivalent) or transdermal estrogen patch (0.05 mg) changed twice weekly
–Taken on calendar days 1-25 each month or every day
–For women without uterus

Continuous Combined Hormone Therapy
–Oral estrogen (0.625 mg CE or equivalent) or transdermal estrogen patch (0.05 mg) changed twice weekly, taken with
–Progestin (2.5 mg-5 mg MPA or equivalent) ~~Lack spotting or BTB~~
–Daily continuous use for women with intact uteri to avoid withdrawal bleeding, minimize progestational side effects

Continuous ET with Intermittent Progestin
–Oral estrogen (0.625 mg CE or equivalent) or transdermal patch (0.05 mg) changed twice weekly
–Estrogen taken 365 days a year or transdermal patch equivalent
–Progestin (5 mg-10 mg MPA or equivalent) taken on calendar days 1-12 (or 14-25)
–10 mg dose more well studied with relation to endometrial protective effects

Cyclical Combined Hormone Therapy
–Oral estrogen (0.625 mg CE or equivalent) or transdermal estrogen patch (0.05 mg) changed twice weekly, taken with
–Progestin (5 mg-10 mg MPA or equivalent)
–ET taken on calendar days 1-25 and progestin taken days 1-12 (or 14-25)
–10 mg dose more well studied with relation to endometrial protective effects

Vaginal Estrogen Cream
–Manufacturer recommendation: 2 g-4 g per vagina daily for 3 wks/1 wk off
–Clinical use: 1 g-2 g per vagina daily for 1 wk, then tapering doses until maintenance doses biweekly

Combined ET with Androgens
–Oral methyltestosterone (1.25 mg-2.5 mg) in combination with ET or in combined formula with estrogen; see ET dosing above
–Progestin added as above on cyclical or continuous regimen

- known or suspected estrogen-dependent neoplasia.
- undiagnosed abnormal genital bleeding.
- active thrombophlebitis or thromboembolic disorders.
- relative contraindications—i.e., may make certain conditions worse (*PDR* 1993):
  - cardiovascular disease.
  - impaired liver function.
  - gallbladder disease.
  - hyperlipidemia.
  - asthma.
  - migraine headaches.
  - epilepsy.
  - uterine fibroids.
  - diabetes.
  - metabolic bone disease.
  - kidney disease.
  - hypertension.
  - depression.

→ Helping the individual woman with decision making: The National Women's Health Network (NWHN) has suggested a series of questions that women should ask their health care providers before starting HT.

- These questions can be used by womens' health care providers as guidelines for discussion and for assistance with personal decision to use or not use hormones for perimenopausal symptom management or disease prevention (NWHN 1989).
- Why would HT be prescribed for me?
  - Am I at risk for osteoporosis?
  - Do I have severe symptoms?
  - What about natural or non-drug methods for coping with these symptoms?
- What are the contraindications to HT? How do they apply to me?
- What kinds of tests are preliminary to starting HT?
- Is the lowest possible dosage prescribed?
- If I have surgically induced menopause, are the HT regimens different?
- If I take HT, what additional diagnostic tests will I need and how often?
- What will the cost for HT be initially and for necessary follow-up care?
- What is the expected duration of treatment and dosage?
- What are the alternatives to HT?

Non-hormonal therapy

→ Antihypertensives:
- less effective than androgens; sometimes useful, but not FDA-approved, for control of hot flashes, especially in women with severe hypertension or heart disease (Notelovitz 1989); short-term therapy of less than 1 year recommended.
- often given in very low doses, which do not affect blood pressure.
- types/dosages/side effects:
  - alpha-adrenergics: clonidine (Catapres®) 0.1 mg p.o. BID, increasing to 0.2 mg p.o. BID if no side effects occur; side effects may include dizziness, dry mouth, drowsiness, constipation, sedation. See *PDR*.
  - beta-adrenergics: Propranlol (Inderal®) 25 mg p.o. every day; side effects may include dry mouth, sexual dysfunction, constipation, depression. See *PDR*.

→ Psychotropics: Tranquilizers, sedatives, and antidepressants:
- often prescribed for emotional lability (no clinical trials); not FDA-approved.
- consult *PDR* for types/dosages.

NOTE: Antihypertensives and psychotropics should be prescribed in consultation with a physician.

→ NSAIDs:
- used for control of headaches or vasomotor instability.
- see **Dysmenorrhea** Protocol for types/dosages/side effects.

→ Bellergal (combination drug containing belladonna, phenobarbital, and ergotamine):
- only non-hormonal drug that is FDA-approved for treatment of menopausal disorders.
- used for relief of hot flashes, restlessness, insomnia.
- potentially addictive since it contains belladonna and phenobarbital. See *PDR*.
- dose: 1 tablet p.o. BID.
- side effects: dizziness, dry mouth, sedation.

Non-drug strategies

→ Natural remedies for symptoms associated with menopause include dietary changes, nutritional supplements, exercise, vitamins, herbs, stress management, biofeedback, acupuncture, massage, and support groups.
- Unfortunately, the efficacy of non-drug therapies is largely unknown and, like hormone or pharmacological therapy, clinical trial data are not available.
- However, non-drug therapies can provide an alternative or complement to HT for many women who do not experience distressing perimenstrual symptoms or are not at high risk for osteoporosis.
- Furthermore, perimenstrual symptom management strategies can be a component of health promotion for the midlife woman.

→ Self-help strategies and general health practices:
- changing harmful health practices:
  - stop smoking.
  - decrease alcohol.
  - reduce caffeine.
  - reduce total fat in diet to 20 percent or less of daily caloric intake:
    - high-fat animal foods, whole milks, and cheeses.
    - hydrogenated fats, coconut oil, palm oil, cocoa butter.
  - avoid high-protein diets that may increase the excretion of calcium, bone loss (Weiss et al. 1981).
- general physical activity:
  - regular, vigorous physical activity 3-5 times a week lasting 15-60 minutes (Shangold 1982).
  - weight-bearing exercise for osteoporosis prevention, such as walking, jogging, stair climbing, rope jumping, dancing, upper body workouts, aerobics.
- vitamins/minerals:
  - calcium: 1000 mg-1500 mg elemental/day:
    - dietary calcium in vegetable form preferred.
    - calcium carbonate provides highest usable calcium.
    - calcium citrate improves absorption.
  - magnesium: $2 \times Ca^{++}$ to Mg for better calcium absorption.
  - vitamin D: Low-fat milk, fish, sunlight.
  - vitamin B-complex and Vitamin C (500 mg/day).
- diet/good nutrition:
  - high-protein diets have been shown to decrease calcium levels and bone density.
    - Red meats are high in protein and phosphorus, which also decrease calcium levels.
    - Lacto-ovo vegetarians lose less bone mass in postmenopausal period than meat eaters.
  - fresh fruit and vegetables 5 times a day:

–fresh produce contains magnesium and boron that aid in calcium retention.

–boron is in apples, pears, grapes, leafy vegetables, nuts, legumes.

▪ decreasing vaginal dryness:
  • almond, coconut, or Vitamin E oil reduces discomfort (should not contain perfumes).
  • vitamin E capsules by mouth (400 mIU/day).
  • water-soluble products such as Astro-Glide®, Replens®, glycerin, KY® jelly.
  • sexual activity, vaginal massage, masturbation.
  • avoid douching (may aggravate vaginal dryness).

▪ self-help for hot flashes:
  • tracking to determine a pattern.
  • reduction of certain foods:
    –stimulants—caffeine, sugar, cola, chocolate.
    –alcohol, spicy foods, hot foods, large meals.
  • vitamins: B-complex (25 mg) and E (up to 400 IU/day):
    –initially, 600 IU-800 IU Vitamin E plus 2 g-3 g Vitamin C for 1-2 weeks.
    –decrease Vitamin E to 400 IU/day after hot flashes subside; no more than 1200 IU/day.
    –women with hypertension or diabetes should take no more than 100 IU/day of Vitamin E.
  • remain calm, loosen clothing, breathe deeply and slowly, use cold compress, carry a fan.
  • for night sweats, open a window, use cotton bedding and nightclothes.
  • stress reduction strategies.
  • yoga exercises: see Lark 1990 in "Bibliography."
  • herbs: Although not rigorously researched, these combinations have been recommended by herbalists:
    –black cohash, licorice root, sarsaparilla, thistle, false unicorn root, red raspberry leaves, elder, squaw vine.
    –chamomile and valerian root tea (reduces insomnia).
    –herbs containing natural estrogen: black cohash, sarsaparilla, false unicorn root, elder, licorice.
    –use cautiously under the guidance of an experienced herbalist.
    –see Boston Women's Health Collective (1987), Lark (1990); and Weed (1992) in "Bibliography."

▪ urinary control and improving orgasmic response:
  • Kegel exercises.
  • see **Sexual Dysfunction** Protocol.

▪ peer support/education:
  • menopause self-help groups with or without professionals can help women educate themselves and provide support and mutual guidance for perimenopausal symptoms (MacPherson 1985).
  • self-help books:
    –*Women of a Certain Age: The Midlife Search for Self* (1979), Lillian Rubin
    –*Menopause: A Positive Approach* (1982), Rosetta Reitz
    –*Menopause: Me and You* (1984), Ann Voda
    –*The Crone: Women of Age, Wisdom and Power* (1985), Barbara Walker
    –*Ourselves, Growing Older: Women Aging with Knowledge and Power* (1987), Boston Women's Health Collective
    –*Menopause Naturally: Preparing for the Second Half of Life* (1988), Sadja Greenwood
    –*The Black Women's Health Book: Speaking for Ourselves* (1990), E.C. White
    –*Menopause: A Well Woman Health Book* (1990), Montreal Health Press
    –*The Menopause Self-Help Book: A Woman's Guide to Feeling Wonderful for the Second Half of Her Life* (1990), Susan Lark
    –*Transformation through Menopause* (1991), M. Van Eyk McCain
    –*Wise Woman Ways: Menopausal Years* (1992), S.S. Weed.
  • menopause newsletters:
    –*A Friend Indeed: For Women in the Prime of Life.* A Friend Indeed Publications, Inc.; Box 515, Place du Parc Station, Montreal, Quebec, Canada H2W2P1; (514) 843-5730.
    –*Hot Flash: Newsletter for Midlife and Older Women.* National Action Forum for Midlife and Older Women; c/o Dr. Jane Porcino, Box 816, Stony Brook, NY 11790-0609.
    –*Menopause News.* 2074 Union St., San Francisco, CA 94123, 800-241-MENO.
    –*PMZ: Postmenopausal Zest Newsletter,* c/o Volcano Press; 330 Ellis St., San Francisco, CA 94102.
    –*The Network News.* National Women's Health Network; 1325 G St., NW, Washington, DC 20005, (202) 347-1140.

CONSULTATION

→ Co-management with physician colleagues may be recommended after data collection is complete for

women who are at very high risk for certain diseases:
- rapid bone demineralization or previous unexplained fractures.
- existing cardiac disease or family history of early CVD.
- other pathology (physical/psychological).

→ Consultation with physician specialists for women on HT/ET:
- irregular uterine bleeding.
- indications for endometrial biopsy.
- abnormal endometrial biopsy.
- suspicious or abnormal mammogram.

→ Consultation with a physician is indicated when considering less commonly used routes of hormone administration (e.g., injectables, implants, percutaneous) and/or less well-established HT regimens (e.g., every-three-month progestins). (These alternative forms are not addressed in this protocol.)

→ As needed for prescription(s).

PATIENT EDUCATION

→ Many women express a lack of knowledge about their bodies or menstrual transitions. Often, clear information is all a woman needs during the perimenopausal transition to relieve her concern about a particular symptom.

→ Patients should be encouraged to participate in their own care and assume a self-care attitude. Providers should take care not to transmit their own biases to patients.

→ It will be important for health care providers for midlife women and women moving through the perimenopausal transition to participate in the following activities:
- adopting cross-cultural, nonracist approaches to assessment and care.
- reducing stereotyped or negative attitudes toward aging women.
- becoming informed about community and local resources for midlife and older women.
- participating in the development of networks where women can obtain and share knowledge about menopause.

→ Providers should offer clear information about all self-care remedies and activities as well as about the risks and benefits of hormone and pharmacological therapy. Women should be encouraged to ask questions about any therapy they are using, whether it is a hormone or a non-drug therapy.

→ Advise women to:
- keep a record of any treatments or therapeutic regimens.
- record any side effects or new symptoms while using a treatment.
- notice both positive and negative effects of any treatment.
- record regular visits for therapeutic maintenance on a calendar.

→ Discuss contraceptive options for the sexually active midlife woman and her partner until menopause is clearly established, i.e., amenorrhea of 12 months duration or longer.
- Methods may include barriers/spermicides, hormonal contraception (oral contraceptives provided nonsmoker with no contraindications; Norplant®/Depo-Provera®, if without contraindications), sterilization, IUD, vasectomy.

→ Address safer sex issues as indicated. See **Table 13A.2, Safer Sex Guidelines**, p. 13-9.

FOLLOW-UP

→ Follow-up will vary depending on the severity of perimenopausal symptoms, health risks, and the woman's therapeutic decisions.
- No HT or symptom management therapy:
  • monitor using health risk screening guidelines.
  • individualize for each woman.
- HT or other drug therapy:
  • assess at three months initially, then every year thereafter (more often as indicated).
  • monitor for reproductive cancers (breast, uterine).
  • monitor other health risks.
  • monitor proper drug use, side effects.

→ Follow up on abnormal lab tests as indicated.

→ If Pap smear indicates atypia, may treat with vaginal estrogen cream and repeat in four to 12 weeks. See **Table 12M.2** for dosing regimens.

→ Document in progress notes and problem list.

Bibliography

American Cancer Society. 1991. *Cancer facts and figures—1991*. Atlanta: the Author.

Adams, C. 1970. Aging and reproduction in the female mammal with particular reference to the rabbit. *Journal of Reproduction and Fertility* 12(suppl):1–16.

Archer, D. 1982. Biochemical findings and medical management of the menopause. In *Changing perspectives on menopause*, eds. A. Voda, M. Dinnerstein, and S. O'Donnell. Austin, TX: University of Texas Press.

Avis, N.E., and McKinlay, S.M. 1991. A longitudinal analysis of women's attitudes toward the menopause: Results from the Massachusetts Women's Health Study. *Maturitas* 13:65–79.

Bachman, G.A. 1985. Correlates of sexual desire in postmenopausal women. *Maturitas* 7:211–216.

———. 1990. Hysterectomy: A critical review. *Journal of Reproductive Medicine* 35(9):839–862.

Bain, C., Willett, W., Hennekens, C.H., Rosner, B., Belanger, C., and Speizer, F.E. 1981. Use of postmenopausal hormones and risk of myocardial infarction. *Circulation* 64:42–46.

Ballinger, S.E. 1985. Psychosocial stress and symptoms of menopause: A comparative study of menopause clinic patients and nonpatients. *Maturitas* 7:315–327.

———. 1990. Stress as a factor in lowered estrogen levels in the early postmenopause. *Annals of the New York Academy of Sciences* 592:95–113.

Barger, M.K. 1988. Care of the menopausal woman. In *Protocols for gynecologic and obstetric health care*, ed. M.K. Barger. Philadelphia: W.B. Saunders.

Bergkvist, L., Adami, H.O., Persson, I., Hoover, R., and Schairer, C. 1989. The risk of breast cancer after estrogen and estrogen-progestin replacement. *New England Journal of Medicine* 321:293–297.

Bohr, H., and Schaadt, O. 1983. Bone mineral content of femoral bone and the lumbar spine measured in women with fracture of the femoral neck by dual photon absorptiometry. *Clinical Orthopedics* 179:240–245.

Boston Women's Health Collective. 1987. *Ourselves, growing older: Women aging with knowledge and power.* New York: Touchstone.

Brenner, P.F., and Mishell, D.R., Jr. 1991. Menopause. In *Infertility, contraception, and reproductive endocrinology*, eds. D.R. Mishell, Jr., V. Davajan, and R.A. Lobo. Boston: Blackwell Scientific Publications.

Brinton, L.A., Hoover, R.N., and Fraumeni, J.F. 1986. Menopausal estrogens and breast cancer risk: An expanded case-control study. *British Journal of Cancer* 54:825–832.

Brinton, L.A., Hoover, R.N., Szklo, M., and Fraumeni, J.F. 1981. Menopausal estrogen use and risk of breast cancer. *Cancer* 47:2517–2522.

Bush, T.L., Cowan, L.D., Barrett-Connor, E., Criqui, M.H., Karon, J.M., Wallace, R.B., Tyroler, H.A., and Rifkind, B.M. 1983. Estrogen use and all cause mortality: Preliminary results from the lipid research clinics program follow-up study. *Journal of the American Medical Association* 249(7):903–906.

Bush, T.L., and Miller, V.T. 1987. Effects of pharmacologic agents used during menopause: Impact on lipids and lipoproteins. In *Menopause physiology and pharmacology*, ed. E.R. Mishell. Chicago: Year Book Medical.

Casper, R., Yen, S., and Wilkes, M. 1979. Menopausal flushes: A neuroendocrine link with pulsatile lutenizing hormone secretion. *Science* 205:823–825.

Chakravarti, S., Collins, W.P., Newton, J.R., Oram, D.H., and Studd, J.W. 1977. Endocrine changes and symptomatology after oophorectomy in premenopausal women. *British Journal of Obstetrics and Gynaecology* 84(10):769–775.

Chetkowski, R.J., Meldrum, D.R., Steingold, K.A., Randle, D., Lu, J.K., Eggena, P., Hershman, J.M., Alkjaersig, N.K., Fletcher, A.P., and Judd, H.L. 1986. Biologic effects of transdermal estradiol. *New England Journal of Medicine* 314(25):1615–1620.

Christiansen, C., Christensen, M.S., and Transbol, I. 1981. Bone mass in postmenopausal women after withdrawal of oestrogen/gestagen replacement therapy. *Lancet* 1:459–461.

Cobb, J.O. 1989. *Understanding menopause.* Toronto: Key Porter Books.

Colditz, G., Stampfer, M., and Willett, W. 1990. Prospective study of estrogen replacement therapy and risk of breast cancer in post-menopausal women. *Journal of the American Medical Association* 264(20):2648–2653.

Colditz, G.A., Willett, W., Stampfer, M., Rosner, B., Speizer, F.E., and Hennekens, C.H. 1987. Menopause and the risk of coronary heart disease in women. *New England Journal of Medicine* 316(18):1105–1110.

Corson, S.L. 1992. Physiology of menopause and update on hormonal replacement therapy. *Clinical Issues in Perinatal and Women's Health Nursing* 2(4):483–496.

Daling, J. 1990. Testimony before the Fertility and Maternal Drug Advisory Committee, Food and Drug Administration, February 1–2.

Dennerstein, L., Burrows, G., Hyman, G., and Wood, C. 1978. Menopausal hot flushes: A double-blind comparison of placebo, ethinyl estradiol and norgestrel. *British Journal of Ob-Gyn* 85:852–856.

Dyrenfurth, I. 1982. Endocrine functions in the woman's second half of life. In *Changing perspectives on menopause*, eds. A. Voda, M. Dinnerstein, and S. O'Donnell. Austin, TX: University of Texas Press.

Elam, M.B., Lipscomb, G.E., Chesney, C.M., Terragno, D.A., and Terragno, N.A. 1980. Effect of synthetic estrogen on platelet aggregation and vascular release of PGI2-like material in the rabbit. *Prostaglandins* 20(6):1039–1051.

Ettinger, B., Genant, H.K., and Cann, C.E. 1987. Postmenopausal bone loss is prevented by treatment with low-dosage estrogen with calcium. *Annals of Internal Medicine* 106(1):40–45.

Ewertz, M. 1988. Influence of noncontraceptive exogenous and endogenous sex hormones on breast cancer risk in Denmark. *International Journal of Cancer* 42:832–838.

Food and Drug Administration. 1986. Estrogens to be labeled for osteoporosis. *Talk Paper.* (April 14). Washington, DC: U.S. Government Printing Office.

———. 1990. Fertility and Maternal Health Drug Advisory Committee, February 1–2.

———. 1991. Fertility and Maternal Health Drug Advisory Committee, June 20–21.

Frank, M.V. 1992. Transition into midlife. *Clinical Issues in Perinatal and Women's Health Nursing* 2(4):421–428.

Freedman, R., Woodward, S., and Sabharwal, S. 1990. Alpha 2-adrenergic mechanism in menopausal hot flushes. *Obstetrics and Gynecology* 76(4):573–578.

Gambrell, R. 1989. Clinical use of progestins in the menopausal patient: Dosage and duration. *Journal of Reproductive Medicine* 27(8):531–538.

———. 1994. Management of hormone replacement therapy side effects. *Menopause* 1:2, 67–72.

Gambrell, R., Maier, R., Sanders, B. 1983. Decreased incidence of breast cancer in post-menopausal estrogen-progestogen users. *Obstetrics and Gynecology* 62(4):435–443.

Genant, H.K., Baylink, D.J., Gallagher, J.C., Harris, S.T., Steiger, P., and Herber, M. 1990. Effect of estrone sulfate on postmenopausal bone loss. *Obstetrics and Gynecology* 76(4):579–584.

Ginsburg, J., Swinhoe, J., and O'Reilly, B. 1981. Cardiovascular responses during the menopausal hot flush. *British Journal of Ob-Gyn* 88:925–930.

Goodman, M., Stewart, C., and Gilbert, F. 1977. Patterns of menopause. *Journal of Gerontology* 32:291–298.

Gosden, R.G. 1985. *Biology of menopause.* London: Academic Press.

Gosden, R.G., Sadler, I.H., Reed, D., and Hunter, R.H. 1990. Characterization of ovarian follicular fluids of sheep, pigs and cows using proton nuclear magnetic resonance spectroscopy. *Experientia* 46(10):1012–1015.

Gosden, R.G., Telfer, E., Faddy, M.J., and Brook, D.J. 1989. Ovarian cyclicity and follicular recruitment in unilaterally oophorectomized mice. *Journal of Reproduction and Fertility* 87(1):257–264.

Greenwood, S. 1988. *Menopause naturally: Preparing for the second half of life.* San Francisco: Volcano Press.

Grossman, M., and Bart, P. 1978. Taking the men out of menopause. In *The woman as patient*, eds. M. Notman and C. Nadelson. New York: Plenum Press.

Guice, E. 1991. Assumptions underlying two hypotheses of hot flash initiation and evidence pertaining to their validity. In *Menstruation, health and illness*, eds. D. Taylor and N. Woods. New York: Hemisphere.

Hargrove, J.T., Maxson, W.S., Wentz, A.C., and Burnett, L.S. 1989. Menopausal hormone replacement therapy with continuous daily oral micronized estradiol and progesterone. *Obstetrics and Gynecology* 73(4):606–612.

Harper, D.C. 1990. Perimenopause and aging. In *Gynecology: Well-woman care*, eds. R. Lichtman and S. Papera. Norwalk, CT: Appleton & Lange.

Harris, S.T., Genant, H.K., Baylink, D.J., Gallagher, J.C., Karp, S.K., McConnell, M.A., Green, E.M., and Stoll, R.W. 1991. *Archives of Internal Medicine* 151(10):1980–1984.

Hasselquist, M., Goldberg, N., Schroeter, A., and Spelsberg, T. 1980. Isolation and characterization of the estrogen receptor in human skin. *Journal of Clinical Endocrinology and Metabolism* 50(1):76–82.

Helgason, S. 1982. Estrogen replacement therapy after the menopause. Estrogenicity and metabolic effects. *Acta Obstetricia et Gynecologica Scandinavica* 107(Suppl):1–29.

Henderson, B.E. 1989. The cancer question: An overview of recent epidemiologic and retrospective data. *American Journal of Obstetrics and Gynecology* 161(6, Pt. 2):1859–1864.

Henrik, E. 1982. Neuroendocrine mechanisms of reproductive aging in women and female rats. In *Perspectives on menopause*, eds. A. Voda, M. Dinnerstein, and S. O'Donnell. Austin, TX: University of Texas Press.

Hirvonen, E., Malkonen, M., and Manningen, V. 1981. Effects of different progestogens on lipoproteins during postmenopausal replacement therapy. *New England Journal of Medicine* 304(10):560–563.

Honore, L.H. 1980. Increased incidence of symptomatic cholesterol cholelithiasis in perimenopausal women receiving estrogen replacement therapy: A retrospective study. *Journal of Reproductive Medicine* 25(4):187–190.

Hoover, R., Gray, L.A., Cole, P., and MacMahon, B. 1976. Menopausal estrogens and breast cancer. *New England Journal of Medicine* 295(8):401–405.

Hulka, B.S. 1990. Hormone replacement therapy and the risk of breast cancer. *CA—A Cancer Journal for Clinicians* 40(5):289–296.

Hunter, M.S. 1990. Emotional well-being, sexual behaviour, and hormone replacement therapy. *Maturitas* 12(3):299–314.

Hutchinson, T., Polansky, S.M., and Feinstein, A. 1979. Postmenopausal estrogens protect against fractures of hip and distal radius: A case-control study. *Lancet* 2:705–709.

Johannson, B.W., Kaij, L., Kullander, S., Lenner, H.C., Svanberg, L., and Astedt, B. 1975. On some late effects of bilateral oophorectomy in the age range 15–30 years. *Acta Obstetricia et Gynecologica Scandinavica* 54(5):449–461.

Kannel, W.B., Wolf, P.A., and Garrison, R.J. 1987. The Framingham Study. Some risk factors related to the annual incidence of cardiovascular disease and death using pooled repeated biennial measurements. In *Framingham Heart Study: 30 Year Followup*. Bethesda, MD: National Institutes of Health.

Kaufman, D.W., Miller, D.R., Rosenberg, L., Helmrich, S.P., Stolley, P., Schottenfeld, D., and Shapiro, S. 1984. Noncontraceptive estrogen use and the risk of breast cancer. *Journal of the American Medical Association* 252(1):63–67.

Kelsey, J., and Berkowitz, G. 1988. Breast cancer epidemiology. *Cancer Research* 48:5615–5623.

Krauss, R.M., Lindgren, F.T., Wingerd, J., and Bradley, D.D. 1979. Effects of estrogens and progestins on high density lipoproteins. *Lipids* 14:113–118.

Kudrow, L. 1975. The relationship of headache frequency to hormone use in migraine. *Headache* 15(1)36–40.

Lang, W., and Aponte, G. 1967. Gross and microscopic anatomy of the aged female reproductive organs. *Clinical Ob-Gyn* 10:454–465.

Lark, S. 1990. *The menopause self-help book: A woman's guide to feeling wonderful for the second half of her life.* Berkeley, CA: Celestial Arts.

Leaf, A. 1989. Management of hypercholesterolemia: Are preventive interventions advisable? *New England Journal of Medicine* 321:680–683.

Lindsay, R., Hart, D.M., MacLean, A., Clark, A.C., Kraszewski, A., and Garwood, J. 1978. Bone response to termination of oestrogen treatment. *Lancet* 1:1325–1327.

Lobo, R. 1987. Prevention of postmenopausal osteoporosis. In *Menopause: Physiology and pharmacology*, ed. D.R. Mishell, Jr., pp. 165–186. Chicago: Year Book Medical.

Lobo, R., McCormick, W., Singer, R., and Roy, S. 1984. DepoProvera compared with conjugated estrogens for the treatment of post-menopausal women. *Obstetrics and Gynecology* 63:1–5.

Longcope, C., Herbert, P.N., McKinlay, S.M., and Goldfield, S.R. 1990. The relationship of total and free estrogens and sex hormone-binding globulin with lipoproteins in women. *Journal of Clinical Endocrinology and Metabolism* 71(1):67–72.

Mack, T.M., Pike, M.C., Henderson, B.E., Pfeffer, R.I., Gerkins, V.R., Arthur, M., and Brown, S.E. 1976. Estrogens and endometrial cancer in a retirement community. *New England Journal of Medicine* 294(23):1262–1267.

MacPherson, K. 1985. Osteoporosis and menopause: A feminist analysis of the social construction of a syndrome. *Advances in Nursing Science* 7(4):11–22.

Makila, U., Wahlberg, L., Vlinikka, L., and Ylikorkala, O. 1982. Regulation of prostacyclin and thromboxane production by human umbilical vessels: The effect of estradiol and progesterone in a superfusion model. *Prostaglandins, Leukotrienes and Medicine* 8(2):115–124.

Martin, P.L., Yen, S.S., Burnier, A.M., and Hermann, H. 1979. *Journal of the American Medical Association* 242(24):2699–2700.

Matthews, K.A. 1989. Interactive effects of behavior and reproductive hormones on sex differences in risk for coronary heart disease. *Health Psychology* 8:373–387.

McBride, A.B., and McBride, W. 1981. Theoretical underpinnings for women's health: *Women and Health* 6:(1–2):37–55.

McCain, M. 1991. *Transformation through menopause.* New York: Bergin and Garvey.

McKinlay, S.M., Brambilla, D.J., and McKinley, J.B. 1991. Women's experiences of menopause. *Current Ob-Gyn* 1:3–7.

McKinlay, S.M., Brambilla, D.J., and Posner, J.G. 1992. The normal menopause transition. *American Journal of Biology* 4:37–46.

McKinley, J.B., McKinlay, S.M., and Brambilla, D.J. 1987. The relative contributions of endocrine changes and social circumstances to depression in middle-aged women. *Journal of Health and Social Behavior* 28:345.

Medical Economics. 1993. *Physicians' desk reference*, 47th ed. Montvale, NJ: the Author.

Merson, J. 1876. The climacteric period in relation to insanity. *West Riding Lunatic Asylum Reports (London)* 6:85–107.

Mishell, D. 1990. Contraceptive options for women in their 40s. *Journal of Reproductive Medicine* 35(4):448–477.

Montreal Health Press. *Menopause: A well woman health book.* Montreal: the Author.

Moyer, D.L., de Lignieres, B., Driguez, P., and Pez, J.P. 1993. Prevention of endometrial hyperplasia by progesterone during long-term estradiol replacement: Influence of bleeding pattern and secretory changes. *Fertility and Sterility* 59(5):992–997.

National Institutes of Health. 1979. *Consensus Development Conference Summaries*, Vol. 2. Washington, DC: U.S. Government Printing Office.

National Institutes of Health, National Institute on Aging. 1992. *Menopause.* Washington, DC: U.S. Government Printing Office.

National Institutes of Health Consensus Conference. 1984. Osteoporosis. *Journal of the American Medical Association* 252(6):799–802.

National Women's Health Network (NWHN). 1989. *Taking hormones and women's health*. Washington, DC: the Author.

Neugarten, B., and Kraines, R. 1965. Menopausal symptoms in women of various ages. *Psychosomatic Medicine* 27:266–273.

Nilas, L., and Christianson, C. 1989. The pathophysiology of peri- and post-menopausal bone loss. *British Journal of Obstetrics and Gynaecology* 96:580–587.

Notelovitz, M. 1982. Carbohydrate metabolism in relation to hormonal replacement therapy. *Acta Obstetricia et Gynecologica Scandinavica* 106(suppl):51–56.

———. 1986. Interrelations of exercise and diet on bone metabolism and osteoporosis. *Current Concepts in Nutrition* 15:203–227.

———. 1987. The role of the gynecologist in osteoporosis prevention: A clinical approach. *Clinical Obstetrics and Gynecology* 30(4):871–882.

———. 1989. Estrogen replacement therapy: Indications, contraindications, and agent selection. *American Journal of Ob-Gyn* 161(6, Pt. 2):1832–1841.

Notelovitz, M., Gudat, J., Ware, M., and Dougherty, M. 1982. Oestrogen-progestin therapy and the lipid balance of post-menopausal women. *Maturitas* 4(4):301–308.

Notelovitz, M., Kitchens, C., Ware, M. 1984. Coagulation and fibrinolysis in estrogen-treated surgically menopausal women. *Obstetrics and Gynecology* 63(5):621–625.

Notelovitz, M., Kitchens, C., Ware, M., Hirschberg, K., and Coone, L. 1983. Combination estrogen and progestogen replacement therapy does not adversely affect coagulation. *Obstetrics and Gynecology* 62(5):596–600.

Notelovitz, M., Martin, D., Tesar, R., Khan, F., Probart, C., Fields, C., and McKenzie, L. 1991. Estrogen therapy and variable-resistance weight training increase bone mineral in surgically menopausal women. *Journal of Bone and Mineral Research* 6(6):583–590.

Odell, W., and Swerdloff, R. 1968. Progestogen-induced LH and FSH surge in post menopausal women: A simulated ovulatory peak. *Proceedings of the National Academy of Sciences USA* 61:529–536.

Office of Technology Assessment. 1992. *The menopause, hormone therapy, and women's health*: U.S. Congress background paper. Washington, DC: U.S. Government Printing Office.

Page, J. 1977. *The other awkward age*. Berkeley, CA: Ten Speed Press.

Petitti, D.B., Sidney, S., and Perlman, J.A. 1988. Increased risk of cholecystectomy in users of supplemental estrogen. *Gastroenterology* 94(1):91–95.

Porcino, J. 1983. *Growing older, getting better*. Reading, MA: Addison-Wesley.

Ramey, E.R. 1982. The national capacity for health in women. In *Women: A developmental perspective*, eds. P.W. Berman and E.R. Ramey (NIH Publication No. 82–2298). Washington, DC: U.S. Government Printing Office.

Ranney, B., and Abu-Ghazaleh, S. 1977. The future function and fortune of ovarian tissue which is retained in vivo during hysterectomy. *American Journal of Obstetrics and Gynecology* 128(6):626–634.

Reader, S., Robertson, W., and Diczfalusy, E. 1983. Microheterogeneity of LH in pituitary glands from women of pre- and postmenopausal age. *Clinical Endocrinology* 19:355–363.

Reitz, R. 1982. *Menopause: A positive approach*. New York: Penguin Books.

Research Advances in Osteoporosis. February, 1990. National Osteoporosis Conference Summary Statement. Arlington, VA.

Resnick, N.M., and Greenspan, S.L. 1991. Senile osteoporosis reconsidered. *Journal of the American Medical Association* 261(7):1025–1029.

Resnik, R. 1976. The effect of progesterone on estrogen-induced uterine blood flow. *Gynecologic Investigation* 128:251–254.

Riggs, B.L. 1987. Pathogenesis of osteoporosis. *American Journal of Obstetrics and Gynecology* 156:1342–1346.

Riggs, B.L., and Melton, L.J. 1986. Involutional osteoporosis. *New England Journal of Medicine* 314:1676–1686.

Riggs, B.L., Wahner, H.W., Seeman, E., Offord, K.P., Dunn, W.L., Mazess, R.B., Johnson, K.A., and Melton, L.J. 1982. Changes in bone mineral density of the proximal femur and spine with aging: Differences between the postmenopausal and senile osteoporosis syndromes. *Journal of Clinical Investigation* 70:716–723.

Rongaglioni, M.C., di Minno, G., Reyers, I., de Gaetano, G., and Donati, M.B. 1979. Increased prostacyclin-like activity in vascular tissues from rats on long-term treatment with an oestrogen-progestogen combination. *Thrombosis Research* 14(4–5):793–797.

Rosenberg, L., Hennekens, C., Rosner, B., Belanger, C., Rothman, K., and Speitzer, R. 1981. Early menopause and the risk of myocardial infarction. *American Journal of Ob-Gyn* 139:47–51.

Ross, R.K., Paganini-Hill, A., Gerkins, V.R., Mack, T.M., Pfeffer, R., Arthur, M., and Henderson, B.E. 1980. A case-control study of menopausal estrogen therapy and breast cancer. *Journal of the American Medical Association* 243:1635–1639.

Rubin, L. 1979. *Women of a certain age: The midlife search for self.* New York: Harper & Row.

Ruggiero, R.J. 1992. Currently used estrogen preparations. *Hormone Replacement 1992: New Attitudes.* San Francisco: East Bay Institute for Research and Education.

Seltzer, V., Benjamin, F., and Deutsch, S. 1990. Perimenopausal bleeding patterns and pathologic findings. *Journal of the American Medical Women's Association* 45(4):132–134.

Semmens, J., and Wagner, G. 1982. Estrogen deprivation and vaginal function in postmenopausal women. *Journal of the American Medical Association* 248:445–448.

Shangold, M.M. 1982. How exercise benefits older women. *Contemporary Ob-Gyn* 19(3):81–86.

Sherman, B., West, J., and Korenman, S. 1976. The menopausal transition: Analysis of LH, FSH, estradiol and progesterone concentrations during menstrual cycles of older women. *Journal of Clinical Endocrinology and Metabolism* 42:629–636.

Sherwin, B.B. 1985. Changes in sexual behavior as a function of plasma sex steroid levels in postmenopausal women. *Maturitas* 7:225–233.

Sherwin, B.B., Gelfand, M.M., and Brender, W. 1985. Androgen enhances sexual motivation in females: A prospective, crossover study of sex steroid administration in the surgical menopause. *Psychosomatic Medicine* 47:339–351.

Smith, D.C., Prentice, R., Thompson, D.J., and Hermann, W.L. 1975. Association of exogenous estrogen and endometrial carcinoma. *New England Journal of Medicine* 293(23):1164–1167.

Smith, P. 1972. Age changes in the female urethra. *British Journal of Urology* 44:667–676.

Speroff, L., Glass, R.H., and Kase, N.G. 1989. *Clinical gynecologic endocrinology and infertility*, 4th ed. Baltimore: Williams & Wilkins.

———. 1994. *Clinical gynecologic endocrinology and infertility*, 5th ed. Baltimore: Williams & Wilkins.

Stampfer, M.J., and Colditz, G.A. 1991. Estrogen replacement therapy and coronary heart disease: A quantitative assessment of the epidemiologic evidence. *Preventive Medicine* 20:47–63.

Steinberg, K.K., Thacker, S.B., Smith, J., Stroup, D.F., Zack, M.M., Flanders, W.D., Berkelman, R.L. 1991. A meta-analysis of the effect of estrogen replacement therapy on the risk of breast cancer. *Journal of the American Medical Association* 265(15):1985–1990.

Stout, R. 1987. Aging and atherosclerosis. *Age and Aging* 6(2):65–72.

Strickland, B.R. 1988. Sex-related differences in health and illness. *Psychology of Women Quarterly* 12:381–399.

Stumpf, W., Sar, M., and Keefer, D. 1975. Atlas of estrogen target cells in rat brain. In *International conference on neurobiology of CNS-hormone interactions*, eds. W. Stumpf and D. Grant. Basel: S. Karger.

Sturdee, D., Wilson, K., Pipili, E., and Crocker, A. 1978. Physiologic aspects of menopausal hot flush. *British Medical Journal* 2:79–80.

Thom, T.J. 1987. Cardiovascular disease mortality among U.S. women. In *Coronary heart disease in women*, eds. E. Eaker, B. Packard, N. Wenger, T. Clarkson, and H. A. Tyroler. New York: Haymarket Doyma.

Treloar, A. 1974. *Predicting the close of menstrual life.* Presentation at Third Annual Society for Menstrual Cycle Conference, April 26–27. Tucson, AZ.

———. 1982. Predicting the close of menstrual life. In *Changing perspectives on menopause*, eds. A. Voda, M. Dinnerstein, and S. O'Donnell. Austin, TX: University of Texas Press.

Treloar, A., Boynton, R., Behn, B., and Brown, B. 1967. Variation in the human menstrual cycle through reproductive life. *International Journal of Fertility* 12:77–126.

U.S. Department of Commerce, Bureau of the Census. 1982. Money, income, and poverty of families and persons in the United States. *Current population reports,* ser. P–60, no. 134, 1–34. Washington, DC: U.S. Government Printing Office.

———. 1989. Projections of the population of the United States, by age, sex, and race: 1988 to 2080. *Current population reports,* ser. P–25, no. 1018. Washington, DC: U.S. Government Printing Office.

U.S. Department of Labor, Bureau of Labor Statistics. 1982. *Linking employment problems of economic status,* Bulletin 2123, table 2, p. 11. Washington, DC: U.S. Government Printing Office.

Utian, W.H. 1975. Effect of hysterectomy, oophorectomy and estrogen therapy on libido. *International Journal of Gynecology and Obstetrics* 13(3):97–100.

———. 1989. Biosynthesis and physiologic effects of estrogen deficiency: A review. *American Journal of Ob-Gyn* 161(6, Pt. 2):1828–1831.

VanKeep, P., Brand, P., and Lehert, P. 1979. Factors affecting the age at menopause. *Journal of Biosocial Science* 6(Suppl.):37–55.

VanLook, P., Lothian, H., Hunter, W., Michie, E., and Baird, D. 1977. Hypothalamic-pituitary-ovarian function in perimenopausal women. *Clinical Endocrinology* 7:13–31.

Voda, A.M. 1981. Climacteric hot flash. *Maturitas* 3:73–90.

————. 1982. Perimenopausal transition. In *Changing perspectives on menopause*, eds. A. Voda, M. Dinnerstein, and S. O'Donnell. Austin, TX: University of Texas Press.

————. 1984. *Menopause: Me and you*. Salt Lake City: University of Utah School of Nursing.

————. 1992. Menopause: A normal view. *Obstetrics and Gynecology* 35(4):923–933.

Voda, A.M., and Eliasson, M. 1983. Menopause: The closure of menstrual life. *Women and Health* 8(2/3):137–156.

Voda, A.M., and George, T. 1986. Menopause. *Annual Review of Nursing Research* 4:55–75.

Walker, B. 1985. *The crone: Women of age, wisdom and power*. New York: Harper & Row.

Wallace, R., Hoover, J., and Barrett-Connor, E. 1979. Altered lipid and lipoprotein levels associated with oral contraceptive and estrogen use: Report from the Medications Working Group of the Lipids Research Clinics Program. *Lancet* 2:111–115.

Walsh, B.W., Schiff, I., Rosner, B., Greenberg, L., Ravnikar, V., Sacks, F. M. 1991. Effects of postmenopausal estrogen replacement on the concentrations and metabolism of plasma lipoproteins. *New England Journal of Medicine* 325(17):1196–1204.

Watkins, B., Meites, J., and Riegle, G. 1975. Age-related changes in pituitary responsiveness to LhRH in the female rat. *Endocrinology* 19:331–338.

Weed, S.S. 1992. *Wise woman ways: Menopausal years*. Woodstock, NY: Ashtree.

Weiss, R.E., Gorn, A., Dux, S., Nimni, M.E. 1981. Influence of high protein diets on cartilage and bone formation in rats. *Journal of Nutrition* 111(5):804–816.

Weiss, N., Ure, C., Ballard, J., and Daling, J. 1980. Decreased risk of fractures of the hip and lower forearm with post-menopausal use of estrogen. *New England Journal of Medicine* 303:1195–1198.

Weissman, M.M., and Klerman, G. 1977. Sex differences, and the epidemiology of depression. *Archives of General Psychiatry* 34:98–111.

White, E.C. 1990. *The black women's health book: Speaking for ourselves*. Seattle: Seal Press.

Whitehead, M.I., Siddle, N., Lane, G., Padwick, M., Ryder, T.A., Pryse-Davies, J., and King, R.J.B. 1987. The pharmacology of progestins. In *Menopause: Physiology and pharmacology*, ed. D.R. Mishell, Jr., pp. 317–334. Chicago: Year Book Medical.

Wide, L., Hobson, B. 1983. Qualitative difference in follicle-stimulating hormone activity in the pituitaries of young women compared to that of men and elderly women. *Journal of Clinical Endocrinology and Metabolism* 56(2):371–375.

Wide, L., and Wide, M. 1984. Higher plasma disappearance rate in the mouse for pituitary FSH of young women compared to men and women. *Acta Endocrinologica (Copenhagen)* 74:1–58.

Williams, A., Weiss, N., Ure, C., and Daling, J. 1982. Effect of weight, smoking and estrogen use on the risk of hip and forearm fractures in postmenopausal women. *Obstetrics and Gynecology* 60:695–699.

Wilson, R.A. 1966. *Feminine forever*. New York: Evans.

Wilton, J., and Noonan, M. 1991. A menopause center: Bridging the midlife gap. In *Clinical Issues in Perinatal and Women's Health Nursing* 2(4):533–538.

Wingard, D.L. 1984. The sex differential in morbidity, mortality, and lifestyle. *Annual Review of Public Health* 5:433–458.

Wingo, P.A., Layde, P.M., Lee, N.C., Rubin, G., and Ory, H.W. 1987. The risk of breast cancer in postmenopausal women who have used estrogen replacement therapy. *Journal of the American Medical Association* 257:209–215.

Wise, A., Gross, M., and Schalch, D. 1973. Quantitative relationships of the pituitary-gonadal axis in postmenopausal women. *Journal of Laboratory and Clinical Medicine* 81:28–36.

Wolfe, S.M. 1991. *Women's health alert*. Reading, MA: Addison-Wesley.

Woods, N. 1982. Menopausal distress: A model for epidemiologic investigation. In *Changing perspectives on menopause*, eds. A. Voda, M. Dinnerstein, and S. O'Donnell. Austin, TX: University of Texas Press.

World Health Organization. 1981. *Research on menopause*, WHO Technical Report, serial no. 670. Geneva: the Author.

The Writing Group for the PEPI Trial. 1995. Effects of estrogen or estrogen/progestin regimens on heart disease risk factors in post-menopausal women. *Journal of the American Medical Association* 273(3):199–208.

Young, R.L., Kumar, N.S., and Goldzieher, J.W. 1990. Management of menopause when estrogen cannot be used. *Drugs* 40(2):220–230.

Ziel, H.K., and Finkel, W.D. 1975. Increased risk of endometrial carcinoma among users of conjugated estrogens. *New England Journal of Medicine* 293(23):1167–1170.

Diana Taylor, Ph.D., R.N., F.A.A.N.

12-N

Perimenstrual Symptoms and Premenstrual Syndrome

The term *perimenstrual symptoms* refers to the cyclic symptom experience in relation to menstruation. Although the majority of women experience one or more perimenstrual symptoms, they do not experience distress or disability associated with them. Very few women experience perimenstrual symptoms to such a degree of severity that it would be considered a syndrome. In this section, the distinction between perimenstrual symptoms and perimenstrual syndromes is explored, along with assessment and therapeutic directions.

Premenstrual syndrome (PMS), a diagnosis that characterizes multiple symptom clusters, is the cyclical recurrence of distressing physical, affective, and behavioral changes that result in the deterioration of interpersonal relationships and personal health (Brown and Zimmer 1986). In addition to these more provocative associations, a woman's experience with perimenstrual symptoms has been found to reduce work efficiency, increase absenteeism, and have an impact on family and personal relationships (Bergsjo, Jenssen, and Vellar 1975; Bickers and Woods 1951; Brown and Zimmer 1986; Parker 1960).

PMS, popularly considered a means for discounting or excusing women's behavior, is not socially or culturally confined (Janiger, Riffenburgh, and Kersh 1972; WHO 1981). In the United States, black and white women have equal frequencies of various premenstrual symptoms, with frequency of symptom reporting peaking in the 25- to 34-year-old group. The prototypical woman seeking professional help for perimenstrual symptoms is a working woman in her early to mid-30s with one or more children (Steege, Stout, and Rupp 1987; Taylor and Bledsoe 1986).

While the majority of women experience a few symptoms associated with the menstrual cycle, approximately eight percent to ten percent of menstruating women, representing eight million American women, experience multiple symptoms to a severe degree (Woods, Dery, and Most 1982a; Woods et al. 1987). Prevalence estimates indicate that 25 percent to 40 percent of women in the general population report mild to moderate perimenstrual symptoms, and two percent to eight percent report extreme or severe symptoms. This estimate is much more conservative than estimates in previous studies (Woods, Dery, and Most 1982b).

Cultural variations exist, according to two cross-cultural studies: fatigue and tension (42 percent) in Japanese women; headache and breast tenderness (80 percent to 90 percent) in Nigerian women; tension, mood swings, bloating (60 percent to 80 percent) in Turkish women; compared with irritability in 70 percent of American women (Janiger, Riffenburgh, and Kersh 1972). Positive perimenstrual symptom experiences have received little attention but have been found to be more prevalent (50 percent to 60 percent) than negative symptom experiences in a community sample of women (Woods et al. 1987).

The definition of PMS includes the delineation of symptom clusters, symptom severity patterns, and the degree of impact on a woman's functional status. The classic form of PMS includes symptom clusters that are severe during the premenstrual phase but decline after menses onset, with mild or no symptom severity experienced during the postmenstrual phase. Premenstrual magnification of physical or negative affect symptoms that continue in severity during the postmenstrual phase can be considered a syndrome separate from PMS. Often, premenstrual magnification (PMM) reflects an underlying condition that worsens with the premenstrual phase.

The majority of women who seek professional help come with the self-made diagnosis of PMS. Of these women, 30 percent to 40 percent will have a relatively classic form of PMS, 30 percent to 40 percent will have a premenstrual exacerbation of an underlying disorder (i.e., PMM), and 20 percent to 30 percent will have a chronic problem without premenstrual exacerbation.

Perimenstrual Symptoms and Typologies

While the most commonly reported perimenstrual symptoms may be complaints of physical discomfort (bloating, skin changes, cramping), the reports of mood change or negative affect symptoms are often the most distressing. Many investigators have confirmed that negative affect symptoms, rapid mood changes, and arousal emerge as the prominent factors accounting for much of the distress experienced by women in the perimenstruum (premenstrual and menstrual phases) (Abraham 1980; Futterman et al. 1988; Halbreich et. al. 1982; Moos 1968; Taylor and Woods 1991; Woods, Dery, and Most 1982a; Woods et al. 1987). This prominent and most distressing symptom cluster is referred to as perimenstrual negative affect (PNA) (Taylor and Woods 1991).

With more than 100 reported symptoms attributed to menstrual cyclicity, delineation of symptoms into subtypes is an important step in understanding women's perimenstrual symptom experience. Several investigators have systematically addressed the differentiation of perimenstrual symptom subtypes (Moos 1968; Abraham 1980; Halbreich et al. 1982; Taylor 1988; Woods 1985). Taylor and Woods (1991) classified symptom clusters of women experiencing severe symptoms using factor and cluster analysis.

→ **PNA** (perimenstrual negative affect) is the most common symptom cluster and has been found to account for 60 percent of the variance in symptom severity: anger, tension, irritability, hostility, anxiety, mood swings, irritability, guilt, impatience, depression, feeling out of control, tearfulness.

→ **PPD** (perimenstrual pain/discomfort) includes symptoms of abdominal/pelvic pain, headache, joint aches/pains.

→ **PDS** (perimenstrual dysphoric symptoms) includes depression, decreased sexual desire, fatigue, decreased energy, decreased appetite, fluid retention.

Symptom Patterns

Patterns of symptom severity or symptom cluster severity are important components of the diagnostic process. Symptom severity patterns are determined by calculating the difference in severity of symptoms or symptom clusters between menstrual cycle phases (Mitchell, Woods, and Lentz 1991). Symptom severity patterns that have been investigated most include the classic PMS severity pattern, with low-severity symptoms occurring postmenstrually and high-severity symptoms occurring premenstrually, and a PMM severity pattern, with moderate- to high-severity symptoms occurring in the postmenses phase and increasing in the premenstrual phase (Harrison et al. 1984; Mitchell, Woods, and Lentz 1991).

While clinicians and researchers generally agree that PMS is not a psychiatric disorder, the National Institute of Mental Health (NIMH) Premenstrual Syndrome Workshop developed criteria that are included in the *Diagnostic and Statistical Manual for Psychiatric Disorders (DSM-IV)*. In 1986, the American Psychiatric Association voted to include "Premenstrual Dysphoric Disorder" (PDD) in the appendix of the DSM, based on the argument that perimenstrual symptoms are considered a psychiatric disorder and therefore are stigmatizing to women. While it is sometimes difficult to differentiate premenstrual symptoms from symptoms of psychiatric disorders, women properly classified do not have significant psychiatric diagnoses (APA 1994).

PMS Etiology

The underlying mechanisms for menstrually related mood syndromes have been poorly understood because of the predominance of a biomedical conceptualization of PMS as a unidimensional or pathological condition. Menstrually related syndromes are complicated biobehavioral conditions requiring a broad biopsychosocial framework to effectively organize clinical data. Perimenstrual symptoms and syndromes may act as modulators or entrainers of other disorders or they may be an abnormal response to normal biological rhythms (e.g., the menstrual cycle, circadian rhythms, adrenocortical pulses).

To date, none of the proposed etiological theories have been substantiated. Biomedical theories have included hypotheses about estrogen excess, estrogen/progesterone imbalance, aldosterone increase, vitamin deficiencies, hypoglycemia, hyperprolactinemia, and psychogenic factors. Current alternative hypotheses have suggested stress as well as endogenous opiate withdrawal as causal factors (Lewis 1992; Reame et al. 1984; Reid and Yen 1983). PMS, in particular, is most likely a psychoneuroendocrine disorder whereby psychosocial variables become influential in lowering the individual's threshold to experience perimenstrual symptoms in response to normal or abnormal biological changes of the menstrual cycle.

Adding stress to the explanatory model of PMS has been proposed by a number of investigators and can be considered a mediator or a causative agent in PMS etiology. Many of the neuroendocrine secretions associated with the human stress response are associated with initiating or aggravating PMS. During the stress response, secretion of aldosterone, antidiuretic hormone, adrenocorticotropic hormone (ACTH), glucocorticoids, and epinephrine is increased (Girdano and Everly 1979; Ganong 1983; Katz and Romfh 1972; Marinari, Leshner, and Doyle 1976; Selye 1956). The stress response may also further disrupt the balance between estrogen and progesterone (Yen and Jaffe 1986).

ACTH increases the amount of estrogen produced by the adrenal glands (Abplanalp et al. 1977; Ganong 1983). High levels of cortisol, representing a chronic stress response, may operate to amplify the reactivity of behavioral and symptom response. Labeling stress responses as PMS may be an acceptable avenue for women to seek professional and/or self-help (Taylor and Woods 1991).

Stress as an antecedent or a physiological response cannot be considered independent from the environment or life context of each individual woman. A woman's psychological and health status may act in concert with her biological processes to determine the ultimate expression of her symptoms and their impact on her life (Brooks-Gunn 1985; Reid 1988; Taylor and Woods 1991; Woods 1985). The manifestation of PMS, particularly PNA, may result from a combination of multiple stressors, a heightened stress response, few supports, and a vulnerable period of biological reactivity.

Treatment for PMS

Treatment for PMS has ranged from the dangerous (ovarian irradiation) to the ridiculous (hiding in one's room) (Delaney, Lupton, and Toth 1976; Frank 1931). Since no singular etiology for PMS has been identified, singular pharmacological therapies have been tried without success. To date, most of the treatments in the pharmacological trials have been as effective as the placebo (Dennerstein et al. 1985; Freeman et al. 1990; Sampson 1979). Clinical research suggests that a combination of treatments may be more satisfactory than a single treatment (Keye 1988; Taylor 1988; Taylor and Woods 1991).

Although support for a nutritional etiology for PMS is lacking in the scientific literature, nutritional ther-

apy for PMS remains common (dietary changes, vitamin and mineral supplementation) (Abraham 1980, 1983; Biskind and Biskind 1942). Research on exercise and the neuroendocrine system suggests that biopsychosocial benefits of a regular exercise program may directly alleviate some of the symptoms of PMS, as well as indirectly mediate symptoms through healthy coping behavior (Farrell et al. 1982; Prior and Vigna 1987).

A clinical trial of the using of relaxation for treating of PMS found a 58 percent reduction in PNA after three months of daily relaxation (Goodale, Domar, and Benson 1990). Support groups have been described as helpful in relieving PMS severity (Robertson 1991; Taylor and Bledsoe 1985); however, most women find the peer support helpful only after initiation of treatment (Taylor 1988; Taylor and Bledsoe 1985). In a survey of women receiving pharmacological treatment for PMS, all women reported using two or more self-care or nonpharmacological strategies in addition to the drug treatments (Mills 1988).

DATABASE

SUBJECTIVE

→ It is critical to listen to the woman's story—her description of symptoms, symptom clusters, symptom severity, symptom patterns, as well as the effect of the perimenstrual symptom experience on her life, her personal functioning, and her environment (relationships, family, work).

→ *General characteristics* of women seeking professional help for perimenstrual symptoms:
- age early to mid-30s.
- one or more children.
- working outside the home.
- experiencing high levels of stress and distress.
- experiencing significant marital discord.
- diminished libido during premenstrual phase.
- symptoms decline in severity as menopause approaches.

→ Reproductive events *not* substantiated as associated with the onset of PMS:
- menarche.
- childbirth.
- oral contraceptive (OC) use.
- abortion.
- pre-eclampsia.

→ Perimenstrual symptom history: If a woman does not identify herself as having PMS, begin by asking her about the nature of her symptoms:
- which symptoms are the most severe or distressing?

- timing of the symptoms throughout the menstrual cycle?
- does anything worsen or alleviate the symptoms?
- presence of symptoms during or after menstruation?
- time and events surrounding onset or exacerbation of symptoms?

→ PMS history: If the woman has been self-identified as having PMS, initially focus on the following questions:

- why do you think you have PMS?
- PMS severity? Rate from minimal to extreme.
- five most distressing *premenstrual* symptoms?
- five most distressing *menstrual* symptoms?
- how long have you experienced PMS?
- age at onset of PMS?
- do you associate an event with PMS onset (childbirth, OC use, tubal ligation, menarche, stressful event)?
- has PMS severity decreased or increased since onset?
- describe the quality of change in PMS severity?
- what makes the symptoms worse or better?
- what forms of treatment have you tried (pharmacological, self-help)?
- work absenteeism or decreased work productivity due to PMS?
- seasonal changes in PMS?
- what are the negative or positive effects of PMS on your life?
- how has PMS affected your family or close relationships?
- what do you think causes PMS?
- what are your treatment goals or outcomes?

→ Additional historical data: In addition to the usual health history data, specific historical data that assist with perimenstrual symptom classification include:

- menstrual regularity.
- marked fluctuations in weight in the non-pregnant state.
- premenstrual alcohol intolerance.
- positive feelings/changes associated with menstruation/menstrual cycle.
- mother's/sister's experiences with perimenstrual symptoms.
- intolerance to OCs, symptoms associated with sterilization procedure.
- postpartum symptoms, perimenstrual symptoms associated with pregnancy.

- inquire about menstrual cycle variation related to any chronic condition, such as upper respiratory or allergy symptoms, asthma, arthritis, migraines, dermatological conditions, eating disorders, depression, vulvovaginitis, fibroids, endometriosis, or chronic PID.

→ Complete personal function, lifestyle, and health status history (e.g., well-being, sleep, exercise, stress, nutrition):

- current health status: how healthy have you felt in the past six months (1-10 scale)?
- general level of well-being by menstrual cycle phase, season, or life events.
- sleep patterns: sleep onset, difficulty falling asleep, difficulty staying asleep, early morning awakening, use of sleeping medications/remedies, feeling rested, naps.
- physical activity: level of physical activity, type and amount of exercise or physical activity.
- stress: general level of stress over the past three months (1-10 scale), types of stressors (personal health, work, family life, personal life), level of stress created by the stressors, stress management strategies.
- nutrition: weight, perception of weight, diet patterns, use of stimulants, vitamins/nutritional supplements, food cravings, eating binges, how often food controls your life.

→ Symptom assessment: The PMS history will provide general information about the woman's symptom experience, but prospective ratings are critical to a precise diagnosis and to ruling out other chronic illness.

- Retrospective symptom severity reports are likely to overestimate severity and do not provide data about symptom patterns.
- Ask if the woman has monitored her symptom severity using a calendar or a symptom checklist.
- PMS calendar (see **Figure 12N.1, Perimenstrual Symptom Calendar**):
  - a menstrual or PMS calendar is useful for women who are able to describe their unique symptoms and symptom clusters and to visualize symptom severity patterns.
  - women fill in their most distressing symptoms, beginning on the first day of their last menstrual period (LMP), using a five-point rating scale (0—no severity, 1—minimal severity, 2—mild severity, 3—moderate severity, 4—extreme severity).

Figure 12N.1.   PERIMENSTRUAL SYMPTOM CALENDAR

Name: _____

ID#: _____

Last Menstrual Period: _____

Instructions:
Record the date of the **first day of your menstrual period** (*first day of bleeding*) in the box above day one. List those physical and emotional symptoms you find most bothersome in the blanks below. Estimate the severity of the symptom(s) (0-4) and write that number in the box opposite the symptom(s) and below the appropriate date. If you can, try to fill out the questionnaire about the same time every day.

Grading of Symptoms
0   Not Present
1   Minimal
2   Mild
3   Moderate
4   Extreme
X   Menses/Bleeding

1st day of menstruation ↓																																			
DATE																																			
DAY OF CYCLE	1	2	3	4	5	6	7	8	9	10	11	12	13	14	15	16	17	18	19	20	21	22	23	24	25	26	27	28	29	30	31	32	33	34	35
MOST BOTHERSOME SYMPTOM(S)																																			

SOURCE: Reprinted with permission from Menstrual Disorder Clinic. 1989. Portland, OR: Oregon Health Sciences University.

■ *Menstrual Symptom Severity Checklist* (MSSL) (see **Table 12N.1, The Menstrual Symptom Severity List**):
  • the MSSL is a 33-item symptom list developed from other menstrual symptom questionnaires and tested and revised through multiple studies (Mitchell et al. 1992; Mitchell, Woods, and Lentz 1991).
  • women rate the symptoms daily using the same severity rating scale as for the menstrual or PMS calendar (0-4).
  • the MSSL is useful for delineating perimenstrual symptom clusters.

→ Family-partner evaluation: Using the MSSL or the menstrual calendar, ask the woman's partner to rate her symptoms for one complete cycle.
  ■ This component of the evaluation reveals both the involvement of the partner in the therapeutic process and the impact of the perimenstrual symptom experience on the relationship.
  ■ Having the partner complete a separate evaluation provides some privacy if the partner is reluctant to directly communicate an assessment.
  ■ Discrepancies between the assessments of the patient and her partner can be used to query the woman about particular symptoms or behavior (e.g., alcohol and drug use, sexual response or behavior, marital discord).
  ■ Many partners experience higher levels of distress and marital discord related to the patient's perimenstrual symptom experience than the patient herself.
  ■ The partner's assessment can be used to develop a complete treatment plan that may include marital counseling.

Table 12N.1. THE MENSTRUAL SYMPTOM SEVERITY LIST (MSSL) EMBEDDED IN THE ORIGINAL SYMPTOM LIST OF THE WASHINGTON WOMEN'S HEALTH DIARY

Daily Experience List

Please read the list of feelings and behaviors. Please fill in the blank next to the number that best describes how you felt today. Fill in 0 for each day if not present.

0 Not present	1 minimal	2 mild	3 moderate	4 extreme

1. *Abdominal pain, discomfort	_____	30. *Hostility	_____
2. *Anger	_____	31. *Hot flashes or sweats	_____
3. *Anxiety	_____	32. *Impatience, intolerance	_____
4. *Awakening during the night	_____	33. Impulsiveness	_____
5. *Backache	_____	34. In control	_____
6. *Bloating or swelling of abdomen	_____	35. Increased activity	_____
7. Blurred or fuzzy vision	_____	36. Increased appetite	_____
8. Bursts of energy or activity	_____	37. Increased food intake	_____
9. Confusion	_____	38. *Increased sensitivity to cold	_____
10. Cramps–uterine or pelvic	_____	39. Increased sexual desire	_____
11. *Craving for specific foods or tastes	_____	40. *Increased sleeping	_____
12. Craving for alcohol	_____	41. Intentional self-injury	_____
13. Decreased appetite	_____	42. *Irritability	_____
14. *Decreased food intake	_____	43. *Loneliness	_____
15. *Decreased sexual desire	_____	44. Lowered coordination/clumsiness	_____
16. *Depression (feel sad or blue)	_____	45. *Lowered desire to talk/move	_____
17. *Desire to be alone	_____	46. Nausea	_____
18. Diarrhea	_____	47. Nervousness	_____
19. *Difficulty concentrating	_____	48. *Out of control	_____
20. *Difficulty in getting to sleep	_____	49. *Painful or tender breasts	_____
21. *Difficulty making decisions	_____	50. *Rapid mood changes	_____
22. Dizziness or lightheadedness	_____	51. Restlessness	_____
23. *Early morning awakening	_____	52. *Sensation of weight gain	_____
24. Fatigue or tiredness	_____	53. *Skin disorders	_____
25. *Feelings of guilt	_____	54. Suicidal ideas or thoughts	_____
26. Feelings of well-being	_____	55. *Swelling of hands or feet	_____
27. Forgetfulness	_____	56. *Tearfulness, crying easily	_____
28. General aches and pains	_____	57. *Tension	_____
29. *Headache	_____		

*The 33 symptoms used to create severity level and cycle phase difference criteria. Copyright © 1990 by N. F. Woods, E. S. Mitchell, and M. J. Lentz.

Source: Reprinted with permission from Woods, N. F., Mitchell, E.S., and Lentz, M. J. 1990. Center for Women's Health Research. Seattle: University of Washington.

- It is important to first describe this process to the patient as a usual component of the evaluation process.
  - If the partner is not present for the evaluation, send the forms home with the patient with specific instructions on filling out the menstrual calendar or MSSL.

OBJECTIVE

→ Physical examination: A general physical examination is important to detect any signs of anatomical change or disease, with specific focus on:
- vital signs as indicated.
- weight (may weigh in luteal phase and after menses to document edematous changes) (Barger 1988).
- assessment of affect, mental health.
- skin examination.
- thyroid examination.
- breast examination.
- abdominal examination.
- complete pelvic examination.
- additional physical examination components as indicated by history.

→ Defining symptom clusters: Group the symptoms recorded on the MSSL or PMS calendar into clusters and rate their severity:
- **PNA**: anger, tension, irritability, hostility, anxiety, mood swings, guilt, impatience, depression, feeling out of control, tearfulness.
- **PPD**: abdominal/pelvic pain, headache, joint aches/pains.
- **PDS**: depression, decreased sexual desire, fatigue, decreased energy, decreased appetite, fluid retention.
- **other** symptoms and symptom clusters.

→ Identifying symptom patterns: Determine symptom severity patterns for total perimenstrual symptoms or for symptom clusters by using DSM-IV criteria or Mitchell-Woods criteria (Mitchell, Woods, and Lentz 1991). See **Table 12N.2, Perimenstrual Symptom Classification Using DSM-IV and Mitchell-Woods Criteria** for criteria.
- The most common symptom patterns include:
  - classic PMS pattern: increasing symptom severity from postmenses (low severity) to premenses (high severity), with at least a 30 percent cycle phase difference.
  - PMM pattern: increasing symptom severity from postmenses (moderate to high severity) to premenses (high to higher severity), without a 30 percent cycle phase difference.
  - other patterns: decreasing symptom severity from postmenses to premenses, with or without a cycle phase difference (this pattern has received little attention and has yet to be typed).

ASSESSMENT

→ Perimenstrual symptoms
→ PMS—symptom clusters classified as:
- PNA subtype
- PPD subtype
- PDS subtype
- other (describe specific symptom cluster)

→ PMM
→ R/O underlying chronic illness with menstrual cycle exacerbation
→ R/O chronic illness (physical/psychological) without cyclical exacerbation
→ R/O menstrual/ovarian dysfunction
→ R/O sexual dysfunction
→ R/O dysmenorrhea
→ E/O endometriosis
→ R/O chronic pelvic pain
→ R/O STDs
→ R/O urinary tract infection/vaginitis
→ R/O endocrine disorder (e.g., hyperprolactinemia, hypothyroidism)
→ R/O breast pain and nodularity (fibrocystic changes)
→ R/O situational stress reaction
→ R/O anxiety
→ R/O depression
→ R/O other psychiatric illness

PLAN

DIAGNOSTIC TESTS

→ Comprehensive symptom, PMS, and health history: described in "Subjective" section.
→ Define symptom clusters and identify symptom patterns. See "Objective" section.
→ Affective disorders may be ruled out using measures of anxiety and depression questionnaires, which can assist in assessment and need for psychiatric referral. Many women

Table 12N.2. PERIMENSTRUAL SYMPTOM CLASSIFICATION USING *DSM-IV* AND MITCHELL-WOODS CRITERIA

Prospective Rating	Symptom occurrence confirmed by prospective daily self-ratings in at least two cycles. Define premenstrual and postmenstrual days to use as comparisons (one to three days of menses can be included in premenstrual phase calculations).
Regularity	Premenstrual phase-specific symptom occurrence in at least two sequential cycles.
Severity	Symptom or symptom cluster severity must cause marked distress or marked impairment in social or occupational function. Sum severity level by symptom cluster (PNA, PDS, PPD) or total symptoms for each phase.
Symptom Pattern	Symptoms display a particular temporal characteristic: symptoms or symptom cluster severity increasing or decreasing from postmenses to premenses.
Cycle Phase Difference	Compare premenstrual symptom severity with postmenstrual symptom severity baseline to determine increasing or decreasing symptom pattern. Symptom cluster severity is present for most of the time during the last week of the luteal phase, begins to remit within a few days after the onset of the follicular phase, and becomes absent in the week post-menses (APA 1994).

attribute all of their symptom distress to PMS, and the results from the questionnaires can provide evidence of a possible psychiatric condition.

- The SCL-90 provides a total distress score as well as scores on eight subscales, including anxiety and depression. Developed by Derogatis (Derogatis and Cleary 1977), the instrument can be scored by hand or entered into the computer and compared with normative, standard scores.
- A number of depression inventories exist, in addition to the subscale for depression in the SCL-90. The Beck Depression Inventory (BDI) (Beck et al. 1961) was developed for use in primary care settings.

→ Laboratory tests: As yet, there is no physiological or hormonal test that confirms the diagnosis of PMS. However, some laboratory studies may be useful for ruling out other conditions:

- serum thyroid stimulating hormone (TSH) (preferably a radioimmunoassay) and thyroxine (free T_4) as indicated to rule out hypothyroidism.
- CBC or Hgb/Hct as indicated to rule out anemia.
- prolactin levels as indicated for galactorrhea or chronic menstrual irregularity.
- serum follicle stimulating hormone (FSH) to rule out menopausal status if a woman is reporting regular hot flashes and menstrual irregularity.

NOTE: Measuring estrogen and progesterone is not recommended for routine assessment.

- wet mounts and genital cultures as indicated to rule out vaginitis/STDs.
- urinalysis as indicated to rule out cystitis.

TREATMENT/MANAGEMENT

→ The goal is to understand each individual's perimenstrual symptoms experience and to help her define and manage the symptoms and their concomitant problems.

→ Biomedical treatments: The following treatments are pharmacological, and only those that have been found to be useful are described. Although it can be argued that vitamin therapy is pharmacological, it will be discussed as part of the symptom management strategies.

- Progesterone: Regardless of the lack of evidence confirming progesterone deficiency as a causal mechanism for PMS, large doses of progesterone have a sedative effect on both men and women.
  - Anecdotal reports of progesterone treatment suggest dramatic relief of PNA.
    - However, randomized controlled clinical trials of progesterone therapy have failed to demonstrate a significant difference between the effects of progesterone and placebo (Adolphe, Dorsey, and Napoliello 1977; Backstrom, Boyle, and Baird 1981; Maddocks et al. 1986; Sampson 1980).
  - Progesterone therapy for treatment of PMS has not received FDA approval (adequate informed consent is mandatory), yet many clinicians consider it useful for some women with severe PNA in the luteal phase to reduce arousal sensations.

- micronized progesterone: 100 mg 1-3 times/day (oral capsules):
  - –non-brand name in powder form must be capsulized by local pharmacist.
  - –may also be obtained (with prescription) from "Health Pharmacies" (608) 277-0407 or 800-373-6704, or "Madison Pharmacy Associates," (608) 833-7046 or 800-558-7046. (Both organizations will send written information and price lists on request.)
  - –micronized progesterone rectal/vaginal suppositories: 50 mg-400 mg 1-4 times/day:
    - ▸ absorption is more rapid via the vaginal or rectal route.
    - ▸ suppositories available through local pharmacist or mail order.
  - –Micronized progesterone sublingual liquid: 25 mg-100 mg 1-6 times/day:
    - ▸ sublingual liquid available through mail order.
- Regimen for progesterone: begin using at ovulation or 2-3 days before symptom onset, gradually decreasing at time of menses:
  - –side effects include dizziness and sleepiness. Although long-term sequelae of natural progesterone are unlikely, the chronic effects of cyclical levels of progesterone and its metabolites remain unknown.

- Ovarian suppression: A number of investigators have found that temporarily suppressing ovulation can reduce both PMS and PPD in women who have been properly classified (Bancroft et al. 1987; Hammarback and Backstrom 1988; Taylor and Harrison-Hohner 1991; Walker and Bancroft 1990).
  - For women who experience symptoms that begin at ovulation or marked perimenstrual pain (dysmenorrhea, endometriosis, menstrual migraines), suppression of ovarian function can bring relief of symptom severity. For most women, a low-dose OC regimen is safest, with few side effects.
  - Combination estrogen/progestin OCs:
    - –any low-dose (30 mcg-35 mcg estrogen) OC with standard administration.
    - –if pelvic pain or cyclical headaches are part of the symptom complex, continuous administration of the OC is necessary.
    - –side effects: common nuisance symptoms include breakthrough bleeding and nausea, which resolve with use.
      - ▸ Gradually introducing the continuous regimen may eliminate the bleeding

episodes (i.e., 5, 3, 1 day break from OC until continuous dose in the third month).
    - –danger signs associated with OCs should be monitored.
  - Synthetic progesterone:
    - medroxyprogesterone acetate (Provera®): 10 mg-20 mg/day p.o. administered continuously to suppress ovulation temporarily.
    - side effects: the dose necessary to suppress ovulation may cause intolerable side effects— breakthrough bleeding, depressive symptoms, decreased libido, weight gain; elevated serum cholesterol and triglycerides may also occur.
      - –Perimenstrual symptoms may be exaggerated in some women.
    - Depo-Provera® has not been used for control of perimenstrual symptoms.
  - Synthetic androgens (17-alpha ethinyl testosterone derivative—Danazol®) and GnRH analogs (nafarelin acetate—Synarel®, leuprolide acetate—Lupron®) may be considered for women who continue to experience cyclical pelvic pain in addition to other perimenstrual syndromes and do not respond to OC regimens or Provera®.

NOTE: Consultation and comanagement are recommended since these women are likely to need additional evaluation (laparoscopy, pelvic imaging).

- Aldosterone inhibitors: Since plasma aldosterone levels are known to rise during the luteal phase of the normal menstrual cycle, interest in the hypothesis that excessive aldosterone secretion could account for premenstrual fluid retention has received clinical attention but has never been confirmed.
  - While most women experience a shift in body fluids during the premenstruum, few will actually increase their total body weight.
  - A few women will experience marked discomfort related to fluid retention in their extremities, breasts, and abdomen.
  - Marked fluid retention may be responsible for premenstrual headaches.
  - Spironolactone (Aldactone®) is both an aldostrone inhibitor and a potassium-sparing, mild diuretic.
  - Dose: 50 mg p.o. BID starting 2-3 days before the anticipated symptoms until menses.
  - Combine with natural forms of diuretic foods (asparagus, apple cider vinegar, herbal teas).

- No adverse reactions except in women with impaired renal function, who may experience hyperkalemia.
- Avoid concurrent use of furosemide and ethacrynic acid because of the precipitation of rebound edema on abrupt withdrawal.
- May be used with thiazides if an additive diuretic action is desired.
▪ Prostaglandin inhibitors: Studies of prostaglandins and their essential fatty acid precursors in women with PMS have suggested lower circulating levels of certain prostaglandins as well as gamma linolenic acid and arachidonic acid (Brush et al. 1984).
  - Both elevated and reduced levels of prostaglandins have been suggested as an etiology for PMS, and treatments based on these hypotheses have involved 2 seemingly opposite approaches: 1) administering an enriched preparation of gamma linolenic acid (derived from oil of evening primrose) to enhance prostaglandin production and, 2) administering prostaglandin synthetase inhibitors to prevent the effects of excessive prostaglandin action.
    –Both approaches have been reported effective in reducing perimenstrual symptoms (which raises questions about patient selection and methodology).
  - NSAIDs may be helpful for reducing PPD:
    –each NSAID has specific side effects as well as a recommended dosage that should be followed. See **Dysmenorrhea** Protocol.
  - Oil of evening primrose is marketed under a number of different brand names, and anecdotal evidence suggests that it reduces PMS severity. Women may try this product prior to professional evaluation and subsequently may want professional guidance.
    –It is important to tell women that:
      ‣ evening primrose oil is an essential fatty acid, gamma-linoleic acid, sometimes marketed under the trade name Efamol®.
      ‣ no long-term side effects are known, but reported short-term side effects are skin blemishes, nausea, soft stools or diarrhea, headache.
      ‣ dose: 1-2 capsules p.o. BID/TID from midcycle to menses, taken on a full stomach.
▪ Psychotropics: Psychotropic medications, such as antidepressants or tranquilizers, have no place in the initial treatment of PMS.

Pharmacological treatment with psychotropics should be considered only for women who have been classified with PMM or who have a dual diagnosis.
→ Symptom management program for PMS therapy: Only women with the most extreme manifestations are likely to require pharmacological therapy.
  ▪ A biopsychosocial approach to PMS treatment can often result in a complete or marked reduction to bothersome perimenstrual symptoms.
  ▪ If pharmacological treatment is necessary, a nonpharmacological approach can be complementary and decrease the dose and duration of the pharmacological therapy. Perimenstrual symptom management is one such biopsychosocial, nonpharmacological approach to PMS therapy.
  ▪ Self-monitoring: Self-awareness of symptom severity and symptom patterns is the first step to treatment. For symptom self-monitoring, methods have been described previously.
    • For some women, self-monitoring alone may be enough to assist them in making the necessary therapeutic changes.
    • Monitoring stress in relationships and work and the individual's reaction to stressors are as important as symptom self-monitoring.
  ▪ Personal choice: Symptom management includes using multiple nonpharmacological treatments that will involve time and energy on the part of the woman experiencing PMS.
    • Previous studies indicate that women want to be in control of their treatment by choosing 2 or more types of nonpharmacological therapy.
    • Allowing choice among treatments provides women control over treatments that may be time-consuming.
    • An individualized treatment plan should be established initially and updated regularly until PMS severity is reduced and stabilized.
    • The treatment plan provides a "treatment contract" between the health care provider and the patient and should include evaluation criteria.
  ▪ Self-modification: Clinical evidence suggests a relationship between dietary changes, vitamin supplementation, and exercise and relief from PMS.
    • These approaches involve a modification of personal behaviors: dietary change, nutritional

supplementation, physical activity and/or exercise.

- Diet and nutritional therapy: Lack of certain vitamins, minerals, and nutrients has been found to be related to menstrual cycle hormones.
  - While little proof exists that dietary change alone reduces PMS severity, a healthy diet promotes general good health and minimizes other stresses and diseases.
  - Furthermore, a typical American diet includes a great deal of simple sugars, processed foods, additives, salt, and stimulants, which further deplete the natural stores of vitamins and minerals.
  - General recommendations include:
    - following a diet high in fruits, vegetables, and complex carbohydrates.
    - following a low-sodium diet in the premenstrual phase.
    - reducing intake of all sugars, including sucrose, fructose, glucose, honey, and brown sugar.
    - avoiding alcohol completely or in the premenstruum.
    - reducing caffeine intake, especially premenstrually.
    - selecting snacks high in nutrients and low in sugars, salt, and fat.
    - selecting whole foods (not refined or processed) such as whole grain breads, brown rice, nuts, seeds.
    - reducing fats by decreasing meat intake, using unsaturated fats such as cold-pressed unhydrogenated vegetable oils, and using low-fat dairy products in moderation.
    - drinking 1 to 2 quarts of water daily along with fruit juices (in moderation) and herbal teas.
    - eating frequent small meals (every 2 hours) during the premenstruum.
    - for women experiencing severe PNA, reducing all forms of caffeine (chocolate, cola, black tea, coffee), especially during the premenstrual phase:
      * caffeine withdrawal symptoms may be avoided by gradually reducing caffeine or by mixing decaffeinated with caffeinated coffee.
      * women experiencing PD may actually find caffeine therapeutic and can tolerate moderate amounts of caffeine, which may improve their mood.
      * sugar, candy, and chocolate can act in the same way as caffeine causing exacerbation of symptoms.
- Nutritional supplements: Vitamins, minerals, amino acids, and PMS-formula supplements have been suggested as nutritional therapy for PMS. Vitamin B_6 and magnesium have been studied more thoroughly than other supplements.
  - Vitamin B_6 (pyridoxine): This vitamin is involved in converting the amino acid tryptophan to serotonin and levodopa (L-DOPA) to dopamine. Both dopamine and serotonin are related to mood and affect.
    - Unfortunately, Vitamin B_6 is not a harmless placebo and can cause irreversible nerve damage and sensory neuropathy at doses of 500 mg daily (Schaumberg et al. 1983).
    - For women who want to try Vitamin B_6, these recommendations should be followed:
      * start with 100 mg-200 mg/day p.o., midcycle to menses.
      * do not take more than 500 mg/day and take only cyclically.
      * side effects of Vitamin B_6 excess include numbness and tingling in arms and legs, shooting pain, headaches, fatigue, dizziness, and weakness.
      * take with a multiple vitamin or PMS-formula vitamin (see p. 12-152).
  - Magnesium: While the theory that women with PMS suffer from a magnesium deficiency has not been substantiated, increasing magnesium has been found to reduce premenstrual constipation.
    - Constipation will increase premenstrual pelvic pain and abdominal bloating.
    - Food sources high in magnesium include whole grains, seeds, and vegetables.
    - Magnesium supplements can be taken in doses of 100 mg-250 mg p.o. during the pre-menstrual week, along with increasing amounts of water.
  - Other vitamins: No other individual vitamin has been found to be effective in reducing PMS severity. Vitamin A, while having no effect on PMS, may be useful in acne treatment. Vitamin E (tocopherol) is present in evening primrose oil and has had mixed results as an individual treatment for PMS.
  - Amino acids: Amino acids are precursors to brain neurotransmitters such as dopamine and serotonin; therefore, amino acid

supplements have been suggested to decrease PNA and PD.

▸ Tryptophan, an amino acid precursor to serotonin, has received the most attention. Dosages as high as 8 g-10 g have been studied with mixed results. Most recently, however, irreversible blood dyscrasias have been associated with tryptophan use (Harrison et al. 1984; Jones 1987).

▸ Increasing foods high in tryptophan is the recommended method for attempting to increase tryptophan (turkey, complex carbohydrates, low-fat dairy products).

▸ Increasing these foods is most appropriate for PNA symptom severity since they have a mild tranquilizing effect.

–Multivitamin and mineral supplements— PMS formulas: A variety of PMS supplements are on the market. Some contain extremely high levels of vitamins or require a woman to take 10 to 15 pills daily to reach the recommended level.

▸ However, many women find it easier to take a vitamin and mineral supplement that contains Vitamin B_6, magnesium, and a combination multivitamin.

▸ A few cautionary recommendations can help a woman to choose an appropriate supplement:

  * choose a PMS supplement that contains approximately 200 mg-300 mg of Vitamin B_6 in 4-6 pills/day (no more than 500 mg/day).

  * avoid supplements that have excessive amounts of fat-soluble vitamins (Vitamins A, E).

  * take PMS-formula vitamins for half the month, switching to a regular multi-vitamin for the remainder of the month.

• Exercise: Research on exercise and the neuroendocrine system suggests that biopsychosocial benefits of a regular exercise program may directly alleviate some of the symptoms of PMS and also indirectly mediate symptoms through healthy coping behavior.

–Most studies have investigated aerobic exercise as a treatment for PMS (Canty 1984; Prior and Vigna 1987), and 1 study indicated a lowered incidence of PMS among women who ran 1 mile to 1.5 miles per day (Jones 1987).

–Aerobic exercise: While daily exercise is good for all-around health, increasing activity levels 1 to 2 weeks premenstrually is helpful for the woman experiencing PNA since moving muscles prompts the brain to produce endogenous opiates.

▸ Assessing current forms of aerobic exercise and pleasurable forms of physical activity is critical to the success of this symptom management strategy.

▸ Set realistic short- and long-term goals.

▸ Plan for warm-up or cool-down periods (one or both, depending on the type of exercise).

▸ Plan aerobic exercise, such as walking, jogging, walking-jogging, swimming, bicycling, skipping rope.

▸ Plan time of day and specific place to exercise and keep exercise log initially.

▸ Work up to a 20-minute session, 3 to 5 times per week.

–Exercise modification and nonaerobic exercise: Many women find it difficult to continue aerobic exercise during the premenstruum because of breast tenderness, abdominal bloating, or cyclical headaches. One of the easiest and most effective modifications is yoga, a series of gentle poses that involves stretching, breathing, and visualization.

▸ Yoga videotapes and classes are often available in the community.

▸ Specific yoga poses—e.g., the sponge, the bow, and the plow—are particularly helpful for PNA symptoms as well as for the physical symptoms accompanying menstruation.

▸ Yoga or stretching exercises can also be incorporated into an aerobic exercise plan.

■ Self-regulation: Although little is known about stress management and PMS, extensive evidence exists on the effects of stress reduction strategies and psychophysiological response.

• Therapeutic effects of cognitive and behavioral stress reduction activities have been demonstrated for headaches, sexual problems, neurodermatitis, hypertension, cardiac disease, depression, anxiety, cancer, and Raynaud's disease (Hamberger and Lohr 1984).

• A clinical trial of the use of relaxation for treatment of PMS found a 58 percent reduction in PNA after 3 months of daily relaxation (Goodale, Domar, and Benson 1990).

- Both cognitive and behavioral stress reduction strategies have been found to be important for self-regulation in women (Taylor 1988; Taylor and Woods 1991).
  - Behavioral strategies for stress reduction:
    - assess specific areas of stress for each individual.
    - use counter-conditioning to avoid physiological arousal:
      - progressive relaxation using tension-relaxation.
      - progressive relaxation without using tension.
    - combine nonaerobic exercise with counterconditioning exercise.
    - instructions for these exercises can be found in Pender's *Health Promotion in Nursing Practice* (1987) and Bulechek and McCloskey's *Nursing Interventions* (1992).
  - Cognitive strategies for stress reduction: Many women have difficulty using behavioral stress reduction strategies to relax because of cognitive tension. Women may describe their minds racing or feeling as if they "can't stop certain thoughts."
    - To take advantage of the physiological effects of the behavioral stress reduction strategies, these women will need instruction on cognitive stress reduction.
    - Identify negative thought patterns and critical self-assessments.
    - Introduce thought-stopping exercises.
    - Change critical or negative self-images by introducing positive images.
    - Enhance self-esteem as a method to reduce cognitive stress: identify real versus ideal body image and performance; identify positive self-image; visualize high and low self-esteem; perform thought-stopping exercises for negative comparisons and perfectionist thinking; and prioritize and set goals for change.
- Environmental modification: Stress is complex and usually includes external as well as personal aspects. Focusing only on the woman may emphasize her role as the "victim" or as being "sick."
  - A combination of personal and environmental change is usually necessary to reduce the effects of stress.
  - Physical or structural environment: Women have difficulty saying "no" to requests or needs from their family, friends, or co-workers,

or they don't pay attention to stress-inducing situations. Recommendations for changing stress related to daily activities include:
  - minimize the frequency of stress-inducing situations.
  - stabilize daily routines.
  - assess responsibility for stress (self or others).
  - schedule change to minimize stress-inducing situations.
  - set specific goals for change.
- Social and relationship environment: Relationships with family members, intimates, or coworkers have been identified as a major source of stress for most women. This area of stress reduction includes enhancement of personal and social competency.
  - Assess relationships:
    - identify areas of stress in particular relationships.
    - identify standards for certain relationships (marital, intimate, friendships).
    - assess relationship patterns and choices.
  - Assess communication patterns.
  - Assess verbal and nonverbal expressions of feeling.
  - Assess stress in particular expressions of feeling.
  - Identify strategies for healthy expression of feeling.
  - Practice assertive behaviors.
  - Balance work/family/love: Identify areas of importance.
  - Demonstrate time management strategies: Prioritize time in each area.
  - Modify social, relationship, and work environments:
    - identify areas of personal control in work and social situations.
    - prioritize change strategies and set goals.
- Peer support and professional guidance: Previous studies of women with severe PMS have found that peer support groups alone are not satisfactory for reducing PMS severity (Taylor 1988; Taylor and Woods 1991).
  - Women with a long duration of severe PMS report a lack of trust in other women with similar symptom severity.
  - Professional guidance is necessary in the early phases of treatment. Furthermore, much of the symptom management education can be administered in a group format with individual follow-up.

- Once women have begun to individualize their symptom management regimens, they can continue in a peer support group to individualize and reinforce treatment success further.
- Specific components of professional guidance and peer support include:
  - professional guidance: prior to being able to access support from other women experiencing PMS, women need professional expertise and information, combined with caring and facilitation of an individualized treatment program. These factors have been identified by women seeking professional help.
  - peer support: once a woman has begun the treatment process and experiences symptom relief, she is able to take advantage of help from other women suffering from PMS.
    - ▸ Factors identified as important to peer support include mutual nurturance, emotional attachment, reassurance of self-worth, and practice at social integration and behavior change.

CONSULTATION

- → Consultation with a PMS specialist is indicated when the patient's symptoms can not be successfully managed by the primary care provider.
  - Many communities have clinics specializing in the assessment and treatment of menstrual disorders.
  - Contact a local nurse practitioner (NP) or nursing organization for listings.
- → Consultation with or referral to a mental health provider may be necessary if the symptom severity is determined to be affective in nature.
- → Consultation with a physician may be indicated for an identified underlying medical problem.
- → As needed for prescription(s).

PATIENT EDUCATION

- → Education begins with the evaluation and self-monitoring process. By monitoring daily health and perimenstrual symptoms, women become aware of internal and external process over the course of their menstrual cycle.
  - For some women, treatment is only symptom management and self-monitoring.
  - However, for most women, education in the form of verbal, written, or audiovisual information will follow the diagnosis.

- → Providing the woman with written and verbal information about the specific diagnosis (PMS, PMM) is the next step in the education process.
  - Explain to her that diagnosis will be followed by an individualized treatment plan and a preliminary contract, starting with the use of the symptom management strategies.
  - Developing of the treatment program will take two or more sessions and can be accomplished in a group format.
- → Books and audiotapes can be an important supplement to the education process. One of the better publications on PMS self-help is Bender and Kelleher's *PMS: A Positive Program to Gain Control* (1986). Stress management audiotapes are helpful to some women.
- → Education in a group format is an efficient method for introducing symptom management strategies.
  - Self-modification strategies can be introduced at one session, with each woman completing her own self-modification plan.
  - Subsequent group sessions can add the self-regulation and environmental modification strategies with practice time.
  - A final session can be used to develop an individualized treatment plan and personal contract (Menstrual Disorder Program 1989).

FOLLOW-UP

- → The initial evaluation will take one to two hours, depending upon individual complexity, and can be divided into two sessions, or history forms can be mailed to the woman prior to her visit.
  - Once the diagnosis has been made, two additional visits will be necessary, with or without group sessions.
  - A post-treatment session should be scheduled at three months to assess treatment success. Women should be advised to monitor their symptoms using a menstrual calendar for at least two treatment cycles.
- → Refer patient to specialty clinic or health care provider with expertise in PMS as indicated. Use community mental health resources if patient requires ongoing psychosocial support.
- → Follow up on abnormal laboratory tests. Refer patient's partner for evaluation/treatment of identified STDs.

→ Treat or refer for treatment/management as indicated for any identified underlying medical condition.

→ Document in progress notes and problem list.

Bibliography

Abplanalp, J. 1983. Psychologic components of the premenstrual syndrome: Evaluating the research and choosing the treatment. *Journal of Reproductive Medicine* 28:517.

Abplanalp, J., Livingston, L., Rose, D.M., and Sandwisch, D. 1977. Cortisol and growth hormone responses to psychological stress during the menstrual cycle. *Psychosomatic Medicine* 39:158.

Abraham, G. 1980. Premenstrual tension. *Current Problems in Obstetrics and Gynecology* 3:723.

———. 1983. Nutritional factors in the etiology of the premenstrual tension syndromes. *Journal of Reproductive Medicine* 28:446–464.

Abraham, G., and Hargrove, J. 1980. Effect of vitamin B_6 on premenstrual symptomology in women with premenstrual tension syndrome: A doubleblind crossover study. *Infertility* 3:155.

Abraham, G. and Lubran, M. 1981. Serum and red cell magnesium levels in patients with premenstrual tension. *American Journal of Clinical Nutrition* 34:2364–2366.

Adolphe, A., Dorsey, E., and Napoliello, M. 1977. The neuropharmacology of depression. *Diseases of the Nervous System* 38:341.

American Psychiatric Association. 1994. *Diagnostic and Statistical Manual of Mental Disorders*, 4th ed. Washington, DC: the Author.

Andersch, B. 1983. Bromocriptine and premenstrual tension: A clinical and hormonal study. *Pharmatherapeutica* 3:107–113.

Backstrom, T., Boyle, H., and Baird, D., 1981. Persistence of symptoms of premenstrual tension in hysterectomized women. *British Journal of Obstetrics and Gynaecology* 88:530.

Bancroft, J., Sanders, D., Warner, P., and Loudon, N. 1987. The effects of oral contraceptives on mood and sexuality: A comparison of triphasic and combined preparations. *Journal of Psychosomatic Obstetrics* 7:1–8.

Barger, M.K. 1990. *Protocols for gynecological and obstetric health care.* Philadelphia: W.B. Saunders.

Beck, A., Ward, C., Mendelson, M., Mock, J., and Erbaugh, J. 1961. An inventory measuring depression. *Archives of General Psychiatry* 4:561.

Bender, S., and Kelleher, K. 1986. *PMS: A positive program to gain control.* Tucson, Ariz.: HP Books.

Bergsjo, P., Jenssen, H., and Vellar, O. 1975. Dysmenorrhea in industrial workers. *Acta Obstetrica Gynecologica Scandinavia* 54:355–359.

Bickers, W., and Woods, M. 1951. Premenstrual tension, a rational treatment. *Texas Journal of Reproduction and Biological Medicine* 9:406.

Biskind, M., and Biskind, G. 1942. Effect of vitamin B complex deficiency on activation of estrone in the liver. *Endocrinology* 31:109–112.

Brooks-Gunn, J. 1985. The salience and timing of the menstrual flow. *Psychosomatic Medicine* 47:363–371.

Brown, M., and Zimmer, P. 1986. Personal and family impact of premenstrual symptoms. *Journal of Obstetrical, Gynecological and Neonatal Nursing* 15:31–38.

Brush, M., Watson, S., Horrobin, D., and Manku, M. 1984. Abnormal essential fatty acid levels in plasma of women with premenstrual syndrome. *American Journal of Obstetrics and Gynecology* 150:363–369.

Bulechek, G., and McCloskey, J. 1992. *Nursing interventions.* Philadelphia: W.B. Saunders.

Canty, A. 1984. Can aerobic exercise relieve the symptoms of premenstrual syndrome? *Journal of Occupational Science and Health* 54:410–411.

Dalton, K. 1954. Similarity of symptomatology of premenstrual syndrome and toxaemia of pregnancy and their response to progesterone. *British Medical Journal* 2:1071–1077.

———. 1959. Menstruation and acute psychiatric illness. *British Medical Journal* 1:148–149.

———. 1960. Menstruation and accidents. *British Medical Journal* 2:1425–1426.

———. 1961. Menstruation and crime. *British Medical Journal* 2:1752–1753.

———. 1964. The influence of menstruation on health and disease. *Proceedings of the Royal Society of Medicine* 57:262–264.

Day, J. 1979. Danazol and the premenstrual syndrome. *Postgraduate Medical Journal* 55:87.

Delaney, J., Lupton, M., and Toth, E. 1976. The storm before the calm: The premenstrual syndrome. In *The curse: The cultural history of menstruation*, eds. J. Delaney, M. Lupton, and E. Toth. New York: E.P. Dutton.

Dennerstein, L., Spencer-Gardner, C., Gotts, G., Brown, J., Smith, M., and Burrows, G. 1985. Progesterone and the premenstrual syndrome: A double blind crossover trial. *British Medical Journal* 290:1617–28.

Derogatis, L., and Cleary, P. 1977. Confirmation of the dimensional structure of the SCL-90: A study in construct validation. *Journal of Clinical Psychology* 33:981–989.

Farrell, P., Gates, W., Maksud, M., and Morgan, W. 1982. Increases in plasma beta-endorphin/beta-lipotropin immunoreactivity after treadmill running in humans. *Journal of Applied Physiology* 52:5.

Frank, R. 1931. The hormonal causes of premenstrual tension. *Archives of Neurologic Psychiatry* 26:1031.

Freeman, E., Rickels, K., Sondheimer, S., and Polansky, M. 1990. Ineffectiveness of progesterone suppository treatment for premenstrual syndrome. *Journal of the American Medical Association* 264:349–353.

Futterman, L., Jones, J., Miccio-Fonseca, L., and Quiqley, T. 1988. Assessing premenstrual syndrome using the premenstrual experience assessment. *Psychological Reports* 63:19–34.

Ganong, W. 1983. *Review of medical physiology*, 11th ed. Los Altos, CA: Lange Medical.

Girdano, D., and Everly, G. 1979. *Controlling stress and tension: A holistic approach*. Englewood, NJ: Prentice-Hall.

Goodale, I., Domar, A., and Benson, H. 1990. Alleviation of premenstrual syndrome symptoms with the relaxation response. *Obstetrics and Gynecology* 75:649–655.

Halbreich, U., Endicott, J., Schach, S., and Nee, J. 1982. The diversity of premenstrual changes as reflected in the premenstrual assessment form. *Acta Psychiatrica Scandinavia* 62:177–180.

Hamberger, L., and Lohr, J. 1984. *Stress and stress management*. New York: Springer.

Hammarback, S., and Backstrom, T. 1988. Induced anovulation as treatment of premenstrual tension syndrome. *Acta Obstetrics and Gynecology Scandinavia* 67:159–166.

Harrison, W., Endicott, J., Rabkin, J., and Nee, J. 1984. Treatment of premenstrual dysphoric changes: Clinical outcome and methodological implications. *Psychopharmacology Bulletin* 20:118–122.

Haskett, R., Steiner, M., Osmun, J., and Carroll, B. 1980. Severe premenstrual tension: Delineation of the syndrome. *Biological Psychiatry* 15:121–139.

Hudson, W. 1982. *The clinical measurement package: A field manual*. Chicago: Dorsey Press.

Janiger, O., Riffenburgh, M., and Kersh, M. 1972. A cross-cultural study of premenstrual symptoms. *Psychosomatics* 13:226–235.

Jones, J. 1987. Nutritional therapies for PMS. *The Melpomene Report* 6:10–14.

Katz, F., and Romfh, P. 1972. Plasma aldosterone and renin activity during the menstrual cycle. *Journal of Clinical Endocrinology and Metabolism* 34:819–821.

Keye, W. 1988. The clinical approach to management and treatment. In *The premenstrual syndrome*, ed. W.R. Keye. Philadelphia: W.B. Saunders.

Lewis, L. 1992. PMS and the progesterone controversy. In *Menstrual health in women's lives*, eds. A. Dan and L. Lewis. Chicago: University of Illinois Press.

Maddocks, S., Hahn, P., Moller, F., and Reid, R. 1986. A double-blind placebo-controlled trial of progesterone vaginal suppositories in the treatment of premenstrual syndrome. *American Journal of Obstetrics and Gynecology* 154:573–581.

Marinari, K., Leshner, A., and Doyle, M. 1976. Menstrual cycle status and adrenocortical reactivity to psychological stress. *Psychoneuroendocrinology* 1:22–36.

Menstrual Disorder Program. 1989. *Menstrual Calendar*. Portland: School of Nursing, Oregon Health Services.

Mills, S. 1988. *The impact of stress on PMS severity for women in couple relationships: Summary of the principal results*. Presentation handout, Women's Health Conference, Portland, OR.

Mitchell, E., Lentz, M., Woods, N., Lee, K., and Taylor, D. 1992. Methodologic issues in the definition of premenstrual symptoms. In *Menstrual health in women's lives*, eds. A. J. Dan and L. L. Lewis. Chicago: University of Illinois Press.

Mitchell, E., Woods, N., and Lentz, M. 1991. Perimenstrual symptoms and perimenstrual syndromes. In *Menstruation, health and illness*, eds. D. Taylor and N. Woods. New York: Hemisphere.

Moos, R. 1968. Psychological aspects of oral contraceptives. *Archives of General Psychiatry* 19:87–94.

O'Brien, P. 1985. The premenstrual syndrome. A review. *Journal of Reproductive Medicine* 30(2):113–26.

Parker, A. 1960. The premenstrual tension syndrome. *Medical Clinics of North America* 44:339.

Pender, N. 1987. *Health promotion in nursing practice*. Norwalk, CT: Appleton-Century-Crofts.

Prior, J., and Vigna, Y. 1987. Conditioning exercise decreases premenstrual symptoms. *European Journal of Applied Physiology* 55:349–355.

Reame, N., Sauder, S.E., Kelch, R., and Marshall, J. 1984. Pulsatile gonadotropin secretion during the human menstrual cycle: Evidence of altered frequency of gonadotropin-releasing hormone secretion. *Journal of Clinical Endocrinology and Metabolism* 59:328–337.

Reid, R. 1988. PMS: Etiologic medical theories. In *The premenstrual syndrome*, ed. W. Keye. Philadelphia: W.B. Saunders.

Reid, R., and Yen, S. 1983. The premenstrual syndrome. *Clinical Obstetrics and Gynecology* 26:710–718.

Robertson, M. 1991. A survey of multidisciplinary and interdisciplinary approaches to premenstrual syndrome. In *Menstruation, health and illness*, eds. D. Taylor and N. Woods. Washington, DC: Hemisphere.

Rubinow, D.R., Roy-Byrne, P., and Hoban, M.C. 1985. Menstrually related mood disorders. In *Premenstrual syndrome*, eds. H. Osofsky and S. Blumenthal. New York: American Psychiatric Association.

Sampson, G. 1979. Premenstrual syndrome: A double-blind controlled trial of progesterone and placebos. *British Journal of Psychiatry* 135:209–215.

———. 1980. Progesterone fluid and electrolytes in premenstrual syndrome. *British Medical Journal* 281:227.

Sampson, G., and Prescott, P. 1981. The assessment of the symptoms of premenstrual syndrome and their response to therapy. *British Journal of Psychiatry* 138:399.

Schaumberg, H., Kaplan, J., Windebank, A., Vick, N., Rasmus, S., Pleasure, D., and Brown, M. 1983. Sensory neuropathy from pyridoxine abuse: A new megavitamin syndrome. *New England Journal of Medicine* 309:445.

Selye, H. 1956. *The stress of life*. New York: McGraw-Hill.

Steege, J., Stout, A., and Rupp, S. 1987. Clinical features. In *The premenstrual syndrome*, ed. W. Keye. Philadelphia: W.B. Saunders.

Stokes, J., and Mendels, J. 1972. Pyridoxine and premenstrual tension. *Lancet* 1:1177–1181.

Taylor, D. 1988. *Nursing interventions for perimenstrual turmoil: A longitudinal therapeutic trial*. Unpublished dissertation, University of Washington, Seattle.

Taylor, D., and Bledsoe, L. 1985. PMS, stress and social support: A pilot study and therapeutic hypotheses. In *Culture, society, and menstruation*, eds. V. Oleson and N. Woods. Washington, DC: Hemisphere.

———. 1986. Peer support, PMS, and stress: A pilot study. *Health Care Women International* 7:159–71.

Taylor, D., and Harrison-Hohner, J. 1991. *Proceedings of the American Society for Psychosomatic Ob-Gyn*. Houston, TX.

Taylor, D., and Woods, N., eds. 1991. *Menstruation, health and illness*. New York: Hemisphere.

Walker, A., and Bancroft, J. 1990. Relationship between premenstrual symptoms and oral contraceptive use: A controlled study. *Psychosomatic Medicine* 52:86–96.

Woods, N. 1985. Self-care practices among young adult married women. *Research in Nursing and Health* 8:227–233.

Woods, N., Dery, G., and Most, A. 1982a. Stressful life events and perimenstrual symptoms. *Journal of Human Stress* 8:23–31.

———. 1982b. Estimating the prevalence of perimenstrual symptoms. *American Journal of Public Health* 72:1257–1264.

———. 1982c. Toward a construct of perimenstrual distress. *Research in Nursing and Health* 5:123–136.

Woods, N., Lentz, M., Mitchell, E., Lee, K., and Taylor, D. July-August 1987. Premenstrual symptoms: Another look. *Public Health Reports* (Suppl.) 106–112.

Woods, N.F., Mitchell, E.S., and Lentz, M.J. 1990. Center for Women's Health Research. Seattle: Univerity of Washington.

World Health Organization. 1981. A cross-cultural study of menstruation. *Studies in Family Planning* 12:3–16.

Yen, S., and Jaffe, R. 1986. *Reproductive endocrinology*. Philadelphia: W.B. Saunders.

Winifred L. Star, R.N., C., N.P., M.S.

12-O

Polyps—Endocervical, Cervical, and Endometrial

Endocervical and cervical polyps are the most common benign neoplastic lesions of the cervix occurring in about 4 percent of all gynecological patients. They are most common in multiparous women in their 40s and 50s. Polyps usually occur because of local inflammation with resultant focal cellular hyperplasia and proliferation. Malignant change within a polyp is extremely rare. Sometimes, microglandular endocervical hyperplasia will present as a 1- to 2-centimeter polyp, representing an exaggerated histologic response, usually to oral contraceptives (Herbst et al. 1992).

Endometrial polyps are localized overgrowths of endometrial glands and stroma projecting beyond the endometrial surface. Etiology is unknown. Since endometrial polyps are often associated with hyperplasia, unopposed estrogen may be the cause. The presence of numerous small polyps scattered throughout the endometrial cavity is referred to as *polypoid hyperplasia*. Polyps of endometrial origin are found in all age groups, with the peak incidence between ages 40 years and 49 years. One in four women with abnormal uterine bleeding will have endometrial polyps. Malignant change in an endometrial polyp is estimated to be as high as 0.5 percent. A woman with endometrial polyps has a twofold risk of subsequent endometrial carcinoma, most often of low stage and grade (Herbst et al. 1992).

DATABASE

SUBJECTIVE

→ Classic symptom of an endocervical/cervical polyp is intermenstrual bleeding, especially after intercourse, douching, or a pelvic examination;

leukorrhea may be present if the cervix is inflamed.

→ Majority of endometrial polyps are asymptomatic. If present, symptoms may include a wide range of abnormal bleeding patterns, with premenstrual and postmenstrual spotting being the most usual presentations.

OBJECTIVE

→ Endocervical/cervical polyps (terms may be used interchangeably):
  ▪ endocervical (arising from endocervical canal)—more common than cervical and seen more often in reproductive-age women; reddish-purple to cherry red, with a long, narrow pedicle; cervical (arising from ectocervix)—more often seen in postmenopausal women; cervical—greyish-white, with short, broad base.
  ▪ single or multiple; few millimeters to 4 cm in diameter.
  ▪ smooth, soft, friable to touch.
  ▪ if large, may dilate cervix.
  ▪ most often first recognized on routine speculum examination; may not be palpable because of soft consistency.

→ Endometrial polyps:
  ▪ most arise from uterine fundus.
  ▪ velvety, grey, tan, red, or brown.
  ▪ few millimeters to several centimeters in diameter; single large polyp may fill entire uterine cavity.
  ▪ may have broad base (sessile) or slender pedicle (pedunculated).

- may protrude from external cervical os if on long pedicle; otherwise, not usually visible on exam.
→ Pap smear may show inflammatory or atypical cells.

ASSESSMENT

→ Endocervical/cervical polyp
→ R/O endometrial polyp, small prolapsed myoma, retained products of conception, sarcoma, cervical malignancy, squamous papilloma

PLAN

DIAGNOSTIC TESTS

→ Diagnosis of endometrial polyps generally made during evaluation of abnormal uterine bleeding, i.e., via hysterectomy, hysteroscopy, or hysterosalpingography. If discovered, other endometrial pathology should be ruled out.
→ Endocervical/cervical and endometrial polyps should be sent to pathology after removal. See "Treatment/Management" section.
→ Additional lab studies/procedures as indicated: may include Pap smear, cervical cultures, wet mounts, CBC, endometrial biopsy.

TREATMENT/MANAGEMENT

→ Most endocervical/cervical polyps can be removed safely in the office.
  - Grasp the base of the polyp with an appropriate size clamp and avulse it with a twisting motion.
  - Some clinicians gently curet the base after removal.
  - Send the specimen to pathology for an histological diagnosis.
  - Bleeding may be controlled with pressure, ferric subsulfate (Monsel's solution), electrocautery, or cryocautery.

- If the polyp does not dislodge easily or if the patient has excessive pain—STOP. Refer to physician for further management.
→ Endometrial polyps are generally removed by curettage or hysteroscope after diagnosis by the physician.

CONSULTATION

→ For patients with abnormal bleeding when the diagnosis is uncertain.
→ Referral to physician is indicated if endometrial polyps are suspected and, in some cases, for removal of endocervical/cervical polyps.
→ For prolonged bleeding immediately after polyp removal.

PATIENT EDUCATION

→ Discuss the (usually) benign nature of the condition and methods for polyp removal. Advise that polyps may reoccur.
→ Ask the patient to return for reassessment if abnormal vaginal bleeding continues after polyp removal.

FOLLOW-UP

→ Based on case presentation.
→ Review pathology results.
→ If abnormal bleeding continues after polyp removal, evaluate the patient for endometrial hyperplasia or carcinoma; an endometrial biopsy is usually performed as a first step. Patient may require physician referral at this time.
→ Document in progress notes and problem list.

Bibliography

Herbst, A.L., Mishell, D.R., Stenchever, M.A., and Droegemueller, W. 1992. *Comprehensive gynecology*, 2d ed. St. Louis: Mosby Year Book.

Toni Ayres, Ed.D., R.N., M.F.C.C.

12-P

Sexual Dysfunction

Sexual dysfunction is generally categorized into one of the three phases in which it occurs—desire phase, arousal phase, or orgasm phase of sexual response (Kaplan 1979). Additional categories covered in this protocol include dyspareunia and vaginismus. Sexual dysfunction should be categorized as lifelong or acquired, general or situational, and affecting one or both partners (Schover et al. 1982).

Desire Phase Disorder

Hypoactive sexual desire

Desire phase dysfunctions include *hypoactive sexual desire* (HSD) and sexual aversion. HSD is defined as "persistently or recurrently deficient or absent sexual fantasies and desire for sexual activity" (American Psychiatric Association [APA] 1987). HSD is a very prevalent sexual dysfunction. Kaplan (1979) has described sexual desire as an appetite that originates in the sex center of the brain (hypothalamus) and, in both men and women, is dependent on hormones (testosterone, luteinizing hormone-releasing hormone [LH-RH]) and influenced by emotions (fear, anger). The suppression of the sexual appetite can be a learned survival skill, as when a sexual situation is perceived as dangerous, either emotionally or physically.

HSD is diagnosed when the disturbance is not caused exclusively by organic factors and is not symptomatic of another psychiatric syndrome such as major depression. The term is used when the etiology of low libido has not been determined. Clients with HSD tend to have deeper and more intense sexual anxieties, greater amounts of hostility and/or resentment in their relation-

Table 12P.1. PSYCHIC FACTORS ASSOCIATED WITH INHIBITED SEXUAL DESIRE (ISD)

- Milder sources of anxiety
  - Performance fears (including body image concerns)
  - Anticipation of lack of pleasure in the act
  - Mild residual guilt about sex and pleasure
  - Simple overconcern for pleasing the partner
  - Failure to communicate one's own needs
  - Repeated non-pleasurable, ungratifying sexual experiences
  - Insensitive or inept partner
  - Anxious and pressuring partner
  - Residues of anti-sexual injunctions from childhood
- Mid-level sources of anxiety
  - Unconscious fear of romantic success
  - Unconscious fear of intimacy
  - Unresolved grief following miscarriage or stillbirth
  - Unresolved feelings regarding abortion
  - Fear of pregnancy
  - Fear of contracting HIV/AIDS
  - Relationship problems (intimacy, power struggles, territoriality)
- Deeper sources of anxiety
  - Complex intrapsychic conflicts involving early emotional development
  - Early learning to inhibit sexual feeling in response to destructive, intrusive, or abusive family interaction
  - Unresolved hostility and resentment in the relationship

Source: Adapted from Kaplan, H.S. 1979. *Disorders of sexual desire*, pp. 78-92. New York: Simon & Schuster.

ships, and more tenacious defense mechanisms than do clients with arousal or orgasm phase problems.

The term "inhibited sexual desire" (ISD) is applied by Kaplan (1979) to cases of low libido for which an etiological diagnosis has been made—e.g., psychic factors inhibiting sexual desire (see **Table 12P.1, Psychic Factors Associated with Inhibited Sexual Desire**). In practice, the two most common etiologies are sexual trauma (sexual abuse, assault, incest) or relationship dynamics that have built up resentment and hostility. Physical causes most commonly include depression, severe stress states, certain drugs and illnesses, and low testosterone levels.

HSD may be further broken down into: 1) primary HSD—total lack of sexual desire throughout a person's life; 2) secondary HSD—loss of previously present desire, e.g., as after childbirth; 3) situational HSD—lack of desire in particular situations but not in others; and 4) global HSD—current lack of desire regardless of situational variables.

Sexual aversion disorder

Sexual aversion disorder is defined as "persistent or recurrent extreme aversion to, and avoidance of, all or almost all, genital sexual contact with a sexual partner" (APA 1987). This disorder is the most severe form of sexual inhibition. The diagnosis is made when the disturbance is not part of another psychiatric disorder such as major depression. History often includes severely negative parental attitude(s) toward sex; sexual trauma (incest, rape); constant pressuring, coercion, or bargaining for sex; repeated unsuccessful attempts to please a sexual partner; relentless unsuccessful attempts to overcome a sexual dysfunction; and/or unresolved conflicts in sexual identity or orientation (Crooks and Bauer 1987).

Arousal Phase Disorder

Sexual arousal disorder

A sexual arousal disorder is diagnosed when either or both of the following conditions are present: 1) "persistent or recurrent partial or complete failure to attain or maintain the lubrication/swelling response of sexual excitement until completion of sexual activity" or 2) "persistent or recurrent lack of a subjective sense of sexual excitement and pleasure during sexual activity" (APA 1987).

Physiologically, arousal response in women is characterized by the development of lubrication, which is pushed through the semipermeable membrane of the vagina as a result of increased vasocongestion. Lubrication is the same psychophysiological response as erection in the male and is governed by the same neurophysiological pathways (primarily the parasympathetic part of the autonomic nervous system). The same psychic factors that are associated with inhibited sexual desire can cause anxiety in the arousal stage and block sexual response and lubrication (see **Table 12P.1**).

Orgasm Phase Disorder

Three basic elements are necessary for orgasm to occur: effective stimulation, sufficient relaxation, and absence of learned inhibition of orgasmic response. An orgasm phase disorder is diagnosed by a "persistent or recurrent delay in, or absence of, orgasm in a female following a normal sexual excitement phase during sexual activity that the clinician judges to be adequate in focus, intensity, and duration" (APA 1987).

Whether or not lack of orgasm (anorgasmia) is a problem should be decided by the client. Some women who are anorgasmic enjoy their sexual experiences. Others view lack of orgasm as sexual failure and feel frustrated and ashamed. Anorgasmia does not preclude arousal, lubrication, and enjoyment of the sexual experience. Orgasm phase disorder may be broken down into four categories.

Primary anorgasmia

The woman has never experienced orgasm by any means, including masturbation or with a partner. It is estimated that approximately six percent to ten percent of women have never had an orgasm. These women often lack knowledge of their own sexuality, including their response patterns and anatomy. While orgasmic women usually learn through self-stimulation, few women with primary anorgasmia masturbate. Often they fear loss of control.

Secondary anorgasmia

The woman has had orgasms at one time but no longer does. A physical component may be associated; thus, a general health history is important to rule out conditions such as diabetes or multiple sclerosis. (It is doubtful, however, that anorgasmia would be the first symptom of these conditions.) Use of the antidepressant Prozac® is known to cause lack of orgasm in some people. Often, the development of anorgasm reflects a major change in the woman's life, such as marriage, a new full-time job, a new or deteriorating relationship, or extreme stress.

Additional contributing factors may include concern that family members will overhear the sexual encounter, lack of sufficient arousal time for orgasm to occur, or preoccupation with fear of losing the ability to achieve orgasm. It is important for the health care provider to inquire about changes which occurred around the time that orgasm response stopped.

Situational anorgasmia

The woman has orgasms only in certain situations (e.g., with masturbation but not with a partner, with coitus only and no other forms of stimulation, or with a certain partner only). It is important to determine the conditions under which the client is orgasmic and her requirements for orgasm.

Coital anorgasmia

This woman is orgasmic with manual or oral stimulation from a partner but not from intercourse alone. This condition is so common that health practitioners must be careful not to consider it a dysfunction unless it is a problem for the patient. According to the Hite Report (1976), only about 30 percent of women routinely experience orgasm during intercourse without additional simultaneous stimulation of the clitoral area. Another 30 percent are orgasmic with simultaneous clitoral stimulation.

Dyspareunia

Dyspareunia is defined as "recurrent or persistent genital pain in either a male or a female before, during, or after sexual intercourse" (APA 1987). The most common cause is lack of lubrication due to insufficient arousal. Intercourse with insufficient lubrication irritates the vaginal walls and increases the possibility of vaginal infection. Foam, sponges, spermicidal jelly or cream, condoms, condom lubricant, nonoxynol-9, and diaphragms also may cause irritation in sensitive women. If a physical cause for the pain goes untreated, ongoing attempts at penetration can result in vaginismus.

Vaginismus

Vaginismus is defined as "recurrent or persistent involuntary spasm of the musculature of the outer third of the vagina that interferes with coitus" (APA 1987). Contraction of the vaginal muscles is the physical manifestation of an emotional response; the psychological association of pain is a result of some kind of trauma. Traumatic associations may include sexual abuse, a first-time sexual experience, a painful vaginal examination, tampon insertion, chronically painful intercourse, strong religious taboos about sex, repeated attempts at penetration by a partner with erectile difficulties, or pain associated with physical problems such as PID or endometriosis. An additional factor is fear—of cancer, pregnancy, HIV infection, STDs, or lesbian orientation.

The vagina "closes off" in an attempt to avoid further pain, even after the cause has been resolved. Desire, arousal, lubrication, and orgasm may be unaffected by vaginismus. Inability to have intercourse may cause distress, shame, and feelings of inadequacy. Some women may not desire intercourse but seek treatment only because they desire pregnancy.

Vaginismus is considered primary if the woman has never been able to tolerate penetration. In secondary vaginismus, a woman has previously enjoyed intercourse but developed spasms after some type of traumatic penetration. Situational or selective vaginismus happens with a specific partner only. Vaginismus is considered rare but is probably under-reported.

Desire Phase Dysfunctions

DATABASE

SUBJECTIVE

Hypoactive sexual desire (HSD)

→ Patient usually complains of having no interest in sexual contact or sexual experience.

→ Patient rarely entertains thoughts of having sex, and if those thoughts occur, she rapidly dismisses them.

→ Lubrication and orgasm may occur on a reflexive level; only desire for a sexual encounter is inhibited.

→ Low sexual desire may be associated with (LoPicolo 1980):
  ▪ history or current complaints of depression.
  ▪ Catholicism.
  ▪ presence of sexual dysfunction.
  ▪ aversion to oral-genital contact.
  ▪ aversion (in both males and females) to female genitals.
  ▪ no history of masturbation or discontinued masturbation.
  ▪ history of relationship problems assessed by the clinician but denied by the couple.

Sexual aversion

→ Patient may report feelings ranging from disgust to extreme, irrational fear of sexual activity (Schover et al. 1982).

→ Patient may experience intense anxiety at the mere thought of having sexual contact.

→ Patient may report physiological symptoms such as sweating, increased heart beat, nausea, or diarrhea.

→ Patient may describe the sexual experience as an ordeal—disgusting or repulsive.

→ Patient rarely has orgasms, and often has no desire to change the condition.

→ History to evaluate desire phase disorders should include:

- complete medical/surgical history:
  - surgical removal of adrenals, ovaries, or pituitary; disfiguring surgery; acquired disability; epilepsy; pituitary tumor; thyroid deficiency; Addison's disease; Cushing's disease; hepatitis; advanced malignancies; degenerative diseases; pulmonary diseases; chronic fatigue syndrome; HIV positivity.
- obstetrical/gynecological/contraceptive history.
- medication history:
  - illicit drug use/abuse; antihypertensives (especially beta-blockers, reserpine, and alpha-methyldopa); sedative-hypnotics, antianxiety drugs, narcotics, phenothiazines, amphetamines, and adrenal steroids in high doses; neurotoxic industrial agents; oral contraceptives.
- psychosocial history to assess current life situation for severe stress/depression:
  - loss of job, death of family member, first six to eight months postpartum, strict breast-feeding.
- review of systems—especially weight gain, weight loss; vegetative symptoms of depression, such as not eating or sleeping.
- sexual history:
  - situational or global lack of desire.
  - severity of lack of desire.
  - couple's and individual's actual sexual behavior, including types of behaviors (coital, manual, oral-genital) and frequency of behaviors; couple's and individual's desired sexual behavior, including interest in and frequency of behaviors not currently engaged in.
  - couple's and individual's motivation to change the situation.
  - frequency of and subjective reaction to sexual thoughts, masturbation, sexual fantasies, erotic dreams, erotic books, magazines, films.
  - extramarital sexual behaviors.
  - relationship factors that keep one or both partners from feeling sexual, including degree of hostility and resentment.
  - past experiences of sexual trauma (incest, molestation, sexual assault, date rape); associated dyspareunia, lack of orgasm.
- see **Appendix 12P.1, General Assessment Questions for Sexual Functioning**, p. 12-171, for more general questions regarding sexual functioning.
  NOTE: Detailed sexual history taking may be beyond the scope of practice of the primary care

provider unless he or she has received training in human sexuality.

OBJECTIVE

→ Complete pelvic examination if complaint or history of pelvic pain or dyspareunia.
→ Additional physical examination components based on history.

ASSESSMENT

→ Desire phase dysfunction: primary, secondary, situational, or global
→ R/O hypoactive sexual desire
→ R/O sexual aversion
→ R/O concomitant sexual dysfunction
→ R/O concomitant medical, psychiatric illness
→ R/O prescription and/or recreational drug effects
→ Assess contributing stress factors
→ Assess motivation and readiness for referral for therapy

PLAN

DIAGNOSTIC TESTS

NOTE: Desire disorders are difficult to diagnose. The key diagnostic issue is the distinction between HSD as the primary diagnosis versus HSD as secondary to a medical, psychiatric, or other sexual dysfunction diagnosis.

→ Laboratory tests may include:
  - plasma testosterone levels on at least 2 different occasions.
  - estradiol, prolactin.
  - estrogen/testosterone ratio.
  - percentage of circulating unbound testosterone.
  - fasting blood sugar.
  - thyroid function tests.
  - additional laboratory tests based on history.

TREATMENT/MANAGEMENT

→ Judge the extent of the dysfunction, taking into account factors affecting sexual functioning, such as age, sex, occupation, and context of the individual's life.
  - Simple behavioral intervention is generally not sufficient to reawaken sexual feelings.
→ Treat identified underlying physiological causes. Desire will often return when feelings of well-being return.

→ Treatment of a primary sexual dysfunction (e.g., dyspareunia, anorgasmia) will often alleviate lack of desire.

→ Progress in treating desire phase dysfunctions is relatively slow and prognosis much less successful than for arousal and orgasm phase dysfunctions.
  ▪ If there has been no sexual interaction for many years in a relationship, the prognosis for therapy is very poor.

→ Refer for sex therapy as indicated. Do not refer during crisis period.
  ▪ Sex therapy referrals for HSD, when the cause is physiological, often have a poor prognosis.
  ▪ Sex therapy is not appropriate when HSD is secondary to depression.

→ If underlying depression is suspected, refer to psychiatrist for medication and/or psychotherapy.

→ Refer for individual psychotherapy as indicated.

→ Refer for couple therapy as indicated.

→ See "Bibliotherapy" in "Patient Education" section.

CONSULTATION

→ Refer for sex therapy, individual psychotherapy, or couple therapy as indicated.

→ Consult with psychotherapist as needed to evaluate signs of depression or anxiety.

→ Consult with pharmacist as needed to clarify effects of various drugs on sexual desire.

→ Primary provider may be serving as a consultant to therapist who refers client for physical and gynecological examinations.

PATIENT EDUCATION

→ Introduce idea of alternate ways for male partner to have orgasmic outlet besides intercourse (e.g., self-masturbation, partner masturbation, rubbing penis on outside of client's body).

→ Reassure patient with underlying depression or severe stress that sexual desire often returns when depression or stress is alleviated.

→ Discuss loss of desire as an adaptive response which may provide an opportunity for self-reflection.

→ Loss of desire is common after childbirth, and desire usually returns after cessation of breast-feeding. Teach client to focus on ways to maintain touching while awaiting return of desire.

→ Bibliotherapy is indicated in cases that appear to stem from mild to mid-level sources of anxiety:
  ▪ Barbach, L. 1975. *For Yourself: The Fulfillment of Female Sexuality*. New York: Doubleday. Easy-to-read self-help book with basic information about taking responsibility for one's own sexuality. Discusses orgasm, the sexual response cycle, sources of sexual confusion, masturbation, and partner exercises.
  ▪ Barbach, L. 1982. *For Each Other: Sharing Sexual Intimacy*. New York: Signet. Easy-to-read self-help book that provides excellent information and exercises. Chapters 11, 12, and 13 focus on normal sexual desire, lack of sexual interest, and reconnecting.
  NOTE: These paperbacks could be sold at practice site.
  ▪ Loulan, J.A. 1984. *Lesbian Sex*. San Francisco: Spinsters/Aunt Lute. About female sexuality in general. Originally written for lesbians but applicable to heterosexuals as well. Book is full of self-help exercises to do alone or with a partner and discusses desire issues on pages 87-89.

FOLLOW-UP

→ Individualized, based on case presentation and needs of the client.

→ Document in progress notes and problem list.

Arousal Phase Disorder: Female Sexual Arousal Disorder

DATABASE

SUBJECTIVE

→ Symptoms may include:
  ▪ lack of lubrication or lack of subjective feeling of arousal.
  ▪ pain during intercourse (dyspareunia).
  ▪ vaginal discomfort/irritation or dysuria following intercourse.

→ Several physical conditions may contribute to lack of lubrication:
  ▪ lack of effective stimulation.
  ▪ chronic use of antihistamines.
  ▪ chronic yeast infections.
  ▪ acute or chronic bacterial vaginosis or trichomoniasis.
  ▪ marijuana use prior to a sexual experience.
  ▪ hysterectomy.

- lack of estrogen resulting from surgical removal of the ovaries, chemotherapy, or menopause.
- adhesions/scarring resulting from vaginal/pelvic surgery.
- endometriosis.
- intact/tight hymen.
- fatigue.

→ Complete medical, surgical, obstetrical, gynecological, contraceptive, medication, habits, and psychosocial history should be obtained.

- Specific history to assess arousal phase disorders should include the following:
  - alcohol use in association with sex.
  - if lack of arousal is situational or general.
  - client's awareness regarding effective stimulation and her ability to communicate her needs to partner.
  - partner cooperation.
  - mutually consensual sexual encounters.
  - stress level.
  - preoccupation with other aspects of life.
  - if coitus is prolonged.

→ See general assessment questions in **Appendix 12P.1**, p. 12-171.

OBJECTIVE

→ Complete pelvic examination to assess for evidence of infections, lesions, or other pathology.

→ Bimanual examination to note any tenderness in introitus, vagina, or pelvis.

→ Additional physical examination components based on history.

ASSESSMENT

→ Arousal phase disorder

→ R/O vaginal/pelvic pathology

→ R/O additional physical/psychic causes

PLAN

DIAGNOSTIC TESTS

→ Wet mount of vaginal secretions.

→ Endocervical cultures for *N. gonorrhoeae* and *C. trachomatis*.

→ Additional laboratory tests as indicated.

TREATMENT/MANAGEMENT

→ Discuss and encourage using artificial water-based lubricants, which may be all that is needed to stimulate the client's own lubrication. Brand

names include Probe®, Astroglide®, PrePair Personal Lubricant®, Wet®, Lubrin®, Replens®.

→ Bibliotherapy—indicated in cases that appear to stem from milder sources of anxiety. See Barbach (1975, 1982).

→ Probe for feelings of apathy, anger, fear, boredom.

→ Kaplan (1979, p. 79) suggests the following behavioral model for sexual tasks:

- sensate focus I—taking turns at pleasuring or caressing the other's body without genital stimulation.
- sensate focus II—taking turns at pleasuring the other's body with gentle, nondemanding genital stimulation which does not proceed to orgasm.
- slow, teasing genital stimulation by partner. The vulva, clitoris, vaginal entrance, and nipples are caressed. This stimulation is interrupted if the woman feels near orgasm and continued a little later, when arousal has diminished somewhat.
- coitus is withheld until the woman is well lubricated.
- slow, teasing, nondemanding intromission in the female superior position under client's control for the purpose of focusing on her vaginal sensations.

→ Refer for sex therapy as indicated.

→ Refer for individual psychotherapy therapy as indicated.

→ Refer for couple therapy as indicated.

CONSULTATION

→ Refer for sex therapy, individual psychotherapy, or couple therapy as indicated.

→ Primary provider might be serving as a consultant to psychotherapist who refers patient for physical or gynecological examination.

PATIENT EDUCATION

→ Encourage patient to take responsibility for her arousal by learning specifically what she needs to become aroused and communicating this information to her partner.

→ See "Bibliotherapy" referral (Barbach 1975, 1982).

→ Reassure patient that using artificial lubricant is not an indicator of failure.

→ Explain the similarities and differences between the male and female sexual response cycle.

→ Make available brief, informative patient-education flyers.

■ May be obtained from Planned Parenthood, 1357 Oakland Boulevard, Walnut Creek, CA 94596, (510) 935-3010.
  • "Excitement and Orgasm: The Sexual Response Cycle."
  • "Sex: The First Time or Anytime."
  • "Have You Ever . . ." (deals with sexual assault/abuse, date rape).

FOLLOW-UP

→ Individualized, based on case presentation and needs of the patient.

→ Document in progress notes and problem list.

Orgasm Phase Disorder

DATABASE

SUBJECTIVE

→ See introductory section for subcategories of disorder and contributing factors.

→ A complete medical, surgical, obstetrical, gyneco-logical, contraceptive, medication, habits, and psychosocial history should be obtained.
  ■ Specific history of orgasm phase disorder should include:
    • evaluation of whether lack of orgasm is primary, secondary, situational, or coital.
      –If patient says she is anorgasmic, ask if she has ever had an orgasm by *any* means.
      –Does she know what an orgasm is?
    • primary anorgasmia:
      –patient's experiences with masturbation; knowledge of location of clitoris; history of masturbation (does she stop stimulation before orgasm?); outcome of becoming orgasmic; partner pressure for orgasm; responsible party for arousal and orgasm; breath holding, teeth gritting during arousal; tightening of stomach and pelvis to produce orgasm.
    • secondary anorgasmia:
      –changes in relationship, health, stress level; medications; stress reduction or relaxation practices; past events that did arouse patient to orgasm; ability to communicate needs to partner; partner receptivity; preoccupation with losing the ability to achieve orgasm.
    • situational anorgasmia:
      –under what circumstances patient is orgasmic and nonorgasmic (manual, oral,

vibrator, self, partner); orgasm relationship to certain partner and/or partner technique.
    • coital anorgasmia:
      –history of orgasm during intercourse, with or without additional clitoral stimulation; partner pressure to have coital orgasms; expectation for simultaneous orgasms with partner.

→ See general assessment questions in **Appendix 12P.1**, p. 12-171.

OBJECTIVE

→ Complete pelvic examination to assess for genital neuropathy.

→ Assess for physical signs associated with diabetes or multiple sclerosis.

ASSESSMENT

→ Orgasm phase disorder: primary, secondary, situational, or coital

→ R/O concomitant medical illness such as diabetes, multiple sclerosis

→ R/O prescription and/or recreational drug effects

→ Assess contributing stress factors

PLAN

DIAGNOSTIC TESTS

→ Pelvic examination to assess for genital neuropathy.

→ Appropriate diagnostic tests to assess for diabetes or multiple sclerosis as indicated.

→ Additional laboratory tests based on history.

TREATMENT/MANAGEMENT

Primary anorgasmia

→ Give permission for self-exploration.

→ Refer for bibliotherapy. See Barbach (1975, 1982).

→ Recommend using water-based lubricant for self-exploration and partner stimulation.

→ Recommend taking plenty of private time to explore genitals, noting which parts when stimulated feel more pleasurable than others. Have patient locate the clitoris and stimulate it in various different ways until she finds the way that feels best (Barbach 1975).

→ Recommend reading a romantic or erotic fantasy for stimulation and distraction from performance anxiety.

→ Introduce the idea that arousal is ultimately the patient's responsibility.

→ Teach relaxation and pelvic breathing so client can breathe deeply as she approaches orgasm. Remind patient to relax jaw muscles.

→ Suggest using vibrator if patient requires more intense stimulation.

→ Refer for psychotherapy as indicated to resolve unconscious fears of orgasm.

Secondary anorgasmia

→ Remind patient that stress can be a sexual inhibitor; advise that stress reduction is beneficial.

→ Discuss the importance of setting aside a special, unhurried time for sex.

→ Demonstrate deep pelvic breathing and jaw relaxation. Instruct patient to use slow, deep pelvic breathing to prevent blocking of orgasm.

→ Give permission for self-exploration and leisurely sexual experimentation.

→ Refer for bibliotherapy. See Barbach (1975, 1982). Patient should note information on risk taking, communication, blocks to orgasm, orgasm expanding potential, and orgasm with a partner.

→ Recommend using water-based lubricant for self-exploration and partner stimulation.

→ Introduce the idea that the patient's arousal is ultimately her own responsibility.

→ Suggest using vibrator if client requires more intense stimulation.

→ Suggest using fantasy for distraction from performance anxiety during stimulation.

Situational anorgasmia

→ Give permission to have any kind of orgasm. Help patient increase self-esteem about her sexuality without pressure for orgasm through intercourse.

→ Introduce idea of communicating with partner about preferences for stimulation.

→ Refer for bibliotherapy. See Barbach (1975, 1982).

Coital anorgasmia

→ Suggest heightened arousal prior to intercourse.

→ Teach Kegel exercises to enhance vaginal sensations.

→ Suggest combining clitoral stimulation (manual or vibrator) with intercourse.

→ Suggest having intercourse in a position in which clitoris can be reached by hand or vibrator or tilting female pelvis upward to maximize contact during intercourse.

CONSULTATION

→ Consult with physician as indicated to assess whether physical illness may be a contributing factor.

→ Consult with pharmacist as indicated to determine if medications might be implicated.

PATIENT EDUCATION

Primary anorgasmia

→ Reassure patient that nothing is "wrong" with her, that she needs to explore herself more.

→ Use pictures or handheld mirror to educate patient in female anatomy. Discuss need for clitoral stimulation.

→ See "Treatment/Management" section.

Secondary anorgasmia

→ See "Treatment/Management" section.

Situational anorgasmia

→ See "Treatment/Management" section.

Coital anorgasmia

→ See "Treatment/Management" section.

FOLLOW-UP

→ Individualized based on case presentation and needs of the patient.

→ Document in progress notes and problem list.

Dyspareunia

DATABASE

SUBJECTIVE

→ History to include pain specifics, such as quality, quantity, location, duration, aggravating/relieving factors.

→ Complete medical, surgical, obstetrical, gynecological, contraceptive, medications, habits, and psychosocial history.
  ▪ Question client specifically about previous vaginal or pelvic surgeries or other pelvic trauma, such as rape.

→ See **Table 12P.2, Dyspareunia**.

Table 12P.2. DYSPAREUNIA

When	Where	Rule Out	Management
Precoital foreplay	External genitalia	Dermatosis Vulvovaginitis Inept male technique Associations with abuse Arthritis in adjacent structures	Treatment Treatment Education & communication Therapy (indiv. or group) Treatment
As penis enters	Introitus	Lack of lubrication Infection Position (angle of penis) Urethritis & cystitis Postmenopausal changes Scar tissue Subluxation of symphysis Rigid hymen	Education Treatment Education Treatment Treatment Medical or surgical Education Education & surgical
Penis in midvagina	Vaginal canal and adjacent viscera	Cystitis Vaginitis Post-menopausal changes Scars Position of penis Anorectal problems	Treatment Treatment Treatment Medical or surgical Education Medical or surgical
Deep penetration with thrusting	Deep in pelvis Lower back Lower abdomen	Varices of broad ligament Endometriosis Position of penis Post-trauma scars Post-menopausal changes Orthopedic problems PID residue	Medical or surgical Hormonal or surgical Education Medical or surgical Treatment Medical or surgical Medical or surgical
During orgasm	Deep in pelvis Lower back Lower abdomen	Varices of broad ligament Endometriosis Scars at vaginal vault or abdomen	Medical or surgical Hormonal or surgical Medical or surgical
Postcoitus	Deep in pelvis Lower back Lower abdomen	Varices of broad ligament Endometriosis Vaginal vault scars Abdominal scars	Medical or surgical Hormonal or surgical Medical or surgical Medical or surgical

Source: Adapted from Arbanel, A.R. 1993. Lecture handout, the Fertility Institute, Los Angeles, CA.

OBJECTIVE

→ Bimanual examination to note any tenderness in introitus, vagina, or pelvis.

→ Assess for unstretched or rigid hymen.

ASSESSMENT

→ Dyspareunia

→ See **Table 12P.2** for differential diagnoses

PLAN

DIAGNOSTIC TESTS

→ Wet mount of vaginal secretions.

→ Endocervical cultures for *N. gonorrhoeae* and *C. trachomatis*.

→ Additional laboratory tests as indicated by history.

TREATMENT/MANAGEMENT

→ Specific to underlying cause(s). See appropriate protocols.

CONSULTATION

→ Primary care provider may act as consultant to mental health professional who is referring client with dyspareunia for physical and gynecological examination.

→ Consult with physician as indicated for difficult case.

PATIENT EDUCATION

→ Specific to underlying cause(s). See appropriate protocols.

→ Discuss ways to avoid positions or movements that aggravate the pain.

→ Individualized, based on case presentation and needs of the patient.

→ Document in progress notes and problem list.

Vaginismus

SUBJECTIVE

→ The degree of vaginal spasm is on a continuum— partial (penetration is possible but painful) to complete (nothing can penetrate).

→ Complete medical, surgical, obstetrical, gynecological, contraceptive, medications, habits, and psychosocial history.

■ Specific questions regarding the presence of desire, arousal, lubrication, and orgasm; history of previous pain related to penetration; fear of penetration, "ripping"; partner sensitivity to client's pain; client's ability to communicate needs to partner; erectile difficulty in partner; use of lubricant; attempts to penetrate virginal hymen.

OBJECTIVE

→ Vaginismus is diagnosed primarily by pelvic examination. Past or present pelvic examination may be connected to the trauma. Discuss this possibility with the patient. Work together to make examination as comfortable as possible.

→ See "Objective" section of "Dyspareunia" section.

→ Assess for involuntary contraction of vaginal muscles upon touching vulva or digitally entering vagina.

ASSESSMENT

→ Vaginismus: primary, secondary, or situational

→ See "Dyspareunia" section

PLAN

DIAGNOSTIC TESTS

→ See "Dyspareunia" section.

TREATMENT/MANAGEMENT

→ Treatment can be protracted, especially when vaginismus is associated with trauma.

→ Treatment is threefold: 1) education and behavioral deconditioning techniques until vaginal spasms disappear; 2) psychodynamic therapy to resolve the phobic elements; and 3) couples therapy to gain essential partner cooperation and communication.

→ Provider may be able to initiate educational and behavioral deconditioning aspects; however, patient should be referred to sex therapist, marriage counselor, social worker, or psychologist with special training in resolving sexual dysfunction.

→ Dispel myths about anatomy, sexual response cycle, intercourse.

→ Discuss the meaning of intercourse for patient and partner.

→ Give patient permission to say "no" to intercourse verbally rather than physically.

→ Reassure patient that because the vaginal muscle reaction is a learned response to the fear of pain, it can be unlearned.

→ Clarify for the patient and partner that while patient can learn to prevent the contractions, she does not consciously will them to occur (Kaplan 1979).

→ Teach Kegel exercises and ask patient to perform approximately 100 per day.

■ She should concentrate on a final squeeze of the muscles of the pelvic floor (pubococcygeus) so that she can get maximum relaxation after the squeeze.

• She should consciously try to relax the muscles of the pelvic floor even further after initially relaxing them.

→ Behavioral deconditioning includes:

■ teaching relaxation and pelvic breathing.

■ gentle self-insertion of graduated dilators to allow adaptation to vaginal penetration and to associate it with feeling calm and in control. **NOTE:** The general principle is to start with very thin objects and work up to an object the size of the partner's penis. Often the patient's or the partner's finger is used instead of an object, starting with the smallest finger. The patient is in total control of the timing, depth, and movement. (Partner can act as a coach for relaxation breathing if patient is comfortable with this.) An inexpensive dilator object is the plastic outside casing of a syringe, which comes in a variety of sizes. USE LOTS OF LUBRICANT (water-based, nonirritating). The step-by-step insertion process is generally as follows:

• perform relaxation and deep pelvic breathing.

• lubricate the vagina.

- insert the smallest object and remain in a prone position for a while. If anxiety comes up, talk about it. Stop at any time. Do not do anything that is painful. The whole point is to become relaxed and comfortable.
- repeat above steps with each graduated object. Patient determines readiness.
- partner inserts smallest finger. Work up to insertion of larger finger, possibly two fingers. When patient is ready, she can signal her partner to begin very slight movement of his finger.
- insert penis (most difficult part). When patient feels ready for penis insertion, she should be in total control. It is helpful to hold her hand on the partner's penis and to direct it inside herself. She should hold the penis inside her with no movement by either partner. When she feels ready for movement, she can move slightly or direct her partner to gently move his penis.

CONSULTATION

→ Primary care provider may act as consultant to mental health professional who is referring client with dyspareunia for physical and gynecological examination.

→ Consult with physician as indicated for difficult case.

PATIENT EDUCATION

→ See "Treatment/Management" section.

FOLLOW-UP

→ Individualized, based on case presentation and needs of the patient.

→ Document in progress notes and problem list.

Bibliography

American Psychiatric Association. 1987. *Diagnostic and statistical manual of mental disorders*, 3d ed., revised. Washington, DC: the Author.

Arbanel, A.R. 1993. Los Angeles: The Fertility Institute.

Barbach, L. 1975. *For yourself: The fulfillment of female sexuality*. New York: Doubleday.

———. 1982. *For each other: Sharing sexual intimacy*. New York: Signet.

Crooks, R., and Bauer, K. 1987. *Our sexuality*, 3d ed. Menlo Park, CA: Benjamin/Cummings.

Hite, S. 1976. *The Hite report: A nationwide study of female sexuality*. New York: Dell Books.

Kaplan, H.S. 1979. *Disorders of sexual desire*. New York: Simon & Schuster.

Leiblum, S.R., and Rosen, R.C. 1989. *Principles and practice of sex therapy*, 2d ed. New York: Guilford Press.

LoPicolo, L. 1980. Low sexual desire. In *Principles and practice of sex therapy*, eds. S.R. Leiblum and L.A. Pervin, pp. 27–64. New York: Guilford Press.

Loulan, J.A. 1984. *Lesbian sex*. San Francisco: Spinsters/Aunt Lute.

Schover, L., Friedman, J., Weiler, S., Heinman, J., and LoPicolo, J. 1982. Multiaxial-problem oriented system for sexual dysfunction. *Archives of General Psychiatry* 39:614–619.

APPENDIX 12P.1

General Assessment Questions for Sexual Functioning

Following is a list of questions that are useful in bringing up the topic of sexual functioning:

GENERAL PROFILE (sexual problem history)

- Which sexual problems, if any, have concerned you in the past or are current concerns?
  - What is the specific problem?
  - What is the onset, course, duration, and severity?

GET SPECIFICS:

- When did the problem start? Have you always had it?
- Why did you come in about it now?
- How frequently do you have sex? What percentage of the time do you have the problem?
- Is it different with different partners? If so, have you any idea why?
- Are you usually fairly turned on when you have the problem? Or does the problem appear after you get turned on and then turned off? Or does the problem arise because you are just not that turned on?
- What do you think contributes to the problem?
- When is there no problem?
- What other attempts have either or both partners made to solve the problem in the past? How did they work? (Gives clinician an idea of what didn't work. Clinician should note attempts that have worsened the problem.)
- What do you think is the ideal way for you and your partner to function in bed, in your daily living, in other aspects of the relationship?

FOLLOW-UP QUESTIONS as indicated:

- What do you consider a sexual stimulus?
- What do you consider a sexual response?
- What reinforces your sexual response?
- What inhibits your sexual response?
- What would be a complete or satisfying sexual experience?
- How does using birth control affect your sexual response?
- How does using safer sex practices affect your sexual response?
- How does your concern for HIV/AIDS affect your sexual response?
- Are there symptoms of PMS (in you or your partner) that affect your sexual response?
- How does your or your partner's monthly cycle affect your sexual response?
- What have been the effects of pregnancy on your sexual response? (Includes three trimesters of pregnancy and postpartum up to 2+ years.)
- Is infertility an issue? How does it affect your feelings about yourself as a sexual person? How has it affected the sexual dynamics between you and your partner?
- How do you feel emotionally about foreplay (amount, kinds, partner communication)?
- How would you describe your ability to let go into your arousal?
- How has your sexuality been different in different stages of development (teen, young adult, adult, older adult)?
- What would increase your willingness to have sexual relations?
- How does focus on your biological clock affect your sexual responses and behaviors?

Maureen Shannon, C.N.M., F.N.P., M.S.

12-Q

Toxic Shock Syndrome

In 1978 the first description of *toxic shock syndrome* (TSS) was reported in the scientific literature. TSS was described as an acute, severe, multisystem disease occurring in seven children and adolescents who presented with a sudden onset of high fever, sore throat, headache, diarrhea, an erythematous rash with subsequent desquamation, liver abnormalities, renal failure, and central nervous system symptoms (e.g., confusion) (Todd et al. 1978). The disease was associated with strains of staphylococci that produced an epidermal toxin.

The unique characteristics of TSS were subsequently noted in seven patients in Wisconsin. Six of the seven patients were menstruating women. In response to this clustering of cases, a statewide TSS surveillance system began in Wisconsin, and 38 cases were reported between 1975 and mid-1980. Of these cases, 37 occurred in women. Of the 37 women, 35 had symptoms during menses, and 97 percent of the menstruating women reported tampon use during the onset of the illness. In addition, *Staphylococcus aureus* (*S. aureus*) was cultured from vaginal and cervical sites in 74 percent of the women from whom specimens were collected. Recurrent TSS episodes were noted in 28 percent of the 35 menstruating women, with all recurrences reportedly during menses (Davis et al. 1980).

In 1980, the CDC began a national TSS surveillance to monitor trends, assess the magnitude, and determine risk factors associated with the disease (CDC 1980). Initial results from this surveillance noted that more than 90 percent of TSS cases were reported in menstruating women of childbearing age (CDC 1990). A mortality rate of five percent was also noted. Continuing investigations discovered several risk factors associated with TSS, including menstruation, tampon use (es-

pecially continuous use of tampons for 24 hours during menstruation), young age, *S. aureus* colonization of the genital tract, and a low-level antibody titer to toxic shock syndrome toxin-1 (TSST-1).

Studies further delineated a number of tampon characteristics that were associated with an increased risk of TSS, including super absorbency, the use of carboxymethylcellulose or polyacrylate rayon in tampon fibers, vaginal/cervical microabrasions resulting from tampon use, and the capacity of the tampon to bind to magnesium (Berkeley et al. 1987; Kass 1989; Kass and Parsonnet 1987; Lanes and Rothman 1990). Although these characteristics were implicated as possible causes, the exact mechanism by which TSST-1 production is facilitated by tampon use is still unknown (CDC 1990).

In 1980, the CDC developed a case definition delineating specific signs and symptoms required for the diagnosis of TSS (see **Table 12Q.1, CDC Case Definition for Toxic Shock Syndrome**). Between 1980 and 1990 a total of 3,295 definite cases of TSS were reported to the CDC, with the majority of cases occurring between mid-1979 and 1981. A significant decline in reported cases was recorded late in 1981 after a particular tampon product (Rely®) was withdrawn from the market.

National incidence of TSS continued to decline. This decline was attributed to several factors, including changes in the composition of remaining tampon products (i.e., decreased absorbency and removal of polyacrylate material from tampon fibers); education of professionals and the public about TSS; labeling of tampon packages regarding product absorbency and early signs of TSS; and the possible change in the use of catamenial products by women (e.g., more women choosing not to use tampons or not to use tampons continuously). Con-

TABLE 12Q.1. CDC CASE DEFINITION FOR TOXIC SHOCK SYNDROME

Following are CDC criteria used for the diagnosis of toxic shock syndrome:
1. Fever: temperature $\geq$ 38.9°C (102°F)
2. Rash: diffuse macular erythroderma
3. Desquamation: 1–2 weeks after the onset of the initial rash, especially involving palms and soles
4. Hypotension: systolic blood pressure < 90 mm Hg for adults or < 5th percentile by age for children, or orthostatic syncope
5. Involvement of three or more of the following organs:
   Gastrointestinal system: vomiting or diarrhea at the onset of symptoms
   Musculoskeletal system: severe myalgia or CPK > 2 times normal levels
   Mucous membranes: vaginal, oropharyngeal, or conjunctival hyperemia
   Renal system: serum BUN or creatinine $\geq$ 2 times normal levels or > 5 WBC/HPF on microscopic urinalysis in the absence of a urinary tract infection
   Hepatic system : bilirubin or transaminase levels $\geq$ 2 times normal levels
   Hematological system: platelets < 100,000/mm^3
   CNS system: disorientation or altered consciousness without focal neurological signs when fever and neurological signs are absent
6. Negative results for the following tests (if obtained):
   Cultures of blood, throat, cerebrospinal fluid
   Serology for Rocky Mountain spotted fever, leptospirosis, or measles

Source: Centers for Disease Control. 1980. Toxic shock syndrome—United States. *Morbidity and Mortality Weekly Report* 29:229.

current with the significant decline in reported TSS cases was a decline in mortality rates, with no deaths associated with TSS cases reported in 1988 and 1989 (CDC 1990).

Nonmenstrual TSS cases have been documented in men and women. TSS can occur in any patient with a possible foci of *S. aureus* infection (e.g., surgical sites, wounds, nasal packing). However, most of these nonmenstrual cases are not associated with TSST-1 production. Although rare, TSS in women using diaphragms and cervical caps has been documented (Schwartz et al. 1989). The exact mechanism by which diaphragm and cervical cap use results in TSS is unknown.

Since 1987 a toxic-shock-like syndrome caused by group A streptococcus has been reported in the literature (Gallo and Fontanarosa 1990). Symptoms similar to TSS are noted in this condition, including shock, renal failure, and adult respiratory distress syndrome (ARDS). However, bacteremia, which is uncommon in *S. aureus* TSS, reportedly also occurs in 50 percent or more of the patients (Chambers 1993; Gallo and Fontanarosa 1990), and the symptoms are not related to menses in women. This syndrome should be included in the differential diagnosis of patients suspected of having TSS.

DATABASE

SUBJECTIVE

→ Predisposing factors may include:
- menses with tampon use (usually within five days of symptom onset).
- history of TSS.
- history of recent surgery, wound, or nasal packing.

→ Patient may report one or more of the following symptoms (Chambers 1993; Chesney 1989):

- sudden onset of high fever ($\geq$ 38.9°C/102°F).
- headache.
- erythema of conjunctiva and/or oropharynx.
- myalgias/arthralgias.
- muscle weakness.
- nausea.
- vomiting.
- frequent, profuse diarrhea.
- chills.
- lightheadedness.
- syncopal episode(s).
- dermatological manifestations:
  - early manifestations that may be reported during first few days of illness include transient generalized erythematous rash, red palms and soles, petechiae (uncommon), generalized nonpitting edema, and/or vesicles/bullae (uncommon).
  - late manifestations that may be reported one week or more after initial symptoms include generalized pruritic, erythematous, maculopapular rash (one to two weeks after initial symptoms); scaling of skin, which may be generalized or specific to fingers, palms, toes, soles (10 to 21 days after initial symptoms); loss of hair and/or nails (one to six months after initial symptoms).

OBJECTIVE

→ Physical examination may reveal the following (Chambers 1993; Chesney 1989; Davis et al. 1980; Ferrante 1990):
- elevated temperature ($\geq$ 38.9°C/102°F).
- hemodynamic signs associated with shock, including decreased blood pressure (systolic

< 90 mm Hg) and increased pulse and respirations.
- patient may appear disoriented or confused.
- erythema of conjunctiva, tongue, pharynx, tympanic membranes, and/or vagina.
- subconjunctival hemorrhages.
- ulcerations of mouth and/or vagina.
- dermatological findings may vary depending upon the stage of illness and may include the following:
  - early findings noted during the acute phase of the illness including:
    –generalized erythematous macular rash.
    –generalized nonpitting edema.
    –erythema of palms and soles.
    –petechiae (uncommon).
    –vesicles/bullae (uncommon).
    –possible evidence of a surgical or traumatic wound (usually not inflamed and often without purulent discharge).
  - dermatological findings noted after acute phase of illness including:
    –generalized, maculopapular rash usually occurring one to two weeks after acute phase.
    –desquamation of fingers, palms, toes, and soles (may be generalized) usually occurring 10 to 21 days after acute phase.
    –evidence of hair and nail loss usually occuring one to six months after acute illness.
→ In ARDS with pleural effusion, initial pulmonary assessment of patients with dehydration may be WNL. However, once the patient is hydrated, pleural effusion may be evident (decreased breath sounds, fremitus, and dullness to chest percussion).
→ Pelvic examination may reveal erythema of vaginal mucosa, vaginal ulceration(s), blood, and/or presence of tampon in vaginal vault.

ASSESSMENT

→ TSS
→ R/O streptococcal TSS
→ R/O ARDS
→ R/O acute renal failure
→ R/O myocardial dysfunction
→ R/O cerebral edema
→ R/O disseminated intravascular coagulation (DIC)

→ R/O gastroenteritis from other causes (e.g., bacterial, viral pathogens)
→ R/O septic shock from other causes (e.g., meningococcus)

PLAN

DIAGNOSTIC TESTS

→ The diagnosis of TSS is based on clinical manifestations that meet the CDC case definition (see **Table 12Q.1**).
- No specific laboratory test is available for confirming a TSS diagnosis.
- However, the following laboratory tests will provide information about the status of the patient and possibly isolate the pathogen responsible for the patient's symptoms, lending support to a TSS diagnosis.
- If TSS is suspected, these tests should be ordered in consultation with a physician:
  - CBC with differential—will reveal >90 percent mature and immature neutrophils and may demonstrate decreased hematocrit.
  - ferritin level—will be decreased.
  - clotting studies—may reveal the following:
    –platelet count—decreased if DIC present.
    –prothrombin time (PT)—prolonged if DIC present.
    –partial thromboplastin time (PTT)— prolonged if DIC present.
    –fibrin split products (FSP)—increased if DIC present.
  - serum chemistry panel—will be abnormal with the following results reported:
    –elevated liver enzymes (alanine aminotransferase [ALT], aspartate aminotransferase [AST]).
    –increased creatinine phosphokinase (CPK).
    –decreased protein and albumin.
    –decreased calcium.
    –decreased phosphorous.
    –elevated BUN.
    –elevated creatinine.
  - cultures:
    –blood cultures are negative because TSS is caused by *S. aureus* toxin (Chambers 1993).
    –cultures obtained from genital and extragenital sites may reveal *S. aureus*, which would support a TSS diagnosis.
  - serum antibody testing for presence of TSST-1—a significant increase in titer in patients with a history of clinical manifestations of TSS would support a TSS

diagnosis. However, the presence of antibody to TSST-1 can occur in asymptomatic patients, and negative or low TSST-1 antibody titers have been reported in patients with nonmenstrual TSS (Chesney 1989; Jacobson, Kasworm, and Daly 1989).
- urinalysis—will reveal pyuria with > 5 leukocytes per high-power field (HPF).
- serial antistreptolysin O (ASO) titers—will not demonstrate rising titers in patients with *S. aureus* TSS (a positive result indicates streptococcal infection).
- streptozyme assay for streptococcal antibodies—will not be positive in patients with *S. aureus* TSS (a positive result indicates streptococcal infection).
- EKG—will demonstrate decreased voltage throughout the precordium, nonspecific ST-T wave changes, and flattened T waves.
- hemodynamic monitoring—should be performed when the patient is admitted to the hospital and will reveal:
  –increased pulmonary wedge pressure, CVP, left ventricular end-diastolic pressure.
  –decreased cardiac index.

TREATMENT/MANAGEMENT

→ The major cause of morbidity and mortality associated with TSS is hypovolemia and shock. Therefore, the immediate treatment of a suspected TSS patient is establishing a peripheral intravenous line to provide hydration and prevent further hemodynamic collapse (Ferrante 1990).

→ Any potentially infected foreign body (e.g., tampon, nasal packing) should be identified and removed immediately.

→ Necessary drainage and irrigation of identified infected sites should be managed by the consulting physician.

→ The decision regarding antibiotic therapy should be made by the consulting physician who is admitting the suspected TSS patient to the hospital. Antibiotic therapy should include agents that are effective against *S. aureus* and beta-lactamase–resistant organisms.

→ The decision regarding corticosteroid therapy should be made by the attending physician admitting the suspected TSS patient to the hospital.

→ The need for immediate hospitalization should be explained to the patient and take place with

individual(s) accompanying the patient to the ambulatory setting.
- If the patient's nearest relative (or significant other) is not accompanying the patient, that person should be notified as soon as possible because of the morbidity and mortality associated with TSS.

CONSULTATION

→ TSS is a life-threatening disease.
- Delays in diagnosis and interventions are associated with an increased risk of mortality.
- Immediate consultation with a physician is warranted for *all* patients suspected of having TSS. The consulting physician is responsible for the patient's treatment plan.

PATIENT EDUCATION

→ When appropriate, the patient and family should be educated in the immediate treatment of TSS (i.e., the need for stabilization and hospitalization of the patient).

→ The cause of TSS, as well as diagnostic tests, therapeutic options, possible complications, strategies for preventing future episodes, and follow-up care, should be discussed by the consulting physician and the patient. Reviewing and/or reiterating these points may be necessary when the patient returns for follow-up care.

→ Education of all menstruating women, and other patients at risk of TSS, about signs and symptoms of TSS and ways to prevent its occurrence (e.g., avoiding using high-absorbency tampons, using tampons for a limited period of time [≤ 18 hours per day] during menses, using diaphragm/cervical cap properly) should be included in primary health care visits.

FOLLOW-UP

→ Follow-up of the patient should be per recommendation of the consulting physician.
→ Document in progress notes and problem list.

Bibliography

Berkeley, S.F., Hightower, A.W., Broome, C.V., and Reingold, A.L. 1987. The relationship of tampon characteristics to menstrual toxic shock syndrome. *Journal of the American Medical Association* 258(7):917–920.
Centers for Disease Control. 1980. Toxic-shock syndrome—United States. *Morbidity and Mortality Weekly Report* 29:227–229.

———. 1990. Reduced incidence of menstrual toxic-shock syndrome—United States, 1980–1990. *Morbidity and Mortality Weekly Report* 39(25):421–423.

Chambers, H.F. 1993. Infectious diseases: Bacterial and chlamydial. In *Current medical diagnosis and treatment*, eds. L.M. Tierney, Jr., S.J. McPhee, M.A. Papadakis, and S.A. Schroeder, 32d ed., p. 1064. Norwalk, CT: Appleton & Lange.

Chesney, P.J. 1989. Clinical aspects and spectrum of illness of toxic shock syndrome: Overview. *Reviews of Infectious Diseases* 11(Suppl. 1):S1–S7.

Davis, J.P., Chesney, P.J., Wand, P.J., La Venture, M., and the Investigation and Laboratory Team. 1980. Toxic-shock syndrome: Epidemiologic features, recurrence, risk factors, and prevention. *The New England Journal of Medicine* 303(25):1429–1435.

Ferrante, J.A. 1990. Infectious skin diseases. *Primary Care* 17(4):867–881.

Gallo, U.E., and Fontanarosa, P.B. 1990. Toxic streptococcal syndrome. *Annals of Emergency Medicine* 19(11):1332–1334.

Jacobson, J.A., Kasworm, E., and Daly, J.A. 1989. Risk of developing toxic shock syndrome associated with toxic shock syndrome toxin 1 following nongenital staphylococcal infection. *Reviews of Infectious Diseases* 11(Suppl. 1):S8–S13.

Kass, E.H. 1989. Magnesium and the pathogenesis of toxic shock syndrome. *Reviews of Infectious Diseases* 11(Suppl. 1):S167–S175.

Kass, E.H., and Parsonnet, J. 1987. On the pathogenesis of toxic shock syndrome. *Reviews of Infectious Diseases* 9(Suppl. 5):S482–S489.

Lanes, S.F., and Rothman, K.J. 1990. Tampon absorbency, composition and oxygen content and risk of toxic shock syndrome. *Journal of Clinical Epidemiology* 43(12):1379–1385.

Reingold, A.L., Broome, C.V., Gaventa, S., Hightower, A.W., and the Toxic Shock Syndrome Study Group. 1989. Risk factors for menstrual toxic shock syndrome: Results of a multistate case-control study. *Reviews of Infectious Diseases* 11(Suppl. 1):S35–S42.

Schwartz, B., Gaventa, S., Broome, C.V., Reingold, A.L., Hightower, A.W., Perlman, J.A., Wolf, P.H., and the Toxic Shock Syndrome Study Group. 1989. Nonmenstrual toxic shock syndrome associated with barrier contraceptives: Report of a case-control study. *Reviews of Infectious Diseases* 11(Suppl. 1):S43–S49.

Todd, J., Fishaut, M., Kapral, F., and Welch, T. 1978. Toxic-shock syndrome associated with phage-group-I staphylococci. *Lancet* 2:1116–1118.

Sandra L. Norman, R.N., N.P., M.S.

12-RA   URINARY TRACT DISORDERS
Urinary Tract Infection

Urinary tract infection (UTI) refers to the invasion of microbial uropathogens in the lower or upper urinary tract, or both. Infection may be divided into lower urinary tract infection, commonly referred to as a *bladder infection* or *cystitis*, and upper urinary tract infection, referred to as a *kidney infection* or *pyelonephritis*. Lower urinary tract infection refers to the inflammation of the bladder mucosa caused by the presence of urinary pathogens in the bladder and is often characterized by urinary frequency, dysuria, urgency, suprapubic discomfort, and malodorous urine. Lower urinary tract infections are often recurrent; however, they are usually uncomplicated, easily treated, and no threat to future health.

Pyelonephritis is an infection of the pelvis and parenchyma of the kidney and is usually the result of an infection that has ascended from the lower urinary tract. Clinical manifestations include those of lower tract infections as well as severe flank pain, fever, chills, malaise, nausea, and vomiting. One-third of patients with symptoms of uncomplicated lower tract infections may also have unrecognized infection of the upper urinary tract (Johnson and Stamm 1987; Rubin, Beam, and Stamm 1992). Unlike lower urinary tract infection, pyelonephritis may result in significant and permanent renal damage, urosepsis, and death.

Lower urinary tract infections are the most common infection affecting women. Twenty-five percent to 35 percent of women will experience a lower urinary tract infection at least once in their lifetimes (Stamm et al. 1989). It has been estimated that $1 billion are spent in the United States annually on the evaluation and treatment of ambulatory cases of lower urinary tract infections (Johnson and Stamm 1987).

There are three possible routes by which bacteria can invade and spread within the urinary tract—the lymphatic, hematogenous, and ascending pathways. Ascent of bacteria within the urethra is the most common pathway of infection. Intestinal flora are almost invariably the source of pathogens. *Escherichia coli* is the most common uropathogen and accounts for 80 percent to 85 percent of UTIs. *Staphylococcus saprophyticus* is the pathogen responsible for approximately 20 percent of UTIs in young women (Stamey 1980). Other uropathogens include *Klebsiella* species, *Proteus mirabilis*, *Pseudomonas*, *Staphylococcus aureus*, *Staphylococcus epidermidis*, and Group D enterococcus.

Colonization of the vaginal epithelium, followed by colonization of the urethral epithelium, are the most important events in the pathogenesis of UTIs in women (Fowler 1989; Stamey 1980; Thomas and Bhatia 1989). This dynamic, noninflammatory process is characterized by the attachment of uropathogen pili onto host cell receptors in the vaginal and periurethral mucosa. The normal bacterial flora of the vaginal introitus and periurethral mucosa interfere with attachment of uropathogens by competing for receptor sites. Lactobacilli inhibit the attachment of uropathogens to introital and uroepithelial cells (Reid and Sobel 1987; Thomas and Bhatia 1989).

Immunoglobulins secreted by the cervix have an inhibitory action on bacterial adherence and colonization of the introital mucosa (Iravani 1990). Vaginal pH also influences colonization. Vaginal fluid is bactericidal at a pH of 4.0. Vaginal pH of 6.5 or greater supports the growth of all gram-negative bacilli (Iravani 1990; Stamey 1980). Vaginal colonization with uropathogens is greater during the first half of the menstrual cycle and is more common in postmenopausal women (Stamey 1980).

The combination of diaphragm and spermicide is associated with profound disturbances of normal vaginal flora. There appears to be a marked increase in *E. coli* colonization, an increase in vaginal pH, and a decrease in lactobacilli with diaphragm use (Stamey 1980; Stamm et al. 1989). There is no association between colonization and personal habits (Chow, Percival-Smith, and Bartlet 1986).

The role of sexual activity in the pathogenesis of urinary tract infections has long been the subject of investigation. If uropathogens have not colonized the urogenital epithelium, intercourse alone will not cause an infection. Therefore, the importance of intercourse as a precipitant of urinary tract infections is limited to women who are inherently susceptible to urogenital colonization (Fowler 1989).

Ascending colonization of the proximal urethra and inoculation of the urine comprise the subsequent steps in the pathogenesis of urinary tract infections. The lower urinary tract exhibits several defense mechanisms that increase its resistance to bacterial invasion. The flushing action of urination removes uropathogens, and the urine acidity, osmolality, organic acids, and urea content inhibit bacterial growth (Iravani 1990).

The lower urinary tract secretes tissue factors such as oliogosaccharides, uromucoids, immunoglobulins (IgA, IgG, and secretory IgA), and bladder mucopolysaccharides that inhibit, prevent, or detach bacterial attachments to the urothelial mucosal cells. These factors appear to be deficient in women susceptible to UTIs (Iravani 1990; Thomas and Bhatia 1989).

Pyelonephritis most commonly occurs secondary to infected urine flowing back up through the ureters into the renal pelvis. Patients at risk for pyelonephritis are those infected with uropathogens with chromosomal virulence factors enabling them to infect the upper urinary tract or bloodstream (Stamm et al. 1989) or the presence of congenital ureterovesical reflex, urinary obstruction, urinary calculi, neurogenic bladder, and diabetes.

Traditionally, the diagnosis of a lower urinary tract infection was based on a urine culture with a uropathogen greater than or equal to 10^5 colony forming units (CFU) per ml from a clean-catch midstream urine specimen (Stamey 1980). However, only 40 percent to 80 percent of women with symptoms of a lower urinary tract infection will demonstrate this quantity of bacteriuria (Fowler 1989; Kellogg, Manzella, and Shaffer 1987; Stamey 1980). The remaining symptomatic patients will have urine cultures that may contain colony counts of 10^2 CFU/ml to 10^5 CFU/ml or may contain no identifiable pathogen.

Low colony counts are frequently found in infections caused by *E. coli, Staphylococcus saprophyticus,*

enterococci, *Klebsiella* species, and *S. aureus* (Thomas and Bhatia 1989). Urine cultures with low colony counts may result from early or subsiding infections, previous use of antibiotics, bacteriostatic agents in the urine, hydration, or diuresis (Stamey 1980; Thomas and Bhatia 1989). It is currently recommended that urine cultures with a uropathogen of 10^2 CFU/ml or greater from a symptomatic women be considered sufficient for the diagnosis of a lower urinary tract infection (Fowler 1989; Stamey 1980; Thomas and Bhatia 1989). The recommended microbiological criterion for diagnosis of suspected acute pyelonephritis is $\geq 10^4$ CFU/ml (Rubin, Beam, and Stamm 1992).

Antibiotic therapy is usually initiated for the treatment of presumptive or documented urinary tract infections. Antimicrobials used to treat urinary tract infections should have the following characteristics: excellent gram-negative coverage, high urinary excretion in active form, minimal effect on the bowel and vaginal flora, low potential to develop bacterial resistance, ease of administration, good patient tolerance, and low cost (Iravani 1990). In addition to the preceding characteristics, antibiotics used to treat pyelonephritis must achieve adequate renal tissue levels. Community resistant patterns should also be considered. For example, more than 25 percent of urinary pathogens of non-nosocomial urinary tract infections are now resistant to ampicillin and amoxicillin (Iravani 1987).

Recently there has been extensive investigation of the appropriate length of treatment for urinary tract infections. Conventional duration of therapy has been seven to ten days of antimicrobial therapy. Recent studies, however, have shown that more than 90 percent of women with lower urinary tract infections are cured within three days of antibiotic therapy (Bump 1990; Norby 1991; Sheehan, Harding, and Ronald 1984).

Advantages of short-course therapy (one to five days) include decreased incidence of side effects and adverse reactions, increased patient compliance, less development of bacterial resistance, less effect on the vaginal flora, less effect on bladder mucopolysaccharides, and lower cost. Short-course therapy is recommended for the treatment of nonpregnant women with acute, uncomplicated lower urinary tract infections. Renal infections will not respond to short-course therapy. Consequently, short-course therapy may be a screening mechanism for unsuspected upper urinary tract infections (Iravani 1990).

Contraindications to short-course therapy include pyelonephritis, known structural or functional abnormalities, and use of indwelling catheters. Short-course therapy in pregnancy continues to be under investigation. A minimum of ten to 14 days of antibiotic therapy is required to treat pyelonephritis and complicated urinary tract infections.

Following the initial episode, recurrent infections are frequent—two to six per year in 85 percent of women (Iravani 1990; Stamey 1980). Susceptibility to recurrent infections is a lifelong phenomenon and is related to biologic deficiencies that allow bacteria to adhere to vaginal and uroepithelium. Urogenital epithelium of women susceptible to recurrent urinary tract infections has been shown to have more attachment sites for uropathogens than does urogenital epithelium of women resistant to infections (Fowler 1989; Thomas and Bhatia 1989). Anatomical or functional abnormalities of the urinary tract are found in fewer than five percent of women with recurrent infections (Stamey 1980; Stamm et al. 1989).

Depending on the frequency and nature of infections, women with recurrent urinary tract infections require special antibiotic treatment, which may include continual prophylaxis, postcoital prophylaxis, or self-treatment.

DATABASE

SUBJECTIVE

→ Risk factors include:
- patient is sexually active.
- increased frequency of coitus.
- childbearing age.
- postmenopausal.
- use of barrier methods of contraception/spermicides.
- recent urogenital instrumentation.
- diabetes.
- urinary stones or history of stones.
- immunosuppressive conditions.
- history of hysterectomy.
- history of cystocele repair.
- history of urethral dilatations.
- childhood urinary tract infections.
- indwelling catheter.
- neurogenic bladder.

→ Symptoms may include:

Lower urinary tract infection
- urinary frequency with small voids.
- dysuria/internal burning with urination.
- poor sensation of emptying.
- suprapubic tenderness.
- gross hematuria.
- urinary urgency.
- stress/urge incontinence.
- nocturia.
- tenesmus.
- malodorous urine.
- cloudy urine.

Upper urinary tract infection
- any of the above symptoms plus:
  - fever ≥38.3°C/101°F.
  - severe flank pain.
  - nausea/vomiting.
  - chills.
  - malaise.

OBJECTIVE

Lower urinary tract infection

→ Abdominal examination: patient may have suprapubic tenderness.

→ Pelvic examination: absence of vulvar erythema, excoriation, or abnormal vaginal discharge (unless concomitant vaginal/cervical infection).

→ Urine microscopy:
- 10+ WBCs/high power field (HPF).
- +RBCs.
- +bacteria.

→ Urine dipstick:
- +WBCs.
- +RBCs.
- +nitrites.
- +leukocyte esterase.

→ Urine culture with a single uropathogen at ≥10².

→ Temperature <37.8°C/100°F.

→ Absence of costovertebral angle (CVA) tenderness.

Upper urinary tract infection

→ Abdominal examination: may have suprapubic tenderness, abdominal tenderness.

→ Back examination: may have CVA tenderness.

→ Urine microscopy:
- 10+ WBCs.
- +RBCs.
- +bacteria.

→ Urine dipstick:
- +WBCs.
- +RBCs.
- +nitrites.
- +leukocyte esterase.

→ Urine culture with a urinary pathogen at ≥10⁴.

→ Temperature ≥38.3°C/101°F.

ASSESSMENT

→ Lower or upper urinary tract infection

→ R/O vaginitis/STD

→ R/O urinary stone

→ R/O interstitial cystitis

→ R/O neurogenic bladder

→ R/O musculoskeletal strain

→ R/O congenital anomalies

PLAN

DIAGNOSTIC TESTS

→ Obtain urine culture and sensitivity for:
  - first urinary tract infection.
  - recurrent urinary tract infection without a culture in past year.
  - previous urine culture with pathogen other than *E. coli/S. saprophyticus.*
  - resistance pattern on previous sensitivities.
  - suspicion of pyelonephritis.
  - subjective/objective data equivocal.
  - gross hematuria.

→ Vaginal/cervical cultures and vaginal wet mount as indicated to rule out vaginitis/STD.

→ Women experiencing recurrent urinary tract infections may also require additional diagnostic tests based on their history and presentation. These additional tests include:
  - kidney, ureters, and bladder (KUB) x-ray.
  - KUB to rule out stones:
    - previous stone or family history.
    - pathogen other than *E. coli/Staphylococcus.*
    - young patients with a positive urine culture and gross hematuria.
  - renal ultrasound to assess kidney size, rule out hydronephrosis, or renal tumor:
    - flank discomfort.
    - young nonsmoker with positive urine culture and gross hematuria.
    - history of urinary tract infections/ pyelonephritis in childhood/early childhood.
  - postvoid residual:
    - patient relates feeling of inability to completely empty bladder.
    - patient relates changes in stream or obstructive symptoms.
    - history of bladder repair.
    - large cystocele on examination.
    - use of antihistaminics, anticholinergics.
    - history of urethral dilatations.

  - wheelchair-confined patients.
  - diaphragm users with diaphragm in place.
  - women with medical illness such as diabetes, neurological conditions (e.g., multiple sclerosis) and lower back problems, which can cause peripheral neuropathy.
- cystogram to rule out vesicoureteral reflux:
  - history of childhood urinary tract infections.
  - history of pyelonephritis.
  - large cystocele.
- cystoscopy to rule out bladder tumors/stones, cystitis cystica:
  - gross hematuria (especially without positive urine culture).
  - numerous urinary tract infections (more than 6 per year).
- IVP to rule out renal tumors, stones, or hydronephrosis:
  - anyone with gross hematuria and a negative urine culture.
  - smokers with gross hematuria regardless of culture result.
  - high suspicion of stone.
  - hydronephrosis.

TREATMENT/MANAGEMENT

The following medication regimens are taken from Fowler 1989; Iravani 1990; Johnson 1991; Norby 1990; and Thomas and Bhatia 1989.

Lower urinary tract infections

→ Medication regimens:
  - trimethoprim and sulfamethoxazole (Septra® DS) 1 p.o. BID for 3 to 5 days.
  - trimethoprim 100 mg, 1 p.o. BID for 3 to 5 days (good alternative for patients with sulfa allergy).
  - nitrofurantoin (Macrodantin®) 50 mg, 1 p.o. TID for 3 to 5 days. (This is a lower dosage than recommended in the *PDR.*)
  - nitrofuration monohydrant (Macrobid®) 100 mg, 1 p.o. BID for 3 to 5 days. (Macrobid®/ Macrodantin® do not reach adequate renal tissue levels; therefore, do not use these drugs if pyelonephritis is suspected. Also, do not use Macrobid® or Macrodantin® in patients with G6PD deficiency.)
  - cephradine (Velosef®) 250 mg-500 mg, 1 p.o. QID for 3 to 5 days.
  - ciprofloxacin (Cipro®) 250 mg-500 mg, 1 p.o. BID for 3 to 5 days.
  - amoxicillin/clavulanate potassium (Augmentin®) 250 mg-500 mg, 1 p.o. TID for 3 to 5 days.

- ampicillin 500 mg, 1 p.o. QID for 3 to 5 days. (This drug is recommended less frequently for the treatment of UTIs secondary to a high number of resistance patterns.)
- phenazopyridine hydrochloride (Pyridium®) for bladder discomfort: 100 mg-200 mg BID-TID prn.

Pyelonephritis

→ Medication regimens:
NOTE: A portion of patients with pyelonephritis will require hospitalization for parenteral antibiotics/fluid replacement, pain management, and antiemetics. The following list of medications may be used to treat pyelonephritis in ambulatory settings; however, these patients will require close follow-up.
- trimethoprim and sulfamethoxazole (Septra® DS) 1 p.o. BID for 10 to 14 days.
- trimethoprim 100 mg, 1 p.o. BID for 10 to 14 days.
- ciprofloxacin (Cipro®) 500 mg, 1 p.o. BID for 10 to 14 days.
- amoxicillin/clavulanate potassium (Augmentin®) 500 mg, 1 p.o. QID for 10 to 14 days.
- garamycin (Gentamicin®) 80 mg-120 mg I.M. plus any of the above regimens.

Recurrent urinary tract infections

→ Medication regimens:
- continual prophylaxis—Used in women experiencing more than 4 to 6 lower urinary tract infections/year or after 1 pyelonephritis.
  - Nitrofurantoin (Macrodantin®) 50 mg, 1 p.o. at bedtime.
  - Trimethoprim 100 mg, 1 p.o. at bedtime.
  - Cephradine (Velosef®) 250 mg, 1 p.o. at bedtime.
  - Cefuroxime (Ceftin®) 250 mg, 1 p.o. at bedtime.
  - Pen Vee® K 250 mg, 1 p.o. at bedtime.
- postcoital prophylaxis—Used for women in whom infections are directly related to coital activity. Any of the above medications taken within 30 minutes before or after intercourse. Must consider frequency of intercourse.
- self-treatment—Used for women experiencing urinary infections less than 6 times/year. Patient self-treats with any of the above medications for 1 to 3 days.

→ Other management considerations:
- vaginal pH—Consider estrogen vaginal cream or Acigel® for patients with increased vaginal pH. Also screen for and treat bacterial vaginosis.
- consider alternative method of birth control in women using diaphragms.

CONSULTATION

→ For presence of urinary stones, hydronephrosis.
→ For abnormal findings on cystogram, renal ultrasound, IVP.
→ For postvoid residuals greater than 50 cc.
→ For cystoscopy.
→ For diagnosis of pyelonephritis.
→ For gross hematuria with negative urine culture.
→ For recurrent infections in wheelchair-confined patients.
→ As needed for prescription(s).

PATIENT EDUCATION

→ Discuss compliance with prescribed medication therapy.
→ Advise patient to avoid alcohol, caffeine, chocolate, hot spicy foods, and citrus while symptomatic.
→ Advise patient to prevent constipation and diarrhea (see **Constipation, Diarrhea** protocols).
→ Advise patient to have vaginal symptoms assessed and treated.
→ Advise patient to avoid vaginal douching.
→ Advise patient to urinate six to eight times/day.
→ Advise patient to urinate 30 to 60 minutes after intercourse.
→ Advise patient to avoid the use of artificial sweetners (adversely affects bladder mucopolysaccharides).
→ Discuss factors that may help in control of recurrent bacterial vaginosis (see **Bacterial Vaginosis** Protocol).

FOLLOW-UP

→ Post-treatment cultures are not usually recommended except in cases of pyelonephritis.
→ If first or occasional lower urinary tract infection, follow-up on prn basis only.
→ Follow-up for ambulatory pyelonephritis should include phone contact with patient early in course to assess response to treatment and after completion of antibiotic therapy to discuss possible referrals, diagnostic tests, and prophylaxis.

→ For patients with recurrent lower urinary tract infections, follow up initially every two to three months while on continual prophylaxis, then every four to six months depending on medication regimen and frequency of infections.

→ Explore other contraceptive options if patient uses diaphragm.

→ Document in progress notes and problem list.

Bibliography

Bergman, A. 1991. Urinary tract infections in women. *Current Opinion in Obstetrics and Gynecology* 3:541–544.

Bump, R.C. 1990. Urinary tract infections in women: Current role of single dose therapy. *Journal of Reproductive Medicine* 35:785–791.

Chow, A.W., Percival-Smith, R., Bartlet, K.H. 1986. Vaginal colonization with *E. coli* in healthy women. *American Journal of Obstetrics and Gynecology* 154:120–126.

Fowler, J.E. 1989. *Urinary tract infections and inflammation*, pp. 13–35, pp. 71–91. Chicago: Yearbook Medical Publishers.

Iravani, A. 1987. Urinary tract infections: Epidemiology and therapeutic approaches. *International Congressional Symposium Series Royal Society of Medicine* 117(25):1–43.

———. 1990. Advances in the understanding and treatment of urinary tract infections in young women. *Urology* 37(6):503–511.

Johnson, J.R. 1991. Urinary tract infection: Selecting the optimal agent. *Drug Therapy* 42:27–46.

Johnson, J.R., and Stamm, W.E. 1987. Diagnosis and treatment of acute urinary tract infections. *Infectious Disease Clinics of North America* 1:773–778.

Kellogg, J.A., Manzella, J.P., Shaffer, S.N., and Schwartz, B.B. 1987. Clinical relevance of culture versus screens for the detection of microbial pathogens in urine specimens. *American Journal of Medicine* 83:739–745.

Norby, S.R. 1990. Short-term treatment of uncomplicated lower urinary tract infections in women. *Reviews of Infectious Diseases* 12(3):458–467.

———. 1991. Efficacy and safety of antibiotic treatment and treatment time. *Scandinavian Journal of Infectious Disease* 74:262–269.

Reid, G., and Sobel, J.D. 1987. Bacterial adherence in the pathogenesis of urinary tract infections: A review. *Reviews of Infectious Diseases* 9:470–482.

Rubin, R., Beam, T., and Stamm, W. 1992. An approach to evaluating antibacterial agents in the treatment of urinary tract infections. *Clinical Infectious Diseases* 14:S246–S251.

Sheehan, G., Harding, G.K.M., and Ronald, A.R. 1984. Advances in the treatment of urinary tract infections. *American Journal of Medicine* 76:141–146.

Stamey, T.A. 1980. *Pathogenesis and treatment of urinary tract infections*. Baltimore: Waverly.

Stamm, W.E., Hooton, T.M., Johnson, J.R., Johnson, C., Stapleton, A., Roberts, P.L., Mosley, S.L., and Fihn, S.D. 1989. Urinary tract infections: From pathogenesis to treatment. *Journal of Infectious Diseases* 159(3):400–406.

Thomas, S., and Bhatia, N.N. 1989. New approaches in the treatment of urinary tract infections. *Urogynecology* 16:897–909.

U.S. Department of Health and Human Services. 1981. Patients' reasons for visiting physicians: National ambulatory medical care survey United States 1977–1978. *Vital Health Statistics* 13:26, 42.

12-RB URINARY TRACT DISORDERS
Urinary Incontinence

Urinary incontinence is defined by the International Continence Society as a condition in which involuntary loss of urine is a "social or hygienic problem and is objectively demonstrated" (Bates et al. 1979). Among women 15 years to 64 years old, the prevalence of urinary incontinence is 10 percent to 25 percent (Thomas et al. 1980). For noninstitutionalized women older than 60 years, the prevalence of urinary incontinence ranges from 30 percent to 60 percent (Diokno et al. 1986). Prevalence of incontinence in the institutionalized elderly is 50 percent and greater (Resnick 1992).

A conservative estimate of the annual monetary costs of managing urinary incontinence in the community is $7 billion, and $3.3 billion in nursing homes (Hu 1990). Significant psychosocial sequelae are associated with incontinence. Depression, embarrassment, fear, guilt, lowered self-esteem, a sense of dependency, social isolation, and abstinence from sexual activity are frequently reported by women with urinary incontinence (Wyman 1988).

An intact bladder, urethra, and neurological system as well as competent urethral sphincter mechanisms are necessary to achieve continence. The detrusor, a smooth muscle that is under voluntary control, is the external layer of the muscular coat of the bladder. In normal conditions, a stable detrusor will relax and expand in response to increasing bladder volumes without involuntary contractions or sensory symptoms. The urethral sphincter mechanism consists of the following: an intrinsic urethral smooth muscle sphincter that extends from the bladder outlet through the pelvic floor, a distal intrinsic urethral striated sphincter that surrounds the urethra, and an extrinsic periurethral striated muscle.

As the bladder fills with urine, the intrinsic urethral sphincter provides the resistance to keep the intraurethral pressure greater than that of the bladder to prevent urine leakage. The extrinsic periurethral muscles strengthen the resistance of the intrinsic mechanisms when bladder or intra-abdominal pressures increase. Continence is maintained as long as the intraurethral pressure remains greater than the bladder pressure. During micturition, a voluntary contraction of the detrusor increases the bladder pressure so it exceeds the intraurethral pressure. Voiding occurs when a voluntary contraction of the detrusor is synchronized with voluntary relaxation of the urethral sphincter mechanisms (Robertson and Hebert 1987; Wyman 1988).

The parasympathetic nervous system is responsible for the majority of detrusor innervation. The detrusor increases its contractile force and frequency in response to cholinergic activity. The bladder base and proximal urethra are innervated by the sympathetic nervous system primarily through alpha receptors that contract the bladder neck and urethra when stimulated. Innervation of the striated urethral sphincter is through the somatic nervous system, although the striated sphincter is thought to receive other innervation as well (Resnick 1992; Wyman 1988).

There are seven classifications of urinary incontinence, which may occur alone or in combination. The most common types are transient, stress, urge, and mixed incontinence.

Transient incontinence is often secondary to existing reversible conditions and is always alleviated by treatment of the condition. Transient causes of incontinence are implicated in up to one-third of elderly in the community (Resnick 1992). The mnemonic DIAPPERS is used to recall the etiologies of transient incontinence: Delirium/confusional state, Infection, Atrophic urethritis/vaginitis, Pharmaceuticals, Psychological, Excessive excretion (congestive heart failure, hyperglycemia), Restricted mobility, and Stool impaction (Resnick 1992). Medications that may precipitate incontinence include anticholinergics, diuretics, antidepressants, antipsychotics, sedatives/hypnotics, narcotic analgesics, alcohol, calcium channel blockers, and alpha adrenergic blockers/agonists (Resnick 1992; Walters 1992; Wyman 1988).

Stress incontinence is an involuntary loss of urine during activities that increase intra-abdominal pressure, such as coughing, laughing, sneezing, and jumping. Among ambulatory women, stress incontinence is the most common type of incontinence, accounting for 50 percent to 70 percent of incontinent cases (Walters and Shields 1988). Stress incontinence may be caused by urethral sphincter deficiency; however, it is usually attributed to pelvic floor and/or abdominal laxity and urethral hypermobility. These anatomical changes allow increases in intra-abdominal pressure to exceed the intraurethral pressure, thereby allowing urine leakage. (Resnick 1992; Ruff and Reaves 1989). Urine leakage is intermittent and usually occurs in small quantities. Stress incontinence is not usually associated with urinary frequency, urgency, dysruia, or nocturia except in the presence of concomitant conditions.

Urge incontinence is an involuntary loss of urine associated with a sudden, strong urge to void. It is the second most common cause of incontinence, affecting one percent to two percent of adult females (Robertson and Hebert 1987). Urge incontinence is usually due to involuntary detrusor contractions and is often referred to as detrusor hyperactivity (Walters 1992). This type of incontinence is associated with certain neurological disorders; however, it also occurs in neurologically intact individuals. In the presence of neurological conditions such as stroke, Parkinson's disease, multiple sclerosis, and injuries of the lower lumbar and sacral spine, urge incontinence is referred to as *detrusor hyperreflexia*.

When there is no associated neurological condition, the terms *unstable bladder* or *detrusor instability* are commonly used to describe this type of incontinence. Potential etiologies of detrusor instability include urinary tract infection, atrophic vaginitis, anxiety, bladder calculi, bladder neoplasm, consumption of bladder irritants or large volumes of fluids, and use of diuretics (Resnick 1992; Ruff and Reaves 1989). Urine leakage is usually intermittent, in larger amounts, associated by a strong urge to void, and often accompanied by urinary frequency and nocturia.

It is not unusual for women to present with *mixed incontinence*, a combination of urge and stress incontinence. Approximately one-third of women with urge incontinence also have stress incontinence (Robertson and Hebert 1987). Mixed incontinence may present as two separate conditions, or the conditions may be causally related.

DATABASE

SUBJECTIVE

→ Risk factors include:
  - confusional state.
  - use of sedative hypnotics, diuretics, anticholinergics, alpha-adrenergic agents, calcium channel blockers.
  - restricted mobility.
  - stool impaction.
  - neurological conditions.
  - urinary tract infection/inflammation.
  - obesity.
  - atrophic urethritis/vaginitis.
  - pelvic floor relaxation.
  - excessive urine production.

→ Symptoms may include:

Stress incontinence
  - patient reports involuntary leakage of urine, precipitated by events that increase intra-abdominal pressure, e.g., cough, laugh, sneeze, exercise.

Urge incontinence
  - patient reports involuntary leakage of urine associated with strong urge to void.
  - patient may report precipitating events such as the sound of running water, hands in warm water, anxiety, or coitus.
  - patient may report urinary frequency and/or nocturia.

Mixed incontinence
  - patient reports symptoms associated with both stress and urge incontinence (see previous discussion).

OBJECTIVE

→ Pelvic examination:

Stress incontinence
  - may observe the effects of hypoestrogenemia on vulvar and vaginal tissues.
  - may observe presence of cystocele, rectocele, prolapsed uterus or urethra.
  - decreased strength of pubococcygeal muscle.
  - positive Q-tip test—With the patient in a supine position, a lubricated cotton-tipped

applicator is placed in the urethra at the urethrovesical junction.

- The angle formed by the applicator and the floor is measured while the patient is resting and during a Valsalva maneuver.
  - An angle of less than 15° during the Valsalva maneuver indicates good anatomic support.
  - An angle of more than 30° indicates poor anatomical support.
  - An angle of 15° to 30° is considered inconclusive (Robertson and Hebert 1987).

- positive stress test—Urine leakage is observed when patient is asked to cough.
  - This maneuver may be performed in the lithotomy or standing position.

- normal postvoid residual—Postvoid residuals are easily determined by straight catheteriztaion immediately after the patient has voided.
  - A normal postvoid residual is 0 cc-50 cc of urine.
  - Postvoid residuals greater than 50 cc should be considered abnormal and may be indicative of other less common types of incontinence such as overflow or reflux.

Urge incontinence

- anatomical support of vagina and urethra may be good or poor.
- strength of pubococcygeal muscle may be good or poor.
- may observe the effects of hypoestrogenemia on vulvar and vaginal tissues.
- normal postvoid residual.

→ Neurological examination: Neurological signs are usually absent, but may be present with detrusor hyperreflexia.

Urge incontinence

- Observe general coordination, mobility, and orientation.
- May examine sacral reflex by stroking skin adjacent to anus, which should result in reflex contraction of external anal sphincter.
- May test patellar, ankle, and plantar reflexes.
- May test sensory function of sacral dermatomes using light touch and pinprick on perineum and around thigh and foot.

Mixed incontinence

→ Objective findings may be any combination of those found with stress and urge incontinence.

ASSESSMENT

→ Stress urinary incontinence

→ Urge incontinence

→ Mixed urinary incontinence

→ R/O transient incontinence

→ R/O neurological conditions

→ R/O abnormal postvoid residual

PLAN

DIAGNOSTIC TESTS

→ Diagnostic tests may include:
- urinalysis.
- urine culture and sensitivities.
- 48- to 72-hour bladder diary.
- Q-tip test.
- stress test.
- postvoid residual.
- cystourethroscopy/cystometrics.

TREATMENT/MANAGEMENT

→ Treatment options taken from Newman 1989; Resnick 1992; Urinary Incontinence Guideline Panel 1992.

Transient incontinence

→ Treat or refer for treatment, etiologies of transient incontinence.

Stress incontinence

→ Oral or topical estrogen for women with vulvar or vaginal hypoestrogenic states in whom estrogen therapy is not contraindicated.
- Estrogen supplementation may increase urethral vascularity, tone, and the alpha-adrenergic responsiveness, which may increase bladder outlet resistance.

→ Kegel exercises—To strengthen voluntary periurethral and pelvic muscles and pelvic visceral structures.

→ Vaginal weights—Sold under trade name Femina® by Dacomed. Set of 5 graduated conical weights (lightest is 20 grams, heaviest is 70 grams) worn intravaginally twice a day for 15 minutes.
- Strengthens pelvic floor muscles, insures proper Kegel, provides sensory biofeedback, provides measure of patient progress.

→ Vaginal pessaries—Mechanical devices of various shapes made of latex rubber. Worn intravaginally to stabilize ureterovesical junction and increase urethral closure pressures.

- Especially helpful in patients with a cystocele who are not candidates for surgery.
- Devices must be fit properly so as not to make incontinence worse.

→ Pharmacological therapy—Based on high concentration of alpha-adrenergic receptors in bladder neck, bladder base, and proximal urethra. Sympathomimetic drugs with alpha-adrenergic agonist activity cause muscle contraction of bladder neck, bladder base, and proximal urethra, thereby increasing bladder outlet resistance.
- Pharmacological therapy for stress incontinence results in significant reduction of stress incontinence in 19 percent to 60 percent of patients (Urinary Incontinence Guideline Panel 1992).
- Therapeutic regimens include:
  - phenylpropanolamine (Ornade®), 1 p.o. BID.
  - psuedoephedrine (Sudafed®), 30 mg-60 mg, 1 p.o. BID.
  - phenylpropanolamine/guaifenesin (Entex® LA), 1 p.o. BID.

→ Surgical intervention—The primary goal of surgical intervention is to elevate the bladder neck, restoring normal urethrovesical anatomy.
- There are many surgical procedures to correct stress incontinence, most of which suspend the bladder neck and urethra with a tissue sling made of the anterior vaginal wall.
  - Approaches may be vaginal or abdominal depending on the type of repair.
- Repairs commonly used to correct stress incontinence are the Marshal-Marchetti-Krantz, Raz, Burch, Stamey, and Peregra procedures.
- Success rates of surgical interventions range from 75 percent to 90 percent for 5 years, with the highest success rates occurring in younger patients (Newman 1989).
- Other surgical interventions less commonly used are artificial sphincters, teflon or collagen injections, and urinary diversion. Teflon®, GoreTex®, or fascial grafts may be used as suburethral slings.

Urge incontinence

→ Habit training—Also known as timed voiding, habit training is the establishment of a routine voiding schedule. The patient is asked to void, usually every 2 to 4 hours, whether or not she feels the need to void.
- The goal of this strategy is to keep the patient dry rather than to improve bladder function.

→ Bladder training—Also known as bladder retraining, this strategy consists of a voiding schedule with progressively increased intervals between mandatory voidings with concomitant distraction/relaxation techniques.
- The goal of bladder training is to restore normal bladder function.

→ Relaxation training—The patient is taught relaxation techniques to use when the sensation of urinary urgency occurs to allow her to make it to the bathroom to void. Relaxation techniques include slow, deep breathing and imagery (Newman 1989).

→ Biofeedback and electrical stimulation—The efficacy of newer treatment options continues to be investigated.

→ Pharmacological therapy:
- oxybutynin chloride (Ditropan®) 5 mg, 1 p.o. BID-QID.
  - Anticholinergic and direct smooth muscle relaxant.
  - Contraindicated in patients with narrow-angle glaucoma.
  - Most common side effects include constipation, dry mouth, dry skin, and blurred vision.
- propantheline bromide (Pro-Banthine®) 7.5 mg-30 mg, 1 p.o. BID-QID.
  - Smooth muscle relaxant and ganglionic-blocking effects.
  - High incidence of side effects, which include visual blurring, xerostomia, nausea, constipation, tachycardia, drowsiness, confusion, urinary retention; the most common is dry mouth.
  - Also contraindicated in narrow-angle glaucoma.
- imipramine (Tofranil®) 10 mg-25 mg, 1 p.o. at bedtime or BID.
  - A tricyclic antidepressant with both anticholinergic and alpha-agonist properties, thereby decreasing bladder contractions and increasing urethral resistance to outflow.
  - Side effects include postural hypotension, fatigue, dry mouth, and dizziness, as well as cardiac conduction disturbances in the elderly.

Mixed incontinence

→ Treatment for mixed incontinence should be contingent on which component of incontinence is most problematic for the patient. A combination of the above options may be used. Often treatment of one component, either stress or urge incontinence, will result in improvement or resolution of the second component.

CONSULTATION

→ Some patients presenting with urinary incontinence may need to be referred to or comanaged with a urologist for additional diagnostic work-up.
  ▪ Specialized diagnostic tests may include cystoscopy, uroflowmetry, cystometrogram, cystogram, and urethral pressure profile.
→ Referral to a urologist is indicated in the following situations:
  ▪ persistent diagnostic uncertainty that may affect therapy.
  ▪ high morbidity associated with non-specific therapy.
  ▪ failed empiric therapy.
  ▪ suspicion of obstruction.
  ▪ postvoid residuals greater than 50 cc.
  ▪ patients with known neurological condition.
  ▪ impending surgical intervention.

PATIENT EDUCATION

→ Explain basic anatomy and physiology of bladder and urethra, normal bladder function, and probable etiology of patient's incontinence.
→ Explore how the patient's urinary incontinence is affecting her life.
→ Discuss treatment options, their success rates, and potential side effects.
→ Teach the correct method of practicing Kegel exercises through palpation and verbal feedback.
  ▪ Kegels should be performed in series of ten, sustaining the contraction for three to ten seconds with equal periods of relaxation.
  ▪ Instruct patient to increase the number of Kegels performed daily until performing 100 per day.
  ▪ It is also helpful to explore times for patients to practice Kegels, such as standing in grocery lines, stopping at traffic stop signs or red lights, or watching television commercials.
→ Teach skills necessary to practice behavioral interventions, i.e., bladder training, habit training, relaxation training.

FOLLOW-UP

→ Follow-up visits are used to evaluate the response to treatment and to reconsider treatment options if necessary.
→ Follow-up should be at four- to 12-week intervals depending on the severity of incontinence and type of treatment.
→ Document in progress notes and problem list.

Bibliography

Bates, P., Bradley, W.E., Glen, E., Griffith, D., Melchoir, M., Rowan, D., Sterling, A., Zinner, N., and Halt, T. 1979. The standardization of terminology of lower urinary tract function. *Journal of Urology* 12:551–554.

Diokno, A.C., Brock, B.M., Brown, M.B., and Herzog, A.R. 1986. Prevalence of urinary incontinence and other urological symptoms in the noninstitutionalized elderly. *Journal of Urology* 136(5):1022–1025.

Hu, T.W. 1990. Impact of urinary incontinence on health care costs. *Journal of American Geriatrics Society* 38(3):292–295.

Newman, D.K. 1989. The treatment of urinary incontinence in adults. *Nurse Practitioner* 14:21–35.

Resnick, N.M. 1992. Urinary incontinence in older adults. *Hospital Practice* (October 15):139–184.

Richardson, D. 1991. Investigative procedures in urogynecology. *Current Opinion in Obstetrics and Gynecology* 3:513–519.

Robertson, J.R., and Hebert, D.B. 1987. Gynecologic urology. In *Current obstetrics and gynecologic diagnosis and treatment*, 6th ed., eds. M.L. Pernoll and R.C. Benson, pp. 770–781. Norwalk, CT: Appleton & Lange.

Ruff, C.C., and Reaves, E.L. 1989. Diagnosing urinary incontinence in adults. *Nurse Practitioner* 14:8–18.

Thiede, H. 1989. The prevalence of urogynecologic disorders. *Urogynecology* 16:709–715.

Thomas, T.M., Plymat, K.R., Blannin, J., and Meade, T.W. 1980. Prevalence of urinary incontinence. *British Medical Journal* 28(6250):1243–1245.

Urinary Incontinence Guideline Panel. 1992. *Urinary incontinence in adults: Clinical practice guideline*. AHCPR Pub. No. 92-0038. Rockville, MD: Agency for Health Care Policy and Research, Public Health Service, U.S. Department of Health and Human Services.

Walters, M.D. 1992. Steps in evaluating the incontinent woman. *Contemporary Obstetrics & Gynecology* 37:9–22.

Walters, M.D., and Shields, L.E. 1988. The diagnostic value of history, physical examinations, and the Q-tip cotton swab test in women with urinary incontinence. *American Journal of Obstetrics and Gynecology* 159:145–151.

Wyman, J.F. 1988. Nursing assessment of the incontinent geriatric outpatient population. *Nursing Clinics of North America* 23(1):169–181.

Sandra L. Norman, R.N., N.P., M.S.

12-RC URINARY TRACT DISORDERS

Interstitial Cystitis

Interstitial cystitis (IC) is a chronic inflammatory condition of the lower urinary tract. IC is commonly referred to as *urgency and frequency syndrome* and *painful bladder*. The exact incidence of IC is unknown, although its prevalence and incidence are increasing. Currently there are approximately 500,000 women in the United States diagnosed with IC; however, only 20 percent of the patients with IC symptoms undergo evaluation for the possible diagnosis of IC (Stamey 1991). The median age of onset is 43 years, and 85 percent of patients diagnosed with IC are women (Parsons 1990).

IC is manifested by a symptom complex of urinary frequency with small voids, dysuria, nocturia, urinary urgency, suprapubic/pelvic/perineal pain, dyspareunia, and anterior vaginal wall discomfort (Stamey 1991). Most patients with IC suffer from the condition years before the diagnosis is made. They are often treated repeatedly for urinary tract infections despite negative urine cultures.

The exact etiology of IC is unknown. It is thought to be multifactorial and, clinically speaking, a syndrome rather than a specific disease (Theoharides and Sant 1991). It is widely accepted that a dysfunctional bladder epithelium plays a role in the pathogenesis of IC (Hurst et al. 1993). The dysfunctional epithelium becomes permeable, allowing irritating substances into the subepithelial tissues. It is unclear why the uroepithelium becomes permeable. Postulated etiologies include an autoimmune process, inflammatory mediators, bladder mastocytosis, neurogenic or psychosomatic conditions, and undefined viral illnesses (Parsons 1990; Theoharides and Sant 1991).

Diagnosis of IC is made only through direct visualization of the bladder mucosa following hydrodistension under anesthesia (Parsons 1990). Immediately following hydrodistension, a bloody effluent and petechial hemorrhages distributed throughout the bladder suggest the diagnosis. The bladder capacity is abnormally small. Hunner's ulcers may be present in the bladder mucosa of some patients with IC (Parsons 1990). Microscopic examination of the bladder mucosa reveals absent surface epithelium, chronic granulation tissue, and marked leukocytosis within the capillaries (Stamey 1991).

DATABASE

SUBJECTIVE

→ Risk factors include:
  ▪ patient is female.

→ Symptoms may include:
  ▪ urinary frequency with small voids.
  ▪ urinary urgency.
  ▪ nocturia.
  ▪ burning with urination.
  ▪ suprapubic discomfort, which is often related to bladder filling and relieved by voiding.
  ▪ deep dyspareunia.
  ▪ pelvic/perineal/anterior vaginal wall pain.
  ▪ exacerbation of symptoms by certain foods, substances, or stress.
  ▪ chronicity of symptoms with periods of exacerbations and remissions.
  ▪ symptoms unrelieved by antibiotic therapy.

OBJECTIVE

→ Patient may present with:
  ▪ negative urine cultures.
  ▪ suprapubic tenderness.

- anterior vaginal wall or perineal discomfort.
- absence of vaginitis or cervicitis, unless there is concomitant infection.

ASSESSMENT

→ Probable interstitial cystitis. (Definitive diagnosis can only be made through cystoscopy.)

→ R/O urinary tract infection

→ R/O vaginitis/STD

→ R/O bladder tumor

PLAN

DIAGNOSTIC TESTS

→ Diagnostic tests may include:
  - urinalysis.
  - urine culture and sensitivities.
  - vaginal wet mount.
  - vaginal and cervical cultures.
  - bladder hydrodistension and cystoscopy under anesthesia.

TREATMENT/MANAGEMENT

→ All patients in whom interstitial cystitis is suspected should be referred to a urologist with experience in treating this condition.

→ The majority of patients with IC experience relief of their symptoms, although treatment modalities are nonspecific and usually noncurative.
  - Symptom relief, however, is often partial and intermittent.
  - The treatment options that follow are taken from Fowler 1989; Parsons 1990; and Stamey 1991.

→ Treatment options include:
  - systemic therapy:
    - antihistaminines—Block H_1 histamine receptor sites. The release of histamine causes bladder pain, hyperemia, and fibrosis.
    - cimetidine (Tagamet®)—Histamine H_2 antagonist.
    - anti-inflammatories—Inhibit mast cell degranulation, which releases prostaglandins.
    - anticholinergics and antispasmodics—Inhibit bladder smooth muscle contraction.
    - heterocyclic antidepressants—Exert analgesic action by inhibiting serotonin uptake at presynaptic neurons. The prolonged availability of serotonin at neuronal synapses increases threshold.
      - The tricyclics have some anticholinergic activity and block pain arousal.

    - heparin—Given subcutaneously or intravenously restores defective mucus layer of the bladder wall.
    - urine alkalinization—i.e., 2 Tums® TID buffers acidic urine.
    - Transcutaneous Electrical Nerve Stimulation (TENS)—Application of high-frequency, conventional TENS is based on gate theory of pain control, in which counterstimulation of the nervous system modifies the perception of pain.
  - intravesical pharmacotherapy—Mainstay of treatment and the standard against which treatments are measured.
    - Silver nitrate—Used for its caustic, antiseptic, and astringent properties.
    - Dimethyl sulfoxide (DMSO)—Pharmacological properties include anti-inflammatory, analgesic, muscle relaxant, and collagen dissolution.
    - Heparin—Restores defective mucus layer of the bladder wall, has anti-allergic and anti-inflammatory activity.
    - Chlorpactin—Used less frequently due to adverse reactions.
  - surgery.
    - Simple hydrodistension—Diagnostic as well as therapeutic. Causes ischemia or mechanical damage to submucosal nerve plexus and stretch receptors, resulting in a decrease in pain and urinary frequency.
    - Most patients with IC respond to nonsurgical treatment.
    - Surgery is the last resort after various forms of conservative treatment have failed.
    - Currently, less than 1 percent to 2 percent of patients require any of the following surgical procedures:
      - transurethral resection of ulcers.
      - laser photoirradiation of ulcers/fissures.
      - bladder denervation.
      - enterocystoplasty—Aim is to replace most of diseased bladder with healthy bowel.
      - urinary diversion—Last resort. A continent pouch and catheterizable stoma are created from bowel; the entire bladder and urethra may be removed.

CONSULTATION

→ Referral required for all patients with suspected IC.

PATIENT EDUCATION

→ Teach patient to avoid foods that appear to incite or aggravate IC symptoms: ethyl alcohol, caffeine, citrus fruits/juices, hot spicy foods, chocolates, berries, processed tomato products.

→ Teach patient to avoid foods and products that contain artificial sweeteners, which affect the bladder epithelium.

→ Explore impact of IC on patient's life.

→ Explore methods of stress reduction.

FOLLOW-UP

→ Patients with interstitial cystitis require easy access to care and close collaboration with their care provider.

→ Frequent assessment of symptoms and evaluation of treatment is important.

→ Follow-up is more frequent during periods of exacerbations and depends on the severity of the patient's symptoms.

→ Document in progress notes and problem list.

Bibliography

Fowler, J.E. 1989. *Urinary tract infection and inflammation*, pp. 294–301. Chicago: Yearbook Medical Publishers.

Hurst, R.E., Parsons, C.L., Roy, J., and Young, J.L. 1993. Urinary glycosaminoglycan excretion as a laboratory marker in the diagnosis of interstitial cystitis. *The Journal of Urology* 149:31–35.

Parsons, L. 1990. Managing interstitial cystitis. *Contemporary Urology* 2(2):45–49.

Stamey, T.A. 1991. Interstitial cystitis. *Monographs in Urology* 12:37–63.

Theoharides, T.C., and Sant, J.R. 1991. Bladder mast cell activation in interstitial cystitis. *Seminars in Urology* 9(2):74–87.

Winifred L. Star, R.N., C., N.P., M.S.

12-SA VAGINITIS
Atrophic Vaginitis

The *atrophic vagina* is a result of decreasing estrogen levels, which lead to incomplete maturation and gradual loss of the glycogen-rich squamous epithelium. When estrogen levels fall below a certain physiological level, atrophy ensues. Consequently, the protective vaginal microflora are not supported or maintained, *Lactobacilli* disappear, and reduced lactic-acid production leads to an increased pH. The epithelium is thus rendered susceptible to the overgrowth of various opportunistic bacterial organisms (e.g., streptococci, staphylococci, coliforms, diptheroids), which may induce superficial infection. The majority of afflicted women are symptom free, however.

By far the largest proportion of atrophism is a result of natural menopause. The degree of vaginal atrophy varies widely according to the individual woman and the status of her hormones. Peripheral conversion of androstenedione provides a source of estrogen and some ovarian estrogen secretion for years after menopause. In many cases, women produce sufficient estrogen to maintain a mature vaginal epithelium. Other causes of estrogen loss that result in atrophy include radiation therapy, ovariectomy, ovarian failure of any cause, antagonistic drug therapy, disease processes, or the postpartum state (Kaufman, Friedrich, and Gardner 1989).

DATABASE
See **Table 12SF.1, Vaginal Infections,** p. 12-214.

SUBJECTIVE
→ History may include any of the factors presented in the previous introductory section.
→ Symptoms may include:
  ▪ pruritus.
  ▪ vulvar irritation, burning.
  ▪ dysuria, frequency, urgency.
  ▪ dyspareunia.
  ▪ abnormal vaginal discharge (watery, or with characteristics as described in "Objective" section).
  ▪ vaginal spotting/bleeding.
→ Patient may be asymptomatic.

OBJECTIVE
→ External genitalia: Sparse, brittle pubic hair; lax, wrinkled labia majora; thinning and shrinking of labia minora; fusing of labia minora with labia majora; atrophic clitoris; eversion of mucosa of urethral meatus.

→ Vagina: Narrowed introitus; smooth, flat, thin rugae; dry, initially pale walls, later with diffuse erythema. Discharge may be odorous, thin, watery, thick, purulent, serosanguineous or bloody, gray, yellow, or green; ecchymosis, petechial hemorrhages may be present; advanced atrophy may result in adhesions or occlusion (kraurosis).

→ Cervix: Small, pale, or erythematous; petechial hemorrhages may be present.

→ Uterus: Small or nonpalpable.

→ Adnexa, rectovaginal examination: WNL unless coexistent pathology.

NOTE: Virginal speculum may be required.

ASSESSMENT

→ Atrophic vaginitis

→ R/O concomitant vaginitis/STD

→ R/O urinary tract infection

→ R/O urethral caruncle/prolapse

→ R/O endometrial hyperplasia

→ R/O uterine cancer

→ R/O squamous intraepithelial lesion/cervical cancer

PLAN

DIAGNOSTIC TESTS

→ Wet-mount microscopy (10× and 40× power) may be performed.
- saline:
  - intermediate/parabasal/basal squamous epithelial cells.
  - increased WBCs.
  - lactobacilli absent.
  - assess for clue cells, *Trichomonas*.
- KOH:
  - WNL unless concomitant infection.
  - assess for amine odor, hyphae, spores.

→ pH 5.5–7.0.

→ Maturation index: Increased intermediate and parabasal cells identified.

→ Gram stain: Intermediate/parabasal/basal cells, numerous bacteria identified.

→ Pap smear, genital cultures as indicated. (Pap smear may show atypia.)

→ Urinalysis with culture and sensitivities as indicated.

→ Endometrial biopsy as indicated by history and physical examination.

→ Additional labs may include but are not limited to: CBC, RPR or VDRL.

TREATMENT/MANAGEMENT

→ Estrogen therapy is the mainstay of treatment. Various creams have been used: conjugated estrogen (Premarin®), estradiol (Estrace®), estropipate (Ogen®), etc. Dosage is usually ½-1 applicator nightly for 1 to 2 weeks (or until relief of symptoms), tapering to ¼-½ applicator once or twice/week.

→ With the above therapy, vaginal estrogen absorption is not likely to produce significant systemic effects; however, some clinicians will offer medroxyprogesterone acetate (Provera®) 5 mg p.o. for at least 12 days every other month to counteract endometrial buildup. Withdrawal bleeding is unlikely but may occur.
- Regimens vary. Consult with physician.

→ Oral estrogen replacement therapy may be used alternatively, especially when systemic estrogen effects are desired. Therapeutic regimens differ and may include:
- conjugated estrogen (Premarin®) 0.3 mg-1.25 mg

OR

estradiol (Estrace®) 1 mg-2 mg on days 1-25 each month along with medroxyprogesterone acetate (Provera®) 5 mg-10 mg for at least 12 days (may be taken days 1-12 or 14-25).
- continuous therapy: Conjugated estrogen (Premarin®) 0.3 mg-1.25 mg

OR

estradiol (Estrace®) 1 mg-2 mg every day along with medroxyprogesterone acetate (Provera®) 2.5 mg-5.0 mg every day.
- see **Perimenopausal Symptoms and Hormone Therapy** Protocol.

NOTE: Full vaginal tissue restoration may not occur for 18 to 24 months with oral hormone replacement therapy. The minimal effective dose for maintenance therapy should be utilized (*PDR* 1993).

→ Tapering doses of vaginal estrogen may be used in a postpartum, breast-feeding woman as indicated without adverse effects on breast milk or the infant (Kaufman and Faro 1994).

→ It should be noted that when estrogen therapy is used to treat atrophic vaginitis, *Candida* and *Trichomonas* that were previously unable to survive in a glycogen-poor vagina may be incited to proliferate and a symptomatic infection may ensue. Treat accordingly.

→ When estrogen replacement therapy is contraindicated, vaginal lubrication with Lubrin® or Replens® may be tried. Lubricants for coitus include Astroglide® (superior product), K-Y Jelly®, or Surgilube®.

→ Treat concomitant identified vaginitis and STDs as indicated. See appropriate protocols.

CONSULTATION

→ As indicated.

→ As needed for prescription(s).

PATIENT EDUCATION

→ Discuss the etiology and nature of the condition.

→ Encourage sexual intercourse as tolerated and appropriate. Lubricants such as Astroglide® are helpful.

→ Dilation of the vagina may be helpful in alleviating some of the atrophic changes. A well-lubricated finger, dildo, or candle may be used. Sitting in a warm tub may help relaxation during the dilation process.

FOLLOW-UP

→ As necessary to the individual case.

→ If an STD is identified, treat appropriately. See appropriate protocols. Refer patient's partner for evaluation and therapy. Discuss safer sex practices (see **Table 13A.2, Safer Sex Guidelines**, p.13-9).

→ Document in problem list and progress notes.

12-SB VAGINITIS

Candida Vaginitis

Among vaginal infections, *Candida (yeast) vaginitis* is the second to *bacterial vaginosis* and three times more frequent than *Trichomonas vaginitis* (Sobel 1990). Yeasts are ubiquitous fungal organisms; they exist everywhere in nature. In the human, yeast is present in the mouth, GI tract, rectum, and vagina. Other places where yeast may grow are the intertriginous areas: vulva, groin, axilla, skin under the breasts, and, in the male, the coronal sulcus of the penis (most often in uncircumsized men). About 20 percent to 40 percent of women harbor yeast in the genital tract as a harmless commensal for months to years without symptoms (Sobel 1989; Weisberg 1990).

A delicate ecosystem exists in the vagina whereby physiological amounts of estrogen induce the formation of mature squamous epithelium rich in glycogen. In turn, the lactobacilli of the vagina metabolize the glycogen into lactic acid, which maintains a pH between 3.5 and 4.5 and keeps pathogenic bacteria in check. Yeast organisms gain access to the vagina mostly from the nearby perianal area, but other methods of inoculation are possible (e.g., sexual transmission [oral and genital] and via fomites).

In the colonization phase, which is usually asymptomatic, yeast and resident vaginal flora exist as commensal organisms. Infection may develop when specific changes in host response or the local environment occur. It is estimated that 75 percent of women will experience at least one episode of yeast vulvovaginitis during their lifetime, and 40 percent to 45 percent will experience at least two episodes (CDC 1993). About five percent of women will suffer from recurrent bouts. *Candida* infection combined with *Trichomonas vaginalis* or bacterial vaginosis occurs in approximately four to six percent and 10 percent of cases, respectively (Horowitz

and Mardh 1991; Kaufman and Faro 1994; Kaufman, Friedrich, and Gardner 1989; Melzer and Marx 1985; Sobel 1989; Sobel 1990).

In the United States, *Candida albicans* is the species most often associated with infection, but other *Candida* organisms such as *Candida (Torulopsis) glabrata* and *Candida tropicalis* have been encountered with increasing frequency in recent years. Studies indicate that these species are more resistant to treatment and more difficult to eradicate. One reason for the increased selection of resistant strains is the shortening of antifungal treatment regimens, which suppress *C. albicans* but cause overgrowth of other species. Yeast's adaptable nature and ability to alter its biochemical pathways (genetic switching) has also contributed to the decrease in its susceptibility to standard therapies (Cauwenbergh 1990; Soll 1988).

Chronic yeast vaginitis—three or more clinically proven infections/year—is a perplexing, frustrating problem. Many factors have been implicated: the intestinal reservoir, fecal contamination of the vagina, mucosal persistence, sexual transmission/practices, virulence and resistance of the organism, type of therapy, patient compliance with therapy, zinc deficiency, and immune system factors. It is interesting to note that non-*Candida* strains are not usually associated with chronic infections and no increase has been found in the usual predisposing factors (see "Subjective" section for discussion of predisposing factors).

At one time, yeast vaginitis was not thought to be sexually transmitted, but newer research has shown that identical yeast species can be isolated from the mouth, seminal fluid, and rectum of partners of infected women. Thus, sexual transmission should be considered in women with recurrent infection.

Cellular immune system dysfunction as a cause for recurrent infection has received a lot of attention recently. It has been shown that women with chronic reinfection have a reduced lymphocytic response to the *Candida* antigen, mediated by an excess of prostaglandin production by abnormal macrophages. Hypersensitivity reactions may trigger the events leading to suppressed cell-mediated immunity via release of histamines. Immune system research continues to unfold the forces responsible for recurrent infection (Kaufman and Faro 1994; Kaufman, Friedrich, and Gardner 1989; Horowitz and Mardh 1991; Sobel 1985; Syntex 1989).

Therapeutic agents used to treat yeast vaginitis can be classified into four groups: dyes (gentian violet) and miscellaneous compounds (potassium sorbate, boric acid, 5-flucytosine); polyenes (Amphotericin B, nystatin, candicidin); imidazoles (clotrimazole, miconazole, butoconazole, tioconazole, ketoconazole); and triazoles (terconazole, fluconazole). The last group is the first in a relatively new generation of azoles for which *in vitro* studies have shown excellent activity against *C. glabrata* and *C. tropicalis* (Rinaldi 1988); however, more data in humans are needed to determine whether these products offer any advantage over the imidazoles.

DATABASE

SUBJECTIVE

→ Predisposing factors include:
- endogenous factors: The intestinal reservoir is a constant reservoir for fungal organisms and thus a possible source of vaginal contamination.
  • Facilitators are poor hygiene, sexual practices, and bowel habits (i.e., constipation) that prolong fecal passage time and allow for increased yeast growth.
- pregnancy: High estrogen levels increase glycogen content of vagina, providing a favorable climate for yeast overgrowth and enhancing vaginal cell affinity for yeast. Incidence increases throughout gestation.
- antibiotics: Broad-spectrum agents (e.g., tetracyclines, cephalosporins, and penicillin/ampicillin-like compounds) reduce the protective lactobacilli of gut/vagina, allowing resident yeast proliferation.
- diabetes, uncontrolled: Increased urinary/vaginal glucose provides enriched medium for yeast growth.
- diet: Dairy products, sweets, and artificial sweeteners encourage yeast proliferation through

increased amounts of lactose/glucose in GI tract.
- immunocompromise conditions and metabolic factors: AIDS, endocrinopathies (diabetes, hypothyroidism, Cushing's syndrome, etc.), anemia, hematological malignancies (lymphoma, leukemia, Hodgkin's disease), autoimmune diseases (lupus, rheumatoid arthritis, temporal arteritis) (Summers and Sharp 1993), zinc deficiency, and corticosteroid/other immunosuppressive drugs.
  • These conditions/factors increase susceptibility to fungal infection (probably) by altering cell-mediated immunity.
- allergens: Pollens and dust, chemicals, detergents, spermicides, and specific properties of seminal fluid may all precipitate the hypersensitivity reaction and affect cell-mediated immunity.
- synthetic fabrics, tight clothing: Increase moisture, providing rich medium in which resident yeast may flourish.
- sexual transmission: Usually seen more frequently in women with recurrent infection.
  • Partner may harbor same-strain yeast in mouth, seminal fluid/ejaculate, rectum, and penile skin, especially with intact foreskin.
  • Thus, oral-genital contact and intercourse may transmit yeast. Anal-vaginal intercourse, digital anal-vaginal manipulation, and use of anal-vaginal dildo may also predispose to vaginal contamination.
- oral contraceptives (controversial): Pharmacological doses of hormones may affect glycogen status of vaginal epithelium, leading to enriched substrate for yeast growth. High-estrogen pills implicated more often.
- other possible precipitating factors: Stress, obesity, menses, trauma, poor hygiene, fomites, warm weather, fever, contraceptive sponges, commercial douches, and feminine hygiene deodorant products.
  • These factors may alter the symbiotic relationship between resident flora in the vagina.
  • Irritants such as perfumed soap and toilet paper, chlorinated pools, and topical anesthetics may cause a reactive vulvitis that can be confused with yeast infection.

→ Symptoms may include:
- pruritus: Primary symptom, located in the vulva; may be mild to severe; may be

exacerbated in evening hours; usual onset in the premenstruum; may improve during menstruation.
- burning: Often accompanies pruritus; may follow intercourse or be secondary to excoriation from scratching (semen itself also may cause postcoital burning).
- dysuria (external); urinary urgency, frequency (reflexogenic).
- dyspareunia.
- leukorrhea: Not a classic symptom and rarely the presenting complaint. However, most patients have slight discharge at some stage of infection. May be thin, creamy, thick/curd-like (occurs more often in pregnancy); usually odorless or may smell sour or "yeast-like."
- dryness in vulvovaginal area.
- swelling of vulvovaginal area.
- woman reporting partner complaints of penile "rash," redness, pruritus, or burning following intercourse.
→ History should include:
- gynecological history.
- sexual history (including sexual orientation, practices, number of partners, partner signs and symptoms); contraceptive history.
- medical history.
- allergies (foods, medications, products, environmental factors); medications.
- habits (drugs, alcohol); exercise; nutrition; stress.
- review of systems.
- family history (diabetes, allergies).
- onset, timing of symptoms, relation to menstrual cycle/sexual activity.
- location of pruritus: Mons, vulva, vaginal, perineum, perianal, generalized.
- characteristics of discharge: Color, quantity, quality, odor.
- associated symptoms.
- aggravating/relieving factors.
- other: Use of self-treatment measures and home remedies; OTC medication; use of spermicides, feminine hygiene deodorant products, douches, bath additives, etc.; type of soap, detergent, toilet paper; use of pads or tampons, sexual paraphernalia; type of undergarments and clothing.

OBJECTIVE

→ Ideally, examination is performed when patient is symptomatic, has not douched for two to three days, has not applied intravaginal cream or contraceptive spermicide for several days to one week, and is not menstruating.
→ Vital signs as indicated (usually unnecessary in uncomplicated infection).
→ Abdominal examination, including inguinal lymph nodes, as indicated.
→ A systematic, thorough examination of the vulvovaginal area should be performed, keeping in mind other potential causes of genital infection.
- Vulva: May see erythema, edema, excoriation, discharge; erythema may extend to perianal area, crural folds, inner thighs, buttocks; satellite pustules may appear at edges of affected area.
- Bartholin's, urethral, Skene's glands: Usually WNL; assess for discharge.
- Vagina: May see thin, creamy, or thick/curd-like white or yellow discharge, erythema; a pseudomembrane may cover the vaginal walls.
- Cervix: May see adherent thin, creamy, or thick/curd-like white or yellow discharge, erythema.
→ Uterus, adnexa, rectovaginal examination: Usually WNL unless concomitant pathology.

ASSESSMENT

→ Yeast vaginitis
→ Yeast vulvitis
→ Yeast vulvovaginitis
→ Recurrent yeast (vulvo)vaginitis
→ R/O physiological leukorrhea
→ R/O other causes of vaginitis: Bacterial vaginosis, *T. vaginalis* vaginitis, cytolytic vaginitis, atrophic vaginitis, chemical/mechanical causes
→ R/O foreign body
→ R/O contact (reactive) vulvitis
→ R/O diabetic vulvitis
→ R/O allergic reaction
→ R/O cutaneous candidiasis of the vulva
→ R/O tinea cruris
→ R/O other vulvar dermatoses (e.g., psoriasis, seborrheic dermatitis, eczemoid dermatitis)
→ R/O STD
→ R/O urinary tract infection
→ R/O infection in partner
→ Assess psychosomatic factors

PLAN

DIAGNOSTIC TESTS

→ Wet-mount microscopy (10× and 40× power) is principle diagnostic method.
- Potassium hydroxide (KOH) 10 percent to 20 percent:
  - spores or branching/budding pseudomycelia (hyphae) may be identified.
    - *C. glabrata* spores are of variable size, spherical-ovoid, in groups or clusters (but may appear singly), and smaller than a red blood cell. Budding (or non-budding) yeast without pseudohyphae is strongly suggestive of *C. glabrata*.
    - *C. albicans* spores, in contrast, are uniform in size, isolated, and almost always associated with hyphae (Kaufman and Faro 1994).
  - amine odor may be present in cases of bacterial vaginosis/*T. vaginalis* vaginitis.

  NOTE: Obtain specimen from more than 1 area. Half of women culture-positive for yeast will have a negative KOH wet mount. Cotton fibers, scratches on slide, and *Leptothrix* (nonfungal vaginal commensal) all appear as long, string-like filaments and thus may be confused with hyphae.
- Saline:
  - lactobacilli are usually present.
  - WBCs may be increased.
  - assess for clue cells, motile trichomonads.

  NOTE: If excessive WBCs identified—think trichomoniasis, other STD.

→ pH: 4.0-4.7 (4.5 most common).

  NOTE: Collect specimen from mid-third of lateral vaginal wall. Tap water, cervical mucus, presence of bacterial vaginosis/*Trichomonas* may result in alkaline readings.

→ Gram stain: Spores and budding hyphae may be seen.

→ Cultures for yeast: May be performed to evaluate recurrent/resistant cases and with suspected candidiasis when KOH prep is negative. Nickerson's, Sabouraud's, Mycosel, or blood agar media may be used. Yeast can be grown at room temperature; some non-*Candida* species may take 10 days to grow out.

  NOTE: In cases of recurrence, the mouths of both patient and partner(s) and the ejaculate of the partner(s) may need to be evaluated by culture.

→ Slide latex agglutination monoclonal antibody test: Used as an adjunctive diagnostic tool when microscopy inconclusive; can detect non-*C. albicans* species; not available everywhere; limited appeal, sensitivity 72 percent to 81 percent; may also test for *Trichomonas*.

→ Pap smear: May identify *Candida* if present in large numbers.

→ Ideally, genital cultures for *Chlamydia trachomatis* and *Neisseria gonorrhoeae* should be performed in all cases of vaginitis.

→ Additional labs as indicated may include but are not limited to: CBC, herpes culture, urinalysis, urine culture and sensitivities, VDRL or RPR, etc.

TREATMENT/MANAGEMENT

→ Identification of *Candida* in an asymptomatic woman does not require treatment (CDC 1993).

→ It has been recommended that definitive therapy be deferred until a specific diagnosis of vaginitis has been made (Friedrich 1988).

→ In some situations, a presumptive diagnosis of yeast vulvovaginitis may lead to empirical antifungal therapy.

→ Avoid overtreatment of leukorrhea without other symptoms and in the absence of clinical pathology.
- Repetitive use of an antifungal agent in the presence of a normal vaginal examination may precipitate a vicious cycle of iatrogenic overtreatment syndrome (Hammill 1989).
- Mild baking soda/H_2O douches (1 tbsp/quart) may be tried every third or fourth day as indicated to lessen amount of vaginal discharge (not recommended in pregnancy, during menses, or if patient is at increased risk for PID).

→ Acute therapy.
- 1-day therapy.
  - Clotrimazole (Mycelex®-G) 500 mg tablet. 1 vaginal application at bedtime once.
  - Tioconazole (Vagistat®-1) 6.5 percent ointment. 1 vaginal application at bedtime once. Use prefilled applicator. (Oil-based formulation; may weaken latex condoms and diaphragms.)
  - Fluconazole (Diflucan®) 150 mg p.o. once.
- 3-day therapy.
  - Miconazole nitrate (Monistat®3) 200 mg suppository. 1 vaginal application at bedtime for 3 days. (Oil-based formulation; may weaken latex condoms and diaphragms.)

- Butoconazole nitrate (Femstat®) 2 percent cream. 1 vaginal application at bedtime for 3 days. Available in prefilled applicator. (Oil-based formulation; may weaken latex condoms and diaphragms.)
- Terconazole (Terazol®3) 0.8 percent cream. 1 vaginal application at bedtime for 3 days.
- Terconazole (Terazol®3) 80 mg suppository. 1 vaginal application at bedtime for 3 days. (Oil-based formulation; may weaken latex condoms and diaphragms.)
  - 7-day therapy.
- Clotrimazole (Mycelex®-7) 1 percent cream or 100 mg inserts; (Mycelex®-G) 1 percent cream; (Gyne-Lotrimin®) 1 percent cream or 100 mg inserts. 1 vaginal application at bedtime for 7 days. OTC.
- Miconazole nitrate (Monistat®-7) 2 percent cream or 100 mg suppository. 1 vaginal application at bedtime for 7 days. (Oil-based formulation; may weaken latex condoms and diaphragms.) OTC.
- Terconazole (Terazol®7) 0.4 percent cream. 1 vaginal application at bedtime for 7 days.
  - 14-day therapy.
- Clotrimazole (Mycelex®-G) 1 percent cream. 1 vaginal application at bedtime for 14 days. OTC.

NOTE: The clinician must decide between 1-, 3-, 7-, or 14-day antifungal therapy based on history and clinical presentation. Single- and/or 3-day therapies are indicated for patients with infrequent, episodic infection of mild to moderate severity and may not be effective for chronic cases and during pregnancy (Sobel 1990). Single-dose oral fluconazole has been shown to be comparable in efficacy to topical azole therapy in many studies (Langdon 1994). For the occasional infection unresponsive to a single course of standard therapy, treat with a second course (Sparks 1991). High relapse rates after therapy can be controlled by continuing treatment for at least 2 weeks or longer (Kaufman and Faro 1994). According to Eschenbach (1991) antifungal agents may be used in any trimester of pregnancy; however, some manufacturers do not recommend their use at all except with medical supervision or only in the second and third trimesters of pregnancy. Refer to the *PDR* or package insert for more specific information.

→ Yeast vulvitis.

- Mild: Use vaginal antifungal cream to vulvar area BID-TID.
- Severe/extensive: Use vaginal antifungal preparations both vaginally and to the affected vulvar areas.
- See **Red Lesions of the Vulva** Protocol.

→ Pruritus/inflammation control.
- Low- to mid-potency corticosteroid cream or ointment sparingly BID-TID to affected area.
  - Options include:
    - hydrocortisone 1 percent (Nutracort®) (non-fluorinated).
    - nystatin and triamcinolone acetonide (Mycolog-II®).
    - triamcinolone acetonide 0.1 percent (Kenalog® or Aristocort®).
    NOTE: Avoid use of fluorinated steroids for extended periods as skin atrophy may result. See **Table 12TB.1, Potency Ranking of Topical Corticosteroids**, p. 12-228.

→ Alternative acute therapies.
- Gentian violet 1 percent: Painted on vulva and in vagina once; may repeat treatment at weekly or monthly intervals depending on response (Kaufman and Faro 1994); may use vaginal antifungal treatment daily for the week after treatment (Friedrich 1983). Effective treatment for *C. albicans* and *C. glabrata*. Do not use either solution or tampons in presence of vulvar excoriation or ulceration.
- Boric acid powder in 0 size gelatin capsule: 600 mg intravaginally once/day for 14 days; may be followed by 600 mg twice/week for 3 weeks (Eschenbach 1991; Jovanovic, Congema, and Nguyen 1991; Kaufman and Faro 1994; Van Slyke, Michel, and Rein 1981).
  - Contraindicated in pregnancy and in patients with poor renal function.
- Potassium sorbate 3 percent aqueous solution: Douche as indicated for treatment/prevention (Friedrich 1993; Kaufman and Faro 1994).
  - Douching contraindicated in patients at risk for PID and not recommended in pregnancy or during menses.
- Vinegar, yogurt (active lactobacillus culture), or lactobacillus douches: 1 tbsp. to 2 tbsp./quart H₂O, douche once a day for 7 days (see above regarding douching); yogurt may also be applied directly into the vagina with a cervical cap, diaphragm, or tampon (Grist 1988).
  - These therapies have not been supported scientifically.

→ Partner therapy.
  ▪ In the presence of balanitis (erythema, pruritis, or irritation of glans penis) or penile dermatitis, a topical antifungal agent may be beneficial (CDC 1993).

→ Therapy for recurrent yeast.
  ▪ The following *general principles* may be applied to manage recurrent infection (Kaufman and Faro 1994; Kaufman, Friedrich, and Gardner 1989; Sobel 1990; Sparks 1991):
    • identify and attempt to eradicate all predisposing factors, if possible.
    • make no assumptions regarding efficacy of previously used therapies.
    • when patient does not respond to antifungal therapy, consider other causes of vulvo-vaginitis, such as *T. vaginalis* vaginitis, bacterial vaginosis, cytolytic vaginitis, atrophic vaginitis, contact vulvitis, lichen sclerosus, vestibulitis, essential vulvodynia, or lichen planus.
    • oral corticosteroids, immunosuppressive drugs, and high-dose estrogen hormones should be discontinued if possible.
    • establish species identity via culture. Consider culturing mouth and ejaculate of partner.
    • treat all patients for a minimum of *2 weeks* regardless of choice of intravaginal antifungal agent.
    • consider labs: Fasting blood sugar, HIV antibody, and serum zinc level.
    • if patient is diabetic, advocate good control.
    • enhance diet with vitamin/mineral supplement.
    • see "Patient Education" section regarding health maintenance and additional general principles.
  ▪ Topical suppressive therapy may include:
    • intravaginal antifungal cream at bedtime for 14 days followed by use every 3 to 4 nights for 6 to 12 months (Eschenbach and Mead 1992b).
    • alternative therapy may include:
      –boric acid 600 mg in 0 size gelatin capsule intravaginally every third night for 6 to 12 months (Eschenbach and Mead 1992b)
          OR
      –may be used intravaginally once/day during menstruation for 4 months following initial dosing BID for 2 weeks (Jovanovic, Congema, and Nguyen 1991).

  ▸ Contraindicated in pregnancy and in patients with poor renal function.
  ▪ Consider systemic suppressive therapy.
  NOTE: Various treatment regimens have been suggested. Infections tend to recur after suppressive therapy is discontinued.
    • Options include:
      –ketoconazole (Nizoral®) 100 mg p.o. once a day for up to 6 months (CDC 1993).
      –ketoconazole (Nizoral®) 400 mg/day for 14 days initially, followed by maintenance dose of 100 mg/day for 6 months
          OR
      –prophylactic doses of 400 mg/day for 1 month followed by 400 mg/day for 5 days at onset of menses for 6 months (Eschenbach 1991; Sobel 1986).
  NOTE: Ketoconazole may be hepatotoxic (estimated to appear in 1:10,000 to 1:15,000 exposed persons [CDC 1993]). Refer to *PDR* and consult with physician prior to prescribing. Liver function tests should be performed prior to initiating therapy and every 3 to 4 months during therapy. Contraindicated in pregnancy and not for use in uncomplicated, infrequent/acute vaginal yeast infections.
      –nystatin orally TID for 1 to 3 months (Kaufman and Faro 1994) (most studies have not shown clear-cut evidence regarding efficacy with this regimen).
→ Additional considerations.
  ▪ Other options for intravaginal antifungals in recurrent cases and for prevention may include:
    • use at bedtime for 3 nights prior to menses for 6 months (Meltzer and Marx 1985).
    • use at bedtime for 3 to 7 days at symptom onset.
    • single-dose cream for episodic postcoital flares.
    • prophylactic use during course of broad-spectrum antibiotic.
    • empiric change to triazole if antifungal resistance suspected clinically (Summers and Sharp 1993).
  ▪ Treat concomitant vaginal infections appropriately. See specific protocols.
  ▪ Additional approaches to therapy in chronic cases or with resistant *Candida* strains may include:
    • flucytosine—14 oral capsules of 500 mg compounded into 45 g hydrophilic cream base (compounded by pharmacist), one 6.4 g

vaginal application at bedtime for 7 days—has been used for resistant *Candida* strains such as *C. tropicalis* (Kaufman and Faro 1994; Horowitz 1986b).

- gentian violet as above.
- treating male with azole antifungal agent to penis, especially under foreskin.
  - Condom therapy for 6 months and avoidance of oral-genital contact may be indicated. May suggest clotrimazole oral troches or nystatin oral suspension to eradicate oral yeast if culture-positive. A new toothbrush is also advisable (Kaufman and Faro 1994). **NOTE:** Routine partner treatment may not influence female recurrence rate, and opinions differ regarding its efficacy.
- antiprostaglandin agents, H_2 receptor antagonists, and antihistamines are drugs being considered for future use (SYNTEX 1989).
- medroxyprogesterone acetate (Depo-Provera®) 150 mg I.M. every 12 weeks has been used to decrease endogenous estrogen levels (Dennerstein 1986).

- Nonmedical approaches to recurrent cases may include:
  - lactobacillus tablets or yogurt: Use intra-vaginally every day when yeast seems likely to occur.
  - ingestion of lactobacilli supplements (capsule or powder), natural yogurt, vitamin/mineral supplements, or garlic has been suggested as a dietary adjunct.
    - For specifics, refer to a book on natural approaches to therapy of vaginitis (Grist 1988).
  - homeopathy, herbs, or acupuncture: Refer patient to practitioner skilled in these techniques if she expresses interest in alternative approaches to treatment of recurrent yeast vaginitis (Grist 1988).

CONSULTATION

- → As needed for prescription.
- → For recurrent infection as indicated.
- → When considering systemic therapy.

PATIENT EDUCATION

- → Discuss cause, precipitating factors, and possible transmission of infection.
- → In cases where no pathology is identified and the only complaint is leukorrhea, reassurance

regarding absence of infection and education regarding normality of cyclical discharge are all that are required.

- → Advise patient that self-treatment with OTC products should be reserved for women who have been previously diagnosed with yeast vulvovaginitis and who are experiencing a recurrence of the same symptoms (CDC 1993).
- → Review/discuss vulvovaginal health and hygiene:
  - all-cotton underwear, loose clothing, avoidance of panty hose.
  - proper wiping technique, i.e., front to back.
  - white, unscented toilet paper.
  - avoidance of chemical irritants such as strong bath or laundry soap, feminine hygiene products, bath additives, plastic-covered or scented peripads, scented tampons, talcum powder, commercial douches, chlorinated swimming pools.
  - avoidance of mechanical irritants such as tight clothing, excessive use of tampons, dildos, vibrators, bicycles.
  - ideally, use only water to wash vulva (if necessary, Aveeno® or other hypoallergenic soap may be used with thorough rinse); pat area dry or use hair dryer on low setting; avoid over-cleaning (woman may do this to attempt to eradicate vaginal infection/STD).
  - hand wash undergarments with mild soap and thorough rinse; line drying preferable.
  - corn starch (not talcum powder) may be used in crural folds if excessive sweating is a problem. Avoid in presence of acute or recurrent yeast infection.
    - Topical antifungal dusting powder (Mycostatin®) may be tried (see *PDR*).
  - for recurrent infection, "sterilize" underclothing in microwave for five minutes on high while garment is still wet from laundering or soak in bleach overnight and rinse thoroughly. Alternately, boiling or washing at temperatures exceeding 70°C may sterilize undergarments (Kaufman and Faro 1994). Disposable panties or panty liners may be used.
  - change tampon frequently (every two to four hours).
- → Stress importance of completing full course of prescribed medication; continue intravaginal medications throughout menses (use with peripad instead of tampon).
- → Advise abstinence from sexual intercourse during course of treatment for infection.

→ Provide guidelines on safer sex practices (see **Table 13A.2, Safer Sex Guidelines,** p. 13-9).

- Encourage condom use with new, multiple, nonmonogamous partners.
- Advise that anal-vaginal sex without interceding wash or oral-genital sex may precipitate infection and may need to be curtailed. Clean fingers may need to be substituted for oral sex during masturbation by partner.

→ Sex toys, douche tips, diaphragms, cervical caps, etc., may act as fomites and thus should be cleaned properly after use.

→ Discuss risk factors for recurrent infections with affected individuals (e.g., diabetes, immuno-suppression, antibiotic or corticosteroid use, HIV infection). Most women will have no predisposing conditions (CDC 1993).

- When treating with systemic medication, advise patient regarding potential side effects (refer to *PDR*) and explain that although recurrent vaginal candidiasis may occur from GI tract carriage, treatment with oral antifungal agents may afford only short-term relief.

→ Suggest that women with recurrent infection avoid tampon use until symptom-free for three to six months. When antibiotics are taken, prophylactic antifungal cream should be used.

→ Encourage good health maintenance: Well-balanced diet with avoidance of excessive simple sugars, starch, dairy products, alcohol, yeast-containing foods; adequate fluids and fiber to encourage good bowel habits; adequate rest and exercise; stress reduction (Burnhill 1990; Horowitz 1986a).

- Other food prohibitions may include malted products, foods containing monosodium glutamate, artificial sweeteners containing lactose, vinegar, smoked products, coffee, and tea (Grist 1988).

→ Systemic allergic reactions to certain foodstuffs—especially citrus fruits, milk, fermented products, corn, and refined sugars—may precipitate yeast-like symptoms.

- Eliminating these substances may alleviate the problem.

- Advise patient to keep a diary of foods that may precipitate vulvovaginal reactions.

→ Environmental allergens, such as pollen, dust, and animal hair, may inadvertently enter the vagina and result in allergic-type vaginal reactions. Ask patient to explore this possibility.

→ When gentian violet is used, advise the patient to wear old panties or use pads or liners because the product stains. Intercourse should be avoided for three to four days post-treatment.

→ Advise patient to keep boric acid capsules, which look like jelly beans, out of reach of children; may cause esophageal ulcers if swallowed.

FOLLOW-UP

→ Acute, uncomplicated cases require no follow-up. Advise patient to return for re-evaluation if symptoms do not abate after therapy.

→ With the advent of OTC antifungal agents (miconazole, clotrimazole), a patient may opt to self-treat "yeast" vaginitis symptoms. If the patient remains symptomatic after OTC-therapy, she should be instructed to see a health care provider for thorough investigation of signs and symptoms, identification of the infectious agent(s) involved, and therapy based on specific clinical findings.

→ Patients treated for recurrent infection should be monitored for compliance with treatment regimens and assessed regularly to monitor effectiveness of therapy and occurrence of side effects (CDC 1993).

→ Sexual transmission should be considered in recurrent cases. The male partner, in general, is affected in only 20 percent of cases. Treatment should be individualized. Sexual partner(s) should be referred to a health care provider for evaluation and treatment as indicated.

→ Follow up cervical cultures and treat identified concomitant STDs (see specific protocols). Discuss importance of partner evaluation and treatment if STD identified.

→ Address additional medical concerns as indicated.

→ Document in progress notes and problem list.

12-SC VAGINITIS

Cytolytic Vaginitis

Lactobacilli-overgrowth syndrome, also known as *cytolytic vaginitis* or *Döderlein's cytolysis,* is a condition caused by accelerated exfoliation and increased turnover of squamous epithelial cells in the vagina. Stress may be a precipitating factor. The condition may also arise in women who have been treated or overtreated for vaginal discharge with a variety of antibiotics and antifungal agents. The resultant overgrowth of lactobacilli, which then become the predominant microorganism, breaks down the vaginal mucosa through increased acid production and lysis of the epithelial cells' cytoplasm (Burnhill 1987; Kaufman and Faro 1994; Kaufman, Friedrich, and Gardner 1989).

DATABASE
See **Table 12SF.1, Vaginal Infections,** p. 12-214.

SUBJECTIVE

→ Symptoms may include:
  - nonodorous, increased, or profuse discharge of thick, pasty, or "flaky" quality.
  - mild burning sensation of the vulva, worse after intercourse.
  - dyspareunia.
  - pruritus (usually absent).
→ Symptoms may be more pronounced in luteal phase.

OBJECTIVE

→ Vulva usually within normal limits (WNL); may see increased presence of thick, white discharge.

→ Vagina may demonstrate increased presence of a nonodorous, thick, white, opaque discharge.

→ Cervix, uterus, adnexa, and rectovaginal exams are WNL unless there is coexistent pathology.

ASSESSMENT

→ Cytolytic vaginitis or Döderlein's cytolysis.
→ R/O *Candida* vaginitis
→ R/O other causes of vaginitis
→ R/O STD
→ R/O squamous intraepithelial lesion

PLAN

DIAGNOSTIC TESTS

→ Wet mounts (10× and 40× power).
  - Saline:
    • increased number of epithelial cells and cellular debris from squamous cell disintegration.
    • large number of rods (lactobacilli) of varying lengths.
    • "false clue cell" (stippled appearance of epithelial cell due to adherence of lactobacilli).
    • few or no white blood cells.
  - Potassium hydroxide:
    • no hyphae; no amine odor.
→ pH: 4.0-4.5.
→ Gram stain: Many lactobacilli and gram-positive rods of varying lengths, fragments of cytoplasm, "stripped" nuclei, lack of significant pathogenic bacteria or yeast.
→ Vaginal cultures: Normal flora or lactobacilli; not normally performed.

TREATMENT/MANAGEMENT

→ Alkaline douches: 1 tsp baking soda/pint of warm H_2O, douche once or twice. May be repeated as needed during symptomatic periods without resorting to excessive use (Kaufman and Faro 1994).
NOTE: This therapy is designed to reduce the lactobacillus population.

→ Avoid overtreatment of normal vaginal discharge.

CONSULTATION

→ As indicated.

PATIENT EDUCATION

→ Discuss proposed mechanisms for the condition.

→ Reassure patient that, without clinical evidence of infection, leukorrhea is usually physiological. Discuss cyclical changes in normal vaginal discharge.

→ Advise patient against seeking over-the-phone treatment by provider and self-overtreating of vaginal symptoms, which may lead to improper therapy of vaginitis or treatment of normal vaginal discharge.

→ Stress good health maintenance: Proper nutrition, rest, exercise, stress reduction.

FOLLOW-UP

→ Individualized according to case presentation.

→ Document in progress notes and problem list.

12-SD   VAGINITIS
Trichomonas Vaginalis Vaginitis

Trichomonas vaginalis is a single-celled anaerobic protozoan, not found as a normal vaginal commensal. Three species infect humans: *T. tenax* (oral cavity), *Pentatrichomonas hominis* (intestinal tract), and *T. vaginalis* (lower genitourinary tract). These species are site-specific and do not survive outside their own environs. Some strains of *T. vaginalis* are more virulent than others, with specific host antibody production, but laboratory tests utilizing antibody titers have been of little importance in diagnosing infection.

Size of the organism varies, with smaller diameter associated with a more intense inflammatory reaction. The rare giant sizes have been associated with the elderly and asymptomatic individuals. The vaginal bacterial flora in trichomoniasis is predominantly lactobacilli-deficient and anaerobic-dominant (Kaufman, Friedrich, and Gardner 1989; Thompson and Gelbart 1989).

T. vaginalis is responsible for about 25 percent of all vaginal infections and is a distant third behind BV and *Candida* vaginitis (Kaufman and Faro 1994). More than 180 million people are infected worldwide annually, including 2.5 million to 3 million women in the United States (Rein and Muller 1990). Prevalence varies with the population studied, with five percent to 50 percent rates reported. Trichomoniasis is sexually transmitted; nonsexual routes of transmission are possible but rare. The organism can survive 24 hours on wet towels and clothes and in chlorinated swimming pools, six hours in soapy or bubble-bath water, and 45 minutes on a toilet seat (Kaufman and Faro 1994).

Sexual transmission rates are high. In women, the incubation period is four to 28 days following exposure (Rein and Muller 1990). Female partners of infected men harbor the organism 80 percent to 100 percent of the time, and male partners of infected women, 13 percent to 85 percent of the time (Meltzer and Marx 1985). About one-third of initially asymptomatic women develop symptoms within six months if left untreated, possibly as a result of changes in the vaginal microenvironment (Rein and Muller 1990). Men are usually asymptomatic, with 36 percent to 50 percent of cases resolving spontaneously within two weeks of exposure (Meltzer and Marx 1985).

In women, sites of infection include the vagina, urethra, Skene's glands, and endocervix. In men, the organism lives in the urethra and prostate gland and under the foreskin. *T. vaginalis* may coexist with gonorrhea in about 20 percent to 50 percent of cases and with BV in about 35 percent of cases. Because *T. vaginalis* is highly motile it is thought that other pathogenic organisms (e.g., *N. gonorrhoeae, C. trachomatis*) can attach to its surface and be swept up the genital tract to cause PID (Kaufman and Faro 1994; Meltzer and Marx 1985; Sweet and Gibbs 1990; Thompson and Gelbart 1989). Recent evidence implicates a possible relationship with trichomoniasis and adverse pregnancy outcomes, in particular preterm rupture of membranes and preterm delivery (CDC 1993).

Three clinical presentations of *T. vaginalis* exist: acute, with all the classic signs and symptoms; chronic, the most common type, with abnormal discharge, possible symptoms, and no gross tissue changes; and asymptomatic carrier state, with no symptoms, normal physical findings, and trichomonads identified in vaginal discharge (Meltzer and Marx 1985).

Failure to eradicate *T. vaginalis* has been identified in some women with resistant strains, making it necessary to increase the drug dosages used in treatment. Other possible causes of treatment failure include pharmacokinetic problems of malabsorption of drug, inactivation of drug by vaginal bacteria, interference by other drugs, noncompliance, drug intolerance, and reinfection (Sweet and Gibbs 1990)

Sequelae specific to *T. vaginalis* infection are minimal. Changes in vaginal pH may facilitate further anaerobic overgrowth and the development of BV with its possible attendant risk for PID. Vaginal symptomatology is bothersome for the client, and concern regarding STDs is common. Infections, both symptomatic and asymptomatic, should be treated to prevent further spread of the organism (Thompson and Gelbart 1989).

DATABASE

See **Table 12SF.1, Vaginal Infections,** p. 12-214.

SUBJECTIVE

→ Predisposing/risk factors include:
- multiple sexual partners.
- infected sexual partners.
- concomitant STD/BV.
- menstrual blood/cervical mucorrhea.
- maternal-fetal transmission during birth process (infant infection usually transitory).
- contaminated fomites.
- black race.

→ Symptoms may include:
- vaginal discharge: Cardinal symptom, may be profuse, foul-smelling.
- vulvar pruritus.
- vulvar tenderness, soreness, irritation, erythema.
- dysuria, frequency.
- dyspareunia.
- lower abdominal discomfort or pain.
- tender inguinal lymph nodes.
- abnormal spotting or bleeding.
- male partner with penile discharge.
- symptom exacerbation during or following menses.
- symptoms may be most acute during pregnancy.
- patient may be asymptomatic.

OBJECTIVE

→ Vital signs as indicated (usually unnecessary in uncomplicated infection).

→ Abdominal examination, including lymph nodes, as indicated.

→ Pelvic examination:
- vulva: Abnormal discharge; erythema of vestibule, labia minora; edema, usually of labia minora; abrasions, excoriations of interlabial sulci, perineum; intertrigo of labia majora, crural folds, inner thighs; chronic irritation may

produce lichenification and pigment changes of the skin.
- urethra, Bartholin's, or Skene's glands: Abnormal discharge may be milked from meatus or duct openings.
- vagina: yellow-gray-green, creamy, purulent, thin, watery, or frothy discharge; foul odor; erythema; granular-appearing or feeling surface; swollen papillae; ecchymosis, petechiae; pseudomembrane formation—small, thin, gray areas that are spottily distributed or an uninterrupted membrane that cannot be wiped off.
- cervix: Punctate hemorrhages ("strawberry cervix," < two percent to three percent); abnormal discharge.
- uterus/adnexa, rectovaginal examination: WNL unless concomitant infection/pathology.

ASSESSMENT

→ *T. vaginalis* vaginitis

→ R/O concomitant BV, *Candida* vaginitis

→ R/O concomitant STD/PID

→ R/O urinary tract infection

→ R/O vaginitis emphysematosa

→ R/O vaginal streptococcal infection

PLAN

DIAGNOSTIC TESTS

→ Wet-mount microscopy ($10\times$ and $40\times$ power) is principal diagnostic method; most cost-effective.
- Saline:
  NOTE: Slide should be kept warm and viewed promptly after collection.
  - motile trichomonads (elongated, slightly larger than WBC); flagella noted; may congregate in a mass and appear quiescent.
  - increased WBCs (usually >10/HPF).
  - predominance of mature squamous epithelial cells.
  - reduced lactobacilli.
  - clue cells may be present with concomitant BV.
- Potassium hydroxide (KOH) (10 percent to 20 percent):
  - amine or "fishy" odor (related to anaerobes present).
  - hyphae of *Candida* may be present.

→ pH: ≥ 6.0. ColorpHast® recommended; collect specimen from lateral vaginal wall or lateral fornix.

→ Pap smear may reveal trichomonads or inflammatory atypia. Confirmatory wet mount should be performed prior to treatment.

→ Cultures–the most sensitive and specific diagnostic method—may be performed in selected cases where *T. vaginalis* is suspected but the saline wet mount is negative.
- Media used: Feinberg-Whittington, Stenson's, Diamond's, Kupferberg's, or Hollander's.
- Disadvantages: Expense, limited availability, up to 7-day waiting period for diagnosis.

→ Immunofluorescence tests and enzyme-linked immunosorbent assays are utilized in research protocols, but are expensive and not practical or available in everyday clinical practice.

→ Microscopic urinalysis may show evidence of *T. vaginalis*.

→ Endocervical cultures for *N. gonorrhoeae* and *C. trachomatis* should be performed. In the absence of a cervix, urethral cultures may substitute.

→ Additional laboratory tests should be individualized and may include but are not limited to: RPR or VDRL, CBC, urinalysis, urine culture and sensitivities, Hepatitis B testing, serological HIV testing.

TREATMENT/MANAGEMENT

→ Both symptomatic and asymptomatic women should be treated to prevent sexual transmission. Therapy is also advised for the male partner.

→ Recommended regimen (CDC 1993):
- metronidazole (Flagyl®) 2 grams p.o. single dose.
  NOTE: Some clinicians prescribe 1-gram doses BID to lessen potential gastrointestinal side effects.

→ Alternate regimen (CDC 1993):
- metronidazole (Flagyl®) 500 mg p.o. BID for 7 days.
  NOTE: Metronidazole should not be used in the first trimester of pregnancy. After the first trimester, a 2-gram dose may be used (CDC 1993). Prophylactic vaginal antifungal agents may be administered with longer course therapy as indicated. See **Candida Vaginitis** Protocol.

→ Treatment failures:
- if failure occurs with either of the above regimens, retreat with metronidazole 500 mg p.o. BID for 7 days. In cases of repeated failure treat with metronidazole single 2 gram p.o. dose daily for 3 to 5 days (CDC 1993).

- consider adding simultaneous metronidazole vaginal cream (Policar 1993).
- patients with culture-proven infection who fail to respond to the above therapies and in whom reinfection has been ruled out should be managed in consultation with an STD expert. Included in the evaluation of these patients should be a determination of the susceptibility of *T. vaginalis* to metronidazole (CDC 1993).

→ Additional treatment approaches to resistant strains:
- susceptibility testing is utilized to determine drug therapy. Cultures may need to be sent to a special laboratory. Resistance can be stratified as follows (Lossick 1990):
  - low-level resistance: Aerobic minimum lethal concentration (MLC) <100 mg/l. Treat with metronidazole 2 grams/day for 3 to 5 days.
  - intermediate resistance: Aerobic MLC 100 mg/l to 200 mg/l. Treat with metronidazole 2.0 grams to 2.5 grams/day for 7 to 10 days.
  - high-level resistance: Aerobic MLC >200 mg/l. Treat with metronidazole ≥3 grams/day for 14 to 21 days.

NOTE: Significant nausea may develop when doses exceed 2 grams/day. Thus, patient motivation must be strong to continue treatment. An antiemetic may be necessary—refer to *PDR*. Patients should be informed that larger doses are experimental and that long-term oncogenic effects are not known, although the risk is considered to be small. In addition, adverse effects such as seizures and peripheral neuropathy have been reported in patients treated with metronidazole. Consult with physician prior to larger-dose therapy. Intravenous therapy is reserved for patients who are unable to tolerate larger p.o. doses; details on this treatment are beyond the scope of this protocol.

→ Other therapeutic alternatives:
- topical therapy should be reserved for cases in which systemic therapy is contraindicated. Options include:
  - metronidazole gel (MetroGel-Vaginal®) has been approved for the treatment of BV but has not been studied for use in trichomoniasis (CDC 1993).
  - metronidazole vaginal tablets (Flagyl®) 1 gram BID-TID for 7 days (limited availability) (Kaufman, Friedrich, and Gardner 1989).

- imidazole antifungal agents: See ***Candida* Vaginitis** Protocol (Kaufman, Friedrich, and Gardner 1989; Rein and Muller 1990).
- 20 percent saline douche (Kaufman and Faro 1994).
- vaginal acidification with commercially available douching agents (e.g., vinegar): may relieve discomfort but does not generally eradicate infection.

→ Partner therapy.
  - Sex partners of infected women should be treated with metronidazole.

CONSULTATION

→ As needed for prescription(s).

→ For resistant infection when considering larger-dose therapy. Consider consultation with an STD expert for culture-documented treatment failures.

PATIENT EDUCATION

→ Discuss etiology and transmission of infection, lifestyle behaviors that put client at risk, and methods to reduce risk and spread of infection.
  - In rare cases, nonsexual transmission may need to be addressed.
  - In addition, asymptomatic carriage may occur for long periods of time; thus, the current partner should not necessarily be implicated. Treatment of both sexual partners is, however, advisable.

→ Provide guidelines on safer sex practices (see **Table 13A.2,** p. 13-9). Encourage condom use with new, multiple, and nonmonogamous partners. Nonoxynol-9 intravaginally has been suggested to be efficacious for trichomoniasis; may try nightly for one week (Eschenbach and Mead 1992b).

→ Discuss vaginal health and hygiene as indicated. See ***Candida* Vaginitis** Protocol.

→ Stress importance of completing full course of prescribed medication.

→ Advise regarding desirability of sexual abstinence or at least use of condoms during course of treatment for infection.

→ Review the common side effects of metronidazole: Metallic taste, nausea, occasional vomiting, diarrhea, and headache.
  - Advise against ingestion of alcohol during and for 24 hours after medication usage as a disulfiram (Antabuse®)-like reaction may occur.
  - Rarely, hematological effects of a transient leukopenia may occur.

→ Advise of possibility of *Candida* vaginitis secondary to oral antibiotic and discuss indications for prophylactic therapy.

→ Allow patient to ventilate her feelings of surprise, shame, fear, or anger when discussing this infection as an STD.

FOLLOW-UP

→ Advise the patient to return for further evaluation if the signs and symptoms of infection have not cleared after the week of treatment, and for recurrent infection.
  - Assess compliance with medication regimen.
  - Therapeutic failures may result if the patient is taking phenobarbital or phenytoin, as these medications may interfere with the pharmacokinetics of metronidazole.

→ Follow up on cervical cultures and treat identified concomitant STDs—see appropriate protocols. Discuss importance of partner evaluation and treatment if STD is identified.

→ HIV-positive persons should be referred to the appropriate provider or agency for early intervention services.

→ Hepatitis B antigen-positive individuals should have liver function tests and receive counseling regarding the implications of their positive status and the need for immunoprophylaxis of sex partners and household members. See **Hepatitis— Viral** Protocol.

→ Address additional medical concerns as indicated.

→ Continue to encourage safer sex practices.

→ Document in progress notes and problem list.

12-SE   VAGINITIS

Bacterial Vaginosis

Bacterial vaginosis (BV) has been defined as "a replacement of the lactobacilli of the vagina by characteristic groups of bacteria accompanied by changed properties of the vaginal fluid" (Westrom 1984, 259). The syndrome is attributed to a synergism between naturally occurring polymicrobes—facultative and anaerobic organisms—the majority of which are *Gardnerella vaginalis, Mobiluncus, Bacteroides, Peptococcus,* and *Peptostreptococcus* sp., some species of viridans streptococci, *Eubacterium, Fusobacterium, Prevotella* sp., and *Mycoplasma hominis.* These bacteria are present at one hundred- to one thousand-fold greater concentrations among women with BV than in normal women, but no one organism is to blame for the problem.

Host characteristics have yet to be determined and factors that initiate the cycle of anaerobic overgrowth are still being investigated. It is postulated that a relative absence of normally occurring, peroxide-producing lactobacilli alters the ecosystem of the vagina, thus allowing anaerobes to predominate and producing metabolic by-products that raise the pH. Amines, the end products of anaerobic metabolism, produce a malodorous discharge that is the hallmark of BV, most noticeable upon alkalinization (after intercourse or with the addition of potassium hydroxide [KOH]). The predominant amines are putrescine, cadaverine, and trimethylamine. Concomitant infection with yeast is estimated at 10 percent and coinfection with *Trichomonas vaginalis* at five percent, but this requires further study (Kaufman and Faro 1994; Kaufman, Friedrich, and Gardner 1989; Hillier and Holmes 1990; Mead 1989; Thomason, Gelbart, and Broekhuizen 1989).

Incidence and prevalence rates for BV are largely lacking, but estimates are in the range of five percent to 60 percent depending on the population studied, with higher prevalence among women attending sexually transmitted disease (STD) clinics. Of the three main categories of vaginitis—yeast, *T. vaginalis,* and BV—BV is the most common form in a general practice, accounting for 40 percent to 50 percent of cases. Many women with this condition are asymptomatic, a state attributed to lower concentrations of vaginal anaerobes than are found in symptomatic women. If left untreated, a large proportion of asymptomatic women may spontaneously resolve an abnormal discharge within six months (Kaufman and Faro 1994; Kaufman, Friedrich, and Gardner 1989; Mead 1989; Spiegel 1991; Thompson, Gelbart, and Scaglione 1989).

BV as an STD has received much attention. Originally, it was thought that BV was exclusively sexually transmitted; however, studies of virginal women have shown its existence in this population (Bump and Buesching 1988). BV-associated organisms have also been isolated from the rectum, suggesting that the female intestinal tract may act as a reservoir for vaginal contamination. The sexual transmission of BV is commuted in a more complex way than other common STDs caused by a single organism. In studies of male partners of infected women, some but not all males are colonized with *Gardnerella, Mycoplasma,* and/or anaerobes. An exchange of these microorganisms may occur during intercourse.

It should be recognized, however, that many authorities no longer consider BV an STD, and that a clinical counterpart in the male has not been recognized. Friedrich (1983) notes that coitus with ejaculation creates an alkaline-dominant vaginal pH for two to three hours, with gradual lowering over an eight-hour period. The higher vaginal pH is detrimental to normal lactobacilli whose role is to keep pathogenic bacteria in check. Most women can adapt to this changing milieu, but, in the predisposed, the alteration in the delicately balanced ecosystem may facilitate overgrowth of the vaginal anaerobes.

Treatment of the male partner has not been shown to affect the recurrence rate for BV infection in the female (CDC 1993). Since the BV organisms are surface inhabitants, male urethral colonization may be short-lived and spontaneously cleared. "Condom therapy" allows for clearance of alkaline semen from the vagina and may enable the woman to restore her normal lactobacilli-dominant environment. Males with underlying genitourinary pathology such as prostatitis or epididymitis may harbor larger quantities of bacteria, which could more easily reinfect their partners; thus in this group of men, therapy may be considered.

Up to 30 percent of women have recurrences of BV. Possible causes include resistant, less susceptible, or persistent organisms; relapse; the failure to reestablish a lactobacillus-dominant flora after therapy; reinfection by the male who harbors the bacterial-vaginosis associated microorganisms; and the persistence of an as yet unidentified host factor rendering a woman more susceptible to infection. Recurrent BV has also been associated with both asymptomatic colonization and symptomatic *Candida* superinfection (CDC 1991; Friedrich 1983; Hillier and Holmes 1990; Kaufman, Friedrich, and Gardner 1989; Mead 1986, 1989; Redondo-Lopez et al. 1990; Thompson, Gelbart, and Scaglione 1991).

Bacterial vaginosis may cause serious infection in some cases. Sequelae may include postcesarean section and postpartum endometritis/wound infection, posthysterectomy cuff cellulitis, and chorioamnionitis. BV has also been implicated in premature labor and delivery, premature rupture of membranes (PROM), PID, subclinical endometritis, urinary tract infection, nonpuerperal breast abscesses, umbilical and mastectomy wounds, abnormal Pap smears, and menorrhagia.

It has been suggested that presurgical candidates, women with a history of preterm labor or PROM, and women at risk for PID be treated when asymptomatic BV exists. However, treatment of asymptomatic women remains controversial (Blanco and Gonik 1991; CDC 1993; Mead 1989; Thompson, Gelbart, and Broekhuizen 1989).

DATABASE
See **Table 12SF.1, Vaginal Infections,** p. 12-214.

SUBJECTIVE

→ Predisposing factors may include:
  - low oxidation reduction potential of vagina.
  - elevated vaginal pH.
  - reduction in H_2O_2-producing lactobacilli.
  - multiple partners, especially in month prior to diagnosis.
  - uncircumcised partners.
  - frequent intercourse.
  - excessive douching.
  - antibiotic therapy.
  - menses.
  - foreign body or retained tampon.
  - rectal reservoir of anaerobic bacteria.
  - poor hygiene.
  - low socioeconomic status.
  - immunological status.
  - hormonal factors.
  - IUD.
  - concomitant vaginal infection/STD.
  - stress.

→ Symptoms may include:
  - none in 40 percent to 50 percent of cases.
  - malodorous discharge (most common symptom, described as "fishy," most evident after sexual intercourse).
  - increased milky discharge.
  - burning, pruritus, external dysuria in some cases.
  - intermenstrual spotting (rare), pelvic pain, infertility (in subclinical endometritis).
  - partner usually asymptomatic.

→ History should include:
  - gynecological history.
  - sexual history, including sexual orientation, sexual practices, number of partners, recent change in partner, partner signs and symptoms; contraceptive history.
  - medical history.
  - allergies to foods, medications, products, or environmental factors; medications.
  - drug and alcohol habits; exercise; nutrition; stress.
  - review of systems; family history of diabetes and allergies.
  - onset, timing of symptoms, relation to menstrual cycle and sexual activity.
  - characteristics of discharge: Color, quantity, quality, odor.
  - location of pruritus if present: Mons, vulva, vaginal perineum, perianal, generalized.
  - associated symptoms.
  - aggravating or relieving factors.
  - other: Use of self-treatment measures and home remedies; over-the-counter medication;

spermicides; feminine hygiene deodorant products, douches, bath additives, etc.; type of soap, detergent, toilet paper; use of pads or tampons; sexual paraphernalia; type of undergarments and clothing.

OBJECTIVE

→ Vital signs as indicated (usually unnecessary in uncomplicated infection).

→ Abdominal examination, including lymph nodes, as indicated.

→ Pelvic examination:
  ▪ external genitalia: Thin, homogeneous, gray-white discharge pooling at introitus (yellow-green tints may also be seen); erythema may be present.
  ▪ Bartholin's, urethral, Skene's (BUS) glands: Assess or palpate for abnormal discharge, masses.
  ▪ vagina: Thin, homogeneous gray-white discharge adherent to walls; bubbles present in 10 percent to 15 percent of cases; erythema absent unless concomitant infection present.
  ▪ cervix: Thin discharge covering ectocervix; os clear; erythema rare; cervical motion tenderness absent in uncomplicated cases.
  ▪ uterus, adnexa, rectovaginal examination WNL unless coexistent pathology.
  NOTE: Since BV is not a tissue pathogen, signs of acute inflammation are usually absent.

→ Additional examination components, depending on case presentation, may include skin, oral cavity, lymph nodes, pubic hair.

ASSESSMENT

→ Bacterial vaginosis
→ R/O physiological leukorrhea
→ R/O other/concomitant vaginal infection
→ R/O STD/PID
→ R/O urinary tract infection

PLAN

DIAGNOSTIC TESTS

NOTE: Symptoms alone are unreliable for a diagnosis. Four criteria to assess BV have been established: abnormal discharge, amine odor, increased pH, and clue cells. Three of the four must be present to make the diagnosis.

→ Discharge: Usually thin, homogeneous gray-white (weakest sign due to subjectivity of examiner).
→ Wet-mount microscopy (view under 10× and 40× power).
  ▪ KOH (10 percent to 20 percent):
    • amine or "fishy" odor (sniff the slide when odor not apparent).
    • assess for presence of hyphae (indicative of concomitant yeast vaginitis).
  ▪ Saline:
    • clue cells—epithelial cell stippled with bacteria, 10 percent to 15 percent of sample. Must be distinguished from "false clue cell," an epithelial cell covered with small numbers of normal lactobacilli. Clue cells are highly suggestive for BV, but by themselves not pathognomonic (Kaufman and Faro 1994).
    • decreased/absent lactobacilli.
    • intercellular fluid with many microorganisms exhibiting corkscrewlike or twitching motility.
    • usually no or few WBCs, but this varies (if a large number of WBCs are found—think concomitant vaginal infection/STD).
    • assess for presence of motile trichomonads (indicative of concomitant *T. vaginalis* vaginitis).
→ pH: >4.5, usually >5.0-6.0 range. ColorpHast® strips are most reliable brand of pH paper. Swab from posterior and lateral fornices of vagina and place sample directly on pH paper *or* place pH paper on discharge from speculum after removal.
  NOTE: Elevated pH may also result from lubricant, tap water, cervical mucus, semen, amniotic fluid, trichomonas, or recent douche.
→ Gram stain may identify the presence of *G. vaginalis* and other bacterial morphotypes.
→ Culture *not* advised to establish diagnosis or as a test-of-cure as *G. vaginalis* may be isolated from 40 percent to 50 percent of normal women. Selective cultures may be utilized to assist in diagnosing other vaginal infections. See specific protocols.
→ Pap smears unreliable.
→ Biochemical tests (e.g., gas-liquid chromatographic analysis, proline aminopeptidase activity) and deoxyribonucleic acid (DNA) probes are other diagnostic tests which have been used to identify BV, mostly in research protocols. They are not generally available in clinical laboratories.
→ Endocervical cultures for *Neisseria gonorrhoeae* and *Chlamydia trachomatis* should be performed

in women at risk for STD. In the absence of a cervix, urethral cultures may be substituted.

→ Additional laboratory tests should be individualized and may include but are not limited to RPR or VDRL, CBC, urinalysis, urine culture and sensitivities, Hepatitis B testing, serological HIV testing, pregnancy test.

TREATMENT/MANAGEMENT

→ Treatment is generally advised only for symptomatic women with a confirmed diagnosis (CDC 1993). It is reasonable to consider treatment of asymptomatic woman prior to surgical abortion (CDC 1993) or prior to upcoming gynecological surgery or invasive procedures (Thompson, Gelbart, and Scaglione 1991).

→ Recommended regimen (CDC 1993):
- metronidazole (Flagyl®) 500 mg p.o. BID for 7 days (95 percent cure rate).

→ Alternative regimens (CDC 1993):
- metronidazole (Flagyl®) 2 grams p.o. in a single dose (84 percent cure rate) (some clinicians prescribe 1 gram BID to lessen potential GI side effects).
- metronidazole vaginal gel 0.75 percent (MetroGel-Vaginal®) 1 vaginal application BID for 5 days.
- clindamycin 2 percent cream (Cleocin® Vaginal Cream) 1 vaginal application at bedtime for 7 days. Contains mineral oil; avoid condoms or diaphragm for at least 72 hours after last use.
- clindamycin (Cleocin®) 300 mg p.o. BID for 7 days.

NOTE: Both oral and dermal clindamycin have been associated with pseudomembranous colitis, which is characterized by severe, persistent diarrhea; severe abdominal cramps; and passage of blood or mucus. Symptoms may begin up to several weeks following therapy. The drug should be discontinued if significant diarrhea develops (*PDR* 1993; Zambrano 1991).

→ Other alternative and adjunctive therapies:
- metronidazole intravaginal sponges: 1000 mg once/day for 24 hours for 3 days (Edelman and North 1989). Still under investigation.
- amoxicillin plus clavulanic acid (Augmentin®) 500 mg p.o. TID for 7 days (Symonds and Biswas 1986).
- ampicillin/amoxicillin 500 mg p.o. QID for 7 days (Malouf 1981; Secour 1988).

- lactic acid-containing gel: Intravaginally once or twice per day for 7 days; has also been used as monthly treatment after menses for 6 months (Andersch et al. 1986; Andersch et al. 1990).
- vinegar douche: 1 tbsp/quart H_2O, douche once/day for 5 to 7 days (Mead 1986).
- hydrogen peroxide douche: 3 percent diluted half strength with H_2O, douche with 1 pint once/day for 7 days; should not be used concomitantly with metronidazole since the drug is most effective under anaerobic conditions; may be used as an adjunctive measure after antibiotic (Kaufman and Faro 1994).

NOTE: The above 3 therapies are probably ineffective in curing BV but have been tried as attempts to restore lactobacilli or acidify the vagina. Douching is not recommended during pregnancy, during menses, or if patient is at increased risk for PID.

→ Recurrent infection:
- switch drug of choice or use local therapy if oral therapy has failed (Eschenbach and Mead 1992b; Mead 1989).
- one-time oral or local regimen at time of intercourse if recurrences are coitus-related or if symptomatic with menses: 500 mg metronidazole BID for several days. Untested prophylactic therapy (Eschenbach and Mead 1992b; Mead 1989).
- periodic acidification of the vagina with vinegar douches is generally ineffective to treat or prevent recurrences (Eschenbach and Mead 1992b).

→ Male partner therapy:
- "condom therapy" is advisable for 4 to 6 weeks in all cases of acute BV. May need to use condoms indefinitely in recurrent cases.
- treatment of the male partner does not seem to influence the response to therapy or the relapse/recurrence rate in the female (CDC 1993).
  - Despite this fact, clinicians have offered partner therapy.
  - See recommended and alternative oral therapies above.
- if the male has acute symptoms of an STD, a history of prostatitis, or epididymitis, refer for evaluation and therapy.

→ Treatment during pregnancy:
- treatment of the asymptomatic woman during pregnancy is not routinely recommended but should be individualized according to case

presentation and risk factors. Consult with physician as indicated.

- metronidazole is contraindicated in the first trimester; clindamycin vaginal cream is the preferred treatment during this time (CDC 1993).
  - In the second and third trimesters, oral metronidazole may be used, although metronidazole gel or clindamycin cream may be preferable (CDC 1993).

→ Additional considerations:
- in the presence of a positive urine culture for *G. vaginalis* in a symptomatic individual—with or without clinical evidence of BV—treat with one of the recommended or alternative oral treatment regimes listed above (Josephson et al. 1988).

CONSULTATION

→ For refractory cases.

→ For treatment during pregnancy as indicated.

→ If the male has acute symptoms of an STD, a history of prostatitis, or epididymitis, refer for evaluation and therapy.

→ In cases of pseudomembranous colitis secondary to clindamycin.

→ As needed for prescription(s).

PATIENT EDUCATION

→ Explain that many factors are related to changes in vaginal flora predisposing to BV: menstruation, hygienic habits, rectal carriage of associated microorganisms, contraceptive methods, immunological status, medications, and hormonal factors.

→ Explain that evidence of sexual transmission remains unclear. Explain how intercourse may introduce BV-associated organisms into the vagina, and that alkaline semen may promote vaginal microbial overgrowth as well. Recommend use of condoms to prevent BV.

→ When BV is diagnosed in asymptomatic patients, discuss the finding. Upon further questioning, a woman may recognize the symptom-complex and opt for treatment.

→ Stress the importance of completing the full course of medication unless severe side effects occur.

→ Review the common side effects of metronidazole: Metallic taste, nausea, occasionally dark urine, vomiting, diarrhea, and headache.
- Advise against ingestion of alcohol during and for 24 hours after medication as a disulfiram (Antabuse®)-like reaction may occur.
- Rarely, hematological effects of a transient leukopenia may occur.

→ Discuss vaginal health and hygiene measures. See *Candida* Vaginitis Protocol. Emphasize proper wiping techniques, as rectal organisms gaining entry to the vagina may precipitate BV. It should be understood that a foul odor in the vulvovaginal area is not normal unless infection is present. Reassure that some vaginal discharge is normal and discuss characteristic cyclical changes.

→ Advise of possibility of *Candida* vaginitis secondary to oral antibiotic and discuss indications for prophylactic therapy (history of antibiotic-induced candidiasis).

→ Provide guidelines on safer sex practices. (See Table 13A.2, Safer Sex Guidelines, p. 13-9, and Table 12I.1, Recommendations for Individuals to Prevent STD/PID, p. 12-96.) Encourage condom use with new, multiple, nonmonogamous partners. "Condom therapy" is probably the best prevention for BV.

→ Routine health maintenance issues should be addressed as indicated.

FOLLOW-UP

→ Advise the patient to return for further evaluation if signs and symptoms of infection have not cleared after the week of treatment, or if infection recurs. Assess compliance with medication regimen.

→ Follow up on all identified concomitant STDs. Refer to specific protocols for treatment and follow-up. Discuss importance of partner evaluation and treatment if STD is identified. Continue to encourage safer sex practices.

→ HIV-positive persons should be referred to the appropriate provider or agency for early intervention services.

→ Hepatitis B antigen-positive individuals should have liver function tests and receive counseling regarding the implications of their positive status and the need for immunoprophylaxis of sex partners and household members. See Hepatitis— Viral Protocol.

→ Therapeutic failures may result if the patient is taking phenobarbital or phenytoin, as these medications may interfere with the pharmaco-kinetics of metronidazole. Advise a return visit to evaluate if symptomatic after treatment.

→ Document in progress notes and problem list.

Table 12SF.1. VAGINAL INFECTIONS

Findings	Candidiasis	Trichomoniasis	Bacterial Vaginosis	Atrophic Vaginitis	Cytolytic Vaginitis
Causative organism	*Candida albicans* *Candida glabrata* *Candida tropicalis*	*Trichomonas vaginalis*	Polymicrobial	Nonspecific atropic changes caused by ↓ estrogen	↑ Exfoliation/turnover of squamous epithelium
Characteristics of discharge	Mild → profuse Thin → thick White, curd-like discharge; adherent to vagina/cervix	Yellow → gray → green odorous discharge; consistency varies; ± bubbles	White → gray/-yellow-green Thin, homogenous, odorous discharge; adherent to walls and at introitus; ± bubbles	Yellow or blood-tinged Thin, scant, watery discharge; variable discharge	Thick white discharge
Vulvovaginal findings	May see erythema, excoriation, edema	May see erythema and edema ± "strawberry patches"	White → gray/yellow-green Thin, homogenous discharge poling at introitus; ± erythema	Atrophic changes, erythema, petechial hemorrhage	Within normal limits; may see ↑ thick, white discharge
Diagnostic tests	pH: 4.0 to 4.7; KOH wet mount: hyphae, spores; Saline wet mount: ↑ WBCs; Gram stain: budding *Candida* Culture: Nickerson's, Sabouraud's, Mycosel or blood agar media	pH: ≥6.0; Saline wet mount: motile trich, ↑ WBCs, ↓ lactobacilli; KOH wet mount: amine odor; Pap smear; Culture: Diamond's, Hollander's, Feinberg-Whittington, or Stenton's media	pH: 5.0 to 6.0; Saline wet mount: clue cells, ↓ lactobacilli ± WBCs; KOH wet mount: amine odor; Gram stain: *G. vaginalis*, *Mobiluncus*, other bacterial morphotypes	pH: 5.5 to 7.0; Saline wet mount: ↑ parabasal cells, ↑ WBCs, ↓ lactobacilli; Gram stain: parabasal cells, + bacteria	pH: 4.0 to 4.5; Saline wet mount: ↑ epithelial cells, ↑ lactobacilli, "false clue cells," ± WBCs; Gram stain: lactobacilli, gram + rods
Treatment regimens	Antifungal therapy, boric acid, gentian violet, potassium sorbate	Metronidazole, clotrimazole	Metronidazole, clindamycin	Estrogen therapy	Baking-soda douches; avoid overtreating normal leukorrhea

Copyright © 1995 by W. Star.

12-SG VAGINITIS
Bibliography

Andersch, B., Forssman, L., Lincoln, K., and Torstensson, P. 1986. Treatment of bacterial vaginosis with an acid cream: A comparison between the effect of lactate-gel and metronidazole. *Gynecology and Obstetrics Investigation* 21:19–25.

Andersch, B., Lindell, D., Dahlen, I., and Brandberg, A. 1990. Bacterial vaginosis and the effect of intermittent prophylactic treatment with acid lactate gel. *Gynecology and Obstetrics Investigation* 30:114–119.

Bistoletti, P., Fredricsson, B., Hagstrom, B., and Nord, C. 1986. Comparison of oral and vaginal metronidazole therapy for nonspecific bacterial vaginosis. *Gynecology and Obstetrics Investigation* 21:144–149.

Bump, R.C., and Buesching, W.J. 1988. Bacterial vaginosis in virginal and sexually active adolescent females: Evidence against exclusive sexual transmission. *American Journal of Obstetrics and Gynecology* 158(4):935–939.

Burnhill, M.S. 1986. Taking a serious approach to vulvovaginitis. *Contemporary Ob/Gyn* 28(3):69–79.

———. 1986b. The immunocompromised patient. *The Female Patient* 1(sp. ed.):29–32.

———. 1987. Sorting out the major vaginal infections. *Contemporary Ob/Gyn* 29(4):47–62.

———. 1990. Clinician's guide to counseling patients with chronic vaginitis. *Contemporary Ob/Gyn* 35(1):37–44.

Cauwenbergh, G. 1990. Vaginal candidiasis: Evolving trends in the incidence and treatment of non-*Candida albicans* infections. In *New directions in diagnosis and therapy of vulvovaginal candidiasis*, eds. B.J. Horowitz, M. Weisberg, G. Cauwenbergh, J.L. Thomason, J.A. James, N. Scaglione, J. Utrie, F.F. Broekhuizen, and E. Weismeier. *Current Problems in Obstetrics, Gynecology, and Fertility* 13(6):241–245.

Centers for Disease Control. 1989. 1989 Sexually transmitted disease treatment guidelines. *Morbidity and Mortality Weekly Report* 38(S–8):1–43.

———. 1993. 1993 Sexually transmitted disease treatment guidelines. *Morbidity and Mortality Weekly Report* 42(No. RR-14):1–102.

Dennerstein, M.B. 1986. Depo-Provera in the treatment of recurrent vulvovaginal candidiasis. *The Journal of Reproductive Medicine* 31:801

Edelman, D.A., and North, B.B. 1989. Treatment of vaginosis with intravaginal sponges containing metronidazole. *The Journal of Reproductive Medicine* 34(5):341–344.

Eschenbach, D.A. 1989. Bacterial vaginosis: Emphasis on upper genital tract complications. *Obstetrics and Gynecology Clinics of North America* 16(3):593–610.

———. 1991. Treatment of vaginitis. In *Vaginitis and vaginosis*, eds. B.J. Horowitz and P.-A. Mardh. New York: Wiley-Liss.

Eschenbach, D.A., and Hillier, S.L. 1989. Advances in diagnostic testing for vaginitis and cervicitis. *The Journal of Reproductive Medicine* 34(8):555–565.

Eschenbach, D.A., Hillier, S., Critchlow, C., Stevens, C., DeRouen, T., and Holmes, K.K. 1988. Diagnosis and clinical manifestations of bacterial vaginosis. *American Journal of Obstetrics and Gynecology* 158(4):819–827.

Eschenbach, D.A., and Mead, P.B. 1992a. Vaginitis: Varying management appropriately. *Contemporary Ob/Gyn* 37(1):25–32.

———. 1992b. Vaginitis update. *Contemporary Ob/Gyn* 37(12):54–70.

Friedrich, E.G., Jr. 1983. *Vulvar Disease*, 2d ed. Philadelphia: W.B. Saunders.

———. 1988. Current perspectives in candidal vulvovaginitis. *American Journal of Obstetrics and Gynecology* 158(4):985–986.

Gardner, H.L., and Dukes, C.D. 1955. *Haemophilus vaginalis* vaginitis: A newly defined specific infection previously classified 'nonspecific' vaginitis. *American Journal of Obstetrics and Gynecology* 69:962–976.

Greaves, W.L., Chungafung, J., Morris, B., Haile, A., and Townsend, J.L. 1988. Clindamycin versus metronidazole in the treatment of bacterial vaginosis. *Obstetrics and Gynecology* 72(5):799–802.

Grist, L. 1988. *A woman's guide to alternative medicine.* Chicago: Contemporary Books.

Hammill, H.A. 1989a. *Trichomonas vaginalis. Obstetrics and Gynecology Clinics of North America* 16(3):531–541.

———. 1989b. Unusual causes of vaginitis. *Obstetrics and Gynecology Clinics of North America* 16(2):337–345.

Hillier, S., and Holmes, K.K. 1990. Bacterial vaginosis. In *Sexually transmitted diseases*, 2d ed., eds. K.K. Holmes, P.-A. Mardh, P.F. Sparling, P.J. Wiesner, W. Cates, Jr., S.M. Lemon, and W.E. Stamm, pp. 547–559. New York: McGraw-Hill.

Hillier, S., Krohn, M.A., and Eschenbach, D.A. 1990. Microbiological efficacy of intravaginal clindamycin cream for the treatment of bacterial vaginosis. *Obstetrics and Gynecology* 76:407–413.

Horowitz, B. 1986a. Role of diet in candidiasis. *The Female Patient* 1(sp. ed.):23–28.

———. 1986b. Topical flucytosine therapy for chronic recurrent *Candida tropicalis* infections. *Journal of Reproductive Medicine* 31:821.

Horowitz, B.J., and Mardh, P.-A. 1991. *Vaginitis and vaginosis.* New York: Wiley-Liss.

Jeffcoate, T.N.A. 1966. Chronic vulvar dystrophies. *American Journal of Obstetrics and Gynecology* 95:61–71.

Josephson, S., Thomason, J., Sturino, K., Zabransky, R., and Williams, J. 1988. *Gardnerella vaginalis* in the urinary tract: Incidence and significance in a hospital population. *Obstetrics and Gynecology* 71(2):245–250.

Jovanovic, R., Congema, E., and Nguyen, H.T. 1991. Antifungal agents vs. boric acid for treating chronic mycotic vulvovaginitis. *The Journal of Reproductive Medicine* 36(8):593–597.

Kaufman, R.H. 1988. Establishing a correct diagnosis of vulvovaginal infection. *American Journal of Obstetrics and Gynecology* 158(4):986–988.

Kaufman, R.H., Friedrich, E.G., and Gardner, H.L. 1989. *Benign diseases of the vulva and vagina*, 3d ed. Chicago: Year Book Medical.

Kaufman, R.H., and Faro, S. 1994. *Benign diseases of the vulva and vagina*, 4th ed. St. Louis: Mosby Year Book.

Langdon, S. November 1994. *Vaginitis.* Outline presented at the STD intensive for clinicians. San Francisco STD/HIV Prevention Training Center, San Francisco.

Lossick, J.G. 1990. Treatment of sexually transmitted vaginosis/vaginitis. *Reviews of Infectious Diseases* 12(suppl. 6):S665-S681.

Lugo-Miro, V.I., Green, M., and Mazur, L. 1992. Comparison of different metronidazole therapeutic regimens for bacterial vaginosis. *Journal of the American Medical Association* 268(1):92–95.

Malouf, M., Fortier, M., Morin, G., and Dube, L. 1981. Treatment of *Hemophilus vaginalis* vaginitis. *Obstetrics and Gynecology* 57(6):711–714.

Marquez-Davila, G., and Martinez-Barreda, C.E. 1985. Predictive value of the 'clue cells' investigation and the amine volatilization test in vaginal infections caused by *Gardnerella vaginalis. Journal of Clinical Microbiology* 22(4):686–687.

Mead, P.B. (moderator). 1986. Establishing bacterial vaginosis. *Contemporary Ob/Gyn* Feb.:186–203.

———. 1989. Reconsidering bacterial vaginosis. *Contemporary Ob/Gyn* 34(6):76–89.

Medical Economics Data. 1993. *Physician's Desk Reference.* Montville, N.J.: the Author.

Meltzer, R.M., and Marx, P. 1985. Adult vulvovaginitis. *Current Problems in Obstetrics, Gynecology, and Fertility* 8(10):4–60.

Pheiffer, T.A., Forsyth, P.S., Durfee, M.A., Pollock, H.M., and Holmes, K.K. 1978. Nonspecific vaginitis. *The New England Journal of Medicine* 298(26):1429–1434.

Platz-Christensen, J., Larsson, P., Sundstrom, E., and Bondeson, L. 1989. Detection of bacterial vaginosis in Papanicolaou smears. *American Journal of Obstetrics and Gynecology* 160:132–133.

Policar, M. 1993. Preview of the 1993 CDC STD treatment guidelines. In *Lecture Notes: Fall Ob/Gyn Update.* Campbell, CA: Education Programs Associates.

Purdon, A., Hanna, J.H., Morse, P.L., Paine, D.D., and Engelkirk, P.G. 1984. An evaluation of single-dose metronidazole for *Gardnerella vaginalis* vaginitis. *Obstetrics and Gynecology* 64(2):271–274.

Rajakumar, R., Lacey, C.J.N., Evans, E.G.V., and Carney, J.A. 1987. Use of slide latex agglutination test for rapid diagnosis of vaginal candidosis. *Genitourinary Medicine* 63:192–195.

Redondo-Lopez, V., Meriwether, C., Schmitt, C., Optiz, M., Cook, R., and Sobel, J.D. 1990. Vulvovaginal candidiasis complicating recurrent bacterial vaginosis. *Sexually Transmitted Diseases* 17(1):51–53.

Rein, M.F., and Muller, M. 1990. *Trichomonas vaginalis* and trichomoniasis. In *Sexually transmitted diseases*, 2d. ed., eds. K.K. Holmes, P.-A. Mardh, P.F. Sparling, P.J. Wiesner, W. Cates, Jr., S.M. Lemon, and W.E. Stamm, pp. 481–492. New York: McGraw-Hill.

Rinaldi, M.G. 1988. The microbiology of terconazole: Results of *in vitro* studies. In *Clinical perspectives: Terconazole, an advance in vulvovaginal candidiasis therapy*, ed. J.D. Sobel. New York: BMI/McGraw Hill.

Secor, R.M. 1988. Bacterial vaginosis: A comprehensive review. *Nursing Clinics of North America* 23(4):865–875.

Sobel, J.D. 1985. Epidemiology and pathogenesis of recurrent vulvovaginal candidiasis. *American Journal of Obstetrics and Gynecology* 152:924–935.

———. 1986. Recurrent vulvovaginal candidiasis: A prospective study of the efficacy of maintenance ketoconazole therapy. *New England Journal of Medicine* 315(23):1455–1458.

———. ed. 1988. *Clinical perspectives: Terconazole, an advance in vulvovaginal candidiasis therapy*. New York: BMI/McGraw-Hill.

———. 1989. Pathophysiology of vulvovaginal candidiasis. *The Journal of Reproductive Medicine* 34(8):572–579.

———. 1990. Vaginal infections in adult women. *Medical Clinics of North America* 74(6):1573–1601.

Soll, D.R. 1988. High-frequency switching in *Candida albicans* and its relations to vaginal candidiasis. *American Journal of Obstetrics and Gynecology* 158(4):997–1001.

Sparks, J.M. 1991. Vaginitis. *The Journal of Reproductive Medicine* 36(10):745–752.

Spiegel, C.A. 1991. Bacterial vaginosis. *Clinical Microbiology Reviews* 4(4):485–502.

Star, W. 1992. *Vaginitis Lecture Outline*. University of California, San Francisco, School of Nursing, Women's Primary Care Program.

Summers, P.R., and Sharp, H.T. 1993. The management of obscure or difficult cases of vulvovaginitis. *Clinical Obstetrics and Gynecology* 36(1):206–214.

Sweet, R.L., and Gibbs, R.S. 1990. *Infectious diseases of the female genital tract*, 2d ed. Baltimore: Williams & Wilkins.

Syntex Laboratories. 1989. *Recurrent vulvovaginal candidiasis*. Palo Alto, CA: the Author.

Syverson, R.E., Buckley, H., Gibian, J., and Ryan, G.M. 1979. Cellular and humoral status in women with chronic *Candida* vaginitis. *The American Journal of Obstetrics and Gynecology* 134(6):624–627.

Thomason, J.L., Gelbart, S.M., Wilcoski, L.M., Peterson, A.K., Jilly, B.J., and Hamilton, P.R. 1988. Proline aminopeptidase activity as a rapid diagnostic test to confirm bacterial vaginosis. *Obstetrics and Gynecology* 71(4):607–611.

Thompson, J.L., and Gelbart, S.M. 1989. *Trichomonas vaginalis*. *Obstetrics and Gynecology* 74(3):536–541.

Thompson, J.L., Gelbart, S.M., and Broekhuizen, F.F. 1989. Advances in the understanding of bacterial vaginosis. *The Journal of Reproductive Medicine* 34(8):581–586.

Thompson, J.L., Gelbart, S.M., and Scaglione, N.J. 1989. Bacterial vaginosis. *Contemporary Ob/Gyn* 34(5):21–26.

———. 1991. Bacterial vaginosis: Current review with indications for asymptomatic therapy. *American Journal of Obstetrics and Gynecology* 165(4, Pt. 2):1210–1217.

Thompson, J.L., James, J.A., Scaglione, N., Utrie, J., and Broekhuizen, F.F. 1990. Prototype triazole antifungal for vulvovaginal candidiasis: U.S. studies. In *New directions in diagnosis and therapy of vulvovaginal candidiasis*, eds. B.J. Horowitz, M. Weisberg, G. Cauwenbergh, J.L. Thompson, J.A. James, N. Scaglione, J. Utrie, F.F. Broekhuizen, and E. Weismeier. *Current Problems in Obstetrics, Gynecology, and Fertility* 13(6):246–249.

Van Slyke, K.K., Michel, V.P., and Rein, M.F. 1981. Treatment of vulvovaginal candidiasis with boric acid powder. *American Journal of Obstetrics and Gynecology* 141(2):145–148.

Vontver, L.A., and Eschenbach, D.A. 1981. The role of *Gardnerella vaginalis* in nonspecific vaginitis. *Clinical Obstetrics and Gynecology* 24(2):439–460.

Watson, R.A. 1985. *Gardnerella vaginalis*: Genitourinary pathogen in men. *Urology* 25(3):217–221.

Weaver, C.H. 1988. Bacterial vaginosis. *The Journal of Family Practice* 27(2):207–215.

Zambrano, D. 1991. Clindamycin in the treatment of obstetric and gynecologic infections: A review. *Clinical Therapeutics* 13(1):50–58.

12-TA   VULVAR DISEASE
Red Lesions of the Vulva

The normal flesh color of the skin of the vulva is due in part to superficial capillary blood flow muted by the epidermal skin cell layers. When skin becomes erythematous, the capillaries are more visible; the degree of redness depends on dilatation and engorgement of the capillary bed and thickness of the overlying epidermis. Local immune inflammatory responses cause vasodilatation—with diffuse erythema usually signaling a benign process.

With carcinomatous lesions, a tumor angiogenesis factor (development of blood vessels) increases the number of surface capillaries. This "neovascularization" process occurs in all overt squamous cell carcinomas. Localized red lesions of the vulva are more suspicious for a neoplastic process. Redness may also be due to fewer cell layers between the surface skin and underlying vasculature, as is seen with Paget's disease and acute reactive vulvitis.

In summary, red lesions of the vulva result from inflammation, neovascularization of a neoplasm, or thinning of the epidermal surface (Friedrich 1983). This protocol will cover *cutaneous candidiasis, contact dermatitis (reactive vulvitis)* and *Paget's disease.* See **Dermatological Disorders, Folliculitis, Psoriasis, Fungal Infections,** protocols.

Cutaneous Candidiasis

Yeast, or *Candida,* vaginal infections may produce symptoms in vulvar tissues secondary to local reactions to allergenic/endotoxic substances from vaginal organisms (Kaufman and Faro 1994). A primary cutaneous candidiasis may, however, arise de novo, affecting the keratinized superficial epidermal layers of the vulva. *Candida albicans* is the most commonly encountered species, but infection with other candidal types may occur (e.g., *T. cruris*). Common reasons for overgrowth of the organism—normally found in the gut, mouth, and vagina—include vaginal pH changes and antibiotics, which deplete the normal lactobacilli of the GI tract, allowing resident yeast to flourish. However, any change in a woman's health status may put her at risk for infection. Vulvar *Candida* is especially prevalent in diabetics and may be the first sign of the disease. Occasionally, oral contraceptives may predispose a woman to *Candida* infections. Dietary factors—e.g., simple sugars, alcohol, and yeast-containing foods—may also play a role (Friedrich 1983; Gomel, Munro, and Rowe 1990).

DATABASE

SUBJECTIVE

→ *Candida* vaginitis may co-exist.

→ Symptoms include:
- intense pruritus.
- burning.
- bleeding of vulvar skin secondary to scratching/ excoriation.
- swelling.
- external dysuria.
- dyspareunia.

→ History to include: Complete gynecological, contraceptive, sexual history; vaginitis or STD history; feminine hygiene products and douching history; clothing history (e.g., type of panties, tight pants); type of soap, detergent, toilet paper used; partner symptomatology; general medical history and state of health; recent systemic illness;

recent use of antibiotics; other regular medications; stress; family history of diabetes.

OBJECTIVE

→ Areas affected may include: mons pubis, labia majora, perianal area, genitocrural folds, inner aspects of thighs (Kaufman and Faro 1994).

→ External genitalia may evidence:
- erythema, edema, excoriation.
- fine, gray sheen overlying erythema.
- fissuring of interlabial sulci.
- intertriginous areas thick and white.
- satellite pustules at edges of lesion.

→ Vagina may evidence:
- normal or abnormal discharge.
- vaginal walls WNL or erythematous.

→ Cervix:
- may be WNL or adherent white, thick discharge may be present; ± erythema.

→ Uterus, adnexa, rectovaginal examination WNL unless coexistent pathology.

ASSESSMENT

→ Cutaneous candidiasis of the vulva
→ R/O *tinea cruris*
→ R/O concomitant vaginal candidiasis
→ R/O reactive vulvitis
→ R/O Paget's disease
→ R/O other dermatoses (e.g., psoriasis, seborrheic dermatitis, eczemoid dermatitis [Kaufman and Faro 1994])
→ R/O diabetes
→ R/O concomitant STD

PLAN

DIAGNOSTIC TESTS

→ 10 percent to 20 percent potassium hydroxide (KOH) wet prep of scrapings from affected skin surface.
NOTE: Use moist saline cotton swab or spatula to obtain sample from vulvar skin, spread on clean glass slide, add 1 drop to 2 drops KOH, cover, and examine under microscope. Both spores and hyphae indicate candidal infection; hyphae alone suggest tineal infection (Kaufman and Faro 1994).

→ KOH and saline wet preps of vaginal discharge to rule out concomitant vaginitis.

→ For further confirmation, cultures for *Candida* can be done. See **Candida Vaginitis** Protocol.

→ FBS to rule out diabetes may be indicated with recurrent infection.

→ Cervical cultures and additional laboratory tests as indicated to rule out concomitant infection/STD.

TREATMENT/MANAGEMENT

→ Vaginal antifungal agents should be used concurrently when treating cutaneous vulvar candidiasis.

→ Antifungal creams for *Candida* plus corticosteroids for inflammation/pruritus are the mainstays of treatment. Some examples include:
- miconazole nitrate 2 percent (Monistat-Derm®): Apply to affected BID for 14 days. Use sparingly in intertriginous areas.
- nystatin and triamcinolone acetonide (Mycolog II®): Apply sparingly to affected area BID. Discontinue if symptoms persist after 25 days (fluorinated steroid—may cause atrophy, striae with prolonged use).
- hydrocortisone cream (Nutracort®) (1 percent to 2.5 percent): Apply sparingly to affected area TID-QID (this product does not contain an antifungal; anti-inflammatory/antipruritic agent only).

→ Alternative therapy may consist of gentian violet 1 percent aqueous solution: Painted on vulvovaginal area once a week for 2 to 3 weeks. Do not use in presence of severe vulvar excoriation/ulceration.

→ For soothing of the vulva, especially with weeping lesions, Burow's (Domeboro®, Bluboro®) solution may be tried: Wet dressings or sitz baths 15 to 30 minutes TID as necessary (Sauer 1991). See **Table 12TA.1, Tips for Treating Skin Lesions.**

→ For severe pruritus, hydroxyzine hydrochloride (Atarax®) or diphenhydramine hydrochloride (Benadryl®): 25 mg p.o. TID may be prescribed (Friedrich 1983). Caution patient about possible side effect of drowsiness. See *PDR*.

CONSULTATION

→ As indicated for assessment of lesion.
→ As needed for prescription(s).
→ Referral to appropriate health care provider as indicated if diabetes diagnosed.

12TA.1. TIPS FOR TREATING SKIN LESIONS

1. Start with *mild* agents, increase potency as acuteness subsides. DO NOT begin with the most potent variety of topical corticosteroid.
2. Most products should be massaged in gently for 5 to 10 seconds.
3. For many conditions, instruct patient to continue treating the skin for 4 to 10 days after the dermatosis has cleared.
4. Ointment bases should be used more often than cream bases. The greasiness allows the medicine to penetrate the skin better, and may alleviate dryness and remove scales.
5. Cream bases are indicated when treating intertriginous and hairy areas.
6. Long-term use of fluorinated steroids should be avoided because of the potential of skin atrophy, striae, and telangiectasia, especially on intertriginous areas, the face, and the anal area. Some commonly prescribed fluorinated topical steroids are: betamethasone, fluocinolone, fluocinonide, and triamcinolone.
7. Agents containing neomycin (e.g., Mycolog®) may precipitate allergy. Mycolog II® does not contain neomycin.
8. Strong topical steroids should not be prescribed for generalized body use. The potent steroids have a definite systemic effect.
9. Long-term use of local steroids may result in diminished effectiveness.
10. Become familiar with all agents prescribed: their indications, use, and possible side effects. Refer to the *PDR*.
11. Wet dressings or sitz baths (warm, hot, or cold) may be used to treat any pruritic, oozing, or crusting dermatosis. Burow's solution (aluminum sulfate, calcium acetate, and boric acid) is often the prescribed agent. Wet dressings should be applied with a clean, soaked gauze, with additional solution added via bulb syringe so gauze does not dry out. The dressing should be left on for 15 to 20 minutes and may be applied TID. The solution should be made fresh every time. Sitz baths may be substituted for wet dressings. The same general principles regarding timing and frequency apply.

Source: Adapted with permission from Sauer, G.C. 1991. *Manual of skin diseases*, 6th ed. Philadelphia: J.B. Lippincott.

PATIENT EDUCATION

→ Discuss etiology and nature of infection.

→ Advise patient that although relief of symptoms may occur in two to three days, topical anti-fungals should be used for two weeks to reduce possibility of recurrence (*PDR* 1993).

→ Review and discuss vulvovaginal health and hygiene:
  ■ Use of all-cotton underwear and loose clothing; proper wiping technique; white unscented toilet paper; avoidance of strong bath or laundry soap; thorough rinsing of underclothes after washing with line drying; avoidance of feminine hygiene deodorant products and excessive douching.
  ■ Ideally, wash vulvar area with water only; may use Aveeno® or other hypoallergenic soap; pat

dry or use hair dryer on low setting. See *Candida* Vaginitis Protocol.

→ For recurrent yeast, advise to "sterilize" panties in microwave after laundering or soak in bleach overnight.

→ Encourage good health maintenance: Well-balanced diet without excessive simple sugars, dairy and yeast products, and alcohol; adequate rest, exercise; stress reduction.

→ Advise regarding desirability of sexual abstinence during course of treatment.

FOLLOW-UP

→ Patient to return as necessary if symptoms not improved with treatment.

→ Review all laboratory work as indicated. Treat all concomitant STDs. If diabetes diagnosed, refer patient to appropriate health care provider.

→ Address additional medical concerns as indicated.

→ Refer sexual partner(s) to health care provider for evaluation and treatment as indicated.

→ Document in progress notes and problem list.

Contact Dermatitis (Reactive Vulvitis)

Reactive changes in the skin of the vulva can be due to a wide variety of physical and chemical stimuli. Most cases are secondary to either a nonimmunological irritant or a cell-mediated allergic response to a circulating antigenic substance. The clinical presentation of primary irritant versus allergic reaction is often indistinguishable and may mimic other dermatoses; thus pinpointing the specific etiology is difficult and good history-taking is important. In most vulvovaginal reactions the contactant is a primary irritant. Perspiration, friction, heat, and pressure are all factors that aggravate the reaction.

Many factors and substances can cause reactive vulvitis, including: scratching, rubbing, bicycle or horse-back riding, coitus, saliva, seminal fluid, vaginal discharge, lubricants, spermicides, synthetic fabrics, fabric dyes, detergents, soap, perfumed oils, feminine hygiene deodorant products, bath oils and additives, OTC remedies, bromine compounds in hot tubs and swimming pools, cytotoxic agents such as fluorouracil (Efudex®), topical medication, and oleoresin, as in poison oak or ivy.

Allergic sensitization may occur with repeated use of fluorouracil and certain topical medications. Plant contact produces classic allergic contact dermatitis (Friedrich 1983; Gomel, Munro, and Rowe 1990; Hammill 1989; Kaufman and Faro 1994).

DATABASE

SUBJECTIVE

→ A good history is the key to diagnosis. Ask about exposure to all of the aforementioned potential irritants as well as systemic medication being taken.

→ Symptoms include:
- pruritus.
- burning.
- tenderness, pain.
- irritation.
- urinary retention in severe cases.

OBJECTIVE

→ Intertriginous areas, e.g., interlabial, genitocrural folds, and the groin are most susceptible to reactions.

→ Diffuse or localized vulvar erythema; may be symmetrical.

→ Edema, exudate, weeping of the area may occur.

→ Excoriation, ulceration may occur.

→ Papulovesicular lesions or bullae may develop.

→ Affected epithelium may appear raised above normal skin.

→ Scaling, thickening, white plaques, or lichenification may occur (features of chronic contact dermatitis).

→ With allergic reactions, redness and wheals at the point of contact are the initial signs; in 24 to 48 hours vesicles and bullae form; lesions may be arranged in linear streaks.

→ Vagina, cervix, uterus, adnexa, and rectovaginal examination will be WNL unless there is coexistent pathology.

NOTE: Lesion distribution may give a clue as to etiology. For example:
- localized introital erythema can be due to coital trauma, vaginal discharge, hygiene products (e.g., deodorant suppositories, douches), lubricants.
- diffuse reaction can be due to fabric irritants, dyes, soap, detergent, perfumed oils, "saddle burn" (Friedrich 1983).

ASSESSMENT

→ Reactive vulvitis (contact dermatitis)

→ R/O *Candida* vulvitis or vulvovaginitis

→ R/O *T. cruris*

→ R/O other dermatoses (e.g., seborrheic dermatitis, psoriasis)

→ R/O concomitant STD

→ R/O squamous cell hyperplasia

→ R/O herpes simplex virus infection

PLAN

DIAGNOSTIC TESTS

→ None specific.

→ Pap smear, genital cultures, wet mounts as indicated to rule out concomitant vulvitis, vaginitis, or STD.

TREATMENT/MANAGEMENT

→ Elimination and avoidance of the precipitating irritant once identified is crucial.

→ Symptomatic relief measures and treatment of inflammation include:
- cool baths or wet dressings with Burow's solution (Domeboro®, Bluboro®) 15 to 30 minutes BID-QID. Works well for acute oozing, crusting lesion.
- low-potency topical corticosteroid (e.g., hydrocortisone ointment or cream) 1 percent to 2.5 percent. Small amount on pad of index finger gently massaged into affected areas BID-TID until skin is restored to normal. Topical therapy may be continued for 4 to 10 days after the dermatosis is cleared. See **Table 12TA.1**. **NOTE:** An ointment base is most useful for penetrating the steroid and removing dryness and scales. A cream base is indicated if the lesion affects a hairy or intertriginous area; however, it may be too drying (Sauer 1991).

→ Topical anesthetics should be avoided.

→ Oral antihistamines, e.g., hydroxyzine hydrochloride (Atarax®) or diphenhydramine hydrochloride (Benadryl®) 10 mg to 25 mg p.o. TID may be necessary for severe pruritus (Friedrich 1983). Caution patient about possible side effect of drowsiness. See *PDR*.

→ Systemic corticosteroids are indicated for severe allergic reactions and are used in decreasing doses over about 3 weeks. Consult with physician.

CONSULTATION

→ As indicated for assessment of condition or when systemic corticosteroids are indicated.

→ As needed for prescripton(s).

→ Discuss elimination of predisposing substances.

→ Be sure patient understands how to apply wet dressings and topical steroid medication.

→ Advise patient that contact dermatitis usually resolves within a few days with sitz baths and emollients; allergic reactions may take weeks to resolve.

→ Suggest hair dryer on low setting after bath and wet dressings to dry vulvar area thoroughly.

→ Advise patient to keep hands off affected area except to apply wet dressings and topical steroid. The itch-scratch cycle is detrimental to resolution of dermatitis. Suggest wearing white cotton gloves at bedtime.

→ Advise patient to limit or avoid certain foods that stimulate pruritus: chocolate, nuts, cheese, coffee, and spicy foods (Sauer 1991).

→ See above "Patient Education" section for particulars on vulvovaginal health and hygiene.

FOLLOW-UP

→ Return visit in one to four weeks or prn for reassessment.

→ Document in progress notes and problem list.

Paget's Disease

Paget's disease of the vulva is a slowly progressive intra-epithelial neoplasia, histologically identical to Paget's disease of the breast. The disease affects areas of the body that contain numerous apocrine glands and represents an unusual differentiation of the primitive stem cell of the epidermis. There appear to be two varieties of Paget's disease: Intraepithelial extramammary Paget's and pagetoid changes within the skin associated with an underlying adenocarcinoma such as the apocrine gland, found in less than 20 percent of cases. Intraepithelial Paget's disease tends to recur locally without propensity for invasion.

Paget's disease with underlying apocrine carcinoma can be aggressive with regional lymph-node metastases. An underlying carcinoma of the breast or GI tract may exist concomitantly with Paget's disease. Primary carcinoma of the rectum, urethra, or bladder may also be present, especially when Paget's affects the perineum. The prognosis for Paget's disease is good if it occurs without underlying adenocarcinoma or lymph node metastasis (DiSaia and Creasman 1989; Friedrich 1983;

Kaufman and Faro 1994; Kaufman, Friedrich, and Gardner 1989).

DATABASE

SUBJECTIVE

→ Affects white women most commonly.

→ Median age at onset is 65 years.

→ May be asymptomatic.

→ Condition may persist for months to years prior to patient seeking attention or diagnosis.

→ Symptoms generally include:
  ▪ itching.
  ▪ soreness or tenderness.

OBJECTIVE

→ Clinical features may include:
  ▪ variable lesion size.
  ▪ localization to one labium or entire vulva.
  ▪ sharp, well-defined borders.
  ▪ erythema with superficial white coating ("cake-icing effect," almost pathognomonic).
  ▪ velvety-red or bright-pink, scaly lesions of variable size; alternately grayish-white, speckled lesions.
  ▪ moist, oozing, friable ulcers.
  ▪ excoriation, induration.
  ▪ mass below epithelium.
  ▪ spread to perineum, perianal area, thigh, or vagina.

→ Since the disease process is multifocal, not all lesions may be clinically evident. "Silent" areas of involvement at various sites account for a high recurrence rate (Friedrich 1983).

→ Vagina, cervix, uterus, adnexa, and rectum are WNL unless there is coexistent pathology.

→ A good description and diagram of the lesion is helpful.

ASSESSMENT

→ Paget's disease

→ R/O squamous cell carcinoma in situ (vulvar intraepithelial neoplasia [VIN] III)

→ R/O malignant melanoma

→ R/O squamous cell hyperplasia

→ R/O *Candida* infection

→ R/O acute or chronic reactive vulvitis

→ R/O coexistent carcinoma(s)

PLAN

DIAGNOSTIC TESTS

→ Biopsy of the lesion for histopathology is the definitive method of assessment. An adequate margin of normal-appearing tissue must be obtained (Kaufman and Faro 1994).

→ Fine needle aspiration (FNA) to evaluate subcutaneous masses for adenocarcinoma.

→ Certain histochemical staining techniques and monoclonal antibodies can distinguish Paget's disease from VIN III and malignant melanoma.

→ Work-up to exclude concomitant carcinoma may include barium enema; computerized tomographic scan; clinical breast examination; mammography; proctosigmoidoscopy; Pap smear; and colposcopy of the vulva, vagina, and cervix.

→ Pap smear, genital cultures, wet mounts, and other diagnostic tests as indicated.

→ A delay in diagnosis may occur if lesion is mistaken for dermatitis.

TREATMENT/MANAGEMENT

→ Primary therapy includes (Kaufman and Faro 1994):
- wide local excision of the lesion.
- for larger areas, superficial "skinning" vulvectomy with wide margins to a depth inclusive of all adnexal structures.

→ Secondarily, more extensive vulvectomy and inguinal lymphadenectomy is performed if invasive carcinoma is identified.

→ As an adjunct to surgical management, Misas (1991) has advocated use of intravenous fluorescein followed by ultraviolet light exposure to the vulva in order to localize areas of disease not grossly visualized (Kaufman and Faro 1994).

→ Wide local excision, laser therapy, 5-FU, and bleomycin have been used for recurrent disease.

CONSULTATION

→ As necessary for initial observation of the lesion.

→ Referral to a physician for biopsy procedure and FNA per site-specific policy.

→ Due to nature of the disease, patient should be referred to a gynecologist or gynecological oncologist for management.

PATIENT EDUCATION

→ Explain etiology of the disease, treatment, and potential sequelae. The physician responsible for care of the patient will detail the particulars.

→ Paget's disease may require disfiguring surgery resulting in sexual dysfunction. Provide counseling prior to surgery.

→ Patients need social and psychological support through phases of treatment for this disease. Refer to appropriate support services.

FOLLOW-UP

→ As recurrence is common, patients will require visits every six months indefinitely. Examination includes careful visual inspection, mammography, stool for guaiac, Pap smear, and colposcopic evaluation.

→ Patients should be instructed to report promptly any recurrent itching, pain, or soreness of the vulva.

→ Biopsies of all suspicious lesions should be undertaken promptly.

→ For recurrent disease, repeated local excisions may be necessary.

→ Document in progress notes and problem list.

12-TB   VULVAR DISEASE
White Lesions of the Vulva

Factors contributing to the appearance of *white lesions of the vulva* include hyperkeratosis (i.e., overgrowth of the horny layer of the epidermis), depigmentation, and relative avascularity. There has been a lack of uniform terminology and classification for these lesions; however, in 1987 the International Society for the Study of Vulvar Disease (ISSVD) reclassified the most common white vulvar lesions, the vulvar dystrophies, into *nonneoplastic epithelial disorders of skin and mucosa.* Categories include *lichen sclerosus, squamous cell hyperplasia* (formerly hyperplastic dystrophy), and other dermatoses (Committee on Terminology of the ISSVD 1990).

The etiology of these various disorders is still unclear. Technically, *dystrophy* means defective nutrition or metabolism, but the definition adds little to the understanding of the phenomenon. Factors that may contribute to the pathogenesis of the nonneoplastic disorders include chronic trauma (scratching), contact irritants, chronic vulvovaginal infections (candidiasis, particularly in diabetics), allergic responses, nutritional deficiencies (folic acid deficiency, Vitamin A deficiency secondary to achlorhydria/poor diet), metabolic disturbances (5 alpha-reductase deficiency), autoimmune disorders, familial disposition, and psychoneuroses. Further research is needed to establish cause-and-effect relationships (Kaufman and Faro 1994).

One controversial issue is these disorders' potential for malignant transformation. It was originally thought that all white lesions of the vulva were premalignant, but this is now known to be untrue. Most researchers believe there is little or no threat that lichen sclerosis will progress to invasive carcinoma; however, both pathologies may exist within the same vulva. Recent prospective studies indicate progression from chronic vulvar dystrophy to cancer on the order of one percent to five percent. A lesion which contains atypical hyperplasia on initial biopsy (two percent to three percent incidence) presents a risk for carcinoma (Jeffcoate 1966). A "mixed" lesion—squamous cell hyperplasia superimposed on a background of lichen sclerosus—is at slightly increased risk for atypicality and development of invasive cancer.

Cases of atypia are now all placed in the category of vulvar intraepithelial neoplasia (VIN). Women at greater risk for cancer progression are those whose lesions do not respond to standard therapy and who continue to have severe itching with resultant chronic scratching (Kaufman and Faro 1994; Rodke, Friedrich, and Wilkinson 1988).

This protocol will cover assessment and management of lichen sclerosus and squamous cell hyperplasia. See also **Vulvar Intraepithelial Neoplasia** Protocol.

Lichen Sclerosus

Lichen sclerosus accounts for about 70 percent of nonneoplastic disorders. Former names included lichen sclerosus et atrophicus, atrophic leukoplakia, kraurosis vulvae, senile atrophy, and atrophic vulvitis. The epithelium in lichen sclerosus is, however, metabolically active, not atrophic. The cause is unknown, but associated factors include autoimmune disease, heredity, achlorhydria, and decreased testosterone levels. Areas of hyperplastic epithelium, often caused by scratching, may coexist with lichen sclerosus. This condition was once called "mixed dystrophy" (Friedrich 1983; Kaufman and Faro 1994).

DATABASE

SUBJECTIVE

→ May occur at any age; majority of women are more than 50 years old.

→ Affected children may have spontaneous resolution in adolescence, but most have persistent disease into adulthood.

→ Affected women of reproductive age often have remission during pregnancy with postpartum reexacerbation.

→ Patient may be asymptomatic.

→ Symptoms may include:
  ▪ pruritus (primary symptom but may not be acutely present, may be sporadic or only mild, may not correlate with the size and severity of lesions).
  ▪ soreness, pain.
  ▪ dyspareunia.
  ▪ excoriations, ulcerations, bruising, skin thickening.

→ History to include: Vaginal infections; allergies; use of feminine hygiene products; history of diabetes, nutritional deficiencies; family history, especially with regard to diabetes, cancer, and skin disorders.

OBJECTIVE

→ Affected skin may appear on trunk, neck, forearm, axilla, under breasts, vulva, skin folds adjacent to thighs, inner aspects of buttocks approximating the anus (Kaufman and Faro 1994).

→ Clinical features (Kaufman and Faro 1994):
  ▪ location on vulva variable and pattern often bilaterally symmetrical.
  ▪ initially low, irregular lesion.
  ▪ white maculopapules that may progress to well-defined plaques.
  ▪ associated "blackhead-like" plugs or depressions.
  ▪ splitting of skin in midline (between clitoris and urethra, in perineum, or especially at fourchette).
  ▪ fissures in skin folds.
  ▪ small hematoma/telangiectasia of skin or mucosa.
  ▪ blisters or ulcers in some cases.
  ▪ "crinkled" or "parchment-like" appearance (commonly extends to anal area in keyhole configuration).
  ▪ adhesion of labia minora to majora.
  ▪ edema or agglutination of prepuce and frenulum that may bury clitoris (early diagnostic sign).
  ▪ contraction of the vaginal introitus (kraurosis).
  ▪ vagina, cervix, uterus, adnexa, and rectum WNL unless coexistent pathology.

→ A diagram and good description of the lesion is helpful.

ASSESSMENT

→ Lichen sclerosus

→ R/O squamous cell hyperplasia

→ R/O vitiligo

→ R/O VIN

→ R/O concomitant invasive cancer

→ R/O other dermatoses (e.g., psoriasis, lichen planus)

→ R/O *Candida* infection

→ R/O condyloma acuminata

PLAN

DIAGNOSTIC TESTS

→ Multiple punch biopsies from selected areas of the vulva—especially from fissured, indurated, ulcerated, or thickened-appearing areas—are mandatory for diagnosis, as areas of hyperplasia and atypia cannot be determined by visual inspection alone.
  ▪ If the appearance of the abnormal areas are all similar, only one biopsy is necessary.
  ▪ Ulcerations can be biopsied at different sites of lesion border or, preferably, entire ulcer should be excised.

→ Pap smear, genital cultures, wet mounts, and other diagnostic tests as indicated.

TREATMENT/MANAGEMENT

→ Treat any associated vulvovaginal infection as indicated.

→ Malignancy must be ruled out prior to local therapy.

→ Local measures for relief of pruritus, ulcerations, and excoriations include (Friedrich 1983):
  ▪ wet dressings: 5 percent aluminum acetate (Burow's solution [Domeboro®, Bluboro®]): dilute 1:10 to 1:20, saturate gauze, apply/reapply for 20 to 30 minutes every day or more often as necessary; alternately may use

Domeboro® tablets or powder (follow directions on product); keep solution refrigerated.

- sitz baths (versus wet dressings) may be tried with Burow's solution or with natural or artificial sea water (prepackaged powders available at aquarium supply stores); the soothing effect on skin is similar.

→ Medications for specific treatment of the disorder include (Kaufman and Faro 1994):

- testosterone propionate 2 percent in petrolatum (mixed by pharmacist): small amount gently massaged into affected areas BID-TID for 3 to 6 months; gradual reduced frequency of application for 1 to 2 years until maintenance therapy of 1 to 2 times per week achieved.
  NOTE: Testosterone may cause clitoromegaly and enhanced libido.
- progesterone 10 ml in oil (50 mg/ml) in 40 g petrolatum may be used for occasional woman unresponsive to testosterone.
- clobetasol propionate (Temovate®) 0.05 percent cream: small amount to affected areas BID for 1 month, once daily for 2 months, then twice weekly for 3 months; therapy may be continued with small amounts over 2 to 3 years (Dalziel and Wojnarowska 1991; Kaufman and Faro 1994).
- for pruritus: Hydrocortisone 1 percent to 2.5 percent; may be used in conjunction with testosterone; severe pruritus may require stronger corticosteroids. (See "Treatment/Management," "Squamous Cell Hyperplasia" section.)

→ Wide local excision for lesions with atypia.

→ Vulvectomy reserved for persistent or extensive disease or progressive atypicality (recurrence rate after vulvectomy high).

→ Nonbeneficial, unproven therapies (Kaufman and Faro 1994):

- estrogen cream (no or weak atrophic effect on skin).
- topical anesthetics (may cause dermatitis).
- oral retinoids (mixed reviews).
- oral chloroquine (dangerous to eye; avoid).
- vitamin A and dilute hydrochloric acid with meals (unpredictable results).
- radiation therapy (not recommended).

→ Lichen sclerosus plus squamous cell hyperplasia are treated with corticosteroids to entire area for 6 weeks followed by testosterone or corticosteroid and testosterone on alternate days, which gives a slower response. (See "Squamous Cell Hyperplasia" section.)

CONSULTATION

→ As indicated for initial assessment.

→ Referral to physician as indicated for biopsy and/or therapy depending on policies of the practice setting.

→ For wide local excision and more extensive surgery, refer to physician.

→ As needed for prescription(s).

PATIENT EDUCATION

→ Explain that the disease has no definitive etiology.

→ In some cases, lesions will not disappear, but continued testosterone will slow disease progression and prevent skin-tearing.

- Symptoms may persist despite improvement in skin appearance.
- Topical corticosteroids can be continued for pruritus relief.
- Additional relief measures for pruritus should be outlined. (See "Treatment/Management" section.)

→ Factors that may be associated with or aggravate the condition should be explored, e.g., hygiene, nutrition, allergies, vaginal infections. Advocate wearing of cotton underwear.

→ Discuss steps to improve overall health—e.g., proper diet, stress reduction, exercise.

→ Assess patient's coping strategies, with suggestions for improvement as indicated—e.g., stress reduction techniques, relaxation, exercise.

→ Ingestion of acidic foods may exacerbate symptoms; antacids may offer relief in this case.

→ Refer for psychosocial support as indicated.

FOLLOW-UP

→ As with many vulvar diseases, ongoing evaluation of the treated areas for disease recurrence is of utmost importance. Lichen sclerosus has been known to recur in 50 percent of cases after excision.

→ Examinations should be performed on a regular basis (i.e., every three to six months) initially. After stabilization, patient visits may be semi-annual.

→ Biopsies of all progressive, recurrent, persistent, or suspicious lesions should be performed, especially from ulcerated, granular, or nodular areas.

→ Instruct patients to report any changes in vulvar tissue and encourage them to continue regular visits even if symptom-free.

→ Document in progress notes and problem list.

Squamous Cell Hyperplasia

This condition was formerly called leukoplakia and hyperplastic dystrophy. Kaufman and Faro (1994) state that most hyperplastic lesions represent variants of lichen simplex chronicus (neurodermatitis). Squamous cell hyperplasia is associated with epithelial thickening and parakeratosis, or overgrowth of the horny layer of the epidermis. Thus the lesion has a white appearance known as leukoplakia. Other dermatoses also have these nonspecific features (e.g., chronic reactive vulvitis and eczema).

   As with lichen sclerosus, etiology of this disorder is unclear. Hyperplasia may represent an epidermal reaction to chronic itching and scratching and be superimposed on a background of lichen sclerosus. Cancerous potential is related to associated cellular atypia of the lesion. This then becomes known as VIN. Although some similarities in appearance exist and the two may lie side by side in the same vulva, squamous cell hyperplasia and lichen sclerosus are separate diseases (Friedrich 1983; Kaufman and Faro 1994). See "Lichen Sclerosus" section.

DATABASE

SUBJECTIVE

→ Age usually less than 50 years.

→ Symptoms include:
- pruritus, usually more severe than with lichen sclerosus.
- excoriations, skin thickening.
- soreness, pain.

OBJECTIVE

→ Variations in lesions may occur due to moisture conditions of vulva, scratching, medication.

→ Clinical features include (Kaufman and Faro 1994):
- range in lesion size from small to extensive; often bilaterally symmetrical.
- localized, raised, well-delineated lesion.
- dusky red vulva.
- white patches or both red and white areas at different sites.

- areas most frequently involved: clitoral hood, labia majora, interlabial grooves, outer labia minora.
- lesion may extend to thighs.
- lichenification (i.e., thickening, hardening), fissures, excoriation.
- isolated involved areas more frequent than with lichen sclerosus.
- clitoral and labial derangement usually absent.

→ Squamous cell hyperplasia may coexist with lichen sclerosus. Thus features of both will appear on same vulva. (See "Objective," "Lichen Sclerosus" section.)

→ Vagina, cervix, uterus, adnexa, rectum WNL unless coexistent pathology.

→ A diagram and good description of the lesion is helpful.

ASSESSMENT

→ Squamous cell hyperplasia
→ R/O lichen sclerosus
→ R/O VIN
→ R/O invasive cancer
→ R/O other dermatoses (See "Assessment," "Lichen Sclerosus" section.)

PLAN

DIAGNOSTIC TESTS

→ See "Diagnostic Tests," "Lichen Sclerosus" section.

TREATMENT/MANAGEMENT

→ Malignancy must be ruled out prior to local therapy.

→ See "Treatment/Management," "Lichen Sclerosus" section for discussion of symptomatic relief measures, e.g., wet dressings, sitz baths.

→ Corticosteroids are the treatment of choice. Options include (Friedrich 1983; Kaufman and Faro 1994):
- hydrocortisone cream/ointment 1 percent—small amount to affected areas BID-TID
OR
- fluocinolone acetonide (Synalar®) cream/ointment 0.025 percent to 0.01 percent—small amount to affected areas BID-TID
OR

- triamcinolone acetonide (Aristocort®, Kenalog®) cream/ointment 0.01 percent—small amount to affected areas BID-TID.
- for severe pruritus, 7:3 combination of betamethasone valerate (Valisone®) 0.1 percent and crotamiton (Eurax®) in cream base—small amount to affected areas BID for 2 to 6 weeks
  OR
- clobetasol propionate (Temovate®) 0.05%. See "Lichen Sclerosus" section.

NOTE: Fluorinated steroids may cause skin atrophy. Once severe pruritus is controlled, fluorinated steroid should be replaced with nonfluorinated variety, e.g., hydrocortisone. See **Table 12TB.1, Potency Ranking of Topical Corticosteroids**.

→ Testosterone is of no value in this condition.

→ Adjunctive therapy with oral hydroxyzine hydrochloride (Atarax®), 25 mg p.o. TID or at bedtime, may be tried for relief of agitation, anxiety, and severe itching. Prescribe with caution; may cause drowsiness. See *PDR*. Consult with physician.

→ Severe pruritus unresponsive to topical therapy may require intradermal injections of triamcinolone, 10 mg/ml diluted 2:1 in saline, or subcutaneous injections of absolute alcohol (a last resort—complications include tissue sloughing, ulceration, severe vulvar pain). The latter treatment is an inpatient procedure performed under anesthesia; refer patient to physician (Kaufman and Faro 1994).

→ Wide local excision for lesions with atypia.

→ Vulvectomy reserved for persistent or extensive disease or progressive atypicality (recurrence rate after vulvectomy high).

→ Lichen sclerosus plus squamous cell hyperplasia is treated with: corticosteroids to entire area for 6 weeks followed by testosterone or corticosteroid and testosterone on alternate days, which produces a slower response. See "Lichen Sclerosus" section.

Table 12TB.1. POTENCY RANKING OF TOPICAL CORTICOSTEROIDS

Group I (Super Potent)
Diprolene® cream/ointment 0.05% (betamethasone dipropionate, in optimized vehicle)
Psorcon® ointment 0.05% (diflorasone diacetate)
Temovate® cream/ointment 0.05% (clobetasol propionate)

Group II (Potent)
Cyclocort® ointment 0.1% (amcinonide)
Diprosone® ointment 0.05% (betamethasone dipropionate)
Florone® ointment 0.05% (diflorasone diacetate)
Halog® cream 0.1% (halcinonide)
Lidex® cream/ointment/gel 0.05% (fluocinonide)
Maxiflor® ointment 0.05% (diflorasone diacetate)
Topicort® cream/ointment 0.25% (desoximethasone)

Group III (Potent)
Aristocort® cream 0.5% (triamcinolone acetonide)
Cyclocort® cream/lotion 0.1% (amcinonide)
Diprosone® cream 0.05% (betamethasone dipropionate)
Florone® cream 0.05% (diflorasone diacetate)
Halog® ointment 0.1% (halcinonide)
Lidex® E cream 0.05% (fluocinonide)
Maxiflor® cream 0.05% (diflorasone diacetate)
Valisone® ointment 0.1% (betamethasone valerate)

Group IV (Mid-strength)
Aristocort® ointment 0.1% (triamcinolone acetonide)
Benisone® ointment 0.025% (betamethasone benzoate)
Cordran® ointment 0.05% (flurandrenolide)
Kenalog® ointment 0.1% (triamcinolone acetonide)
Synalar® cream 0.2%/ointment 0.025% (fluocinolone acetonide)

Group V (Mid-strength)
Benisone® cream 0.025% (betamethasone benzoate)
Cordran® cream 0.05% (flurandrenolide)
Diprosone® lotion 0.05% (betamethasone dipropionate)
Kenalog® cream/lotion 0.1% (triamcinolone acetonide)
Locoid® cream/ointment 0.1% (hydrocortisone butyrate)
Synalar® cream 0.025% (fluocinolone acetonide)
Valisone® cream/lotion 0.1% (betamethasone valerate)
Westcort® cream 0.2% (hydrocortisone valerate)

Group VI (Mild)
Aclovate® cream/ointment 0.05% (alclometasone dipropionate)
DesOwen®, Tridesilon® cream 0.05% (desonide)
Synalar® cream/solution 0.01% (fluocinolone acetonide)

Group VII (Mild)
Nutracort® cream/lotion 1% (hydrocortisone)
Other topicals with hydrocortisone, dexamethasone, flumethalone, prednisolone, and methyl prednisolone

NOTE: Groups are arranged alphabetically. Trade names appear first; generic names are in parentheses. Potency descends with each group. There are no significant differences between agents in Groups II–VII. In Group I, Temovate® is more potent than Diprolone® or Psorcon®.

Sources: Adapted with permission from Cornell, R.C., and Stoughton, R.B. 1984. The use of topical steroids in psoriasis. *Dermatologic Clinics* 2(3):397–409; Sauer, G.C. 1991. *Manual of skin diseases*, 6th ed. Philadelphia: J.B. Lippincott.

CONSULTATION

→ See "Consultation," "Lichen Sclerosus" section.

→ When considering adjunctive oral therapy for relief of agitation, severe pruritus, etc.

→ For surgical procedures and intradermal or subcutaneous injections to control pruritus, refer to physician.

→ As needed for prescription(s).

PATIENT EDUCATION

→ See "Patient Education," "Lichen Sclerosus" section.

→ Advise removal of chemical irritants from patient's life to ameliorate this condition. Tips include:
  ▪ no soap to vulvar area, plain water for bathing.
  ▪ all-cotton panties.
  ▪ mild laundry soap to clean underwear, rinse well, line dry.
  ▪ no feminine hygiene deodorant products on vulvar area.
  ▪ white, unscented toilet paper.

FOLLOW-UP

→ Refer to "Follow-Up," "Lichen Sclerosus" section.

→ Recurrent squamous cell hyperplasia must be treated as new lesion.

→ Document in progress notes and problem list.

12-TC VULVAR DISEASE
Dark Lesions of the Vulva

Any stimulus that increases the number or production of melanocytes or melanin results in color changes or hyperpigmentation of vulvar skin. The vulva's skin color is darker than the rest of the body's due to the large number of melanocytes concentrated there. Ten percent of all vulvar lesions are *dark lesions*. Their features are dissimilar, and benign-appearing lesions may actually be cancer. Ideally, all dark lesions of the vulva should be biopsied for a histological diagnosis (Friedrich 1983). Dark lesions of the vulva to be covered in this chapter are *lentigo, nevi, seborrheic keratoses,* and *melanoma*. Vulvar intraepithelial neoplasia (VIN), which also may present as a dark lesion, is detailed in a separate protocol. Information on consultation, patient education, and follow-up for dark lesions is combined at the end of this chapter. Other conditions that may present as dark lesions are *Pediculosis pubis* and scabies. See **Dermatological Disorders** Protocol.

Lentigo

A lentigo is an area of the skin where melanocytes produce excess amounts of melanin. No malignant potential is associated with this lesion.

DATABASE

SUBJECTIVE

→ Appears in mid-adult life.

→ No relationship to sun exposure.

→ Patient may be asymptomatic.

OBJECTIVE

→ Clinical features include:
- lesion located anywhere on vulva.
- circumscribed, macular lesion; resembles a freckle.
- light brown color.
- size varies from 1 mm to 10 mm.

→ Atypical cells may exist above basal layer.

→ Vagina, cervix, uterus, adnexa, rectum WNL unless coexistent pathology.

→ A good description and diagram of the lesion are helpful.

ASSESSMENT

→ Lentigo

→ R/O junctional nevi

→ R/O melanoma

→ R/O basal cell carcinoma

→ R/O VIN

→ R/O other dermatoses

PLAN

→ Biopsy—diagnostic and curative.

→ No other specific therapy indicated.

→ Pap smear, genital cultures, wet mounts, other diagnostic tests as indicated.

Nevi

Nevi, or moles, are clusters of "neural crest cells" derived from melanocytes in the epidermis and Schwann cells of the dermal nerves. Three main groups develop—junctional, compound, and intradermal nevi—as maturation from the basal layer of the epithelium occurs. With this transformation over time comes a diminished potential for melanoma transformation (i.e., junctional and compound nevi have greater malignant potential). About 30 percent to 50 percent of melanomas arise from preexisting nevi.

Dysplastic nevi (usually many more lesions present; not commonly found on the vulva) and *congenital* nevi (present since birth) carry increased risks for malignant melanoma development. The dysplastic type usually appears in adolescence and may continue to appear even after 35 years of age; it may be inherited or sporadic (Friedrich 1983; Kaufman and Faro 1994). Congenital nevi have a lifetime malignancy potential of five percent to 20 percent especially if the lesion is larger than 2 centimeters (Consensus Conference 1984).

DATABASE

SUBJECTIVE

→ Not usually recognized until after puberty, when lesions tend to darken.

→ Asymptomatic generally; may report raised area of vulvar skin or irritation.

→ Lesion may be stable for years or slowly enlarge.

OBJECTIVE

→ Five clinical types of nevi have been described (Lever 1990):
  ▪ flat: Usually junctional nevi, looks like lentigo.
  ▪ slightly elevated: Usually compound nevi.
  ▪ papillomatous: Majority intradermal, some compound nevi.
  ▪ dome-shaped: Usually intradermal nevi.
  ▪ pedunculated: Intradermal nevi.

→ Clinical features include:
  ▪ oval or cuboidal shape.
  ▪ size varies 1 mm to 2 cm.
  ▪ depth of color varies from flesh-colored to light tan to dark brown to black.

→ Vulvar melanosis often confused with nevi: usually presents as pigmented patch, flat and smooth; may be either a focal, pigmented area or large, diffuse, macular, pigmented area. Similar vaginal pigments may also exist (Kaufman and Faro 1994).

→ Vagina, cervix, uterus, adnexa, rectum WNL unless co-existent pathology

→ A good description and diagram of the lesion are important.

ASSESSMENT

→ Nevi

→ R/O lentigo

→ R/O melanoma

→ R/O melanosis

→ R/O VIN

→ R/O basal cell carcinoma

→ R/O seborrheic keratosis

→ R/O accessory breast tissue

→ R/O other dermatoses

PLAN

DIAGNOSTIC TESTS

→ Biopsy to establish histopathological diagnosis.

→ Pap smear, genital cultures, wet mounts, other diagnostic tests as indicated.

TREATMENT/MANAGEMENT

→ Pigmented nevi should be removed under the following conditions (Kaufman and Faro 1994):
  ▪ if subject to irritation, as on vulva.
  ▪ if smooth, dark brown, blue, or black.
  ▪ with increased growth or pigmentation.
  ▪ with associated ulceration, bleeding, or pain.
  NOTE: Increased growth, bleeding, ulceration, or "satellite lesions" may indicate malignancy and should be excised promptly.

→ Excision should include 0.5 cm to 1 cm of normal skin and subcutaneous tissue.

→ Destructive techniques are not advisable as they make histological evaluation impossible.

→ Benign vulvar melanosis is generally managed conservatively, but a biopsy is necessary to establish an accurate diagnosis.

→ Papular or hairy moles have a low malignant potential, thus removal is not urgent unless pain or bleeding exists.

→ Some sources recommend excision of congenital hairy nevi (Lerner 1972).

Seborrheic Keratosis

In the postmenopausal years, seborrheic keratosis is the most common tumor of the skin, though it is relatively unusual on the vulva. The lesion comprises proliferative basal epidermal cells and melanocytes that grow in an upward, controlled manner. Malignant potential is rare but has been reported (Friedrich 1983; Kaufman and Faro 1994).

DATABASE

SUBJECTIVE

→ Patient may be asymptomatic or may report raised lesion.

OBJECTIVE

→ Similar lesions elsewhere on body.

→ Appear singly or in clusters.

→ Size varies from tiny to several centimeters.

→ Appear flesh-colored or black, majority dark brown and greasy.

→ Papular lesion with flat top.

→ Appears as if lesion could be picked or shaved off.

→ Lesion may also be macular.

→ Sudden onset of multiple lesions may signal unrelated internal malignancy.

→ Vagina, cervix, uterus, adnexa, rectum WNL unless coexistent pathology.

→ A good description and diagram of the lesion are helpful.

ASSESSMENT

→ Seborrheic keratosis
→ R/O nevi
→ R/O melanoma
→ R/O VIN
→ R/O other dermatoses

PLAN

DIAGNOSTIC TESTS

→ Biopsy to establish histopathological diagnosis if lesion removed.

→ Pap smear, genital cultures, wet mounts, other diagnostic tests as indicated.

TREATMENT/MANAGEMENT

→ No treatment necessary unless lesion is large, disfiguring, or painful.

→ Simple excision may remove entire lesion and is diagnostic and curative.

→ Lesion may be scraped off with dermal curet after freezing with ethyl chloride; send specimen to pathology.

Table 12TC.1. CLARK'S STAGING CLASSIFICATION BY LEVELS

Level	Definition
I	In-situ melanoma: all demonstrable tumor is above the basement membrane in the epidermis.
II	Melanoma extends through the basement membrane into the papillary dermis.
III	The tumor fills the papillary dermis and extends into the reticular dermis but does not invade it.
IV	The tumor extends into the reticular dermis.
V	The tumor extends into the subcutaneous fat.

Source: Reprinted with permission from DiSaia, P.J., and Creasman, W.T. 1989. *Clinical gynecologic oncology*, 3rd ed., p. 267. St. Louis: C.V. Mosby.

→ Postsurgical bleeding may be controlled with ferric subsulfate (Monsel's solution) (Kaufman and Faro 1994).

Melanoma

Melanoma is a rare, malignant tumor that makes up 10 percent of all vulvar cancers. In women, five percent of melanomas arise in the vulva. Three varieties exist: lentigo maligna, superficial spreading (the most common), and nodular melanoma. Melanomas may arise de novo or from preexisting junctional or compound nevi (30 percent of cases). Prognosis for survival primarily depends on the depth or level of tumor invasion rather than the size of the tumor. (See **Table 12TC.1, Clark's Staging Classification by Levels**.) Ten-year survival rates for Levels I to II, III, IV, and V tumors are 100 percent, 83 percent, 65 percent, and 23 percent, respectively. Other factors influencing survival are urethral and vaginal extension, presence or absence of regional lymph nodes, and distant metastases (Barclay 1991; DiSaia and Creasman 1989; Friedrich 1983; Morrow and Townsend 1981).

DATABASE

SUBJECTIVE

→ Mostly found in women over age 50 years.

→ Caucasian usually only race affected.

→ Patient may be asymptomatic.

→ Symptoms may include:
  ▪ a "lump."
  ▪ pruritis.
  ▪ bleeding.
  ▪ irritation.
  ▪ enlargement of a "mole."
  ▪ change in "mole" pigmentation.
  ▪ "mole" with irregular borders.

→ Lesion may be present for variable amounts of time prior to discovery.

→ High-risk categories for developing melanoma include (DiSaia and Creasman 1989):
  ▪ family history of melanoma.
  ▪ poor or no tanning ability.
  ▪ moles that are blue-black, speckled, splotchy, or jagged on the border.
  ▪ change in size, shape, color of mole.
  ▪ mole larger than dime.

→ Family history of "moles."

OBJECTIVE

→ Labia majora, labia minora, clitoris are involved sites in most cases.

→ Vagina, cervix, uterus, adnexa, rectum WNL unless coexistent pathology.

→ A good description and diagram of the lesion are important.

Lentigo maligna

→ Rare on vulva.

→ Resembles flat freckle.

→ Has speckled appearance.

→ May be extensive, although superficial.

Superficial spreading

→ Most common type affecting vulva.

→ Usually elevated.

→ May be ulcerated.

→ May be 2 cm to 3 cm in diameter.

→ Fairly good prognosis if detected early.

Nodular melanoma

→ Has raised, irregular surface.

→ Small diameter but deep involvement.

→ Variable degrees of pigmentation.

→ Some amelanotic varieties.

→ Increased frequency of nodal metastasis.

→ Has poor prognosis.

ASSESSMENT

→ Melanoma

→ R/O lentigo

→ R/O nevi

→ R/O seborrheic keratosis

→ R/O VIN

→ R/O furuncle

→ R/O basal cell carcinoma

→ R/O other dermatoses

PLAN

DIAGNOSTIC TESTS

→ Biopsy to establish histopathological diagnosis.

→ Pap smear, genital cultures, wet mounts, other diagnostic tests as indicated.

TREATMENT/MANAGEMENT

→ If presenting lesion is small, punch biopsy may be performed; larger lesions require excision of greater areas.

→ Definitive therapy by physician after histopathological diagnosis established. Treatment selection depends on the consulting gynecological oncologist. Management remains controversial. Options include:
  ▪ wide local excision: Trend is toward greater use of this therapy for varying depths of tumor invasion.
  ▪ radical vulvectomy with bilateral inguinal (and in some cases pelvic) lymphadenectomy may be necessary for deep tumor invasion.
  ▪ exenteration for urethral or bladder extension.
  ▪ radiation in selected cases.

CONSULTATION (pertinent to all dark lesions)

→ For all suspicious-appearing lesions.

→ Refer to physician for biopsy procedure per site-specific policy.

→ Refer to physician for surgical procedures and treatment regimens that fall outside scope of clinician's practice.

→ Refer to physician, preferably gynecological oncologist, all patients with melanoma.

PATIENT EDUCATION and FOLLOW-UP
(pertinent to all dark lesions)

→ Advise patient to inspect her vulva periodically and report significant changes in skin appearance and increased pain and/or bleeding of vulvar lesion(s). Frequency of self-examination and clinical examinations is individualized according to case presentation.

→ Serial photographs may be helpful in lesion follow-up.

→ Depending on initial pathology, decision to biopsy similar, recurring, benign-appearing lesions should be individualized. Consult with physician. If there is any doubt, biopsy.

→ Patients with malignant melanoma need more aggressive management. Education and psychological support are paramount. The physician responsible for the patient's care will educate her regarding nature of the disease, necessary treatment, surgical alternatives, potential complications, and required follow-up.

→ Sexual dysfunction is a common complication of radical vulvar surgery. Psychosexual support is extremely important for the patient's successful recovery. Referral for counseling may be necessary if patient undergoes major surgical intervention.

→ Document in progress notes and problem list.

12-TD VULVAR DISEASE
Small Lesions of the Vulva

Small lesions of the vulva rarely exceed 1 centimeter in diameter. They may be white, red, dull blue, or variegated in color. In general, small vulvar lesions have little in common. Etiologies differ and may include viruses, embryological remnants, trauma, duct blockage, or neoplasia. Although some lesions have a classic, textbook appearance, others can be diagnosed only by histopathology. Some growths are more prone to occur only in specific anatomic locations of the vulva (Friedrich 1983).

This protocol will cover several of the more common small lesions of the vulva, including *epidermal cysts (sebaceous cysts), acrochordon (skin tags), hemangiomas, caruncles (urethral),* and *Fox-Fordyce disease.* Condylomata acuminata is covered in the **Sexually Transmitted Diseases** Protocols. Molluscum contagiosum and furuncles and carbuncles are under the **Dermatological Disorders** Protocols.

Epidermal Cysts

Epidermal cysts are the most common small lesions of the vulva. Often erroneously called "sebaceous cysts," they are lined with keratinizing squamous epithelium and contain cellular debris with a sebaceous appearance and odor. The majority of these cysts arise from pilosebaceous ducts that have become occluded (Kaufman and Faro 1994). True sebaceous cells, however, are rarely found. Infection, fibrosis, or calcification may develop in an epidermal cyst (Friedrich 1983).

DATABASE

SUBJECTIVE

→ Patient is seldom symptomatic unless secondarily infected.

→ Patient may be aware of a lump, bump, or "knobby" sensation of vulva; cyst may slowly enlarge.

OBJECTIVE

→ Lesions:
- usually arise on labia majora.
- usually multiple (but may be single lesion), round, nontender, yellow.
- size ranges 5 mm to 2 cm in diameter; usually <1 cm.
- solid, firm to palpation; feels like a "BB shot."
- caseous, gritty, foul-smelling material inside.
- possible signs of secondary infection.

ASSESSMENT

→ Epidermal cyst
→ R/O syringoma
→ R/O hidradenoma
→ R/O accessory breast tissue
→ R/O fibroma
→ R/O lipoma

PLAN

DIAGNOSTIC TESTS

→ Excision for histopathological diagnosis when larger, isolated epidermal cyst cannot be recognized by inspection alone.

TREATMENT/MANAGEMENT

→ None unless cyst is annoying or cosmetically unacceptable to patient.

→ Removal can be done under local anesthesia. Alternately, a 20-gauge needle can be inserted into cyst and the contents expressed under gentle pressure. This treatment usually offers only temporary relief, as cyst contents tend to reaccumulate.

→ Acutely infected cysts may be treated with warm soaks or packs and incision and drainage (I & D). Excision may be performed to prevent recurrence.

CONSULTATION

→ Usually not indicated.

→ Refer patient to physician for removal under local anesthesia or in cases of infection for I & D.

PATIENT EDUCATION

→ Reassure and explain benign nature of the condition. Treatment is not usually advocated unless patient is bothered by cyst(s).

FOLLOW-UP

→ None specific unless secondarily infected.

→ Have patient return for reassessment after therapy as indicated.

→ Document in progress notes and problem list.

Acrochordon

These soft, fibroepithelial polyps are fleshy growths that are usually referred to as skin tags. The cause is unknown, and there is no malignant potential.

DATABASE

SUBJECTIVE

→ Usually asymptomatic.

→ Patient may be aware of bump or small, fleshy growth on vulva, adjacent medial aspect of the thigh, or perianal area.

OBJECTIVE

→ Structure is usually solitary, flesh-colored (though tip may be lighter), soft, wrinkled, polypoid. Usually on a pedicle but occasionally sessile. Resembles empty sac of skin. Multiple skin tags are usually widely separated.

→ Size ranges from several millimeters to more than 1 centimeter. Giant acrochordons may exist.

→ Repeated trauma or irritation may lead to swelling, ecchymosis, or ulceration. Twisting of the stalk may cause infarction (Friedrich 1983; Kaufman and Faro 1994).

ASSESSMENT

→ Acrochordon (also called skin tags)

→ R/O intradermal nevi

→ R/O accessory breast tissue

→ R/O hidradenoma

→ R/O neurofibroma

PLAN

DIAGNOSTIC TESTS

→ Excisional biopsy may be indicated when lesion is larger than 1 cm or if there is doubt about diagnosis (Friedrich 1983).

TREATMENT/MANAGEMENT

→ None indicated unless patient is disturbed by lesion, or in cases of chronic irritation.

→ Lesion may be removed by a variety of methods:
- under local anesthesia, cut lesion close to surface and apply ferric subsulfate (Monsel's solution), silver nitrate, or a single suture to control bleeding as indicated (Kaufman and Faro 1994).
- electrocautery, cryosurgery, laser (Friedrich 1983).

CONSULTATION

→ Referral to a physician may be necessary for removal.

PATIENT EDUCATION

→ Reassure and explain benign nature of condition. Treatment is not usually advocated unless patient is bothered by lesion.

FOLLOW-UP

→ None specific. Have patient return for reassessment after therapy as indicated.

→ Document in progress notes and problem list.

Hemangiomas

Unlike true neoplasms, hemangiomas are malformations of blood-vessel origin. Three forms affect the adult vulva: the cherry angioma, the angiokeratoma, and the pyogenic granuloma (Friedrich 1983).

DATABASE

SUBJECTIVE

Cherry angioma

→ Generally asymptomatic, but may bleed as a result of surface trauma.

→ Commonly appears in fourth or fifth decade of life.

→ May present as source of postmenopausal bleeding.

Angiokeratoma

→ Most develop during childbearing years.

→ Associated with or aggravated by pregnancy.

→ Usually asymptomatic unless irritated or ulcerated as result of trauma.

Pyogenic granuloma

→ More rare than cherry angioma and angiokeratoma.

→ Usually arises during pregnancy (analogous to gingival granuloma); may regress postpartum, but usually lingers and recurs.

→ Most symptomatic of vulvar hemangiomas, commonly with bleeding and chronic purulent exudate.

OBJECTIVE

Cherry angioma

→ Tiny, compressible papules, usually <2 mm to 3 mm; frequently multiple; located mostly on labia majora.

→ Bright-red to dark-blue color.

→ Can demonstrate blanching by running fingernail over lesion in linear fashion; may help differentiate this lesion from others.

Angiokeratoma

→ May be single or multiple; slightly lobulated, irregular, or papular with verrucous surface; located mostly on labia majora.

→ Dark-bright red, brown, blue, purple, or black color.

→ Size range 0.2 cm to 2.0 cm; usually not as abundant as cherry angioma.

Pyogenic granuloma

→ Usually single lesion with beefy red surface, often with raised collar of skin surrounding base; crust may cover lesion; may be sessile or pedunculated; located mostly on labia majora.

→ Dull-red to reddish-brown color, friable if traumatized.

→ May be tender to palpation with underlying induration.

→ Size range 0.5 cm to 2.0 cm; usually largest of vulvar hemangiomas.

ASSESSMENT

Cherry angioma

→ Assess as source of postmenopausal bleeding

Angiokeratoma

→ R/O melanoma, nevi, condyloma

Pyogenic granuloma

→ R/O basal cell carcinoma, malignant melanoma, hidradenoma

PLAN

DIAGNOSTIC TESTS

→ Excisional biopsy is warranted with angiokeratoma or pyogenic granuloma when diagnosis uncertain or with rapid lesion growth or bleeding.

TREATMENT/MANAGEMENT

Cherry angiomas

→ Usually requires no therapy but may be treated with excision, cryosurgery, electrocautery, or laser in cases of repeated bleeding (Friedrich 1983; Kaufman and Faro 1994).

Angiokeratomas

→ Can be treated with local excision if trauma causes pain or bleeding or if nature of the tumor cannot be determined on clinical grounds (Kaufman and Faro 1994).

Pyogenic granulomas

→ Should be treated with wide excision. If patient is pregnant, treatment may be deferred until postpartum (Friedrich 1983; Kaufman and Faro 1994).

CONSULTATION

→ As indicated for assessment of lesion.

→ Referral to physician may be necessary for biopsy and treatment.

PATIENT EDUCATION

→ Discuss benign nature of lesions and indications for treatment.

FOLLOW-UP

→ As indicated following therapy, if any.

→ Pyogenic granulomas may recur.

→ Document in progress notes and problem list.

Caruncle (urethral)

Although not a disorder of the vulva per se, a urethral caruncle is commonly found during pelvic examination. Urethral caruncles develop from ectropion of the posterior urethral wall, incident to postmenopausal shrinkage of vaginal mucosa, with subsequent mucosal changes caused by trauma and environmental conditions. Other causes for caruncle development are chronic irritation and infection of the urethral meatus. The term *caruncle* has been used to describe various urethral lesions, with prolapse of the urethral mucosa the entity most often mistaken for a caruncle. Urethral mucosal prolapse is a "sliding out" of the mucosa through the external meatus and is common during premenarchal or postmenopausal years due to estrogen deficiency (Kaufman and Faro 1994).

DATABASE

SUBJECTIVE

→ Patient is usually asymptomatic.

→ Patient may notice growth or lump.

→ Pain, bleeding, dysuria, or hematuria may be present.

→ Undergarments or coital activity may be prohibitive due to exquisite tenderness in some cases.

→ Lesion size does not always correspond to degree of discomfort, i.e., small lesions may be extremely tender.

→ In contrast, prolapse of urethral mucosa causes little pain or discomfort. Voiding difficulties may be present if edema occurs.

OBJECTIVE

→ Appears as red, friable, fleshy tumor in distal portion of urethral mucosa, usually at posterior meatus.

→ Usually single and sessile but may be pedunculated.

→ Size ranges from a few millimeters to one centimeter.

→ Carcinoma should be suspected if there is tenderness, induration, swelling, or masses along entire length of urethra, together with enlarged inguinal lymph nodes (Kaufman and Faro 1994).

ASSESSMENT

→ Urethral caruncle

→ R/O prolapse of the urethral mucosa

→ R/O hemangioma

→ R/O varices

→ R/O condyloma

→ R/O polyps

→ R/O carcinoma

PLAN

DIAGNOSTIC TESTS

→ Biopsy is rarely indicated but should be performed when carcinoma is suspected. Topical anesthesia may be applied prior to sampling. A small sample is sent for histopathological diagnosis.

TREATMENT/MANAGEMENT

→ Topical or oral estrogen may be prescribed. See **Perimenopausal Symptoms and Hormone Therapy** Protocol for dosage schedules.

→ Large or pedunculated lesions may be fulgurated or treated with laser (under local anesthesia) or cryotherapy.

→ Surgery may be required for large lesions.

CONSULTATION

→ As indicated for biopsy and/or therapy.

PATIENT EDUCATION

→ Discuss benign nature of condition and indications for treatment.

→ Discuss medication regimen.

FOLLOW-UP

→ As indicated by treatment plan.

→ Urethral caruncles may recur.

→ Document in progress notes and problem list.

Fox-Fordyce Disease

This entity is a disorder of the apocrine-gland duct at its opening into the hair follicle. It is characterized by chronic, multiple microcyst formation caused by retention of sweat in the ducts and excessive keratinization of the follicular epithelium. Etiology is unknown. Leakage of apocrine secretion into the dermis and epidermis causes intense pruritus, the hallmark of the disease (Friedrich 1983; Kaufman and Faro 1994).

DATABASE

SUBJECTIVE

→ Occurs in postpubertal, premenopausal women.

→ May affect vulva, axilla, or both.

→ Symptoms include intense pruritus, exacerbated with menstrual cycle.

→ Pregnancy ameliorates condition, which generally resolves after menopause.

OBJECTIVE

→ Mons pubis most often affected; axillary involvement helps establish diagnosis.

→ Closely grouped, discrete lesions; multiple, tiny, flesh-colored papules ranging in size from 1 mm to 3 mm in diameter.

→ No surrounding erythema or induration; normal skin overlying and separating papules.

→ Scratch marks may be present.

ASSESSMENT

→ Fox-Fordyce disease

→ R/O syringoma

→ R/O pediculosis pubis

PLAN

DIAGNOSTIC TESTS

→ None.

TREATMENT/MANAGEMENT

→ Topical estrogen: 1 mg estrone in peanut oil (Theelin®)/oz. petrolatum, applied TID (Friedrich 1983).

→ High-estrogenic oral contraceptives.

→ Anti-acne measures. See **Acne Vulgaris** Protocol.

→ Topical corticosteroids: Mild to mid-strength for relief of pruritus. See **Table 12TB.1, Potency Ranking of Topical Corticosteroids,** p. 12-228.

→ Ultraviolet lamp treatment; topical tretinoin (Retin-A®).

CONSULTATION

→ Refer to dermatologist if warranted.

→ As needed for prescription(s).

PATIENT EDUCATION

→ Discuss nature of condition and different therapies. Chronicity of the condition may be frustrating for patient. Offer support as indicated.

FOLLOW-UP

→ As indicated by treatment modality and symptom recurrence.

→ Document in progress notes and problem list.

12-TE VULVAR DISEASE
Large Lesions of the Vulva

Large lesions of the vulva most often start as small ones and thus may go unnoticed until they reach a significant size. Embarrassment and fear may prolong the delay in presenting to a clinician for care. This protocol covers *Bartholin's cysts/abcess* and *verrucous carcinoma*. Squamous cell carcinoma and lymphogranuloma venereum (LGV) begin as ulcerative conditions and may progress to large vulvar lesions. These entities are detailed in other vulvar disease protocols and in the **Sexually Transmitted Diseases** Protocols.

Bartholin's Cyst/Abscess

The Bartholin's glands are two mucus-secreting, glandular structures within the vulva, located on either side of the fourchette, which drain into the posterior introital area. Cysts of the gland arise within the duct system as a result of duct occlusion, resulting in subsequent mucus retention. The majority of cysts are unilocular and involve the main duct; however, deeper, multilocular cysts may also form. Mucus accumulation is, in part, a function of sexual stimulation. Thus the size of a cyst may vary in response to a given individual's degree of sexual activity.

The cause of most cysts remains unknown, but obstruction is postulated to result from various factors: congenital stenosis or atresia of the duct, thickened mucus near the duct opening, mechanical trauma, and, occasionally, improperly placed episiotomies and sutures. Primary Bartholin's cyst formation in a woman over age 40 years should arouse suspicion for a neoplasm (Friedrich 1983; Kaufman and Faro 1994).

An abscess forms when cystic fluid becomes infected. It was originally thought that abscesses were primarily caused by gonorrheal infection, but further re-search has shown a wide spectrum of organisms to be involved. The majority of infections occur secondary to any number of anaerobic, aerobic, or facultative organisms including *E. coli*, bacteroides, proteus, and peptostreptococcus species. *Chlamydia trachomatis* has also been identified as an involved pathogen, usually recovered from the cervix. Screening for sexually transmitted infections of the abscess and the cervix remains an important part of assessment. There has been one case report in the literature of bartholinitis-associated, toxic shock-like syndrome secondary to streptococcal exotoxin (Cort 1991; Kaufman and Faro 1994; Shearin, Boehlke, and Karanth 1989).

DATABASE

SUBJECTIVE

Cysts

→ Patients are mostly asymptomatic.

→ Symptoms may include:
  ▪ minor discomfort during intercourse.
  ▪ larger lesions that may interfere with walking, sitting, or intercourse.

Abscess

→ Multiple sexual partners increase the risk for STD-associated infection.

→ Usually develops rapidly within two to three days.

→ May rupture spontaneously within 72 hours.

→ Symptoms may include:
  ▪ varying degrees of pain or tenderness.
  ▪ difficulty sitting or walking.
  ▪ dyspareunia.

■ few systemic symptoms unless extensive inflammation.

OBJECTIVE

Cysts

→ May be incidental finding on routine pelvic examination.

→ Clinical features include:
- visible round or ovoid mass causing crescent-shaped vestibular entrance (posterior part of labia majora).
- nontender but tense, palpable swelling; usually unilateral.
- size varies from usually 1 cm to 4 cm; may reach 8 cm to 10 cm.

Abscess

→ Clinical features include:
- very tender, fluctuant mass; usually unilateral.
- edema, erythema of overlying skin.
- labial edema, distortion of labia on affected side.
- size rarely larger than 5 cm.
- impending rupture evidenced by area of softening or "pointing."

→ Bilateral abscess formation suggestive of gonorrheal infection.

ASSESSMENT

→ Bartholin's cyst

→ Bartholin's abscess

→ R/O carcinoma of Bartholin's gland

→ R/O STD

PLAN

DIAGNOSTIC TESTS

→ Cultures of purulent abscess fluid and cervix for *Neisseria gonorrhoeae* and *Chlamydia trachomatis* to rule out associated STD.

→ Additional tests may include:
- CBC for severe gland infection or inflammation.
- VDRL or RPR as indicated.

TREATMENT/MANAGEMENT

→ Most small, asymptomatic Bartholin's cysts require no therapy.

→ Treatment is indicated for:
- rapid cyst enlargement.
- increased pain, pressure, introital obstruction.
- hemorrhage into cyst cavity.

■ abscess formation.

→ The aim of therapy for both cysts and abscesses is to create a fistulous tract from the dilated duct to the vestibule (Friedrich 1993). Options include:
- I & D and insertion of Word catheter (single-lumen #10 catheter with 1-inch stem and inflatable balloon, sealed stopper on one end) is treatment for symptomatic cysts and acute abscess formation:
  - under local anesthesia, a small incision is made into the cyst/abscess. Purulent fluid is allowed to drain out. The balloon tip is inserted into cyst cavity, filled with 2 to 4cc of H_2O, and left in place for 30 days, with catheter stem up in vagina.
    - This "fistulization" method allows for patency of incision until epithelialization ensures a permanent ostium. Sitz baths several times a day initially may speed healing process (Cort 1991; Kaufman and Faro 1994). See **Figures 12TE.1, Word Catheter Ready for Insertion and After Inflation,** and **12TE.2, Inflatable Bulb-Tipped Catheter Used to Treat Bartholin's Cysts and Abscesses**.
    - Marsupialization for cysts with tendency for recurrent abscess formation: Under local or general anesthesia, a vertical incision is made in the vaginal mucosa over the cyst. The cyst wall is then sutured to the vaginal mucosa medially and skin of the introitus laterally, inferiorly, and superiorly.
      - ▸ A permanent outlet for gland secretions remains.
      - ▸ When general anesthesia is necessary, patient is admitted to come-and-go surgery.
      - ▸ This procedure is not performed on acutely infected cysts (Cort 1991; Kaufman and Faro 1994).

→ An acute abscess treated with sitz baths may spontaneously rupture within 72 hours, however, recurrence is likely.

→ Broad-spectrum antibiotics may be utilized for early treatment of bartholinitis; however, this approach may delay ripening of the abscess.

→ Excision of the gland (bartholinectomy) is not recommended due to increased morbidity (cellulitis, hemorrhage, hematoma, incomplete removal and subsequent recurrence, painful scar-tissue formation).

Figure 12TE.1.   WORD CATHETER READY FOR INSERTION (TOP) AND AFTER INFLATION (BOTTOM)

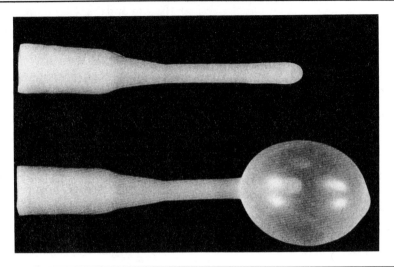

Source: Reprinted with permission from Friedrich, E.G., Jr. 1983. *Vulvar disease*, 2nd ed., p. 71. Philadelphia: W.B. Saunders.

- This procedure is reserved for patients with huge, multilocular, or recurrent painful cysts.
→ A recently developed procedure called the *window operation* has been advocated as a more effective way to treat Bartholin's cysts and recurrent abscesses. Under local anesthesia, a small piece of skin, including the cyst wall, is excised in an oval shape. Suturing is performed along the excised margin.
  - A new mucotaneous junction forms within 4 weeks.
  - Postoperative antibiotics are given in cases of acute inflammation (Cho, Ahn, and Cha 1990).
→ CO_2 laser has been used for treatment of cysts and abscesses.
→ Women over the age of 40 years with primary Bartholin's cyst formation should be referred to a physician for cyst removal to rule out a neoplasm.

CONSULTATION

→ Refer to physician as indicated for I & D procedure and placement of Word catheter.
→ Patients with recurrent symptomatic cysts and recurrent abscess formation should be referred to a gynecologist for marsupialization.
→ Women over the age of 40 years with primary Bartholin's cyst formation should be referred to a physician for cyst removal to rule out a neoplasm.

PATIENT EDUCATION

→ Reassure patients with asymptomatic cysts found on routine pelvic examination as to benign nature of condition. Advise them to report increased growth of cyst, pain, and/or obstruction interfering with daily activities and sexual intercourse.
→ Discuss etiology and nature of acute abscess.
→ Advise regarding STD potential and need for genital cultures and cultures of abscess.
→ Reinforce that, ideally, the Word catheter is to be left in place for 30 days. It is very difficult to replace the catheter once it falls out.
→ Detail symptom-relief measures after I & D or marsupialization. These include sitz baths, OTC analgesics (e.g., acetaminophen 325 mg p.o. every four hours prn pain), and rest.
→ After marsupialization, physician should discuss follow-up measures with patient.
→ Advise women with multiple sexual partners regarding safer sex practices. See **Table 13A.2, Safer Sex Practices,** p. 13-9.

FOLLOW-UP

→ Follow-up appointment prn and in 4-6 weeks for reassessment and removal of the Word catheter.
→ Document in progress notes and problem list.

Figure 12TE.2. INFLATABLE BULB-TIPPED CATHETER USED TO TREAT BARTHOLIN'S CYSTS AND ABSCESSES

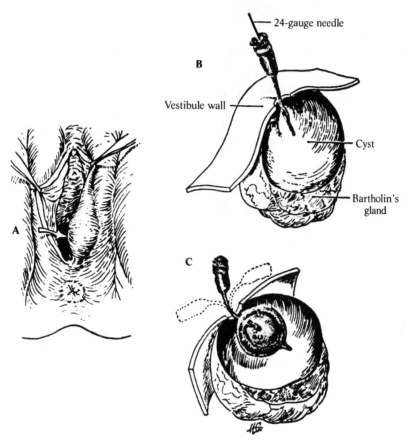

A. An arrow indicates the location for a stab wound in a cyst or abscess. **B.** Insertion of the catheter in the stab wound. **C.** Inserted catheter initiated with 2 ml to 4 ml water.

Source: Reprinted with permission from Word, B. 1964. New instrument for office treatment of cysts and abscesses of Bartholin's glands. *Journal of the American Medical Association* 190:777–778. Copyright 1964, American Medical Association.

Verrucous Carcinoma

Verrucous carcinoma is a lesion that clinically resembles a giant condyloma, except that verrucous cells have inversion or downward growth into the dermis. This carcinoma is an unusual variant of squamous cell carcinoma; it is slow-growing and locally invasive with a tendency for local recurrence despite radical excision. The disease does not spread by lymphatic or hematological channels; thus distant metastases do not occur. Etiology is unknown. Invasive squamous cell carcinoma and VIN may co-exist with verrucous carcinoma (DiSaia and Creasman 1989; Friedrich 1983; Kistner 1986; Morrow and Townsend 1981).

DATABASE

SUBJECTIVE

→ Seen more commonly in older women.

→ Symptoms may include:
- large, "cauliflower-like" growth.
- pruritus, bleeding.

OBJECTIVE

→ Clinical features may include:
- large/gigantic condyloma-like lesion.
- dramatic appearance.
- may involve oral cavity and extensive areas of the vulva.
- may resemble invasive cancer.

→ Vagina, cervix, uterus, adnexa, rectum WNL unless other pathologies coexist.

ASSESSMENT

→ Verrucous carcinoma

→ R/O condyloma acuminata

→ R/O granuloma inguinale

→ R/O lymphogranuloma venereum

→ R/O VIN

→ R/O invasive squamous cell carcinoma

PLAN

DIAGNOSTIC TESTS

→ Biopsy must be done to establish histopathological diagnosis.

→ Pap smear, genital cultures, wet mounts, VDRL, or RPR, and other diagnostic tests as indicated.

TREATMENT/MANAGEMENT

→ Refer to physician for wide local excision.

→ Radiation contraindicated (may convert lesion to highly malignant cancer).

→ Podophyllin, trichloroacetic acid, bichloroacetic acid have no effect.

CONSULTATION

→ Usually sought due to dramatic appearance of lesion. Refer to physician, as needed, for biopsy procedure.

→ Refer to gynecologist or gynecological oncologist for treatment.

PATIENT EDUCATION

→ Physician should discuss nature of disease and management with patient.

→ Psychological support is needed due to dramatic nature of disease presentation.

FOLLOW-UP

→ Lesion tends to recur locally; additional surgery warranted.

→ Semi-annual gynecological visits should be maintained.

→ Advise patient to inspect vulvar area carefully on a regular basis.

→ Document in progress notes and problem list.

12-TF VULVAR DISEASE
Ulcerative Lesions of the Vulva

Ulcers form as a result of a defect in skin integrity caused by localized destruction of the epidermis. Most ulcerative lesions of the vulva are the result of an infectious process, with STDs heading the list. Carcinomas of the vulva may also present as ulcerative lesions and should be considered, especially when the appearance of the lesion changes little over time (Friedrich 1983). This protocol will cover *squamous cell carcinoma* and *basal cell carcinoma*. Additional ulcerative lesions affecting the vulva—such as herpes simplex, syphilis, chancroid, lymphogranuloma venereum, and granuloma inguinale—are covered in the **Sexually Transmitted Diseases** Protocols.

Squamous Cell Carcinoma

Malignancies of the vulva account for three percent to five percent of all genital cancers in women and one percent to two percent of all female cancers in general. There are various histologies and wide differences in the biological behaviors of these tumors. The largest group is made up of squamous cell carcinomas. Other carcinomas of the vulva include basal cell carcinoma, verrucous carcinoma, and malignant melanoma. See **Large Lesions of the Vulva** and **Dark Lesions of the Vulva** protocols.

Invasive squamous cell carcinoma arises from the squamous epithelium of the skin and mucous membrane of the vulva (between the vaginal introitus and the outer labia majora). The cancer affects mainly women over age 60 years; however, the disease has recently occured in younger age groups (15 percent in women under age 40 years). Environmental factors, smoking, and viral infection—especially with HPV—may play a role in the etiology of the disease. In many cases, the initial lesion appears to arise from an area of VIN (DiSaia and

Creasman 1989). Fifteen percent to 20 percent of patients may have an antecedent, concomitant, or subsequent cervical carcinoma that is either in situ or invasive (Morrow and Townsend 1981).

Vulvar squamous cell carcinoma, if left untreated, has potentially disabling and fatal consequences, but early diagnosis and treatment may mean a cure. Unfortunately, the disease state is advanced at the time of diagnosis in most cases. Local extension of the malignancy to the urethra, perineum, vagina, and anorectum is common. In more advanced stages, the pubic bone, skin of the leg, and bladder may become involved. The hallmark of the disease is lymphatic spread that is systematic and predictable, first to the superficial groin nodes and then to the deeper pelvic-wall lymphatics (Morrow and Townsend 1981).

Several different methods have been devised to determine the depth of tumor invasion in superficially invasive disease. Microinvasive squamous cell carcinoma (Stage Ia) has been defined by the International Society for the Study of Vulvar Disease (ISSVD) as a lesion ≤2 cm in diameter with ≤1 mm of stromal invasion (Wilkinson, Kneale, and Lynch 1986). Since risk of lymph-node metastasis in these cases is minimal, radical therapy can be avoided (Richart et al. 1988).

A risk-scoring formula developed by the Gynecology Oncology Group (GOG) has also been utilized to identify patients at low risk for metastases or recurrence, allowing for more conservative therapy. The GOG criteria include patients with no clinically suspicious nodes, no tumor in lymphatic spaces, no tumor at a midline location, a grade 1 lesion no thicker than 5 mm, or a grade 2 lesion no thicker than 2 mm (Sedlis et al. 1988).

For advanced tumors, staging of vulvar cancer is done utilizing the FIGO (International Federation of Gynecology and Obstetrics) system, which incorporates a TNM (tumor-node-metastasis) classification. Patients are divided into stages based on the size and location of the lesion, the clinical status of groin nodes, and the presence or absence of demonstrable metastases (Friedrich 1983). (See **Table 12TF.1, International Federation of Gynecology and Obstetrics Classification of Gynecological Carcinomas.**) The prime factor determining the patient's prognosis is the presence or absence of inguinal-node metastasis. About 20 percent of patients with positive groin nodes will have pelvic lymph-node metastases; the pelvic nodes are almost never affected without groin-node involvement (Jones, Wentz, and Burnett 1988).

Survival depends on the extent of disease at the time of diagnosis. The five-year survival rate after complete surgical intervention—radical vulvectomy plus inguinal and pelvic lymphadenectomy—for Stages I and II disease is approximately 90 percent.

In contrast, only 20 percent of patients with pelvic-node metastases will survive five years or more (DiSaia and Creasman 1989). Recurrences are usually seen within one to two years after therapy. Local recurrences are more common than distant ones and are usually near the site of the primary lesion. The incidence of local recurrence after radical vulvectomy for Stage I cancer is reported to be about 10 percent (Richart et al. 1988).

Surgical treatment of the disease varies and depends on clinical staging. The undesirable effects of radical vulvectomy include sex-organ removal, potential wound-healing complications, and lymphedema. Psychosexual alterations may be a major component of recovery, and ongoing support is vital for patient acceptance of her changed being.

DATABASE

SUBJECTIVE

→ Risk factors may include:
  - chronic vulvar irritation.

Table 12TF.1. INTERNATIONAL FEDERATION OF GYNECOLOGY AND OBSTETRICS CLASSIFICATION OF GYNECOLOGICAL CARCINOMAS

Classification—Carcinoma of the Vulva

T-Primary Tumor

Tis	Preinvasive carcinoma (carcinoma in situ).
T 1	Tumor confined to the vulva and/or perineum; 2 cm or less in greatest dimension.
T 2	Tumor confined to the vulva and/or perineum; more than 2 cm in greatest dimension.
T 3	Tumor of any size with adjacent spread to the urethra and/or vagina and/or anus.
T 4	Tumor of any size infiltrating the bladder mucosa and/or the rectal mucosa, including the upper part of the urethral mucosa and/or fixed to the bone.

N-Regional Lymph Nodes

N 0	No lymph node metastasis.
N 1	Unilateral regional lymph node metastasis.
N 2	Bilateral regional lymph node metastasis.

M-Distant Metastasis

M 0	No clinical metastases.
M 1	Distant metastasis (including pelvic lymph node metastasis).

Definitions of Clinical Stages—Carcinoma of the Vulva

Stage 0	Tis	Carcinoma in situ, intraepithelial carcinoma.
Stage I	T1 N0 M0	Tumor confined to the vulva and/or perineum; 2 cm or less in greatest dimension; no nodal metastasis.
Stage II	T2 N0 M0	Tumor confined to the vulva and/or perineum; more than 2 cm in greatest dimension; no nodal metastasis.
Stage III	T3 N0 M0	Tumor of any size with
	T3 N1 M0	adjacent spread of lower urethra and/or vagina, or the anus, and/or
	T1 N1 M0	unilateral regional lymph node metastasis.
	T2 N1 M0	
Stage IVA	T1 N2 M0	Tumor invades any of the following: upper urethra, bladder mucosa, rectal mucosa, pelvic bone, and/or bilateral,
	T2 N2 M0	regional node metastasis.
	T3 N2 M0	
	T4 Any N M0	
Stage IVB	Any T	Any distant metastasis including pelvic lymph nodes.
	Any N	
	M1	

Source: Reprinted with permission from DiSaia, P.J., and W. T. Creasman. 1989. *Clinical gynecologic oncology*. 3d ed., p. 653. St. Louis: C.V. Mosby.

- VIN.
- HPV infection.
- obesity, diabetes, hypertension, arteriosclerosis; may reflect increased incidence with aging.
- low socioeconomic status.
- immunodeficiency; may exist in younger subsets of women.

→ Classically occurs in women 60 years to 70 years old; 15 percent of cases are in women less than 40 years old; no racial predilection.

→ No remission or exacerbation.

→ Woman may have had symptoms for two to 16 months prior to seeking attention; medical therapy for lesion may have occurred for 12 months or longer without biopsy or referral for definitive diagnosis.

→ Asymptomatic in up to 20 percent of cases.

→ Symptoms may include:
- chronic, long-term pruritus.
- lump, mass (more than 50 percent of cases), ulcer, warty growth.
- external dysuria.
- contact bleeding.
- pain.

→ A complete health history should be taken.

OBJECTIVE

→ Majority of lesions on labia majora, labia minora, clitoris, but any vulvar site possible.

→ One-third of tumors are bilateral or midline (increased incidence of nodal spread).

→ Lesions may have *widely* variable presentation:
- size varies from <1 cm to huge.
- usually localized, unifocal, well demarcated.
- may be multifocal or confluent (less often).
- white, pink, red, or pigmented.
- flat, nodular, papular, or exophytic.
- edges sharply rolled with underlying induration.
- dry or exudative.
- ulcerated (one-third of cases).
- friable; bleeding.
- painless or tender.
- possible secondary infection.

→ Physical examination should include careful assessment of:
- extent of lesion: Visual inspection—note proximity to urethra, vagina, labial-crural folds, and anus.
- mobility of lesion: Palpate well.

- skin of inguinal area, mons pubis, perineum: Palpate for associated lesion, nodules.
- inguinal lymph nodes: Inspect and palpate well—note enlargement, fixation, ulceration, suppuration (indicates advanced disease); classify as not palpable, palpable but not clinically suspicious, palpable and clinically suspicious, fixed, or ulcerated (Jones, Wentz, and Burnett 1988).
- integrity of pelvic floor.
- peripheral pulses.
- uterus, adnexa, rectum for abnormalities.

→ A good description and diagram of the lesion is important.

ASSESSMENT

→ Squamous cell carcinoma
→ R/O VIN
→ R/O non-neoplastic epithelial disorder (vulvar dystrophy)
→ R/O granuloma inguinale
→ R/O lymphogranuloma venereum
→ R/O syphilis
→ R/O herpes genitalis
→ R/O condyloma acuminata
→ R/O tuberculosis of the vulva
→ R/O concomitant vaginal/cervical neoplasia

PLAN

DIAGNOSTIC TESTS

→ Biopsy must be done to establish histopathological diagnosis. Punch biopsy (under local anesthesia) from center of lesion may be undertaken if lesion is small. Lesions ≤1 cm may be totally excised under local anesthesia; consult with or refer to physician.

→ Pap smear, genital cultures, wet mounts, VDRL or RPR, other diagnostic tests as indicated

→ Colposcopy of the vagina and cervix should be performed to rule out concomitant neoplasia.

→ Cystoscopy and/or anoscopy should be performed if bladder or rectal involvement is suspected.

→ Preoperative studies vary and depend on the extent of disease and general health of patient. Additional tests may include complete blood count, urinalysis, complete biochemical profile, chest x-ray, EKG, proctoscopy, barium enema, intravenous pyelogram, bone scan, CT scan.

TREATMENT/MANAGEMENT

→ Refer patient to gynecological oncologist.

→ Treatment is individualized based on lesion size and location, depth of tumor invasion, lymphatic involvement, health and wishes of patient, condition of unaffected vulva, presence or absence of other gynecological problems, other signs of genital tract neoplasia (Morrow and Townsend 1981).

→ Treatment options include (DiSaia and Creasman 1989):
- wide local excision.
- wide local excision with superficial inguinal lymphadenectomy.
- simple (unilateral) vulvectomy with unilateral or bilateral inguinal lymphadenectomy.
- radical vulvectomy with unilateral or bilateral inguinal lymphadenectomy.
- radical vulvectomy with unilateral or bilateral inguinal and pelvic lymphadenectomy.
- combined radiation and surgery. Radiation alone is not used as primary therapy but may be used for inoperable, locally recurrent disease.
- exenteration for advanced disease.
- chemotherapy (under investigation).

CONSULTATION

→ As necessary for initial assessment.

→ Referral to physician for initial biopsy procedure may be necessary.

→ Referral to gynecologist or gynecological oncologist for treatment.

PATIENT EDUCATION

→ The physician responsible for the patient's care should discuss etiology and nature of condition with patient, and outline the details of management. Components include surgical alternatives and potential complications, recovery, and sexuality issues.

→ Despite potential overwhelming nature of the disease, successful treatment with acceptable morbidity and long-term survival is possible. Hope is an important message.

→ Psychosocial support is extremely important for the patient's ongoing health and well-being. A clinical nurse specialist in oncology may be utilized for patient education and support. Referrals for psychosexual counseling may be necessary for successful recovery and ability to cope.

→ Since HPV has been implicated in carcinoma of the vulva, safer sex practices are important for the prevention of STD. See **Table 13A.2, Safer Sex Guidelines,** p. 13-9.

FOLLOW-UP

→ Patient will generally be followed by the physician responsible for her care. Specific return visit will be set up according to individual patient's needs and will vary from site to site.

→ Biopsy of all recurring, suspicious-appearing lesions should be undertaken promptly.

→ Document in the progress notes and problem list.

Basal Cell Carcinoma

Basal cell carcinoma is a locally invasive malignancy that generally does not metastasize. It is commonly found on exposed body surfaces but is rare on the vulva, accounting for only two percent to three percent of all vulvar cancer. General cure rates are 100 percent, and if margins are tumor-free, the prognosis is excellent. Regional lymph nodes and lungs have been affected in some cases. Local recurrences are common, about 20 percent of cases. A mixed basal-squamous cell carcinoma may also exist; this lesion has a poorer prognosis than pure basal cell carcinoma alone (Kaufman, Friedrich, and Gardner 1989).

Multiple theories exist regarding the histogenesis of the disorder and discussion is beyond the scope of this protocol. The tumor's origin is thought to be immature, incompletely differentiated "pluripotential" cells of the basal epithelium, hair shaft, or glands (Kaufman and Faro 1994).

DATABASE

SUBJECTIVE

→ Most often affects Caucasian women in the postmenopausal years; median age 63 years.

→ Patient may be asymptomatic.

→ Symptoms may include:
- pruritus.
- irritation.
- burning.
- chronic ulceration.
- presence of nodule or mass.
- bleeding or discharge if lesion is large.

OBJECTIVE

→ Lesions usually found on labia majora; other sites may include labia minora, clitoris, mons pubis, fourchette.

→ Clinical presentation may include:
  - pearly, "rolled edge," or "rodent" ulcer (one-third of basal cell carcinomas present as ulcers).
  - polypoid or nodular lesion; usually <2 cm in diameter.
  - red or brown pigmentation; can present as freckle-like lesion.
  - necrotic debris or crusts may appear at lesion base.
  - secondary infection with inguinal adenopathy may occur.

→ Lesion may extend beyond limits of physical borders. Good description and diagram of lesion are important.

→ Vagina, cervix, uterus, adnexa, rectum WNL unless other pathologies coexist.

ASSESSMENT

→ Basal cell carcinoma

→ R/O mixed basal-squamous cell carcinoma

→ R/O concomitant squamous cell carcinoma

→ R/O nevus

→ R/O melanoma

→ R/O herpes genitalis

→ R/O syphilis

→ R/O hidradenitis

PLAN

DIAGNOSTIC TESTS

→ Biopsy must be done to establish histopathological diagnosis. Consult with or refer to physician.

→ Pap smear, genital cultures, wet mounts, VDRL or RPR, other diagnostic tests as indicated.

TREATMENT/MANAGEMENT

→ Wide and deep local excision, including area of normal-appearing tissue, is treatment of choice. Multiple sections through tumor should be excised to rule out concomitant squamous cell carcinoma or melanoma. Refer to physician.

→ Lymph-node dissection usually not necessary due to low potential for metastasis.

→ 5-Fluorouracil (Efudex®) not recommended; may mask invasive basal cell cancer.

CONSULTATION

→ As necessary for initial assessment of lesion.

→ Refer to physician for biopsy procedure as necessary.

→ Refer to gynecologist or gynecological oncologist for treatment.

PATIENT EDUCATION

→ The physician responsible for the patient's care should discuss both the etiology and the nature of the condition with the patient, and detail the particulars of management.

FOLLOW-UP

→ Since recurrence is fairly common, ongoing clinical observation of vulvar area should be done at least semi-annually.

→ Advise patient to inspect her vulvar area regularly.

→ Recurrent tumors may require more aggressive therapy.

→ Document in progress notes and problem list.

12-TG VULVAR DISEASE

Vulvar Intraepithelial Neoplasia

Vulvar intraepithelial neoplasia (VIN) is a premalignant condition characterized by a disorientation of epithelial architecture that extends throughout its full thickness. By definition, VIN is confined to the basement membrane of the epidermis with no extension to the underlying dermis. Intraepithelial disorders have been grouped as follows (Committee on Terminology of the International Society for the Study of Vulvar Disease 1990):

   I. Squamous (may include HPV change).
     A. VIN I (mild dysplasia).
     B. VIN II (moderate dysplasia).
     C. VIN III (severe dysplasia or carcinoma in situ).
   II. Other.
     A. Paget's disease (intraepithelial).
     B. Melanoma in situ, level I.

In the past, the condition was referred to by various names: Bowen's disease, Bowenoid papulosis, erythroplasia of Queyrat, carcinoma in situ simplex, and squamous cell carcinoma in situ. Today the more commonly used terminology is VIN.

Neoplasia results from cellular changes precipitated by an oncogenic stimulus, which is then modified by the host reaction. The chromosomal makeup of the epithelial cell's deoxyribonucleic acid is altered, new cell properties emerge, and uncontrolled replication occurs. The incidence of VIN has dramatically increased over the past 20 years. The disease now affects younger women, the majority of whom are under the age of 50 years. VIN is closely associated with the presence of HPV, especially HPV-16, and HPV-18. Carcinoma in situ of the cervix is an associated finding in approximately 20 percent of patients with VIN. Vaginal and anal neoplasia may also coexist (Friedrich 1983; Kaufman and Faro 1994).

Early invasive disease is seen in six percent to ten percent of patients with VIN, with elderly and immunocompromised women at increased risk. Progression of VIN to invasive carcinoma may occur over time but the frequency is unknown. Aggressiveness of the lesions cannot be based on clinical factors such as symptoms, lesion location, and past history. Depending on host defense mechanisms, there is a possibility that VIN will *not* progress to an invasive disease state if left untreated (Chafe et al. 1988; DePetrillo et al. 1987; Friedrich 1983; Kaufman and Faro 1994; Morgan and Wilkinson, 1988). See **Red Lesions of the Vulva**, "Paget's Disease," and **Dark Lesions of the Vulva**, "Melanoma" protocols.

DATABASE

SUBJECTiVE

  → Risk factors may include:
    ■ HPV infection.
    ■ HSV infection.
    ■ multiple sexual partners.
    ■ smoking.
    ■ immunodeficiency.
    ■ oral contraceptives.
    ■ chronic vulvar irritation.
    ■ lighter skin pigmentation.

  → Onset generally in women under age 50 years; can occur in teenagers and women in their 20s.

  → Fifty percent of women asymptomatic.

  → Symptoms may include:
    ■ pruritus (most common symptom).
    ■ pain, soreness, burning, swelling.
    ■ warts, lumps, nodules, presence of tumor.

- bleeding, discharge, ulceration.
- discoloration.

OBJECTIVE

→ Lesions may first be noted during routine pelvic examination; may be subtle.

→ Distribution of lesions in decreasing order of frequency (Chafe et al. 1988):
- labia minora.
- perineum.
- perianal.
- labia majora.
- clitoris.

→ Multifocal distribution more common in 30-year-to 50-year-olds; malignant transformation rare unless immunocompromised.

→ Unifocal distribution more common in post-menopausal women, especially those over 60 years old; greater incidence of superficial invasion.

→ VIN I-II lesions (Kaufman and Faro 1994):
- well localized and delineated.
- slightly elevated, white, and rough.
- red-brown hue, and/or red and white patches less commonly.

→ VIN III lesions (Kaufman and Faro 1994):
- widely variable appearance.
- majority are multifocal; extensive areas may be involved.
- red, moist, crusted, sharply demarcated.
- small, isolated red or white patch.
- distinct white patch; may have distinct red appearance.
- combination of red and white areas with superficial scaling.
- condyloma-like.
- hyperpigmented, entirely or at legion margins.

→ Lesions that are ulcerated, indurated and/or granular, raised and irregular may indicate invasive disease.

→ Vagina, cervix, uterus, adnexa, and rectum within normal limits unless co-existent pathology.

→ A good description and diagram of the lesion is important.

ASSESSMENT

→ VIN

→ R/O condyloma

→ R/O invasive cancer

→ R/O other dermatological conditions

PLAN

DIAGNOSTIC TESTS

(Kaufman and Faro 1994):

→ Early diagnosis depends on regular, careful examination of vulva. Index of suspicion for VIN is important parameter. White, ulcerated, nodular, fissured, or abnormally raised areas should be biopsied.

→ Histological evaluation of biopsy specimen from suspicious lesions will render definitive diagnosis. Delineation of extent of disease is critical and invasion must be ruled out. The use of toluidine blue may be of value in determining biopsy sites, especially with a single extensive lesion or with multiple ones. Multiple biopsy samples with the Keye's punch may be necessary.

→ Colposcopy of the vulva after three percent to five percent acetic acid application may be used to identify sites for biopsy. Colposcopy of vagina, cervix, anus may also be performed to rule out concomitant intraepithelial neoplasia.

→ Careful inspection of the anal canal via proctoscopy is indicated when carcinoma in situ involves the perineum.

→ Determination of skin appendage involvement must be made.
NOTE: Diagnostic evaluation is usually performed by the physician in most settings; however, practices may vary. Biopsy and colposcopic procedures should be performed by a properly trained, experienced practitioner.

→ Pap smear, genital cultures, wet mounts, other diagnostic tests as indicated.

TREATMENT/MANAGEMENT

→ If VIN is confirmed, refer patient to physician for treatment.

→ Treatment should be individualized based on patient's age and wishes, location and extent of lesion, and risk factors that may increase risk of invasive disease.

→ Treatment options include (DiSaia and Creasman 1989; Kaufman and Faro 1994; Roy 1988):
- wide local excision used when VIN diagnosis indefinite or when invasion cannot be ruled out.
- CO_2 laser vaporization: Performed under local anesthesia with colposcopic guidance; most popular therapeutic modality after invasion definitely ruled out; may be carried out in

stages if lesion large; general anesthesia may be necessary if treating large areas at one time.
- skinning vulvectomy (with or without skin graft): Indicated when VIN extensive; refer patient to gynecological oncologist skilled in this technique.
→ Alternate (but less acceptable) therapeutic modalities:
- topical 5-fluorouracil 2 percent to 5 percent (Efudex®): Thoroughly massaged into affected vulvar tissue TID for up to 1 month (DiSaia and Creasman 1989). Rarely used due to extreme patient discomfort, poor efficacy, and high recurrence rates.
- cryotherapy.
- electrocautery.
NOTE: Occult, invasive squamous cell carcinoma must be ruled out prior to any local destructive therapy.

CONSULTATION

→ Referral to physician will usually be necessary for lesion evaluation, and for biopsy procedure.
→ Referral to gynecologist or gynecological oncologist will be necessary to accomplish specific therapeutic modalities.

PATIENT EDUCATION

→ Primary health-care provider may discuss etiology and nature of disease with patient. The physician responsible for care of patient should detail the particulars of management and necessary follow-up.
→ As HPV infection is associated with this condition, advise safer sex practices to prevent sexually transmitted diseases. See **Table 13A.2, Safer Sex Guidelines,** p. 13-9.

FOLLOW-UP

→ Long-term follow-up is necessary due to the relatively high risk of recurrence.
→ Site-specific guidelines for follow-up may vary. In general, follow-up examinations include careful visual inspection; colposcopy of the vulva, vagina, and cervix; and Pap smear every three to six months for two years.
→ Psychosexual counseling may be indicated for the patient undergoing significant vulvar surgery.
→ Document in progress notes and problem list.

12-TH VULVAR DISEASE
Vulvodynia

The International Society for the Study of Vulvar Disease (ISSVD) defines *vulvodynia* as chronic vulvar discomfort often characterized by burning, stinging, irritation, or rawness (ISSVD Committee 1991). The incidence and prevalence are unknown, and many etiologies have been implicated. The parameters of vulvodynia, established originally in 1977 by Dodson and Friedrich, included persistent symptoms of long-standing duration, lack of demonstrable pathology, sexual inactivity as a result of symptoms, unsuccessful consultation with multiple physicians, "allergy" to common vaginal preparations, reluctance to accept a psychophysiological cause, and emotional lability or dependency (Lynch 1986).

The approach to vulvodynia has changed since the initial parameters were set up, and continued investigation attempts to establish more appropriate definitions of the disorder. McKay (1992) established subsets of vulvodynia, including dermatoses, infection, vestibulitis, iatrogenic factors, and dysesthetic (essential) vulvodynia. *Vulvar dermatoses* include inflammatory dermatoses—irritant dermatitis, lichen planus, and other erosive conditions—and lichen sclerosus. *Infectious causes* include *Candida*, HPV, and HSV. Of these, *Candida* is the most significant infectious agent to consider in the evaluation of a patient with vulvodynia, as it may cause a cyclical vulvitis, which is defined as episodic vulvodynia with symptom-free periods between recurrences. Immune response factors, allergy or hypersensitivity to the *Candida* organism, or changes in the vaginal ecosystem may be responsible for these cyclical recurrences.

HPV was once thought the most likely cause of vulvodynia; however, it is now considered significant only in certain cases. Acute, recurring herpes simplex lesions

may cause episodic burning. Nonlesional, recurrent infection may produce symptom patterns associated with pudendal neuralgia.

Vulvar vestibulitis is a syndrome of unknown etiology, characterized by chronic, nonspecific inflammation of the area around the minor vestibular glands in the superficial stroma of the vestibular tissue. The condition may be acute but is generally chronic and persistent, with resultant severe dyspareunia and vulvodynia. Researchers have attempted to demonstrate many causes: acute or chronic vulvovaginal infectious processes (especially *Candida* and HPV), altered vaginal pH balance (e.g., in association with estrogen-deficient states, bacterial vaginosis, decreased or absent lactobacilli), autoimmune reactions, irritants (e.g., soaps, douches, and sprays), chemical therapeutic agents, topical medications, postinflammatory tissue damage, and hypersensitivity reactions to an undetermined agent. Recent data suggest a disorder of the urogenital sinus-derived epithelium.

All in all, the etiology of this condition remains obscure; however, vestibulitis represents the most significant component to evaluate in vulvodynia of multifactorial origin (Dotters and Droegemueller 1989; ISSVD 1991; Kaufman and Faro 1994; Marinoff and Turner 1991; McKay 1988, 1989a,b, 1992; Turner and Marinoff 1988).

Iatrogenic factors include side effects of topical steroids (secondary or periorificial dermatitis due to a rebound inflammatory reaction after steroid medication is withdrawn), complications of CO_2 laser therapy, and sequelae of alcohol injections (McKay 1992).

Dysesthetic (essential) vulvodynia refers to a burning-type pain that is constant, diffuse, and unremitting. Its etiology may lie in a neurological problem

Table 12TH.1. DIFFERENTIAL DIAGNOSIS OF VULVODYNIA: PATTERNS OF DISCOMFORT

Symptom Pattern	Dyspareunia	Physical Findings	"Typical Patient"	Diagnosis	Treatment
Cyclical itching and burning, often related to menses; responds to anticandial agents but recurs; topical drugs may irritate	Irritation after coitus; severe with flares	Variable erythema and edema, minimal vaginal discharge; fissures may occur with intercourse; episodic scaling and pustules	Premenopausal or receiving estrogen replacement, history of frequent *Candida* infection; frequent use of antibiotics for sinus condition, urinary tract infection, or acne; usually better on anticandidal drugs but recurrence frequent	Cyclical vulvovaginitis seems related to *Candida* infection but exact mechanism unknown	4-6 months of low-dose systemic ketoconazole or vaginal anticandidal agents
"Irritated" mucosa; poor tolerance of topical medications; corticosteroids may help, then flare symptoms	Often irritated after coitus	Variable erythema; mucosal telangiectasias, sebaceous hyperplasia, or papular eruption over labia majora	History of frequent or chronic use of fluorinated or full-strength topical steroid; often culture-positive *Candida*	Periorificial dermatitis due to topical steroids or irritant reaction; *Candida* infection common	Taper steroids, treat with anticandidal drugs every other day while patient takes steroids; avoid irritating topical agents
"Irritated mucosa," relieved after treatment for HPV but recurrent	Discomfort at entry, after coitus, or both	Papillomatous appearance of mucosal surfaces; ± condyloma; erythema and hyperemia variable	History of HPV infection or koilocytosis in some; others are simply reaction pattern	Vestibular papillomatosis; HPV (condyloma)	Do not treat papillomatosis unless proven related to HPV; recurrent HPV (condyloma) may be treated with BCA/TCA, laser, ± 5-FU
Pain mainly with intercourse	Specific pain at entry; may prevent intercourse	Point tenderness to cotton-swab palpitation of vestibular gland orifices	Usually sexually active until onset of pain; previous inflammatory episodes likely (including following laser surgery)	Vulvar vestibulitis	Multiple therapies tried: sitz baths, low-potency steroids, coital lubricants, topical anesthetics, interferon, surgery, etc.
Constant burning, not related to touch or pressure	Not necessarily	Variable or no erythema; often other perineal symptoms	Usually postmenopausal, often not receiving estrogen replacement	Dysesthetic vulvodynia, pudendal neuralgia	Low-dose amitriptyline to control symptoms

Note: HPV = human papillomavirus infection; 5-FU = 5-fluorouracil; TCA = tricholoracetic acid.

Source: Adapted with permission from McKay, M. 1992. Vulvodynia: Diagnostic patterns. *Dermatology Clincs* 10(2):423-433.

related to altered cutaneous perception or damaged sensory nerves. When considering a diagnosis of dysesthetic vulvodynia, one should attempt to differentiate sensory input (pudendal neuralgia) from nerve injury (reflex sympathetic dystrophy). In pudendal neuralgia, sensory input factors may cause pain that radiates out from the vulva to the perineum, groin, or thighs, similar to the pain found in postherpetic neuralgia. Reflex sympathetic dystrophy (RSD) is an umbrella term for superficial, burning-type pain thought to be due to a previous nerve injury, though difficult to prove in most cases. The pain of a sympathetic nerve injury tends to spread beyond its original dermatomal pattern.

Proposed etiologies for dysesthetic vulvodynia include HSV, orthopedic problems of the back (osteoporosis, back injury, disk herniation, space-occupying lesion), postsurgical or nonsurgical trauma and sports

trauma, and, more rarely, neurofibroma and multiple sclerosis (Kaufman and Faro 1994; McKay 1988, 1989a,b, 1992; Turner and Marinoff 1991). (See **Table 12TH.1, Differential Diagnosis of Vulvodynia: Patterns of Discomfort.**)

The patient with vulvodynia has often sought out many health care providers in search for a diagnosis and cure. In some cases, she exhibits much frustration and anger toward the medical establishment for its limited success in diagnosis and treatment. Though often told her problem is primarily psychological, "the patient with vulvodynia is no more psychologically unbalanced than one with atopic dermatitis or acne" (McKay 1992, 432). These women present a diagnostic challenge, and psychological support is paramount in their care.

DATABASE

SUBJECTIVE

→ Woman is typically white, 20 years to 30 years old (except in essential vulvodynia, where woman is generally postmenopausal); may have long-standing history of vulvodynia (months to years) and many provider visits.

→ Primary psychological disease may be present in a select group of women. Symptoms of depression are common.

→ Initial episode of acute pain may be traced to specific event: vulvovaginitis, allergic or irritant reaction to topical agent (e.g., soap, steroid, podophyllin or bi- or trichloroacetic acid, or 5-fluorouracil [Efudex®]).

→ Exposure (known or unknown) to HPV may have occurred within the preceding three to nine months or longer.

→ May have history of recurrent candidiasis, herpes genitalis, HPV, allergies, general or gynecological surgery, orthopedic problems, and/or trauma to the genital area.

→ Symptom constellation may include:
 - vulvodynia (burning, stinging, irritation, or rawness). Pain may be intermittent or constant, localized, bilateral and/or symmetrical; almost always in vulvar vestibule (posterior fourchette most commonly involved).
   • Symptoms most common in vestibulitis; may also be reported in dermatoses and cyclical infections (*Candida*, HSV).
   • May also report swelling, redness at posterior fourchette.
 - itching, erythema, edema, "split" skin, irregularity or roughness of skin surface, fissures, vaginal discharge.
   • Symptoms more common in dermatoses, cyclical infections.
 - symptom recurrence at menses or postcoitally.
   • Symptoms mostly associated with cyclical *Candida* infection.
 - dysuria, urgency, frequency; absence of lubrication.
   • Symptoms associated with vestibulitis.
 - precipitation of symptoms by sexual intercourse or pressure exerted at vestibular area, e.g., tampon insertion, bicycle or horseback riding, tight clothing.
   • Symptoms most common in vestibulitis.
 - sensation of pins and needles, "crawling"; episodic superficial burning radiating from vulva to perineum, groin, thighs; deep aching; itch-burn sensation; lancinating or stabbing pain; burning pain with light touch (clothing, water, pubic-hair motion); dyspareunia with both intromission and deep penetration.
   • Symptoms mostly associated with essential vulvodynia due to pudendal neuralgia or RSD.
 - redness and generalized burning when topical steroid withdrawn from use on vulva (rebound inflammatory reaction, periorificial dermatitis).
 - dyspareunia, decreased coital frequency (may be associated with vulvodynia of any cause).
   • Entry dyspareunia more common in vestibulitis.
   • Dyspareunia with penile penetration, and during and after intercourse more common with pudendal neuralgia.

→ Aggravating factors may include:
 - sexual activity: Intromission, masturbation.
 - recurrent vulvovaginitis.
 - physical activities.
 - sweating.
 - rubbing of clothing, tampons.
 - topical creams, ointments (lubricants, steroids, anesthetics).

→ Relieving factors may include:
 - tub baths.
 - ice packs.
 - bed rest.

→ History should include:
 - thorough symptom evaluation (onset, location, duration, course, quality and quantity of pain, associated symptoms, aggravating and relieving factors).
 - menstrual cycle history.
 - previous vulvovaginal infections (e.g., candidiasis, trichomonas, bacterial vaginosis, condyloma, other STDs).
 - careful search for mechanical and chemical irritants, use of topical or systemic medication.
 - contraceptive history.
 - sexual history, including history of sexual abuse/trauma and sexual dysfunction.
 - sexual-partner history and symptomatology.
 - past and present dermatological and orthopedic conditions.
 - surgical history.
 - habits (drugs, alcohol, exercise, nutrition etc.).
 - stress level, psychological history.

OBJECTIVE

→ A thorough, systematic examination of the genitalia from labia majora inward must be performed to assess all potential etiologies of vulvodynia. Diagrams are helpful in detailing anatomic distribution of involved areas(s).

→ Clinical features may include:
- pelvic examination:
  - labia majora: Erythema, edema, papules, pustules, architectural skin changes, fissuring, herpetic lesions may be present; satellite pustules may appear at edges of vulva; interlabial fissures may occur.
    - Diagnostic considerations include inflammatory dermatoses, lichen sclerosus, infectious states (*Candida*, HPV, HSV), periorificial dermatitis, postalcohol scarring.
  - labia minora/vestibule: Multiple, small cutaneous papillae and acetowhitening (see "Diagnostic Tests" section); papillomatosis may be present normally or in subclinical HPV infection; herpetic lesions may be present; interlabial fissures may occur.
    - Diagnostic considerations include HPV/papillomatosis, HSV, lichen sclerosus.
  - vestibule: Erythematous foci may be present at 5 o'clock and 7 o'clock (at ducts of Bartholin's glands); exquisite pain to light touch with saline-moistened cotton swab may be present at base of hymen or fourchette, parameatal, or subfrenular areas of vestibule; erythema at introitus; shallow ulcers adjacent to hymenal ring; fissuring of posterior fourchette, or herpetic lesions may also be present.
    - Diagnostic considerations include vestibulitis, *Candida* infection, HSV.
  - perineum: Thickened surgical scar, palpable nodule, herpetic lesions, or fissures may be present. Diagnostic considerations include pudendal neuralgia, HSV, lichen sclerosus.
  - vagina: Erythema, abnormal discharge may be present when infectious states exist; thickened surgical scar, palpable nodule may be present.
    - Diagnostic considerations include *Candida* infection, HSV, pudendal neuralgia.
  - cervix, uterus, adnexa, rectovaginal examinations are usually WNL unless there is coexistent pathology.
- additional examination components:

- sensory testing with cotton swab and sharp pin in vestibule and labial areas may be utilized to assess pudendal neuralgia, as other physical findings are nonspecific. May need to consult with or refer patient to neurologist. Any of the following may be found (McKay 1992; Taber 1985; Turner and Marinoff 1991):
  - allodynia—pain elicited by stimulus that does not normally cause pain (e.g., light touch).
  - hyperalgesia—exaggerated response to painful stimulus.
  - hyperpathia—increased reaction to repetitive stimulus; delayed reaction; radiating sensation; after sensation.
  - hypoesthesia—decreased sensitivity to stimuli.
  - hyperesthesia—increased sensitivity to sensory stimuli such as pain or touch; may extend from mons to upper inner thighs and posteriorly across ischial tuberosities.

→ See also "Diagnostic Tests" section.

ASSESSMENT

→ Vulvodynia

→ R/O inflammatory/erosive vulvar dermatoses: irritant dermatitis, lichen planus, lupus erythematosus, bullous dermatoses, apthosis, Behçet's syndrome

→ R/O infectious states (*Candida*, HSV, HPV)

→ R/O subclinical HPV infection

→ R/O papillomatosis

→ R/O vulvar vestibulitis

→ R/O iatrogenic vulvodynia

→ R/O dysesthetic (essential) vulvodynia

→ R/O concomitant STDs

→ R/O VIN

→ R/O cervical squamous intraepithelial lesion (SIL)

→ R/O urinary tract infection

→ R/O interstitial cystitis

PLAN

DIAGNOSTIC TESTS

→ Diagnostic tests should primarily be directed to documentation of infectious disease states.

→ Potassium hydroxide (KOH) and saline wet mounts of vaginal secretions should be performed to assess for *Candida*, *Trichomonas*, or bacterial vaginosis.

→ Scrapings from affected skin may be taken, placed on glass slide, mixed with KOH, and viewed microscopically for presence of *Candida*.

→ Vaginal and vulvar cultures for *Candida* should be performed.

→ pH testing of the vagina may be performed.

→ Pap smear, genital cultures, blood chemistries, HIV testing, FBS, other diagnostic tests as indicated.

→ Acetic acid 3 percent to 5 percent may be applied to vulva for HPV assessment. Several minutes after application, acetowhitening of affected area may appear, and small, cutaneous papillae with associated vascular pattern may be identified on mucous membrane of labia minora, vestibule, or posterior fourchette (papillomatosis). These changes can be seen with the naked eye, a hand-held lens, or colposcope.
NOTE: Acetowhitening is suggestive but not diagnostic of HPV infection. Papillomatosis may be present normally or in subclinical HPV infection. Acetowhitening may also be due to tissue inflammation, trauma, allergic or contact dermatitis, lichen sclerosus, pantyhose, or tight pants.

→ Colposcopy of entire vulva, vagina, and cervix may be utilized for assessment of HPV and SIL.

→ Tissue biopsy of anogenital areas may be done for histopathological confirmation of HPV. Biopsies of suspicious or questionable areas should be done to rule out VIN and other dermatoses.
  ■ Biopsy for direct immunofluorescence should be considered in the differential diagnosis of erosive vulvovaginal conditions (e.g., lichen planus, lupus erythematosus, bullous dermatoses, apthosis, Behçet's syndrome. (McKay 1992).

→ Serum testing for herpes antibodies are of limited value. If negative, herpes infection can be ruled out; positive tests indicate circulating antibodies but do not assist in determining of the date or time of exposure.

→ Molecular hybridization techniques (Southern blot, dot blot, polymerized chain reaction) are specific diagnostic techniques utilized to assess the presence of HPV DNA. These tests have limited availability and may only be available for research purposes.

→ For vulvar vestibulitis, specific criteria for diagnosis include (Friedrich 1987):
  ■ severe pain on vestibular touch or attempted vaginal entry.
  ■ tenderness to pressure localized within vulvar vestibule.
  ■ physical findings confined to vestibular erythema of various degrees.
  NOTE: Biopsies are not usually beneficial in diagnosis of vestibulitis. If performed, histological findings may show a nonspecific chronic inflammation of submucosal tissue surrounding the minor vestibular glands.

→ Sensory testing as described in "Objective" section to assess pudendal neuralgia.

→ Orthopedic and additional neurological assessment, x-ray, CT scan, MRI can be utilized as necessary to evaluate orthopedic and other causes of essential vulvodynia.

TREATMENT/MANAGEMENT

→ Treatment of *specific* underlying cause, if identified, is key. See specific treatment modalities below.

→ Psychological support to help patient deal with the chronicity of the condition and to support her coping mechanisms is an important component of care. Refer to appropriate resources: social service, psychological or sexual counseling, stress management.

→ Psychiatric evaluation may be indicated in certain cases.

Vulvar dermatoses

→ Treat underlying dermatological disorders as identified. See specific protocols.

Cyclical *Candida* infection

→ Culture-positivity need not be a criterion for treatment.

→ Long-term (4 to 6 months) maintenance therapy with local or systemic antifungal agents may be employed in patients with a variable symptom pattern and those who have had relief of symptoms from anticandidal measures in the past. (Key to success is consistent, low-dose *Candida* suppression.) Options include (McKay 1992):
  ■ local therapy:
    • antifungal cream (azole): one-half applicator every night at bedtime.
  ■ systemic therapy:

- ketoconazole (Nizoral®): 100 mg/day for 1 to 2 months tapering to 100 mg every other day for 2 months. Alternately, may be used 100 mg/day for 5 days prior to menses. Antifungal cream may be used every other day or every third day at bedtime in conjunction with systemic therapy (McKay 1989a).
  NOTE: Nizoral® is hepatotoxic. See *PDR*. Consult with physician prior to use. Regimens may vary.

→ It is important to rule out chronic illness such as diabetes, HIV infection.

Herpes simplex virus infection

→ Oral acyclovir (Zovirax®) may be offered (ACOG 1988; McKay 1992):
- primary infection: 200 mg p.o. every 4 hours 5 times/day for 10 days.
- recurrent infection: 200 mg p.o. every 4 hours 5 times/day for 5 days.
- frequent infection (chronic suppressive therapy, at least 6 outbreaks/year): 400 mg p.o. BID for up to 12 months.

→ See **Genital Herpes Simplex Virus** Protocol.

HPV

→ Spontaneous regression is possible; thus aggressive therapy should be reserved for intractable symptoms (Bergeron et al. 1990; McKay 1992).

→ Well-localized, small lesions respond well to 85 percent bi- or trichloroacetic acid; larger areas might best be treated with laser therapy or cryotherapy followed by adjuvant topical 5-fluorouracil cream (5-FU) (Efudex®): small amount rubbed in thoroughly to affected area 2 consecutive days a week for 10 weeks (Moscicki 1990). **NOTE:** 5-FU therapy may result in a sore, painful vulva.

→ Avoid treatment of asymptomatic papillomatosis.

→ See **Human Papillomavirus** Protocol for details on therapy of condyloma acuminata.

Vestibulitis

→ In cases where specific etiology cannot be found, many symptomatic women improve with time and/or are able to adjust satisfactorily to discomfort. Thus specific therapy may not be necessary.

→ There are no firmly established treatment guidelines, and multiple therapies have been tried to alleviate vestibulitis, including:

- warm sitz baths (for recent onset, mild signs or symptoms).
- coital lubricants.
- topical lidocaine hydrochloride (Xylocaine®) 2 to 5 percent: applied with cotton swab prn and/or 10 to 15 minutes prior to intercourse (McKay 1992; J. Stern, personal communication, December 11, 1990).
- topical corticosteroids (low potency): Small amount to affected areas BID regularly (may need to be used for weeks to months) (McKay 1989b, 1992; J. Stern, personal communication, December 11, 1990). See **Table 12TB.1, Potency Ranking of Topical Corticosteroids,** p. 12-228.
- local or systemic antifungal agents for chronic, recurrent candidiasis. See "Cyclical *Candida* Infection" section.
- treatment of specific vaginal infections (e.g., BV, atrophic vaginitis), and cervicitis as indicated.
- alpha-interferon (for subset of patients with biopsy or hybridization evidence of HPV): 1,000,000 U intradermally to vulvar vestibule 3 times/week for 4 weeks (Horowitz 1989; Umpierre et al. 1991). Beta-interferon I.M. has also been tried. Consult with or refer to physician. May only be available as part of a research protocol in certain centers. See **Human Papillomavirus** Protocol.
- dexamethasone 8 mg with equal volume of 1 percent lidocaine or bupivacaine (2 ml) injected into reddened areas of vestibule once/week for 3 weeks (Eschenbach and Mead 1992). Consult with or refer to physician.
- surgical resection of vestibule (perineoplasty) has been successful (60 percent to 90 percent) in alleviating the condition (Dotters and Droegemueller 1989; McKay et al. 1991, 1992; J. Stern, personal communication, December 11, 1990). This is a radical approach and should be reserved for patients with severe levels of dyspareunia: defined as dyspareunia that completely prevents intercourse at times, has lasted at least 6 months, has not responded to 6-month trial of conservative therapy, or for which no cause can be identified (McKay 1992; Marinoff and Turner 1991). Refer to experienced physician.

→ Avoid overtreatment with antibiotics, topical irritants (potent steroids and other local medications and products), and local destructive measures.

→ Prevention of repeated inflammation may include concomitant use of topical antifungal agents when systemic antibiotics are prescribed and avoidance of potent topical steroids or irritating topical medications (McKay 1992).

Iatrogenic factors

→ Prevention is the key.

→ Avoid use of potent steroids on vulva for chronic vulvar dermatoses. A popular offender is combination betamethasone (steroid) with clotrimazole (antifungal) (McKay 1992).

→ Gradual tapering is necessary to withdraw patient from chronic topical steroid use. Rebound steroid irritant reactions may be treated with hydrocortisone ointment 1 percent, or bland emollients such as diaper salve and vegetable shortening (McKay 1991).

→ Avoid use of alcohol injection as a treatment for vulvar pruritus.

→ Recently, a low oxalate diet plus calcium citrate (200 mg calcium + 950 mg citrate, 2 tablets p.o. TID) has been tried to reduce symptoms (Solomons, Melmed, and Heitler 1991).
NOTE: Foods high in oxalates include: rhubarb, spinach, celery, and peanuts.

Dysesthetic (Essential) vulvodynia

→ Topical lidocaine ointment (Xylocaine®) 5% may be applied prn for local relief (McKay 1992).

→ Pudendal neuralgia may be treated with tricyclic antidepressants: Prevent reuptake and degradation of neurotransmitters to allow pain impulses to modulate (Eschenbach and Mead 1992; Kaufman and Faro 1994; McKay 1992; Turner and Marinoff 1991).
  ▪ Amitriptyline (Elavil®) 10 mg p.o. BID. If tolerated, dose is gradually increased every 2 to 4 weeks until pain relief achieved. (As much as 100 mg/day may be required). Once pain relief achieved, dosage should be maintained for 4-8 weeks, then gradually decreased until maintenance level established. If symptom-free for 3-6 months, dose may be gradually decreased until medication no longer required (Kaufman and Faro 1994, 300).
  NOTE: Dosage regimens vary in treating vulvodynia. Management by physician experienced with use of these drugs advised. See *PDR* for side effects of antidepressants.

  ▪ Alternate medications may include desipramine, trazodone, or clonazepam. Management by physician advised. See *PDR*.

→ Anticonvulsants or antiviral drugs may be used in postherpetic neuralgia (Turner and Marinoff 1991):
  ▪ phenytoin (Dilantin®) 300 mg-400 mg/day p.o. in 2 divided doses; discontinue if no relief in 3 weeks; higher doses may lead to toxicity. Consult with or refer to physician.
  ▪ carbamazepine (Tegretol®) 100 mg/day p.o. increased by increments of 100 mg every 2 days up to 600 mg/day, as needed for pain control. Consult with or refer to physician. Hematological, dermatological, hepatic toxicities may occur; close monitoring necessary.
  ▪ acyclovir (Zovirax®) 1200-1600 mg p.o./day for 6 to 8 weeks (Kaufman and Faro 1994).
  NOTE: Large doses—consult with physician.

→ Additional alternative therapies for essential vulvodynia have been tried with inconsistent results. These include NSAIDS, hormones, antibiotics, retinoids, acupuncture, transcutaneous electrical stimulation, regional blocks, and surgical nerve resection (Kaufman and Faro 1994; Turner and Marinoff 1991).

CONSULTATION

→ See "Objective" and "Treatment/Management" sections.

→ For severe, unremitting cases unresponsive to local measures, refer patient to gynecologist or dermatologist skilled in assessment and management of patients with vulvodynia.

→ For cases in which antidepressant or anticonvulsant therapy is being considered, it may be necessary to consult with or refer to psychiatrist or neurologist.

→ As needed for prescription(s).

PATIENT EDUCATION

→ Discus proposed etiologies of various subsets of vulvodynia and possibility of long-term therapy toward resolution. Inform patient that a continued search for more definitive etiologies and treatment modalities is under way. Explain that vulvodynia is not contagious (as long as communicable disease agents have been ruled out).

→ Discuss the importance of a healthy immune system and its role in disease prevention.

→ Encourage patient to keep a diary of all offending substances and, ideally, eliminate their use. See *Candida* **Vaginitis** Protocol for patient education regarding vulvovaginal health and hygiene measures.

→ Excessive douching or use of potent topical steroids should be avoided, as these may result in dermatitis.

→ In women with known antibiotic-induced cyclical *Candida* infection, prophylactic topical antifungals should be utilized. The patient should ask her health care provider for prescription as necessary, or OTC products should be used at the onset of taking medication.

→ Make sure patient understands how to properly apply topical steroid medication when used for treatment of vestibulitis. See **Table 12TA.1, Tips for Treating Skin Lesions**, p. 12-220.

→ Lubricants may be used with intercourse (e.g., Astroglide®) to ease penile entry.

→ Explain that even after surgery, vulvodynia may return.

FOLLOW-UP

→ Support is essential for patient's psychological health.

→ Psychological or psychosexual counseling may be necessary in refractory cases. Provide appropriate referrals. Communicate with patient on how she is coping.

→ Arrange return-visit schedule that best meets needs of patient; varies with case presentation.

→ Document in progress notes and problem list.

12-TI VULVAR DISEASE
Bibliography

American College of Obstetricians and Gynecologists. 1988. *Gynecologic herpes simplex virus infections*, ACOG Technical Bulletin No. 119. Washington, DC: the Author.

Barclay, D.L. 1991. Premalignant and malignant disorders of the vulva and vagina. In *Current obstetric and gynecologic diagnosis and treatment*, 7th ed., ed. M.L. Pernoll, pp. 923–936. Norwalk, CT: Appleton & Lange.

Bergeron, C., Ferenczy, A., Richart, R.M., and Guralnick, M. 1990. Micropapillomatosis labialis appears unrelated to human papillomavirus. *Obstetrics and Gynecology* 76(2):281–286.

Chafe, W., Richards, A., Morgan, L., and Wilkinson, E. 1988. Unrecognized invasive carcinoma in vulvar intraepithelial neoplasia. *Gynecologic Oncology* 31:154–162.

Cho, J.Y., Ahn, M.O., and Cha, K.S. 1990. Window operation: An alternative treatment method for Bartholin's gland cysts and abscesses. *Obstetrics and Gynecology* 76:886–888.

Committee on Terminology of the International Society for the Study of Vulvar Disease. 1990. New nomenclature for vulvar disease. *The Journal of Reproductive Medicine* 35:483–484.

Consensus Conference. 1984. Precursors to malignant melanoma. *The Journal of the American Medical Association* 251:1864–1866.

Cornell, R.C., and Stoughton, R.B. 1984. The ranking of topical steroids in psoriasis. *Dermatologic Clinics* 2(3):399.

Cort, M.B. 1991. Bartholin's gland cyst and abscess. In *Ob/Gyn secrets*, eds. H.L. Frederickson and L. Wilkins-Haug. Philadelphia: Hanley & Belfus.

Dalziel, K.L., and Wojnarowska, F. 1991. The treatment of vulvar lichen sclerosus with a very potent topical steroid (clobetasol propionate 0.05%) cream. *British Journal of Dermatology* 124:461–464.

DePetrillo, A., Krepart, G., Roy, M., and Wilkinson, E.J. 1987. Less radical surgery for vulvar cancer. *Contemporary Ob/Gyn* 30(1):160–175.

DiSaia, P.J., and Creasman, W.T. 1989. *Clinical gynecologic oncology*, 3d ed. St. Louis: C.V. Mosby.

Dotters, D.J., and Droegemueller, W. 1989. Vulvar vestibulitis: Common cause of vulvar pain. *Clinical Advances in the Treatment of Infections* 3(1):1–12.

Eschenbach, D.A, and Mead, P.B. 1992. Vaginitis update. *Contemporary Ob/Gyn* 37(12):54–70.

Friedrich, E.G., Jr. 1983. *Vulvar disease*, 2d ed. Philadelphia: W.B. Saunders.

Friedrich, E.G. 1987. Vulvar vestibulitis syndrome. *The Journal of Reproductive Medicine* 32:110–114.

Gomel, V., Munro, M.G., and Rowe, T.C. 1990. *Gynecology: A practical approach*. Baltimore: Williams & Wilkins.

Hammill, H.A. 1989. Unusual causes of vaginitis. *Obstetrics and Gynecology Clinics of North America* 16(2):337–345.

Horowitz, B.J. 1989. Interferon therapy for vulvitis. *Obstetrics and Gynecology* 73(3):446–448.

International Society for the Study of Vulvar Disease. 1991. Vulvar vestibulitis and vestibular papillomatosis. Report of the ISSVD committee on vulvodynia. *The Journal of Reproductive Medicine* 36(6):413–415.

Jones, H.W., Wentz, A.C., and Burnett, L.S. 1988. *Novak's textbook of gynecology*, 11th ed. Baltimore: Williams & Wilkins.

Kaufman, R.H., Friedrich, E.G., Jr., and Gardner, H.L. 1989. *Benign diseases of the vulva and vagina,* 3d ed. Chicago: Year Book Medical.

Kistner, R.W. 1986. *Gynecology: Principles and practice,* 4th ed. Chicago: Year Book Medical.

Lerner, A.B. 1972. Pigmented nevi. *Modern Medicine* 17:131.

Lever, W.F. 1990. *Histopathology of the skin,* 7th ed. Philadelphia: J. B. Lippincott.

Lynch, P.J. 1986. Vulvodynia: A syndrome of unexplained vulvar pain, psychologic disability and sexual dysfunction. *The Journal of Reproductive Medicine* 31(9):773–780.

Mann, M.S., Kaufman, R.H., Brown, Jr., D., and Adam, E. 1992. Vulvar vestibulitis: Significant clinical variables and treatment outcome. *Obstetrics and Gynecology* 79(1):122–125.

Marinoff, S.C., and Turner, M.L.C. 1991. Vulvar vestibulitis syndrome: An overview. *American Journal of Obstetrics and Gynecology* 165(4, Pt. 2):1228–1232.

McKay, M. 1988. Subsets of vulvodynia. *The Journal of Reproductive Medicine* 33:695–698.

———. 1989a. Vulvodynia: A multifactorial clinical problem. *Archives of Dermatology* 125:256–262.

———. 1989b. Vulvodynia and pruritus vulvae. *Seminars in Dermatology* 8(1):40–47.

———. 1991. Vulvitis and vulvovaginitis: Cutaneous considerations. *American Journal of Obstetrics and Gynecology* 165(4, Pt. 2):1176–1182.

———. 1992. Vulvodynia: Diagnostic patterns. *Dermatology Clinics* 10(2):423–433.

McKay, M., Frankman, O., Horowitz, B.J., Lecart, C., Micheletti, L., Ridley, C.M., Turner, M.L.C., and Woodruff, J.D. 1991. Vulvar vestibulitis and vestibular papillomatosis. Report on the ISSVD committee on vulvodynia. *The Journal of Reproductive Medicine* 36(6):413–415.

Medical Economics Data. *Physicians' Desk Reference.* 1993. Montvale, NJ: the Author.

Misas, J.E., Cold, C.J., and Hall, F.W. 1991. Vulvar Paget's disease: Fluorescein-aided visualization of margins. *Obstetrics and Gynecology* 77(1):156–159.

Morgan, L.S., and Wilkinson, E.J. 1988. Meeting the challenge of superficially invasive carcinoma. *Contemporary Ob/Gyn* 31(5):181–185.

Morrow, C.P., and Townsend, D. 1981. *Synopsis of gynecologic oncology,* 2d ed. New York: John Wiley.

Moscicki, A-M. 1990. Genital human papillomavirus infections. *Adolescent Medicine* (3):451–469.

Reid, R., Greenberg, M.D., Daoud, Y., Husain, M., Selvaggi, S., and Wilkinson, E. 1988. Colposcopic findings in women with vulvar pain syndromes. A pre-

liminary report. *The Journal of Reproductive Medicine* 33(6):523–533.

Richart, R., Boronow, R.C., Hacker, N., Monaghan, J.M., and Thomas, G.M. 1988. Microscopic vulvar Ca: A new concept. *Contemporary Ob/Gyn* 32(4):117–136.

Rodke, G., Friedrich, E.G., and Wilkinson, E.J. 1988. Malignant potential of mixed vulvar dystrophy (lichen sclerosus associated with squamous cell hyperplasia). *The Journal of Reproductive Medicine* 33(6):545–550.

Roy, M. 1988. VIN: Latest management approaches. *Contemporary Ob/Gyn* 31(5):170–179.

Russel, P., and Bannatyne, P. 1989. *Surgical pathology of the ovaries.* Edinburgh, Scotland: Churchill Livingstone.

Sauer, G.C. 1991. *Manual of skin diseases,* 6th ed. Philadelphia: J.B. Lippincott.

Sedlis, A., Homesley, H., Marshall, R., and Bundy, B.N. 1988. Evaluating risk factors for vulvar cancer. *Contemporary Ob/Gyn* 32(3):67–74.

Shearin, R.S., Boehlke, J., and Karanth, S. 1989. Toxic shock-like syndrome associated with Bartholin's gland abscess: Case report. *American Journal of Obstetrics and Gynecology* 160:1073–1074.

Solomons, C.C., Melmed, M.H., and Heitler, S.M. 1991. Calcium citrate for vulvar vestibulitis. A case report. *The Journal of Reproductive Medicine* 36(12):879–882.

Stewart, D.E., Psych, D., Whelan, C.I., Fong, I.W., and Tessler, K.M. 1990. Psychosocial aspects of chronic, clinically unconfirmed, vulvovaginitis. *Obstetrics and Gynecology* 76(5, Pt. 1):853–856.

Thomas, C.L., ed. 1989. *Taber's cyclopedic medical dictionary,* 16th ed. Philadelphia: F.A. Davis.

Turner, M.L.C., and Marinoff, S.C. 1988. Association of of human papillomavirus with vulvodynia and the vulvar vestibulitis syndrome. *The Journal of Reproductive Medicine* 33(6):533–537.

———. 1991. Pudendal neuralgia. *American Journal of Obstetrics and Gynecology* 165(4, Pt. 2):1233–1236.

Umpierre, S.A., Kaufman, R.H., Adam, E., Woods, K.V., and Adler-Storthz, K. 1991. Human papillomavirus DNA in tissue biopsy specimens of vulvar vestibulitis patients treated with interferon. *Obstetrics and Gynecology* 78(4):693–695.

Wilkinson, E.J., Kneale, B., and Lynch, P.J. 1986. Report of the International Society for the Study of Vulvar Disease, Terminology Committee. *The Journal of Reproductive Medicine* 31:973.

Wilkinson, E.J. 1987. *Pathology of the vulva and vagina.* New York: Churchill Livingstone.

Word, B. 1964. New instrument for office treatment of cysts and abscesses of Bartholin's gland. *The Journal of the American Medical Association* 190:777–778.

SECTION 13

Sexually Transmitted Diseases

Winifred L. Star, R.N., C., N.P., M.S.

13-A

Chancroid

Chancroid (or "soft chancre") is a sexually transmitted disease (STD) caused by the facultative gram-negative bacillus *Hemophilus ducreyi*. The disease is most prevalent in the developing countries of Africa, Asia, and Latin America but rare in the United States. However, epidemics have occurred in Los Angeles, Boston, Dallas, New York City, and parts of Georgia and Florida. A continued rise in the number of cases since 1985 has been reported.

Prostitutes appear to be the reservoir for disease in outbreak areas. Approximately 5,000 thousand cases were reported in the United States in 1987. Worldwide incidence of chancroid may now exceed that of syphilis, and in limited areas it is more common than gonorrhea.

Men are affected more than women by a ratio of ten to one (10:1), but it is unclear whether women have lower rates of infection, or asymptomatic lesions, or whether they are carriers of *H. ducreyi* without lesions. The incidence is higher in tourists, military personnel, and seafarers, and among drug users there has also been an apparent increase. Coinfection with *T. pallidum* or herpes simplex virus (HSV) may occur in as many as ten percent of patients (CDC 1993a).

The major means of disease acquisition is sexual. Autoinoculation of fingers or other sites occasionally is reported. Trauma or an abrasion is necessary for the organism to penetrate the epidermis. Transmission by fomites does not play a role (Blanco and Gonik 1991; Jessamine and Ronald 1990; Piot and Plummer 1990; Ronald and Albritton 1990; Sweet and Gibbs 1990; Willis 1990). Although the incubation period in women has not been well-established, it may be between two to 10 days, and usually four to seven days. Prodromal symptoms and systemic illness are not part of the clinical manifestation of chancroid.

Studies in Africa have provided evidence that chancroid is a major risk factor for heterosexual transmission of the human immunodeficiency virus (HIV). Genital ulcers in women render them more susceptible to HIV infection, and in an HIV-infected woman the presence of a genital ulcer increases the chance that a sexual partner will become infected.

It is thought that a genital ulcer enhances the passage of HIV into vaginal secretions; and, indeed, chancroid has been established as a cofactor for HIV transmission (CDC 1993a). A high rate of HIV infection among chancroid patients has been reported in the United States and elsewhere (CDC 1993a). Treatment failures of chancroid are more common if the individual has asymptomatic HIV (Ronald and Albritton 1990).

H. ducreyi has demonstrated plasmid-mediated antibiotic resistance for a variety of antibiotics, and a large proportion of isolates are beta-lactamase positive (Jessamine and Ronald 1990; Ronald and Albritton 1990).

DATABASE

SUBJECTIVE

→ Prostitutes are major carriers.

→ Patient may have history of travel to areas where chancroid is endemic.

→ Occurs predominantly among blacks, Hispanics, and lower socioeconomic groups.

→ Most affected individuals are heterosexual.

→ Asymptomatic subclinical lesions may exist, although unlikely.

→ Extent of female role as asymptomatic reservoirs/carriers unclear.

→ Chancroid may be a risk factor for HIV acquisition/transmission.
  ▪ Cofactors include other STDs.
  ▪ Genital herpes may increase susceptibility.

→ Use of systemic/local antibiotics and topical steroids, and an immunodeficient state may modify the clinical presentation of genital ulcers.

→ Symptoms may include:
  ▪ vaginal discharge.
  ▪ external dysuria.
  ▪ pain on defecation.
  ▪ rectal bleeding.
  ▪ dyspareunia.
  ▪ a "hernia."
  ▪ painful ulcer(s) or may be unaware of an ulcer; there is no prodrome.
  ▪ mild constitutional symptoms.

→ A gynecological and medical history should be obtained including:
  ▪ menstrual cycle.
  ▪ contraception.
  ▪ description of symptoms:
    • onset.
    • duration.
    • quality/quantity.
    • frequency.
    • course.
    • aggravating/relieving factors.
    • associated symptoms.
  ▪ previous history of same/similar problem.
  ▪ STD history (including dates/treatment).
  ▪ sensitive questioning regarding recent sexual activity, including date of last exposure, sex practices, sites of exposure, number of partners in past month, use of condoms.
  ▪ sex partner history.
  ▪ acute/chronic illness.
  ▪ general health.
  ▪ medications.
  ▪ allergies.
  ▪ habits.
  ▪ history of laboratory tests for syphilis, Hepatitis B, HIV.
  ▪ review of systems (CDC 1991).

OBJECTIVE

→ Examination may be individualized based on case presentation.

→ Thorough STD examination includes:

▪ vital signs as indicated.
▪ general skin inspection of face, trunk, forearms, palms, and soles for lesions, rashes, discoloration.
▪ inspection of pharynx and oral cavity for infection, lesions, discoloration.
▪ abdominal inspection and palpation for masses, tenderness, rebound tenderness.
▪ inspection of pubic hair for lice, nits.
▪ inspection of external genitalia for discharge, masses, lesions.
▪ inspection and palpation of Bartholin's, urethral, and Skene's glands for discharge, masses.
▪ inspection of vagina for discharge, lesions.
▪ inspection of cervix for lesions, discharge, eversion, erythema, edema, friability; assessment for cervical motion tenderness (CMT).
▪ uterine assessment for size, shape, consistency, mobility, tenderness.
▪ palpation of adnexa for masses, tenderness.
▪ inspection of perianus, anus for lesions, bleeding, discharge.
▪ rectal examination as indicated.
▪ assessment for presence or absence of associated lymphadenopathy (CDC 1991).

→ Chancroid ulcers most often involve the labia, fourchette, vestibule, clitoris, vaginal introitus, or perineum.
  ▪ Periurethral and vaginal ulcers may also occur.

→ Extragenital lesions of the breasts, thighs, mouth, and fingers may occur.

→ Characteristics of chancroid lesion:
  ▪ single or multiple lesions may appear.
  ▪ starts as erythematous papule, becomes pustular → eroded → ulcerated over 24 to 48 hours with an outer zone of erythema. Alternately, papule may persist as pustule ("dwarf chancroid").
  ▪ deep, ragged with undermined edges.
  ▪ sharply demarcated.
  ▪ little or no induration (soft chancre).
  ▪ base is a gray or yellow necrotic purulent exudate; very friable.
  ▪ little surrounding inflammation.
  ▪ usually painful or tender to touch.
  ▪ may become 2 cm to 3 cm in diameter; may coalesce and erode through tissue planes resulting in fistulas.

→ Progression of disease affects inguinal lymph node area, usually unilaterally with erythema of overlying skin forming an acute, painful, tender

bubo (more than 50 percent of cases in seven to ten days, unilateral in two-thirds of cases, less common in females).
  - Occasionally a "groove sign" appears when both inguinal and femoral nodes are involved, divided by the inguinal ligament.
→ Bubo may continue to enlarge and spontaneously rupture through skin (especially if larger than five cm) with extrusion of thick, creamy, viscous pus. Sinus tracts may form.
→ Inguinal adenopathy may persist for an indeterminate amount of time after ulcer healed.
→ Superinfection with *Fusobacterium* or *Bacteroides* species may occur. This may lead to gangrene and severe genital tissue destruction.
→ No signs of systemic infection or spread to distant sites.
→ Complete and accurate descriptions of any identified lesions or other pertinent physical findings should be written in the objective section of the progress note.

ASSESSMENT

→ Chancroid
→ R/O syphilis
→ R/O herpes simplex
→ R/O lymphogranuloma venereum (LGV)
→ R/O granuloma inguinale
→ R/O folliculitis
→ R/O superinfection, rectovaginal fistula, labial adhesions (complications of chancroid)
→ R/O HIV
→ R/O concomitant STD (e.g., gonorrhea, chlamydia)
→ R/O noninfectious cause of ulcer: trauma, drug eruption, Crohn's/Beçhet's disease
→ R/O metastatic genital cancer (cervical, vulvar, vaginal)

PLAN

DIAGNOSTIC TESTS

→ Distinguish between chancroid and other causes of genital ulcers. See **Table 13A.1, Clinical Features of Genital Ulcers** and **Figure 13A.1, Sexually Active Patient with Genital Ulcer(s)**.
→ Culture for *H. ducreyi* ulcer confirms diagnosis.
  - Use cotton or calcium alginate swab and obtain specimen from ulcer base after gentle removal of necrotic exudate with saline.
  - Alternately, aspirate from bubo may be sent for culture; however, aspirated fluid from the bubo is almost always sterile. Culture media for chancroid is highly selective (gonococcal agar or Mueller-Hinton agar). Ensure laboratory capabilities.
→ Gram stain of ulcer base may be done, but this test is unreliable.
  - Roll specimen gently onto slide, stain and observe typical "school of fish" or "railroad track" patterns.
→ A probable diagnosis of chanchroid can be made in the presence of painful genital ulcer(s), plus:
  - no evidence of syphilis infection (by dark-field of ulcer exudate *or* serological test at least 7 days after ulcer onset), and
  - either the clinical ulcer(s) presentation is atypical for HSV or the HSV test results are negative (CDC 1993a).
→ A suggestive diagnosis of chancroid includes a combination of painful ulcer(s) with tender inguinal adenopathy. Suppurative inguinal adenopathy is almost pathognomonic of chancroid (CDC 1993a).
→ Diagnostic tests to rule out other causes of genital ulcers and lymphadenopathy include:
  - dark-field or direct immunofluorescence test of serous fluid for *T. pallidum* from genital and non-oral lesion(s) to rule out syphilis. (See **Syphilis** Protocol.)
  - RPR (or VDRL) or treponemal tests to rule out syphilis. (See **Syphilis** Protocol.)
  - Herpes cultures or Tzanck stain to rule out herpes. (See **Genital Herpes Simplex Virus** Protocol.)
  - see "Diagnostic Test" sections of **Lymphogranuloma Venereum** and **Granuloma Inguinale (Donovanosis)** protocols.
→ Endocervical culture for *N. gonorrhoeae* and endocervical diagnostic tests for *C. trachomatis*. (In the absence of a cervix, urethral specimen may be obtained.)
→ HIV antibody testing should be performed at the time of diagnosis (CDC 1993a).
→ Alternative diagnostic tests for chancroid are not widely available but may include: compliment fixation, precipitin, agglutination tests, enzyme-

Table 13A.1. CLINICAL FEATURES OF GENITAL ULCERS

	Syphilis	Herpes	Chancroid	Lymphogranuloma Venereum	Donovanosis
Incubation period	2-4 weeks (1-12 weeks)	2-7 days	1-14 days	3 days-6 weeks	1-4 weeks (up to 6 months)
Primary lesion	Papule	Vesicle	Papule or pustule	Papule, pustule, or vesicle	Papule
Number of lesions	Usually one	Multiple, may coalesce	Usually multiple, may coalesce	Usually one	Variable
Diameter, mm	5-15	1-2	2-20	2-10	Variable
Edges	Sharply demarcated, elevated, round, or oval	Erythematous	Undeminded, ragged, irregular	Elevated, round, or oval	Elevated, irregular
Depth	Superficial or deep	Superficial	Excavated	Superficial or deep	Elevated
Base	Smooth, nonpurulent	Serous, erythematous	Purulent	Variable	Red and rough ("beefy")
Induration	Firm	None	Soft	Occasionally firm	Firm
Pain	Unusual	Common	Usually very tender	Variable	Uncommon
Lymphadenopathy	Firm, nontender, bilateral	Firm, tender, often bilateral	Tender, may suppurate, usually unilateral	Tender, may suppurate, loculated, usually unilateral	Pseudoadenopathy

Source: Reprinted with permission from Piot, P., and Plummer, F.A. 1990. Genital ulcer adenopathy syndrome. In *Sexually transmitted diseases*, 2nd ed., eds. K.K. Homes, P.-A. Mårdh, P.F. Sparling, P.J. Wiesner, W. Cates, Jr., S.M. Lemon, and W.E. Stamm, p. 712. New York: McGraw-Hill.

linked immunosorbent assay (ELISA), and direct immunofluorescence (DFA).

→ Additional tests may include (but are not limited to): wet mounts, Pap smear, CBC, urinalysis, urine culture and sensitivities, Hepatitis B screen, pregnancy test.

TREATMENT/MANAGEMENT

→ Recommended regimens:
- azithromycin (Zithromax®) 1 gram p.o. in a single dose

OR
- ceftriaxone (Rocephin®) 250 mg I.M. in a single dose

OR
- erythromycin base (E-Mycin®) 500 mg p.o. QID for 7 days (CDC 1993a).

NOTE: The 7-day erythromycin course is suggested by some experts as the preferred regimen when treating HIV-infected patients (CDC 1993a). With use of single-dose therapy in these individuals, follow-up must be ensured.

→ Alternative regimens (not evaluated as extensively; neither regimen studied in United States):
- amoxicillin 500 mg plus clavulanic acid 125 mg (Augmentin®) p.o. TID for 7 days

OR
- ciprofloxacin hydrochloride (Cipro®) 500 mg p.o. BID for 3 days.

NOTE: Ciprofloxacin contraindicated in pregnancy, lactation, and in adolescents age 17 years or under (CDC 1993a). The safety of azithromycin during pregnancy and lactation has not been established.

→ Partner therapy.
- All sexual partners exposed within the 10 days preceding patient's symptom onset should be evaluated and treated with one of the above regimens (CDC 1991, 1993a).
  • Provide referrals to provider/facility that offers appropriate STD care as indicated.

→ Additional considerations.
- Fluctuant lymph nodes should be aspirated through adjacent healthy skin to prevent rupture. Do not incise and drain or excise bubos—this delays healing. In some cases repeated aspirations may be necessary.
  NOTE: Bubos may appear to worsen in the 1 to 2 days following therapy.
- A broad-spectrum systemic antibiotic is indicated in cases of severe secondary bacterial infection of the ulcer.

Figure 13A.1. SEXUALLY ACTIVE PATIENT WITH GENITAL ULCER(S)

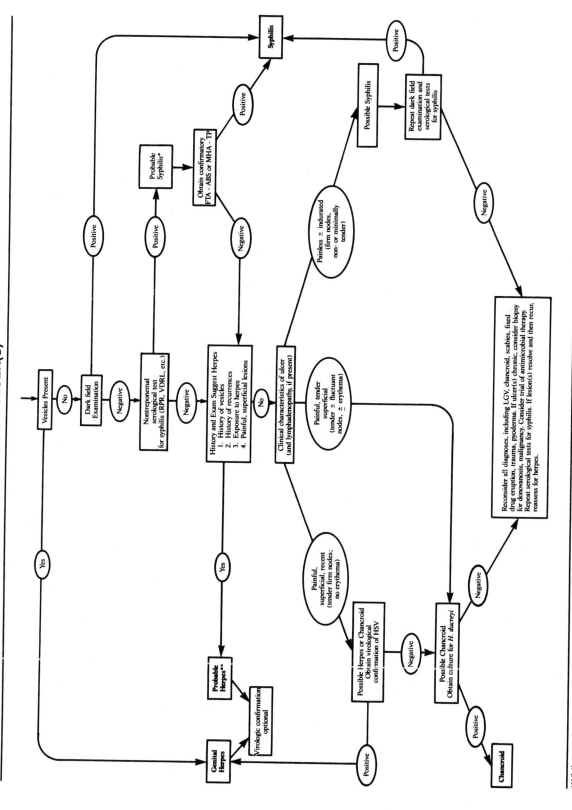

*While awaiting the FTA-ABS test results, most clinicians would initiate syphilis therapy for patients having dark-field-negative, RPR-positive ulcers that resemble chancres.

**Confirmation of probable herpes is desirable. If the confirmation test for herpes is negative, or if the course is atypical, reevaluate the diagnosis, repeat serological test for syphilis in 3 to 4 weeks, consider fixed drug eruption if there is history of recurrent lesions at the same time, and rule out herpes at the next recurrence.

Source: Reprinted with permission from Piot, P., and Plummer, F.A. 1990. Genital ulcer adenopathy syndrome. In *Sexually transmitted diseases*, 2nd ed., eds. K.K. Homes, P.-A. Mårdh, P.F. Sparling, P.J. Wiesner, W. Cates, Jr., S.M. Lemon, and W.E. Stamm, p. 712. New York: McGraw-Hill.

- Good hygiene and saline soaks will promote tissue granulation and ulcer reepithelialization.
- Untreated ulcers will heal in about 5 weeks.

CONSULTATION

→ As indicated for patient evaluation, abnormal lab studies.

→ For patients unresponsive to therapy, refer to a physician.

→ As needed for prescription(s).

PATIENT EDUCATION

→ Discuss etiology and nature of chancroid, including mode of transmission, incubation period, symptoms, potential complications, co-association with HIV infection, and importance of partner examination and treatment.
- Patient-education handouts are a useful adjunct to teaching.

→ Advise patient and partner to finish full course of medication and return for follow-up (see "Follow-Up" section).

→ Explain that healing time is related to the size of the ulcer and may require more than two weeks for a large lesion. Scarring may result in extensive cases. Lymphadenopathy resolution is slower than that of ulcers (CDC 1993a).

→ Advise abstinence from intercourse until patient and partner are treated and cured. If symptoms recur, patient and partner should be instructed to seek care promptly.

→ Address STD prevention and HIV risk reduction, provide guidelines for safer sex practices, encourage careful screening of sex partners and committed use of condoms (especially with new, multiple, non-monogamous partners). See **Table 13A.2, Safer Sex Guidelines** and **Table 12I.1, Recommendations for Individuals to Prevent STD/PID**, p. 12-96.

→ Allow patient to ventilate her feelings of surprise, shame, fear, anger as indicated. Psychological support may be important for the patient in gaining control over her sexual situation and to enable her to prevent future STDs.

FOLLOW-UP

→ Patients should be re-examined three to seven days after initiation of therapy (CDC 1993a). Ulcers will improve within this time if treatment is successful.
- Observe patient at weekly intervals until ulcer has completely resolved.
- Adenopathy may persist and may require needle aspiration through adjacent healthy skin (CDC 1989a).

→ History on follow-up should include symptom status, medication compliance, drug reaction and side effects, partner therapy, sexual exposure, and use of condoms.

→ Treatment failures should arouse suspicion for HIV infection, incorrect diagnosis, noncompliance with medication, resistance to antibiotic, incorrect diagnosis, or coexistent STD (CDC 1993a).

→ Perform antibiotic susceptibility tests on *H. ducreyi* isolates in patients who are unresponsive to therapy.

→ Tests for HIV and syphilis should be repeated in three months if initially negative.

→ HIV-infected patients require close monitoring. Longer courses of therapy may be necessary and healing may be slower. Refer to physician as indicated.

→ Follow-up on all laboratory tests ordered. Treat all concomitant STDs and other identified conditions.

→ HIV-positive results should be conveyed in person and by a provider who has received training in the complexities of test disclosure. HIV-positive persons should be referred to the appropriate provider or agency for early intervention services.

→ Hepatitis B antigen-positive individuals should have liver function tests and receive counseling regarding the implications of their positive status and need for immunoprophylaxis of sex partners and household members. (See **Hepatitis—Viral** Protocol.)

→ Because chancroid is a state-mandated reportable disease, a morbidity report must be filed with the department of public health.

→ Continue to encourage safer sex practices.

→ Document in progress notes and problem list.

Table 13A.2. SAFER SEX GUIDELINES

Behaviors	Safest	Low-Risk (Possible Risk of HIV Exposure)	Possibly Unsafe	High-Risk (Unsafe)
	Abstinence Self-masturbation Monogamous relationship both partners uninfected and not involved in high-risk activities (e.g., needle sharing) Hugging,* massaging,* touching* Dry kissing Mutual masturbation* Drug abstinence	Wet kissing Vaginal intercourse with condom use Anal intercourse with condom use Fellatio interruptus Urine contact with intact skin	Cunnilingus Fellatio	Unprotected receptive anal intercourse Unprotected vaginal intercourse Unprotected anal penetration Oral-anal contact Multiple sexual partners Sharing sex toys or douches Sharing needles for any purpose
Prevention Strategies	Avoid high risk behaviors	Avoid exposure to possibly infected bodily fluids Consistent use of condoms & spermicide with vaginal intercourse Avoid anal intercourse (if engaging in anal intercourse use condom)	Use dental dam or female condom with cunnilingus Use condom with fellatio	Avoid exposure to possibly infected bodily fluids Consistent use of condom & spermicide with vaginal intercourse Avoid anal penetration (penile or hand) (if engaging in anal penetration use condom with anal intercourse, latex glove with hand penetration) Avoid oral-anal contact Do not share sex toys or douching equipment Do not share needles (if sharing needles clean with bleach before and after use)

*If no breaks in skin.

Source: Adapted with permission from Cohen, P.T. 1990. Safe sex, safer sex and the prevention of HIV infection. In *The AIDS knowledge base*, eds. P.T. Cohen, M.A. Sande, and P.A. Volberding, pp. 1–10. Waltham, MA: The Medical Publishing Group; De Ferrari E. 1989. Counseling women regarding high risk behaviors associated with HIV infection. *Journal of Nurse Midwifery* 34(5):276-280.

13-B

Chlamydia Trachomatis

Chlamydiae are a group of obligate intracellular microorganisms differentiated from other bacteria by a unique growth cycle. The organisms lack the ability to synthesize high-energy compounds. Thus, in order to survive and grow, they must completely depend on the host cell for energy and nutrients (Schacter 1990).

Two biological forms of the organism exist: the elementary body, the infectious, extracellular form; and the reticulate body, the replicative, intracellular form (Fraiz and Jones 1988). The entire life cycle for chlamydia lasts about 48 hours and is an involved process of attachment, penetration, and replication (Blanco and Gonik 1991). More detailed discussion of the developmental cycle is beyond the scope of this protocol.

The genus contains two species, *C. psittaci* and *C. trachomatis.* The former causes disease in birds and animals. However, a new *C. psittaci* strain, TWAR, recently has been demonstrated to cause respiratory tract infections in humans.

C. trachomatis can be divided into a number of serovars and biovars which are responsible for a wide spectrum of diseases. Serovars A, B, and C cause hyperendemic trachoma, seen mostly in developing countries. D to K are associated with urethritis, cervicitis, salpingitis, proctitis, inclusion conjunctivitis, epididymitis, and newborn pneumonia. Biovars L1, L2, and L3 are responsible for lymphogranuloma venereum (LGV) (Blanco and Gonik 1991; Schacter 1994). The major modes of transmission of *C. trachomatis* are sexual and congenital; however, with trachoma, child to child is the most common method of transmission in endemic areas. Nonsexual transmission may occur if infected genital secretions are inoculated on to mucous membranes, particularly of the eye.

Genital chlamydial infections have surpassed gonorrhea as the number one STD in western industrialized society. An estimated four million cases occur per year in the United States with a cost of $2.2 billion (Cates and Wasserheit 1991). In this country, chlamydial infections are common among adolescents and young adults (CDC 1993b).

In women, chlamydial infections are often difficult to diagnose due to the high incidence of asymptomatic infections (50 percent to 70 percent). Thus, these infections have become a substantial threat to women's reproductive health. The prevalence of chlamydial infection ranges from three percent to five percent in asymptomatic women to more than 20 percent in women in STD clinics. In sexually active female adolescent populations, prevalence ranges are 15 percent to 28 percent (Schacter 1994).

The incubation period is six to 14 days, but women may harbor the organism for extended periods of time (Sweet and Gibbs 1990). Studies report that *C. trachomatis* can be isolated from the cervix of 60 percent to 70 percent of female sex partners of men with chlamydial urethritis (Stamm and Holmes 1990). An estimated 20 percent to 40 percent of sexually active women have been exposed to *C. trachomatis* and have positive antibodies (Faro 1991). Approximately 40 percent of women with gonorrhea have concomitant chlamydia (Schacter 1987).

C. trachomatis is responsible for 35 percent to 50 percent of nongonococcal urethritis in heterosexual men and the most frequent cause of post-gonococcal urethritis. Forty percent to 50 percent of men with chlamydial infection, however, are asymptomatic (Schacter 1994).

The clinical manifestations caused by chlamydia closely parallel those of *N. gonorrhoeae*. Sites of infection in women include the pharynx (only three percent to six percent); the urethra; Bartholin's glands; the endocervix (the most common site) with extension to the endometrium, salpinx, and peritoneum; and the rectum (only five percent).

Other manifestations of chlamydial infection may include perihepatitis or Fitz-Hugh-Curtis (FHC) syndrome—a complication of chlamydial-associated salpingitis; Reiter's syndrome (urethritis, conjunctivitis, arthritis, and characteristic mucotaneous lesions, usually seen in men); and pneumonia, endocarditis, and meningoencephalitis (all fairly rare) (Stamm and Holmes 1990). Full discussion of these complications is beyond the scope of this protocol. The reader is referred to a current STD textbook.

Knowledge of the natural history of chlamydial infections is still unfolding. However, it seems the infection has the ability to smolder until complications arise. Both *C. trachomatis* and *N. gonorrhoeae* may cause significant tissue damage (e.g., subepithelial inflammation, epithelial ulceration, and scarring), although symptoms of chlamydial infection are usually less severe than those of gonorrhea (Stamm and Holmes 1990).

Asymptomatic or minimally symptomatic infectious states are common. Therefore the disease may persist for years and not be recognized until late in its course. Sequelae of genital chlamydial infection are significant and include acute or chronic pelvic inflammatory disease (PID), tubal infertility, and ectopic pregnancy. (See associated protocols.)

DATABASE

SUBJECTIVE

→ Risk factors include:
- young age.
- highest incidence ages 15 years to 21 years.
- early age at first intercourse.
- multiple sexual partners.
- non-white race.
- single marital status.
- lower socioeconomic status.
- presence of cervical eversion (ectopy).
- use of oral contraceptives (induces cervical eversion).
- use of no or nonbarrier contraception.
- history of concomitant gonorrhea/other STD.
- sexual partner with nongonococcal urethritis (NGU), gonorrhea, or other STD.
- new sexual partner within preceding two months.
- douching (may precipitate upper genital tract infection in women with chlamydia-positive cervix).
- intrauterine device (IUD) use (increases risk for chlamydia-associated endometritis).
- see **Lymphogranuloma Venereum** Protocol.

→ Patient may present with:
- may be asymptomatic.
- endocervicitis:
  - abnormal vaginal discharge.
  - postcoital or intermenstrual vaginal bleeding or spotting.
- urethral syndrome/urethritis:
  - dysuria, frequency.
  - usually no suprapubic tenderness or hematuria.
  - onset of symptoms often occurs with new sexual partner in past month or with exposure to partner with NGU.
  - symptoms may be of longer duration than in acute cystitis (more than seven to ten days).
  - less likely to have history of recurrent urinary tract infection (UTI).
  - often taking oral contraceptives.
- endometritis/salpingitis:
  - intermenstrual spotting/bleeding.
  - menorrhagia.
  - dysmenorrhea.
  - dyspareunia.
  - abdominal/pelvic pain.
  - fever, chills, malaise, nausea, vomiting.
  - symptoms usually less severe than those associated with gonorrheal or anaerobic pelvic infection.
  - late symptoms of undiagnosed infection may include chronic pelvic pain, ectopic pregnancy symptoms (see **Ectopic Pregnancy** Protocol), and/or unexplained infertility.
  - see **Pelvic Inflammatory Disease** Protocol.
- conjunctivitis:
  - conjunctival irritation, redness.
  - see **Conjunctivitis** Protocol.
- pharyngitis:
  - most infections asymptomatic.
  - see **Pharyngitis** Protocol.
- bartholinitis:
  - varying degrees of pain/tenderness in Bartholin's gland.
  - difficulty sitting, walking.
  - dyspareunia.
  - few systemic symptoms unless extensive inflammation.

- see **Vulvar Disease–Large Lesions of the Vulva** Protocol.
  - proctitis:
    - clinical manifestations in women not well-studied. Symptoms may include anal irritation, rectal pain, hematochezia, tenesmus, mucous discharge, constipation, painful defecation.
    - see **Lymphogranuloma Venereum** Protocol.
  - perihepatitis (Fitz-Hugh-Curtis syndrome):
    - severe right upper quadrant (pleuritic) pain (may occur from six days before to 14 days after the onset of lower abdominal pain from salpingitis).
    - other symptoms may include fever, nausea, vomiting, increased vaginal discharge, menorrhagia, dysmenorrhea, or dyspareunia.
  - Reiter's syndrome:
    - spectrum of urogenital inflammation remains to be established in women (Handsfield and Pollock 1990).
    - wide range of articular symptoms or nonspecific rheumatic complaints.
    - skin, mouth, nail lesions.
    - conjunctival irritation, redness.
→ Gynecological and medical history should be obtained including:
  - menstrual cycle.
  - contraception.
  - description of symptoms:
    - onset.
    - duration.
    - quality/quantity.
    - frequency.
    - course.
    - aggravating and relieving factors.
    - associated symptoms.
  - previous history of same or similar symptoms.
  - STD history (including dates/treatment).
  - sensitive questioning regarding recent sexual activity (including date of last exposure, sex practices, sites of exposure, number of partners in past month, use of condoms).
  - sex partner history.
  - acute/chronic illness.
  - general health.
  - medications.
  - allergies.
  - habits.
  - history of laboratory tests for syphilis, Hepatitis B, HIV.
  - review of systems (CDC 1991).

OBJECTIVE
→ Examination may be individualized based on case presentation.
→ Thorough STD examination includes:
  - vital signs as indicated.
  - general skin inspection of face, trunk, forearms, palms, and soles for lesions, rashes, discoloration.
  - inspection of pharynx and oral cavity for infection, lesions, discoloration.
  - abdominal inspection and palpation for masses, tenderness, rebound tenderness.
  - inspection of pubic hair for lice, nits.
  - inspection of external genitalia for discharge, masses, lesions.
  - inspection and palpation of Bartholin's, urethral, and Skene's glands for discharge, masses.
  - inspection of vagina for blood, discharge, lesions.
  - inspection of cervix for lesions, discharge, eversion, erythema, edema, friability; assessment for CMT.
  - uterine assessment for size, shape, consistency, mobility, tenderness.
  - palpation of adnexa for masses, tenderness.
  - inspection of perianus and anus for lesions, bleeding, discharge.
  - rectal examination as indicated.
  - assessment for presence or absence of associated cervical inguinal lymphadenopathy (CDC 1991).
→ Physical examination components and findings specific to assessment of patients with chlamydial infection may include:
  - temperature: may be elevated in patients with PID, UTI, FHC syndrome, tubo-ovarian abscess (TOA).
  - abdomen: usually within normal limits (WNL) in uncomplicated infections:
    - may have right upper quadrant tenderness (or liver tenderness) in FHC syndrome.
    - generalized tenderness and/or rebound tenderness in endometritis, salpingitis, peritonitis.
    - inguinal mass/adenopathy in LGV.
  - external genitalia: usually WNL; erythema, edema, excoriation may be present in concomitant vaginitis.
  - Bartholin's, urethral, Skene's glands: usually WNL.

- Purulent or mucoid exudate (milk the glands, urethra), meatal erythema/swelling may be present in urethritis.
  - Swelling/abscess formation may be present in bartholinitis.
- vagina: abnormal discharge, blood, pus may be present.
- cervix: purulent or mucopurulent discharge, (see "Diagnostic Tests" section), edema/erythema of the zone of ectopy, friability, CMT may be present.
- uterus: usually WNL in uncomplicated infections.
  - Tenderness may be present in endometritis.
- adnexa: usually WNL in uncomplicated infection.
  - Masses/tenderness may be present in salpingitis, FHC syndrome, TOA.
- rectum: usually WNL in uncomplicated infections.
  - Blood or mucus discharge may be present in proctitis (uncommon in women).
  - Masses/tenderness in cul-de-sac area may be present in salpingitis, FHC syndrome, TOA.
→ Additional assessment of Reiter's syndrome may include:
- skin.
  - Lesions of keratodermia blennorrhagica occur most commonly on plantar surfaces of feet—erythematous macules enlarging to hyperkeratotic papules with red halos/central clearing, resembling psoriasis (Handsfield and Pollock 1990).
- mouth.
  - Painless shallow ulcers on palate, tongue, buccal mucosa, lips, tonsillar pillars, or pharynx (Handsfield and Pollock 1990).
- nails.
  - Thickening, brown-yellow discoloration (Handsfield and Pollock 1990).
- extremities.
  - Asymmetrical polyarticular synovitis-tendonitis often seen initially with tendon insertion sites, the common sites of inflammation (e.g., Achilles tendon, plantar fascia).
  - Arthritis of knees, ankles, feet, most commonly with knee effusions and fusiform dactylitis ("sausage digits") of fingers, toes; sacroiliitis (Handsfield and Pollock 1990).
- the HLA-B27 antigen is present in 70 percent to 80 percent of whites and 15 percent to 75 percent of blacks with Reiter's syndrome.

Manifestations of Reiter's syndrome are more severe in these patients (Handsfield and Pollock 1990).

→ Anoscopy may be indicated in women with proctitis. Findings include mucopus and erythematous, friable mucosa.
→ Complete and accurate description of any identified lesion or other pertinent physical manifestation should be noted in the "Objective" section of the progress notes.
→ See "Objective" section of **Lymphogranuloma Venereum** Protocol.

ASSESSMENT

→ *Chlamydia trachomatis* infection
→ Exposure to *C. trachomatis*, other STD
→ Mucopurulent cervicitis
→ R/O chlamydia
→ R/O gonorrhea
→ R/O syphilis
→ R/O other concomitant STD
→ R/O vaginitis
→ R/O urethral syndrome/UTI
→ R/O PID
→ R/O TOA
→ R/O ectopic pregnancy
→ R/O perihepatitis (FHC syndrome). Differentials include: cholecystitis, hepatitis, pleurisy, pneumonia, pyelonephritis, mononucleosis, perforated ulcer, appendicitis, liver/subdiaphragmatic abscess, toxic shock syndrome
→ R/O Reiter's syndrome
→ R/O LGV

PLAN

DIAGNOSTIC TESTS
→ Mucopurulent cervicitis (MPC) is highly indicative of chlamydial infection (may also be present in gonorrhea).
- Characteristics include:
  - yellow or green mucopus on a white cotton-tipped swab of endocervical secretions ("positive swab test").
  - friability, erythema, or edema within a zone of cervical eversion (ectopy).
  - >10 PMNs per oil immersion field (× 1000 magnification) of a gram stain of endocervical

mucus (collected after first gently removing ectocervical vaginal secretions).

NOTE: Some clinicians suggest >5 PMNs/HPF as a cutoff (Moscicki et al. 1987).

→ Selection of most appropriate laboratory test is site-specific and will depend upon availability, lab expertise, and *C. trachomatis* prevalence in the population.

▪ Options include:
- cultures: Considered the "gold standard" for diagnosis of chlamydia, sensitivity 80 percent to 100 percent, specificity near 100 percent; 48-hour to 72-hour turnaround; greatest value in screening low-prevalence populations (Stamm and Mardh 1991). Endocervical cultures for *N. gonorrhoeae* also should be obtained. See **Gonorrhea** Protocol.

  NOTE: Cultures should be obtained *prior* to the use of bacteriostatic lubricant. Endocervical cells are necessary for *C. trachomatis* isolation. Ectocervical secretions should be removed prior to endocervical sampling. Insert swab 1 cm to 2 cm into the cervical os and gently abrade. Rayon or cotton-tipped swabs on plastic shafts or cytological brushes are preferable. Specimen should be placed immediately in proper media, refrigerated, transported on ice, and inoculated within 24 hours (Stamm and Holmes 1990). Depending on clinical presentation cultures may also be taken from:
  –urethra.
    ▸ Insert swab 2 cm into urethra and rotate. (In the absence of a cervix, the urethra should be cultured.)
  –eye.
    ▸ With the eyelid everted, swab vigorously over mucosa.
- rectum.
  –Best obtained by direct visualization via anoscopy, but can be obtained by swabbing 2 cm into the rectum.
  –Bartholin's gland.
    ▸ Strip exudate from gland duct openings.
- Antigen detection methods:
  –direct immunofluorescent monoclonal antibody (DFA) tests (MicroTrak®): sensitivity 70 percent to 90 percent, specificity >90 percent; false positive rate 2 percent to 3 percent; need fluorescence microscope; can be performed in 15 to 30 minutes; less costly than culture, but not

ideal for screening low-prevalence populations; cost-effective for small number of specimens.
  –enzyme-linked immunosorbent assay (EIA) (Chlamydiazyme®): sensitivity 67 percent to 90 percent, specificity > 90 percent; false-positive rate 2 percent to 3 percent; 4 hours to perform, requires less expertise; less costly than culture; less reliable in low-prevalence populations; best utilized in processing large numbers of specimens in high-risk settings.
  –DNA probe assay (Gen-Probe Pace Assay®): identifies genetic blueprint of *C. trachomatis*; results in 24-hours; sensitivity 88 percent to 92 percent, specificity 96 percent to 99 percent; relatively new tool.
  –polymerase chain reaction (PCR), ligation chain reaction (LCR): newer approach, not in widespread use commercially.
- serology is generally not useful for diagnosis of *C. trachomatis* infections (except in LGV, FHC syndrome, and in women with PID) due to the high background rate of antichlamydial antibodies in the population.
- The microimmunofluorescence (Micro-IF) assay detects IgG and IgM antibodies.
  –Extremely high IgG or IgM levels, IgM antibodies, or fourfold rises in IgG titers are considered diagnostic of recent infection (Sweet and Gibbs 1990).
- see **Lymphogranuloma Venereum** Protocol.
- pap smear may show cellular atypia; if present, endocervical cultures for *C. trachomatis* and *N. gonorrhoeae* should be considered.
  –Cytological detection is a reliable means of diagnosis for trachoma and inclusion conjunctivitis (McGregor 1989).
- VDRL or RPR to rule out syphilis to be performed.
- wet mounts in presence of abnormal vaginal discharge.
- urinalysis may reveal pyuria (>10 WBCs/HPF spun urine) and culture may be negative for common urinary pathogens in acute *C. trachomatis*-associated urethral syndrome. Gonorrhea and trichomonal infections also should be ruled out.
- serological HIV testing should be offered.
- additional tests may include (but are not limited to): Pap smear, CBC, liver function

studies, Hepatitis B screen, chest x-ray, ultrasound, pregnancy test.
- laparoscopy is the definitive method of diagnosis for salpingitis and perihepatitis.
- See **Lymphogranuloma Venereum, Pelvic Inflammatory Disease,** and **Pelvic Masses** protocols.

TREATMENT/MANAGEMENT

→ Patients with MPC should await results of *C. trachomatis* and *N. gonorrhoea* cultures prior to treatment, unless there is high suspicion of infection or the patient is unlikely to return for follow-up (CDC 1993b).

→ The CDC (1993b) recommends the following treatment of patients with MPC:
- treat for chlamydia and gonorrhea in populations with a high prevalence of both infections.
- treat for chlamydia only if the prevalence of gonorrhea is low but the likelihood of chlamydia is substantial.
- await culture results if the prevalence of both infections is low and if compliance with follow-up can be ensured.
- sex partners should be notified, examined, and treated based on the patient's culture results. In cases where patients are treated presumptively, partners should receive the same therapy.

→ Recommended treatment regimens for chlamydia:
- doxycycline (Vibramycin®) 100 mg p.o. BID for 7 days

OR
- azithromycin (Zithromax®) 1 gram p.o. in a single dose.
  NOTE: Safety and efficacy of azithromycin for persons 15 years of age and younger have not been established (CDC 1993b).

→ Alternative regimens:
- ofloxacin (Floxin®) 300 mg p.o. BID for 7 days

OR
- erythromycin base (E-Mycin®) 500 mg p.o. QID for / days

OR
- erythromycin ethylsuccinate (E.E.S.®) 800 mg p.o. QID for 7 days

OR
- sulfisoxazole (Gantrisin®) 500 mg p.o. QID for 10 days (inferior efficacy) (CDC 1993b).
NOTE: Ofloxacin contraindicated in pregnancy and in persons 17 years of age and younger; similar efficacy to doxycycline and azithromycin but more expensive (CDC 1993b).

→ Partner therapy:
- all sex partners of *symptomatic* patients in the previous 30 days, and of *asymptomatic* patients in the past 60 days should be evaluated and treated.
- the last sex partner should be treated even if the aforementioned time intervals have been exceeded (CDC 1993b).
- provide referrals to provider or facility which offers appropriate STD care as necessary.

→ Treatment during pregnancy:
- recommended regimen:
  - erythromycin base (E-Mycin®) 500 mg p.o. QID for 7 days (CDC 1993b).
- alternative regimens:
  - erythromycin base (E-mycin®) 250 mg p.o. QID for 14 days

OR
  - erythromycin ethylsuccinate (E.E.S.®) 800 mg p.o. QID for 7 days

OR
  - erythromycin ethylsuccinate (E.E.S.®) 400 mg p.o. QID for 14 days (CDC 1993b).
  - if erythromycin cannot be tolerated: Amoxicillin 500 mg p.o. TID for 7 to 10 days (limited data regarding efficacy) (CDC 1993b).
NOTE: Erythromycin *estolate* is contraindicated in pregnancy. Also, doxycycline and ofloxacin are contraindicated in pregnancy; sulfisoxazole is contraindicated near term and during nursing. Safety and efficacy of azithromycin in pregnancy/lactation not established (CDC 1993b).

→ Additional considerations:
- HIV-infected patients with MPC or identified chlamydial infection should receive the same treatment as outlined above (CDC 1993b).
- mainstay of treatment for Reiter's syndrome is anti-inflammatory drugs, e.g., indomethacin (Indocin®) 75 mg to 150 mg/day p.o. in divided doses, or other nonsteroidal agents.
  - Consult with physician.
  - Underlying chlamydia-associated and/or gonorrhea-associated cervicitis/urethritis should be treated with the recommended drug regimens.
  - See **Gonorrhea** Protocol.
  - Partners of patients with Reiter's syndrome should be referred for treatment.

→ Refer to **Pelvic Inflammatory Disease** Protocol for treatment of FHC syndrome.

→ See **Pelvic Masses, Gonorrhea, Syphilis, Lymphogranuloma Venereum, Pelvic Inflammatory Disease**, and other **Sexually Transmitted Diseases** protocols.

CONSULTATION

→ Consultation with a physician is indicated for patients with PID, TOA, symptoms of ectopic pregnancy, Reiter's syndrome, complicated LGV.

→ As needed for prescription(s).

PATIENT EDUCATION

→ Discuss the etiology and nature of chlamydial infections, including mode of transmission, incubation period, symptoms, potential complications, the possibility of coexistent gonorrhea or other STD, and the importance of partner treatment even if asymptomatic.

▪ Patient education handouts are a helpful adjunct to teaching.

→ Advise patient and partner to finish full course of medication.

→ Advise abstinence from intercourse until patient and partner are treated and cured (i.e., medication completed, free of symptoms). If symptoms recur, patient and partner should be instructed to seek care promptly.

→ Address STD prevention and HIV risk reduction, provide guidelines for safer sex practices, encourage careful screening of sex partners and committed use of condoms (especially with new, multiple, non-monogamous partners).

▪ See **Table 13A.2, Safer Sex Guidelines**, p. 13-9, and **Table 12I.1, Recommendations for Individuals to Prevent STD/PID**, p. 12-96.

→ Allow patient to ventilate her feelings of surprise, shame, fear, anger as indicated. Psychological support may be important for the patient in gaining control over her sexual situation and to enable her to successfully prevent future STDs.

FOLLOW-UP

→ Test of cure is not necessary after treatment with doxycycline or azithromycin unless the patient or partner is symptomatic or reinfection is suspected (CDC 1993b). Retesting may be considered three weeks after treatment completion if erythromycin, sulfisoxazole, or amoxicillin was used (usually not necessary when ofloxacin is used) (CDC 1993b). **NOTE:** Cultures, if performed at sooner than 3 weeks post-therapy completion, may yield false negative results. Nonculture tests at sooner than 3 weeks may be false positive due to continued dead organism excretion (CDC 1993b).

→ In pregnancy, repeat testing—preferably by culture—is recommended after completing therapy. (See previous "NOTE.")

→ Rescreening several months after treatment should be considered to detect reinfection, which in some populations may be high (CDC 1993b).

→ When the patient or partner continues to be symptomatic, a return visit is necessary. History on follow-up should include symptom status, medication compliance, drug reaction and side effects, partner therapy, sexual exposure, and use of condoms.

→ Follow-up on all laboratory tests ordered. Treat all concomitant STDs and other identified conditions.

→ Negative HIV tests may be repeated in three to six months. Continue to encourage safer sex.

→ As indicated, HIV-positive results should be conveyed in person and by a provider who has received training in the complexities of test disclosure. HIV-positive persons should be referred to the appropriate provider or agency for early intervention services.

→ Hepatitis B antigen-positive individuals should have liver function tests and receive counseling regarding the implications of their positive status and need for immunoprophylaxis of sex partners and household members. (See **Hepatitis—Viral** Protocol.)

→ Routine *C. trachomatis* screening is recommended for the following categories: sexually active adolescents; women ages 20 years to 24 years, particularly those who report non-use or inconsistent use of barrier contraceptives; women with new or multiple sex partners (CDC 1991, 1993b).

→ In certain states, because chlamydia may be a mandated reportable disease, a morbidity report may need to be filed with the department of public health.

→ Patients with FHC syndrome may have chronic upper quadrant pain despite adequate antibiotic therapy; laparoscopic lysis of adhesions may be indicated. Refer to physician.

→ Document chlamydia diagnosis and complications/sequelae in progress notes and problem list.

Winifred L. Star, R.N., C., N.P., M.S.

13-C

Gonorrhea

Gonorrhea, the most commonly reported communicable disease, is caused by *Neisseria gonorrhoeae* (gonococcus), a gram-negative diplococci. In the United States, one million cases per year are reported, but it is estimated that about three million occur. The predominant mode of transmission is sexual contact (genital-genital, oral-genital, and anal-genital). Transmission via fomites or nonsexual means is extremely rare. The infection presents more frequently in males than in females (1.5:1), with rates of infection varying among different populations (Fogel 1988). Most men are symptomatic.

In this country, 82 percent of reported cases occur in 15- to 29-year-olds, with the highest rates in the 20- to 24-year-old age group. Blacks are affected 20 to 30 times more often than whites; Hispanics and Native Americans three to five times more often (Handsfield 1991). Incidence appears to be seasonal, with the highest rates in summer and lowest rates in late winter and early spring (Hook III and Handsfield 1990). In clinics providing routine gynecological care, the prevalence of asymptomatic infection cases is one percent to two percent, while in STD clinics, case rates may be as high as 25 percent (Moy and Clasen 1990; Sweet and Gibbs 1990).

Gonorrhea prevalence is sustained by continued transmission via asymptomatically infected individuals and by "core group" transmitters, who are increasingly more likely than others in the population to attain and transmit infection (Hook III and Handsfield 1990). Since 1975, however, there has been a slow, steady decline in gonorrhea in this country (Larsen 1990).

The risk of transmission from an infected male to an exposed female after a single episode of intercourse is estimated to be about 80 percent to 90 percent, with an incubation period of three to five days; the majority

of patients, however, remain asymptomatic (Blanco and Gonik 1991; CDC 1993b; Gibbs and Sweet 1989). Coinfection with *Chlamydia trachomatis* or *Trichomonas vaginalis* occurs in 30 percent to 50 percent of cases (Dallabetta and Hook III 1987).

Common sites of gonococcal infection in women are the endocervix (primary site), urethra, Skene's and Bartholin's glands, and rectum. Colonization of the urethra is present in 70 percent to 90 percent of infected women, although uncommon in the absence of endocervical disease. In hysterectomized women, however, the urethra is the usual site of infection. Gland infection is rare in the absence of endocervical or urethral infection. Infection of the rectum occurs in 35 percent to 50 percent of women with endocervical gonorrhea and may be the only site of infection in about five percent of cases. Most rectal infections result from local spread of infected cervical secretions.

Pharyngeal infection, caused by orogenital contact and transmission (and occasionally by autoinoculation from anogenital infection), occurs in ten percent to 20 percent of heterosexual women with gonorrheal infections. It is the sole site of infection in less than five percent of cases. Infection of the pharynx appears to be transmitted more efficiently by fellatio than cunnilingus (Hook III and Handsfield 1990).

Gonococci infect nonsquamous epithelium-lined mucosal membranes mostly of the urogenital tract and secondarily of the rectum, oropharynx, and/or conjunctivae (Hook III and Handsfield 1990). Once inoculated onto the mucosal surface, the gonococci attach to the villi of the epithelial cell and enter by phagocytosis (Brooks 1988). In approximately three to 21 days after exposure, an endotoxin is produced which results in redness and swelling of the affected tissue. Spread of gonorrhea occurs via direct tissue extension, the bloodstream, or both.

Dilation of the endocervical canal during menstruation facilitates the direct spread of the organism to the endometrium, fallopian tubes, and peritoneal cavity which may result in PID, in 15 percent to 20 percent of cases (Fogel 1988; Sweet and Gibbs 1990). Fitz-Hugh-Curtis (FHC) syndrome, a form of perihepatitis, was initially felt to be secondary to ascending gonococcal infection; however, it is now more often associated with chlamydial disease (Greenblatt 1990). Ascending infection may cause progressive mucosal damage, accompanied by a leukocyte response and submucosal abscess formation. Infertility or ectopic pregnancy are serious sequelae of upper genital tract infection (Hook III and Handsfield 1990).

Disseminated gonococcal infection (DGI) occurs in 0.5 percent to three percent of all patients with untreated gonorrhea. The ratio of affected women to men is four to one (4:1), and primary genital, anorectal, or pharyngeal infection is commonly asymptomatic (Blanco and Gonik 1991; Handsfield and Pollock 1990). Dissemination in women often is associated with menstruation or pregnancy (Buntin et al. 1991). Greater than 80 percent of DGI patients will have a positive culture for *N. gonorrhoeae* from anogenital or pharyngeal sources, or will have a positive contact. DGI occurs in two stages: the first is characterized by a bacteremia (seven to 30 days after infection) with chills, fever, and skin lesions; the second by acute septic arthritis or tenosynovitis. (See "Objective" section of this protocol.)

Uncommon complications of gonococcal bacteremia include: endocarditis, affecting one percent to three percent of individuals with DGI; and meningitis, with less than 25 cases reported (Hook III and Handsfield 1990). Conjunctival infections also may arise. If left untreated, corneal ulceration/perforation, scarring, lens opacification, and eventual blindness may result (Quinones 1990).

Meningococcal infections may mimic gonococcal infections. Colonization with *N. meningitidis* has been documented in the pharynx, urethra, endocervix, and anus. The inherent pathogenicity of anogenital meningococcal infections is unclear, but case reports have linked meningococcal isolation to urethritis, vaginal discharge, salpingitis, and DGI-like syndromes (Hook III and Handsfield 1990).

In recent years, treatment for gonorrhea has been complicated by antibiotic-resistant strains. Resistance can be of three types: penicillinase-producing *N. gonorrhoeae* (PPNG), chromosomally-mediated-resistant *N. gonorrhoeae* (CMRNG), and tetracycline-resistant *N. gonorrhoeae* (TRNG).

"PPNG are gonococcal strains that have acquired an extrachromosomal element which encodes for beta-lactamase, an enzyme that destroys the beta-lactam ring of penicillin" (CDC 1987a, 1S).

By 1988, an estimated less than four percent of all gonococcal infections were penicillinase-producing. In the United States, there is a substantial variance in PPNG prevalence nationwide, with hyperendemic pockets in south Florida, New York City, and San Francisco (more than three percent of reported cases in a two-month period are caused by PPNG) (CDC 1987a; Hook III and Handsfield 1990).

In contrast to PPNG, CMRNG strains do not produce beta-lactamase. Resistance in these cases is not limited to penicillin and can include resistance to tetracycline, cephalosporins, spectinomycin, and other aminoglycosides. Although a quite common form of resistance, in most instances CMRNG strains have not been associated with treatment failure, either because the levels of resistance were not high or the antibiotic in question was not used in treatment (CDC 1987a).

In cases of high-level TRNG, treatment with tetracycline alone will not be effective. Areas of the country most affected by TRNG are the northeastern states and the Baltimore, Maryland, area. The CDC maintains surveillance of gonococcal isolates which demonstrate antimicrobial resistance. No ceftriaxone-resistant strains have been reported (CDC 1993d).

DATABASE

SUBJECTIVE

→ Risk factors include:
- young age.
- early onset of sexual activity.
- unmarried status.
- nonwhite race.
- lower socioeconomic status.
- urban residence.
- prostitution.
- illicit drug use.
- people who trade sex for drugs.
- multiple sexual partners (especially in previous month).
- increased frequency of sexual intercourse.
- exposure to "core group" transmitters (i.e., those who have had repeated episodes of gonorrhea, continue to have sex despite symptoms, engage in high-risk behaviors (e.g., drugs, prostitution/prostitution patronage), live in areas of high population density, are of low socioeconomic status (Dalabetta and Hook III 1987; Hook III and Handsfield 1990).

- partner who has gonorrhea or other STD.
- history of gonorrhea or other STD.
- concomitant STD.
- history of PID.
- no use of or non-barrier contraception.
- hormonal contraception.

→ Symptoms include:
- patient may be asymptomatic or complain of any of the following:
  - vulvar pruritus/irritation.
  - swelling of labia majora.
  - increased or abnormal vaginal discharge.
  - abnormal bleeding.
  - dysuria.
  - urinary urgency/frequency.
  - dyspareunia.
  - dysmenorrhea.
  - menstrual irregularity.
  - lower abdominal/pelvic discomfort, cramping, pain.
  - low-back ache.
  - anal pruritus/discharge.
  - rectal fullness, pressure, pain.
  - mucoid/mucopurulent rectal discharge.
  - tenesmus or painful defecation.
  - constipation or diarrhea.
  - pus or blood in stool.
  - sore throat.
  - nausea, vomiting, diarrhea.
  - fever.
  - malaise.
  - inguinal/cervical adenopathy.
  - skin lesions.
  - joint/tendon pain.
  - migratory polyarthritis.
- symptoms tend to be worse postmenstrually.
- symptoms also will depend upon the site of infection.
- partner(s) may have symptoms of urethral/rectal discharge, dysuria, frequency, redness of urethral meatus, epididymal pain or swelling, lower abdominal pain, rectal pain, tenesmus, pus or blood in stool.
- see **Pelvic Inflammatory Disease, Pelvic Masses** protocols.

→ Gynecological and medical history should include:
- menstrual cycle.
- contraception.
- description of symptoms:
  - onset.
  - duration.
  - quality/quantity.
  - frequency.
  - course.
  - aggravating/relieving factors.
  - associated symptoms.
- previous history of same/similar problem.
- STD history (including dates/treatment).
- sensitive questioning regarding recent sexual activity (including date of last exposure, sex practices, sites of exposure, number of partners in past month, use of condoms).
- sex partner history.
- acute or chronic illness.
- general health.
- medications.
- allergies.
- habits.
- history of laboratory tests for syphilis, Hepatitis B, HIV.
- review of systems (CDC 1991).

OBJECTIVE

→ Examination may be individualized based on case presentation.

→ Thorough STD examination includes:
- vital signs as indicated.
- general skin inspection of face, trunk, forearms, palms, soles for lesions, rashes, discoloration.
- inspection of pharynx and oral cavity for infection, lesions, discoloration.
- abdominal inspection and palpation for masses, tenderness, rebound tenderness.
- inspection of pubic hair for lice, nits.
- inspection of external genitalia for discharge, masses, lesions.
- inspection and palpation of Bartholin's, urethral, and Skene's glands for discharge, masses.
- inspection of vagina for discharge, lesions.
- inspection of cervix for lesions, discharge, eversion, erythema, edema, friability; assessment for CMT.
- uterine assessment for size, shape, consistency, mobility, tenderness.
- palpation of adnexa for masses, tenderness.
- inspection of perianus and anus for lesions, bleeding, discharge.
- rectal examination as indicated.
- assessment of presence or absence of associated cervical or inguinal lymphadenopathy (CDC 1991).

→ Physical examination components and findings specific to assessment of patients with gonorrhea may include:
- temperature: may be elevated in patients with pharyngitis, UTI, DGI, PID, TOA.
- throat/neck: pharyngeal injection, cervical lymphadenopathy (may be present with pharyngitis).
- skin: assess volar aspect of arms, hands, fingers.
  • Cutaneous manifestations of DGI include:
    – 1 mm to 2 mm-2 cm-diameter lesions; usually found on distal portion of extremity, five to 30 lesions average.
    – pinpoint erythematous macule progressing to papules, vesiculopustules, or hemorrhagic bullae.
    – mature lesion usually elevated, slightly umbilicated with grey necrotic center, irregular rim, and surrounding erythema (Buntin et al. 1991; Handsfield and Pollock 1990; Hook III and Handsfield 1990).

NOTE: Primary cutaneous infection with *N. gonorrhoeae* presents with localized ulcer of genitals, perineum, proximal lower extremities, or finger (Hook III and Handsfield 1990).
- extremity examination: assess small hand joints, wrists, knees, and ankles for tenderness, swelling, erythema, effusion associated with DGI.
  • Monoarthritis is present in 30 percent to 40 percent of patients with DGI; the rest have multiple joint involvement (Handsfield and Pollock 1990).
- abdomen: usually WNL in uncomplicated infections; may have tenderness and/or rebound tenderness in PID.
- external genitalia: erythema, edema, excoriation may be present.
- Bartolin's, urethral, Skene's glands: purulent or mucoid exudate (milk the glands, urethra); swelling/abscess formation may be present.
- vagina: abnormal discharge, blood, pus may be present.
- cervix: purulent or mucopurulent discharge may be present.
  • See details in *Chlamydia Trachomatis* Protocol, "Diagnostic Tests" section.
  • Edema/erythema of the zone of ectopy, friability, CMT may be present.
- uterus: usually WNL in uncomplicated infections; may have tenderness in acute PID.
- adnexa: usually WNL in uncomplicated infections; may have tenderness or masses in PID or TOA.

- rectum: usually WNL in uncomplicated infection; blood, mucopurulent discharge may be present in rectal infection; may have tenderness/masses in cul-de-sac area with PID or TOA.

→ Anoscopy, if performed, may reveal erythema, edema, mucopurulent exudate, and friable mucosa usually in the distal 5 cm to 10 cm of rectum.

→ Complete and accurate description of any identified lesion or other pertinent physical finding should be written in the "Objective" section of the progress note.

→ See *Chlamydia Trachomatis* Protocol for discussion of objective findings in FHC and Reiter's syndromes.

→ See **Pelvic Inflammatory Disease, Pelvic Masses, Syphilis**, and other **Sexually Transmitted Diseases** protocols.

ASSESSMENT

→ Gonorrhea (may be endocervical, pharyngeal, rectal)
→ Exposure to gonorrhea, other STD
→ Mucopurulent cervicitis
→ R/O gonorrhea
→ R/O *Chlamydia trachomatis*
→ R/O syphilis
→ R/O other concomitant STD
→ R/O vaginitis
→ R/O UTI/urethral syndrome
→ R/O DGI
→ R/O PID
→ R/O TOA
→ R/O perihepatitis (FHC syndrome)
→ R/O endocarditis/meningitis (rare)
→ R/O *N. meningitidis* infection

PLAN

DIAGNOSTIC TESTS

→ Cultures are considered the "gold standard" for diagnosis of gonorrhea (sensitivity 96 percent to 100 percent).
- Endocervical cultures for both *N. gonorrhoeae* and *C. trachomatis* should be obtained *prior* to use of bacteriostatic lubricant. (Endocervical cells are necessary for *C. trachomatis* culture. See *Chlamydia Trachomatis* Protocol.)

NOTE: For optimum gonococcus yield, *two* consecutive endocervical (or endocervical and rectal) specimens should be obtained, since a single specimen will miss 5 percent to 10 percent of gonococcal infections (Gibbs and Sweet 1989; Mardh and Danielsson 1990). After cleaning the ectocervix of exudate, insert swab 1 cm to 2 cm into endocervical canal and rotate for 10 to 30 seconds. (Samples may be collected from the posterior fornix but this practice is not recommended routinely.) In the absence of a cervix, urethral cultures should be obtained. To obtain a specimen, strip the urethra to express exudate or gently swab inside urethra. Use modified Thayer-Martin media for gonococcus and place promptly in CO_2 incubator, candle jar, or biological chamber system (self-sealing plastic bags—e.g., Bio-Bag®) that use CO_2-generating pills. All gonococcal isolates should be screened for beta-lactamase production.

→ Pharyngeal, rectal, and gland duct cultures as indicated depending upon signs, symptoms, sites exposed.
NOTE: Pharyngeal specimens are obtained from the posterior pharynx, tonsils, tonsillar pillars. Rectal cultures should be obtained by swabbing 2 cm to 4 cm into the anal canal, avoiding feces. Direct visualization via anoscopy should be used for specimen collection in patients with anorectal symptoms. Gland duct cultures are obtained after stripping exudate from gland duct openings.

→ Gram stain of endocervical or urethral secretions may be used as an adjunct to diagnosis in high-prevalence settings.
  ▪ It should not be used for screening of asymptomatic women or for diagnosis of pharyngeal gonorrhea.
  ▪ Positive stains reveal gram-negative diplococci within or closely associated with polymorphonuclear leukocytes; sensitivity 50 percent to 70 percent (Hook III and Handsfield 1990).

→ Direct specimen antigen detection methods (enzyme-linked immunosorbent assays [Gonozyme®], fluorescent antibody techniques, and DNA-hybridization techniques) are now commercially available and may be useful in high-prevalence populations or as alternative or complementary tests (Mardh and Danielsson 1990; Spence 1988).

NOTE: Except for the DNA-hybridization tests, antigen detection tests *do not* determine beta-lactamase production; thus, ideally they should be followed by culture. Complete discussion of the advantages and disadvantages of these tests is beyond the scope of this protocol.

→ Serological tests for *N. gonorrhoeae* antibodies are not recommended for screening or diagnosis but may be used as an adjunct to culture.

→ VDRL or RPR to rule out syphilis to be performed.

→ Serological HIV testing should be offered.

→ Suspected DGI:
  ▪ urogenital, oropharyngeal, and rectal specimens should be obtained for culture.
    • Cultures will be positive in more than 80 percent of patients (Hook III and Handsfield 1990; Mardh and Danielsson 1990).
  ▪ blood culture may be obtained.
  NOTE: Blood cultures should be collected promptly after suspicion of DGI because the incidence of positive cultures decreases quickly after onset of signs, symptoms (Mardh and Danielsson 1990). Positive results may be obtained in up to 50 percent of patients with polyarthritis within 2 days of symptom onset (Handsfield and Pollock 1990).
  ▪ acute and convalescent serum antibody titers may be obtained.
  ▪ culture or gram stain may be obtained from skin lesions, but these are positive in only 10 percent of cases (Dallabetta and Hook III 1987). Skin lesion material (scraped off with scalpel and smeared on glass slide) also may be sent for examination with fluorescent-labeled antigonococcal antibodies (Mardh and Danielsson 1990).
  ▪ synovial fluid may be aspirated from affected joints for culture or gram stain.
  NOTE: Specimen may be sent directly to laboratory in capped syringe for gram stain and culture, or inoculated directly into blood culture bottles (Mardh and Danielsson 1990). Cultures are often positive in cases where synovial leukocyte counts exceed 40,000 WBC/mm³ (Hook III and Handsfield 1990). Gram stain is positive in only 10 percent to 30 percent of cases (Dalabetta and Hook III 1987).
  Proven DGI = positive cultures from joints, blood, skin lesions.
  Probable DGI = arthritis/dermatitis syndrome, positive gonococcal cultures from primary

mucosal site, negative cultures from blood/other sterile-site.
Possible DGI = arthritis/dermatitis syndrome, positive response to therapy, negative cultures (Hook III and Handsfield 1990).

→ Screening for complement deficiency should be considered in patients with recurrent systemic gonococcal or meningococcal infection (Hook III and Handsfield 1990).

→ Additional tests may include (but are not limited to): wet mounts, Pap smear, CBC, urinalysis, urine culture and sensitivities, Hepatitis B screen, pregnancy test.

→ See **Chlamydia Trachomatis**, **Pelvic Inflammatory Disease**, and **Pelvic Masses** protocols.

TREATMENT/MANAGEMENT

→ Patients with MPC should await results of *C. trachomatis* and *N. gonorrhoeae* cultures prior to treatment, unless there is a high index of suspicion for infection or the patient is unlikely to return for follow-up (CDC 1993d).

  ▪ The CDC (1993d) recommends the following regarding treatment of patients with MPC:
    • treat for chlamydia and gonorrhea in populations with a high prevalence of both infections.
    • treat for chlamydia only if the prevalence of gonorrhea is low but the likelihood of chlamydia is substantial.
    • await culture results if the prevalence of both infections is low and if compliance with follow-up can be ensured.
    • sex partners should be notified, examined, and treated based on the patient's culture results.
      –In cases where patients are treated presumptively, partners should receive the same therapy.

→ Many antimicrobials are active against *N. gonorrhoeae*. The treatment regimens below are not intended to be a comprehensive list.

Uncomplicated anal or genital infection

→ Recommended regimens include:
  ▪ ceftriaxone (Rocephin®) 125 mg I.M. in a single dose

OR

  ▪ cefixime (Suprax®) 400 mg p.o. in a single dose
OR
  ▪ ciprofloxacin (Cipro®) 500 mg p.o. in a single dose

OR

  ▪ ofloxacin (Floxin®) 400 mg p.o. in a single dose
PLUS
  ▪ a regimen effective for possible coinfection with *C. trachomatis*, such as doxycycline (Vibramycin®) 100 mg p.o. BID for 7 days (CDC 1993d). (See **Chlamydia Trachomatis** Protocol.)
  NOTE: Quinolones (i.e., ciprofloxacin, ofloxacin) are contraindicated in pregnancy and lactation and in persons 17 years of age or younger; they are not effective against incubating syphilis (CDC 1993d).

→ Alternative regimens include:
  ▪ injectables:
    • spectinomycin (Trobicin®) 2 grams I.M. in a single dose (useful when patients are unable to tolerate cephalosporins/quinolones)
OR
    • ceftizoxime (Cefizox®) 500 mg I.M. in a single dose (the most effective of alternate cephalosporins)
OR
    • cefotaxime (Claforan®) 500 mg I.M. in a single dose
OR
    • cefotetan (Cefotan®) 1 gram I.M. in a single dose
OR
    • cefoxitin (Mefoxin®) 2 grams I.M. in a single dose
PLUS
    • a regimen effective for possible coinfection with *C. trachomatis*, such as doxycycline (Vibramycin®) 100 mg p.o. BID for 7 days (CDC 1993d). (See **Chlamydia Trachomatis** Protocol.)
    NOTE: Above alternate injectable cephalosporins are no more advantageous than ceftriaxone; ceftizoxime is the most effective of the alternates. Spectinomycin is not effective against incubating syphilis and relatively ineffective against pharyngeal gonorrhea (CDC 1993d).
  ▪ Oral cephalosporins:
    • cefuroxime axetil (Ceftin®) 1 g p.o. in a single dose
OR
    • cefpodoxime proxetil (Vantin®) 200 mg p.o. in a single dose
PLUS
    • a regimen effective for possible coinfection with *C. trachomatis*, such as doxycycline

(Vibramycin®) 100 mg p.o. BID for 7 days
(CDC 1993d). (See *Chlamydia Trachomatis*
Protocol.)
NOTE: Neither alternate oral cephalosporin is
very effective against pharyngeal gonorrhea.
- oral quinolones:
  - enoxacin (Penetrex®) 400 mg p.o. in a single
    dose
              OR
  - lomefloxacin (Maxaquin®) 400 mg p.o. in a
    single dose
              OR
  - norfloxacin (Noroxin®) 800 mg p.o. in a
    single dose
              PLUS
  - a regimen effective for possible coinfection
    with *C. trachomatis*, such as doxycycline
    (Vibramycin®) 100 mg p.o. BID for 7 days
    (CDC 1993d). (See *Chlamydia Trachomatis*
    Protocol.)
  NOTE: Above alternate quinolones are no
  more advantageous than ciprofloxacin or
  ofloxacin. Quinolones are not effective against
  incubating syphilis and are contraindicated in
  pregnancy, lactation, and in persons 17 years
  of age or younger (CDC 1993d).
- single-drug therapy for gonorrhea and
  chlamydia:
  - ofloxacin (Floxin®) 400 mg p.o., then 300 mg
    p.o. BID for 7 days (CDC 1993d).
  NOTE: Contraindicated in pregnancy and
  lactation and in persons 17 years of age and
  younger (CDC 1993d).

Uncomplicated pharyngeal infection

→ Ceftriaxone (Rocephin®) 125 mg I.M. in a single
  dose
              OR
→ Ciprofloxacin (Cipro®) 500 mg p.o. in a single
  dose.
NOTE: Quinolones are not effective against
incubating syphilis; contraindicated in pregnancy and
lactation and in persons 17 years of age or younger
(CDC 1993d).
→ The CDC (1993d) recommends that persons
  treated for gonorrhea be treated presumptively
  with a regimen effective for chlamydia.

Adult gonococcal conjunctivitis

→ Ceftriaxone (Rocephin®) 1 g I.M. in a single dose.
  Lavage the infected eye with saline solution once
  (CDC 1993d).

→ Ophthalmological assessment as indicated.
→ Consider coexistent chlamydial infection if
  condition does not respond to therapy.
  - The CDC (1993d) recommends that persons
    treated for gonorrhea be treated presumptively
    with a regimen effective for chlamydia.

Disseminated gonococcal infection (DGI)

→ Hospitalization is recommended for initial
  therapy, especially in unreliable patients. Details
  of treatment are beyond the scope of this protocol.
  Refer to 1993 CDC guidelines (CDC 1993d).

Gonococcal meningitis/endocarditis

→ Hospitalization is recommended. Specific
  treatment regimens for these conditions are
  beyond the scope of this protocol. Refer to 1993
  CDC guidelines (CDC 1993d).

Treatment in pregnancy

→ Use a recommended or alternate cephalosporin
  plus erythromycin to cover possible coexisting
  chlamydia (CDC 1993d). (See *Chlamydia
  Trachomatis* Protocol.)
→ In cases where cephalosporins are not tolerated,
  use spectinomycin 2 g I.M. in a single dose.
  However, spectinomycin is not effective against
  incubating syphilis and relatively ineffective
  against pharyngeal gonorrhea (CDC 1993d).
→ Quinolones and tetracyclines are contraindicated
  during pregnancy.

Partner therapy

→ All sexual contacts of patients with *symptomatic*
  gonorrhea who have been exposed within the 30
  days prior to the onset of the patient's symptoms
  should be evaluated and treated for both
  gonorrhea and chlamydia (CDC 1991, 1993d).
  - Sexual partners of patients with *asymptomatic*
    infections should be evaluated and treated if the
    sexual contact was within 60 days of the
    patient's diagnosis.
  - The most recent sexual partner should be
    treated regardless of the aforementioned time
    periods. Provide referrals to provider or facility
    that offers appropriate STD care as indicated.

Special considerations

→ Cross-reactivity of cephalosporins and penicillin
  in penicilin-allergic patients may occur in up to 10
  percent of patients (*PDR* 1993).
  - Cephalosporins should be withheld in those
    patients with a history of anaphylactic or

histamine response to penicillin (City and County of San Francisco, Department of Public Health 1989; *PDR* 1993).

→ Serious and fatal reactions have been reported in patients receiving ciprofloxacin and theophylline concurrently (*PDR* 1993).

→ For patients sensitive/allergic to cephalosporins, quinolones should be used.
  ▪ If neither can be tolerated, substitute with spectinomycin, except in cases of suspected pharyngeal infection.
    • In this situation trimethoprim/sulfamethox-azole 720 mg/3600 mg p.o. once a day for 5 days may be effective (CDC 1993d).

→ Patients with both gonorrhea *and* syphilis as well as contacts of patients with syphilis should be treated for syphilis according to CDC guidelines.
  ▪ Most patients with *incubating* syphilis will be cured with regimens that include ceftriaxone or a 7-day course of either doxycycline or erythromycin (CDC 1993d).
  ▪ Spectinomycin and the quinolones are not effective against incubating syphilis.
    • If used, a serological test for syphilis should be repeated in 1 month (CDC 1989b). (See **Syphilis** Protocol.)

→ HIV-infected persons should be treated with the same regimens as those for individuals without HIV (CDC 1993d).

→ Observe patients for untoward reactions to I.M. medication for a period of 30 minutes after administration.

→ See **Pelvic Inflammatory Disease, Pelvic Masses, *Chlamydia Trachomatis*, Syphilis,** and other **Sexually Transmitted Diseases** protocols.

CONSULTATION

→ Consultation with a physician is indicated for patients with PID, DGI, FHC syndrome, endocarditis, meningitis.

→ Hospitalization is recommended for initial therapy of DGI and complications thereof and for patients with endocarditis or meningitis. Hospitalization should be considered in patients with PID. (See **Pelvic Inflammatory Disease** Protocol.)

→ As needed for prescription(s).

PATIENT EDUCATION

→ Discuss etiology and nature of gonorrhea, including mode of transmission, incubation period, symptoms, potential complications and possibility of coexistent chlamydia or other STD, and importance of evaluation and treatment of sexual partner(s).
  ▪ Patient-education handouts are a helpful adjunct to teaching.

→ Stress compliance with treatment regimens.

→ Advise abstinence from intercourse until patient and partner are treated and cured. If symptoms recur, patient and partner should be instructed to seek care promptly.

→ Address STD prevention and HIV risk-reduction.
  ▪ Provide guidelines for safer sex practices.
  ▪ Encourage careful screening of sex partners and committed use of condoms/spermicides (especially with new, multiple, nonmonogamous partners).
  ▪ See **Table 13A.2, Safer Sex Guidelines,** p. 13-9, and **Table 12I.1, Recommendations for Individuals to Prevent STD/PID,** p. 12-96.

→ Allow patient to ventilate her feelings of surprise, shame, fear, anger as indicated. Psychological support may be important for the patient in gaining control over her sexual situation and to enable her to prevent future STDs.

FOLLOW-UP

→ Test-of-cure cultures are not essential in cases of uncomplicated gonorrhea treated with the above regimens (CDC 1993d).
  ▪ Patients with persistent symptoms after treatment should have a culture done for *N. gonorrhoeae*, with isolates tested for antimicrobial susceptibility (CDC 1993d).

→ Recurrence of gonorrhea may be due to reinfection.
  ▪ Advise patient to return for evaluation if symptoms of infection recur.
  ▪ History on follow-up should include symptom status, medication compliance, drug reaction or side effects, partner therapy, sexual exposure, and use of condoms.
  ▪ All sexual partners of symptomatic patients should be evaluated.

→ Infection with *C. trachomatis* and other organisms should be considered in cases of persistent cervicitis, urethritis, or proctitis (CDC 1993d).

→ Patients treated with spectinomycin or the quinolones should have a serological test for syphilis in one month (CDC 1989b).

→ Follow up on all laboratory tests ordered. Treat all concomitant STDs and other identified conditions.
  ▪ Continue to encourage safer sex.

→ Negative HIV antibody tests may be repeated in three to six months.

→ HIV-positive results should be conveyed in person and by a provider who has received training in the complexities of test disclosure. HIV-positive persons should be referred to the appropriate provider or agency for early intervention services.

→ Hepatitis B antigen-positive individuals should have liver function tests and receive counseling regarding the implications of their positive status and need for immunoprophylaxis of sex partners and household members. (See **Hepatitis—Viral** Protocol.)

→ Routine gonococcal cultures for screening of asymptomatic women in high-risk groups should be considered—i.e., women with history of repeated gonorrhea or other STD, prostitutes, women with multiple partners or a sexual partner with multiple sexual contacts, partners of male with gonorrhea or urethritis in past three months, teenagers, younger women, drug abusers (Sweet and Gibbs 1990; U.S. Preventive Services Task Force 1990).

→ Because gonorrhea is a state-mandated reportable disease, a morbidity report needs to be filed with the department of public health.

→ See **Pelvic Inflammatory Disease, Pelvic Masses, *Chlamydia Trachomatis*, Syphilis,** and other **Sexually Transmitted Diseases** protocols.

→ Document gonorrhea diagnosis and complications/sequelae thereof in progress notes and problem list.

13-D

Granuloma Inguinale (Donovanosis)

An extremely rare disease in the United States, *granuloma inguinale* is common in central Australia, New Guinea, India, southern China, the Caribbean, Africa, and other subtropical and tropical environments. The Centers for Disease Control and Prevention (CDC) reports fewer than 100 cases in the U.S. annually; an epidemic of 20 cases was reported recently in Texas.

The infectious agent in granuloma inguinale is *Calymmatobacterium granulomatis*, a gram-negative bacterium, also called the Donovan body. Granuloma inguinale is believed to be transmitted both sexually and nonsexually. The most frequent occurrence is in sexually active individuals, and a history of sexual intercourse almost always precedes onset of the primary genital ulcer. Other STDs, such as syphilis and/or gonorrhea, may coexist with granuloma inguinale.

Contagion is generally mild, and repeated exposure is necessary for development of most cases of the disease. Nonsexual transmission may occur via autoinoculation of the genital tract from the rectum. Disease occurrence has been identified in the very young and elderly. In the Caribbean, a high incidence of squamous carcinoma of the vulva has been reported in premenopausal women with granuloma inguinale (Blanco and Gonik 1991; Hart 1990; Richens 1991; Sweet and Gibbs 1990).

Classically, progression of the disease is from a primary genital ulcer to subcutaneous granulomatous spread. The incubation period is generally from eight to 80 days. The inguinal area may become infected (pseudobubo) with overlying skin ulceration. Distant sites of disseminated infection are also possible, including the liver, thorax, lungs, spleen, colon, and bone. Patients often present late in the course of the disease when disfigure-

ment already has occurred. Without treatment, scarring and tissue destruction are common.

In patients with AIDS, *donovanosis* infection may behave differently, and treatment failure may result even after extended courses of antibiotics. In South Africa, sexually active individuals infected with granuloma inguinale have associated HIV seropositivity (Blanco and Gonik 1991; Hart 1990).

In treatment of the disease, a host of antibiotics have been employed, some potentially toxic and others with variable effectiveness. Granuloma inguinale responds best to lipid-soluble antibiotics such as chloramphenicol, erythromycin, lincomycin, quinolones, and tetracyclines (See following "Treatment" section.) (Hart 1990; Richens 1991).

DATABASE

SUBJECTIVE

→ Peak ages for granuloma inguinale are from 20 years to 40 years.

→ Patient has history of sexual contact three to 40 days prior to appearance of initial lesion.

→ Patient may have history of travel to area where granuloma inguinale is endemic.

→ Fifty percent or more of sex partners of patients with disease affected.

→ Coexistent STD common (e.g., gonorrhea, syphilis).

→ Initial lesion may go unnoticed.

→ Symptoms may include:
  ▪ pruritus—may precede or accompany lesion.
  ▪ painless lump in genital area.

- ulceration of genital tissues.
- ulceration may also occur in mouth and on lips, throat, face.
- bleeding from ulcerated lesions.
- swelling in inguinal area.
- vaginal discharge or bleeding.
- perianal "cauliflower-like" tumor.

→ Gynecological and medical history should include:
- menstrual cycle.
- contraception.
- description of symptoms:
  - onset.
  - duration.
  - quality/quantity.
  - frequency.
  - course.
  - aggravating/relieving factors.
  - associated symptoms.
- previous history of same/similar problem.
- STD history (including dates/treatment).
- sensitive questioning regarding recent sexual activity, including date of last exposure, sex practices, sites of exposure, number of partners in past month, use of condoms.
- sex partner history.
- acute/chronic illness.
- general health.
- medications.
- allergies.
- habits.
- history of laboratory tests for syphilis, Hepatitis B, HIV.
- review of systems (CDC 1991).

OBJECTIVE

→ Examination may be individualized based on case presentation.

→ Thorough STD examination includes:
- vital signs as indicated.
- general skin inspection of face, trunk, forearms, palms, soles for lesions, rashes, discoloration.
- inspection of pharynx and oral cavity for erythema, infection, lesions, discoloration.
- abdominal inspection and palpation for masses, tenderness, rebound tenderness.
- inspection of pubic hair for lice, nits.
- inspection of external genitalia for discharge, masses, lesions.
- inspection and palpation of Bartholin's, urethral, and Skene's glands for discharge, masses.
- inspection of vagina for discharge, lesions.

- inspection of cervix for lesions, discharge, eversion, erythema edema, friability; assessment for CMT.
- uterine assessment for size, shape, consistency, mobility, tenderness.
- palpation of adnexa for masses, tenderness.
- inspection of perianus and anus for lesions, bleeding, discharge.
- rectal examination as indicated.
- assessment of presence or absence of associated lymphadenopathy (CDC 1991).

→ Characteristics of granuloma inguinale include:
- lesions generally appearing on the labia, fourchette, crural folds, and perianus.
- lesions of the vagina, cervix, head (mouth, lips, throat, face), and/or axilla may also occur.
- vulvar and cervical changes may mimic carcinomatous growth. (Six percent of cases present with extragenital disease [Greenblatt 1990].)
- initial small, nontender single or multiple papule(s) or nodule(s).
- lesion that erodes through skin, producing clean, sharply defined granulomatous ulcer; beefy red/velvety, friable, slowly enlarging with variable induration.
- spread to inguinal area, producing pseudo-bubo—a subcutaneous granulomatous process not involving the lymph nodes, thus adenopathy absent.
  - Overlying skin usually ulcerates.
- lymphedema of labia and distal tissues that may occur in chronic active disease phase.
  - However, lymphatic blockage and fibrosis are rare.
- secondary infection which may produce necrotic debris at ulcer edge.
  - Cellulitis rare, however.
- verrucous form of disease which may occur in perianal area.
- systemic symptoms, absent except in rare cases of intrapelvic spread, secondary infection, or hematogenous dissemination.
- in some cases, extensive scarring which may accompany active disease.
- depigmented irregular scars that may appear at border of healed lesion.

→ Complete and accurate descriptions of any identified lesions or other pertinent physical findings should be written in the "Objective" section of the progress note.

ASSESSMENT

→ Granuloma inguinale

→ R/O herpes genitalis

→ R/O chancroid

→ R/O LGV

→ R/O carcinoma

→ R/O syphilis

→ R/O condyloma lata

→ R/O ulcerated genital warts

→ R/O genital amebiasis

→ R/O concomitant STDs

→ R/O metastatic genital cancer (cervical, vulvar, vaginal)

PLAN

DIAGNOSTIC TESTS

→ Distinguish between granuloma inguinale and other causes of genital ulcers.
  - See **Table 13A.1, Clinical Features of Genital Ulcers**, p. 13-6, and **Figure 13A.1, Sexually Active Patient with Genital Ulcers**, p. 13-7.

→ Culture is not recommended for diagnosis due to the fastidious nature of the organism and lack of adequate culture methods.

→ Identification of Donovan bodies from lesional material stained with Giemsa or Wright's stain is the "gold standard" of diagnosis.
  NOTE: Good technique in obtaining and preparing slide is important: 1) clean active ulcerated area with saline; 2) with forceps, scalpel blade, punch biopsy instrument, or cotton swab, detach small piece of tissue from edge of ulcer (local anesthesia may be necessary); 3) smear on glass slide or crush specimen between two glass slides; 4) air dry, heat fix, then stain. Donovan bodies appear as "safety-pin," blue-black organisms (Richens 1991).

→ Biopsy is recommended for very early or sclerotic lesions, those with superinfection, and when carcinoma is being ruled out (Richens 1991).

→ Pap smears may have identified Donovan bodies.

→ Complement fixation tests have been used in some settings but are not standardized approaches to diagnosis.

→ Diagnostic tests to rule out other causes of genital ulcers and lymphadenopathy include:

  - dark-field or direct immunofluorescence test of serous fluid for *T. pallidum* from genital and non-oral lesion(s) to rule out syphilis. (See **Syphilis** Protocol.)
  - RPR (or VDRL) to rule out syphilis. (See **Syphilis** Protocol.)
  - herpes cultures or Tzanck stain from genital lesion(s) to rule out herpes. (See **Genital Herpes Simplex Virus** Protocol.)
  - see "Diagnostic Test" sections of **Chancroid** and **Lymphogranuloma Venereum** protocols.

→ Endocervical culture for *N. gonorrhoeae* and endocervical diagnostic tests for *C. trachomatis*. In the absence of a cervix, urethral specimen may be obtained.

→ HIV testing should be offered.

→ Additional tests may include (but are not limited to): wet mounts, CBC, urinalysis, urine culture and sensitivities, pregnancy testing, Hepatitis B screen.

TREATMENT/MANAGEMENT

→ Treatment of choice:
  - tetracycline (Achromycin V®, Sumycin®) 500 mg p.o. QID for 21 days (Hart 1990; Sweet and Gibbs 1990)

  OR

  - doxycycline (Vibramycin®) 100 mg p.o. BID for 21 days (Greenblatt 1990).

→ Treatment alternatives:
  - chloramphenicol (Chloromycetin®) 500 mg p.o. TID for 21 days (best choice in developing countries; reserved for resistant cases).
  - gentamycin (Garamycin®) 1 mg/kg I.M. or I.V. BID for 21 days (reserved for resistant cases).
  NOTE: Toxicity may occur with the above 2 drugs. See *PDR*.
  - ampicillin (Omnipen®) 500 mg p.o. QID for 12 weeks.
  - erythromycin (E-Mycin®) 500 mg p.o. every 6 hours for 21 days.
  - cotrimoxazole (Septrin®) 2 tablets p.o. every 12 hours for 10 days.
  - lincomycin (Lincocin®) 500 mg p.o. QID for 21 days.
  - sulfisoxazole (Gantrisin®) 500 mg p.o. QID for 21 days.
  - spectinomycin (Trobicin®) 1 gram I.M. for 21 days (higher relapse rates) (Blanco and Gonik 1991; Greenblatt 1990; Hart 1990).

→ Treatment of sequelae and complications.

- Strictures and fistulae may require surgery.
- Because extragenital lesions may be refractory to antibiotics, surgical curettage plus antibiotic therapy may be necessary.
- Spread of donovanosis to pelvic organs may occur, mimicking PID or malignancy. Surgical exploration may be indicated for drainage of fluid collections but must be attempted only with antibiotic coverage to prevent dissemination of donovanosis (Richens 1991).

CONSULTATION

→ As indicated for assessment and management of patient.

→ As needed for prescription(s).

→ Physician referral for complicated cases.

PATIENT EDUCATION

→ Discuss etiology and nature of the infection including mode of transmission, incubation period, symptoms, diagnostic tests, potential complications, and possible association with increased risk for HIV acquisition.
  - Explain to the patient that an area of depigmentation may occur at the border of the healed lesion (Hart 1990).
  - Patient-education handouts are a helpful adjunct to teaching.

→ Advise patient to finish full course of medication and return for follow-up (see "Follow-Up" section).

→ Discuss importance of evaluation and treatment of sexual partner(s). Provide referrals to provider or facility offering appropriate STD care.

→ Advise abstinence from intercourse until patient and partner are treated and cured. If symptoms recur, patient or partner should be instructed to seek care promptly.

→ Address STD prevention and HIV risk-reduction.
  - Provide guidelines for safer sex practices.
  - Encourage careful screening of sex partners and committed use of condoms (especially with new, multiple, non-monogamous partners).
  - See **Table 13A.2, Safer Sex Guidelines**, p. 13-9, and **Table 12I.1, Recommendations for Individuals to Prevent STD/PID**, p. 12-96.

→ Allow patient to ventilate her feelings of surprise, shame, fear, anger as indicated. Psychological support may be important for the patient in gaining control over her sexual situation and to enable her to prevent future STDs.

FOLLOW-UP

→ Treatment should be continued for 21 days or until all lesions are healed.
  - Lesions are generally paler/less visible in a few days, shrinking after seven days.
  - Total healing may take three to five weeks.
  - Recurrence rates are higher if antibiotics are discontinued prior to healing of primary lesion.
  - Patients should be seen during the course of treatment for assessment of response to therapy (weekly or individualized until lesions are clearly resolving) (CDC 1991).

→ History on follow-up should include symptom status, medication compliance, drug reaction and side effects, partner therapy, sexual exposure, and use of condoms (CDC 1991).

→ Serological tests for syphilis should be repeated in three months.

→ HIV antibody tests should be repeated in three and six months. Continue to encourage safer sex.

→ Follow up on all laboratory tests ordered. Treat all concomitant STDs and other identified conditions.

→ If ordered, HIV test results should be conveyed in person and by a provider who has received training in the complexities of test disclosure. HIV-positive persons should be referred to the appropriate provider or agency for early intervention services.

→ Hepatitis B antigen-positive individuals should have liver function tests and receive counseling regarding the implications of seropositivity and need for immunoprophylaxis of sex partners and household members. (See **Hepatitis—Viral** Protocol.)

→ Because granuloma inguinale is a state-mandated reportable disease, a morbidity report must be filed with the department of public health.

→ Document in progress notes and problem list.

Joan R. Murphy, R.N., C., M.S., N.P., C.N.S.

13-E

Genital Herpes Simplex Virus

Genital herpes simplex virus (HSV) is a sexually transmitted disease caused by two types of the herpes virus. *Herpes simplex virus type II* (HSV-2) causes the majority of genital infections and infections below the waist. *Herpes simplex virus type I* (HSV-1) is responsible for most oral lesions and infections above the waist, although approximately 15 percent of primary genital HSV infections are caused by HSV-1 (Rose and Camp 1988; Sweet and Gibbs 1990).

Both HSV-1 and HSV-2 can infect mucous membranes and/or abraded skin at any site, but the severity and duration of symptoms with an initial infection are not influenced by virus type. Conversely, virus type and site of infection *do* affect the likelihood of recurrences and their frequency (Mertz 1990).

HSV is the single most common cause of genital ulcers in the United States (Mertz 1990). The infection is transmitted by mucosal contact with HSV-infected secretions, and lesions progress through four stages: vesicular, pustular, ulcerative, and coalescent/crusted (Corey et al. 1983; Mead 1991; Strauss 1985). See **Figure 13E.1, Clinical Course of Primary Genital Herpes Simplex Virus Infection.** Humans are the sole known reservoir for HSV, although survival of HSV on environmental surfaces has been documented. Fomite and aerosol transmission are unlikely, however. The risk of sexual transmission is estimated at 10 percent per year in recent studies of monogamous heterosexual couples with discordant HSV serum antibody status (Safrin 1994).

The incidence of HSV infections is rising, and approximately 500,000 new cases of genital HSV occur annually in the United States (Sweet and Gibbs 1990). The prevalence of genital HSV is estimated to range from 0.3 percent to 22 percent of the population, or approximately 20 million cases. The varying percentages depend on age, race, sex, level of sexual activity, and socioeconomic status (Strauss 1985; Sweet and Gibbs 1990).

Prevalence rates are difficult to estimate due to the fact that HSV is not required to be reported in the United States (Strauss 1985). It has been estimated that approximately 15 percent to 35 percent of Caucasians and 35 percent to 50 percent of non-Caucasians in the general population of the United States are seropositive for HSV-2 antibody (Safrin 1994).

The risk of transmission from an infected male to a female is estimated to be 80 percent to 100 percent (Rose and Camp 1988; Strauss 1985). Higher rates are seen in the third decade of life and in more educated, and married and Caucasian populations (Strauss 1985; Sweet and Gibbs 1990).

Much controversy exists regarding the role HSV plays in the development of cervical cancer. It has been stated that women with HSV develop cervical cancer approximately five times as often as women who do not have HSV, but more recent studies have shown a link with human papillomavirus instead (Davies 1990; Sweet and Gibbs 1990).

There are four distinct presentations of HSV infection (Mead 1991; Sweet and Gibbs 1990).

Primary Herpes

Primary herpes is the first clinical episode of HSV in a patient who does not have antibodies to HSV-1 or HSV-2. The incubation period is one to 45 days, with a mean of 5.8 days (Strauss 1985). Primary HSV is characterized by severe local symptoms with a prolonged duration, commonly with bilateral distribution. Lesions progress

Figure 13E.1. CLINICAL COURSE OF PRIMARY GENITAL HERPES SIMPLEX VIRUS INFECTION

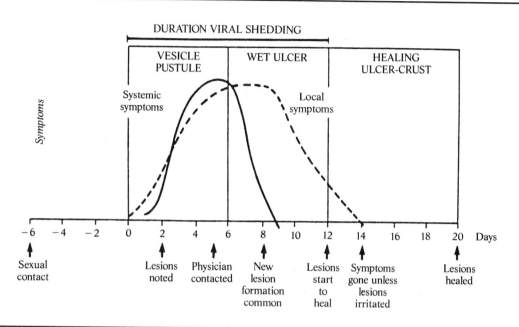

Source: Reprinted with permission from Corey, L.; Adams, H.G.; Brown, Z.A.; and Holmes, K.K. 1983. Genital herpes simplex virus infections: Clinical manifestations, course, and complication. *Annals of Internal Medicine* 98(6):961.

from painful and pruritic pustules to vesicles which often coalesce to form large areas of ulceration. If untreated, new lesions often form by the second week, with healing occurring by the third week after onset (Davies 1990; Mertz 1990). (See **Figure 13E.1.**) Systemic symptoms such as fever, malaise, myalgia, and adenopathy often accompany a primary outbreak (ACOG 1988; Davies 1990; Mead 1991; Mertz 1990; Strauss 1985; Sweet and Gibbs 1990).

Symptoms usually last approximately two weeks, and healing occurs in one to two weeks. Therefore, total time of infection from onset of lesions to complete healing is three to four weeks (ACOG 1988; Mead 1991). Mean duration of viral shedding is 11 to 14 days (Mead 1991; Mertz 1990). Cervical shedding of the virus occurs in 80 percent to 86 percent of women with primary HSV (Sweet and Gibbs 1990). Serum antibody is not present when symptoms appear, then rises in convalescence. However, titer levels may be blunted by acyclovir, if used for therapy (Safrin 1994). (See **Table 13E.1, Characteristics of True Primary and Recurrent Genital Herpes Infection**.)

Concomitant with primary genital infection, HSV ascends peripheral sensory nerves and enters the spinal root ganglia, where it establishes latency. Reactivation is precipitated by multiple factors (Corey 1990; Safrin 1994) (see following "Recurrent Herpes" section).

Possible complications of primary HSV include viral meningitis (four percent to ten percent), HSV encephalitis, temporary autonomic nervous system dysfunction (less than one percent), extragenital lesions, and herpes pharyngitis (ACOG 1988). Concomitant yeast infections are also common (Davies 1990). Primary HSV tends to be more severe in women than in men (Mertz 1990). Disseminated HSV infection is extremely rare in immunocompetent individuals.

Non-Primary First-Episode Herpes

Non-primary first-episode herpes is the initial clinical outbreak of herpes in a patient who has either HSV-1 or HSV-2 antibodies (Mead 1991; Sweet and Gibbs 1990). The infection occurs due to reactivation of the latent virus (ACOG 1988). The clinical course is less severe, and signs and symptoms are of shorter duration, similar to recurrent HSV (ACOG 1988; Davies 1990). The only definitive way to determine whether a patient has had a primary or non-primary outbreak is by serological testing (i.e., in non-primary first episodes antibody present initially, rises in convalescence), although lack of severe clinical signs and symptoms correlates well with non-primary first-episode infections. Cervical shedding of HSV occurs in approximately 65 percent of cases (Safrin 1994; Sweet and Gibbs 1990).

Table 13E.1. CHARACTERISTICS OF TRUE PRIMARY AND RECURRENT GENITAL HERPES INFECTION

Features	True primary	Recurrent
Incubation period	2 to 10 days	
Prodrome		1 to 2 days
Fever	+	
Regional lymphadenopathy	+	
Malaise	+	
Duration of genital symptoms (mean)	Approx. 15 days	Approx. 7 days
Duration of viral shedding (mean)	Approx. 15 days	Approx. 5 days
Number of lesions	Greater	Fewer
Cervical lesions	Common	Uncommon

Reprinted with permission from Sweet, R.L., and Gibbs, R.S. 1990. *Infectious diseases of the female genital tract*, p. 145. Baltimore: Williams & Wilkins.

Recurrent Herpes

Recurrent HSV is characterized by symptoms, signs, and sites of infection localized to the genital region (Corey 1990). Symptoms are usually mild and of shorter duration than with primary HSV (average five to ten days) (ACOG 1988). Systemic symptoms are usually absent.

Most outbreaks are well-localized, with a smaller mean number of lesions occurring and usually unilateral (Mertz 1990). Approximately 50 percent of recurrent HSV outbreaks are preceded by a prodrome. The prodrome occurs several hours to several days before the onset of lesions and is characterized by local symptoms such as paresthesias, itching, and pain (Davies 1990; Mertz 1990; Sweet and Gibbs 1990).

The duration of viral shedding is shorter with recurrent HSV, with a mean duration of four days (Mertz 1990). Cervical shedding of HSV with recurrent outbreaks occurs in only about 12 percent of cases (Sweet and Gibbs 1990). (See **Table 13E.1.**) There is generally no change in antibody titer in convalescence (Safrin 1994).

Certain "triggers" may reactivate the latent virus and cause recurrent outbreaks (e.g., stress, menses, trauma, illness, ultraviolet light). There is no scientific evidence that sexual activity affects the onset of recurrences (Davies 1990). However, some patients may report that sexual intercourse is a factor in triggering outbreaks.

The average rate of recurrence is approximately four times per year for the first few years, with a subsequent gradual decrease in frequency (Davies 1990). Approximately 50 percent of patients with primary HSV will have a recurrent outbreak within six months (Sweet and Gibbs 1990).

Genital HSV-1 infection does not recur as frequently as genital HSV-2 (Davies 1990). In the first year, the median number of recurrences of HSV-2 is four times greater than HSV-1. Recurrence of genital HSV-1 is milder, with a shorter course, than HSV-2 (Sweet and Gibbs 1990). The most frequent recurrences are due to genital HSV-2; the next frequent are due to oral-labial HSV-1; then genital HSV-1; and the least frequent recurrences are due to oral-labial HSV-2 (Mertz 1990). Frequent recurrences happen only in a minority of affected people, and the vast majority of patients infected with HSV-2 are unaware of their infection, which may recur infrequently, if at all (ACOG 1988; Mertz 1990).

Asymptomatic Herpes

Asymptomatic HSV is defined as transmission of HSV in the absence of clinical signs and symptoms. Most commonly, this occurs with patients who do not have a history of genital HSV. Serum antibody is present (Safrin 1994). Women with a positive history of symptomatic genital HSV have been shown to asymptomatically shed HSV four percent to 14 percent of the time, and one-third to two-thirds of women with positive genital cultures do not have clinically evident lesions (Rose and Camp 1988; Sweet and Gibbs 1990).

Rates of asymptomatic shedding seem to be greater with HSV-2 than HSV-1, and the presence of serum antibody to HSV-1 seems to decrease rates of asymptomatic shedding with HSV-2 (Safrin 1994). The rate of asymptomatic infection is unknown, but may be as high as 50 percent (Strauss 1985).

Many cases of genital herpes are acquired from individuals who are unaware that they have a genital infection with HSV or who were asymptomatic at the time of sexual contact (CDC 1993c). It is not known whether there is any difference in asymptomatic shedding between patients who use oral acyclovir and those who do not (ACOG 1988).

DATABASE

SUBJECTIVE

Primary infection

→ The most common etiology of vulvar ulcers is infection with HSV (Mead 1991). Severity of symptoms, duration of viral shedding, and duration of lesions is similar in primary HSV-1 and HSV-2 disease (Corey 1990).

→ Patient may have history of exposure to infected partner.

→ Symptoms may include:
  ▪ multiple painful genital lesions (papules, vesicles, pustules, ulcers, fissures).
    • May be bilateral.
  ▪ itching, burning, and/or tingling at site of infection.
  ▪ flu-like symptoms—malaise, headache, fever, stiff neck, mild photophobia, myalgias, nausea.
    • Systemic symptoms appear early, reach a peak in three to four days after lesion onset, and gradually recede over subsequent three to four days (Corey 1990).
  ▪ dysuria (both external and internal), urinary retention.
  ▪ inguinal adenopathy.
    • Usually appears during second to third week; often last symptom to resolve (Corey 1990).
  ▪ sacral paresthesia.
  ▪ change in vaginal discharge (amount, color, consistency, odor).
  ▪ dyspareunia/pelvic pain.
  ▪ tender inguinal adenopathy.
  ▪ sore throat (in pharyngeal infection; 20 percent of patients with primary HSV-1 or HSV-2).

→ Symptoms last for approximately two to four weeks.

→ See previous discussion of "Primary" and "Non-Primary First-Episode Herpes Infection."

Recurrent infection

→ Approximately 50 percent of patients will have a recurrent infection within six months of the primary outbreak (Sweet and Gibbs 1990), and many HSV infections present with atypical symptoms (Mertz 1990).

→ Patient may be asymptomatic.

→ Patient may present with:
  ▪ history of previous HSV outbreaks.

→ Symptoms may include:

  ▪ prodromal symptoms: pain, itching, burning, tingling, numbness, sensitivity (paresthesias) at site where lesions will develop.
    • Symptoms last from 12 hours to two days, but may come and go for up to one week.
  ▪ painful, well-localized genital sore(s) (single or small clusters).
  ▪ itching, burning, and/or tingling at site of infection.
  ▪ dysuria (usually external).
  ▪ systemic symptoms (usually absent).

→ Symptoms usually resolve within seven to ten days.

→ See previous discussion of "Recurrent Herpes Infection."

OBJECTIVE

→ Patient may present with the following findings:
  ▪ elevated temperature (primary HSV).
  ▪ pharynx: if infected, signs include mild erythema or diffuse ulceration with white exudate. Tender cervical lymph nodes are usually present in association with HSV pharyngitis.
  ▪ external genitalia: papules, vesicles, ulcerations, crusted-over lesions, localized erythema/edema.
    • Bilateral lesions usually indicative of primary HSV; unilateral lesions usually indicative of recurrent HSV).

NOTE: Hurricaine® gel, a numbing compound, may be used to facilitate the pelvic examination when painful lesions are present.

  ▪ vagina: leukorrhea, normal or abnormal discharge.
  ▪ cervix: may be friable, erythematous; watery discharge may be present; may see ulcerative lesions on ectocervix; necrotic mass may be present; may have CMT.

NOTE: Primary herpes cervicitis occurs in approximately 90 percent of primary HSV-2 infection, 70 percent of primary HSV-1 infection, and 70 percent of nonprimary first-episode HSV-2 infection. Only ten percent to 30 percent of women with recurrent lesions have concomitant cervical infection (Corey 1990).

  ▪ inguinal and/or generalized lymphadenopathy (primary HSV); inguinal nodes usually firm, nonfluctuant, tender.
  ▪ extragenital lesions (fingers, eyes, perianal area, buttocks, thighs, oropharynx) (common complication of primary HSV, uncommon in non-primary/recurrent HSV).

→ Wet mount: no pathogens, unless concomitant infection; may see increased WBCs.

→ Pap smear may reveal presence of giant, multinucleated cells (not diagnostic of HSV-2).

→ Results of HSV culture of lesions and/or cervix may be positive (diagnostic of HSV infection or viral shedding).

→ Serological studies reveal fourfold or greater rise in antibody titer (compare acute and convalescent serum).
  ▪ Useful for determination of primary HSV.

→ HSV antibody testing also may be used to document past, asymptomatic, or atypical infection but does not discriminate well between HSV-1 and HSV-2 (Corey 1990). A single positive serum antibody does not indicate new or old infection unless a previous negative test is available (Safrin 1994).

→ See previous discussions of "Primary Herpes," "Non-Primary First-Episode Herpes," and "Recurrent Herpes" infections.

ASSESSMENT

→ R/O herpes genitalis

→ R/O extragenital herpes lesions

→ R/O chancroid

→ R/O syphilitic chancre

→ R/O lymphogranuloma venereum

→ R/O fungal infection

→ R/O eczemoid vulvitis (lichen sclerosus/squamous cell hyperplasia)

→ R/O pemphigus/bullous pemphigoid

→ R/O Beçhet's syndrome

→ R/O aphthous ulceration ("canker sore")

→ R/O squamous/basal cell carcinoma

→ R/O trauma

→ R/O Crohn's disease

→ R/O invasive cervical carcinoma

PLAN

DIAGNOSTIC TESTS

→ Herpes culture of genital lesions and/or cervix. (Tissue culture is the most sensitive and specific diagnostic test) (Mertz 1990; Strauss 1985). **NOTE:** A negative HSV culture *does not prove* that the patient does not have HSV (Davies 1990). Up to 40 percent of HSV lesions test

falsely negative even when cultured on the first or second day after the outbreak occurs (Davies 1990).

→ Tzanck stain of genital lesions (low sensitivity and specificity) (Mertz 1990).
  ▪ Cannot differentiate between HSV-1 and HSV-2, or HSV from varicella zoster virus (VSV).

→ Pap smear (low sensitivity) (Mertz 1990).
  ▪ Cannot differentiate between HSV-1 and HSV-2.

→ Serological assays, complement fixation, neutralization, immunofluorescence, immunoperoxidase, radioimmunoassay, ELISA, detect the presence of antibodies to HSV antigens.
  ▪ May be used for documentation of seroconversion after primary HSV and as a possible screen for past HSV infection.
  ▪ Do not differentiate between HSV-1 and HSV-2 secondary to cross-reactivity of the antibodies (Mertz 1990; Strauss 1985). See "Objective" section.

→ Antigen detection assays are substantially less sensitive than tissue culture and not commonly utilized (Mead 1991).

→ Western blot testing and immunoblot can distinguish HSV-1 and HSV-2 but are only available in research labs (Safrin 1994).

→ Nucleic acid detection—e.g., polymerase stain reaction (PCR)—is under study.

→ RPR or VDRL; dark-field or direct immunofluorescence test of serous fluid for *T. pallidum* to rule out syphilis. (See **Syphilis** Protocol).

→ Distinguish between herpes and other causes of genital ulcers. See **Table 13A.1, Clinical Features of Genital Ulcers**, p. 13-6, and **Figure 13A.1, Sexually Active Patient with Genital Ulcer(s)**, p. 13-7.

→ See "Diagnostic Test" sections of **Chancroid, Granuloma Inguinale (Donovanosis),** and **Lymphogranuloma Venereum** protocols.

TREATMENT/MANAGEMENT

→ There is no known cure for HSV infections.

→ Acyclovir (Zovirax®) interferes with HSV DNA synthesis.
  ▪ Major advantage is high degree of selectivity against HSV-infected cells and lack of activity against normal cells (Baker 1991).

- Acyclovir neither eradicates latent virus nor affects subsequent risk, frequency, or severity of recurrences after it is discontinued (CDC 1993c).

→ **First episodes (primary and non-primary infection):**
  - acyclovir 200 mg p.o. 5 times/day for 7 to 10 days or until clinical resolution attained (should initiate within 6 days of onset of lesions) (ACOG 1988; CDC 1993c; *PDR* 1993).
    - Mean duration of infection decreased by 3 to 5 days; viral shedding by 8 days; time to healing by 7 days.
    - Topical ointment provides marginal benefit and its use is discouraged.

NOTE: Patients with extremely severe episodes (prostration, central nervous system [CNS] involvement, urinary retention) may require hospitalization for more aggressive management/ intravenous therapy (*PDR* 1993).

→ **Recurrent infection (intermittent therapy):**
  - acyclovir 200 mg p.o. 5 times/day for 5 days
    OR
  - acyclovir 400 mg p.o. 3 times/day for 5 days
    OR
  - acyclovir 800 mg p.o. 2 times/day for 5 days (CDC 1993c).
    - When initiated during prodrome or within 2 days of lesion onset, some patients experience limited benefit. Most immunocompetent patients with recurrent disease do not benefit from acyclovir and it is generally not recommended (CDC 1993c).
    - Topical ointment not licensed or indicated for recurrent infection.

→ **Frequent infection (chronic suppressive therapy—at least 6 outbreaks/year):**
  - acyclovir 400 mg p.o. BID
    OR
  - acyclovir 200 mg p.o. 3 to 5 times/day (CDC 1993b).
  - doses up to 800 mg p.o. BID have been used for "nonresponders," e.g., 12 recurrences a year or more, continuous recurrences, or continuous prodrome (Goldberg et al. 1993).
    - Identify lowest dose that provides relief from frequently recurring symptoms.
    - Should not be used for the suppression of recurrent disease in mildly affected individuals (*PDR* 1993).
    - After 1 year of therapy, frequency/severity of infection should be re-evaluated to assess need

for continuation. A trial off acyclovir usually will be required (*PDR* 1993).
  - Patients with very frequent or severe episodes before treatment may warrant uninterrupted suppression for more than 1 year (*PDR* 1993).
    - Daily suppression has been shown to be safe and effective for up to 5 years (CDC 1993c; Goldberg et al. 1993).
    - Data from 6 to 7 year trials are currently being evaluated.
  - Limited information in patients who discontinue acyclovir suggests a variable decrease in the frequency of recurrences after prolonged suppression (Goldberg et al. 1993).
  - No evidence of clinically significant resistance has been reported with suppressive treatment in immunocompetent individuals (Kaplowitz et al. 1991; Mertz 1990).
    - Viruses with decreased sensitivity to acyclovir have been recovered from immunocompromised patients (Burroughs Wellcome Company 1993; Erlich et al. 1989).
  - Questions are still unanswered regarding the relevance to humans of in vitro mutagenicity/ toxicity studies in animals.
    - See *PDR* or package insert information.
    - In a study by Clive et al. (1991), no mutagenicity was observed in patients receiving acyclovir for recurrent genital herpes.
  - Acyclovir is generally well tolerated.
    - The most frequent adverse effects may include nausea, diarrhea, headache, rash, paresthesia.
    - No clinically significant trends indicating cumulative toxicity have occurred with suppressive therapy up to 5 years (Goldberg et al. 1993).
- alternatives to acyclovir:
  - no safe, effective alternatives have been identified (Mertz 1990).
  - currently being studied:
    - vaccines.
    - interferon.
    - other antiviral medications.
- palliative therapy:
  - keep lesions clean and dry.
  - may apply cold milk or witch hazel compresses, Campho-phenique® lotion, Listerine® followed by aloe vera gel, Burow's solution (Domeboro®) to lesions QID for 30 minutes.

- warm/cool sitz baths prn followed by blow dryer on cool setting.
- pain relief: topical Xylocaine® applied to site of lesions; acetaminophen 325 mg, 2 tablets p.o. every 4 hours prn.
- avoid use of most creams and ointments.
- L-lysine 750 mg to 1000 mg p.o./day when lesions are present and 500 mg p.o./day during asymptomatic periods (Lichtman and Duran 1990).
  - –Unknown if actually beneficial (Sacks 1986).
  - –Controlled studies have not shown reduced duration of symptoms or frequency of recurrence.
  - –Has been shown to have an inhibitory effect on HSV replication in cell culture (Lichtman and Duran 1990).

CONSULTATION

→ Consultation with a physician is indicated if patient has signs/symptoms of severe primary infection requiring possible hospitalization for intravenous acyclovir therapy, details of which are beyond the scope of this protocol.

→ Refer to mental health services for psychological support as necessary.

→ As needed for prescription(s).

PATIENT EDUCATION

→ Discuss cause and transmission of infection; primary, non-primary initial, and recurrent outbreaks; dormant states; asymptomatic shedding.
  - Provide with HSV patient-education handouts if available.

→ Allow patient to ventilate feelings regarding the diagnosis.

→ Advise abstinence from oral-genital sex with the onset of prodromal symptoms and/or genital lesions until lesions are completely healed.

→ Emphasize importance of safer sex practices, and use of condoms and spermicide containing nonoxynol-9 (virucidal). See **Table 13A.2, Safer Sex Guidelines**, p. 13-9, and **Table 12I.1, Recommendations for Individuals to Prevent STD/PID**, p. 12-96.

→ Instruct/encourage good perineal hygiene to prevent superimposed infection.

→ Provide instructions for use of acyclovir; discuss intermittent versus chronic suppressive therapy for individuals with recurrences. (See "Treatment/Management" section.)

→ Advise regarding palliative measures. (See "Treatment/Management" section.)

→ Discuss aggravating factors—e.g., illness, stress, fatigue, menses, poor nutrition, irritation/friction, intercourse, excessive heat/sun. Encourage general health maintenance, appropriate rest, adequate nutrition.

→ May advise limitation of arginine-rich foods—i.e., nuts, chocolate, cola, rice, cottonseed meal and oil. Arginine favors the replication of HSV and competes with lysine (Lichtman and Duran 1990).

→ Refer partner(s) for evaluation if any lesions/characteristic symptoms are present.

→ Advise patient to obtain yearly Pap smears.

→ If they become pregnant, women should inform their health care provider of a history of HSV infection in themselves or their sexual partner(s) (ACOG 1988).

→ Refer for psychological support and stress management as indicated.

→ Advise patients to inform prospective partners of risk of HSV exposure.
  - This is an area which can be very difficult for patients to cope with; thus, support and guidance may be necessary.
  - Provide patients with support group/resource information:
    - American Social Health Association
      260 Sheridan Avenue
      Palo Alto, CA 94306
      –Provides directory of HSV self-help chapters in the United States and Canada, and maintains a listing of health care providers/therapists who specialize in the treatment of HSV (American Social Health Association 1983).
    - Herpes Resource Center
      P.O. Box 100
      Palo Alto, CA 94302
      –Publishes a quarterly newsletter called "The Helper" which focuses on a broad range of information pertaining to HSV infection.
    - health care providers can receive a wide range of patient education and support materials from:
      –Wellcome Dialogue
      800-843-8889

FOLLOW-UP

→ If indicated, schedule a follow-up visit after the initial diagnosis to evaluate treatment effectiveness and coping strategies, and to answer any further questions.

→ Annual Pap smears are recommended (ACOG 1988).

→ Re-evaluate suppressive acyclovir therapy annually with a trial off the medication, unless individual case presentation warrants uninterrupted suppression. (See "Treatment/Management" section).

→ May check to see if any significant changes in laboratory values of WBC count, creatinine, bilirubin, SGOT, SGPT, or alkaline phosphatase occurred in patients on long-term suppressive therapy (Goldberg et al. 1993).

■ Consult with physician as indicated regarding ordering of laboratory tests for patients on suppressive therapy.

→ Document in progress notes and problem list.

Jeanette M. Broering, R.N., M.S., C.P.N.P.

13-F
Human Papillomavirus

Human papillomaviruses (HPV) are epitheliotropic viruses that infect surface epithelia and mucous membranes and may produce warts or epithelial growths at the site of infection. In addition to causing genital warts, HPV infection may be associated with later development of cervical cancer. Projected estimates indicate that 10 percent of all women are infected with high-risk types of HPV (e.g., 16 and 18). However, the majority of these women will not develop cervical cancer (Lorincz et al. 1987).

It appears that HPV infection of the genital tract is essential but not alone in causing cervical cancer. Cofactors believed to influence the development of cervical intraepithelial neoplasia (CIN) have been identified, and include smoking and the deleterious influence of nicotine on the cervix (Winkelstein 1990), use of oral contraceptives, early onset of sexual activity, greater number of lifetime sexual partners, and infection with other STDs (Schiffman 1992). Epidemiological studies have demonstrated an association of these factors with the development of CIN. However, definitive data on the causal mechanisms and natural history of HPV infection remain to be studied and interpreted.

Biology

Over 65 known subtypes of HPV have been reported and classified based on DNA sequencing; more are being discovered (Carlson and Twiggs 1992). Greater than 20 subtypes have been associated with lower genital tract infections (ACOG 1994). Knowledge of the viruses' natural history and growth cycle is limited because the virus cannot be propagated in tissue culture. HPV has site-specific affinity, and a variety of epithelial sites for infec-

tion exist (see **Table 13F.1, HPV Types and Common Sites of Infection**).

Incidence/Prevalence

The exact incidence of this disease is unknown since there are no mandatory surveillance mechanisms. Frequency of HPV varies according to detection method used and population screened (ACOG 1994). Data generated from office-based private practitioners in the United States revealed 224,900 newly diagnosed cases of genital warts, representing a 4.5-fold increase between the years 1966 and 1984 (Becker, Stone, and Alexander 1987).

Peak incidence is among women 20 years to 24 years old. Among reproductive-age women, the rate of detection of HPV ranges from approximately six percent in those with normal cervical examination and cytology, to 60 percent in those with cervical neoplasia (ACOG 1994).

With the evolution of the AIDS epidemic and the earlier treatment of women infected with HIV, concern for the development of cervical cancer has risen. However, cancer surveillance data do not support any significant rise in incidence rates to date. Some authors hypothesize that most persons with AIDS die of opportunistic infections before the onset of more aggressive forms of cancer (Palefsky 1991).

Transmission

Most HPV infection is transmitted by sexual exposure. During labor and delivery maternal-fetal transmission may occur in the presence of HPV infection of the birth canal. In a sexually active person who has been exposed

Table 13F.1.   HUMAN PAPILLOMAVIRUS (HPV) TYPES AND COMMON SITES OF INFECTION

Type of HPV	Usual epithelial site of infection	Type of warts/lesion
1	Soles of feet	Deep plantar
2,4,7	Hands	Common
5,8,9,12,14,15,17 19-25,36,37,38 46,47,50	Forehead, arms, and trunk	Epidermodysplasia verruciformis
6,11,42,54	Genital tract and anus	Condyloma acuminatum
6,11,16,18,30,31 33,34,35,39,40,42 43,45,51,52,56,58	Genital tract and anus	Atypical condylomata, papules, and vulvar intraepithelial neoplasia (VIN); genital tract and anal cancers

to the virus, the incubation period ranges from three weeks to eight months. Three months is the average time from viral exposure to the development of clinically apparent warts. Nonsexual routes of transmission remain to be documented conclusively (Schiffman 1992). It is not clear whether subclinical or latent disease is transmissible (ACOG 1994). Coinfection with other STDs is common.

The appearance of clinical warts in the female correlates well with the appearance of clinical warts in her male sexual partner. Fifty percent of the male partners of women with condyloma have clinically apparent lesions and 25 percent have subclinical lesions (ACOG 1994). No data exist on the efficiency of female to female transmission. However, it is reasonable to evaluate any sexual partner of a female presenting with clinical condyloma irrespective of partner's gender (Palefsky 1993).

DATABASE

SUBJECTIVE

→ All sexually active or experienced women are at risk for exposure to HPV; however, the greatest risk factors include:
- history of multiple lifetime sexual partners.
- history of multiple (current or previous) STDs.
- history of contact with a partner with genital warts.
- lack of condom use.
- age of less than 25 years.
- pregnancy.
- altered immune response.

→ Patient is usually asymptomatic or presents with complaint of painless, warty-appearing growth on genitals, most commonly occurring at posterior introitus, adjacent labia minora, and remainder of the vestibule.
- Less commonly reported to occur on the clitoris, perineum, vagina, cervix, anus, and rectum.

→ Additional symptoms may include:
- vulvar pruitus, burning, and/or bleeding.
- vaginal discharge.
- dysparunia.

→ Patient may have a history of abnormal Pap smear(s).

→ Pregnancy may exacerbate lesion(s).

OBJECTIVE

→ Examination may be individualized based on case presentation.

→ Thorough STD examination includes:
- vital signs as indicated.
- general inspection of face, trunk, forearms, palms, soles for lesions, rashes, discoloration.
- inspection of oral cavity for lesions, discoloration.
- abdominal inspection and palpation for masses, tenderness, rebound tenderness.
- inspection of pubic hair for lice, nits.
- inspection of external genitalia for discharge, masses, lesions.
- inspection/palpation of Bartholin's, urethral, and Skene's glands for discharge, masses.
- inspection of vagina for discharge, lesions.
- inspection of cervix for lesions, discharge, eversion, edema, friability, CMT.
- uterine assessment for size, shape, consistency, mobility, tenderness.
- palpation of adnexa for massess, tenderness.
- inspection of perianus, anus for lesions, bleeding, discharge.
- rectal examination and anoscopy as indicated.
- assessment of presence or absence of associated lymphadenopathy (CDC 1991).

→ HPV infection may be categorized utilizing the following method of stratification: clinical, subclinical, and latent (asymptomatic) HPV infections (Ling 1992a).

- Infection may occur anywhere in the anogenitourinary tract including mons pubis, vulva, vagina, urethra, cervix, perianal skin, or rectum.
- Nongenital lesions of the mouth, larynx, or conjunctiva may also occur.

Clinically apparent gross lesions

→ Lesions in the anogenital area are visible to the naked eye without the addition of any appearance-enhancing techniques.

→ Lesions have a broad spectrum of clinical appearance.

→ Condyloma acuminata: typically white or pink, raised, cauliflower, verrucous lesions.
NOTE: Vulvar vestibular papillae may resemble small condylomata, but are rarely associated with HPV (ACOG 1994).

→ Flat lesions may appear as slightly raised, discrete, hyperpigmented brown, white, red, or gray lesions (Sawchuk 1992).

→ Vaginal lesions may appear as raised, granular asperites, or raised spicules.

→ Large lesions may become ulcerated and infected.

→ Condyloma may grow markedly during pregnancy.

Subclinical infection

→ Lesions appear only after the utilization of enhancing techniques.

→ Acetowhite areas within the anogenital tract are evident after the application of three percent to five percent acetic acid; may be seen with the naked eye or with the use of an optical magnifying device such as a colposcope or hand-held magnifying glass. (See "Diagnostic Tests" section.)

→ Abnormal cervical cytology may be classified under this subgroup.

Latent HPV disease

→ There are no visible lesions.

→ Detected only by DNA hybridization for HPV.

→ Biologic significance is unclear (Syrjanen 1992).

→ Eighty percent of patients may go into sustained clinical remission.
- Those remaining continue to have active disease with potential neoplastic transformation (Reid and Greenberg 1991).

ASSESSMENT

→ Condyloma acuminata

→ HPV—subclinical infection; latent infection

→ R/O condyloma lata as a manifestation of secondary syphilis

→ R/O concomitant STDs

→ R/O vaginitis

→ R/O squamous intraepithelial lesion (SIL), also known as site specific lesion such as cervical, vulvar, vaginal, or anal intraepithelial neoplasia (CIN, VIN, VAIN, or AIN, respectively)

→ R/O verrucous carcinoma

PLAN

DIAGNOSTIC TESTS

→ Inspection with unaided eye may reveal exophytic condyloma acuminata.

→ Gross visual inspection after application of 3 percent to 5 percent acetic acid may reveal discrete, flat, subclinical lesions.
- Colposcopy or hand-held magnification may enhance ability to visualize. (Specificity 10 percent to 27 percent [Moscicki 1990].)
NOTE: Acetowhitening may also be due to tissue inflammation, trauma, allergic or contact dermatitis, pantyhose or tight pants, or a variation of normal epithelium.

→ Biopsy of lesion for histopathological diagnosis may be performed in certain cases (e.g., unusual appearance, lesion unresponsive to local therapy).

→ Pap smear should be done.
- Cervical cytology may detect cellular changes as noted by the presence of koilocytes, low or high grade SIL. (Specificity 1 percent to 10 percent.) Definitive diagnosis made only through biopsy and pathology report of lesion severity (Moscicki 1990).

→ Molecular hybridization detects presence of DNA or RNA through multiple techniques (dot blot, Southern blot or polymerized chain reaction [PCR]). PCR is the most sensitive of all the hybridization tests.
- Positive test results cannot be used to determine onset of infection or current status of infectivity.
- Although commercial preparations of these tests have been approved by the Food and Drug Administration (FDA) and are offered by many clinical laboratories, the cost-effectiveness, clinical utility, and implications for clinical

management have yet to be determined (Carlson and Twiggs 1992).

→ Evaluate for concurrent existence of other STDs to include: *N. gonorrhoeae*, *C. trachomatis*, syphilis, and vaginal wet smears to rule out *T. vaginalis*. See specific protocols.

→ Offer HIV testing.

TREATMENT/MANAGEMENT

→ Treat visible warts. Treatment regimens described in **Table 13F.2, Commonly Used Therapies for Treatment of Genital Warts**.
NOTE: Topical therapies such as trichloroacetic acid (TCA) can cause transient discomfort at the time of treatment. Use of topical anesthesia such as 20 percent benzocaine sprayed on the vulva several minutes before application and wiped off before the use of TCA can greatly reduce the immediate pain caused by this substance. Inquiry about patient allergy to benzocaine should precede use of local pain therapy and would be contraindicated in those with known sensitivity. Immediate application of a cold compress to the affected area after treament can be equally beneficial.

→ Thick, keratinized lesions which do not respond to local therapies should be biopsied to rule out verrucous carcinoma (ACOG 1994).

→ Examine sexual partners concurrently and treat visible warts. Referral may be necessary.

→ The evaluation of sex partners in the absence of clinical disease (i.e., female with condylomatous changes on cervical cytology only) is more controversial.
■ The majority of these partners will be asymptomatic and require no treatment.
■ However, all partners should be evaluated if they are extremely worried, if only for purposes of reassurance.

→ Treat concomitant vaginitis/STD.

→ Obtain Pap smear on all women with warts, annually at a minimum, unless other risk factors exist such as concurrent HIV infection.
■ Some authors suggest that HIV-infected women at risk for HPV disease be screened every 6 months by cervical cytology and routine colposcopic examination of the vulva, vagina, and cervix concurrently (Northfelt and Palefsky 1992).
■ Women with abnormalities on cervical cytology should be followed and evaluated per site-

specific protocol (see **Abnormal Cervical Cytology** Protocol).

CONSULTATION

→ Physician consultation is indicated for patients with persistent condyloma not responding to therapy after several treatments or patients with extensive vulvar, vaginal, or cervical disease. Pregnancy may exacerbate HPV and warrant referral to a physician.

→ Refer to a physician for colposcopic evaluation and biopsy any patient with:
■ two consecutive atypical cervical cytologies.
■ SIL or CIN on cervical cytology.
■ visible cervical lesion (leukoplakia).

PATIENT EDUCATION

→ Counsel patient about abstinence during acute treatment phase.
■ Although the use of condoms has not been demonstrated to reduce the risk of reinfection, their use should be emphasized to reduce the risk of acquisition of other STDs (ACOG 1994). (See **Table 13A.2, Safer Sex Guidelines**, p. 13-9, and **Table 12I.1, Recommendations for Individuals to Prevent STD/PID**, p. 12-96.)

→ Discuss importance of partner evaluation and treatment as indicated.

→ Counsel patients with a history of multiple partners, multiple STDs, and high-risk behavior (such as unprotected anal receptive intercourse or intravenous or injection drug use) as to the risk of HIV infection. (See **Human Immunodeficiency Virus [HIV]** Protocol).

→ Counsel as to the need for continued surveillance with Pap smears.

→ Psychological support is important for the well-being of the patient.
■ Advise the patient that although visible lesions can be removed, eradication of HPV from the genital tract can not be guaranteed (ACOG 1994).
■ Reassure and educate the patient that behaviors which promote optimal wellness may enhance the immune system and will aid with resolution of the virus.
■ The American Social Health Association (ASHA) operates an "HPV Support Program" that provides support services and publishes a quarterly newsletter, *HPV News*.

Table 13F.2. COMMONLY USED THERAPIES FOR TREATMENT OF GENITAL WARTS

Therapeutic Modality	Long-Term Cure Rates	Site-Specific Use	Mechanism of Action	Advantages	Disadvantages/ Additional Information
Podophyllin (2.5 percent to 10 percent podofilox in 25 percent preparation of crude podophyllin)	14 percent to 31 percent	External genitalia and perianal region. No use on vagina/cervix. Applied directly to warts with cotton swab weekly for up to 6 weeks.	Local inflammatory response, histologically shows keratinocyte necrosis and abnormal mitoses; causes warts to shrink.	Low cost; convenience.	1. Local adverse reactions include erythema, tenderness, burning, pain, swelling, and superficial erosions. 2. Systemic toxicity and fetal demise reported; therefore, use in pregnancy contraindicated. 3. Low cure rate. 4. Requires series of visits to health practitioner, patient must wash off in 4 to 6 hours after application.
Podophyllotoxin (Podolfilox 0.5 percent topical solution)	18 percent	External genitalia and perianal region. No use on vagina/cervix. Patient applies once in A.M. and P.M. for 3 days in a row followed by 4 days without treatment; repeat cycle up to a total of 4 weeks.	Same as podophyllin.	1. Purity, stable shelf life, negligible systemic absorption. 2. Intended for home treatment by patient, thereby minimizing repeated office visits and associated costs. 3. No need to wash off once applied.	1. Same local reactions as with podophyllin. 2. Contraindicated in pregnancy.
Trichloroacetic acid (TCA) or Bichloracetic acid (BCA) 50 percent or 85 percent strength	50 percent	External genitalia, perianal region, vagina, and anus. Apply with wooden tip of Q-tip onto wart and 5 mm beyond every 7 to 12 days up to 6 weeks. Colposcopic guidance during application will limit area of skin damage.	Immediately upon contact causes superficial destruction of skin lesions and superficial skin necrosis.	1. Convenience, low cost. 2. Approved for use during pregnancy. 3. No need to wash off once applied.	Local pain and tissue necrosis.
5-Fluorouracil (5-FU, Efudex)	57 percent	Topical application to vulva and vagina, primarily. Use with male limited due to severe local reactions. Vulva: small amount to affected area 2 consecutive days a week for 10 weeks. Vagina: ¼ applicator once a week at bedtime for 10 weeks. Zinc oxide to protect vulva. Patient to wash hands after use to avoid getting medication on sensitive areas such as eyes.	Interferes with cellular proliferation by disrupting DNA and RNA synthesis.	1. Adjuvant therapy role mostly following laser therapy or cryotherapy of cervix for treatment of extensive/diffuse vaginal HPV disease. 2. Topical application (vulvar or intravaginal) usually on weekly basis for an extended time interval. Treatment regimens vary by local practice preference.	Complications include acute erosive vulvitis; pain, redness, and discharge are common. Contraindicated in pregnancy.

Continued

Table 13F.2. COMMONLY USED THERAPIES FOR TREATMENT OF GENITAL WARTS (CONTINUED)

Therapeutic Modality	Long-Term Cure Rates	Site-Specific Use	Mechanism of Action	Advantages	Disadvantages/ Additional Information
Cryotherapy with liquid nitrogen or cryoprobe	67 percent to 88 percent	Vulva, cervix, perianal condyloma. Performed by physician or specially trained NP.	Tissue freezing results in membrane rupture and intracellular dehydration, cell death, and localized tissue crushing.	Direct application through a variety of devices based on size and location of lesion (cotton swab or cryosurgical probe). Clinically well tolerated, moderate discomfort. Rarely requires use of local anesthesia; best suited for small lesions.	1. Increased cost for treatment based on usual and customary local fee structure. 2. Post-cervical cryotherapy results in heavy, prolonged vaginal discharge perceived as nuisance to client. Advise no tampons, coitus, or tub baths/hot tubs for 2 weeks post procedure.
Surgical methods: electrosurgery or surgical excision via scissors/blade	64 percent to 72 percent >3 mos. cure rate.	Vulvar and perianal condyloma; performed by physician or specially trained NP.	Destruction of lesion by burning off or physical removal.	Best suited for small numbers and size of warts.	1. Requires local anesthesia. 2. Mild post-operative pain. 3. Hospitalization may be required for extensive lesions.
Laser therapy (carbon dioxide laser)	Variable reports: 43 percent to 99 percent based on extensiveness of disease and goal of therapy.	Cervix, vagina, vulva, anus, distal urethra. Performed by physician.	Direct tissue vaporization; high degree of accuracy in size of area and depth of destruction.	Use in situations where extensive or bulky lesions exist.	1. Complications include short-term pain and swelling, ulceration, infection, or delayed healing. Additional hospital stay may be warranted for pain management for those women who have extensive procedure. Permanent scarring is not infrequent. 2. Cost utility must be weighed, particularly if extensive procedure. Cost of operating room, general anesthesia, and post-operative inpatient stay make this approach very expensive. Outpatient procedures are done depending upon extensiveness of disease and local practice customs. 3. Reservoir of HPV may be contained in areas adjacent to tissue that was treated. Recurrence of disease hypothesized to occur by reinfection of wound area.
Interferon alfa-2b (INTRON A, registered trademark by Schering Pharmaceuticals)	33 percent to 38 percent (genital). Long-term data on relapse not available.	Genital, hand(s), larynx. Intralesional injection of 1.0 million IU (0.1 ml) into each lesion 3 times per week on alternate days, for 3 weeks; maximum of 5 lesions for treatment. Repeat second treatment in 16 weeks if no response to initial therapy.	Interferons have antiviral, immunopotentiating, and antiproliferative activities.	For use with recalcitrant condyloma acuminata not responsive to any of the aforementioned therapies.	1. Systemic administration results in "flu-like" illness including fever, headache, nausea, myalgias, and fatigue. 2. Contraindicated in pregnancy; animal studies report spontaneous abortions among primates exposed to this drug. 3. Costly. 4. This is not to be considered a primary therapy for patients with genital warts. Necessitates referral to specialist, i.e., dermatologist or gynecologist experienced in using agent.

Source: Adapted from Ling, M.R. 1992b. Therapy of genital human papillomavirus infections. Part II: Methods of treatment. *International Journal of Dermatology* 31(11):769–773; Moscicki, A.B. 1990. Genital human papillomavirus infection. *Adolescent Medicine: State of the Art Reviews* 1(3):451–469; Medical Economics Data. 1992. *Physicians' Desk Reference*, 46th ed. Montvale, NJ: the Author.

■ Inquiries regarding these services may be
  forwarded to:
   American Social Health Association/HPV
   P.O. Box 13827
   Research Triangle Park, NC 27709
   (919) 361-8400

FOLLOW-UP

→ See **Table 13F.2**, for frequency of local therapeutic
  measures for condyloma.

→ Recommended time intervals for Pap smears have
  not been established.

  ■ For women without SIL who are known to be
    HPV/DNA positive, Moscicki's group at the
    University of California, San Francisco recom-
    mends cervical cytology every six months for
    two years (Moscicki 1993).

  ■ If these are all negative, annual Pap smears may
    be resumed.

  ■ Regional practice standards may vary, and
    clinicians are advised to seek local consultation
    as indicated.

→ Follow up on laboratory tests and treat
  concomitant STD. Treat/refer partner(s) as
  indicated. See appropriate protocols.

→ HIV-positive results should be conveyed in person
  by a provider who has received training in the
  complexities of test disclosure. HIV-positive
  persons should be referred to the appropriate
  provider or agency for early intervention services.

→ Document in progress notes and problem list.

Winifred L. Star, R.N., C., N.P., M.S.

13-G

Lymphogranuloma Venereum

Lymphogranuloma venereum (LGV) is an STD caused by one of three biovars of the bacterium *Chlamydia trachomatis*: L1, L2, and L3. Although extremely rare in the United States, LGV is prevalent in tropical and semitropical climates of Africa, India, Southeast Asia, South America, and the Caribbean. There are about 500 to 600 hundred cases reported to the Centers for Disease Control and Prevention (CDC) per year. Cluster areas have appeared in Washington, D.C., and central Florida.

Men are more frequently affected than women, with a ratio of 5:1, but late complications of the disease are more common in women. In nonendemic areas, most reported cases occur in soldiers, sailors, and travelers who have frequented or lived in endemic areas.

LGV often has been confused with other ulcerative STDs such as syphilis, herpes, and chancroid. The pathogenesis of the disease is not yet fully understood, and the frequency of isolation after exposure is unknown. It is thought that LGV is less contagious than gonorrhea and that the entrance pathway is through small abrasions/lacerations in skin or mucous membrane (Blanco and Gonik 1991; Burgoyne 1990; Levin et al. 1987; Perine and Osoba 1990).

LGV is an aggressive disease, predominantly of lymphatic tissue, with potential for serious sequelae. There are three stages of infection which are analogous to syphilis: primary, secondary, and tertiary. The primary stage includes an infrequent, painless papule or ulcer with short duration and few symptoms. The incubation period is approximately three to thirty days from exposure. Forty percent of individuals with more advanced disease recall no primary lesion.

In women, the cervix or the urethra are the most common sites of acute primary infection with manifesta-

tions of cervicitis or urethritis. These areas may remain infected for weeks to months. Most patients seeking care no longer have self-limited genital ulcers (Burgoyne 1990; CDC 1991, 1993e; Greenblatt 1990; Levin et al. 1987; Perine and Osoba 1990; Sweet and Gibbs 1990).

Secondary stage disease usually lasts one to four weeks or longer after initial exposure and is characterized by acute suppurative inguinal lymphadenitis with bubo formation (inguinal syndrome) and/or acute hemorrhagic proctitis (anogenitorectal syndrome). In persons exposed via receptive anal intercourse, the most common manifestation of LGV is acute proctocolitis.

Constitutional symptoms including fever, malaise, myalgias, and anorexia are present in the second stage. The inflammatory process may persist for several weeks to months. During this time, lymph nodes may abscess, rupture, and form sinus tracts or fistulas. Other systemic manifestations may include hepatitis, meningitis, pneumonitis, and conjunctivitis. The central nervous system may become infected via systemic spread of the organism.

Host immunity will limit dissemination and local extension of the disease. However, a latent state may ensue when chlamydial replication is slowed but the organism not completely eliminated. Viable chlamydial organisms have been recovered from infected tissue up to 20 years after infection.

The majority of affected individuals will recover from LGV after the second stage but some will develop complications of the tertiary stage characterized by progressive tissue destruction and extensive scarring. Chronic edema and scarring of the vulva results in painful ulcerations (esthiomene), rectovaginal fistula and stricture formation, and lymphedema of the legs and genitals (genital elephantiasis) (Burgoyne 1990; CDC 1991; Greenblatt 1990; Levin et al. 1987; Perine and Osoba 1990; Sweet and Gibbs 1990).

A number of different antimicrobials have been used to treat LGV, and spontaneous remission is possible. Outpatient surgical treatment is limited to aspiration of lymph nodes and incision and drainage of abscesses. Complications of advanced rectal stricture require more sophisticated surgical procedures and hospitalization. Concomitant STDs are likely in patients with LGV and should be treated accordingly (Perine and Osoba 1990).

DATABASE

SUBJECTIVE

→ LGV is more common in third decade of life.

→ LGV is seen more frequently among sexually promiscuous people, in rural areas, and in lower socioeconomic classes.

→ Patient may have history of travel to country where LGV is endemic.

→ Symptomatic early infection less common in women. Late complications (ulceration, rectal strictures, hypertrophy of genitals) more frequent in women.

→ Gynecological and medical history should include:
  ▪ menstrual cycle.
  ▪ contraception.
  ▪ description of symptoms:
    • onset.
    • duration.
    • quality/quantity.
    • frequency.
    • course.
    • aggravating/relieving factors.
    • associated symptoms.
  ▪ previous history of same/similar problem.
  ▪ STD history (including dates/treatment).
  ▪ sensitive questioning regarding recent sexual activity (including date of last exposure), sex practices, sites of exposure, number of partners in past month, use of condoms.
  ▪ sex partner history.
  ▪ acute/chronic illness.
  ▪ general health.
  ▪ medications.
  ▪ allergies.
  ▪ habits.
  ▪ history of laboratory tests for syphilis, Hepatitis B, HIV.
  ▪ review of systems (CDC 1991).

Primary stage

→ Genital lesions are asymptomatic after incubation of from three to 30 days. Lesion heals within few days with no sequelae.

→ Symptoms include those associated with cervicitis, urethritis, and/or proctitis: abnormal discharge or bleeding, pelvic pain; dysuria, urgency, frequency (urethritis may be mild and asymptomatic); diarrhea, rectal discharge.

→ Relatively few patients present in this stage unless lesions are in rectum.

→ See "Objective" section.

Secondary stage

→ Inguinal syndrome.
  ▪ This stage begins one to four weeks after primary lesion develops; may be delayed four to six months.
  ▪ Symptoms include:
    • painful swelling of inguinal lymph nodes, enlarging over one to two weeks (reason most patients seek care).
      −Present in 20 percent to 30 percent of women.
    • constitutional symptoms of fever, malaise, myalgias, arthralgias, headache, anorexia (may precede adenopathy).
    • lower abdominal pain, back pain (one-third of cases, due to involvement of deep pelvic/ lumbar lymph nodes).
  ▪ Rupture of bubo relieves pain, fever. Relapse of buboes may occur in about 20 percent of untreated cases.
  ▪ See "Objective" section.

→ Anogenitorectal syndrome.
  ▪ Early symptoms include anal pruritus, mucous rectal discharge.
  ▪ Later symptoms include fever, tenesmus, rectal pain, mucopurulent rectal discharge (sign of secondary infection), left lower abdominal pain.
  ▪ See "Objective" section.

→ Other manifestations include:
  ▪ lesions in mouth, throat.
  ▪ swollen lymph glands in neck area.
  ▪ symptoms of conjunctivitis.
  ▪ skin manifestations.
  ▪ see "Objective" section.

Tertiary stage

→ Symptoms may include:
  ■ constipation, passage of "pencil stools," colicky abdominal pain, distention, weight loss (indicative of rectal stricture).
  ■ perianal hemorrhoid-like tissue growths (sign of obstruction of lymph/venous drainage of lower rectum, called lymphorrhoids or perianal condylomas).
  ■ "growths," ulceration at urinary meatus with dysuria, frequency, incontinence (urethro-genitoperineal syndrome).
  ■ chronic, painful genital ulcerations.
  ■ edema from clitoris to anus, legs.
  ■ see "Objective" section.

OBJECTIVE

→ Examination may be individualized based on case presentation.

→ Thorough STD examination includes:
  ■ vital signs as indicated.
  ■ general skin inspection of face, trunk, forearms, palms, soles for lesions, rashes, discoloration.
  ■ inspection of pharynx and oral cavity for infection, lesions, discoloration.
  ■ abdominal inspection and palpation for masses, tenderness, rebound tenderness.
  ■ inspection of pubic hair for lice, nits.
  ■ inspection of external genitalia for discharge, masses, lesions; inspection and palpation of Bartholin's, urethral, and Skene's glands for discharge, masses.
  ■ inspection of vagina for discharge, lesions.
  ■ inspection of cervix for lesions, discharge, eversion, erythema, edema, friability; assessment for CMT.
  ■ uterine assessment for size, shape, consistency, mobility, tenderness.
  ■ palpation of adnexa for masses, tenderness.
  ■ inspection of perianus, anus for lesions, bleeding, discharge.
  ■ rectal examination as indicated.
  ■ assessment of presence, absence of associated lymphadenopathy (CDC 1991).

Primary stage

→ Papular, vesicular, shallow ulcerative, or eroded lesion most commonly found on posterior vaginal wall, fourchette, posterior lip of cervix, vulva, or extragenital area (mouth, fingers, nose); heals rapidly with no scar.

■ Primary lesion may be absent in 75 percent to 80 percent of cases.

→ Signs of cervicitis, urethritis (mucopurulent discharge), or salpingitis (lower abdominal tenderness, CMT may be present).

Secondary stage

→ Inguinal syndrome.
  ■ Patient may present with fever.
  ■ Firm, tender inguinal bubo with overlying erythema (unilateral in two-thirds of cases), enlarges over one to two weeks.
    • Occurs in about 20 percent to 30 percent of women.
  ■ In one-third of cases, bubo becomes fluctuant and ruptures; the remainder involute and form firm mass without suppuration.
  ■ In 10 percent to 20 percent of cases, femoral lymph nodes affected and may be separated from inguinal lymph nodes by inguinal ligament (so-called "groove sign").
  ■ In 75 percent of cases, deep iliac lymph nodes involved; large pelvic mass formed, not likely to suppurate.
  ■ Adenopathy of axillary, cervical, and submaxillary nodes may exist if primary lesion in mouth or nasopharynx.
  ■ Follicular conjunctivitis may occur with lymphadenopathy of maxillary and posterior auricular nodes.

→ Anogenitorectal syndrome (or proctocolitis).
  ■ Rectal mucosa friable, hyperemic with superficial, irregular ulcerations; mucopurulent rectal discharge occurs with secondary infection.
  ■ Granulomas and abscesses may form in bowel wall (chronic inflammatory process).
  ■ Abdominal examination may reveal left lower quadrant tenderness, palpable thickened pelvic colon.

Tertiary stage

→ Patient may present with:
  ■ papillary growths, ulceration of urethral meatus.
  ■ rectovaginal erosion with fistula formation.
  ■ lymphorrhoids in perianal area.
  ■ chronic progressive lymphangitis, edema, fibrosis of vulva with induration, enlargement, ulceration of genital tissues (esthiomene); ulcerations mostly on labia majora, perineum, crural folds.
  ■ lymphedema from clitoris to anus, legs (genital elephantiasis).

→ Perirectal abscess formation and anal fissures may occur (may be only manifestation of chronic anogenital LGV).

→ Rectal stricture may form. Rectal examination may reveal normal consistency to mucosa above stricture but ulcerative and granular below (examination quite painful); may palpate moveable lymph nodes under bowel wall.

→ Complete bowel obstruction rare but may cause perforation and peritonitis, usual cause of death in LGV.

Other manifestations

→ Skin manifestations include:
  ▪ erythema nodosum:
    • tender, well-circumscribed erythematous nodules.
    • may become raised, confluent, pruritic.
    • seen mainly on legs, may occur on arms, body; may occur in five percent to ten percent of cases of LGV (Sauer 1991).
  ▪ erythema multiforme:
    • red iris-shaped or bull's-eye-like macules, papules, or bullae confined mainly to the extremities, face, or lip.
    • may occur in five percent to ten percent of cases of LGV (Sauer 1991).

→ Other manifestations may include: mediastinal adenitis, pericarditis, hepatitis, pneumonitis, arthritis, aseptic meningitis, conjunctivitis, papillary edema.

→ Complete and accurate descriptions of any identified lesions or other pertinent physical findings should be written in the "Objective" section of the progress note.

ASSESSMENT

→ (LGV)

→ R/O syphilis

→ R/O chancroid

→ R/O herpes genitalis

→ R/O concomitant STDs

→ R/O other possible causes of inguinal lymphadenitis: metastatic cervical, vulvar, or vaginal cancer; Hodgkin's disease; incarcerated hernia; infected lesions of legs, feet; plague; tularemia; tuberculosis

→ R/O salpingitis

→ R/O appendicitis

→ R/O TOA

PLAN

DIAGNOSTIC TESTS

→ Distinguish between LGV and other causes of genital ulcers.
  ▪ See **Table 13A.1, Clinical Features of Genital Ulcers**, p. 13-6, and **Figure 13A.1, Sexually Active Patient with Genital Ulcer(s)**, p. 13-7.
  ▪ Definitive diagnosis: isolation of *C. trachomatis* (L1, L2, or L3) by tissue culture of lymph node aspirate *or* immunofluorescence of *C. trachomatis* inclusion bodies in leukocytes of inguinal lymph node (bubo) aspirate (CDC 1991).
  ▪ Material for culture may also be obtained from ulcer base or rectal lesions.
  NOTE: Material from infected tissue and/or ruptured buboes poses a health risk to personnel. Universal precautions should be applied.

→ Additional specific diagnostic tests may include:
  ▪ CF test: titers ≥1:64.
  NOTE: Titers usually high initially and do not rise much between acute and 6-week convalescent specimens. High or low titers may persist for years. Titers may also represent levels from other chlamydial infections.
  ▪ microimmunofluorescent (Micro-IF) test: titers ≥1:512; more sensitive than CF test but not readily available.
  ▪ radioisotope precipitation (RIP) test; more sensitive than Micro-IF test but not readily available.
  ▪ cytology: elementary and inclusion bodies of *C. trachomatis* may be identified with fluorescent antibody-staining methods.
  ▪ Giemsa stain.
  ▪ Frei test.
  ▪ radiological procedures: lymphography, barium enema.
  ▪ biopsy of rectal tissue to rule out cancer.

→ CBC shows mild leukocytosis with increased monocytes/eosinophils in early disease, more significant polymorphonuclear leukocytosis if superinfection present.

→ Diagnostic tests to rule out other causes of genital ulcers and lymphadenopathy include:
  ▪ dark-field or direct immunofluorescence test of serous fluid for *T. pallidum* from genital and non-oral lesion(s) to rule out syphilis.
    • See **Syphilis** Protocol.

- RPR (or VDRL) or treponemal tests to rule out syphilis.
  - See **Syphilis** Protocol.
- herpes cultures or Tzanck stain to rule out herpes.
  - See **Genital Herpes Simplex Virus** Protocol.
- see "Diagnostic Test" sections of **Chancroid** and **Granuloma Inguinale** protocols.

→ Endocervical culture for *N. gonorrhoeae* and endocervical diagnostic tests for *C. trachomatis*.
  - In the absence of a cervix, urethral specimen may be obtained.

→ HIV testing should be offered.

→ Additional tests may include (but are not limited to): wet mounts, Pap smear, urinalysis, urine culture and sensitivities, pregnancy test, Hepatitis B screen.

TREATMENT/MANAGEMENT

→ Recommended regimen:
  - doxycycline (Vibramycin®) 100 mg p.o. BID for 21 days (CDC 1993e).

→ Alternate regimens:
  - erythromycin (E-Mycin®) 500 mg p.o. QID for 21 days

OR

  - sulfisoxazole (Gantrisin®) 500 mg p.o. QID for 21 days (or equivalent sulfonamide) (CDC 1993e).

→ Surgical intervention.
  - Antibiotic therapy should precede surgical intervention. Fluctuant lymph nodes should be aspirated through normal adjacent skin to prevent fistula formation (CDC 1991). Occasionally incision and drainage (I and D) is indicated.
    - Consult with or refer to physician.
  - Rectal strictures may require dilation with elastic bougies. Advanced strictures require a variety of surgical procedures.
  - Additional indications for operation include bowel obstruction, persistent rectovaginal fistula, and destruction of anal canal/sphincter or perineum. Refer to surgeon.
    NOTE: Ideally, antibiotics should be given for several months prior to surgery.
  - Patients with chronic or late manifestations of anogenitorectal syndrome (e.g., perirectal abscess, rectovaginal fistula, rectal stricture) should be managed by a physician due to the serious and complex nature of these conditions.

→ Partner therapy.
  - All sexual partners exposed within the 30 days prior to the patient's symptom onset should be examined, tested for urethral or cervical chlamydial infection, and treated (CDC 1993e). Provide referrals to provider or facility which offers appropriate STD care.

→ Special considerations.
  - Pregnant and lactating women should be treated with erythromycin (see previous discussion of "Alternate Regimens") (CDC 1993e).
  - HIV-infected individuals should be treated with the regimens listed previously (CDC 1993e).

CONSULTATION

→ Consultation with a physician as indicated for patient evaluation, abnormal laboratory studies, and management.

→ For advanced cases of LGV, referral to physician is warranted.

→ As needed for prescription(s).

PATIENT EDUCATION

→ Discuss etiology and nature of LGV including mode of transmission, incubation period, symptoms and potential complications, and importance of partner evaluation and treatment.
  - Patient education handouts are a helpful adjunct to teaching.

→ Advise patient to finish full course of medication and return for follow-up (see "Follow-Up" section). After antibiotics have been started, patient's fever and pain should abate, and she should feel markedly better within one to two days.

→ Advise patient that buboes are unlikely to suppurate after medication has begun. However, in some cases it may become necessary to needle-aspirate fluctuant buboes to prevent rupture.
  - Patient may need physician intervention for this procedure.

→ Chronic or late complications of anogenitorectal syndrome may require surgical management. Procedures should be discussed with the patient by the physician responsible for her care.

→ Advise abstinence from intercourse until patient and partner are treated and cured. If symptoms recur, patient and partner should be instructed to seek care promptly.

→ Address STD prevention and HIV risk-reduction.

■ Provide guidelines for safer sex practices.

■ Encourage careful screening of sex partners and committed use of condoms (especially with new, multiple, non-monogamous partners). See **Table 13A.2, Safer Sex Guidelines**, p. 13-9, and **Table 12I.1, Recommendations for Individuals to Prevent STD/PID**, p. 12-96.

→ Allow patient to ventilate her feelings of surprise, shame, fear, anger as indicated. Psychological support may be important for the patient in gaining control over her sexual situation and to enable her to prevent future STDs.

FOLLOW-UP

→ Follow-up visits at one- to two-week intervals should be scheduled for clinical assessment of response to therapy.

→ Advise patient to return for evaluation if symptoms persist or recur after treatment completed.

→ History on follow-up should include symptom status, medication compliance, drug reaction and side effects, partner therapy, sexual exposure and use of condoms, and drug history.

→ Patients with complicated secondary- and/or tertiary-stage disease should be followed by a physician due to the serious and complex nature of the condition. Ongoing medical, surgical, and psychological evaluation and support will be indicated.

→ Serological tests for syphilis should be repeated in three months.

→ HIV antibody tests should be repeated in three and six months. Continue to encourage safer sex.

→ Follow up on all lab tests ordered. Treat all concomitant STDs and other identified conditions.

→ HIV-positive results should be conveyed in person by a provider who has received training in the complexities of test disclosure. HIV-positive persons should be referred to the appropriate provider or agency for early intervention services.

→ Hepatitis B antigen-positive individuals should have liver function tests and receive counseling regarding the implications of their positive status and need for immunoprophylaxis of sex partners and household members. (See **Hepatitis—Viral** Protocol.)

→ Because LGV is a state-mandated reportable disease, a morbidity report must be filed with the department of public health.

→ Document in progress notes and problem list.

13-H

Syphilis

Syphilis is a chronic infectious process caused by the motile spirochete *Treponema pallidum*. In the United States, while incidences of the infection had been declining up through the early 1980s, since 1987 there has been a marked increase in cases—mostly in Texas, Florida, California, and New York City. The current increase appears to be predominantly among heterosexuals and may be attributed to exchanging sex for drugs, drug abuse, and prostitution (CDC 1987b; Wendel and Gilstrap III 1990). Spread of the infection is mainly through sexual contact but may also occur via nonsexual intimate contact, blood transfusion, and transplacental transmission.

T. pallidum enters the body through non-evident breaks in the skin or mucous membrane, usually during sexual intercourse. The risk of acquisition from an infected partner is about 30 percent to 60 percent (Chapel 1984; Thin 1990). The first observable reaction occurs in 10 to 90 days (average 21 days) and consists of a painless papule or chancre at the site of penetration of the organism (Chapel 1984). This marks onset of the primary stage of syphilis. As local replication occurs, simultaneous dissemination via the lymphatics and blood stream begins (Musher 1987).

Associated regional lymphadenopathy appears seven to ten days after chancre development in 60 percent to 80 percent of patients (Chapel 1984). In women, this primary stage often goes unnoticed. Thus, diagnosis generally does not occur at this time. The primary chancre, even without treatment, usually disappears in two to six weeks (Sweet and Gibbs 1990). Relapse of the primary chancre (termed *monorecidive* or *chancre redux*) is rare (Thin 1990).

The secondary stage of syphilis begins from three to six weeks up to six months after primary inocu-

lation (Sweet and Gibbs 1990; Thin 1990). In 30 percent of cases, because there may be a healing chancre at diagnosis of secondary infection, primary and secondary stages of syphilis may overlap (McPhee 1984).

Systemic involvement of all major organ systems occurs in the secondary stage. Flu-like symptoms, a generalized maculopapular skin rash, mucus membrane lesions, and generalized lymphadenopathy usually occur. Untreated, secondary syphilis lesions resolve in approximately two to six weeks (Blanco and Gonik 1991). At this time, the latent stage ensues, in most cases without apparent clinical manifestations.

The latent stage is divided into early latent (<one year duration) and late latent syphilis (>one year duration). Twenty-five percent of affected individuals may have an exacerbation of secondary syphilis in the early latent phase (Sweet and Gibbs 1990). The lesion-free, asymptomatic late-latent stage is not considered infectious, however, but transplacental infection may still occur (Sweet and Gibbs 1990). Approximately 30 percent of untreated individuals in the latent stage of syphilis develop late or tertiary syphilis (Blanco and Gonik 1990).

Late (or tertiary) syphilis occurs one to 20 years after initial infection and is characterized by CNS involvement (although neurosyphilis may occur at any stage), cardiovascular or musculoskeletal system, and gumma formation (late benign tertiary syphilis) (Blanco and Gonik 1991; CDC 1991; Sweet and Gibbs 1990). In-depth discussion of tertiary syphilis is beyond the scope of this protocol. The reader is directed to a current STD textbook.

Coexistence of primary and/or secondary syphilis with AIDS is common (Felman 1989). HIV-infected persons with syphilis may have an increase in syphilis complications, more rapid progression of syphilitic infection to the tertiary stage, and more serious sequelae involving the central nervous system (Blanco and Gonik 1991; Sweet and Gibbs 1990; Zenker and Rolfs 1990). In addition, serological tests may be inaccurate and standard syphilis therapy inadequate in HIV-infected patients (Zenker and Rolfs 1990).

DATABASE

SUBJECTIVE

→ Risk factors include:
- heterosexual.
- young age (15 years to 24 years most common).
- black race.
- low socioeconomic status.
- inner-city dweller.
- trading sex for illegal drugs.
- drug abuse (intravenous drug use [IVDU] and crack).
- prostitution.
- multiple sexual partners.
- concomitant STD.
- prior history of syphilis.
- no condom use.
- HIV infection (may alter course of syphilis infection).

→ Features include:

Primary syphilis:
- patient may be asymptomatic.
- genital lesion:
- usually raised, painless; locations may include vulva, fourchette, vagina, cervix.
- nongenital lesion:
  • usually raised, painless; locations may include anus, lip(s) (most common site), tongue, tonsils, gingiva (rare), finger, eyelid, breast, nipple.
- inguinal or cervical lymphadenopathy.
- vaginal or urethral discharge.
- rectal pain on defecation, rectal bleeding, mucoid or blood-streaked stool.
- no constitutional symptoms.

Secondary syphilis:
- patient may be asymptomatic.
- often subtle symptomatology.
- flu-like symptoms (50 percent of patients):
  • sore throat, malaise, headache, fever, myalgias, arthralgias, hoarseness, anorexia.
  • weight loss.

- skin "rash" of trunk, extremities, palms, and/or soles (this syphiloderm occurs in more than 80 percent of cases):
  • may be pruritic.
- persisting primary chancre (25 percent of cases).
- skin and mucous membrane lesions of vulva, perineum, anus, mouth (condyloma lata, "mucous patches").
- bone pain.
- patchy hair loss.
- neurological complaints:
  • meningitis symptoms, headache, hearing or vision loss, tingling, weakness, mental changes.
- generalized lymphadenopathy.

Latent syphilis:
- patient is usually asymptomatic.
- twenty-five percent of women may have exacerbation of secondary syphilis lesions (Sweet and Gibbs 1990).

Late syphilis and neurosyphilis:
- discussion of symptomatology is beyond the scope of this protocol.

→ Gynecological and medical history should include:
- menstrual cycle.
- contraception.
- description of symptoms:
  • onset.
  • duration.
  • quality/quantity.
  • frequency.
  • course.
  • aggravating/relieving factors.
  • associated symptoms.
- previous history of same/similar problem (including VDRL or RPR results, if known).
- STD history (including dates/treatment).
- sensitive questioning regarding recent sexual activity (including date of last exposure, sex practices, sites of exposure, number of partners in past month, use of condoms).
- sex partner history.
- acute/chronic illness.
- general health.
- medications.
- allergies.
- habits.
- history of laboratory tests for syphilis, Hepatitis B, HIV.
- review of systems (CDC 1991).

OBJECTIVE

→ Thorough STD examination includes:
- vital signs as indicated.
- general skin inspection of face, trunk, forearms, palms, soles for lesions, rashes, discoloration.
- inspection of pharynx and oral cavity for erythema, infection, lesions, discoloration.
- abdominal inspection and palpation for masses, tenderness, rebound tenderness.
- inspection of pubic hair for lice, nits.
- inspection of external genitalia for discharge, masses, lesions.
- inspection/palpation of Bartholin's, urethral, and Skene's glands for discharge, masses.
- inspection of vagina for blood, discharge, lesions.
- inspection of cervix for lesions, discharge, eversion, erythema, edema, friability; assessment for CMT.
- uterine assessment for size, shape, consistency, mobility, tenderness.
- palpation of adnexa for masses, tenderness.
- inspection of perianus, anus, rectum for lesions, bleeding, discharge.
- rectal examination as indicated.
- assessment of presence or absence of associated cervical, inguinal lymphadenopathy (CDC 1991).

→ Physical examinations components and findings specific to assessment of patients with syphilis may include:

Primary syphilis:
- external genitalia chancres (fourchette, vulva):
  - single or multiple lesions may occur.
    - Progress from dull red macule 0.5 cm-1 cm → papule → ulcer (chancre).
    - Chancre round or elongated, covered with grayish exudate, surrounded by indurated margin.
    - May have stippled hemorrhage line or dilated capillaries circling margin.
    - Usually nontender.
- urethral meatus chancres (one percent to three percent of cases): scant serous/sero-sanguineous discharge, induration.
- vaginal chancres (<one percent of cases): eroded papules or nodules.
- cervical chancres (five percent to 44 percent of cases).
  - In majority of cases, lesion surrounds external os, remainder are on anterior or posterior lip.

- nongenital-area chancres (five percent of chancres).
  - May appear on lip(s) (most common site), tongue, tonsils, gingiva (rare), fingers, eyelid, breast, nipple, anus.
  - Extragenital lesions may be atypical.
    - Lip: solitary, eroded or ulcerated papule or nodule.
    - Tongue: smooth, firm, eroded, or ulcerated plaque.
    - Tonsils: unilateral, firm, slightly elevated plaques with grey exudate.
    - Anus: dull red, indurated, eroded; may also appear as an indurated fissure or hemorrhoid; anorectal lesions can be palpated on digital examination (Chapel 1984).
- Regional lymphadenopathy:
  - usually occurs within one week of chancre.
  - nodes nontender, small-moderate size, rubbery, nonsuppurative.
  - bilateral inguinal adenopathy with genital/anal chancre.
  - unilateral submental or anterior cervical adenopathy if chancre in oropharyngeal cavity.
  - in some cases, if chancre on anus, lower two-thirds of vulva, or cervix, inguinal adenopathy will be absent (Chapel 1984).
  - Perform neurological examination as indicated.

Secondary syphilis:
- fever.
- weight loss.
- skin "rash" (more than 80 percent of cases): 0.5 cm-1 cm faint rose-pink macular lesions beginning on trunk and flexor surfaces of upper extremities; become dull red, papular, spreading to whole body, especially palms and soles.
- split papules: eroded, fissured papules affecting intertriginous areas (especially nasolabial fold, angles of mouth, behind ears).
- condyloma lata: characteristically large, raised, broad papules, resembling viral warts, typically on anus, vulva, or other warm, moist areas.
- mucosal lesions: "mucous patch"—7 mm to 10 mm raised, inflammatory papule with oval central erosion and grey membrane.
  - May affect any mucous membrane.
  - Diffuse inflammation may occur on pharynx/tonsils ("syphilitic sore throat").

NOTE: Cutaneous lesions of secondary syphilis heal in two to six weeks without scarring; hypo-

hyper-pigmentation may occur in resolving lesions. Relapsing secondary lesions may occur within five years (Chapel 1984; Thin 1990).
- hair loss (alopecia):
  - patchy loss on scalp, eyelashes, eyebrows. Diffuse thinning also may occur.
- lymphadenopathy:
  - inguinal, suboccipital, posterior cervical, axillary, epitrochlear. Nodes are discrete, nontender, moderately enlarged, rubbery.
- other findings: arthritis, bursitis, osteitis, hepatitis, anterior iritis, choroiditis, nephritis/ nephrotic syndrome, gastritis, gastric ulcer.
- perform neurological examination as indicated. CNS involvement may include aseptic meningitis, cranial nerve palsies, transverse myelitis, deafness.

Latent syphilis:
- clinical findings are usually limited to positive nontreponemal and treponemal tests.
- relapse of secondary signs in 25 percent of cases (e.g., recurrent mucocutaneous lesions, usually within the first year [Hook III and Marra 1992]).

te syphilis and neurosyphilis:
iscussion of manifestations is beyond the scope f this protocol.

SMENT

→ Syphilis—primary, secondary, or latent
→ R/O syphilis
→ R/O other type of genital ulcer disease: herpes simplex, granuloma inguinale, LGV, chancroid, vulvar cancer
→ R/O other types of orogenital ulceration: Reiter's/ Stevens-Johnson's/Behçet's syndromes, etc.
→ R/O other dermatoses
→ R/O concomitant STDs
→ R/O HIV infection
→ R/O mononucleosis
→ R/O Hodgkin's disease
→ R/O lymphoma
→ R/O complications associated with secondary syphilis: arthritis, bursitis, osteitis, hepatitis, nephrotic syndrome, gastritis, gastric ulceration, iritis, choroiditis
→ R/O neurosyphilis

PLAN

DIAGNOSTIC TESTS
→ Index of suspicion is requisite to diagnosis.
→ Types of tests:
- darkfield microscopy (DF): useful in primary and secondary syphilis and provides definitive immediate diagnosis of *T. pallidum* from lesions and tissues (except oral lesions).
- direct fluorescent antibody to *T. pallidum* (DFA-TP) can be used for primary and secondary lesions and biopsy tissue.
- nontreponemal serological testing provides indirect evidence of primary or secondary syphilis and includes one of the following (Larsen, Hunter, and Creighton 1990; Thin 1990):
  - Venereal Disease Research Laboratory (VDRL).
  - Rapid Plasma Reagin (RPR).
  - Reagin screen test (RST).
  - Toluidine red unheated serum test (TRUST).
NOTE: See **Table 13H.1, Important Points in the Interpretation of Syphilis Tests**.
- treponemal serological tests are used for confirmation of nontreponemal tests and for patients with symptoms of late syphilis (Larsen, Hunter, and Creighton 1990). Tests include:
  - fluorescent treponemal antibody-absorption (FTA-ABS).
  - microhemagglutination assay for antibody to *T. pallidum* (MHA-TP).
  - hemagglutination treponemal test for syphilis (HATTS).
  - enzyme immunoassay methods (ELISA).
NOTE: See **Table 13H.1**.
- (PCR) can be used for lesion exudate, CSF, amniotic fluid; not available except in research labs.
→ Criteria for diagnosis.
Primary syphilis:
- definitive diagnosis is via direct microscopic examination utilizing the following modalities:
  - dark-field microscopy of *T. pallidum* from chancre or regional lymph-node aspirate. **NOTE:** Ideal specimen is serous-rich fluid. Clean chancre with sterile saline and then abrade area, squeeze to produce serous exudate then press directly on to microscope slide, and apply cover slip. Lymph node aspirates may also be used: disinfect area, inject 0.2 ml of sterile saline into node and

Table 13H.1.   IMPORTANT POINTS IN THE INTERPRETATION OF SYPHILIS TESTS

Nontreponemal Tests

→ More than a reactive VDRL or RPR is needed to justify the diagnosis of syphilis.

→ Nontreponemal tests should be used for *screening* and to *follow response to treatment*, and should not be used interchangeably for sequential testing.

→ Tests reported as reactive or nonreactive with quantitative results reported as a dilution (i.e., 1:4) or as a reciprocal of the dilutions (i.e., 4 dilutions). A fourfold titer change is equivalent to a change of two doubling-dilution (e.g., from 1:16 to 1:4 or from 1:8 to 1:32) (CDC 1993f).

→ Rising titers indicate infection, reinfection, or treatment failure.

→ May be nonreactive in the primary stage of syphilis; usually do not become reactive until at least 7 to 10 days after the appearance of the chancre (CDC 1991).

→ Initial nonreactive nontreponemal tests should be repeated in 1 week, 1 month, and 3 months in cases where the lesion is suspicious for syphilis and dark-field examination is unavailable (Larsen, Hunter, and Creighton 1990). In addition, with a suspect lesion, a treponemal test (see below) should be performed if the nontreponemal test is nonreactive (Larsen, Hunter, and Creighton 1990).

→ If the patient with secondary syphilis develops a very high titer, the VDRL or RPR could remain nonreactive due to the *prozone phenomenon*.[1] Thus, in all cases where suspicious lesions are present, ask the laboratory to dilute the negative serum and continue the titration.

→ Nonreactive VDRL or RPRs may occur in a patient with late symptomatic syphilis, either acquired or congenital. A negative nontreponemal test does not rule out syphilis. False negative tests may occur in HIV infection.

→ Reactive VDRL or RPR performed on a sample of spinal fluid always represents syphilis unless proved otherwise. CNS involvement (except in cases of tabes dorsalis) also is indicated by elevations of spinal-fluid blood cell count and total protein.

→ A sustained two-tube rise in titer (e.g., 1:2 to 1:8) performed by the same laboratory is considered minimal evidence of the need for re-treatment. The only exception is the adequately treated congenital syphilitic whose titer may fluctuate without any particular significance.

→ When there is any doubt about previous treatment, every *pregnant* woman with a reactive serological test for syphilis should be considered to require treatment. The usual medical and epidemiological follow-up can be performed later to confirm the diagnosis.

→ If a VDRL or RPR performed on the cord blood of a newborn is reactive, it may be due to passive transfer of reagin from the mother. A VDRL or RPR should be performed every month for 3 months to determine whether the titer is rising or falling. If the titer falls rapidly or becomes nonreactive, then passive transfer, not congenital syphilis, is the case.

→ With adequate therapy of primary and secondary syphilis, titers should decline fourfold in 3 months and eightfold in 6 months. In primary syphilis, non-treponemal tests are usually nonreactive 1 year after treatment, and in secondary syphilis, 2 years after treatment (Thin 1990). For early latent syphilis a fourfold decline in titer should occur in 6 months and nontreponemal tests should be nonreactive by 2 years after adequate therapy. In late latent syphilis, decreases in titers are variable after treatment is completed (Bolan 1994).

→ VDRL or RPR may remain positive in low titer (serofast state) or in the high pretreatment titer range for life if the patient receives treatment in the latter part of the infection. In such cases, cure is not based on serological reversal, and treatment need not be repeated unless there is other evidence of reinfection.

→ A reactive VDRL or RPR in the absence of syphilis is called a biological false positive (BFP: 1 percent to 2 percent of cases). A BFP must always be proven to not represent syphilis. BFPs may occur in the following conditions:
  ▪ infectious mononucleosis.
  ▪ leprosy, malaria.
  ▪ lupus erythematosus and other autoimmune diseases.
  ▪ vaccina.
  ▪ viral pneumonia and other viral infections.
  ▪ pregnancy.
  ▪ narcotic addiction.
  ▪ acute febrile illness.
  ▪ Lyme disease.
  ▪ chronic infections.
  ▪ immunizations.

→ Other spirochete infections (e.g., yaws, pinta, bejel) produce positive reactions as well, but this should not be considered as false positive (City and County of San Francisco, Department of Public Health 1992; Jaffe and Musher 1990; Larsen, Hunter, and Creighton 1990).

Continued

Table 13H.1.   IMPORTANT POINTS IN THE INTERPRETATION OF SYPHILIS TESTS (CONTINUED)

Treponemal Tests

→ *Do not* use treponemal tests for screening or to assess response to treatment.

→ Used for confirmation of nontreponemal tests and for patients with symptoms of late syphilis (Larsen, Hunter, and Creighton 1990).

→ FTA-ABS is 90 percent to 95 percent sensitive, first to become reactive; MHA-TP is 80 percent to 85 percent sensitive, reactive about same time as reagin tests (CDC 1991).

→ With a suspect lesion, treponemal test should be performed if the nontreponemal test is nonreactive (Larsen, Hunter, and Creighton 1990).

→ Reactive test indicates past or present infection. In incubating syphilis, however, tests may be negative.

→ One percent false-positive rate in the general population (may be seen in lupus erythematosus, infectious mononucleosis, leprosy).

→ In the majority of cases, once test is positive it remains so for life; thus treponemal tests *cannot* be used to follow response to therapy. Fifteen to 25 percent of cases treated in the early primary stage may revert to nonreactive in 2 to 3 years (CDC 1993f).

---

[1]See protocol for discussion.

then aspirate fluid. Immediate dark-field microscopy by experienced microscopist to identify *T. pallidum* must be performed after specimen collection (Larsen, Hunter, and Creighton 1990). If initial dark-field is negative in a suspect case, repeat test on 2 successive days; advise patient to cleanse lesion with physiological saline between exams and avoid topical substances (CDC 1991; Thin 1990).

• direct fluorescent antibody test for *T. pallidum* (DFA-TP): alternative when dark-field not available or for oral lesions.
  NOTE: Lesion material collected on slide is stained with fluorescein-labelled anti-*T. pallidum* globulin and examined under fluorescent microscope (Larsen, Hunter, and Creighton 1990; Thin 1990).
• silver stain of biopsy material may also be used to identify *T. pallidum* (CDC 1991).
■ presumptive evidence of primary syphilis includes:
  • typical lesion(s) (chancre)
              PLUS
  • reactive nontreponemal test without prior history of syphilis
              OR
  • ≥four-fold titer increase on quantitative nontreponemal test compared with most recent previous test for person with history of syphilis (CDC 1991).
■ suggestive evidence includes:
  • lesion resembling chancre.

• sexual exposure in previous 10 to 90 days to person with primary, secondary, or early latent syphilis (CDC 1991).
■ if signs/symptoms of neurologic disease (e.g., auditory, cranial nerve, meningeal manifestations) or ophthalmic disease are present, CSF analysis and ocular slit-lamp evaluation should be performed (CDC 1993f).

Secondary syphilis:
■ definitive diagnosis includes:
  • identification of *T. pallidum* from skin/mucous membrane lesions or lymph node aspirate via dark-field microscopy or DFA-TP
              OR
  • demonstration of *T. pallidum* on DFA-TP or histological staining of biopsy material from lesions characteristic of secondary syphilis (CDC 1991).
■ presumptive evidence includes:
  • skin/mucous membrane lesions of secondary syphilis, specifically one of the following:
    ▸ skin lesions, bilaterally symmetrical.
    ▸ condyloma lata.
    ▸ mucus patches of cervix or oropharynx,
              PLUS
  • reactive nontreponemal test (≥1:8) in absence of syphilis history
              OR
  • ≥fourfold titer increase on nontreponemal test compared with most recent previous test for person with history of syphilis (CDC 1991).
■ suggestive evidence when serology unavailable includes:

- ≥one skin/mucous membrane lesions suggestive of syphilis
  PLUS
- sexual exposure in previous 6 months to person diagnosed with primary, secondary, or early latent syphilis (CDC 1991).
- additional signs of secondary syphilis which may aid diagnosis may include:
  - alopecia.
  - loss of eyelashes, lateral third of eyebrows.
  - iritis.
  - fever and malaise.
  - generalized lymphadenopathy.
  - hepatomegaly and/or splenomegaly (CDC 1991).
- patients with atypical findings and/or nontreponemal titers <1:16 should have repeat nontreponemal tests and a confirmatory treponemal test (Larsen, Hunter, and Creighton 1990).
  - Less than 2 percent of patients will have a nonreactive nontreponemal test due to the *prozone phenomenon*. Lab should be asked to dilute the sera and continue titration. (Larsen, Hunter, and Creighton 1990; San Francisco City Clinic 1992).

NOTE: The prozone phenomenon occurs when a higher than optimal amount of antibody in the tested sera prevents the flocculation reaction typical of a positive test (Berkowitz, Baxi, and Fox 1990).

- in some cases of coinfection with HIV, treponemal tests have been negative despite biopsy confirmation of secondary syphilis (Felman 1989).
- evaluation of CSF via lumbar puncture usually is not indicated in secondary syphilis but should be considered in patients with signs or symptoms of neurological involvement (e.g., auditory, cranial nerve, meningeal, or ophthalmic manifestations) (CDC 1989d).

Early latent syphilis (<1 year):
- presumptive evidence includes:
  - absence of signs and symptoms
    PLUS
  - reactive nontreponemal and treponemal tests
    PLUS
  - history of nonreactive test in past year
    OR
  - ≥four-fold increase in nontreponemal test titer compared with previous test
    OR

- history of symptoms suggestive of primary/secondary syphilis (CDC 1991).
- suggestive evidence includes:
  - reactive nontreponemal test
    PLUS
  - sexual exposure within preceding year to person diagnosed with primary, secondary, or early latent syphilis (CDC 1991).

Late latent syphilis (>1 year):
- presumptive evidence includes:
  - reactive nontreponemal test
    PLUS
  - reactive treponemal test
    PLUS
  - no history of syphilis or previous tests
    OR
  - symptoms indicative of late syphilis (CDC 1991).
- CSF analysis is suggested in the following instances: duration of syphilis unknown, clinical signs of neurological or ophthalmic involvement present, nontreponemal titer ≥1:32 (unless duration of infection <1 year), evidence of active syphilis (e.g., aoritis, gumma, iritis), nonpenicillin therapy planned (unless duration of infection <1 year), treatment failure, HIV-infection (CDC 1991, 1993f).

Neurosyphilis:
- definitive diagnosis includes:
  - reactive VDRL from CSF (VDRL-CSF) (most definitive test)
    OR
  - *T pallidum* identified in CSF or CNS tissue by dark-field, DFA, histology, or animal inoculation. (CDC 1991)

NOTE: The FTA-ABS test of CSF may be less specific (i.e., more false positives) than the VDRL, but it is very sensitive. When nonreactive, this test provides strong evidence against neurosyphilis (CDC 1991). CSF FTA-ABS and hemagglutination tests cannot be used unless titrated for comparison with serum levels (Musher 1987; Sweet and Gibbs 1990).

- presumptive evidence includes:
  - syphilis diagnosis
    PLUS
  - clinical signs indicative of CNS syphilis
    OR
  - CSF protein or leukocyte count elevation (in absence of other known causes) (CDC 1991).

NOTE: CSF leukocyte count usually elevated

(>5 WBC/mm³) in neurosyphilis (CDC 1991).

→ Additional considerations.

- Distinguish between syphilis and other causes of genital ulcers. See **Table 13A.1, Clinical Features of Genital Ulcers**, p. 13-6, and **Figure 13A.1, Sexually Active Patient with Genital Ulcers**, p. 13-7.

- Diagnostic tests to rule out other causes of genital ulcers and lymphadenopathy include herpes cultures or Tzanck stain to rule out herpes. See **Herpes Simplex Virus** Protocol.

  - See "Diagnostic Test" sections of **Chancroid**, **Lymphogranuloma Venereum**, and **Granuloma Inguinale (Donovanosis)** protocols.

- Endocervical culture for *N. gonorrhoeae* and endocervical diagnostic tests for *C. trachomatis* should be considered to rule out concomitant STDs.

  - In the absence of a cervix, urethral specimen may be obtained.

- Wet mounts of vaginal discharge to rule concomitant vaginitis, especially trichomoniasis. See **Vaginitis** Protocols.

- All patients with syphilis should be tested for HIV (CDC 1993f).

- Additional labs may be ordered as indicated and may include, but are not limited to: CBC, urinalysis, urine culture and sensitivities, Hepatitis B screen, pregnancy test, CD_4+ cell and lymphocyte counts (if patient known to be HIV-positive).

- In an HIV-infected patient, if serological tests are nonreactive or do not seem to fit the clinical picture, alternative diagnostic tests should be employed (e.g., biopsy of lesion, dark-field examination, DFA-TP).

TREATMENT/MANAGEMENT

→ Parenteral penicillin G is the preferred drug in all stages. It is the only therapy with documented efficacy for pregnant women and neurosyphilis patients (CDC 1993f).

Primary and secondary syphilis

→ Benzathine penicillin G, 2.4 million units I.M., in a single dose.

→ Alternative regimens for penicillin-allergic persons:

- doxycycline (Vibramycin®) 100 mg p.o. BID for 2 weeks

OR

- tetracycline (Achromycin®) 500 mg p.o. QID for 2 weeks

OR

- erythromycin (E-Mycin®) 500 mg p.o. QID for 2 weeks (less effective).

→ For penicillin-allergic pregnant patients and in cases where compliance or follow-up cannot be ensured, treatment with penicillin should be given after desensitization (if necessary). Refer to 1993f CDC reference, pp. 44–46. See also additional considerations regarding pregnancy below (CDC 1993f).

Latent syphilis: Early latent

→ Benzathine penicillin G, 2.4 million units I.M. in a single dose (CDC 1993f).

Latent syphilis: Late latent or unknown duration

→ Benzathine penicillin G, 7.2 million units total, administered as 3 doses of 2.4 million units I.M. each, at 1-week intervals (CDC 1993f).

→ Alternative regimens for non-pregnant penicillin-allergic patients include:

- doxycycline (Vibramycin®) 100 mg p.o. BID for 2 weeks (4 weeks if duration of infection is >1 year)

OR

- tetracycline (Achromycin®) 500 mg p.o. QID for 2 weeks (4 weeks if duration of infection is > 1 year).

  NOTE: Non-penicillin therapy is indicated only after CSF exam has excluded neurosyphilis (CDC 1993f).

→ Pregnant patients allergic to penicillin should be desensitized as indicated and treated with penicillin. Refer to 1993f CDC reference, pp. 44–46. See also following additional considerations regarding pregnancy.

Late syphilis (gumma and cardiovascular syphilis, *not* neurosyphilis):

→ a CSF examination should be performed prior to therapy. Complete discussion of management of patients with cardiovascular or gummatous syphilis is beyond the scope of this protocol. Patient should be referred to a physician.

→ non-pregnant, nonallergic patients may be treated with: benzathine penicillin G, 7.2 million units total, administered as 3 doses of 2.4 million units I.M., at 1-week intervals (CDC 1993f).

→ non-pregnant, penicillin-allergic patients should be managed as for late latent syphilis.

→ pregnant, penicillin-allergic patients should be desensitized as indicated and treated with penicillin. Refer to 1993f CDC reference, pp. 44–46. See also additional considerations regarding pregnancy that follow (CDC 1993f).

Neurosyphilis

→ Discussion regarding intravenous therapy for neurosyphilis is beyond the scope of this protocol.

→ If compliance can be ensured, treatment may consist of:
- procaine penicillin, 2.4 million units I.M. daily
  PLUS
- probenecid (Benemid®) 500 mg p.o. QID, both for 10-14 days (CDC 1993f).
  NOTE: The addition of benzathine penicillin G, 2.4 million units I.M. weekly for 3 doses after completion of the above has been recommended (CDC 1989d, 1993f).

→ Penicillin-allergic patients should be treated with penicillin after desensitization as indicated. Refer to 1993f CDC references, pp. 44–46. See also additional considerations regarding pregnancy that follow (CDC 1993f).

Syphilis and HIV-infection: Primary and secondary syphilis

→ Benzathine penicillin G 2.4 million units I.M.
- Some experts recommend additional treatments as suggested for late syphilis or other supplemental antibiotics in addition to benzathine penicillin. In addition, some experts recommend CSF examination prior to therapy (CDC 1993f).

Syphilis and HIV Infection: Latent syphilis

→ CSF examination should be performed.

→ If CSF examination is WNL, benzathine penicillin G 7.2 million units I.M. total, as 3 weekly doses of 2.4 million units each (CDC 1993f).

→ Penicillin-allergic patients with HIV may be skin-tested to confirm allergy, desensitized as indicated, and then treated with penicillin.

→ Close, careful follow-up of HIV-infected syphilis patients is essential.

Partner therapy

→ All sex partners of patients with syphilis should be evaluated both clinically and serologically. Provide referrals to provider or facility which offers appropriate STD care, if necessary.

→ Persons exposed to a patient with primary, secondary, or latent syphilis (of less than 1 year's duration) within the preceding 90 days should be treated presumptively, even if seronegative (CDC 1993f).

→ Persons exposed to a patient with primary, secondary, or latent syphilis (of less than 1 year's duration) more than 90 days prior to examination should be treated presumptively if serological tests are not available immediately and follow-up cannot be ensured (CDC 1993f).

→ For partner notification purposes and presumptive treatment of exposed sex partners, patients who have syphilis of unknown duration and non-treponemal titers ≥1:32 may be considered to be infected with early syphilis (CDC 1993f).

→ Long-term sex partners of patients with late syphilis should be evaluated both clinically and serologically (CDC 1993f).

→ Time periods before treatment used in identifying at-risk sex partners are:
- 3 months plus duration of symptoms for primary syphilis.
- 6 months plus duration of symptoms for secondary syphilis.
- 1 year for early latent syphilis (CDC 1993f).

Additional considerations

→ Lumbar puncture for CSF evaluation is recommended in cases where neurological signs or symptoms are present or if treatment failure is suspected (CDC 1991). See "Diagnostic Tests" section.

→ Syphilis screening during pregnancy should be performed as soon as the patient presents for care.

→ Seropositive pregnant women should be considered infected unless it can be documented that prior treatment has been completed and sequential serological antibody titers have declined appropriately (CDC 1993f).

→ Treatment during pregnancy is as appropriate for the stage of syphilis—see previous discussion.
- It has been recommended by some experts that additional therapy (e.g., second dose of benzathine penicillin 2.4 million units I.M.) be given 1 week after the initial dose, especially during the third trimester and in women with secondary syphilis (CDC 1993f).
- Tetracycline and doxycycline are contraindicated.
- Erythromycin is unreliable in curing an affected fetus (CDC 1993f).

CONSULTATION

→ Consultation with a physician is indicated for complicated or advanced cases and for treatment failures.

→ If neurosyphilis is suspected, refer to a physician for evaluation and management.

→ As needed for prescription(s).

PATIENT EDUCATION

→ Discuss the etiology and nature of syphilis, including mode of transmission, incubation period, symptoms, course of disease, potential complications, possible association with HIV infection, and importance of partner evaluation and treatment.

  ▪ Patient-education handouts are a useful adjunct to teaching.

NOTE: It is important to discuss the *Jarisch-Herxheimer* reaction. This is a self-limited acute febrile reaction which may occur after any therapy for syphilis. It is postulated to occur due to the rapid release of treponemal antigens (Charles 1990). It is common among early syphilis patients (CDC 1993f). Onset may be a few hours after treatment and symptoms may last for 24 hours and include: fever, malaise, headache, musculoskeletal pain, nausea, and tachycardia. The chancre may swell or secondary syphilitic lesions may appear for the first time. Antipyretics may be taken (Thin 1990). Women in the second trimester of pregnancy whose treatment precipitates this reaction are at risk for premature labor and/or fetal distress (CDC 1993f).

→ If patient is on oral medication, advise her to finish full course. When multiple injections are indicated, advise patient of importance of follow-up until therapy completed.

  ▪ Give instructions for follow-up as indicated for stage of disease. See "Follow-Up" section.

→ Advise abstinence from intercourse until patient and partner treated and cured. If symptoms recur, patient and partner should be instructed to seek care promptly.

→ Address STD prevention and HIV risk-reduction.

  ▪ Provide guidelines for safer sex practices.

  ▪ Encourage careful screening of sex partners and committed use of condoms (especially with new, multiple, non-monogamous partners).

  ▪ See **Table 13A.2, Safer Sex Guidelines**, p. 13-9, and **Table 12I.1, Recommendations for Individuals to Prevent STD**, p. 12-96.

→ Educate patients to become aware of their VDRL or RPR results.

  ▪ Suggest they keep a diary to facilitate future management.

→ Allow patient to ventilate her feelings of surprise, shame, fear, anger, as indicated. Psychological support may be important for the patient in gaining control over her sexual situation and to enable her to prevent future STDs.

FOLLOW-UP

→ The importance of follow-up should be stressed. It is especially important in a reproductive-age woman; if inadequately treated, the possibility of congenital syphilis may occur during an ensuing pregnancy. A pregnant woman at high risk for syphilis should be tested initially, during the third trimester, and at delivery (CDC 1993f).

→ History on follow-up should include symptom status, medication compliance, drug reaction and side effects, partner therapy, sexual exposure, and use of condoms.

→ See **Table 13H.1**.

Primary and secondary syphilis

→ Clinical and serological examination at three and six months.

→ Patients with persistent or recurrent signs or symptoms, or a sustained fourfold increase in nontreponemal test titer (over baseline or subsequent test), should be considered treatment failures or reinfected.

  ▪ Evaluate for HIV-infection and re-treat (see following discussion, "Syphilis and HIV Infection").

  ▪ Lumbar puncture should be performed unless reinfection is likely (CDC 1993f). Consult with physician.

→ Persons at risk for treatment failure are identified by failure of nontreponemal test titers to decline fourfold by three months after therapy. Additional clinical and serological follow-up should be performed.

  ▪ Evaluate for HIV infection.

  ▪ Re-treat if further follow-up cannot be ensured (see following discussion, "Syphilis and HIV Infection").

  ▪ Some STD experts recommend CSF evaluation in these situations (CDC 1993f). Consult with physician.

→ Re-treatment regimen: benzathine penicillin G 2.4 million units I.M. once a week for three weeks (unless lumbar puncture indicates neurosyphilis) (CDC 1993f).

→ Patients with primary syphilis who reside in a high HIV prevalence area should be re-screened for HIV in three months (CDC 1993f).

Latent syphilis

→ Quantitative nontreponemal tests should be repeated at six and 12 months (CDC 1993f).

→ If titers increase fourfold, an intially high titer (≥1:32) fails to decline at least fourfold (two dilutions) within 12 to 24 months, or signs or symptoms of syphilis develop, the patient should be evaluated for neurosyphilis and re-treated appropriately (CDC 1993f).

Late syphilis

→ There is little evidence regarding follow-up. Clinical response to therapy dependent upon nature of the lesion(s) (CDC 1993f).

Neurosyphilis

→ CSF examination should be repeated every six months until the CSF cell count is normal. If the cell count has not decreased at six months or is not normal by two years, re-treatment should be considered (CDC 1993f). Consult with physician.

Syphilis and HIV infection

→ Re-examination and quantitative nontreponemal tests at one, two, three, six, nine, and 12 months after treatment (CDC 1993f).

→ CSF examination after therapy (i.e., at six months) suggested by some experts (CDC 1993f).

→ If patient meets criteria for treatment failure, a CSF examination should be performed and re-treatment initiated. CSF examination and retreatment should be strongly considered in those patients who fail to demonstrate a fourfold decrease on nontreponemal titer within three months after treatment for primary or secondary syphilis.
  ▪ If CSF examination is WNL, retreat with benzathine penicillin G 7.2 million units as three weekly doses of 2.4 million units each (CDC 1993f). Consult with physician.

→ Pregnancy.
  ▪ Serological titers should be assessed monthly until treatment adequacy assured (CDC 1993f).

→ Additional considerations.
  ▪ Follow up on all additional laboratory tests ordered. Treat all concomitant STDs and other identified conditions. Continue to encourage safer sex practices.
  ▪ HIV-positive results should be conveyed in person and by a provider who has received training in the complexities of test disclosure. HIV-positive persons should be referred to the appropriate provider or agency for early intervention services.
  ▪ Hepatitis B antigen-positive individuals should have liver function tests and receive counseling regarding the implciations of their positive status and need for immunoprophylaxis of sex partners and household members. See **Hepatitis—Viral** Protocol.
  ▪ Because syphilis is a reportable disease mandated by state law, a report must be filed with the department of public health.
  ▪ Document in progress notes and problem list.

13-1

Bibliography

American College of Obstetricians and Gynecologists. 1988. *Gynecologic herpes simplex virus infections.* Technical Bulletin No. 119. Washington, DC: the Author.

————. 1994. Genital human papillomavirus infections. Technical Bulletin No. 193. Washington, DC: the Author.

American Social Health Association. 1985. *Some questions and answers about herpes.* Palo Alto, CA: United Way.

————. New treatment guidelines for ACV, 1989. *The Helper* (Spring):9–11. Palo Alto, CA: United Way.

Baker, D.A. 1991. Prolonged continuous acyclovir treatment of recurring genital herpes simplex virus infections. *Proceedings of a symposium held at the 91st annual meeting of the American College of Obstetricians and Gynecologists,* pp. 17–20. Intramed Communications.

Becker, T.M., Stone, K.M., and Alexander, E.R. 1987. Genital human papillomavirus: A growing concern. *Obstetrics and Gynecology Clinics of North America* 14(3):389–396.

Berkowitz, K., Baxi, L., and Fox, H.E. 1990. False-negative syphilis screening: The prozone phenomenon, nonimmune hydrops, and diagnosis of syphilis during pregnancy. *American Journal of Obstetrics and Gynecology* 163(3):975–977.

Black, J.R., Long, J.M., Zwickl, B.E., Ray, B.S., Verdon, M.S., Wetherby, S., Hook III, E.W. and Handsfield, H.H. 1989. Multicenter randomized study of single-dose ofloxacin versus amoxicillin-probenecid for treatment of uncomplicated gonococcal infection. *Antimicrobial Agents and Chemotherapy* 33(2):167–170.

Blanco, J.D., and Gonik, B. 1991. Sexually transmitted diseases. *Current Problems in Obstetrics, Gynecology, and Fertility* 14(6):179–233.

Bolan, G. 1994 (Nov). *Syphilis.* Outline presented at the STD intensive for clinicians (Nov. 11–18). San Francisco STD/HIV Prevention Training Center. San Francisco, CA.

Bowie, W.R. 1992. Effective treatment of urethritis. A practical guide. *Drugs* 44(2):207–215.

Brooks, G.F. 1988. Gonococcal infection. Unpublished lecture handout. University of California, San Francisco.

Buntin, D.M., Rosen, T., Lesher, J.L., Plotnick, H., Brademas, M.E., and Berger, T.G. 1991. Sexually transmitted diseases: Bacterial infections. *Journal of the American Academy of Dermatology* 25(2, Pt.1):287–299.

Burgoyne, R.A. 1990. Lymphogranuloma venereum. *Primary Care* 12(1):153–155.

Burroughs Wellcome Company. 1993. *Sensitivity/resistance of herpes simplex virus to zovirax (acyclovir).* ZVR11-Z. Drug Information Department (800-443-6763).

Carlson, J.W., and Twiggs, L.B. 1992. Clinical applications of molecular biologic screening for human papillomavirus: Diagnostic techniques. *Clinical Obstetrics and Gynecology* 35(1):13–21.

Cates Jr., W., and Wasserheit, J.N. 1991. Genital chlamydial infections: Epidemiology and reproductive sequelae. *American Journal of Obstetrics and Gynecology* 164(6, Pt. 2):1771–1781.

Centers for Disease Control. 1985. *Chlamydia trachomatis* infections: Policy guidelines for prevention and control. *Morbidity and Mortality Weekly Report* 34(Suppl. 3S):53S.

———. 1987a. Antibiotic-resistant strains of *Neisseria gonorrhoeae*. *Morbidity and Mortality Weekly Report* 36(Suppl. 5S):1S–18S.

———. 1987b. Increases in primary and secondary syphilis—United States. *Morbidity and Mortality Weekly Report* 36(25):393–397.

———. 1989a. 1989 Sexually transmitted diseases treatment guidelines. *Morbidity and Mortality Weekly Report* 38(S-8):4–5.

———. 1989b. 1989 Sexually transmitted diseases treatment guidelines. *Morbidity and Mortality Weekly Report* 38(S-8):21–27.

———. 1989c. 1989 Sexually transmitted diseases treatment guidelines. *Morbidity and Mortality Weekly Report* 38(S-8):18–21.

———. 1989d. 1989 Sexually transmitted diseases treatment guidelines. *Morbidity and Mortality Weekly Report*. 38(S-8):5–15.

———. 1991. *Sexually transmitted diseases. Clinical Practice Guidelines*. Atlanta: the Author.

———. 1993a. 1993 Sexually transmitted diseases treatment guidelines. *Morbidity and Mortality Weekly Report* 42(RR-14):20–22.

———. 1993b. 1993 Sexually transmitted diseases treatment guidelines. *Morbidity and Mortality Weekly Report* 42(RR-14):49–52.

———. 1993c. 1993 Sexually transmitted diseases treatment guidelines. *Morbidity and Mortality Weekly Report* 42(RR-14):22–26.

———. 1993d. 1993 Sexually transmitted diseases treatment guidelines. *Morbidity and Mortality Weekly Report* 42(RR-14):56–67.

———. 1993e. 1993 Sexually transmitted diseases treatment guidelines. *Morbidity and Mortality Weekly Report* 42(RR-14):26–27.

———. 1993f. 1993 Sexually transmitted diseases treatment guidelines. *Morbidity and Mortality Weekly Report* 42(RR-14):27–46.

Chapel, T.A. 1984. Primary and secondary syphilis. *Cutis* 33(1):4–9.

City and County of San Francisco, Department of Public Health. 1989. *Medical Alert—PPNG in San Francisco*. San Francisco: the Author.

———. 1992. *Macro-vue RPR card test, 18mm circle qualitative*. San Francisco: the Author.

Clive, D., Corey, L., Reichman, R.C., Davis, L.G., and Hozier, J.C. 1991. A double-blind, placebo-controlled cytogenetic study of oral acyclovir in patients with recurrent genital herpes. *Journal of Infectious Diseases* 164(4):753–757.

Cohen, P.T. 1990. Safe sex and the prevention of HIV infection. In *The AIDS knowledge base*, eds. P.T. Cohen, M.A. Sande, and P.A. Volberding, 11.1.4, pp. 1–10. Waltham, MA: The Medical Publishing Group.

Corey, L. 1990. Genital herpes. In *Sexually transmitted diseases*, 2d ed., eds. K.K. Holmes, P.-A. Mardh, P.F. Sparling, P.J. Wiesner, W. Cates, Jr., S.M. Lemon, and W.E. Stamm, pp. 391–413. New York: McGraw-Hill.

Corey, L., Adams, H.G., Brown, Z.A., and Holmes, K.K. 1983. Genital herpes simplex virus infections: Clinical manifestations, course, and complications. *Annals of Internal Medicine* 98(6):958–972.

Corrado, M.L. 1991. The clinical experience with ofloxacin in the treatment of sexually transmitted diseases. *American Journal of Obstetrics and Gynecology* 164(5 Pt. 2):1396–1399.

Dalabetta, G., and Hook III, E.W. 1987. Gonococcal infections. *Infectious Disease Clinics of North America* 1(1):25–55.

Davies, K. 1990. Genital herpes, an overview. *Journal of Obstetric, Gynecologic, and Neonatal Nursing* 19:401–406.

De Ferrari, E. 1989. Counseling women regarding high risk behaviors associated with HIV infection. *Journal of Nurse-Midwifery* 34(5):276–280.

Erlich, K.S., Mills, J., Chatis, P., Mertz, G.J., Busch, D.F., Follansbee, S.E., Grant, R.M., and Crumbacker, C.S. 1989. Acyclovir-resistant herpes simplex virus in patients with the acquired immunodeficiency syndrome. *New England Journal of Medicine* 320(5):293–296.

Faro, S. 1991. *Chlamydia trachomatis*: Female pelvic infection. American Journal of Obstetrics and Gynecology 164(6, Pt. 2):1767–1770.

Faro, S., Mertens, M.G., Maccato, M., Hammill, H.A., Roberts, S., and Riddle, G. 1991. Effectiveness of ofloxacin in the treatment of *Chlamydia trachomatis* and *Neisseria gonorrhoeae* cervical infection. *American Journal of Obstetrics and Gynecology* 164(5, Pt. 2):1380–1383.

Felman, Y.M. 1989. Recent developments in the diagnosis and treatment of sexually transmitted diseases: Infectious syphilis and acquired immunodeficiency syndrome. *Cutis* 44(4):288–290.

Fife, K., et al. 1992. Recurrence patterns of genital herpes after cessation of ≥ 5 years of chronic acyclovir suppression. In Programs and Abstracts VII International Conference on AIDS/III STD World Congress, July 12–24, Amsterdam. VZ p. B240, Abs # POB 3898.

Fogel, C.I.F. 1988. Gonorrhea: Not a new problem but a serious one. *Nursing Clinics of North America* 23(4):885–897.

Fraiz, J., and Jones, R.B. 1988. Chlamydial infections. *Annual Reviews in Medicine* 39:357–370.

Gibbs, R.S., and Sweet, R. 1989. Clinical disorders. In *Maternal-fetal medicine: Principles and practice*, 2d ed., eds. R.K. Creasy and R. Resnik, pp. 704–707. Philadelphia, W.B. Saunders.

Goldberg, L.H., Kaufman, R., Kurtz, T.O., Conant, M.A., Eron, L.J., Batenhorst, R.L., Boone, G.S., and the Acyclovir Study Group. 1993. Long-term suppression of recurrent genital herpes with acyclovir: A five-year benchmark. *Archives of Dermatology* 129(May):582–587.

Greenblatt, R. 1990. Lecture Notes, unpublished. San Francisco STD Prevention Training Center. STD Comprehensive Course for Clinicians.

Handsfield, H.H. 1991. Recent developments in STDs: I. Bacterial diseases. *Hospital Practice* (July 15):47–56.

Handsfield, H.H., and Pollock, P.S. 1990. Arthritis associated with sexually transmitted diseases. In *Sexually transmitted diseases*, 2d ed., eds. K.K. Holmes, P.-A. Mardh, P.F. Sparling, P.J. Wiesner, W. Cates, Jr., S.M. Lemon, and W.E. Stamm, pp. 737–751. New York: McGraw-Hill.

Hart, G. 1990. Donovanosis. In *Sexually transmitted diseases*, 2d ed., eds. K.K. Holmes, P.-A. Mardh, P.F. Sparling, P.J. Wiesner, W. Cates, Jr., S.M. Lemon, and W.E. Stamm, pp. 273–277. New York: McGraw-Hill.

Heine, R.P. and McGregor, J.A. 1992. Quinolones in the gynecologic setting. *The Female Patient* 17:31–37.

Holmes, K.K., Mardh, P.-A., Sparling, P.F., Wiesner, P.J., Cates, W., Jr., Lemon, S.M., and Stamm, W.E., 2d ed., eds. 1990. *Sexually transmitted diseases*. New York: McGraw-Hill.

Hook III, E.W., and Handsfield, H.H. 1990. Gonococcal infections in the adult. In *Sexually transmitted diseases*, 2d ed., eds. K.K. Holmes, P.-A. Mardh, P.F. Sparling, P.J. Wiesner, W. Cates, Jr., S.M. Lemon, and W.E. Stamm, pp. 149–165. New York: McGraw-Hill.

Hook III, E.W., and Marra, C.M. 1992. Acquired syphilis in adults. *The New England Journal of Medicine* 326(16):1060–1069.

Humphrey, L. 1992, May. *Herpes simplex virus infection in women.* Unpublished lecture presented at the Advanced Women's Health Seminar, University of California, San Francisco, School of Nursing.

Jaffe, H.W., and Musher, D.M. 1990. Management of the reactive syphilis serology. In *Sexually transmitted diseases*, 2d ed., eds. K.K. Holmes, P.-A. Mardh, P.F. Sparling, P.J. Wiesner, W. Cates, Jr., S.M. Lemon, and W.E. Stamm, pp. 935–939. New York: McGraw-Hill.

Jessamine, P., and Ronald, A.R. 1990. Chancroid and the role of genital ulcer disease in the spread of human retroviruses. *Medical Clinics of North America* 74(6):1417–1431.

Johnson, R.B. 1991. The role of azalide antibiotics in the treatment of chlamydia. *American Journal of Obstetrics and Gynecology* 164(6 Pt. 2):1794–1796.

Kaiser Permanente Medical Center. 1986. *Genital herpes—Questions and answers.* San Francisco: the Author.

Kaplowitz, L.G., Baker, D., Gelb, L., Blythe, J., Hale, R., Frost, P., Crumpacker, C., Robinovich, S., Peacock, J.E., Herndon, J., Davis, L.G., and The Acyclovir Study Group. 1991. Prolonged continuous acyclovir treatment of normal adults with frequently recurring genital herpes simplex virus infection. *Journal of the American Medical Association* 265(6):747–751.

Kent, G.P., Harrison, H.R., Berman, S.M., and Kennylside, R.A. 1988. Screening for *Chlamydia trachomatis* infection in a sexually transmitted disease clinic: Comparison of diagnostic tests with clinical and historical risk factors. *Sexually Transmitted Diseases* 15(1):51–57.

Kurtz, T., et al., 1990. Safety and efficacy of long term suppressive zovirax treatment of frequently recurring genital herpes: Year 5 results. In Programs and Abstracts 30th Interscience Conference on Antimicrobial Agents and Chemotherapy, Oct. 21–24, Atlanta. Abs #1107 (#18585702/2), p. 270.

Larsen, B. 1990. STD: Assessing the last decade and the next. *Contemporary Ob/Gyn* 35(12):58–70.

Larsen, S.A., Hunter, E.F., and Creighton, E.T. 1990. Syphilis. In *Sexually transmitted diseases*, 2d ed., eds. K.K. Holmes, P.-A. Mardh, P.F. Sparling, P.J. Wiesner, W. Cates, Jr., S.M. Lemon, and W.E. Stamm, pp. 927–934. New York: McGraw-Hill.

Levin, S., Pottage, J.C., Kessler, H.A., Benson, C.A., Goodman, L.J., and Trenholme, G.M. 1987. The office approach to the sexually transmitted diseases: Part II. *Current Problems in Obstetrics, Gynecology, and Fertility* 10(12):567–611.

Lichtman, R., and Duran, P. 1990. Sexually transmitted diseases. In *Gynecology. well-woman care*, eds. R. Lichtman and S. Papera. Norwalk, CT.: Appleton & Lange.

Ling, M.R. 1992a. Therapy of genital human papillomavirus infections. Part I: Indications for and justification of therapy. *International Journal of Dermatology* 31(10):682–686.

———. 1992b. Therapy of genital human papillomavirus infections. Part II: Methods of treatment. *International Journal of Dermatology* 31(11):769–773.

Lorincz, A.T., Temple, G.F., Kurman, R.J., Jenson, A.B., and Lancaster, W.D. 1987. Oncogenic association of specific human papillomavirus types with cervical neoplasia. *Journal of National Cancer Institute* 79:671–677.

Maiti, H., Chowdhury, F.H., Richmond, S.J., Stirland, R.M., Tooth, J.A., Bhattacharyya, M.N., and Stock, J.K. 1991. Ofloxacin in the treatment of uncomplicated gonorrhea and chlamydial infection. *Clinical Therapeutics* 13(4):441–447.

Mardh, P.-A., and Danielsson, D. 1990. *Neisseria gonorrhoeae*. In *Sexually transmitted diseases*, 2d. ed., eds. K.K. Holmes, P.-A. Mardh, P.F. Sparling, P.J. Wiesner, W. Cates, Jr., S.M. Lemon, and W.E. Stamm, pp. 903–916. New York: McGraw-Hill.

Martin, D.H., Mroczkowski, T.F., Dalu, Z.A., McCarty, J., Jones, R.B., Hopkins, S.J., and Johnson, R.B. 1992. A controlled trial of single dose azithromycin for the treatment of chlamydial urethritis and cervicitis. The Azithromycin for Chlamydial Infections Study Group. *New England Journal of Medicine* 327(13):921–925.

McGregor, J.A. 1989. Chlamydial infection in women. *Obstetrics and Gynecology Clinics of North America* 16(3):565–592.

McPhee, S.J. 1984. Secondary syphilis: Uncommon manifestations of a common disease. *The Western Journal of Medicine* 140(1):10–20.

Mead, P.B. 1991. Recognizing vulvar herpes: Clinical diagnosis and laboratory confirmation. *Proceedings, symposium, 91st annual meeting of the American College of Obstetricians and Gynecologists*, pp. 12–16. Intramed Communications.

Medical Economics Data. 1992. *Physicians' Desk Reference*. 46th ed. Montvale, NJ: the Author.

————. 1993. *Physicians' Desk Reference*, 47th ed. Montvale, NJ: the Author.

Mertz, G.J. 1990. Genital herpes simplex virus infections. *Medical Clinics of North America* 74:1433–1454.

Mertz, G.J., Jones, C.J., Mills, J., Fife, K.H., Lemon, S.M., Stapleton, J.T., Hill, E.L., Davis, L.G., and the Acyclovir Study Group. 1988. Long-term acyclovir suppression of frequently recurring genital herpes simplex virus infection. *Journal of the American Medical Association* 260(2):201–206.

Mogabgab, W.J., 1991. Recent developments in the treatment of sexually transmitted diseases. *American Journal of Medicine* 91(6A):140S–144S.

Moscicki, A.B. 1990. Genital human papillomavirus infections. *Adolescent Medicine: State of the Art Reviews* 1(3):451–469.

Moscicki, B., Shafer, M., Millstein, S.G., Irwin, C.E., and Schacter, J. 1987. The use and limitations of endocervical stains and mucopurulent cervicitis as predictors for *Chlamydia trachomatis* in female adolescents. *American Journal of Obstetrics and Gynecology* 157(1):65–71.

Moy, J.G., and Clasen, M.E. 1990. The patient with gonococcal infection. *Primary Care* 17(1):59–83.

Murphy, J.R. 1992. *Herpes genitalis*. Ob/Gyn nurse practitioner protocol (unpublished). San Francisco: Kaiser Permanente Medical Center.

Musher, D.M. 1987. Syphilis. *Infectious Disease Clinics of North America* 1(1):83–95.

Nelson, A.L. 1992. Sexually transmitted diseases. Unpublished lecture notes. Education Programs Associates—Ob/Gyn Update. San Francisco, CA.

Northfelt, D.W., and Palefsky, J.M. 1992. Human papillomavirus-associated anogenital neoplasia in persons with HIV infection. *AIDS Clinical Review* 241–259.

Ossewaarde, J.M., Plantema, F.H., Rieffe, M., Nawrocki, R.P., de Vries, A., and van Loon, A.M. 1992. Efficacy of single-dose azithromycin versus doxycyline in the treatment of cervical infections caused by *Chlamydia trachomatis*. *European Journal of Clinical Microbiology and Infectious Diseases* 11(8):693–697.

Palefsky, J. 1991. Human papillomavirus infection among HIV-infected individuals. *Hematology/Oncology Clinics of North America* 5(2):357–370.

————. 1993. Personal communication, June 2.

Perine, P.L., and Osoba, A.O. 1990. Lymphogranuloma venereum. In *Sexually transmitted diseases*, 2d ed., eds. K.K. Holmes, P.-A. Mardh, P.F. Sparling, P.J. Wiesner, W. Cates, Jr., S.M. Lemon, and W.E. Stamm, pp. 195–204). New York: McGraw-Hill.

Peters, D.H., Friedel, H.A., and McTavish, D. 1992. Azithromycin. A review of its antimicrobial activity, pharmacokinetic properties and clinical efficacy. *Drugs* 44(5):750–799.

Piot, P., and Plummer, F.A. 1990. Genital ulcer adenopathy syndrome. In *Sexually transmitted diseases*, 2d ed., eds. K.K. Holmes, P. Mardh, P.F. Sparling, P.J. Wiesner, W. Cates, Jr., S.M. Lemon, and W.E. Stamm, pp. 711–716. New York: McGraw-Hill.

Quinones, R. 1990. Unpublished lecture notes. San Francisco STD Prevention Training Center. STD Comprehensive Course for Clinicians.

Reid, R., and Greenberg, M.D. 1991. Human papillomavirus related disease of the vulva. *Clinical Obstetrics and Gynecology* 34(3):630–650.

Richens, R. 1991. The diagnosis and treatment of donovanosis (granuloma inguinale). *Genitourinary Medicine* 67:441–452.

Ronald, A.R., and Albritton, W. 1990. Chancroid and *Haemophilus ducreyi*. In *Sexually transmitted diseases*, 2d ed., eds. K.K. Holmes, P.-A. Mardh, P.F. Sparling, P.J. Wiesner, W. Cates, Jr., S.M. Lemon, and W.E. Stamm, pp. 263–271. New York: McGraw-Hill.

Rose, F.B., and Camp, C.J. 1988. Genital herpes: How to relieve patients' physical and psychological symptoms. *Postgraduate Medicine* 84(3):81–86.

Sacks, S.L. 1986. *The truth about herpes.* Vancouver, BC: Verdant Press.

Safrin, S. 1994 (Nov.) Genital and perirectal herpes simplex virus infection. Outline presented at the STD Intensive for Clinicians. San Francisco STD/HIV Prevention Training Center. San Francisco. Nov. 14–18.

San Francisco City Clinic 1992. Important points in the interpretation of the VDRL. Internal document.

Sauer, G.C. 1991. *Manual of skin diseases,* 6th ed. Philadelphia: J.B. Lippincott.

Sawchuk, W.S. 1992. Vulvar manifestation of human papillomavirus infection. *Dermatology Clinics* 10(2):405–414.

Schacter, J. 1987. Breaking the chain of chlamydial infection. *Contemporary Ob/Gyn* 30(1):146–159.

———. 1990. Biology of *Chlamydia trachomatis.* In *Sexually transmitted diseases,* 2d ed., eds. K.K. Holmes, P.-A. Mardh, P.F. Sparling, P.J. Wiesner, W. Cates, Jr., S.M. Lemon, and W.E. Stamm, pp. 167–180. New York: McGraw-Hill.

———. 1994 (Nov.) *Chlamydia trachomatis.* Outline presented at the STD Intensive for Clinicians. San Francisco STD/HIV Prevention Training Center. San Francisco. Nov. 14–18.

Schiffman, M.H. 1992. Recent progress in defining the epidemiology of human papillomavirus infection and cervical neoplasia. *Journal of the National Cancer Institute* 84(6):394–398.

Shannon, M.T. 1990. Genital herpes simplex viral infections. In *Ambulatory obstetrics: Protocols for nurse practitioners/nurse-midwives,* 2d ed., eds. W.L. Star, M.T. Shannon, L.N. Sammons, L.L. Lommel, and Y. Gutierrez. San Francisco: University of California, School of Nursing.

Spence, M.R. 1988. The treatment of gonorrhea, syphilis, chancroid, lymphogranuloma venereum, and granuloma inguinale. *Clinical Obstetrics and Gynecology* 31(2):453–465.

Stamm, W.E. 1991. Azithromycin in the treatment of uncomplicated genital chlamydial infections. *American Journal of Medicine* 91(3A):19S–22S.

Stamm, W.E., and Holmes, K.K. 1990. *Chlamydia trachomatis* infections of the adult. In *Sexually transmitted disease,* 2d ed., eds. K.K. Holmes, P.-A. Mardh, P.F. Sparling, P.J. Wiesner, W. Cates, Jr., S.M. Lemon, and W.E. Stamm, pp. 181–193. New York: McGraw-Hill.

Stamm, W.E., and Mardh, P.-A. 1990. *Chlamydia trachomatis.* In *Sexually transmitted diseases,* 2d ed., eds. K.K. Holmes, P.-A. Mardh, P.F. Sparling, P.J. Wiesner, W. Cates, Jr., S.M. Lemon, and W.E. Stamm, pp. 917–925. New York: McGraw-Hill.

Steingrimsson, O., Olafsson, J.H., Thorarinsson, H., Ryan, R.W., Johnson, R.B., and Tilton, R.C. 1990. Azithromycin in the treatment of sexually transmitted disease. *Journal of Antimicrobial Chemotherapy* (Suppl A) (January):109–114.

Strauss, S.E. (moderator). 1985. Herpes simplex virus infections: Biology, treatment, and prevention. *Annals of Internal Medicine* 103(3):404–419.

Sweet, R.L., and Gibbs, R.S. 1990. *Infectious diseases of the female genital tract,* 2d ed. Baltimore: Williams & Wilkins.

Syrjanen, K. 1992. Long-term consequences of genital HPV infections in women. *Annals of Medicine* 24(4):233–235.

The Medical Letter on Drugs and Therapeutics. 1992. Drugs for viral infections 34(867):31–32.

Thin, R.N. 1990. Early syphilis in the adult. In *Sexually transmitted diseases,* 2d ed., eds. K.K. Holmes, P.A. Mardh, P.F. Sparling, P.J. Wiesner, W. Cates, Jr., S.M. Lemon, and W.E. Stamm, pp. 221–230. New York: McGraw-Hill.

U.S. Department of Health and Human Services. 1991. Herpes simplex virus (HSV) infection. *Sexually transmitted diseases, clinical practice guidelines.* Atlanta: Centers for Disease Control.

U.S. Preventive Services Task Force. 1990. Screening for sexually transmitted diseases. *American Family Physician* 42(3):691–702.

Watley, J.D., Thin, R.N., Mumtaz, G., and Ridgway, G.L. 1991. Azithromycin versus doxycycline in the treatment of non-gonococcal urethritis. *International Journal of STD and AIDS* 2(4):248–251.

Wendel, G.D., and Gilstrap, L.C. III. 1990. Syphilis rise calls for accurate diagnosis. *Contemporary Ob/Gyn* 35(6):37–46.

Willis, S.E. 1990. Chancroid. *Primary Care* 17(1):145–153.

Winkelstein, W. 1990. Smoking and cervical cancer—Current status: A review. *American Journal of Epidemiology* 131(6):945–960.

Wright, T.C., and Richart, R.M. 1990. Role of human papillomavirus in the pathogenesis of genital tract warts and cancer. *Gynecologic Oncology* 37(2):151–164.

Zenker, P.N., and Rolfs, R.T. 1990. Treatment of syphilis, 1989. *Reviews of Infectious Diseases* 12(Suppl. 6): S590–S609.

SECTION 14

Behavioral Disorders

Marty Jessup, R.N., M.S.

14-A

Alcoholism and Other Drug Dependencies

Alcohol and other drug dependency is a chronic and progressive disease characterized by compulsion, loss of control, and continued use in spite of adverse consequences (Smith 1990). With early intervention and treatment, the prognosis is positive and full recovery is possible. Without treatment, addiction is usually ultimately fatal.

Addiction is a family disease and has an impact on each member of the family. Children of addicts/alcoholics are especially affected by the chaotic objective and emotional conditions of their parents. When the child of an alcoholic or drug-dependent parent becomes an adult, she is usually faced with myriad problems as a result of childhood neglect and possibly abuse. There are clear links between violence and addiction in women. Almost 70 percent of women in treatment for addictive disease have experienced rape, incest, or other sexual abuse (Roth 1990).

Women who either abuse or are dependent upon alcohol or another drug (see **Table 14A.1, Criteria for Substance Abuse** and **Table 14A.2, Criteria for Substance Dependence**) require assessment and a treatment-oriented intervention. Since women with alcohol or other drug dependencies present frequently to the health care system, health care providers are in an excellent position to act as facilitators of recovery from addiction and adoption of a clean and sober lifestyle by their patients.

Among teenage girls, drug and alcohol use is increasing. Approximately 26 percent of teenage girls have used an illegal drug (National Institute of Drug Abuse [NIDA] 1989). According to the National Council on Alcoholism and Drug Dependence (NCADD), 55 percent of women aged 18 years and over drink moderately, five percent drink heavily, and 40 percent do not drink at all.

Table 14A.1. CRITERIA FOR SUBSTANCE ABUSE

A. A maladaptive pattern of substance use leading to clinically significant impairment or distress, as manifested by one (or more) of the following, occurring within a 12-month period:

 1. Recurrent substance use resulting in a failure to fulfill major role obligations at work, school, or home (e.g., repeated absences or poor work performance related to substance use; substance-related absences, suspensions, or expulsions from school; neglect of children or household).

 2. Recurrent substance use in situations in which it is physically hazardous (e.g., driving an automobile or operating a machine when impaired by subtance use).

 3. Recurrent substance-related legal problems (e.g., arrests for substance-related disorderly conduct).

 4. Continued substance use despite having persistent or recurrent social or interpersonal problems caused by/exacerbated by the effects of the substance (e.g., arguments with spouse about consequences of intoxication, physical fights).

B. The symptoms have never met the criteria for Substance Dependence for this class of substance.

Source: Reprinted with permission from the American Psychiatric Association. 1994. *Diagnostic and statistical manual of mental disorders,* 4th ed. Washington, DC: the Author.

Moderate drinking is defined as less than 60 drinks per month and *heavy drinking* as *more than that amount.* (NCADD 1990). Women receive two-thirds of all legally prescribed mood-altering drugs (Sandmeier 1984), and alcohol and drug use among women ages 14 years to 44 years is currently considered widespread (NIDA 1989). Among women over 55 years, 85 percent use alcohol at least once a month (Hoffman and Harrison 1989). Approximately thirty-four percent of the membership of Alcoholics Anonymous is female (Alcoholics Anonymous 1986).

Addiction is thought to be the result of a probable biogenetic predisposition combined with environmen-

Table 14A.2.   CRITERIA FOR SUBSTANCE DEPENDENCE

A maladaptive pattern of substance use, leading to clinically significant impairment or distress, as manifested by three (or more) of the following, occurring at any time in the same 12-month period:

1. Tolerance, as defined by either of the following:
   a. A need for markedly increased amounts of the substance to achieve intoxication or desired effect.
   b. Markedly diminished effect with continued use of the same amount of the substance.
2. Withdrawal, as manifested by either of the following:
   a. The characteristic withdrawal syndrome for the substance (refer to Criteria A and B of the criteria sets for withdrawal from the specific substances). Refer to *DSM IV* for further information.
   b. The same (or a closely related) substance is taken to relieve or avoid withdrawal symptoms.
3. The substance is often taken in larger amounts or over a longer period of time than was intended.

4. There is a persistent desire or unsuccessful efforts to cut down or control substance use.
5. A great deal of time is spent in activities necessary to obtain the substance (e.g., chain smoking) or recover from its effects.
6. Important social, occupational, or recreational activities are given up or reduced because of substance use.
7. The substance use is continued despite knowledge of having a persistent or recurrent physical or psychological problem that is likely to have been caused or exacerbated by the substance (e.g., current cocaine use despite recognition of cocaine-induced depression, or continued drinking despite recognition that an ulcer was made worse by alcohol consumption).

Source: Reprinted with permission from the American Psychiatric Association. 1994. *Diagnostic and statistical manual of mental disorders*, 4th ed. Washington, DC: the Author.

tal stressors (Wallace, J. 1990). Biogenetic predisposition suggests that there is an increased risk for children of addicts/alcoholics to develop the disease of alcoholism or another drug dependency. Approximately 60 percent of all persons with an addiction have one or both parents with an alcohol or other drug dependency. Landmark research in the 1980s examined the presence of actual genetic markers that are correlated to the later development of alcoholism (Schuckit 1985).

Some stressors that women experience which may contribute to addiction or drug abuse include family or spousal discord; death of a spouse, child, or family member; poverty; unemployment; role changes; racism; sexism; sexual and/or physical abuse as a child; domestic violence; the stresses of single parenting; homelessness; and being raised in a family affected by alcohol or drug dependency.

Often, women who are drug- or alcohol-dependent seek social services and are either rejected as a recipient of those services because of their addiction, or their alcohol or drug dependency is accepted as "normal" or "expected" and ignored. With health care providers' and institutions' increased reporting of addicts and alcoholics to child protective services, many women are fearful and therefore seek health care via emergency rooms or through a variety of different providers and agencies (Nelson and Jessup 1992).

Women of any ethnic group, socioeconomic class, or age can develop the disease of addiction (Richardson and Williams 1990; Wallace, B.C. 1990; Glick and Moore 1991; Mora and Gilbert 1991). Though there are different drugs of choice and varying manifestations of the disease process as well as differing treatment approaches, women of differing racial and socioeconomic groups do develop essentially the same disease.

Currently, the majority of women who are frequent users of drugs or alcohol are *poly-drug* (more than one) *users* and use either on a daily maintenance basis or in a binge pattern of use. Because addiction in women is more highly stigmatized, shame, embarrassment, and fear of the criminal justice system are frequent characteristics of addicted women (Roth 1990).

In the course of alcoholism, women develop physical problems in response to alcohol consumption more quickly than do men. Women are more likely to develop liver disease even when they drink less alcohol than their male counterparts. Women alcoholics are at greater risk for circulatory disorders and anemias, and are more likely to commit suicide (Hill 1984). When women and men consume equal amounts of beverage alcohol, the women reach higher peak blood alcohol levels (Jones and Jones 1976).

More than half of all women who are HIV-positive have become so through the self-administration of intravenous drugs (Mitchell 1990). Approximately 80 percent of pediatric cases of AIDS may be attributed to maternal intravenous drug use or the drug-using mother's partner infecting the mother (CDC 1990).

All women who use alcohol and drugs are at risk for HIV/AIDS because of the resultant disinhibition of sexual behavior and the potential for unsafe sex. Since treatment for addiction has been shown to decrease rates of seropositivity in opiate-dependent populations significantly, efforts to identify and provide referrals for addiction treatment should be intensified (Chaisson et al. 1989; U.S. Department of Health and Human Services 1990).

Only recently have programs begun to be designed with the specific needs of women in mind. Historically, treatment centers for addiction have been established based on traditional male models of recovery.

Traditional coed therapy groups or programs mostly directed at men have prevented women from confronting issues of rape, incest, abuse, and other violence by men. As many drug- and alcohol-dependent women have poor self-esteem and difficulty asserting themselves, attention to their issues is frequently secondary. In addition, transportation and child care have been noted historically as barriers to women seeking treatment (Soman 1992).

Referral for treatment needs to be made to the most appropriate program in the woman's region. Many programs (especially in urban areas) are now tailored to a particular population. Providers should consider the financial status, drug of choice, age, sexual preference, and ethnicity of the woman prior to making a referral.

Any referral for addiction treatment should include a referral to a 12-Step program such as Alcoholics Anonymous, Narcotics Anonymous, or Cocaine Anonymous. Most communities now have a 12-Step meeting; many have language-appropriate or women's meetings as well.

Treatment for addiction varies based on the individual patient's problem and ability to participate in an outpatient, inpatient, or residential program (see **Appendix 14A.3, Treatment for Addiction**, p. 14-11). Recovery is, however, a lifelong process and the actual treatment is only the beginning. Ongoing recovery requires abstinence and participation in activities of recovery (see **Appendix 14A.4, Recovery from Addiction**, p. 14-12).

DATABASE

SUBJECTIVE

→ Essentially all women are at risk, although there is a greater risk for those with a family history of alcoholism or other drug dependency.

→ The presence of "past history" suggests the patient should be either in recovery currently or that the active phase of the disease has returned—she currently is using and drinking (i.e., relapsed).

→ Specific behavioral and historical indicators (see **Table 14A.3, Indicators of Addiction**).

→ Patient states, "My drinking/using is out of control. I need help." Variations of this statement can include other articulated requests for help or denial of the existence of a problem.

→ Denial: "I don't have a problem" or "I used to have a problem, but that's all over now...." (accompanied by subjective and objective evidence of a drug dependency).

→ Minimization: "It's not that bad, I only drink on the weekends...."

Table 14A.3. INDICATORS OF ADDICTION

Behavioral	Historical
▶ depression	▶ family dissolution
▶ history of childhood neglect	▶ alcohol- or drug-abusing partner
▶ intense daily drama	▶ placement of children outside the home
▶ family and personal chaos	▶ family history of alcoholism or another drug dependency
▶ inappropriate behavior	▶ psychiatric treatment or hospital admissions
▶ mood swings	▶ child with drug-/alcohol-related effects
▶ outbursts of anger	▶ many physician contacts
▶ difficulty concentrating	▶ many emergency room contacts
▶ irritability or agitation	▶ frequent physician prescriptions
▶ unreliability	
▶ unpredictable behavior	
▶ impulsive actions	
▶ signs of intoxication	
▶ alcohol on breath	
▶ slurred speech	
▶ staggering gait	
▶ suicidal thoughts, gestures, or attempts	
▶ conflicts with significant other/ spouse	
▶ domestic violence	
▶ decreased job performance	
▶ missed appointments	
▶ cited for driving under the influence	
▶ vague history regarding personal or medical problems	

Source: Adapted with permission from Jessup, M. 1990. The treatment of perinatal addiction: Identification, intervention, and advocacy. *Western Journal of Medicine* 152:553-558.

→ Rationalization: " I have so much stress in my life, I have to do something to calm down...."

→ Drug and alcohol history to include:
  ▪ psychoactive substances used and year of first use.
  ▪ route of administration.
  ▪ tolerance.
  ▪ past treatment attempts or 12-Step meetings.
  ▪ negative consequences of addiction (past and present).
  ▪ codependency issues.
  ▪ adult child of alcoholic, other family history.
  ▪ motivation for abstinence and recovery.
  ▪ ability to access treatment (i.e., disability, financial status, intellectual level).

→ Complete medical history should be obtained.

OBJECTIVE

→ Patient may present with:
  ▪ hair loss.
  ▪ dilated or pinpoint pupils, bloodshot or glassy eyes, yellow sclera, toxic amblyopia.
  ▪ rhinitis, perforation of nasal septum, epistaxis.
  ▪ poor dental hygiene, gum disease, abscesses.
  ▪ hypertension, mitral valve disease, anemias, bacteremias, myocarditis.

- tuberculosis, asthma, chronic cough, rales, sinusitis, bronchitis, angiothrombotic pulmonary hypertension, noncardiogenic pulmonary edema, tracheobronchial epithelial disease, other acute pulmonary effects.
- abscesses, cellulitis, septic thrombophlebitis, edema and erythema and/or scars on the hands, palmar erythema, track marks, thrombosed veins, traumatic burns, subdural hemorrhage, bruising, loss of muscle mass.
- gastritis, esophagitis, ulcers, acute and/or chronic hepatitis, hepatomegaly, pancreatitis, chronic constipation or diarrhea, ascites, malabsorption syndrome.
- abnormal vaginal bleeding, decreased vaginal lubrication.
- sexually transmitted diseases (STDs), HIV seropositivity.
- overdose, withdrawal symptoms, seizures, tremors, delirium tremens (DTs), blackouts, "grayouts," cognitive and sensory impairment, memory lapses and losses.
- alcoholic myopathy, ataxia.

ASSESSMENT

→ Alcohol and/or other drug dependency

→ Concomitant physical and/or psychiatric illness

PLAN

DIAGNOSTIC TESTS

→ Laboratory tests may include:
  - blood alcohol level.
  - toxicology screen.
  - glucose tolerance test (GTT).
  - aspartate aminotransferase (AST), alanine aminotransferase (ALT).
  - MCH and MCV (elevated with excessive alcohol consumption with or without folic acid or B_{12} deficiency).
  - uric acid (elevated with excessive alcohol consumption).
  - albumin (decreased).
  - total protein (decreased).
  - serum magnesium and potassium (decreased).

→ Administer CAGE Questionnaire and MAST (see **Tables 14A.4, Cage Questionnaire** and **14A.5, Short Michigan Alcoholism Screening Test**).

Table 14A.4. CAGE QUESTIONNAIRE

1. Have you ever felt you should **CUT DOWN** on your drinking?
2. Have people **ANNOYED** you by criticizing your drinking?
3. Have you ever felt bad or **GUILTY** about your drinking?
4. Have you ever had a drink first thing in the morning to get rid of a hangover (**EYE-OPENER**)?

Source: Reprinted with permission from Mayfield, D., McLeod, G., and Hall, P. 1974. The CAGE questionnaire: Validation of a new alcoholism screening instrument. *American Journal of Psychiatry* 131:1121-1123.

TREATMENT/MANAGEMENT

→ A statement of concern to the patient is important: "I am concerned that you may have a problem with alcohol/cocaine/marijuana/etc."

→ Evidence of drug use should be presented to patient: "These are the kinds of problems that are usually associated with drug/alcohol use:
  - your history of pancreatitis, blackouts, palmar erythema, marital problems;
  - your arrest for driving under the influence (DUI) in 1990;
  - your history of being an adult child of an alcoholic; and your feeling more depressed as your drinking has escalated."

→ Patient education: provide information regarding the potential negative physical, emotional, financial, spiritual, and psychological consequences of continued use of the substance(s).

→ Refer patient for treatment to local program.
  - Give list of local 12-Step meetings—e.g., Alcoholics Anonymous, Narcotics Anonymous, Cocaine Anonymous.
    - Ideally, patient should call local AA or other 12-Step group for list of meetings (see **Appendixes 14A.3** and **14A.4**, pp. 14-11 and 14-12, respectively).

CONSULTATION

→ Physician (psychiatric) consultation recommended and required for evaluation for dual-diagnosis issues (see **Appendix 14A.1, Dual-Diagnosis Disorders**, p. 14-9) that may or may not result in prescription of psychotropic or psychoactive medications.

→ Physician (addiction medicine specialist) consultation required for prescription of mood-altering drugs to a recovering person (see **Appendix 14A.2, The Use of Mood-Altering Medications by Recovering Persons**, p. 14-10).

Table 14A.5.   SHORT MICHIGAN ALCOHOLISM SCREENING TEST[1]

1. Do you feel you are a normal drinker? (By normal we mean you drink less than or as much as most other people.) (No)	8. Have you ever gotten into trouble at work because of drinking? (Yes)
2. Does your wife or husband, a parent, or other near relative ever worry or complain about your drinking? (Yes)	9. Have you ever neglected your obligations, your family, or your work for more than two days in a row because you were drinking? (Yes)
3. Do you ever feel guilty about your drinking? (Yes)	10. Have you ever gone to anyone for help about your drinking? (Yes)
4. Do friends or relatives think you are a normal drinker? (No)	11. Have you ever been in a hospital because of drinking? (Yes)
5. Are you able to stop drinking when you want to? (No)	12. Have you ever been arrested for drunken driving, driving while intoxicated, or driving under the influence of alcoholic beverages? (Yes)
6. Have you ever attended a meeting of Alcoholics Anonymous? (Yes)	13. Have you ever been arrested, even for a few hours, because of other drunken behavior? (Yes)
7. Has drinking ever created problems between you and your wife or husband, a parent, or other near relative? (Yes)	

[1]The responses in parentheses indicate the presence of alcoholism.

Source: Reprinted with permission from Selzer, M., Vinokur, A., and van Rooijen, L. 1975. A self-administered short Michigan Alcoholism Screening Test. *Journal of Studies on Alcohol* 36:117-126. Adapted from the original MAST: Michigan Alcoholism Screening Test. 1971. *American Journal of Psychiatry* 127:1653-1654.

→ Addiction-treatment program staff person may provide consultation to determine appropriate referral—i.e., residential, inpatient, outpatient, methadone maintenance, sober living setting.

→ Consultation with any other persons providing health care services or counseling to addicted person is recommended as alcohol- and drug-dependent persons may "hospital hop" and/or have multiple persons providing prescriptions or services. Collaboration is recommended.

PATIENT EDUCATION

→ Review all previous physical, emotional, financial, spiritual, and psychological effects of the primary drug(s) of abuse to date.

→ State the expected and possible physical effects that may ensue with continued abuse of these drug(s).

→ Ask the patient to describe what she thinks may be the potential negative impact of continued drug abuse on the emotional, financial, spiritual, and psychological realms of her life.

→ Describe the probable impact of continued drug use on the emotional, financial, spiritual, and psychological realms of the patient's life.

→ State that with treatment and application of 12-Step programs, abstinence and recovery are possible.

FOLLOW-UP

→ Ask patient if she sought and completed course of treatment for addiction.
  ▪ If yes, support and commend efforts.

Table 14A.6.   RELAPSE THINKING IN THE CLIENT

▶ Return of rationalizing, denial, and minimization	▶ High index of anger much of the time
▶ Stops attending 12-Step meetings	▶ Feels like a victim and/or is "stuck" there
▶ Secretive and vague about life and feelings	▶ Afraid of health and well-being
▶ Increased impulsive behavior	▶ Unsure if recovery is really what she wants
▶ Unable to have life organization and plans	▶ Much idle time
▶ Hungry, angry, lonely, and tired with no action to remedy	▶ Immaturity about problem resolution; seeks quick solutions
▶ Frustration and immobility	▶ Begins to believe she can return to occasional drinking/using with few consequences
▶ Self-pity	
▶ Anxiety	
▶ Self-blaming	
▶ Defensive	

Source: Adapted with permission from Gorski, T.T., and Miller, M. 1986. *Staying sober: A guide for relapse prevention.* Independence, MO: Independence Press.

  ▪ If no, refer again for treatment and to 12-Step meetings or other self-help support groups.

→ Check on recovery efforts when patient is seen subsequently.

→ Observe for all physical and behavioral signs of resumed drinking or drug use or just "relapse thinking" (see **Table 14A.6, Relapse Thinking in the Client**).

→ If relapse is imminent or has occurred, repeat steps under "Treatment/Management" section (if relapse is imminent, use examples of relapse thinking as evidence of concern).

→ On the rare occasion that a mood-altering drug is indicated, advise patient of issues concerning the use of these drugs by persons in recovery from an addiction (see **Appendix 14A.2**, p. 14-10).

→ See **Appendix 14A.4**, p. 14-12.

→ Document in progress notes and problem list, as appropriate, the status of the patient's alcohol or other drug dependency.

APPENDIX 14A.1

Dual-Diagnosis Disorders

Definition and Demographics:

- The co-morbidity of psychiatric illness and alcohol or another drug dependency.

- Approximately 20 percent to 60 percent of addicted persons may have a co-existing psychiatric problem (Meyer 1986).

- Seventy percent of individuals with an antisocial personality disorder abuse alcohol. Other research suggests a 20 percent rate of alcohol abuse among persons with a diagnosis of bipolar disorder (Schukit 1986).

- Drug and alcohol abuse in the young, chronically mentally ill may exceed 50 percent (Safer 1987).

- Frequently misdiagnosed and then prescriptive drugs used inappropriately in a misguided attempt to treat the psychiatric patient who is also addicted to psychoactive drugs.

- Misperception that an "ordinary" addict/alcoholic may not also have significant psychopathology.

- Patient inability to seek or tolerate conventional modes of treatment for addiction without significant provider input and case management.

Diagnosis and Treatment:

- Long-term evaluation is usually indicated to differentiate between signs of intoxication, signs of alcohol and other drug withdrawal, organic brain damage, developmental disability, and psychiatric symptom re-emergence after detoxification.

- Patient must be clean and sober prior to the designation of a psychiatric diagnosis.

- Prognosis improved if the individual is treated in a setting that has treatment experience in both psychiatric illness and alcohol and other drug dependencies.

APPENDIX 14A.2

The Use of Mood-Altering Medications by Recovering Persons

- Generally contraindicated.
- Fractures, dental work, surgical procedures, or psychiatric problems may require legitimate prescription of analgesics, anesthesia, or medications.
- Prescription of or advocacy for prescription of these drugs should be done by those providers knowledgeable in addiction medicine and cognizant of the behavioral, medical, and pharmacological issues in the treatment of addicted persons.
- Deprivation of these medications for a bona fide medical indication would be inhumane and inappropriate and could lead to relapse.
- Consultation with addiction treatment specialist prior to prescription is necessary to ensure that medication is essential and to determine safe and effective non-pharmacological alternatives to be tried first.

- A minimum number of doses should be prescribed. Automatically refillable prescriptions are never recommended.
- Patient should notify persons in her support system (family, friends, 12-Step sponsor) that she will be taking the drug and should create an agreement regarding the discontinuance of the drug and actions she will take if relapse occurs. This should constitute a plan shared by patient, support system members, and prescribing health care provider.
- If medications for a psychiatric illness are prescribed, careful follow-up and dual management by a psychiatrist knowledgeable in addiction is strongly recommended.

APPENDIX 14A.3

Treatment for Addiction

- Assistance to achieve abstinence, introduction to the 12-Step programs, and education about the disease of alcoholism and other drug dependencies.

- Process may include an initial treatment for physiological detoxification depending on patient's physical condition, chronicity of addiction, and number and types of drugs of choice.

- Detoxification—the very first step in the treatment continuum—can occur in either an outpatient or inpatient setting.

- Treatment provides tools to maintain sobriety and an introduction to a clean and sober support system.

- Programs focus on relapse prevention and identification of psychological issues that might require long-term attention. Some programs provide intervention and assistance to the family as a whole.

- Women-sensitive programs include women-oriented outreach strategies, health care information and services, child and family services, vocational rehabilitation, skills training to enhance self-esteem, drug and alcohol education, legal assistance, and processes to address sexuality and intimacy (Reed 1987).

- Modalities for treatment include outpatient, day treatment, residential, sober living homes, methadone maintenance, in-hospital 21-day programs (inpatient), and therapeutic communities (long-term). These programs vary in length of stay, extent of services, and mode of payment.

APPENDIX 14A.4

Recovery from Addiction

- Is a life-long process initiated by treatment or going to a 12-Step meeting.
- Abstinence from all mood-altering drugs is required for a true recovery.
- Requires adherence to a daily program of activities that foster, support, and educate about the recovery process.
- Recovery occurs in the physical, emotional, psychological, and spiritual realms.
- Characterized by a reduction of chaos, resumption of self-esteem, healing of the physical and emotional wounds, and a willingness, openness, and honesty about the emotional work to be done.

- The first year in recovery is spent developing the tools to help the person stay free from alcohol and other drugs one day at a time. As recovery progresses, other issues may be addressed in long-term psychotherapy.
- Variables that foster recovery include a clean and sober lifestyle and support system, assistance with material problems (e.g., employment, child care, financial security), good role models, obtaining a sponsor in a 12-Step program, and having a health care provider who understands the nature and treatment of addiction.

Pilar Bernal de Pheils, R.N., M.S., F.N.P.

14-B
Anxiety Disorders

Anxiety can be an appropriate response to a real and threatening situation. It can be framed as a positive phenomenon that helps "mobilize and direct all available energy toward solving problem abilities and achievement" (Hodiamont 1991). Anxiety can also represent a mental health disorder and is the dominant feature in *panic disorder, phobic disorder,* and *generalized anxiety disorder (GAD)*.

Anxiety disorders are the most common psychiatric disorders, surpassing even the depressive and substance abuse disorders. The lifetime prevalence of anxiety disorders is 14 percent (Reiger et al. 1988). When evaluating anxiety, it is important to identify whether the anxiety is a normal response or a pathological entity. As a pathological condition, anxiety can be categorized into a specific disorder. It can be precipitated by a general medical condition or be substance-induced. It can present with psychiatric disorders.

→ Medical conditions causing anxiety may include:
- ■ thyroid disease.
- ■ hypoglycemia.
- ■ pheochromocytoma.
- ■ mitral valve prolapse.
- ■ cardiac arrhythmias.
- ■ chest pain.
- ■ complex partial seizures.
- ■ alcoholism.

→ Drugs known to cause anxiety states include:
- ■ stimulant intoxication:
  - • bronchodilators.
  - • B-agonists.
  - • thyroid preparations.
  - • caffeine.
  - • cocaine.
- ■ depressant withdrawal:
  - • alcohol.
  - • anti-anxiety agents.
  - • sedative hypnotics.

Anxiety presenting with other psychiatric disorders (e.g., major depression, adjustment disorder with anxious mood, eating disorders, and psychotic disorders) is usually related to the psychiatric illness (Edwards 1991). This is most common when a depressive disorder is present. Thirty to 70 percent of patients with primary anxiety disorders may also suffer depression (Berrier, Charney, and Heninger 1985).

This protocol addresses the most common specific anxiety disorders in women as they are defined in the *Diagnostic and Statistical Manual of Mental Disorders* (American Psychiatric Association 1994).

Panic disorder is characterized by a series of recurrent and unexpected panic attacks, followed by at least one month of persistent fear of having another attack, and worry about its possible consequences or implications, or having a significant behavioral change related to the attacks. During the attack episode, internal fear develops suddenly and peaks within 10 minutes; and this fear is accompanied by at least four characteristic associated symptoms of anxiety (see "Database" section) and is usually accompanied by a sense of imminent danger and urge to escape. The definition of panic disorder includes at least two attacks.

Individuals with panic disorders also commonly suffer from limited symptom attacks where fewer than four of the associated symptoms of anxiety are present. The criterion of panic attacks should not be considered when they are a direct physiological effect of a substance, or a general medical condition, and are not better accounted for by another medical disorder. Panic disorder is diagnosed with or without agoraphobia depending on whether the criterion is met (see following discussion on agoraphobia).

Patients suffering from panic disorders will frequently visit primary health care providers (Katon 1986). They respond well to appropriate treatment in which the disorder is recognized and managed appropriately, helping to avert phobic avoidance (Brown et al. 1991).

Agoraphobia is characterized by marked fear of being in public places (e.g., elevators, crowds, lines, bridges), or fear of situations from which escape may be difficult or embarrassing or help may be difficult able if a panic attack occurs. As a result of this fear, the person increasingly restricts activities outside her home, must have a companion if away from home, or endures agoraphobia despite intense anxiety. Agoraphobia is usually considered a complication of panic disorders. In most cases panic attacks precede agoraphobia.

Specific phobia is characterized by a persistent (and recognized as excessive) fear of specific objects (most commonly animals, e.g., dogs, mice) or situations (e.g., closed spaces [*claustrophobia*], heights [*acrophobia*], or air travel). The level of anxiety or fear varies as a function of the degree of proximity to the phobic stimulus and the degree to which escape from the phobic stimulus is limited.

Generalized anxiety disorder is characterized by excessive anxiety and worry difficult to control for a number of events or activities occuring during a period of at least six months. The anxiety and worry are associated with the presence most of the days of at least three of the following symptoms: restlessness or feeling keyed up or on edge, being easily fatigued, difficulty concentrating or mind going blank, irritability, muscle tension, sleep disturbance. This anxiety fluctuates, is present more days than not.

The course of this disorder generally is intermittent, with exacerbations and remissions throughout many years. Significant distress or social, functional, and occupational impairment can be caused by the anxiety, worry or physical symptoms. This disorder does not develop into panic attacks or phobias, is not due to the physiological effects of a substance (drug or abuse of medication) or a general medical condition and does not occur exclusively during a mood disorder, psychotic disorder, or a pervasive developmental disorder.

DATABASE

SUBJECTIVE

→ Panic disorder:
- average age of onset late 20s.
- more common in females.
- patient reports at least four of the following symptoms developed during at least one of the attacks:
  - dyspnea or smothering sensation.
  - dizziness, unsteady feelings, or faintness.
  - palpitations or tachycardia.
  - trembling or shaking.
  - sweating.
  - choking.
  - nausea or abdominal distress.
  - depersonalization or derealization.
  - paresthesias.
  - hot flashes or chills.
  - chest pain or discomfort.
  - fear of dying.
  - fear of going crazy or doing something uncontrollable.
- may complain of nervousness and apprehension between panic attacks, usually focused on the fear of having another attack.
- possible predisposing factors include:
  - separation anxiety disorder in childhood.
  - sudden loss of social supports.
  - disruption of important interpersonal relationships.
- medical history may include:
  - mitral valve prolapse (incidence increases from five percent in the general population to 20 percent in panic disorders [Savage et al. 1983).
  - depression.
- personal/health history may include:
  - substance abuse, particularly alcohol and anxiolytics.
  - limited impairment in social or occupational functioning.
- family history may include panic attacks.

→ Agoraphobia:
- average age of onset 20s or 30s.
- more common in women and married people.
- characteristics include:
  - fear of being in places or situations from which escape might be difficult, i.e., closed spaces (e.g., elevators, tunnels), crowds (e.g., churches, theaters, malls), transportation vehicles or facilities (e.g., planes, trains, highways).

- fear of being in places or situations in which help might not be available in case a panic attack develops.
- fear resulting in restriction of activities outside the home, needing a companion for activities outside the home, or endurance of agoraphobic situations despite intense anxiety.
  - agoraphobia is usually associated with panic attacks.
  - personal/health history may include:
    - severe social, occupational impairment.
    - early traumatic separation from parents.

→ Specific phobia:
  - age of onset varies. Animal phobias usually begin in childhood, blood/injury phobias (i.e., witnessing blood or tissue injuries) in adolescence, circumscribed phobias most frequently in fourth decade of life.
  - more common in females.
  - phobic stimulus unrelated to obsessive compulsive disorder (OCD) or to PTSD, separation anxiety disorder, social phobia, panic disorder with agoraphobia, or agoraphobia without a history of panic disorder.
  - characteristics may include:
    - marked, persistent, excessive, or unreasonable fear of a circumscribed stimulus, other than fear of having a panic attack, or humiliation or embarrassment in certain social situations (social phobia).
    - anxiety response during exposure to stimuli.
    - avoidance or endurance with extreme anxiety of object or situation.
    - recognizing fear as be excessive or unreasonable.
  - symptoms may include:
    - feeling panicky.
    - sweating.
    - tachycardia.
    - dyspnea.
    - vasovagal fainting if blood injury-related phobias.
  - personal/health history may include:
    - social or occupational impairment if the phobic object cannot be avoided.
    - panic disorder with agarophobia.
    - family history may include same type of phobia (i.e., fear of blood and injury, fear of animals).

→ Generalized Anxiety Disorder (GAD):
  - age of onset most commonly in the 20s and 30s.
  - characteristics may include:

- fluctuating unrealistic or excessive anxiety or worry about at least two life circumstances for a period of at least six months.
- anxiety that is not the result of a panic disorder, social phobia, obsessive-compulsive behavior or anorexia nervosa.
  - reports at least six of the following symptoms:
    - motor tension:
      - trembling, shaking, or feeling shaky.
      - muscle tension, aches, or soreness.
      - restlessness.
      - easy fatigability.
    - autonomic hyperactivity:
      - dyspnea or smothering sensation.
      - palpitations, tachycardia.
      - sweating, or cold, clammy hands.
      - dry mouth.
      - dizziness or lightheadedness.
      - nausea, diarrhea, or other abdominal distress.
      - hot flashes or chills.
      - frequent urination.
      - trouble swallowing or "lump in throat."
    - hyper-vigilance:
      - feeling keyed up or on edge.
      - exaggerated startle response.
      - difficulty concentrating or mind going blank.
      - trouble falling asleep or staying asleep.
      - irritability.
  - medical history may include:
    - major depressive episode (considered a predisposing factor).
    - peptic ulcer.
    - migraine.
    - ulcerative colitis.
  - personal/health history may include mild social and occupational impairment.

OBJECTIVE

→ During an acute anxiety attack, the patient may present with:
  - elevated blood pressure.
  - tachycardia.
  - tachypnea.
  - restlessness.
  - trembling.
  - screaming.
  - erythema or pallor.
  - sweating.
  - cold and clammy hands.
→ Other physical findings WNL.

→ Common finding in panic disorders is a mid-systolic apical and/or late systolic murmur on auscultation (an indication of mitral valve prolapse). (See **Mitral Valve Prolapse** Protocol.)

ASSESSMENT

→ Panic disorder

→ Panic disorder with agoraphobia

→ Agoraphobia:
  ▪ mild
  ▪ moderate
  ▪ severe

→ Specific phobia

→ Generalized anxiety disorder

→ R/O anxiety disorder due to a general medical condition

→ R/O substance-induced anxiety disorder

→ R/O other underlying mental health disorders

→ R/O somatoform disorders (hypochondriasis and somatization disorder)

PLAN

DIAGNOSTIC TESTS

→ No specific diagnostic tests used in clinical practice.

→ Additional diagnostic tests as indicated by database to rule out organic causes of anxiety.

→ Echocardiogram if signs of mitral valve prolapse. (See **Mitral Valve Prolapse** Potocol).

TREATMENT/MANAGEMENT

→ If anxiety present during visit:
  ▪ remain with patient during period of anxiety.
  ▪ approach patient in a calm, matter-of-fact manner.
  ▪ place patient in safe, non-stimulating environment.
  ▪ encourage patient to express feelings, describe symptoms, and relate behaviors that relieve this condition.

→ Anxiety disorders—psychological therapy.
  ▪ All clients with anxiety disorders can benefit from psychological therapy. Of these, *psychotherapy, behavioral therapy,* and *cognitive therapy* have been used extensively.
    • Psychotherapy:
      –supportive therapy; counseling to accept responsibility for behavior and actions and, if possible, to work out solutions (Edwards 1991).
      ▸ Simple, brief technique with limited objectives.
      ▸ Can be given to couples, families, and groups.
    –guidelines for supportive therapy include:
      ▸ showing concern.
      ▸ listening sympathetically.
      ▸ allowing client to release/verbalize emotions or unconscious fears if necessary.
      ▸ giving reassurance.
      ▸ giving suggestions and advice on ongoing problems.
      ▸ providing encouragement.
      ▸ discussing methods of coping with stress.
  • Behavioral therapy:
    –relaxation; attempting to break the vicious cycle of anxiety.
      ▸ Can be used in groups.
      ▸ May be aided by tape recording.
      ▸ Encouragement of daily practice of technique at home.
      ▸ Through sessions, encouragement to talk about difficulties in achieving relaxation.
      ▸ Electromyographic biofeedback facilitation of relaxation by reduction in frontalis muscle potential (Silver and Blanchard 1978).
    –guidelines to behavior therapy include:
      ▸ having a quiet room, with dim lights, and a comfortable chair.
      ▸ asking the client to focus initially on her own breathing.
      ▸ directing the client to move slowly through tension and relaxation for each major muscle group.
      ▸ directing the client to maintain tension for ten seconds and release it instantaneously on cue; at least 2 repetitions of the tension-relaxation cycle.
      ▸ giving instructions very slowly, allowing client to enjoy feelings of relaxation.
      ▸ technique to be taught in a progressive manner, encouraging client toward independent practice of relaxation.
    –exposure treatment; used mostly for phobic anxiety states:
      ▸ client persuaded to repeatedly confront the feared object or situation.
      ▸ exposure trials to progress for longer periods of time.

  ▸ exposure to be determined by level of anxiety and the presence of other medical complications—e.g., asthma, heart disease.
  ▸ therapist may not be present for the phobic situation.
  ▸ client to keep a diary monitored by the therapist.
  ▸ significant improvement seen within 4 to 20 sessions; often maintained for up to 2 to 4 years.
  ▸ therapy to be discontinued if client fails to habituate within 2 weeks.
  –systematic desensitization:
  ▸ client to draw up a hierarchy of feared stimuli or situations that provoke anxiety, initially controlled in imagination, while in pleasant relaxed state.
  ▸ extension of feared stimuli or situation to real-life situations.
  –social skill training and assertiveness training. More effective and satisfying behaviors are substituted through rehearsal with other patients and then practiced in real-life situations. Guidelines include (Edwards 1991):
  ▸ instructing patient in these behaviors.
  ▸ coaching.
  ▸ modeling.
  ▸ role reversal.
• Cognitive therapy:
  –combines exposure with cognitive behavior, restructuring, and distraction techniques (Edwards 1991).
  ▸ Identification of illogical thoughts (e.g., of failure, disease, or death) and objective discussion of evidence for and against the belief.
  ▸ Patient recognition of the irrationality and damaging effects of her ideas.
  ▸ Encouragement to substitute healthier ideas with the help of positive self-commentaries.
  ▸ In panic disorder, attempt at substituting of normal, rational explanation for abnormal, catastrophic interpretation.
→ Panic disorder and agoraphobia—pharmacotherapy.
  ▪ Consultation with a mental health care provider is indicated (particularly in cases in which short-term psychological treatment has failed).
  ▪ Pharmacotherapy is recommended on a short-term basis as an adjunct to psychotherapy

(Brown et al. 1991). Medication categories include tricyclic antidepressants, benzodiazepines, monoamine oxidase (MAO) inhibitors, and beta-adrenergic blocking agents.
• Tricyclic antidepressants (TCAs):
  –imipramine hydrochloride (Trofanil®) often used to start treatment. Dose varies from as low as 25 mg/day to 150 mg/day to as high as 300 mg/day.
  –hyperstimulation reaction—characterized by intensification of anxiety symptoms, agitation, tachycardia, and insomnia—may result. It may be experienced in 20 percent of patients. Beginning with a low dose (10 mg to 25 mg/day) and gradually increasing the dosage is helpful in minimizing this effect.
  –resolution of panic symptoms takes from 2 to 6 weeks.
  –TCA treatment is effective with mild depressive symptoms often associated with panic disorders. (see also **Depression** Protocol for a more thorough review in antidepressant therapy).
  –B-adrenergic blocking agents are recommended to decrease tachycardia, but used alone, are not effective therapies for panic disorders.
• Benzodiazepines (BZDs):
  –alprazolam (Xanax®) 2 mg to 3 mg/day, in multiple daily dosing (at least TID to QID) is recommended as an adjunctive therapy to an antidepressant—until the antidepressant exerts its full effect—in patients who can not tolerate tricyclic antidepressants, or when MAO inhibitors are contraindicated.
  –other benzodiazepines also recommended: lorazepam (Ativan®), diazepam (Valium®), clonazepam (Klonopin®). See *PDR* for dosing. Probably not as effective as alprazolam for low-grade depression that oftens accompanies panic disorder.
  –patients who self-medicate at 2 to 3 times the therapeutic dose can experience physical dependence in 2 to 3 weeks. Dependence at therapeutic dose can occur if taken for more than 6 months. Gradual tapering of dose should be initiated after 4 to 16 weeks and adjunctive therapy may be required (i.e., sedating antidepressants, B-blockers, carbamazepine).

–sedation, the most common side effect, usually subsides with dose reduction or continued administration.

–other adverse effects: ataxia, slurred speech, and amnesia if dose is too high or mixed with sedatives and alcohol.

→ Generalized anxiety disorder—pharmacotherapy.
- Consultation with a mental health care provider is indicated (particularly in cases in which short-term psychological treatment has failed).
- Pharmacotherapy is recommended on a short-term basis and as an adjunct to psychotherapy (Brown et al. 1991).
  - BZDs:
    –effective in treatment of GAD.
    –decrease psychic and somatic symptoms of anxiety.
    –quick onset of action and relative safety with overdose.
    –for chronic anxiety consider long-acting BZDs—diazepam (Valium®), chlordiazepoxide (Librium®), clorazepate (Tranxene®), prazepam (Centrax®), halazepam (Paxipan®), clonazepam (Klonopin®). See PDR for dosages and side effects.
    –when anxiety limited to a particular situation or to brief, stressful periods, consider short acting BZDs—oxazepam (Serax®), lorazepam (Ativan®), alprazolam (Xanax®).
    –anterograde amnesia is a significant side effect of short-acting BZDs, particularly if combined with alcohol.
    –patients who self-medicate at 2 to 3 times the therapeutic dose can experience physical dependence in 2 to 3 weeks. Dependence at therapeutic dose can occur if taken for more than 6 months. Gradual tapering of dose should be initiated after 4 to 16 weeks and adjunctive therapy may be required (i.e., sedating antidepressants, B-blockers, carbamazepine).
  - Buspirone (Buspar®):
    –first non-BZD introduced in the market with no anticonvulsant, muscle relaxant, or hypnotic properties.
    –as effective as diazepam (Valium®) at equipotent doses (i.e., 10 mg to 60 mg/day).
    –side effects include: dizziness, nausea, gastrointestinal upset, headache, and insomnia.

–dysphoria if higher doses (i.e., higher than 30 mg/day).
–advantage to use of Buspar® over BZDs include: non-sedating, minimal impairment of cognitive and psychomotor skills, low abuse and dependence potential, no withdrawal effects after discontinuation, and does not interact with alcohol.
–disadvantages compared to BZDs include: slow onset of action, lower satisfaction in patients with chronic anxiety if previous use of BZDs.
- Antidepressants:
  –efficacy not as clear as with panic disorders.
- B-adrenergic blockers:
  –still in use despite no proof of efficacy, probably due to fewer side effects and no abuse potential.
  –useful in ameliorating somatic symptoms (e.g.: tremor, tachycardia, palpitations).
- Antihistamines:
  –play a minor role in management of anxiety. Since no addictive potential used in patients with history of drug abuse and alcoholism.
  –hydroxyzine (Atarax®), (Vistaril®), provides sedation at expense of anticholinergic effect.
- Barbiturates and non-barbiturates:
  –rarely used due to low margin of safety, potential for addiction, development of tolerance, lethality in overdose, potential for drug interactions.
- Antipsychotics:
  –limited to anxiety associated with psychotic disorders.

CONSULTATION

→ See "Treatment/Management" section.
→ Consultation with or referral to a mental health care provider as indicated.
→ If patient fails to respond to short-term psychological treatment, refer to mental health professional.
→ Patients receiving MAO inhibitors are usually managed by a mental health professional.

PATIENT EDUCATION

→ Educate the client regarding the role that the autonomic nervous system plays in initiating symptoms.
→ Teach patients and their families that anxiety disorders are distinct conditions that can be appropriately treated like other illnesses.

→ Teach client relaxation techniques. Client may obtain a tape recording of these techniques. Explain to the patient that relaxation will break the vicious cycle of anxiety.

→ Engage the family in management of patients with anxiety disorders.

→ Encourage client to use the self-help manual "Living with Fear," which has been proven to speed recovery in patients with anxiety disorders (Sorby, Reavley, and Huber 1991).

- A copy of this booklet can be requested from W. Reavley, Department of Clinical Psychology, Graylingwell, Chicester, West Sussex, PO 1Y 48Q, Great Britain.

- Assist client in recognizing anxious feelings and their precipitating events.

- Discuss with client appropriate techniques to alleviate anxiety behavior and deal with feelings (see "Treatment/Management" section).

FOLLOW-UP

→ Make sure that patient has access to care on a 24-hour basis for crisis management, should need arise.

→ Health care provider should be aware of community resources for mental health care referral.

→ Patient to be followed at weekly intervals to monitor psychological management.

→ Document in progress notes and problem list.

14-C

Battering/Domestic Violence

Battering occurs among all ethnic and socioeconomic groups. Although the actual incidence is unknown, domestic violence is undoubtedly one of our most pervasive public health problems. It is estimated that up to six million women are abused each year by their current or former male partners—one every 7.4 seconds (McLear et al. 1989; Slade, Daniel, and Heisler 1991). Battering is the single most common injury to women—surpassing rape, muggings, and motor vehicle accidents combined (Randall 1990). In addition, approximately 30 percent of all female homicide victims are killed by their male partners (Slade, Daniel, and Heiser 1991).

The health consequences for the victim of battering are profound, since it may lead to low self-esteem, depression, increased drug or alcohol abuse, multiple injuries, permanent physical or emotional damage, and death by suicide or homicide. Women are not the only ones affected. Children living in homes where battering takes place experience emotional problems, increased fears and anger, and increased risk of abuse, injuries, and death (Helton 1986).

Battering's cost to society is enormous, contributing to increased legal, police, prison, medical, and counseling efforts and expenditures. The health care costs alone are staggering. It is believed that battering accounts for 998,000 days of hospitalization, 28,700 emergency room visits, and 39,900 physician visits, with total medical costs approaching $44 million annually (Warshaw 1989).

Approximately 95 percent of cases of domestic violence involve men battering intimate female partners (Dickstein 1988), although there have been reported incidents of women battering men and women battering other women. This protocol addresses only the cases of

battering that involve violence between a woman and a male partner. The term itself implies physical abuse, but the woman is often the target of psychological, emotional, and financial abuse as well.

There was little research on domestic violence until the 1970s. Currently, no single predictive, comprehensive theory of battering exists to explain its cause. Theories related to alcohol and substance abuse, social learning, social stratification and powerlessness, cultural support, and our patriarchal society have all been explored.

It has been suggested that there are two types of violent relationships. One involves partners who experience psychological conflicts, arising from the relationship itself, that eventually lead to abuse. The second is involved in the majority of domestic violence cases and involves a man with a violence-prone personality (Moss 1991).

For the latter group, Walker (1984) described a cycle of violence consisting of three stages:

→ the *tension-building phase* in which conflicts and verbal abuse increase,

→ the *acute battering episode*, and

→ the *honeymoon phase* in which the man expresses remorse and often promises that he will never hurt his partner again.

Research shows that for 75 percent of abused women the frequency and severity of battering episodes only increase (McLear et al. 1989).

There have been many explanations put forth as to why women stay in such relationships. Walker (1984) described the concept of *learned helplessness* in which the victim becomes depressed and hopeless after her attempts to end the violence fail. Researchers are now attempting to understand battered women in the broader context of victims' reaction to catastrophe, violent crime, and prolonged captivity (Packer 1990; Moss 1991).

Reasons for staying with an abusive partner include lack of family support, the high social approval accorded marriage, lack of assistive community resources, religious beliefs, financial considerations, and concern for her own safety as well as the safety of her children and other relatives (Moss 1991). This last reason is getting much more attention as the number of battered women who kill their spouses increases. Close to one-half of families with battered women have children who have also been abused (by the same abuser) (McLear et al. 1989).

In one study of 218 battered women, one-third were not living with their attacker at the time (Berrios and Grady 1991). Thus, in many instances, leaving the situation does not end the abuse. In fact, the risk of homicide tends to increase when the woman threatens to leave (Campbell 1986).

Despite these shocking statistics, health care providers rarely ask women about battering, identifying as few as one out of 20 abused women (Flitcraft 1990). Warshaw (1987) studied 52 emergency room patients who were known to have been in an altercation with another person. In 90 percent of the interactions, the physician did not obtain a psychosocial history, did not inquire about abuse, and did not assess the woman's safety. Nurses did no better. Although protocol established that they were responsible for providing referral information to these women, in over 90 percent of cases they did not.

Explanations for this lack of identification include sex bias, misinformation, the structure of the prevailing medical model, and lack of training (Moss and Taylor 1991). Training is especially important since sex bias and misinformation can be decreased with appropriate instruction.

To meet the needs of battered women, health care providers must assess *all* women for this problem and recognize battering for what it is—a potentially *life-threatening condition* no less dangerous than cancer, cardiovascular disease, or any other major health problem.

DATABASE

SUBJECTIVE

→ All women are at risk for battering regardless of age, race, or socioeconomic status.

→ Client may describe episodes of physical, sexual, psychological, or verbal abuse directed at herself or others.

→ Client may present with injuries that are inconsistent with the history described.

→ Client may have a history of frequent visits to health care providers where she presents with multiple injuries or vague somatic complaints including headaches, gastrointestinal (GI) complaints, fatigue, sleeplessness, sexual dysfunction, chest pain, palpitations, allergic skin reactions, musculoskeletal aches, and anxiety.

→ Client may report history of:
- missed appointments or presenting for treatment days after an injury.
- alcohol or substance use in client or partner.
- eating disorders, depression, panic attacks, suicidal ideation, or suicide attempt(s).
- pre-term labor or low birth-weight infant in previous pregnancies.

→ Client may be accompanied by male partner who is overprotective and does not want the client to be left alone with the health care provider.

OBJECTIVE

→ Client may appear restless, angry, defensive, tearful, evasive, or anxious. May also exhibit an inappropriate affect or avoid eye contact.

→ Patient may present with:
- patchy alopecia.
- cigarette burns; human bites; multiple injuries in various stages of healing; wounds to the face, head, neck, breasts, or abdomen; wounds from a knife or firearm.
- foreign object(s) in ear, nose, vagina, or rectum.
- conditions associated with stress including hypertension, obesity, weight loss, and GI ulcers.
- signs or symptoms consistent with sexual assault (see **Sexual Assault** Protocol).
- signs or symptoms indicative of post-traumatic stress disorder:
  - nightmares, exaggerated startle responses, guilt, fearfulness, and the inability to concentrate (APA 1994).

ASSESSMENT

→ Physical assault

→ Abusive partner, domestic violence

→ R/O potential for death by suicide or homicide

→ R/O substance or alcohol abuse

→ R/O coexisting psychological disorder in client and partner

→ R/O coexisting child abuse

→ If violent behavior is atypical for the male partner, rule out organic origin in the abuser (e.g., brain metastasis, subdural hematoma, drug reaction)

PLAN

DIAGNOSTIC TESTS

→ No specific diagnostic tests are required.

→ Necessary tests will depend upon the nature of any injury.

→ X-rays may reveal presence or history of multiple fractures.

TREATMENT/MANAGEMENT

→ Screen *all* women for domestic violence regardless of age, race, or socioeconomic or marital status.

→ Assess the client's safety as well as her children's or other family/household members' who may be at risk for injury or death.
  ▪ Inquire specifically about threats of homicide or suicidal intent.

→ Assess living arrangements and support systems (family, friends, community).

→ Refer woman and her family to community resources including legal services, shelters, law enforcement agencies, and counseling services.

→ Specific legal guidelines exist regarding the reporting of domestic violence, child abuse, and suicidal or homicidal intent.
  ▪ Notify police only at the request of the client *or* when the law requires it.

→ Use caution when prescribing sedatives, tranquilizers, or antidepressants. They could be used by the client in a suicide attempt.

→ Assist client with the development of an escape plan (see "Patient Education" section).

→ Guard client confidentiality and never give out information pertaining to client's whereabouts, health care, or appointment times.

→ Incorporate into your practice health promotion/ health maintenance strategies aimed at reducing domestic violence.
  ▪ Utilize empowerment strategies to build self-esteem in female clients of all ages (see "Patient Education" section).
  ▪ Assist males—especially children and adolescents—in identifying alternative ways to express anger and to improve communication with females.

CONSULTATION

→ Physician consultation required in cases involving serious injuries/medical conditions.

→ Social service referral should be made in cases involving child abuse or to identify additional legal, law enforcement, housing, financial, and counseling services.

→ Referral to psychological/psychiatric services should be made in suspected cases of psychological disorders or substance abuse.

→ Assistance should be sought with emergency mental health and/or law enforcement services in instances of suicidal or homicidal intent.

PATIENT EDUCATION

→ Encourage all women clients to pursue education, employment, and other means of self-actualization to empower themselves and build self-esteem.

→ Teach women to control their fertility through available methods of contraception and abortion services.
  ▪ This can have an empowering effect as well as help them avoid an unwanted pregnancy which could lead to more episodes of abuse.

→ Inform teens and young women that violence and abuse are not a normal part of intimate relationships.
  ▪ Help them avoid potential abusers—men who seem very jealous, overprotective, or controlling; have a history of substance or alcohol abuse; or exhibit violent behavior toward animals, objects, or other people.

→ Let client know she is free to discuss this issue with you and encourage her to do so.

→ Assure client that she is not alone and that many women share this problem.
  ▪ Explore the health consequences of battering for her, her children, and other family/household members.

→ Educate client about the cycle of violence and explain that without intervention violent episodes will likely increase in both frequency and severity.

→ Provide client with referral information for legal, law enforcement, shelter, financial, and counseling services.
  ▪ The Michigan Coalition against Domestic Violence provides information to health care providers and operates a national hotline:

Table 14C.1. ESCAPE PLAN

▸ Pack a change of clothes for yourself and your children. Include toilet articles, medications, and keys to the house and car.

▸ Include cash, checkbook, savings account book, credit cards, and ATM card.

▸ Collect identification papers such as birth certificates, social security card(s), voter registration card(s), passport(s), visas, immigration papers, and driver's license(s). These will be useful for traveling, enrolling children in school, and seeking financial assistance.

▸ Take a special book or toy for each child.

▸ If available, gather financial records, utility bills, mortgage papers, rent receipts, and automobile title. These items may be kept with a friend or neighbor. Decide exactly where you will go, day or night, and make a plan.

▸ Safety is the most important issue. If no items can be collected, leave without them.

Source: Adapted with permission from Helton, A. 1986. *Protocol of care for the battered woman.* Houston, TX: March of Dimes Birth Defects Foundation.

800-333-SAFE; telecommunications device for the deaf 800-873-6363.

■ The National Coalition against Domestic Violence provides a network of shelters and counseling programs: P.O. Box 34103 Washington, DC 20043-4103, (202) 638-6388.

→ Assist client with the development of an escape plan such as the one proposed by Helton (1986). (See **Table 14C.1, Escape Plan**).

→ Caution client about documents that the abuser may see inadvertently—e.g., referrals, health education materials, work/school excuses, or discharge materials.

FOLLOW-UP

→ See "Consultation" section.

→ Continue to monitor at future visits. Consider these clients to be high risk and follow them with more frequent visits and telephone contact.

→ Be aware that changes in life situation (e.g., unemployment, pregnancy, leaving the abusive relationship) may increase the chances of the client being abused.

→ On rare occasions, the health care provider may be required to testify if the client decides to pursue legal action against her batterer.

→ Document findings in progress notes and problem list in a clear, precise, and comprehensive fashion using diagrams, measurements, and photographs (if the client consents).

■ Since this information might be used for legal purposes, adhere to state and local requirements including those regarding documentation, consent, and specimen collection.

Pilar Bernal de Pheils, R.N., M.S., F.N.P.

14-D

Depression

Depression is a mental health problem commonly encountered in primary care practice (Martin and Davis 1989). Epidemiological studies show that five percent of male adults and ten percent of female adults have at least one depressive illness in their lifetimes. Current theories concerning the etiology of major depression are multifactorial, involving the interaction of biochemical, genetic, and environmental factors (Calarco and Krone 1991; Smith 1986).

The assessment of depression is a complex process since patients present frequently with somatic complaints rather than dysphoria. This leads to under-recognized depression in the ambulatory care setting (Dreyfus 1987). An additional concern with the assessment of depression in an ambulatory medical care setting is the issue of suicide. Forty-five percent of suicides have a history of depressive disorders (Pokorny 1977).

Types of Depression

Depression is categorized as a mental disorder by the American Psychiatric Association in the *Diagnostic and Statistical Manual of Mental Health Disorders (DSM-IV)* (APA 1994). According to this classification, depression can occur as a part of:

1. a mood disorder (e.g., major depression, dysthymia and depressive disorders not otherwise specified [patient does not meet the criteria for any specific mood disorder or adjustment disorder with depressed mood]),

2. a predominant symptom in adjustment disorder (adjustment disorder with depressed mood),

3. a non-mood psychotic disorder (e.g. schizoaffective disorder),

4. a mood disorder due to a general medical condition, or

5. a substance-induced mood disorder.

This protocol addresses depression as a mood disorder and as a predominant symptom in adjustment disorder.

A *major depression episode* is characterized by the DSM-IV (APA 1994) as a condition in which the essential feature is either depressed mood or *anhedonia* (loss of interest or pleasure) in all, or almost all, activities. It also includes the presence of at least four associated symptoms, most of them of the neurovegetative type, for a period of at least two weeks (see "Database" section).

A major depressive disorder is characterized by one or more major depressive episodes and can be classified as either *mild*—few if any symptoms in excess of those required to make the diagnosis and mild impairment in occupational and social functioning; *moderate*—symptoms and impairment between mild and severe; and *severe*—several symptoms in excess required to make the diagnosis and marked interference with occupational or social functioning.

A severe depressive episode is also specified as without psychotic features or with psychotic features. If the diagnostic criteria for major depressive episode is not currently met it may indicate that the major depressive episode is in partial remission (the patient does not have dysthymia, and the symptoms are currently less than those of mild depression) or in full remission (no significant signs or symptoms of depression in the past six months).

The onset of a major depressive episode may develop over weeks to months. Its duration may be six months or longer, with an eventual complete remission of symptoms in the majority of the cases. However, in five percent to ten percent of patients, some symptoms persist for two years or longer. These cases are specified as chronic.

Suicide is the major complication of major depression. A patient with this disorder is 30 times more likely to commit suicide than a non-depressed person (Lowenstein 1985).

When assessing the patient for major depression it is important to rule out a mood disturbance due to a physiological consequence of a specific general medical condition, a substance-induced mood disorder, or other psychiatric disorders that can masquerade as depression. The following etiologies from a general medical condition and a substance-induced condition should be considered:

→ Drug-induced: anti-hypertensive agents such as reserpine, methyldopa, or clonidine; corticosteroids, cholinergic drugs, benzodiazepines, or barbiturates.

→ Drug abuse: alcohol, sedative hypnotics, cocaine or other psycho-stimulant (e.g., amphetamines, barbiturates, narcotics, nicotine) withdrawal.

→ Toxic metabolic disorders: hyperthyroidism (especially in elderly), hypothyroidism, Cushing's syndrome, diabetes mellitus, hypercalcemia, hyponatremia, or renal disease.

→ Neurological disorders: stroke, subdural hematoma, multiple sclerosis, brain tumors, Parkinson's and Huntington's diseases, syphilis, dementia, or uncontrolled pellagra.

→ Other: recent surgery (including but not limited to hysterectomy), pancreatic carcinoma, or viral infections (especially mononucleosis and influenza).

Dysthymia, also known as *depressive neurosis*, is a chronic disturbance of mood involving depressed mood most of the days for at least two years. In addition to depressed mood, two of the following symptoms must also be present: poor appetite or overeating, insomnia or hyperinsomnia, low energy or fatigue, low self-esteem, poor concentration or difficulty making decisions, and feelings of hopelessness. To fit the diagnosis of dysthymia, the person may be symptom free for no longer than two months, and only if the initial two-year period of the disorder is free of major depressive episode. Major depressive episodes may be superimposed on the dysthymic disorder after two initial years of the latter.

The differential diagnoses of dysthymia and major depression may be difficult since both disorders share similar symptoms and differ only in duration and severity, dysthymia being less severe but chronic. Dysthymia usu-

ally begins without a clear onset and usually has superimposed major depression which increases the possibility that the patient will seek treatment.

Adjustment disorder with depressed mood (not in *DSM-IV*) is characterized by the *DSM-IV* (APA 1994) as a maladaptive reaction in which the predominant manifestations are symptoms of depressed mood, tearfulness, and feelings of hopelessness. Symptoms occur as a response to a single or multiple, recurrent, or continuous psychosocial stressor such as divorce, work difficulties, or chronic illness. This disorder begins within three months of onset of the stressor and lasts no longer than six months. It is usually self-limited and resolves when the stress ceases or a new level of adaptation is achieved. Adjustment disorder with depressed mood can occur at any age, and the intensity of the stressor does not necessarily reflect the severity of the reaction. This disturbance is not a result of uncomplicated bereavement, nor does it meet the criteria for any specific mental disorder.

DATABASE

SUBJECTIVE

→ Major depression.
- Precipitating factors include:
  • substance abuse.
  • chronic physical illness.
  • psychosocial stressor.
  • childbirth.
- Medical health history may reveal:
  • recent surgery (especially within the last year).
  • depression.
- Personal/health/ social history may reveal:
  • difficult social situation, social isolation (lack of family, friends or other social supports).
  • stress related to unemployment, poverty, adolescence.
  • recent loss or unresolved grief.
  • marital conflicts or dysfunctional family patterns.
  • variable social and occupational impairment. May be so severe that the individual is not functional even in the routine of daily living (e.g. feeding or clothing herself).
- Family history may be positive for:
  • depression.
  • bipolar disorder.
  • suicide.
- Age of onset usually late 20s, but may begin at any age.
- Symptoms develop suddenly or over weeks or months.

- Reports at least one of the following symptoms most of the day, and nearly every day:
  - depressed mood—i.e., feeling of sadness, being "blue" or gloomy—ormarkedly diminished interest or pleasure—i.e., loss of interest in friends, family, and work (anhedonia).
- Reports at least four of the following associated symptoms during a two-week period, representing a change from previous functioning:
  - appetite disturbance—most commonly loss of appetite but can be increased appetite.
  - sleep disturbances—most frequently insomnia. (These symptoms are usually the ones that bring patient into treatment.)
  - psychomotor agitation or retardation—being unable to remain still if agitated, or slow speech with more pauses than normal and slow body movements.
  - fatigue and loss of energy.
  - feelings of worthlessness and/or excessive guilt that may be delusional.
  - decreased cognitive functioning—having difficulty in concentration, thinking, and memory loss.
  - suicidal ideation or attempts—may believe that she or others may be better off dead.
- May also complain of:
  - feeling of helplessness, hopelessness, and inadequacy.
  - heaviness in head or chest pains.
  - headache, backache, constipation.
- Common associated features may include:
  - tearfulness.
  - anxiety.
  - anger or irritability.
  - brooding or obsessive rumination.
  - excessive concern with physical health.
  - panic attacks.
  - phobias.
- Some women mask their sadness or despair, affecting a cheerful manner or even a kind of hectic gaiety. More commonly, however, the affect is flat.

→ Dysthymia.
- Personal/health/social history may include:
  - mild to moderate social and occupational functioning impairment.
  - psychoactive substance dependence or abuse (degree of severity increased by the chronicity of the disorder).

- Family history may include major depression in first-degree relative(s).
- Onset: childhood through early adulthood (For this reason, has often been referred to as *depressive personality*.).
- Reports at least two of the following symptoms during periods of depressed mood:
  - eating disturbances.
  - sleeping disturbances.
  - low level of energy or fatigue.
  - low self-esteem.
  - feeling of hopelessness.
  - cognitive difficulties.
  - poor concentration or difficulty making decisions.

→ Adjustment disorder with depressed mood.
- Medical health history may reveal chronic illness.
- Personal/health/social history may reveal:
  - social and occupational impairment.
- Age of onset variable.
- Symptoms begin within three months of an identifiable psychosocial stressor(s) onset, and last no longer than six months.
- May report symptoms of:
  - depressed mood.
  - tearfulness.
  - feelings of hopelessness.
- Symptoms are in excess of a normal and expected reaction to stressor.

OBJECTIVE

→ General appearance may include:
- lack of care in grooming.
- slumped posture.
- sad face expression.
- smiling in the presence of denial or repression (*masked depression*).

→ Mental status may include:
- psychomotor retardation or agitation.
- long periods of hesitation before answering or slow speech.
- affect that is sad, irritable, anxious, angry, tearful, or despondent.
- thought that is clear and coherent or tangential, circumstantial, or nonsensical.
- ideas of worthlessness, helplessness, hopelessness, guilt, suicidal thoughts, homicide. With severe depression, delusions and hallucinations may be present.

ASSESSMENT

→ Major depression
- Mild, moderate, or severe
- Single episode or recurrent
- Chronic
- In partial or full remission
- R/O uncomplicated bereavement
- R/O mood disorder due to a general medical condition
- R/O substance-induced mood disorder
- R/O bipolar disorder, depressed phase
- R/O schizophrenia
- R/O primary degenerative dementia of the Alzheimer's type and multi-infarct dementia (more common in elderly)

→ Dysthymia
- R/O major depression
- R/O major depression in partial remission

→ Adjustment disorder with depressed mood

→ Depressive disorder not otherwise specified

PLAN

DIAGNOSTIC TESTS

→ There are no useful chemical tests to confirm a diagnosis of depression.

→ Additional diagnostic tests as indicated to rule out organic causes of depression.

The Beck Depression Inventory (BDI) (either long form or short form) may be used for suspicion of depression (Dreyfus 1987).

→ The BDI is useful for monitoring treatment response and changes in affective status over time.

→ A baseline EKG should be obtained for all patients over 40 years old when initiating tricyclic antidepressant medication.

→ Blood pressure measurements (lying and standing) and pulse should be obtained when patient initiates tricyclic antidepressant medication.

MANAGEMENT/TREATMENT

→ Treatment of depression depends on the type of depression, severity of symptoms, personal and social impairments related to the depression, and availability of treatment resources (Abraham, Neese, and Westerman 1991).

→ Major depression.

- With mild depression, psychotherapy is the first choice of treatment (Dreyfus 1988). Counseling, group therapy, self-help group, diet and exercise programs, and instruction in coping skills can be of benefit (Smith 1986).
- If moderate or severe depression, medical consultation is indicated. Pharmacotherapy and psychotherapy are recommended. Pharmacotherapy is effective in management of neurovegetative symptoms, psychotherapy approach may enhance social functioning.

→ Dysthymia disorders.
- Consultation with a mental health care provider is indicated.
- Education, supportive counseling, antidepressant therapy, psychotherapy, and family therapy are recommended.
- Antidepressive pharmacotherapy may help relieve symptom but overall is less effective than for symptoms associated with major depression (Laage 1988).

→ Adjustment disorder with depressed mood.
- May be co-managed with mental health care provider.
- Treatment includes supportive psychotherapy and education—particularly the latter—if disorder precipitated by a medical illness (Perry and Anderson 1992).
- If moderate sleep and eating disturbances are present, heterocyclic antidepressants may be effective.

→ Pharmacological guidelines.
- Heterocyclic antidepressants:
  - first-line therapy for depression.
  - benefit 65 percent to 80 percent of depressed patients (Shen 1990).
  - drug choice should be decided on with patient based on side effects, mechanisms of action, and presenting symptoms.
  - tricyclic antidepressants include:
    −imipramine (Tofranil®, Sk-pramine®), amitriptyline (Elavil®, Endep®), nortriptyline (Pamelor®, Aventil®), desipramine (Norpramin®, Pertofrane®), doxepin (Adapin®, Sinequan®), protriptyline (Vivactil®), trimipramine (Surmontil®) (Consult *PDR* for dosage and administration.).
  - new-generation antidepressants include:
    −maprotiline (Ludiomil®), amoxapine (Asendin®), fluoxetine (Prozac®), trazadone (Desyrel®), alprazolam (Xanax®),

clomipramine (Anafranil®), bupropion (Wellbutrin®), sertraline (Zoloft®), Paroxetine (Pacil®). See *PDR* for dosage and administration.

- the new-generation antidepressants have fewer side effects, but have not been proven to act faster or relieve depression better than the standard tricyclic antidepressants such as amitriptyline (Elavil®), and doxepin (Sinequan®).

- risk of dependency increases with prolonged use of alprazolam, a mild antidepressant and an excellent anti-anxiety drug.

- major side effects for all heterocyclic antidepressants include:
  - cardiotoxicity. Patients with recent cardiac disease must have a consultation with a cardiologist before initiating heterocyclic medication.
  - hypotension. Elderly patients and patients with cardiovascular disease are more vulnerable. Fluoxetine, bupropion, and alprazolam have no orthostatic effects.
  - sedation. May be beneficial in anxious, agitated or insomniac patients. Can be counterproductive in patients with somnolence and psychomotor retardation. Consider lowering dose, administer total dose at bedtime, or change to a less-sedating antidepressant. Amitriptyline is highly sedative.
  - reduction of seizure threshold. May cause seizures in up to 4 percent of patients. Desipramine, trazadone, and MAO inhibitors lower seizure threshold the least (Brasfield 1991).
  - weight gain. Not associated with fluoxetine or bupropion.
  - sexual dysfunction.
  - anticholinergic effects. Central (i.e., poor concentration, memory loss, confusion and temperature fluctuation), or peripheral (i.e., dry mouth, constipation, tachycardia, urinary hesitance or retention, increase or decrease in sweating, nasal stuffiness, and blurred vision).
    ‣ Fluoxetine, trazadone, and buboprion do not have anticholinergic effects.
    ‣ Desipramine has low anticholinergic effect. Consider reducing dose or changing to less anticholinergic antidepressant. If antidepressants are discontinued abruptly, dose is reduced drastically, or a change to a

less anticholinergic drug is made, rebound cholinergic effects may ensue (i.e., dizziness, nausea, diarrhea, malaise, anxiety, insomnia, and restlessness).
  - memory loss or lack of concentration. Can be either an anticholinergic effect or a result of depression.
  - constipation. Consider stool softener (see **Constipation** Protocol).

- to minimize side effects of heterocyclic antidepressants, begin with a low dose, and slowly titrate upward every 3 to 4 days until a therapeutic dosage without intolerable side effects is reached. (Consult *PDR* for dose ranges of heterocyclic antidepressants.) (Hyman and Jenike 1987).

- total prescribed dose at bedtime is recommended to improve compliance and tolerance of side effects.
  - Exceptions to this recommendation are desipramine and fluoxetine which can cause insomnia if dosed at bedtime.
  - Trazadone requires multiple dosing for maximum effectiveness.

- blood plasma concentrations of some tricyclic antidepressants are recommended to monitor therapeutic doses and toxic levels.
  - Plasma concentration monitoring of imipramine, amitriptyline, desipramine, and nortriptyline are useful in patients:
    ‣ who do not respond to therapy.
    ‣ who do not comply with therapy.
    ‣ with side effects.
    ‣ who are elderly.
    ‣ who are taking other medications. (Consult *PDR*.)
  - Obtain plasma levels within 5 to 10 days of initiating antidepressant and 8 to 12 hours after the patient has taken the medication to establish therapeutic levels.
  - Other agents (e.g., alcohol, tobacco) may alter plasma levels.

- antidepressant drugs interact with other medications, causing increased side effects and anxiety and reduced antidepressant activity and effectiveness. The reader is directed to a pharmacology text to review medications that interact with antidepressants.

- continue antidepressant medication for 6 to 12 months after depression is successfully treated to reduce risk of relapse.

- discontinue antidepressant gradually over several weeks to avoid cholinergic effects.

- first depressive episode may be adequately treated with medication for 3 to 6 months while chronic depression may require several years of therapy.
- elderly patients require special attention including lower doses of antidepressant medication. In elderly individuals the dose should be lowered to one-half or one-third of the adult dose (Hyman and Jenike 1987).
- consultation is indicated when heterocyclic antidepressants are not effective following an adequate trial. Drug trial failure should be considered when a patient has no response after 4 weeks on a full dosage with documented therapeutic blood levels.
- if the patient evidences any potential of suicide risk, or has a history of suicide attempts, it is recommended that no more than 1 week's supply or a total of 1 gram of a heterocyclic antidepressant is prescribed at a time (Hyman and Jenike 1987).
- Other psychoactive drugs:
  - MAO inhibitors, lithium, carbamazepine, and other antiepileptic agents are second-line drugs and should be used in consultation with a psychiatric clinician.
  - these medications are recommended for those who do not respond well to or have medical contraindications to heterocyclic antidepressants.
- Evaluation of suicide.
  - Assess suicide risk in confirmed cases of depression.
  - Assessing risk of suicide requires attention to:
    - thoughts (ideas, wishes, motives).
    - intent (degree of probability that patient intends to act on the thoughts).
    - plans (formulation of a clear, detailed plan).
  - Ask the patient in a straightforward manner if she has any suicide thoughts, intent, or plan. The following questions have been suggested (Buckwalter and Babich 1990):
    - have you thought life is not worth living?
    - have you considered harming yourself?
    - do you have a plan for harming yourself?
    - have you ever acted on a plan?
    - have you ever attempted suicide?
  - If possible, ask patient's family and friends if she has left any clue indicating suicide (i.e., a written note, a spoken threat, or a previous attempt at self-destruction).

- If patient is at high risk for suicide, never leave her alone. Obtain immediate psychiatric consultation (Lowenstein 1985).

CONSULTATION

→ See "Treatment/Management" section.

PATIENT EDUCATION

→ Educate patient and family regarding symptoms of depression. Since mental illness is commonly stigmatized, both patient and family should be counseled and stress placed on the importance of prescribed treatment.

→ Support and validate patient's feelings of sadness and remind her that depression can be treated.

→ Educate the patient about the side effects of the medication prescribed:
  - techniques that decrease incidence of dry mouth and constipation.
    - Use of sugarless gum, ice chips, and drinking adequate amount of fluids.
  - encourage proper daily dental cleaning to prevent tooth decay, mouth ulcers, and gum disease.
  - encourage patient to increase intake of fluids, prune juice, and high-fiber foods to prevent constipation.
  - instruct patient to get up slowly from sitting or lying positions to prevent falls (if medication has a high orthostatic effect).
  - advise patient that full effect of antidepressant medication will not be evident for ten days to three weeks (at adequate therapeutic levels).
  - advise patient that sleep, appetite, and energy levels generally improve within a week.
  - instruct patient to report side effects rather than stop medication.
  - instruct patient to call if suicidal thoughts are present or depressive symptoms worsen.
  - advise patient to consult health care provider before using over-the-counter medications.
  - advise patient to consult health care provider before discontinuing or changing medication.

→ Review patient compliance with medication. Non-compliance may be secondary to cost, adverse side effects, ambivalence regarding the disease, and time lag in effectiveness. (Mejo 1990).

→ Engage family members in the management of depressive patients:
  - to supervise/monitor medication regimen.
  - to keep follow-up appointments.

- to uncover, explore, and modify stressful situations and provide a reassuring, supportive environment.
- to decrease social isolation that results from and exacerbates depression.
- to encourage spouse to express feelings of warmth and compassion in regard to spouse's depressive illness. This has been proven to increase speed of recovery (McLeod, Kessler, and Landis 1992).

→ Teach patient relaxation techniques, if indicated.

→ Encourage patient to participate in a regular exercise program.

→ Educate patient in proper nutrition.

→ Encourage patients to avoid situations in which conflicts may arise. Less rapid recovery from depressive illness has been found to be significant when there is a conflictual relationship with friends (McLeod, Kessler, and Landis 1992).

FOLLOW-UP

→ Assure that the patient and her family have access to care on a 24-hour basis for crisis management, should need arise.

→ Patient to be followed at regular intervals to monitor medications and reinforce psychotherapeutic work.

→ Document in progress notes and problem list.

Pilar Bernal de Pheils, R.N., M.S., F.N.P.

14-E

Eating Disorders

Anorexia nervosa and *bulimia nervosa* are eating disorders characterized by severe disturbances in eating behavior (APA 1994). The age of onset is typically in adolescence or early adult life, with the ratio of females to males 10:1. The etiology of eating disorders is still largely unknown, but both biological and psychological factors appear to play a role (Palmer 1990).

These disorders appear to be related, often occurring concurrently (50 percent of the cases). When they occur concurrently, treatment is more difficult and the prognosis is poorer. The prevalence of these two conditions has increased considerably in the last two decades. For anorexia nervosa the prevalence ranges from 0.5 percent to one percent of females in late adolescence and early adulthood (Herzog and Copeland 1985; APA 1994) and for bulimia nervosa the prevalence ranges from one percent to 4.5 percent of college-age women (Bushnell et al. 1990; APA 1994).

Both conditions are serious, life-threatening disorders. Anorexia nervosa is characterized by self-imposed starvation. The anorexic person becomes obsessed with food, weight, counting calories, and vigorous exercise. Bulimia nervosa is characterized by binge eating usually followed by self-induced vomiting or some other form of purging as a means of controlling weight.

There is a high rate of association of depression with anorexia and bulimia. Feelings of worthlessness and helplessness are present in the anorexic as a result of her obsession with perfection (Garner and Garfinkel 1985). Major depression is more likely to be present in the bulimia patient than in the anorexic; the more severe the bulimia the more likelihood the association with and severity of the depression. Low self-esteem is also characteristic of both disorders and high anxiety levels increase

with purgative behavior. Shame and guilt in relation to eating are experienced in higher levels in anorexics and bulimics than in the normal population (Frank 1991).

Anorexic patients have strong self-control which is manifested in their depriving themselves of food and drinks to avoid gaining weight. On the other hand, bulimics lack control and discipline. Both conditions evidence a negative body image and dissatisfaction with body size.

For a more thorough discussion of the characteristics of these disorders the reader is directed to the "Database" section of the protocol and to an excellent review of the literature by Skok and McLaughlin (1991), listed in the bibliography.

The diagnostic criteria for these conditions are given in the *Diagnostic and Statistical Manual of Mental Disorders (DSM IV)* (APA 1994). All criteria must be present to make the diagnosis (see **Tables 14E.1,** and **14E.2**).

According to the DSM-IV, the mean age of onset for anorexia nervosa is 17 years; it rarely occurs in females over age 40 years. The cause is highly variable. Some women recover fully after one episode, some fluctuate between weight gain and relapse, and others experience unrelenting weight loss resulting in debilitating illness or death. The mortality rate from anorexia nervosa is over 10 percent. The course of bulimia nervosa is usually intermittent over a period of years. While anorexics may need hospitalization to prevent death from starvation, bulimics seldom have an incapacitating disease. Instead, they have a high rate of relapse (Herzog et al. 1991).

Individuals with anorexia nervosa or bulimia nervosa are usually very secretive. Clients rarely volunteer information about their eating patterns. Families and

Table 14E.1. DIAGNOSTIC CRITERIA FOR ANOREXIA NERVOSA, *DSM-IV*

- Refusal to maintain body weight over a minimal normal weight for age and height—e.g., weight loss leading to maintenance of body weight 15% below the expected; or failure to make expected weight gain during period of growth, leading to body weight 15% below that expected.
- Intense fear of gaining weight or becoming fat, even though underweight.
- Disturbance in the way in which one's body weight, size, or shape is experienced—undue influence of body weight or shape on self-evaluation, or denial of the seriousness of the current low body weight.
- In postmenarcheal females, amenorrhea—i.e., the absence of at least three consecutive menstrual cycles. (A woman is considered to have amenorrhea if her periods occur only following hormone administration [e.g., estrogen].)
- Specify type:
  - **Restricting type:** during the current episode of anorexia nervosa, the person has not regularly engaged in binge-eating or purging behavior (i.e., self-induced vomiting or the misuse of laxatives, diuretics, or enemas).
  - **Binge-Eating/Purging type:** during the current episode of anorexia nervosa, the person has regularly engaged in binge-eating or purging behavior (i.e., self-induced vomiting or the misuse of laxatives, diuretics, or enemas.

Source: Reprinted with permission from American Psychiatric Association. 1994. *Diagnostic and statistical manual of mental disorders*, 4th ed., pp. 544-545. Washington, DC: the Author.

Table 14E.2. DIAGNOSTIC CRITERIA FOR BULIMIA NERVOSA, *DSM-IV*

A. Recurrent episodes of binge eating. An episode of binge eating is characterized by both of the following:
   1. eating, in a discrete period of time (e.g., within any two-hour period), an amount of food that is definitely larger than most people could eat during a similar period of time and under similar circumstances.
   2. a sense of lack of control over eating during the episode (e.g., a feeling that one cannot stop eating or control what or how much one is eating).

B. Recurrent inappropriate compensatory behavior in order to prevent weight gain, such as self-induced vomiting; misuse of laxatives, diuretics, enemas, or other medications; fasting or excessive exercise.

C. The binge eating and inappropriate compensatory behaviors both occur, on average, at least twice a week for three months.

D. Self-evaluation is unduly influenced by body shape and weight.

E. The disturbance does not occur excessively during episodes of anorexia nervosa.

   Specify type:

   Purging type: during the current episode of bulimia nervosa, the person has regularly engaged in self-induced vomiting or the misuse of laxatives, diuretics or enamas.

   Nonpurging type: during the current episode of bulimia nervosa, the person has used other inappropriate compensatory behaviors such as fasting or excessive exercise, but has not regularly engaged in self-induced vomiting or the misuse of laxatives, diuretics, or enemas.

Source: Reprinted with permission from American Psychiatric Association. 1994. *Diagnostic and statistical manual of mental disorders*, 4th ed., pp. 549-550. Washington, DC: the Author.

friends may be unaware of their disease for years. Symptoms are often subclinical until the disease is advanced, resulting in significant morbidity and mortality. Anorexics usually are detected earlier than bulimics because of the former's obvious physical condition. On the other hand, bulimics may appear physically healthy with a normal (or close to normal) weight, making the identification of this disorder more difficult.

Important clues when assessing the client history include personal, social, and family health (particularly if there is a longstanding, chronic condition). A thorough history and physical examination may increase case finding at an earlier stage of the disease which will improve recovery rate.

DATABASE

SUBJECTIVE

Anorexia nervosa

→ Age of onset: early to late adolescence.

→ Predominantly in women from educated and prosperous homes.

→ An anorexic is often someone who:
   - denies or refuses to disclose any problems with being underweight.

- is frantically preoccupied with food and eating and has an intense fear of becoming fat.
- restricts her food intake even though her appetite is not decreased.
- tends to have obsessive-compulsive behavior, manifested in some cases in over-involvement in exercise routines.
- has a distorted body image, viewing herself as larger than she is and having negative attitudes towards herself.
- uses eating or refusing to eat as a way of achieving a sense of control and a solution for the problem of feelings of powerlessness, ineffectiveness, and incompetence.
- may fear loss of control over here eating. In this case, may binge (eat large amounts of food) and purge (induce vomiting) like a bulimic, suffering from a combination of anorexia and bulimia symptoms. Fifty percent of anorexic patients may exhibit bulimic behavior, the main differentiating factor is the severe weight loss in anorexia) (Garner and Garfinkel 1985).
- is described by others as a perfectionist, successful individual.

→ Medical/health history may reveal:
- depression (occurs in approximately 50 percent of anorexics).
- fractures (a result of low estrogen levels and calcium depletion; may be compensated for by moderate physical exercise that reduces bone mass loss).
- excessive dieting, fasting and/or exercise for weight loss.
- client requesting advice regarding diet for weight loss or prescription for diuretics or laxatives.
- mildly overweight client prior to onset of anorexia.

→ Personal/social history of client may reveal:
- poor family communication skills.
- non-existent family meals or meals which are no longer an enjoyable experience.
- dieting as an important part of the family ritual.
- high achievement expected in family. Client may feel uncomfortable receiving support/affection needed to achieve excellence expected.
- sexual molestation in early years by a family member or a neighbor.
- decreased interest in sex.
- a recent stressful situation.

→ Family history may be positive for:
- anorexia nervosa in sisters and/or mother.
- higher frequency of depression and bipolar disorder in first-degree biological relatives.
- maternal obesity.

→ Client may complain of:
- feeling of fullness.
- constipation, sometimes accompanied by abdominal pain.
- insomnia and early awakening.
- amenorrhea or irregular menses or delayed menarche.
- feeling cold even on hot days.
- symptoms associated with severe weight loss:
  - dry skin and hair.
  - cold hands and feet.
  - general weakness.
  - nausea.
  - loss of appetite (late in illness, rare).

Bulimia nervosa

→ Age of onset: adolescence or early adult life.

→ A bulimic is often an individual who:
- fears being overweight. This fear manifests itself in either a restrictive eating pattern or a purging behavior.
- has a distorted body image, believes she is overweight, even though is normal or slightly below or above what is expected.
- believes that specific parts of her body is too large—e.g., buttocks, thighs (Herzog et al. 1991).
- is preoccupied with food, weight, and dieting, and has an excessive desire to lose weight.
- has low self-esteem, high anxiety levels, and communication problems.
- lacks control and discipline, blaming symptoms on others.
- has compulsive behaviors which lead to stealing in order to obtain high-calorie foods and laxatives.

→ Medical/health history may reveal:
- weekly weight fluctuations of up to 20 pounds (Yates and Sambrailo 1984).
- depression (most often major depression).
- coexisting personality disorder.
- overweight status in the past.
- excessive exercise (though not as driven as anorexics).
- excessive use of laxatives or diuretics.
- alcohol and drug (particularly amphetamines) abuse.
- in severe cases, history of convulsions (due to electrolyte imbalance, hypoglycemia, or alcohol binges), esophagitis, and pharyngitis (due to repeated vomiting).

→ Personal/social history of client may reveal:
- problematic family interactions, parents over-involved or emotionally detached.
- family member(s) extremely concerned about own weight and/or dieting.
- divorced parents.
- stressful or traumatic situation within six months of disorder onset (e.g., going to college, being criticized for being fat).
- sexual abuse.

→ Family history may be positive for:
- anorexia nervosa or bulimia nervosa in first-degree relative.
- obesity in parents.
- major depression in first-degree biological relative.
- alcoholism.

→ Client may complain of symptoms that are secondary to binge eating, fasting, vomiting, and/or laxative or diuretic use (Herzog et al. 1991):

- fatigue, nervousness, insomnia (all also related to emotional distress).
- sensitivity to cold weather.
- frequent or severe headaches.
- sore throat.
- abdominal pain.
- constipation.
- nausea.
- sensitive teeth.
- menstrual irregularities.
→ Less common complaints (seen with increasing severity of disturbance):
  - changes in skin and hair growth.
  - heartburn.
  - racing, irregular heartbeat.
  - chest pain.
  - salivary gland enlargement.
  - edema in hands.
  - cramping of muscles, feet and legs (due to electrolyte imbalance).
  - muscle weakness (due to hyponatremia).

OBJECTIVE

Anorexia nervosa

→ General appearance: client may be wearing layers of clothing to hide physical appearance and obtain supply of warmth.
→ Body weight 15 percent below normal weight.
→ Early adolescent may have a delay in physical development.
→ The following physical findings may be present as a result of prolonged state of starvation and being underweight:
  - bradycardia: ranging from 44 to 60 beats per minute.
  - hypotension: ranging from 70/40 to 90/50 (Some blood pressure measurements need to be obtained with a pediatric cuff.).
  - hypothermia: rectal body temperatures ranging from 94.9°F to 96.0°F (35.0°C to 35.6°C).
  - decreased respiratory rate.
  - muscular weakness.
→ Cardiovascular system (Kalager, Brubackk, and Bassoe 1978):
  - heart murmurs.
  - mitral valve prolapse.
  - cardiac arrhythmia.
  - decreased peripheral circulation.
  - acrocyanosis.
  - EKG abnormalities.
  - Raynaud's phenomenon.

→ Skin/hair:
  - pale, dry, flaky facial skin.
  - lanugo (fine body hair) around vermillion border of lips, lower border of mandible, and extremities.
  - yellowish or bronze skin color (due to elevated beta-carotene).
  - alopecia.
  - skin lesions.
→ Mental status:
  - thought: dichotomous thinking (all or nothing, black or white).
  - low sense of self-worth.
  - difficulty in thinking clearly.
→ Laboratory findings which may be present as a result of starvation and electrolyte imbalance:
  - mild anemia.
  - leukopenia.
  - elevated beta-carotene levels.
  - mild hypoglycemia.
  - elevated BUN level.
  - hypomagnesemia.
  - hypokalemia.
  - decreased glomerular filtration rate.
  - decreased concentrating capacity of kidneys.
  - urinary calculi.
  - acute renal failure (rate).

Bulimia nervosa

→ Most often bulimics appear healthy.
→ Body weight normal or slightly higher than expected.
→ Physical findings are a product of medical complications that occur from excessive vomiting, binging, or restrictive cycles, or abuse of laxatives, diuretics or emetics:
  - dental enamel erosion.
  - buccal erosion.
  - increased number of cavities.
  - loss of teeth.
  - callus on index and second finger (near or at first knuckle).
  - palatal petechiae (in severe cases).
  - facial ecchymosis and blood vessel hemorrhages in and around the eyes (in severe cases).
  - sore, erythematous tongue.
  - bilateral, non-tender parotid or submandibular gland enlargement.
  - cardiac arrhythmias.
  - hypotension.
  - epigastric tenderness.

- mental status: dichotomous thinking (all or nothing, black or white), low self-esteem.
- → Rare complications of bulimia are cardiac myopathy due to ipecac abuse, cardiac arrest, and esophageal tears and gastric rupture due to induced vomiting.
- → Most laboratory findings are within normal limits unless bulimia nervosa is advanced, in which case findings may include:
  - electrolyte imbalance, which may be evidenced by:
    - metabolic alkalosis/acidosis.
    - hypokalemia.
    - hypocalcemia.
    - hypomagnesemia.
    - hypochloremia.
    - hyponatremia.
  - elevated cholesterol levels.
  - CBC may indicate anemia as a result of malnutrition.
  - increased BUN (indicates volume depletion).
  - urine positive for ketone and protein (indicates deficiency in carbohydrate metabolism).
  - urine specific gravity may be elevated if patient is dehydrated or lowered if patient is over-hydrated with water to temporarily increase weight.
  - EKG revealing flat or inverted T-waves, U-waves, ST-segment depression.
  - stool for occult blood may be positive if esophageal tears or gastric rupture has occurred (rare, but severe complication).

ASSESSMENT

- → Anorexia nervosa
  - R/O physical disorders (e.g., malignancy, malabsorption syndromes, hyperthyroidism, diabetes mellitus)
  - R/O depressive disorder
  - R/O schizophrenia
- → Bulimia nervosa
  - R/O personality disorder (binge eating present, but not full criteria for bulimia nervosa)
  - R/O depressive disorder (commonly major depression)
  - R/O schizophrenia
- → Anorexia nervosa and bulimia nervosa (anorexia nervosa occurring in a person with bulimia nervosa)

PLAN

DIAGNOSTIC TESTS

Anorexia nervosa

- → No specific diagnostic tests used in clinical practice.
- → Additional diagnostic tests as indicated by "Database" section to rule out complications.
- → An **Eating Attitude Test** (Button and Whitehouse 1981) (see **Appendix 14E.1**, p. 14-39) may be helpful to identify high-risk patients, particularly those working in high-risk occupations—e.g., professional dancers, models, actresses.

Bulimia nervosa

- → Urine dipstick for ketones, protein, specific gravity.
- → CBC.
- → Blood chemistry panel for electrolyte values.
- → Additional diagnostic tests as indicated by "Database" section to rule out complications.
- → Eating attitude tests, as for anorexia nervosa, may also be helpful in high-risk populations.

TREATMENT/MANAGEMENT

General measures

- → Initiating treatment of the anorexic or bulimic patient may be very difficult because of *denial*, a key feature of these eating disorders.
  - Many anorexics, as well as their families, do not recognize the severity of the disorder. Discussing the signs, symptoms, and laboratory findings can provide the patient with her first awareness of this condition and motivate her and her family to obtain treatment (Powers 1990).
  - Bulimia patients may respond with anger, shame, and tears as a result of "being discovered."
- → If denial is present and the clinician is highly suspicious of an eating disorder, directing questions to the patient that address the diagnostic criteria of the *DSM-IV* (1994) can help identify those with the disorder.
- → Medical consultation is indicated, and management by a multidisciplinary team experienced in these types of disorders (i.e., physician/nurse practitioner, nutritionist, psychiatrist, social worker, or eating disorder counselor) is recommended for confirmed cases.

→ Patients can benefit from treatment modalities such as individual, group, family, or marital psychotherapy (Garner and Garfinkel 1985).

→ Most of the therapies mentioned above commonly have a psychodynamic and/or cognitive/behavioral orientation, described in depth in Garner and Garfinkel (1985). For simple but very handy suggestions in the behavioral/cognitive approach to the management of bulimia nervosa—which also can be applied to the anorexic patient—the reader is referred to an excellent article by Yanovsky (1991).

→ Evaluate depression and suicide risk in all eating disorder patients (see **Depression** Protocol).

→ Referral to dental care is indicated for evaluation and treatment of patients who purge with vomiting.

→ Discontinuation of diuretics or laxatives may lead temporarily to fluid retention and weight gain. A moderate restriction on sodium intake on a short-term basis may help if patient distressed by the weight gain (Yanovsky 1991).

→ Potassium supplementation is required if hypokalemia present. For values of ≥2.8 mEq, 20 mEq of potassium chloride 80 p.o. every day or BID is recommended. Patients with potassium levels <2.8 mEq should be considered for parenteral treatment and hospitalization (Herzog and Copeland 1985). Mild cases supplement by increasing the intake of foods rich in potassium.

→ For adolescents with a history that indicates high risk of developing eating disorders (i.e., engaging in activities which require a lean figure like dancing, modeling, acting) dietary history and corroboration with family or friends regarding intake may be helpful.

Anorexia nervosa

→ Pharmacotherapy has no place in the first-line approach to the treatment of this disorder. It has been ineffective in the promotion of food intake and weight gain, as well as in the management of anxiety and depression in patients with anorexia (Kennedy and Goldbloom 1991).

- Antidepressant medication is not always indicated in the treatment of depression in anorexics. Instead, ongoing psychotherapy is used instead to explore and change patient's attitudes and beliefs about herself.

Bulimia nervosa

→ Individual therapy under a practitioner who can manage the overall treatment plan is recommended, to allow a treatment relationship to develop. Group, family therapy, and pharmacotherapy then can be introduced as adjunct therapy (Herzog et al. 1991).

→ Antidepressant medications have been found to be effective in treating depression in bulimics.

- Fluoxetine hydrochloride (Prozac®) 20 mg has been recommended (Buckner 1991; Pope and Hudson 1989).

- Compliance is enhanced by lack of weight gain and absence of anticholinergic effects.

- The major side effect is nausea, which subsides after a few days. Anxiety and insomnia occur in 10 percent to 15 percent percent of patients and may require discontinuation of medication (Yanovsky 1991).

- Other antidepressants effective in treating depression in bulimics include imipramine, desipramine and phenelzine (Pope et al. 1983; Walsh et al. 1988).
  - A trial of several antidepressants may be necessary before one is found to be effective.
  - It should be stressed that drug therapy, alone, is less effective than intensive psychological treatment (Freeman and Munro 1988).

→ Monitor for severe constipation in patients who stop abusing laxatives. In severe cases of constipation—to prevent fecal impaction—osmotic laxatives such as lactulose can be used (Yanovsky 1991).

CONSULTATION

→ See "Treatment/Management" section.

→ A list of qualified psychotherapists can be obtained from the American Anorexia/Bulimia Association (AA/BA) 418 E. 76th Street, New York, New York 10021 (212) 734-1114.

PATIENT EDUCATION

→ Eating disorders should be dealt with in a nonjudgmental and supportive manner, with the clinician allowing discussion about emotions and behaviors, but willing to confront the patient.

→ Educate client about medical consequences and psychological effects of weight reduction and eating disorders. Stress importance of follow-up treatment if relapses occur (i.e., binge-purging in the bulimia patient, fasting in the anorexic).

→ Correct inaccurate beliefs about weight control with use of laxatives—i.e., how laxatives exert their effect in large intestine, while most of calories consumed are absorbed into the small intestine.

→ Advise patients to reduce risk of constipation by increasing dietary fiber, ensuring adequate fluid intake, maintaining exercise, and using bulk laxatives as needed (see **Constipation** Protocol).

→ Women with eating disorders need to be re-educated and reconditioned regarding their eating attitudes.

- Encourage patients to follow structured meal planning as an effective way to ensure balanced meals. By planning menu and meal times the patient may be less likely to fast and/or binge when she knows what and when she will be eating. Be firm and direct about meal planning. Many patients will resist, believing they will become overweight quickly (Mitchell 1991).

- Stress importance of eating several times a day at regular intervals to avoid the vicious cycle of fasting/hunger, which results in binge eating and vomiting in bulimic patients.

- Allow patient initially to exclude high-risk binge foods from the diet. It is important that the patient learn that food can be eaten in reasonable amounts.

- Educate patient on proper nutrition. Advise patient that a balanced diet (1800-2400 calories daily, eaten several times during the day) will not cause weight gain (Marshal 1991).

- Discuss modification of eating habits. Encourage client to always sit to eat, to always eat with others, and to plan to do something after the meal such as taking a walk, taking a bubble bath, or calling a friend.

- Encourage patient to keep a food diary to increase her understanding of what she eats and to help her recognize which feelings bring on the urge to eat.

- Assist patient in recognizing when she feels uncomfortable with a situation, person, thought, or feeling which may trigger an urge response (i.e., purge, binge, restrict). Discuss coping mechanisms that will help to avoid this response.

- Encourage patient to avoid trigger situations until there is some progress in recovery.

→ Teach patient that discussion of the above issues with treatment team members will foster self-monitoring of eating patterns and help her uncover exactly which behaviors/situations precipitate maladaptive eating habits.

→ Establish a contract with the patient (and her family) regarding a target body weight, along with a food contract. A food contract will include the amount and timing of food intake.

→ Teach patient an appropriate exercise program. Lead her to understand the compulsiveness of her past behavior and encourage her to exercise in a normal and enjoyable fashion.

→ Engage family members in management of eating disorders.

→ Patients with eating disorders may benefit from educational resources and support groups. These organizations, in addition, provide consultation and a listing of eating disorder professionals.

- Anorexia Nervosa and Related Eating Disorders, Inc.
  P.O. Box 5102
  Eugene, OR 97405
  (503) 344-1144 (24-hour hotline)
- Anorexia, Bulimia Care
  P.O. Box 213
  Lincoln Center, Massachusetts 01773
  (617) 259-9667
- Reader Institute
  800-255-1818

FOLLOW-UP

→ Prolonged outpatient treatment and sometimes hospitalization will be required for the management of anorexic patients. Powers (1990) describes the following criteria for outpatient treatment:

Candidates for outpatient treatment:
- patient has been ill less than a year.
- patient has lost <25 percent of ideal body weight.
- patient does not binge eat or purge.
- patient lives with an intact, family that cooperates with her treatment.

→ Hospitalization will be necessary if:
- medical complications are evident.
- patient has lost >25 percent of ideal body weight, especially if weight loss has been very rapid.
- anorexia is complicated with bulimia nervosa.
- patient is ill longer than a year.
- suicidal ideation is present.
- patient is living in a destructive family environment.

- incest has occurred and has not been discussed openly.
- outpatient treatment fails.

→ Weekly appointments, with the multidisciplinary team, for outpatient treatment of the anorexic/bulimic patient are required on a long-term basis. Relapse is common after any form of treatment.

→ Much of the follow-up care will be given by the eating disorders therapist. The primary care provider, along with the multidisciplinary team, must co-manage the patient's nutritional status, frequently monitoring it and staying alert to medical complications.

→ Ongoing psychological support of the patient and family is essential.

→ Document in progress notes and problem list.

APPENDIX 14E.1

Eating Attitudes Test

	Always	Very often	Often	Sometimes	Rarely	Never
Name: Date:						
1) I am terrified about being overweight.						
2) I avoid eating when I am hungry.						
3) I find myself preoccupied with food.						
4) I have gone on eating binges where I feel that I may not be able to stop.						
5) I cut my food into small pieces.						
6) I am aware of the calorie content of the foods that I eat.						
7) I particularly avoid foods with a high carbohydrate rate (e.g., bread, potatoes, rice, etc.).						
8) I feel that others would prefer if I ate more.						
9) I feel extremely guilty after eating.						
10) I am preoccupied with a desire to be thinner.						
11) I think about burning up calories when I exercise.						
12) Other people think that I am too thin.						
13) I am preoccupied with the thought of having fat on my body.						
14) I take longer than others to eat my meals.						
15) I avoid foods with sugar in them.						
16) I eat diet foods.						
17) I feel that food controls my life.						
18) I display self-control around food.						
19) I feel that others pressure me to eat.						
20) I give too much time and thought to food.						
21) I feel uncomfortable after eating sweets.						
22) I engage in dieting behavior.						
23) I like my stomach to be empty.						
24) I enjoy trying rich new foods.						
25) I have the impulse to vomit after meals.						
26) I vomit after I have eaten.						

Source: Reprinted with permission from Button, E.J. and Whitehouse, A. 1981. Subclinical anorexia nervosa. *Psychosomatic Medicine* 11:509-516. Copyright 1981 American Psychosomatic Society.

Susan L. Adams, R.N., N.P., M.S.

14-F

Sexual Abuse (Minors and Adult Survivors)

Sexual abuse occurs in a variety of forms including child sexual abuse (CSA)—i.e., incest, molestation, child pornography, rape—stranger, date, marital, care provider/client sexual relationships, and sexual harassment (Gise and Paddison 1988). For the purposes of this protocol, CSA as a condition for minors (under the age of 18 years) and for adult survivors will be the focus. Domestic violence, sexual assault, and sexual dysfunction are discussed in other protocols (see **Battering/Domestic Violence, Sexual Assault,** and **Sexual Dysfunction** protocols).

Definitions of CSA in the literature vary. The United States National Center on Child Abuse and Neglect (NCCAN) (1978) proposed the following definition: an act perpetrated upon a child by a significantly older person with the intent to stimulate the child sexually and to satisfy the aggressor's sexual impulses. This includes sexual abuse committed by another minor when that person is either significantly older than the victim or in a position of power or control over that child.

Although numerous definitions have appeared in the literature, Bachmann, Moeller, and Benett (1988) cite four major components that are consistently included: 1) the nature and purpose of the sexual activity; 2) the age and relationship of the perpetrator to the child; 3) the child's understanding of the activity; and, 4) the type of coercion used.

Sexual abuse can be *assaultive*—producing injury and resulting in severe emotional trauma—or *non-assaultive*—causing little if any physical injury and undetermined amounts of emotional stress (Kessler and Hyden 1991). There may only be one occurrence in an individual's life or abuse may be chronic and long-term.

The abuse can be *incestuous* (intrafamilial) or can be perpetrated by strangers.

There is a broad spectrum of sexually abusive behaviors including provocative nudity and disrobing; genital exposure; observation of the child undressing, bathing, excreting, or urinating (especially in older children capable of performing these functions without assistance); kissing in a lingering or intimate way; fondling; masturbation with the child observing; fellatio; cunnilingus; digital penetration of the anus and/or vagina; penile penetration of the anus and/or vagina, and "dry intercourse" (Sgroi, Blick, and Porter 1985). Infants as well as adolescents are victims, although the tendency is for victimization to decrease as the child becomes older and starts to question the appropriateness of the behaviors and is in a position to reject the approaches.

Reported incidences of CSA vary, depending on the setting for study populations and the definitions used to describe sexual abuse. For example, one of the highest rates of reported child sexual abuse (66 percent) was found among a population of pregnant adolescents in a Washington State study (Boyer and Fine 1992), and a 52 percent incest incidence was found among patients in an urban psychiatric emergency facility (Briere and Zaidi 1989). Russell (1983) cited a prevalence of 38 percent of women in a retrospective random San Francisco community sample where at least one occurrence of CSA was reported.

CSA is an international problem. For example, thirty-two percent of women at the University of Costa Rica (Krugman, Mata, and Krugman 1992) and 12 percent of women in Great Britain reported having been sexually abused (Baker and Duncan 1985).

Sexual abuse occurs regardless of socioeconomic class, occupational strata, urban or rural residency, education, religion, or ethnic background (Bachmann, Moeller, and Benett 1988). There appears to be a multigenerational pattern of abuse and dysfunctional family interactions. There have been difficulties in separating the effects of sexual abuse from those of other emotional and/or physical abuses within the family.

A possible profile for a victim of CSA includes: oldest female in a large family (four or more children) where substance abuse co-exists and that female is thrust into the parenting role. The father/stepfather is probably violent, especially toward family members who are not sexually abused. The mother is usually unaware of or dissociated from the abusive relationship and may lack essential mother/child interpersonal skills. The "secrecy factor" makes it possible for only the abuser and victim to be aware of the abuse in many cases (Gilgun 1984).

Survivors of CSA report difficulties with their own parenting skills and attitudes toward their children. Social isolation, disorganization, fear of disintegration, lack of trust, family unhappiness, and frequent conflict characterize the families of incestuous relationships (Bachmann, Moeller, and Benett 1988; Cole and Woolger 1989; Berth-Jones and Graham-Brown 1990; Finkelhor et al. 1990; Cole, et al. 1992).

Long-term sequelae of CSA can include physical complaints. For example Paddison et al. (1990) found a relationship between CSA and premenstrual syndrome (PMS). In a high socioeconomic group, 33 percent of women experiencing PMS were more likely to have been abused by a "friend" when compared with a low socioeconomic group where 52 percent of women (experiencing PMS) were more likely to have been abused by a relative.

Wurtele, Kaplan, and Keairnes (1990) reported a 28 percent incidence of sexual abuse prior to age 14 years in women experiencing chronic pain (back/neck, myofacial, carpal tunnel syndrome, chronic tension headaches). The authors hypothesized support for abuse/muscle tension/chronic pain linkage where musculoskeletal pain syndromes are assumed to be related to chronic and excessive contraction of the involved muscle groups.

Associations have been made between chronic pelvic pain and CSA (Harrop-Griffiths et al. 1988; Reiter et al. 1991). Reiter et al. (1991) found a correlation between sexual abuse and somatization in women with nonsomatic chronic pelvic pain and cautioned against the use of hysterectomy in this population until completion of thorough medical and psychological evaluations.

Psychological sequelae including depression, anxiety, low self-esteem, anger, guilt, self-blame, dissociation, obsessive-compulsive symptoms, panic disorders, phobias, and paranoid ideation have been reported (Brown and Garrison 1990; Cahill, Llewelyn, and Pearson 1991; Kreidler and Hassan 1992; Beitchman et al. 1992; Pribor and Dinwiddie 1992; Hall et al. 1994). There is evidence that incestuous experiences with fathers/stepfathers and the use of violence are more traumatic than non-incestuous ones (Beitchman et al. 1992).

Sexual dysfunction is commonly noted and includes desire dysfunction, arousal problems, adverse feeling states, and anorgasmia (Gise and Paddison 1988; Brown and Garrison 1990; Mackey et al. 1991). Revictimization and promiscuity have also been reported (Bachmann, Moeller, and Benett 1988; Beitchman et. al. 1992) and may predispose CSA survivors to STDs including human papillomavirus (HPV), herpes simplex virus (HSV), and human immunodeficiency virus (HIV) (Zierler et al. 1991).

Victims of CSA present to the clinical setting in a variety of situations. A child victim may enter care immediately after the occurrence for evaluation of injuries, or a grown adult woman may present herself several years later with complaints of physical, psychological, emotional, and/or social conditions where CSA is the underlying problem. Sensitivity from the primary health care provider is necessary.

Often, adults who were sexually abused as children seek therapy in the face of a seemingly unrelated crisis. If the trauma of sexual abuse is to be resolved successfully, therapy is recommended. However, Feinauer (1989) found that the quality of the individual's support system influenced the level of the person's adjustment to the trauma of sexual abuse and was possibly a more important determinant of adjustment than therapy.

Victims of CSA who are minor children must be removed from the unsafe environment. In the case of suspected child abuse, the law requires reporting to child protective services (CPS) agencies.

Scott (1992) studied the impact of CSA on the Los Angeles community's mental health status and determined that a history of CSA significantly increased an individual's odds of developing eight psychiatric disorders in adulthood, including substance abuse/dependence. Results indicated that continued prevention efforts aimed at eliminating CSA from the community hold extensive potential for improving everyone's quality of life. Economic benefits would also accrue because of the elimination of the financial strain of providing care for individuals experiencing the sequelae of CSA.

The primary objective of the physical examination in the case of current abuse is to address the medical needs of the victim. The secondary purpose is to collect samples that can be used later as evidence. Most police agencies, hospitals, and large health care institutions will have prepackaged rape or sexual abuse evidence kits and guidelines are available to assist care providers with performance of a complete and comprehensive examination (Indest 1989; Kessler and Hyden 1991; Muram 1992).

Minor Child—Under 18 Years Old

DATABASE

SUBJECTIVE

→ It is possible that an adolescent will present to a health care setting by herself.

→ Risk factors for CSA include:
- substance abuse in the home.
- coexisting physical/emotional abuse.
- family violence.
- multigenerational factors.

→ An adult may report suspicion of CSA.

→ Child may describe the abuse using sexually explicit terms to describe sexual behaviors.
- Most prepubescent children will not be capable of describing sexual behaviors unless they themselves have been exposed.

→ Child may be able to show sexual behaviors (e.g., fellatio, intercourse, fondling) using anatomically correct dolls.

→ Child may demonstrate hypersexual behavior including compulsive masturbation, promiscuity, prostitution.

→ Child may have nightmares/night terrors, phobic reactions, truancy, withdrawal/depression, clinging behaviors, poor school performance, running away, suicidal ideation, poor peer relationships, and other emotional disturbances.

→ Client may report history of:
- GI complaints—e.g., anorexia, vomiting, abdominal pain, rectal pain.
- genitourinary (GU) complaints—e.g., pelvic pain; urinary symptoms; vaginal itching, discharge, and/or pain; unexplained pregnancies.
- vague somatic complaints—e.g., headaches and muscle aches.

→ Client may report prior trauma, hospitalizations, contact with public health and/or social services (e.g., CPS).

→ Subjective data should be collected using the victim's own terms and direct quotes from any adult person involved with bringing the abuse to the attention of the health care provider.

OBJECTIVE

→ See **Sexual Assault** Protocol.

→ Client may present with:
- poor hygiene.
- extreme anxiety during pelvic examination.
- vaginitis and STDs—past and current (see **Vaginitis, Sexually Transmitted Diseases** protocols).
- unexplained pregnancy.

→ It is also possible that there is no physical evidence of CSA.

ASSESSMENT

→ R/O child sexual abuse

→ R/O coexisting forms of child abuse

→ R/O consensual sexual activity between minors

→ R/O substance abuse

→ R/O illness/injury (e.g., STDs, pregnancy, tissue trauma, psychiatric disorders, neurological disorders)

→ R/O presence of long-term sequelae

PLAN

→ See **Sexual Assault** Protocol (may vary depending on the age of the victim).

→ Consultation involves referral to child protective services for *any* suspected sexual abuse and/or physical abuse of a child under 18 years of age as required by law.
- The client should be advised that a report is being made.
- In California, health care providers who fail to report suspected abuse are guilty of a misdemeanor punishable by up to six months in jail and/or up to a $1,000 fine. He or she may also be found civilly liable for damages, especially if the child-victim or another child is further victimized because of the failure to report (Chaidez 1991).
- It is not necessary to report a minor when there is consensual sexual activity, unless the client and partner are of discrepant age (e.g., ages 12 years and 16 years or older). Review of local legal guidelines is advised.

Adult Survivor of CSA

DATABASE

SUBJECTIVE

→ All women are at risk for CSA regardless of age, race, socioeconomic status, or sexual preference.

→ Client may report history of:
- CSA.
- familial and/or personal substance/alcohol abuse.
- family violence/physical abuse.
- abusive relationships with male partners.
- psychological disorder—e.g., depression, suicide attempts, phobic reactions, borderline personality, eating disorders, panic attacks.
- contact with law enforcement and/or social service agencies—e.g., foster care placement, detention in juvenile hall.
- prostitution and/or multiple sexual partners.
- multiple visits to health care provider, presenting with vague somatic complaints including chronic musculoskeletal problems, headaches, sexual dysfunction, GU and GI complaints, sleep disorders, psychiatric complaints—e.g., depression, anxiety, panic attacks.

→ Client may report early age at first intercourse.

OBJECTIVE

→ There may be no physical evidence of past CSA.

→ Client may evidence conditions associated with stress including alopecia, hypertension, obesity, ulcers, and migraine headaches.

→ Client may appear restless, angry, defensive, anxious, and evasive and may demonstrate inappropriate affect and/or avoidance of eye contact.

→ Client may present with poor hygiene.

→ During the examination, the client may demonstrate a hesitation or refusal to undress and/or *extreme* anxiety reaction or overly compliant behavior.
- Unusual scars—including old cigarette burns, lacerations, pelvic trauma, especially in nulliparous women.
- STDs—e.g., HSV, HPV.

ASSESSMENT

→ R/O CSA .

→ R/O psychological disorder

→ R/O substance and/or alcohol abuse

→ R/O current domestic violence

→ R/O existing medical conditions, illnesses, and/or injuries—e.g., pelvic disease, ulcers, musculoskeletal disorders, STDs

→ R/O potential for death by suicide or homicide

→ R/O presence of long-term sequelae—e.g., sexual depression, panic disorders, promiscuity

PLAN

DIAGNOSTIC TESTS

→ What tests are necessary will depend on the nature of the complaint, condition, or injury.

TREATMENT/MANAGEMENT

→ Clinician should explore own feelings regarding CSA to determine if she or he can approach these women in a holistic, supportive, and nonjudgmental fashion.

→ Screen *all* women for past history of CSA, regardless of age, race, socioeconomic status, marital status, or sexual preference.

→ Assess living arrangements and support systems.

→ Provide service to address the client's chief complaint or concern.
- Usually the client will not present to the clinic with the complaint of CSA.
- The history is elicited after she presents with another need—e.g., STD evaluation, pregnancy, pelvic pain, contraception, annual examination.

→ Integrate the history of CSA into the treatment plan for all medical, social, and psychological services.

→ Communicate history of CSA to the client's other care providers but only with her consent.

→ Referral for psychological counseling/therapy is recommended for individual client and family as indicated.

→ Referral to support groups for incest survivors is recommended.

→ Referral to 12-Step programs is recommended for alcohol abuse, substance abuse, codependency, or adult children of alcoholics (depending on history).

→ Referral to other community agencies depending on client needs (e.g., parenting classes, legal support services, social services) is recommended.

→ Encourage stress management strategies for clients who are feeling the effects of past CSA in their lives—e.g., use of an informed support network (intimate partners, friends), rest, exercise, recreation, adequate nutrition, meditation, contact with the therapist.

CONSULTATION

→ Consult with physician per protocol regarding medical conditions.

→ Consult with social service agents to provide assistance with legal, financial, housing issues.

→ Consult with psychological/psychiatric services in suspected cases of psychological disorders and/or substance abuse.

PATIENT EDUCATION

→ Educate client about CSA—incidence, possible sequelae, multigenerational factors, and risks to her in future relationships, especially with her own children.

→ Assure the client that she is not alone. Many women share this problem and respond to it in a variety of ways.

→ Encourage client to find means of self-actualization to empower herself and build self-esteem—e.g., through education, employment, community outreach, fertility control, assertiveness training.

→ In some situations, education of client about what constitutes abuse and validation of her experience as an abusive event may be necessary.

→ Inform client of the availability of supportive services in the communities to discuss CSA. Encourage her to utilize these services.

→ Explain the rationale for all examination procedures and treatments.
  ▪ Advise the client that if she is experiencing too much discomfort, the examination will be stopped immediately and a reassessment made to evaluate why she is experiencing pain.

→ Counsel client regarding high-risk behaviors that could jeopardize her health—e.g., STDs (including HIV infection, unwanted pregnancy, abusive relationships).

FOLLOW-UP

→ Continue to monitor at future visits.

→ Be aware that life events/changes may predispose the client to crisis—e.g., new relationships, pregnancy, death of the abuser.

→ Document appropriately in progress notes and problem list. The sensitive nature of the subject requires discretion concerning what is written in the medical record.

14-G

Sexual Assault

Sexual assault is defined as any sexual act performed by a person on another person without his or her consent (Moscarello 1991). The term, *rape*, is usually more narrowly defined as sexual intercourse without consent. In contrast, statutory rape occurs when a person is defined by statute as being incapable of consenting because she/he is under a specific age. For the purposes of this protocol, the terms sexual assault and rape will be used interchangeably. Sexually assaulted children, sexually assaulted males, and incest survivors have special needs that will not be addressed in this protocol.

The actual prevalence of rape is unknown, but estimates are that it affects one out of every six women (Beebe 1991). In 1987, 91,000 rapes and attempted rapes were reported (Sampselle 1991). This is probably a gross underestimate of actual numbers, however, since reported assaults are estimated to represent only 10 percent to 30 percent of the total (Glaser et al. 1991).

The majority of rapes are committed by men who are not strangers to their victims—dates, spouses, long-term partners, and relatives (e.g., fathers, uncles, brothers, cousins) (Schwartz 1991). Although marital rape may occur in 10 percent to 14 percent of all marriages, 21 states still have marital exclusion laws (Schwartz 1991).

The etiology of rape is complex and involves many sociocultural factors including acceptance of interpersonal violence, adversarial perception of heterosexual relations, acceptance of rape myths, and sex role stereotyping.

The evidence as to whether or not certain women are more vulnerable to rape is inconclusive. However, studies have shown that women who were sexually abused as children may be at higher risk for rape as adults. In addition, there is research that connects violence portrayed in the media with violent behavior in society (Schwartz 1991).

About 40 percent of sexual assault victims sustain physical injuries. One percent of these require hospitalization, while 0.1 percent are fatal (ACOG 1992). Although most of the physical injuries sustained during sexual assault are minor and resolve fairly soon, the psychological damage is much more likely to last for months or years after the assault.

Burgess and Holmstrom (1974) described the response of women to assault as the *rape trauma syndrome*, a constellation of physical and psychological symptoms. The syndrome consists of two phases: *acute* and *delayed* or *organizational*.

The acute phase may last for hours or days and is characterized by an alteration in coping mechanisms. The woman may appear to be in control of her behavior or completely out of control. She may exhibit disorganization, shock, and disbelief. She may also express fear and anger and have episodes of crying. Other signs and symptoms include anorexia, nausea and vomiting, abdominal pain, pelvic pain, muscle aches, headaches, sleep disturbances such as insomnia and nightmares, vaginal itching and discharge, rectal pain, and emotional problems including anxiety, sexual dysfunction, depression, and mood swings.

The delayed or organizational phase can last for months or years. The woman may experience flashbacks, phobias, nightmares, suicidal ideation, and gynecological and menstrual complaints, and engage in substance abuse.

Today, the responses of sexual assault survivors to their ordeals often are described in the broader context of *post-traumatic stress disorder* (PTSD) (Ruch et al. 1991). This disorder was added to the *Diagnostic and Statistical Manual of Mental Disorders* in 1980 as an anxiety disorder after it was determined that victims of many types of psychological trauma (e.g., terrorism, war, torture, violent crimes, and natural disasters) exhibit similar symptoms.

To meet the diagnostic criteria for PTSD, a person must have experienced an event outside the range of normal experience and have symptoms that last longer than one month in each of the following areas: 1) persistent re-experiencing of the trauma, 2) avoidance of stimuli associated with the trauma or a numbing of general responsiveness, and 3) persistent symptoms of increased arousal and anxiety (Bownes, O'Gorman, and Sayers 1991).

Although after experiencing an assault most women initially meet these criteria, their symptoms usually subside by the fourth month after the rape. However, a proportion of survivors remain symptomatic for years afterward (Bownes, O'Gorman, and Sayers 1991). In one study, Rothbaum et al. (1990) found that 94 percent of rape victims met the criteria for PTSD shortly after the assault, 47 percent still suffered from PTSD three months after the assault, and 16.5 percent had persistent symptoms of PTSD 17 years after the attack.

Women who have a history of depression, suicide attempts, substance abuse, sexual abuse, or sexual assault may have a more severe response to a sexual assault (Moscarello 1991). The nature of the assault, the client's locus of control, coping ability, life stress, personality variables, social networks, and developmental stage also help to determine the intensity of the response (Ruch et al. 1991).

When caring for assault survivors, health care providers must address their medical, legal, and emotional needs. Since the physical injuries sustained are usually minor, many emergency rooms and sexual assault centers are now using specially trained nurses, referred to as *sexual assault nurse examiners* (SANEs), to care for these clients.

SANE programs were developed in response to a lack of experienced health care providers trained to meet the special needs of assault survivors in a sensitive and standardized fashion. For a listing of SANE programs see "Sexual Assault Nurse Examiners: A SANE Way to Care for Rape Victims" (Lenehan 1991), in the bibliography.

SANEs receive specialized training regarding the physical and emotional sequelae of rape, crisis intervention counseling, law enforcement procedures, forensics, evidence collection, colposcopy, and the criminal justice system. They examine victims, collect evidence,

provide counseling and follow-up care, and testify in court.

DATABASE

NOTE: If the assault has occured within the last 72 hours, it is strongly recommended (and, in some communities, required) that the client be referred to a designated sexual assault center or emergency room with trained sexual assault nurse/physician examiners for the completion of an evidentiary examination using a rape kit. The examination may be completed even if the survivor is unsure regarding prosecution. The following material regarding the examination is provided for informational purposes only.

SUBJECTIVE

→ The survivor should be interviewed and examined as soon as possible after the incident in a private, quiet, comfortable environment. She may wish to have a family member, partner, friend, rape crisis counselor, or advocate from a sexual assault organization present.
- Client may describe episode(s) of sexual assault.
- Client may report history of:
  • GI complaints—e.g., anorexia, nausea, vomiting, abdominal, or rectal pain.
  • GU complaints—e.g., vaginal itching, discharge, pelvic pain, menstrual complaints.
  • vague somatic complaints—e.g., headaches, muscle aches.
  • sleep disturbances—e.g., insomnia, nightmares.
  • emotional disturbances—e.g., anxiety, depression, suicidal ideation, mood swings, flashbacks, phobias, sexual dysfunction, substance abuse, diminished interest in usual activities.
- Client may report feeling detached from others.
- Client may be unable to recall important aspects of the trauma.

→ Obtain a *complete* health history from survivor.

OBJECTIVE

→ Use of evidence collection protocol is recommended (see **Appendix 14G.1, Sexual Assault Examination and Forensic Report Form**, p. 14-50).
- Obtain the client's consent for examination and evidence collection.
  • Ideally, all evidence should be collected before the client bathes, urinates, defecates,

douches, washes out her mouth, or cleans her fingernails.

- If the assault occurred in the 72 hours prior to the examination, an evidence collection kit should be used.
- The client should undress standing on paper to catch any fibers or debris that fall from her body or clothing.
  - All clothing is kept in separate paper bags, instead of plastic, to discourage bacterial growth.
  - Any wet stains should be allowed to air dry before bagging.
- A complete physical examination should be performed in all cases of sexual assault, regardless of the length of time which has elapsed since the assault. Note the following:
  - affect: Client may appear fearful, angry, disorganized, seem to be in complete control, or have a restricted range of affect.
  - presence of slurred/incoherent speech or uneven gait.
  - bruises, abrasions, bite marks, lacerations, fractures, restraint or strangulation marks, stab and/or gunshot wounds.
    - The most common sites of trauma include the genitals, mouth, throat, wrists, arms, breasts, and thighs (Beebe 1991).
  - presence of foreign objects in vagina, urethra, rectum, ear, nose, or mouth.
  - lacerations, ecchymosis, and edema in the area of the posterior fourchette (the greatest point of stress associated with forced stretching during penile penetration).
    - These mounting injuries may be enhanced for visualization with the application of toluidine blue or the use of colposcopy (Slaughter and Brown 1992).

ASSESSMENT

- → Sexual assault
- → R/O serious trauma
- → R/O concurrent domestic violence
- → R/O potential for death by suicide or homicide
- → R/O coexisting child abuse
- → R/O substance abuse
- → R/O STDs
- → R/O pregnancy
- → R/O presence of long-term sequelae

PLAN

DIAGNOSTIC TESTS

- → It is essential that the chain of evidence not be broken. All specimens should be labeled, dated, sealed, and locked up until the appropriate law enforcement official takes possession of them.
- → Appropriate tests (e.g., x-rays) should be ordered to rule out physical trauma.
- → If bite marks are present, a forensic odontologist should make a cast and document the findings.
- → The victim's head and pubic hair should be combed while she stands over paper.
  - Obtaining pubic hairs is controversial, but some jurisdictions request that they be collected.
- → The oral cavity may be swabbed to recover seminal fluid/sperm. Oral washings may also be done depending upon the lab facilities available.
  - The client may wash out her mouth with clear water after the samples are taken. She then is instructed not to eat, drink, or smoke for 30 minutes, at which time a saliva sample is taken.
- → Blood and saliva samples are taken to determine the ABO secretor status of the victim.
  - ABO factors are found in everyone's blood but they are also found in other body secretions—semen, saliva, and vaginal secretions—in about 75 percent to 80 percent of the population. The remaining 20 percent to 25 percent are *non-secretors*.
- → A Wood's light is used to check the perineum and thighs for blood or semen.
  - The dried secretions are then collected with saline-moistened cotton swabs.
- → Any semen present is collected from the vagina, cervix, or rectum.
  - Because sperm contain DNA, they can be used to identify the assailant.
  - Motile sperm can be detected in the vagina for up to 8 hours, from cervical mucus for 2 to 3 days, and from the rectum for an undetermined amount of time.
  - Non-motile sperm can be detected in the vagina for up to 24 hours, from the cervix for up to 17 days, and from the rectum for 24 hours (ACOG 1992).
- → If no sperm are present (i.e., the perpetrator had no ejaculation or had undergone a vasectomy), seminal plasma components (prostatic antigen p30 and acid phosphatase) may be found in the vagina, rectum, mouth, skin, or clothing for up to

several hours and can be used to identify semen and the ABO blood type of secretors.

→ Collection of vaginal secretions for DNA fingerprinting is recommended.

→ Collection of saliva to check for major blood group antigens is recommended.

→ Collection of fingernail scrapings to look for the skin and blood of the attacker is recommended.

→ Obtain specimens for blood tests, wet mounts, and cultures for the diagnosis and treatment of existing infections (e.g., candidiasis, gonorrhea, chlamydia, syphilis, herpes, HIV, trichomoniasis, Hepatitis B, and bacterial vaginosis).
NOTE: HIV testing should be done at the time of the initial examination. If this test is negative, advise the woman to have repeat testing at 3 months and 6 months after the initial test.

→ Obtain specimen for pregnancy test if indicated.

→ Toxicology blood/urine screens are *not* routinely performed.

TREATMENT/MANAGEMENT

→ See "Subjective," "Objective," and "Diagnostic Tests" sections.

→ Offer mouthwash, soap, and a clean set of clothes to the client. She might want to shower after the examination.

→ Although the risk of contracting an STD is usually small, prophylactic antibiotics should be provided.
  ▪ The following regimen is effective against gonorrhea, chlamydia, trichomoniasis, bacterial vaginosis, and incubating syphilis (CDC 1993):
  • ceftriaxone 125 mg I.M. in a single dose
    PLUS
  • metronidazole 2 grams p.o. in a single dose
    PLUS
  • doxycycline 100 mg p.o. BID for 7 days.
    NOTE: Warn client not to use alcoholic beverages for 24 to 48 hours after taking metronidazole.

→ Though the risk of pregnancy is only 2 percent to 4 percent, a "morning-after" regimen for pregnancy prevention should be offered as follows: a total of 200 mcg of ethinyl estradiol plus 2.0 mg norgestrel or 1.0 mg levonorgestrel. Regimens include:
  ▪ Ovral® 2 tablets STAT then 2 tablets 12 hours later
    OR

  ▪ Lo/Ovral®, Nordette®, Levlen®, Triphasil®, or Tri-Levlen® (yellow pills only) 4 tablets STAT then 4 tablets 12 hours later (Hatcher et al. 1994).
  ▪ The following may be used for nausea (from the morning-after pill) (Hatcher et al. 1994):
    • non-prescription drugs:
      –dimenhydrenate (Dramamine®) 50 mg tablets, 1 or 2 tablets p.o. every 4 to 6 hours.
      –cyclizine hydrochloride (Marezine®) 50 mg tablets, 1 tablet p.o. every 4 to 6 hours.
    • prescription drugs (Warn client not to drink alcoholic beverages or use dangerous equipment):
      –trimethobenzamide hydrochloride (Tigan®) 250 mg tablets, 1 tablet every 8 hours, or 200 mg rectal suppositories, 1 suppository every 8 hours.
      –promethazine hydrocloride (Phenergan®) 25 mg tablets, 1 tablet every 12 hours, or 25 mg rectal suppositories, 1 suppository every 12 hours.

→ Offer tetanus prophylaxis if indicated.

→ Offer Hepatitis B prophylaxis (CDC 1993):
  ▪ .06 ml/kg of Hepatitis B immune globulin (HBIG) in a single I.M. dose with 14 days of exposure. HBIG should be followed by the standard 3-dose immunization series with Hepatitis B virus (HBV) vaccine beginning at the time of HBIG administration.

→ Provide crisis intervention counseling.

→ Provide informational brochure about sexual assault, if available.
  ▪ Copies may be obtained from:
  Texas Department of Health, Bureau of Emergency Management Sexual Assault Prevention and Crisis Services Program
  1100 West 49th St.
  Austin, TX 78756-3199
  (512) 458-7550

→ If domestic violence is suspected, see **Battering/ Domestic Violence** Protocol.

CONSULTATION

→ Consultation with a physician is required if serious injuries are evidenced or suspected.
  ▪ General guidelines include, but are not limited to:
  • history of loss of consciousness.
  • lack of orientation.
  • chest or abdominal pain.

- head/neck/back injury.
- limited range of motion of extremities.
- history of foreign object insertion, or
- perineal laceration.

→ Consultation with psychological/psychiatric services with special training in sexual assault is necessary if suicidal ideation, substance abuse, or other emotional disturbances are present.

→ Consultation with appropriate law enforcement officials is required regarding the collection, storage, and transportation of evidence. Consultation is also indicated if the assault was part of the broader problem of domestic violence with homicidal intent and/or concurrent child abuse.

→ As needed for prescription(s).

PATIENT EDUCATION

→ Explain the rationale for examination procedures, cultures, and prophylactic medications.

→ Explain side effects of all medications. Refer to *Physicians' Desk Reference (PDR)*.

→ Explain that the examination and evidence collection can be done regardless of whether the woman decides to report the rape to the police.

→ Reassure client that women respond to assault in a variety of ways and that her feelings are normal.

→ Provide client with telephone number of victim assistance program, if available.

→ Explain that in some jurisdictions, a rape survivor can request that her assailant be tested for HIV.

→ Provide client with telephone numbers of law enforcement, psychological and medical services, and HIV hotline.

→ Health promotion/maintenance and prevention for all women:

- since *all* women are at risk for assault, all women should be screened for sexual violence.
- utilize strategies in your practice that empower women—e.g., allowing women to have control over their health care; talking to clients while they are still fully clothed; teaching women about their bodies.
- inform patients that violence is not a normal part of relationships.
- provide clients with alternative methods of conflict resolution.
- discourage rigid sex role stereotyping.
- teach teens the warning signals regarding date rape and tactics for resisting peer pressure.
- encourage assertiveness, leadership skill building, and self-defense in female clients.

FOLLOW-UP

→ The client's emotional status should be re-evaluated 24 to 48 hours after the initial assessment, and, if indicated, long-term counseling offered. Follow-up contacts should be carried out in a very discreet manner.

→ The client should return for medical follow-up in four to six weeks (or sooner as indicated). Evaluation may include repeat STD cultures and syphilis serology (VDRL or RPR) unless prophylaxis was provided. A pregnancy test as indicated.

→ Recommend repeat HIV test in three months (or test assailant then re-test three months later).

→ The sexual assault nurse examiner may be required to testify on behalf of the client if the case goes to trial.

→ Document in progress notes and problem list.
- Events should be recorded accurately and injuries documented with drawings or photographs.

APPENDIX 14G.1

Sexual Assault Examination and Forensic Report Form

SEXUAL ASSAULT EXAMINATION FORM

Please print legibly. To be filled out with medical information gathered from the survivor. Please inform the survivor that, should the case go to court, it may be necessary to gather additional evidence at a later time. Please fill in all spaces with information or N/A.

Name of Survivor: _____ DOB: _____ Sex: _____ Race: _____

Address: _____ Phone: _____

Survivor Brought in by: _____ Agency or Relationship of Escort: _____

Survivor Number: _____ Law Enforcement Case Number: _____

Exam Date: _____ Time of Collection: _____ Date of Assault: _____ Time of Assault: _____

Number of Assailant(s): _____ Sex of Assailant(s): _____ Race of Assailant(s): _____

_____

VITAL SIGNS: Time: _____ Blood Pressure: _____ Pulse: _____

Respiration: _____ Temperature: _____

Known Allergies: _____

Current Medications: _____

HISTORY OF ASSAULT: (Survivor's description of pertinent details of the assault—oral, rectal, vaginal penetration; digital penetration or use of foreign object; oral contact by assailant; oral contact by survivor; ejaculation and location of such, if known by survivor.)

_____

_____

_____

_____

_____

Prior to evidence collection, survivor has: _____ Douched _____ Wiped/Washed _____ Bathed
_____ Showered _____ Urinated _____ Defecated _____ Vomited _____ Had Food or Drink
_____ Brushed Teeth or Used Mouthwash _____ Changed Clothes _____ Other _____ None of the Above

At time of assault, was:
Contraceptive foam or spermicide present?   _____ Yes _____ No _____ Unknown
Lubricant used by assailant?   _____ Yes _____ No _____ Unknown
   What kind? _____
Condom used by assailant?   _____ Yes _____ No _____ Unknown
   During entire assault?   _____ Yes _____ No _____ Unknown
Tampon present?   _____ Yes _____ No _____ Unknown
Survivor menstruating?   _____ Yes _____ No _____ Unknown
Assailant injured during assault?   _____ Yes _____ No _____ Unknown   If so, where _____

Was there penetration?   _____ Oral _____ Vaginal _____ Rectal _____ Other _____ Unknown
Did he ejaculate?   _____ Oral _____ Vaginal _____ Rectal _____ Other _____ Unknown

At time of exam, was tampon present? _____ Yes _____ No   Menstruation at time of exam? _____ Yes _____ No
Was survivor bleeding from any wounds inflicted by assailant? _____ Yes _____ No   If so, where? _____

Where did the assault take place? _____
When was the survivor's most recent sexual contact with a male up to 1 week prior to the assault? _____
Race of that individual _____
If the response is less than 24 hours, inform the survivor of the possibility that blood and semen samples may be requested from that individual at a later date.

SIGNIFICANT PAST MEDICAL HISTORY:
Last normal menstrual period: _____
Has she used vaginal tampons?: _____
Contraceptives?: _____
Vaginal surgical procedures: _____

GENERAL APPEARANCE: (behavior, affect) _____
_____
_____

BODY SURFACE INJURIES: (Include all details of trauma; abrasions, bite marks; presence of blood or other secretions on body.)
_____
_____
_____
_____

BODY DIAGRAMS: Document injuries and observations on the attached body diagrams.

GENITAL EXAMINATION:
Labia Majora _____
Labia Minora _____
Wood's Lamp _____
Hymen _____
Vagina _____
Cervix _____ Penis/Scrotum _____
Uterus, Adnexae _____ Rectum _____
Colposcope _____ Guiac _____
Check for Sperm _____ Positive _____ Negative   Motile _____ Yes _____ No

Document injuries and observations on the attached diagrams of genitalia.

DIAGNOSTIC TESTS: (Do not include in evidence collection kit)
_____ Pregnancy Test: _____ Positive _____ Negative
_____ VDRL/FTA/RPR
_____ GC Cultures: _____ Oral _____ Vaginal _____ Urethral _____ Rectal
_____ Chlamydia Cultures: _____ Vaginal _____ Urethral _____ Rectal
_____ Additional tests

TREATMENT:
Prophylaxis for STD: __ Yes __ No   Medication: _____ Dosage: _____ Time: _____ RN: _____
Prophylaxis for Pregnancy: __ Yes __ No   Medication: _____ Dosage: _____ Time: _____ RN: _____
Other prescribed medication: Medication: _____ Dosage: _____ Time: _____ RN: _____
Condition: _____
Tetanus Toxoid Given: __ Yes __ No
Surgical Procedures: _____

COMMUNICABLE DISEASES OR RISK TO LAB PERSONNEL: (e.g., Hepatitis, TB, Herpes, HIV, etc.) and/or presence of parasites (e.g., head lice, pubic lice, body lice, mites, etc.)
_____

EVIDENCE ITEMS INCLUDED IN KIT

___ # of Oral Swabs (2)   ___ # of External Penile Swabs (2)   ___ Fingernail Scrapings   ___ Tampon, diaper,
___ # of Oral Smears (1)   ___ # of External Penile Smears (1)   ___ Head Hair Combings & Comb   sanitary pad, sponge
___ # of Vaginal Swabs (4)   ___ # of Saliva Swabs (2)   ___ Head Hair Pulled Standards   ___ Dried Blood Stains
___ # of Rectal Swabs (4)   ___ # of Yellow Blood Tube(s)   ___ Pubic Hair Combings & Comb   ___ Foreign Matter
___ # of Rectal Smears (1)   ___ # of Purple Blood Tube(s)   ___ Pubic Hair Pulled Standards
    ___ # of Red Blood Tube(s)   ___ Panties (if they fit in box)

___ Other (Please Specify) _____

EVIDENCE ITEMS NOT INCLUDED IN THE KIT

___ Clothing ___ # of paper bags ___ Photographs ___ x-rays ___ Other _____ (Specify)
(Available)

(Please list clothing or miscellaneous items)

Article	**Description** (tears or stains)
_____	_____
_____	_____
_____	_____
_____	_____

PATIENT FOLLOW-UP CARE/LEGAL CHECKLIST:

____ GYN/Medical/STD follow-up appointment   ____ Yes ____ No
____ Sexual assault counseling referral   ____ Yes ____ No
____ Written and verbal information given to patient   ____ Yes ____ No
____ Medical facility received permission to contact survivor ____ by telephone ____ by mail ___ permission denied
____ Authorization for Release of Evidence to Law Enforcement Agency completed   ____ Yes ____ No
____ Law enforcement/Children's Protective Services notified if suspect child abuse   ____ Yes ____ No

Impressions from exam:
_____
_____
_____
_____

_____   _____
Examining Physician/Nurse Examiner - Signature   Assisting Nurse - Signature

_____   _____
Physician/Nurse Examiner - Printed Name   Assisting Nurse - Printed Name

Name of Hospital _____   Address _____

City _____   State _____ Zip _____

Request for Medical Examination, Treatment, Collection of Forensic Evidence, and Release of Medical Records

I hereby authorize _____ to perform a medical examination, treatment and the
                                 (Name of Hospital)
collection of forensic evidence. I further permit the release of copies of the complete report to include the examination
and tests to the law enforcement agency. I release _____ and its representatives
                                                   (Name of Hospital)
from legal responsibility or liability for the release of this information.

_____
Signature of Survivor or Parent or Guardian

Note: If the parent or guardian is not available for signature, child may be examined for sexual abuse under _____
civil statute.
                                                                     (State)

RECEIPT OF INFORMATION

I have received the following items (check those which apply):

____ One sealed evidence kit ____ x-rays or copies of x-rays ____ Photographs ____ Sealed clothing bag(s)
____ # of bags
____ Other _____

Signature of person receiving
information and/or articles: _____ Date _____ Time _____

ID #/Badge #/Title _____ Agency _____

Name of person releasing articles:

_____   _____
Printed Name   Signature

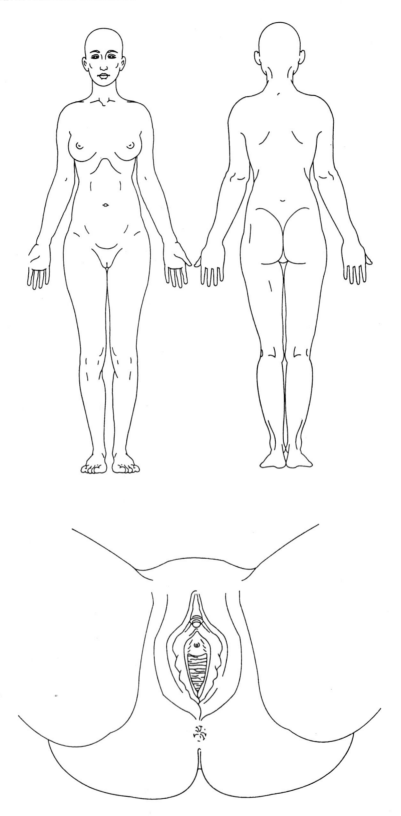

14-H

Smoking Cessation

Despite the recent decline of cigarette smoking, tobacco use remains the single most preventable cause of death and disability in the United States (McGinnis and Foege 1993). One in six deaths is attributable to smoking (Rose 1991). In the United States, smoking causes more deaths each year than the combined deaths from the First World War and the Korean and Vietnam wars (Godenick 1989).

It is estimated that 1,000 people die each day from tobacco-related illnesses—the equivalent of the number of passengers in three jumbo jet crashes without survivors every day. Yet the public perceives greater health risks from nuclear power plants, acquired immune deficiency syndrome (AIDS), handgun injuries, and suicide than from smoking (Houston 1992). In reality, smoking causes more deaths per year than AIDS, motor vehicle accidents, alcohol, homicide, drugs, and suicide combined (Koop 1988).

Eighty-three percent of lung cancer cases and 30 percent of all other cancers are attributed to smoking (American Cancer Society 1990). Smoking causes 85 percent of incidences of chronic obstructive pulmonary disease (COPD), the second leading cause of worker disability in the United States (Frank and Jaen 1993). In terms of health care costs and lost worker productivity, smoking costs an estimated $200 billion a year (Fielding 1985; Rose 1991). Smoking also increases risk for peptic ulcer disease, exacerbates allergies and asthma, and causes premature wrinkling of the skin and periodontal disease. Half of the 5,000 deaths per year from house fires are a result of fires started by someone smoking (Joseph and Byrd 1989).

Women have special concerns regarding reproduction and fertility when they smoke. Infertility is more common in smokers as a result of irregular menses and amenorrhea associated with the hormonal changes related to nicotine. Nicotine interferes with the normal release of gonadotropins which can result in menstrual irregularities as well as hirsutism, early menopause, and accelerated osteoporosis.

It is known that ectopic pregnancy risk is increased by smoking, though exactly why is under investigation (Fredriccson and Gilljam 1992). Miscarriage is almost twice as high in smokers as compared to nonsmokers. There is also increased risk for premature birth, polyhydraminos, placenta previa, and premature rupture of membranes. These complications are thought to be caused by the compensatory hypertrophy of the placenta as it competes for oxygen with the carbon monoxide produced by cigarette smoking.

Smoking reduces birth weight and is the most important factor influencing birth weight when compared to alcohol, caffeine, and socioeconomic variables. With cigarette consumption of greater than 10 per day, there is increased risk of sudden infant death syndrome (SIDS) . Finally, cleft palate malformation has been identified in some studies as occurring more frequently in smoking mothers (Fredriccson and Gilljam 1992).

History of Tobacco

Tobacco is native to the Americas. The ritual of smoking was adopted from Native Americans by American settlers in the 1800s. In 1884, the cigarette rolling machine was invented, allowing the mass production of cigarettes. By World War I, tobacco was considered as indispensable as food and was included in ration packets distributed to Americans on the home front.

The prevalence of smoking continued to increase from the 1920s to 1960s because of advertising strategies and the association of smoking with the glamour and adventure of Hollywood. During World War II, President Franklin D. Roosevelt declared tobacco an essential crop, giving draft deferments to tobacco growers. Seventy-five percent of American tobacco production was consumed by the American military forces. Smoking became an entrenched part of American culture. Even the journals of the American Medical Association (AMA) accepted cigarette advertisements (Houston 1992).

In 1941, the seminal work of two physicians, Oschner and DeBakey, called attention to the similarity of the curve of increased sales of cigarettes to the greater prevalence of lung cancer (Wynder and Graham 1950). Nine years later, Wynder and Graham (1950) published their results of a well-designed study linking cigarette smoking with bronchiogenic carcinoma.

In 1964, the U.S. Surgeon General issued the first public report linking smoking with negative health consequences. Despite more than 60,000 documents proving the relationship between smoking and lung cancer, 30 percent of all other cancers, cardiovascular disease, and COPD, the tobacco industry denies this evidence and claims there exists legitimate scientific controversy regarding these studies (Houston 1992). Spending an estimated $3.5 billion a year on advertising and promotion of its products, the tobacco industry is a powerful political lobby, its clout being the chief reason why it has no regulatory body controlling its advertising or production of cigarettes.

Smoking Cessation

Twenty-eight percent of all Americans smoke, the lowest percentage in years, down from 40 percent in 1965. Though there are now more Americans who have quit smoking than who currently smoke, 46 million Americans still smoke (Kahn 1993). The fastest growing group of new smokers is adolescents, with girls outpacing boys. Most current smokers started to smoke as preteens or adolescents. Among current female smokers, more are likely to be separated or divorced, younger than 25 years old, have less than a high school education, and make less than $20,000 a year (Still 1993).

Seventy percent of smokers see a health care provider at least once a year (Houston 1992). These visits are often a consequence of smoking-related illness, predisposing the smoker to intervention and teaching. Most surveys document that 70 percent to 90 percent of smokers want to quit and that more than half will make at least one serious attempt (Houston 1992; Solberg et al. 1990).

Seventy percent of patients report that a firm, supportive message from their doctor acts as a motivator to quit (Frank and Jaen 1993). Most physicians feel that counseling patients to quit smoking is as important as counseling for weight control or screening for breast cancer, yet approximately one-half of all internists never help the smoker pick a quit date (Cummings, Rubin, and Oster 1989). Fewer than 50 percent of smokers report being advised by their provider to quit smoking, and only four percent report receiving help from their provider to do so.

Minimal contact and limited time strategies are effective in helping clients quit. Interventions of only two minutes duration, long enough to deliver a smoking cessation message along with printed self-help materials, increase one-year cessation rates (Russell 1979). Results improve with longer interventions, follow-up, and written materials, with success rates at one year varying between five percent to 25 percent (Houston 1992; Schwarz 1985). It is important to recognize that though these numbers may seem small, when dealing with large numbers, five percent to 25 percent can make a difference. For example, if only five percent of the 32 million smokers who go to a health care provider this year receive a smoking cessation message with printed self-help materials, as many as 1.6 million smokers might quit.

Cessation is difficult because nicotine is a psychoactive drug with effects that reinforce smoking behavior despite known health risks (Milhorne 1989). Studies have shown nicotine to be more addictive than heroin or cocaine (Koop 1988). Nicotine acts on receptor sites in the peripheral and central nervous systems and has the capacity to both excite and inhibit many neurohormonal pathways.

Nicotine replacement therapies are thought to be useful by reducing the withdrawal symptoms associated with abstinence. Numerous studies of smokers wanting to quit indicate a decrease in the irritability and discomfort of abstinence when using nicotine gum or a patch (Benowitz 1993; Lee and D'Alonzo 1993; Robbins 1993). Initial smoking cessation is dramatic, but at one year relapse rates are 75 percent.

The literature demonstrates cessation rates of 25 percent for either gum or patch, twice the rate of placebo (Benowitz 1993; Gora 1993; Robbins 1993). In contrast to most studies, Gilbert et al. (1989) found no evidence of enhanced quit rates when Nicorette® gum was added to a comprehensive intervention package offered to all smokers in a primary care setting. This study differed from others in that it included all smokers and not just smokers motivated to quit.

Table 14H.1. ONE-YEAR CESSATION RATES WITH INTERVENTION—MINIMUM ONE-YEAR FOLLOW-UP

Intervention	No. of Trials	Range (%)	Median (%)
Self-help	7	12-33	18
Nicotine gum	9	8-38	11
Nicotine gum and counseling	11	12-49	29
Hypnosis	8	13-68	19.5
Acupuncture	6	8-32	27
Physician advice or counseling	12	3-13	6
Physician advice—intensive	10	13-38	22.5
Physician intervention			
Pulmonary patients	6	25-76	31.5
Cardiac patients	16	11-73	43
Rapid smoking cessation technique	6	6-40	21
Group	31	5-71	28
Multiple programs	17	6-76	40

Source: Reprinted from Schwartz, J.L. 1987. Review and evaluation of smoking cessation methods: The United States and Canada, 1978-1985. Bethesda, MD: National Cancer Institute, National Institutes of Health.

Cessation is also difficult because of the variables affecting smoking behavior. There are four categories of forces that drive smoking behavior—the patient, the patient's support network, the value or cultural beliefs of the patient, and the treatment modality chosen (Still 1993). Lennox (1992) reviews the literature to identify these factors and determine which ones result in successful cessation. By recognizing the uniqueness of the patient's smoking behavior, intervention strategies can be individualized and thus more likely to succeed.

In 1985, Schwarz reviewed the literature to compare the available programs and pharmacological aids for smoking cessation. As is evident from **Table 14H.1, One-Year Cessation Rates with Intervention—Minimum One-Year Follow-Up**, no one technique shows long-term cessation rates any more impressive than others. The main markers of success are repeated face-to-face contacts by the smoker, over an extended period of time, with physician and non-physician contacts and use of more than one modality for motivating change (Joseph and Byrd 1989; Lennox 1992).

Nursing has long been a leader in patient education and many studies identify nurses as valuable, cost-effective resources for office-based smoking cessation programs (Hollis et al. 1993). In a study by Taylor et al. (1990), a nurse-managed intervention cessation program increased quit rates up to 70 percent after myocardial infarction, compared to the 30 percent to 50 percent quit rates in the non-intervention group. When nurse practitioners' (NPs) practices were compared to physicians' practices, NPs were found to discuss smoking cessation, arrange follow-up appointments, and distribute printed self-help materials more often (Zahnd et al. 1990). Help-

ing clients quit smoking may be the single most important intervention to improve their health.

DATABASE

SUBJECTIVE

→ Obtain a smoking history. Ask "Do you smoke?" "For how long?" "How much do you smoke?" "Are you interested in quitting?" "Have you ever quit before?" "What made you start again?"

→ If client has quit, ascertain prior smoking history as above.
- Recent cessation (within the year) increases risk for relapse.
- Offer praise and congratulations for quitting.
- If quiting is recent, offer printed self-help materials and referrals to Nicotine Anonymous, American Lung Association, or American Cancer Society (see **Appendix 14H.1, Referral Sources**, p. 14-61).
- Past medical history to include:
  - illnesses specific to cardiorespiratory system— e.g., bronchitis, sinusitis, pneumonia, allergies, asthma, COPD, coronary artery disease, myocardial infarction, peripheral vascular disease, Raynaud's disease, hypertension, hypercholesterolemia, blood clots.
  - cancer—e.g, lung, mouth, larynx, esophagus, bladder, kidney, pancreas, brain, cervix, breast.
  - gynecological history—infertility, abnormal pap smears, use of oral contraceptives, low birth-weight babies, complications of pregnancy.
  - gastritis or peptic ulcer disease.

→ Family history may reveal cancer, coronary artery disease, peptic ulcer disease, asthma, COPD.

→ Psychosocial history may include prior history of depression or substance abuse. In addition:
- identify social supports and living situations in terms of other smokers.
- assess coexistent stressors to determine whether timing is right to introduce a major lifestyle change.
- identify need for possible referrals.

→ Review of systems to include:
- respiratory complaints of shortness of breath, productive or non-productive cough, post-nasal drip, wheezing, decreased exercise tolerance, frequent colds, and allergy symptoms.

- cardiovascular symptoms such as chest pain, leg pain when walking short distances, excessively cold hands, or feet with color change.
- gastrointestinal symptoms such as abdominal burning or pain, acid indigestion, heartburn, constipation, diarrhea; frequent use of antacids; food intolerances.
- cosmetic changes noted—e.g., early skin wrinkling, teeth or finger staining.

OBJECTIVE

→ General appearance may include:
- appears older than stated age.
- increased facial lines.
- yellowish stains on fingers, teeth.
- clothes, hair smelling of tobacco.

→ Vital signs may include increase in blood pressure or heart rate if existent cardiorespiratory symptoms.

→ Head, eyes, ears, nose, throat:
- assess for presence of peridontal disease:
  - include bimanual oral examination.

→ Chest:
- generally few findings unless illness present.
- assess the following:
  - respirations.
  - quality of cough if observed.
  - anterior-posterior diameter (AP diameter).
  - presence of adventitious sounds.
  - office spirometry.

→ Extremities:
- note color, temperature, and pulses.

ASSESSMENT

→ Identify smoking history, relapse history, motivation to quit.

→ Rule out concomitant physical illness.

PLAN

DIAGNOSTIC TESTS

→ Fagerstrom's Addiction Scale may be useful (See **Appendix 14H.2, Measurement of Degree of Physical Dependence on Tobacco Smoking**, p. 14-62).

→ Pulmonary function tests are generally normal unless respiratory illness present.

→ Cholesterol level—if elevated, may be useful as motivator to quit.

→ Additional laboratory tests as indicated by history and physical examination.

TREATMENT/MANAGEMENT

→ Advise client to stop smoking.
- If evidence of concomitant illness or signs of abnormality on physical examination, use this as indication of the harmful effects of tobacco, and need to quit.
- Patient education regarding the negative effects of smoking and the benefits of quitting (See **Appendix 14H.3, Quitting: What Happens When You Stop Smoking**, p. 14-63).

→ Help client pick a quit date.

→ Arrange support, follow-up, and resources. (See **Appendixes 14H.1, Referral Sources**, p. 14-61 and **14H.4, Patient Education Materials**, p. 14-64).

→ Consider consultation if history of major depression, or smoker desires nicotine patch or gum in the presence of cardiovascular disease or pregnancy (Benowitz 1993; Hughes 1993).

Pharmacological Adjuncts

NOTE: Although there is no evidence that the nicotine patch or gum adversely affects coronary artery or peripheral vascular disease, hypertension, or stroke, nicotine replacement therapy is generally not prescribed when a history of these conditions exist. In addition, nicotine replacement therapy usually is not recommended during pregnancy (Benowitz 1993; Hughes 1993).

→ Nicotine patch (Habitrol®, Nicoderm®, Nicotrol®, Prostep®) is a transdermal system absorbed through the skin over 24 or 16 hours, depending on the brand. Use for addicted patients as defined by Fagerstrom's scale (see **Appendix 14H.2.,** p. 14-62).
- Client should start use after quit date. Instructions for use include:
  - apply every morning on a dry area of upper arm, stomach, or buttock.
    - Rotate sites, re-using the same site no more frequently than every 7 days.
  - leave on for 24 hours, unless using a 16-hour brand, Nicotrol®. Taper over 2 to 3 months— e.g., 21 mg/day for 6 weeks, 14 mg/day for 3 weeks, and, finally, 7 mg/day for 3 weeks.
- 21 mg patch is equivalent to trough concentrations (i.e., lowest level of blood nicotine) in smokers averaging 1 to 2 packs per day.

- Generally well tolerated, though 50 percent of users experience some local skin irritation.
- Encourage client enrollment in a smoking cessation class.

→ Nicotine gum.
- Delivers nicotine through transbuccal absorption.
- Client should start use after quit date. Instructions for use include:
  - after drinking any beverage, wait 10 to 15 minutes before using gum. (There is decreased absorption in an acidic environment.)
  - chew slowly, until there is a tingle or peppery taste, then "park" the gum against the cheek.
  - repeat the chewing once the taste disappears, about one minute.
  - the gum lasts 20 to 30 minutes.
- Use on a regular schedule. Most people need 10 to 16 pieces per day.
  - Do not use more than 20 pieces per day.
- Once client has quit for 3 months, she should begin to taper use.
  - Taper gradually over 2 to 3 months.
  - Taper 1 to 2 pieces per week.
- Encourage client enrollment in a smoking cessation class.

CONSULTATION

→ In patients with depression or history of depression, antidepressant agents may be required. Referral for counseling is recommended.

→ In pregnant patients or those with cardiovascular disease, consultation with a physician is advised prior to the use of pharmacological adjuncts for smoking cessation.

→ As needed for prescription(s).

PATIENT EDUCATION

→ Inform client that quitting smoking is the single most important thing she can do for her health.

→ Encourage client to think of quitting smoking as learning a foreign language. Both efforts require practice. If a relapse occurs, encourage client not to give up and to try again.

→ Smoking cessation may take a while to master.
- On average, it takes three attempts before a smoker stays quit for good.
- Encourage the smoker not to feel as if she has a character defect because she did not succeed in the past. Encourage her to try again.

→ Have the smoker write on a 3″ × 5″ file card the three most important reasons she has for quitting. Have her keep this card in the same place she keeps her cigarettes. Once she has quit, have her pull out the card and read it whenever she has an urge.

→ Have client practice quitting a little every day.
- For example, on Monday, advise client not to smoke from 6:00 a.m. until 9:00 a.m.; on Tuesday, not to smoke from 9:00 a.m. until 12 noon; on Wednesday, not to smoke from noon until 3:00 p.m., and so on.
- Once the week is completed, the smoker will learn which cigarettes were most important and why and then will know which cigarettes might prove to be those harder not to have.

→ Have client keep a smoking diary.
- Identifying what triggers smoking is key to determining alternate behaviors to smoking.

→ Give client permission to reward non-smoking behaviors. Rewarded behavior is repeated.

→ Encourage client to join a class on quitting smoking.

→ Ask client to read as much as possible about the health effects of smoking, the benefits of quitting, and the tobacco industry (See **Appendixes 14H.3**, p. 14-63 and **14H.4**, p. 14-64).

→ Encourage plenty of rest, fresh air, exercise.

→ Recommend attention to good nutrition.
- Smokers need an extra amount of folate, beta-carotene, and Vitamins B_6, E, and C (Baron 1993).

→ Ask client to reach out to non-smokers, to find a "buddy" in her quit smoking campaign. People with more social support have higher success rates (Lennox 1992).

→ Tell client to expect a small weight gain, seven pounds to ten pounds is normal.
- Being overweight generally is healthier than smoking.
- Tell client to increase the level and frequency of exercise.

→ Advise client to be wary of relapse. Advise client to avoid high-risk situations initially, and to learn and practice positive imagery meditation or self-hypnosis techniques.

→ Tell client to expect to succeed, to be confident.

→ Once client has quit for six months, encourage community involvement—e.g., volunteer on

"former smoker" panels, teach a quit smoking
class, be a buddy for other "newly quit" smokers.

FOLLOW-UP

→ It is helpful to have a scheduled stop smoking
visit, establish a quit date, and give client
homework (See "Patient Education" section).

→ Establish a "quit day" appointment if possible.
  ▪ Make this a celebratory visit, sign a contract,
    review strategies for urge control, offer referral
    sources.

→ Meet with client once every two weeks for one
month; every month for three months; then at six
months and one year. If the client chooses a
cessation program, then follow up by telephone on
or near quit day to offer ongoing encouragement.
Offer support visit at three months.

→ Ask at every visit about client's efforts. Do not get
discouraged if she has relapsed. Praise her initial
effort, and explore what caused the relapse.

→ Document smoking history and cessation
strategies in progress notes. Identify smoking
status on problem list as appropriate.

APPENDIX 14H.1

Referral Sources

American Lung Association
1740 Broadway
New York, New York 10019
(212) 315-8700
800-LUNG-USA

American Cancer Society
1599 Clifton St., NE
Atlanta, Georgia 30329
(404) 320-3333
800-4-CANCER

Nicotine Anonymous
World Services
3410 Geary Boulevard
San Francisco, California 94117
(415) 750-0328

APPENDIX 14H.2

Measurement of Degree of Physical Dependence on Tobacco Smoking*

Questions	Answers	Points
1. How soon after you wake do you smoke your first cigarette?	Within 30 min After 30 min	1 0
2. Do you find it difficult to refrain from smoking in places where it is forbidden, e.g. in church, at the library, etc.?	Yes No	1 0
3. Which cigarette would you hate most to give up?	The first one in the morning Any other	1 0
4. How many cigarettes a day do you smoke?	15 or less 16-25 26 or more	0 1 2
5. Do you smoke more frequently during the early morning than during the rest of the day?	Yes No	1 0
6. Do you smoke if you are so ill that you are in bed most of the day?	Yes No	1 0
7. What is the nicotine level of your usual brand of cigarettes?	0.9 mg or less 1.0 mg-1.2 mg 1.3 mg or more	0 1 2
8. Do you inhale?	Never Sometimes Always	0 1 2

*High dependence is 8 points or more of the total 11 possible points, and low dependence is 6 points or less.

Source: Reprinted with permission from Fagerstrom, K.O. 1978. Measuring degree of physical dependence on tobacco smoking with reference to individualization of treatment. *Addictive Behavior* 3:235-241.

APPENDIX 14H.3

Quitting! What Happens When You Stop Smoking

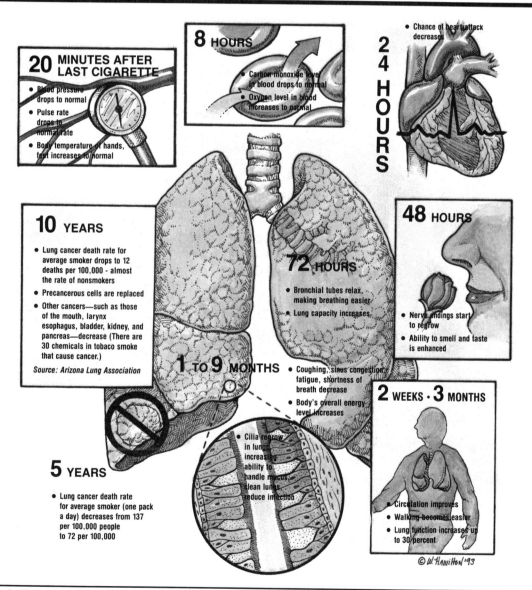

20 MINUTES AFTER LAST CIGARETTE
- Blood pressure drops to normal
- Pulse rate drops to normal rate
- Body temperature of hands, feet increases to normal

8 HOURS
- Carbon monoxide level in blood drops to normal
- Oxygen level in blood increases to normal

24 HOURS
- Chance of heart attack decreases

48 HOURS
- Nerve endings start to regrow
- Ability to smell and taste is enhanced

72 HOURS
- Bronchial tubes relax, making breathing easier
- Lung capacity increases

2 WEEKS · 3 MONTHS
- Circulation improves
- Walking becomes easier
- Lung function increases up to 30 percent

1 TO 9 MONTHS
- Coughing, sinus congestion, fatigue, shortness of breath decrease
- Body's overall energy level increases
- Cilia regrow in lungs increasing ability to handle mucus, clean lungs, reduce infection

5 YEARS
- Lung cancer death rate for average smoker (one pack a day) decreases from 137 per 100,000 people to 72 per 100,000

10 YEARS
- Lung cancer death rate for average smoker drops to 12 deaths per 100,000 - almost the rate of nonsmokers
- Precancerous cells are replaced
- Other cancers—such as those of the mouth, larynx esophagus, bladder, kidney, and pancreas—decrease (There are 30 chemicals in tobacco smoke that cause cancer.)

Source: Arizona Lung Association

© W. Hamilton '93

Source: Reprinted with permission from Timmreck, T.C., and Randolph, J.F. Clinical steps to improve compliance. *Geriatrics* 48(4): Apr. 1993. Art by William Hamilton.

APPENDIX 14H.4

Patient-Education Materials

**Directory of Tobacco Prevention and
    Cessation Services**
City and County of San Francisco, California
Tobacco Free Project
Department of Public Health
Bureau of Health Promotion and Education
(415) 554-9152

Smart Move! A Stop Smoking Guide
American Cancer Society
800-ACS-2345
88-900M-Rev.8/89-No. 2515-LE

**Clearing the Air: How to Quit
    Smoking . . . and Quit for Keeps**
U.S. Department of Health and Human Services
Public Health Service
National Institutes of Health (NIH)
Publication No. 87-1647

Weight Control Guidance in Smoking Cessation
American Heart Association
7320 Greenville Avenue
Dallas, Texas 75231

Catherine M. Kelber, R.N., C., M.S., A.N.P.

14-1

Stress Management

Stress, an unavoidable fact of life, can have both beneficial and negative effects on humans. Despite extensive research, controversy exists as to the exact definition of stress. Selye (1974) first coined the term stress in the 1930s and described a physiological response pattern that occurs when an individual perceives a threat. This response is mediated by adrenaline and other hormones and includes increased blood pressure, heart rate, clotting, and tension of muscles. Stress flows on a continuum between positive, motivating, creative stress and negative, disabling *distress* or *stress overload.* Prolonged distress can cause organ damage leading to disease.

Stressful events have been well documented in the literature and range from daily hassles, annoyances, and irritants (Monroe 1983), to major life changes such as marriage, divorce, changing jobs or residence, death of a spouse, and illness or injury (Holmes and Rahe 1967).

Lazarus and Folkman (1984) devised a transactional model suggesting that an individual's perception of what is stressful and his or her perceived ability to cope with that stressor is key in eliciting the stress response. Stress and coping are affected by environmental, experiential, cognitive, and personality differences. An individual's perceptions and beliefs about the consequences of the actual event determine the level of stress (Ellis 1975).

There are countless reactions to stress including anxiety, depression, somatic symptoms, denial, withdrawal, and substance abuse. Feelings of fear, rage, guilt, shame, and helplessness are common. Symptoms of acute stress can present as restlessness, irritability, fatigue, increased startle reaction, a feeling of tension, sleep dis-

turbances, and an inability to concentrate (Schroeder et al. 1991).

Chronic stress conditions should be suspected if patients present often with multiple somatic complaints and may suggest underlying chronic anxiety or depressive mood disorders. Identified stress-related diseases include hypertension, heart disease, asthma, rheumatoid arthritis, irritable bowel disease, ulcers, headaches, chronic pain, eczema, and recurrent, non-specific vaginal infections (Manderino and Brown 1992).

It is estimated that stress-related complaints account for 75 percent of visits to a medical provider (Charlesworth and Nathan 1984). Women present more often than men with somatic complaints, anxiety, and depression. The stress experienced by women is thought to be related to the increased societal demands women began to face during the last decade. More and more women are juggling careers, family responsibilities, and personal fulfillment and facing other stressors including pregnancy, childbirth, menopause, single parenthood, financial insecurity, and physical and sexual assault (Manderino and Brown 1992).

Stress management is a skill that can be learned. There is, however, no simple overall treatment strategy for stress. An approach consisting of multiple modalities is usually necessary. Attention to sources of stress, stress awareness, cognitive appraisal, coping ability, and patient preferences is imperative when mounting a successful management program. Pender (1987) suggests a multidimensional model for intervention that consists of the following:

→ minimizing the frequency of stress-inducing situations (changing what can be changed in the environment).

→ psychological preparation to increase resistance to stress (changing attitudes).

→ counter-conditioning to avoid physiological arousal resulting from stress (altering physiological responses).

DATABASE

SUBJECTIVE

→ Obtain from client a description of current somatic symptom complex.
  ▪ Clients may sometimes present stating they are "stressed," but more commonly seek care for a particular symptom or constellation of symptoms.

→ Client may present with past history of same symptom or multiple visits for somatic complaints.

→ Assess current and former coping style.
  ▪ Helpful questions include "When you feel this way, what things do you do to make yourself feel better?" or "Have you noticed any changes in your behavior during this period?"

→ Assess current coping level.
  ▪ Is it adequate or is client in crisis? Is client at risk for harm to self or others? Could client benefit from additional coping strategies?

→ Client may present with past history and/or family history of psychiatric disorders:
  ▪ anxiety, depression, psychoses, addictive behaviors, phobias, suicide attempts.

→ Obtain obstetrical/gynecological history:
  ▪ current pregnancy; recent delivery or termination; severe premenstrual syndrome or recent menopause.

→ Assess current employment and job satisfaction:
  ▪ schedule, responsibilities, recent changes, or promotions.

→ Obtain psychosocial history:
  ▪ current/recent/past relationship status and satisfaction; recent major change(s) in life; social support; single parent; history of violence or abuse.

→ Obtain medication history:
  ▪ cold preparations, antihypertensives, bronchodilators, steroids, antidepressants, anti-anxiety agents, and others (may mimic or mask stress-related symptoms).

→ Discuss client's habits:
  ▪ current or increased use of alcohol, drugs, or cigarettes; nutritional status and any change in eating behavior or appetite; sleep pattern or disruption; caffeine use; usual or current exercise pattern.

→ Conduct appropriate review of systems for chief complaint and/or history of weight loss or gain; change in sexual desire; suicidal ideation; mood changes (symptoms of anxiety, panic, or depression); inability to perform normal daily activities; fatigue; heat or cold intolerance; polyuria; polydipsia; polyphagia.

OBJECTIVE

→ Attention should be paid to those systems that:
  ▪ are related to the presenting complaint.
  ▪ may receive target-organ damage from prolonged stress, or
  ▪ may be the cause of stress-related symptoms:
    • blood pressure, pulse.
    • general appearance:
      −sometimes key in diagnosing mood disorders.
      −rapid, pressured speech may indicate mania or a bipolar disorder.
    • thyroid examination:
      −evidence of goiter or nodule.
    • heart examination.
    • mental status examination.

ASSESSMENT

→ Stress syndrome, acute or chronic

→ R/O disorders that may need referral for psychiatric, behavioral, phobia, or medication therapy

→ R/O other common underlying causes for fatigue, depression, anxiety (e.g., thyroid disease, diabetes, anemia)

PLAN

DIAGNOSTIC TESTS

→ Thyroid function tests (TFTs), fasting blood sugar (FBS), and/or CBC if appropriate.

TREATMENT/MANAGEMENT

→ Refer to psychiatrist if appropriate.

→ Consider short-term treatment with alprazolam (Xanax®) or buspirone hydrochloride (Buspar®) for acute situational anxiety.

- Patients should be started on the lowest recommended doses and titrated carefully upward dependent upon relief of symptoms.
- They should be informed that this medication is only for short-term use and should not be used for chronic, everyday stress.
- Xanax® has potential for addiction and withdrawal symptoms.

→ Manage any underlying suspected medication or disease etiologies.

→ Advise adequate nutrition.
  - Discontinue caffeine, limit alcohol use.
  - See **General Nutrition Guidelines.**

→ Advise adequate sleep and rest.

→ Prescribe an exercise regimen—that includes aerobics—at least 4 to 5 days a week.
  - Regular exercise has been shown to decrease anxiety, increase productivity, improve body image and increase psychological well-being (Pender 1987).

→ Refer for "assertiveness" or "time management" training.

→ Offer assistance with "Cognitive Restructuring Techniques."
  - These techniques are intended to help the patient identify and change negative thought patterns that trigger and perpetuate self-defeating and stress-producing thoughts (Pender 1987).

→ Advise use of daily scheduled relaxation techniques.
  - Progressive relaxation, biofeedback, meditation, self-hypnosis, yoga, and guided imagery can be recommended to control physiological responses to stress. (For examples, see **Figure 14I.1, Progressive Deep Muscle Relaxation, Figure 14I.2, Autogenic Training**, and **Figure 14I.3, Diaphragmatic Breathing**.) The use of taped exercises and music enhances the relaxation response in some patients. Choice of technique should depend on patient preference.

→ Consider massage therapy for release of muscular tension.

Figure 14I.1. PROGRESSIVE DEEP MUSCLE RELAXATION

Practice is to be done while sitting in a chair with your back straight, head on a line with your back, both feet on the floor, and hands resting in your lap. Each muscle is to be tightened, held in tightened position for 15-20 seconds, and then slowly let go while studying the difference between tension and relaxation.

Forehead. Wrinkle up your forehead by arching your eyebrows and creasing your forehead, hold the tension, and then slowly let go of the tension.

Eyes. Squeeze your eyes together tightly, hold the tension, and then slowly let go of the tension.

Nose. Wrinkle up your nose and spread your nostrils, hold the tension, and then slowly let go of the tension.

Face. Put a forced smile on your face and spread your face, hold the tension, and then slowly let go of the tension.

Tongue. Push your tongue hard against the roof of your mouth, hold the tension, and then slowly let go of the tension.

Jaws. Clench your jaws together tightly, hold the tension, and then slowly let go of the tension.

Lips. Pucker up your lips and spread them, hold the tension, and then slowly let go of the tension.

Neck. Tighten the muscles of your neck by pulling your chin in and shrugging up your shoulders, hold the tension, and then slowly let go of the tension.

Right Arm. Tense your right arm and hand by stretching it out in front of you and clenching your fist tightly, hold the tension, and then slowly let go of the tension.

Left Arm. Tense your left arm and hand by stretching it out in front of you, and then slowly let go of the tension.

Right Leg. Extend your right leg in front of you (at the height of the chair seat), tense your thigh and leg by pointing your toes inward toward your face, hold the tension, and then slowly let go of the tension.

Upper Back. Tense your back muscles by sitting slightly forward in the chair, bending your elbows and trying to get them to touch each other behind your back, hold the tension, and then slowly let go of the tension.

Chest. Tense your chest muscles by pulling your stomach in and thrusting your chest upward and outward, hold the tension, and then slowly let go of the tension.

Stomach. Tense your stomach muscles, making them hard by pushing your stomach out, hold the tension, and then slowly let go of the tension.

Buttocks and Thighs. Tense your buttocks and thighs by placing your feet squarely on the floor, pointing your toes into the floor and forcing your heels to remain on the floor while pushing forward, hold the tension, and then slowly let go of the tension.

Practice should be engaged in twice daily for a period of 12-15 minutes. Mastery of the technique is after 2-4 weeks of twice-daily practice.

Source: Reprinted with permission from Goroll, A.H., May, L.A., and Mulley, A. 1987. *Primary care medicine*, p. 905. Philadelphia: J.B. Lippincott.

Figure 141.2. AUTOGENIC TRAINING

Practice is to be done while sitting in a soft, comfortable chair with your eyes closed. As attention is called to specific groups of muscles, try to *visualize* and *feel* the relaxation of those muscles. Try to let *happen* what is being suggested. Repeat each formula 2-3 times.

▸ My forehead and scalp feel heavy, limp, loose, and relaxed.

▸ My eyes and nose feel heavy, limp, loose, and relaxed.

▸ My face and jaws feel heavy, limp, loose, and relaxed.

▸ My neck, shoulders, and back feel heavy, limp, loose, and relaxed.

▸ My arms and hands feel heavy, limp, loose, and relaxed.

▸ My chest, solar plexus, and the central part of my body feel quiet, calm, comfortable, and relaxed.

▸ My stomach feels heavy, limp, loose, and relaxed.

▸ My buttocks, thighs, calves, ankles, and toes feel quiet, heavy, limp, loose, and relaxed.

▸ My whole body feels quiet, heavy, limp, and relaxed.

Practice should be engaged in twice daily for a period of 6-8 minutes. Mastery of the technique is after 1-3 weeks of twice-daily practice.

Source: Reprinted with permission from Goroll, A.H., May, L.A., and Mulley, A. 1987. *Primary care medicine*, p. 906. Philadelphia: J.B. Lippincott.

Figure 141.3. DIAPHRAGMATIC BREATHING

While sitting or lying down with a pillow at the small of your back:

1. Breathe in slowly and deeply by pushing your stomach out.
2. Say the word "relax" silently to yourself prior to exhaling.
3. Exhale slowly, letting your stomach come in.
4. Repeat entire procedure 10 times consecutively, with emphasis on slow, deep breaths.

Practice should take place 5 times per day, 10 consecutive diaphragmatic breaths each sitting. Time for mastery is after 1-2 weeks of daily practice.

Source: Reprinted with permission from Goroll, A.H., May, L.A., and Mulley, A. 1987. *Primary care medicine*, p. 906. Philadelphia: J.B. Lippincott.

→ Help client to maintain a sense of humor.
  ▪ Laughter evokes endorphin release and decreases anxiety.
    • Suggest viewing comedy on television or video or reading lighthearted books.

CONSULTATION

→ Physician consultation required for prescribing controlled drugs.

→ Referral to psychiatrist or psychologist as indicated.

PATIENT EDUCATION

→ Help client to understand the concept of stress:
  ▪ what is stress and what causes it?
  ▪ what are the client's sources of stress?
  ▪ what is the relationship between stress and client's somatic symptoms?
  ▪ what are the effects of prolonged stress?
  ▪ what strategies are available to avoid, prevent, and counteract the effects of stress?

FOLLOW-UP

→ Clients usually need several visits to monitor progress.
  ▪ It is unlikely that patients with limited self-awareness will be able to make the connection between symptoms and stress in the first few visits.
  ▪ Usually a safe, trusting relationship needs to be established before clients are willing to make major behavior changes.
  ▪ Stress management is a long-term process and requires ongoing reinforcement from the provider.

→ Document in progress notes and problem list.

14-J
Bibliography

Abrahan, I.L., Neese, J.B., and Westerman, P.S. 1991. Depression: Nursing implications of a clinical and social problem. *Nursing Clinics of North America* 26(3):527–544.

Alcoholics Anonymous, Inc. 1986. *General Services Branch membership survey.* New York: the Author.

Allen, T.W. 1989. Let's join the battle against domestic violence. *Journal of American Osteopathic Association* 89(4):457.

Altshuler, B.D. 1990. Eating disorder patients recognition and intervention. *Journal of Dental Hygiene* 64(3):119–125.

American Cancer Society. 1990. *Cancer facts and figures, 1990.* New York: the Author.

American College of Obstetricians and Gynecologists. 1989. *The battered woman,* Technical Bulletin No. 124. Washington, DC: the Author.

———. 1992. *Sexual assault,* Technical Bulletin No. 172. Washington, DC: the Author.

American Psychiatric Association. 1980. *Diagnostic and statistical manual of mental disorders.* Washington, DC: the Author.

———. 1987. *Diagnostic and statistical manual of mental disorders,* 3rd ed. revised. Washington, DC: the Author.

———. 1994. *Diagnostic and statistical manual of mental disorders,* 4th ed. Washington, DC: the Author.

Andrist, L.C. 1988. Taking a sexual history and educating clients about safe sex. *Nursing Clinics of North America* 23(4):959–973.

Bachmann, G.A., Moeller, T.P., and Benett, J. 1988. Childhood sexual abuse and the consequences in adult women. *Obstetrics and Gynecology* 71(4):631–642.

Baker, A.W., and Duncan, S.P. 1985. Child sexual abuse: A study of prevalence in Great Britain. *Child Abuse and Neglect* 9:457–467.

Baron, R. October 1993. *Antioxidant vitamins and health.* Paper presented at 8th Annual Primary Care Medicine Conference, Principles and Practice. San Francisco: University of California, San Francisco.

Beebe, D.K. 1991. Emergency management of the adult female rape victim. *American Family Physician* 43(6):2041–2046.

Beitchman, J.H., Zucker, K.J., Hood, J.E., DaCosta, G.A., Akman, D., and Cassavia, E. 1992. A review of the long-term effects of child sexual abuse. *Child Abuse and Neglect* 16:101–118.

Benowitz, N.L. 1993. Nicotine replacement therapy: What has been accomplished-Can we do better? *Drugs* 2:157–170.

Berrier, A., Charney, D.S., and Heninger, G.R. 1985. The diagnostic validity of anxiety disorders and their relationship to depressive illness. *A Mexican Journal of Psychiatry* 142:787–797.

Berrios, D.C., and Grady, D. 1991. Domestic violence risk factors and outcomes. *Western Journal of Medicine* 155:133–135.

Berth-Jones, J., and Graham-Brown, R.A.C. 1990. Childhood sexual abuse—A dermatological perspective. *Clinical and Experimental Dermatology* 15:321–330.

Bownes, I.T., O'Gorman, E.C., and Sayers, A. 1991. Assault characteristics and post-traumatic stress disorder in rape victims. *Acta Psychiatrica Scandinavica* 83(1):27–30.

Boyer, D., and Fine, D. 1992. Sexual abuse as a factor in adolescent pregnancy and child maltreatment. *Family Planning Perspectives* 24(1):4–19.

Brasfield, K. 1991. Practical psychopharmacologic considerations in depression. *Nursing Clinics of North America* 16(3):651–663.

Briere, J., and Zaidi, L.Y. 1989. Sexual abuse histories and sequelae in female psychiatric emergency room patients. *American Journal of Psychiatry* 146:1602–1606.

Brown, B.E., and Garrison, C.J. 1990. Patterns of symptomatology of adult women incest survivors. *Western Journal of Nursing Research* 12(5):587–600.

Brown, C.S., Rakel, R.E., Wells, B.G., Downs, I.M., and Akiskal, H.S. 1991. A practical update on anxiety disorders and their pharmacologic treatment. *Archives of Internal Medicine* 151:873–884.

Buckner, E. 1991. Do you have patients with anorexia or bulimia? Understanding is the first step in helping. *Postgraduate Medicine* 89(4):209–215.

Buckwater, K.C., and Babich, K.S. 1990. Psychologic and physiologic aspects of depression. *Nursing Clinics of North America* 25(4):945–954.

Bulik, C.M., Epstein, L.H., and Kaye, W. 1990. Treatment of laxative abuse in a female with bulimia nervosa using an operant extinction paradigm. *Journal of Substance Abuse* 2(3):381–388.

Bullock, L.F., and McFarlane, J. 1989. The birth-weight/battering connection. *American Journal of Nursing* 89(9):1153–1155.

Burge, S.K. 1989. Violence against women as a health care issue. *Family Medicine* 21(5):368–373.

Burgess, A., and Holmstrom, L. 1974. Rape trauma syndrome. *American Journal of Psychiatry* 131:981–986.

Burke, M.E., and Vangellow, J. 1990. Anorexia nervosa and bulimia nervosa: Chronic conditions affecting pregnancy. *NAACOG: Clinical Issues in Perinatal and Women's Health Nursing* 1(2):240–254.

Bushnell, J.A., Wells, E.J., Hornblow, A.R., Oakley-Browne, M.A., and Joyce, P. 1990. Prevalence of three bulimia syndromes in the general population. *Psychological Medicine* 20:671–680.

Button, E.J., Whitehouse, A. 1981. Subclinical anorexia nervosa. *Psychosomatic Medicine* 11:509–516.

Cahill, C., Llewelyn, S.P., and Pearson, C. 1991. Long-term effects of sexual abuse which occurred in childhood: A review. *British Journal of Clinical Psychology* 30:117–130.

Calarco, M.M., and Krone, K.P. 1991. An integrated nursing model of depressive behavior in adults. *Nursing Clinics of North America* 26(3):573–584.

Campbell, J. 1986. Nursing assessment for risk of homicide with battered women. *Annals of Nursing Science* 8:36–51.

Centers for Disease Control. 1989. Education about adult domestic violence in U.S. and Canadian medical schools, 1987-1988. *Morbidity and Mortality Weekly Report* 38(2):17–19.

———. January 1990. Monthly AIDS/HIV surveillance report. Atlanta: the Author.

Chaidez, L., ed. 1991. *The California child abuse and neglect reporting law: Issues and answers for health practitioners.* State of California, Department of Social Services, Office of Child Abuse Prevention.

Chaisson, R.E., Bacchetti, R., Osmond, D., Brodic, B., Sande, M.A., and Moss, A.R. 1989. Cocaine use and HIV infection in intravenous users in San Francisco. *Journal of the American Medical Association* 261:561–565.

Charlesworth, C.A., and Nathan, R.G. 1982. *Stress management—A comprehensive guide to wellness.* Houston: Biobehavioral Press.

Cheadle, M.J. 1991. The screening sexual history: Getting to the problem. *Clinics in Geriatric Medicine* 7(1):9–13.

Cole, P.M., and Woolger, C. 1989. Incest survivors: The relation of their perceptions of their parents and their own parenting attitudes. *Child Abuse and Neglect* 13:409–416.

Cole, P.M., Woolger, C., Power, T.G., and Smith, K.D. 1992. Parenting difficulties among adult survivors of father-daughter incest. *Child Abuse and Neglect* 16:239–249.

Crawshaw, J. 1985. Anorexia and bulimia: The earliest clues. *Patient Care* 19(18):80–95.

Cummings, S.R., Coates, T.J., Richard, R.J., Hansen, B., Zahnd, E.G., VanderMartin, R., Duncan, C., Gerbert, B., Martin, A., and Stein, M.J. 1989. Training physicians in counseling about smoking cessation: A randomized trial of the "Quit for Life" program. *Annals of Internal Medicine* 110:640–647.

Cummings, S.R., Rubin, S.M. and Oster, G. 1989. The cost-effectiveness of counseling smokers to quit. *Journal of the American Medical Association* 261:75–79.

Davis, M., Eshelman, E.R., and McKay, M. 1982. *The relaxation and stress reduction workbook.* Oakland, CA: New Harbinger Publications.

Dickstein, L.J. 1988. Spouse abuse and other domestic violence. *Pediatric Clinics of North America* 11(4):611–629.

Dreyfus, J.K. 1987. The prevalence of depression in women in an ambulatory care setting. *The Nurse Practitioner Journal* 12(4):34–50.

———. 1988. The treatment of depression in an ambulatory care setting. *The Nurse Practitioner Journal* 13(7):14–33.

Edwards, J.G. 1991. Clinical anxiety and its treatment. *Neuropeptides* 19(Suppl):1–10.

Ellis, A.A. 1975. *A new guide to rational living.* North Hollywood, CA: Wilshire Books.

Emergency Nurses Association. Emergency Nurses Association sexual assault nurse examiners' resource list. 1991. *Journal of Emergency Nursing* 17(4):31A–35A, 95.

Fagerstrom, K.O. 1978. Measuring degree of physical dependence on tobacco smoking with reference to individualization of treatment. *Addictive Behavior* 3:235–241.

Feinauer, L.L. 1989. Relationship of treatment to adjustment in women sexually abused as children. *The American Journal of Family Therapy* 17(4):326–334.

Fielding, J.E. 1985. Smoking: Health effects and control. *New England Journal of Medicine* 313:491–498, 555–565.

Finkelhor, D., Hotaling, G., Lewis, I.A., and Smith, C. 1990. Sexual abuse in a national survey of adult men and women: Prevalence, characteristics, and risk factors. *Child Abuse and Neglect* 14:19–28.

Flitcraft, A. 1990. Battered women in your practice? *Patient Care* 24(16):107–118.

Franger, A.L. 1988. Taking a sexual history and managing common sexual problems. *Journal of Reproductive Medicine* 33(7):639–643.

Frank, E. 1991. Shame and guilt in eating disorders. *American Journal of Orthopsychiatry* 6(12):303–306.

Frank, S.H., and Jaen, C. R. 1993. Office evaluation and treatment of the dependent smoker. *Primary Care* 20:251–268.

Fredriccson, B., and Gilljam, H. 1992. Smoking and reproduction: Short- and long-term effects and benefits of smoking cessation. *Acta Obstetrica Gynecologica Scandinavia* 71:580–592.

Freeman, C.P., and Munro, J.K. 1988. Drug and group treatment for bulimia/bulimia nervosa. *Journal of Psychosomatic Research* 32:647–660.

Garner, D.M., and Garfinkel, P.E. 1985. *Handbook of psychotherapy for anorexia nervosa and bulimia nervosa.* New York: Guilford Press.

Gilbert, J.R., Wilson, D.M.C., Best, J.A., Taylor, D.W., Lindsay, E.A., Singer, J., and Wilms, D.G. 1989. Smoking cessation in primary care: A randomized controlled trial of nicotine-bearing chewing gum. *The Journal of Family Practice* 28:49–55.

Gilgun, J.F. 1984. Does the mother know? Alternatives to blaming mothers for child sexual abuse. *Response* Fall Issue:2–4.

Gise, L.H., and Paddison, P. 1988. Rape, sexual abuse, and its victims. *Psychiatric Clinics of North America* 11(4):629–648.

Glaser, J.B., Schacter, J., Benes, S., Cummings, M., Frances, C.A., and McCormack, W.M. 1991. Sexually transmitted diseases in postpubertal female rape victims. *The Journal of Infectious Diseases* 164(4):726–730.

Glick, R., and Moore, J. 1990. Introduction. In *Drugs in hispanic communities,* eds. R. Glick and J. Moore. New Brunswick, N.J.: Rutgers University Press.

Godenick, M.T. 1989. A review of available smoking cessation methods, 1989. *Maryland Medical Journal* 38:277–279.

Gora, M.L. 1993. Nicotine transdermal systems. *The Annals of Pharmacotherapy* 27:742–749.

Goroll, A.H., May, L.A., and Mulley, A., eds. 1987. *Primary care medicine.* Philadelphia: J.B. Lippincott.

Gorski, T.T., and Miller, M. 1986. *Staying sober: A guide for relapse prevention.* Independence, MO: Independent Press.

Guinan, M.E. 1990. Domestic violence: Physicians a link to prevention. *Journal of the American Medical Women's Association* 45(6):231.

Hall, L.A., Sachs, B., Rayens, M.K., and Lutenbacher, M. 1994. Childhood physical and sexual abuse: Their relationship with depressive symptoms in adulthood. *Image. The Journal of Nursing Scholarship* 25(4):317–323.

Harrop-Griffiths, J., Katon, W., Walker, E., Holm, L., Russo, J., and Hickok, L. 1988. The association between chronic pelvic pain, psychiatric diagnoses, and childhood sexual abuse. *Obstetrics and Gynecology* 71:589–594.

Hatcher, R.A., Trussel, J., Stewart, F., Stewart, G.K., Kowal, D., Guest, F., Cates, W., and Policar, M. 1994. *Contraceptive technology,* 16th ed. New York: Irvington Publishers.

Helton, A. 1986. *Protocol of care for the battered woman,* pp. 1–20. Houston, TX: March of Dimes Birth Defects Foundation.

Herzog, D.B., Keller, M.B., Lavori, P.W., and Bradburn, I.S. 1991. Bulimia nervosa in adolescence. *Developmental and Behavioral Pediatrics* 12(3):191–195.

Herzog, D.B., and Copeland, P.M. 1985. Eating disorders. *New England Journal of Medicine* 313(5):295–301.

Hill, S. 1984. Vulnerability to the biomedical consequences of alcoholism and alcohol related problems. In *Alcohol problems in women,* eds. S. Wilsnack and L. Beckman. New York: Guilford Press.

Hodiamont, Q. 1991. How normal are anxiety and fear? *The International Journal of Social Psychiatry* 37(1):43–50.

Hoffman, N.G., and Harrison, P.A. March-April, 1989. Characteristics of the older patient in chemical dependency treatment. *Counselor* 11.

Hollis, J.F., Lichenstein, E., Vogt, T.M., Stevens, V.J., and Biglan, A. 1993. Nurse-assisted counseling for smokers in primary care. *American College of Physicians* 118:521–525.

Holmes, T.H., and Rahe, R.H. 1967. The social readjustment scale. *Journal of Psychosomatic Research* 11:213–218.

Houston, T.P. 1992. Smoking cessation in office practice. *Primary Care* 19:493–507.

Hughes, J.R. 1993. Risk/benefit assessment of nicotine preparations in smoking cessation. *Drug Safety* 8:49–56.

Hunt, D.M. 1990. Spouse abuse care goes beyond the office door. *Postgraduate Medicine* 87(2):130–135.

Hyman, S.E., and Jenike, M.A. 1987. Approach to the patient with depression in primary care medicine. In *Primary care medicine*, 2d ed., eds. A.H. Goroll, L.A. May, and A.G. Mulley. Philadephia: J.B. Lippincott.

Indest, G.F. 1989. Medico-legal issues in detecting and proving the sexual abuse of children. *Medical Science Law* 29(1):33–46.

Jessup, M. 1990. The treatment of perinatal addiction: Identification, intervention and advocacy. *Western Journal of Medicine* 152:553–558.

Jones, B.B., and Jones, M.K. 1976. Women and alcohol: Intoxication, metabolism and the menstrual cycle. In *Alcohol problems in women and children*, eds. M. Greenblatt and M. Schukit. New York: Grune and Stratton.

Joseph, A.M., and Byrd, J.C. 1989. Smoking cessation in practice. *Primary Care* 16:83–98.

Kahn, H. 1993. *Nicotine addiction and smoking cessation.* Unpublished manuscript.

Kalager, R., Brubackk, O., and Bassoe, H.H. 1978. Cardiac performance in patients with anorexia nervosa. *Cardiology* 63(1):1–4.

Katon, W. 1986. Panic disorder: Epidemiology, diagnosis, and treatment in primary care. *Journal of Clinical Psychiatry* 43:21–27.

Kaye, W.H., and Weltzin, T.E. 1991. Neurochemistry of bulimia nervosa. *Journal of Clinical Psychiatry* 52(Suppl. 10):21–28.

Kennedy, S.H., and Goldbloom, D.S. 1991. Current perspectives on drug therapies for anorexia nervosa and bulimia nervosa. *Drugs* 41(3):367–377.

Kent, A. 1991. Advances in bulimia nervosa. *The Practitioner* 235(1502):396–399.

Kessler, D.B., and Hyden, P. 1991. Physical, sexual, and emotional abuse of children. *Clinical Symposia* 43(1):2–32.

Koop, C.E. 1988. *Smoking: Everything you and your family need to know.* Ambrose Video.

Kreidler, M.C., and Hassan, M. 1992. Use of an interactional model with survivors of incest. *Issues in Mental Health Nursing* 13:149–158.

Krejci, R.C., Sargent, R., Forand, K.J., Ureda, J.R., Saunders, R.P., and Durstine, J.L. 1992. Psychological and behavioral differences among females classified as bulimic, obligatory exerciser and normal control. *Psychiatry* 55(2):185–193.

Krugman, S., Mata, L., and Krugman, R. 1991. Sexual abuse and corporal punishment during childhood: A pilot retrospective survey of university students in Costa Rica. *Pediatrics* 90(1):157–161.

Laage, T.A. 1988. Recognizing the drug resistant patient in anxiety and depression. *Medical Clinics of North America* 72:897–909.

Lazarus, R.S., and Folkman, S. 1984. *Stress, appraisal and coping.* New York: Springer.

Lee, E.W., and D'Alonzo, G.E. 1993. Cigarette smoking, nicotine addiction and its pharmacological treatment. *Archives of Internal Medicine* 153:34–48.

Lenehan, G. 1991. Sexual assault nurse examiners: a SANE way to care for rape victims. *Journal of Emergency Nursing* Feb. 17(1):1–2.

Lennox, A.S. 1992. Determinants of outcome in smoking cessation. *British Journal of General Practice* 42:247–252.

Lowenstein, S.R. 1985. Suicidal behavior recognition and intervention. *Hospital Practice* 20:52–71.

Mackey, T.F., Hacker, S.S., Weissfeld, L.A., Ambrose, N.C., Fisher, M.G., and Zobel, D.L. 1991. Comparative effects of sexual assault on sexual functioning of child sexual abuse survivors and others. *Issues in Mental Health Nursing* 12:89–112.

Maddocks, S.E., and Kaplin, A.S. 1991. The prediction of treatment response in bulimia nervosa: A study of patient variables. *British Journal of Psychiatry* 159:846–849.

Manderino, M.A., and Brown, M.C. 1992. A practical, step-by-step approach to stress management for women. *Nurse Practitioner* 17(7):18–28.

Marshal, L. 1991. Eating disorders. In *Psychiatric mental health nursing*, eds. F. Gary and C.K. Kavanagh. Philadelphia: J.B. Lippincott.

Martin, A.C., and Davis, L.L. 1989. Mental health problems in primary care setting: A study of nurse practitioners' practice. *Nurse Practitioner* 4(10):40–50.

Massie, M.E., and Johnson, S.M. 1989. The importance of recognizing a history of sexual abuse in female adolescents. *Journal of Adolescent Health Care* 10(3):184–191.

Mayfield, D., McLeod, G., and Hall, P. 1974. The CAGE questionnaire: Validation of a new alcoholism screening instrument. *American Journal of Psychiatry* 131:1121–1123.

McFarlane, J., and Anderson, E. 1987. Prevention of battering during pregnancy: Focus on behavioral change. *Public Health Nursing* 4(3):166–174.

McGinnis, J.M., and Foege, W.H. 1993. Actual causes of death in the United States. *Journal of the American Medical Association* 270:2207–2212.

McLear, S.V., Anwar, R., Herman, S., and Maquiling, K. 1989. Education is not enough: A systems failure in protecting battered women. *Annals of Emergency Surgery* 18(6):651–653.

McLeod, J.D., Kessler, R.C., and Landis, K.R. 1992. Speed of recovery from major depressive episodes in a community sample of married men and women. *Journal of Abnormal Psychology* 101(2):277–286.

Mehta, P., and Dandrea, L.A. 1988. The battered woman. *American Family Physician* 37(1):193–199.

Mejo, S. 1990. The use of antidepressant medication: A guide for the primary care nurse practitioner. *Journal of the American Academy of Nurse Practitioners* 2(4):153–159.

Meyer, R.E. 1986. How to understand the relationship between psychopathology and addictive disorders: Another example of the chicken and the egg. In *Psychopathology and addictive disorders*, ed. R.E. Meyer. New York: Guilford Press.

Milhorne, H.T. 1989. Nicotine dependence. *American Family Physician* 39:214–224.

Mitchell, J. August, 1990. Treating HIV-infected women in chemical dependency programs. *AIDS Patient Care* 36–37.

Mitchell, J.E. 1991. Bulimia nervosa. *Boletin de la Asociacion medica de Puerto Rico* 83(1):22–24.

Monroe, S. 1983. Major and minor life events as predictors of psychological distress. *Journal of Behavioral Medicine* 6:189–205.

Mora, J., and Gilbert, M.J. 1991. Issues for Latinas: Mexican American women. In *Alcohol and drugs are women's issues*, ed. P. Roth. Metuchen, N.J.: Women's Action Alliance and Scarecrow Press.

Morrison, L.J. 1988. The battering syndrome: A poor record of detection in the emergency department. *Journal of Emergency Medicine* 6(6):521–526.

Moscarello, R. 1991. Post-traumatic stress disorder after sexual assault: Its psychodynamics and treatment. *Journal of the American Academy of Psychoanalysis* 19(2):235–253.

Moss, V. 1991. Battered women and the myth of masochism. *Journal of Psychosocial Nursing* 29(7):19–23.

Moss, V.A., and Taylor, W. 1991. Domestic violence. *Association of Operating Room Nurses Journal* 53(5):1158–1164.

Muram, D. 1992. Child sexual abuse. *Obstetrics and Gynecology Clinics of North America* 19(1):193–207.

National Center on Child Abuse and Neglect. August, 1978. *Child sexual abuse: Incest, assault and exploitation. Special report.* Publication No. (OHDS)79-30166. Washington, DC: U.S. Department of Health, Education and Welfare.

National Council on Alcoholism and Other Drug Dependencies. 1990. *Alcoholism, other drug addictions and related problems among women.* New York: the Author.

National Institute on Drug Abuse. 1989. *National household survey on drug abuse: Population estimates 1988.* USDHHS Pub. No. (ADM)89–1636. Rockville, MD: U.S. Department of Health and Human Services.

Nelson, L., and Jessup, M. 1992. Advocacy, ethics and the law. In *Drug dependency and pregnancy: Managing withdrawal*, ed. M. Jessup. Sacramento, CA.: California Department of Health Services, Maternal and Child Health Branch.

Orioli, E.M., Jaffe, D.T., and Scott, C.D. 1987. *Stress map.* New York: Newmarket Press.

Osborn, M., and Bryan, S. 1989. Patient care guidelines. Evidentiary examination in sexual assault. *Journal of Emergency Nursing* 15(3):284–290.

Packer, I.K. 1990. Domestic violence: The role of the mental health expert. *Medicine and Law* 9(6):1274–1276.

Paddison, P.L., Gise, L.H., Lebovits, A., Strain, J. J., Cirasole, D.M., and Levine, J.P. 1990. Sexual abuse and premenstrual syndrome: Comparison between a lower and higher socioeconomic group. *Psychosomatics* 31(3):265–272.

Palmer, T. 1990. Anorexia nervosa, bulimia nervosa: Causal theories and treatment. *Nurse Practitioner* 15(4):13–21.

Pendelton, L., Tisdale, M., and Mailer, M. 1991. Personality pathology in bulimics versus controls. *Comprehensive Psychiatry* 32(6):516–520.

Pender, N. 1987. *Health promotion in nursing practice.* Los Altos, CA: Appleton & Lange.

Perry, M.V., and Anderson, L.A. 1992. Assessment and treatment strategies for depressive disorders commonly encountered in primary care settings. *The Nurse Practitioner Journal* 17(6):25–36.

Plehn, K.W. 1990. Anorexia nervosa and bulimia: Incidence and diagnosis. *Nurse Practitioner* 15(4):22–31.

Pokorny, A.D. 1977. Suicide and depression. In *Pharmacology and treatment of depression*, ed. N. Fann. New York: Spectrum Publications.

Pope, H.G., Hudson, J.I., Jonas, J.M., and Yurgelun-Todd, D. 1983. Bulimia treated with imipramine: A placebo controlled double-blind study. *American Journal of Psychiatry* 140:554–558.

Pope, H.G., and Hudson, J.I. 1989. Pharmacologic treatment of bulimia nervosa: Research findings and practical suggestions. *Psychiatric Annual* 19:483–487.

Powers, P. 1990. Anorexia nervosa: Evaluation and treatment. *Neuropsychiatry Comprehensive Therapy* 16(2):24–34.

Pribor, E.F., and Dinwiddie, S.H. 1992. Psychiatric correlates of incest in childhood. *American Journal of Psychiatry* 149(1):52–56.

Randall, T. 1990. Domestic violence intervention calls for more than treating injuries. *Journal of the American Medical Association* 264(8):939–944.

———. 1991. Tools available for health care providers whose patients are at risk for domestic violence. *Journal of the American Medical Association* 266(9):1179–1180.

Rath, G.D., Jarratt, L.G., and Leonardson, G. 1989. Rates of domestic violence against adult women by men partners. *Journal of the American Board of Family Practice* 2(4):227–233.

Reed, B. 1987. Developing women-sensitive drug dependence treatment services: Why so difficult? *Journal of Psychoactive Drugs* 19(2):151–164.

Reiger, D.A., Boyd, J.H., Burke, J.D., Rae, D.S., Myers, J.K., Kramer, M., Robins, L.N., George, L.K., Karno, M., and Locke, B.Z. 1988. One-month prevalence of mental disorders in the United States. *Archives of General Psychiatry* 45:577–866.

Reiter, R.C., Shakerin, L.R., Gambone, J.C., and Milburn, A.K. 1991. Correlation between sexual abuse and somatization in women with somatic and nonsomatic chronic pelvic pain. *American Journal of Obstetrics and Gynecology* 165:104–109.

Richardson, T.M., and Williams, B.A. 1990. *African-Americans in treatment: Dealing with cultural differences.* Center City, MN: Hazelden.

Robbins, A.S. 1993. Pharmacological approaches to smoking cessation. *American Journal of Preventative Medicine* 9:31–33.

Rose, M.A. 1991. Intervention strategies for smoking cessation: The role of oncology nursing. *Cancer Nursing* 14:225–231.

Rothbaum, B., Foa, E., Murdock, T., Riggs, D., and Walsh, W. 1990. Post-traumatic stress disorder in rape victims. Unpublished manuscript.

Roth, P. 1990. Introduction. In *Alcohol and drugs are women's issues*, ed. P. Roth. Metuchen, N.J.: Women's Action Alliance and Scarecrow Press.

Ruch, L.D., Amedeo, S.R., Leon, J.J., and Gartrell, J.W. 1991. Repeated sexual victimization and trauma change during the acute phase of the sexual assault trauma syndrome. *Women and Health* 17(1):1–19.

Russell, D. 1983. The incidence and prevalence of intrafamilial sexual abuse of female children. *Child Abuse and Neglect* 7:133–145.

Russell, M.A.H., Wilson, C., Taylor, C., and Baker, C.D. 1979. Effect of general practitioners' advice against smoking. *British Medical Journal* 2:231–236.

Safer, D. 1987. Substance abuse among young chronic patients. *Hospital and Community Psychiatry* 38(5):511–514.

Sampselle, C.M. 1991. The role of nursing in preventing violence against women. *Journal of Obstetric, Gynecologic and Neonatal Nursing* 20(6):481–487.

Sandmeier, M. 1984. Alcohol, mood-altering drugs and smoking. In *The new our bodies, ourselves*, ed. Boston Women's Health Collective. New York: Simon and Schuster.

Satin, A.J., Hemsell, D.L., Stone, I.C., Theriot, S., and Wendel, G.D. 1991. Sexual assault in pregnancy. *Obstetrics and Gynecology* 77(5):710–714.

Savage, P.D., Garrison, R.J., Deveraux, R.B., Castelli, W.P., Anderson, S.J., Levy, D., Thomas, H.E., Kannel, W.B., and Feinelib, M. 1983. Mitral valve prolapse in the general population, I: epidemiological features: The Framingham study. *American Heart Journal* 106:571–576.

Schroeder, S.A., Krupp, M.A., Tierney, L.M., and McPhee, S.J. 1991. *Current medical diagnosis and treatment.* San Mateo, CA: Appleton & Lange.

Schuckit, M. 1985. Genetics of alcoholism. University of California, Davis conference. *Alcoholism: Clinical and Experimental Research* 9(6):475–492.

Schwartz, I.L. 1991. Sexual violence against women: Prevalence, consequences, societal factors and prevention. *American Journal of Preventive Medicine* 7(6):363–373.

Schwarz, J.L. 1985. *Review and evaluation of smoking cessation methods: The United States and Canada, 1978–1985.* (NIH publication 87–2940) Bethesda, MD: National Institutes of Health

Scott, K.D. 1992. Childhood sexual abuse: Impact on a community's mental health status. *Child Abuse and Neglect* 16:285–295.

Selye, H. 1974. *Stress without distress.* New York: Dutton.

Selzer, M., Vinokur, A., and van Rooijen, I. 1975. A self-administered short Michigan Alcoholism Screening Test. *Journal of Studies on Alcohol* 36:117–126. (Adapted from the original MAST: Michigan Alcoholism Screening Test. 1971. *American Journal of Psychiatry* 127:1653–1654).

Sgroi, S.M., Blick, L.C., and Porter, F.S. 1985. *A conceptual framework for child sexual abuse.* As presented at the Education Programs Associates course on Adolescent Sexual Abuse, Reporting & Counseling. 12/8/92, Berkeley, CA.

Silver, B.V., and Blanchard, E.B. 1978. Biofeedback and relaxation training in the treatment of psychophysiological disorders: Or are the machines really necessary? *Journal of Behavioral Medicine* 1:217–239.

Shen, N. 1990. Pharmacotherapy of depression: The American current status. *Kelo Journal of Medicine* 39(4):237–241.

Skok, R.L., and McLaughlin, T.F. 1991. Characteristics common to females who exhibit anorectic or bulimic behavior: A review of current literature. *Journal of Clinical Psychology* 47(6):846–853.

Slade, M., Daniel, L.J., and Heisler, C.J. 1991. Application of forensic toxicology to the problem of domestic violence. *Journal of Forensic Sciences* 36(3):708–713.

Slaughter, L., and Brown, C.R. 1992. Colposcopy to establish physical findings in rape victims. *American Journal of Obstetrics and Gynecology* 166(1)(pt. 1): 83–86.

Smith, D.E. 1990. Introduction. *Western Journal of Medicine* 152:(5).

Smith, L.S. 1986. In *Psychologic concerns in contemporary women's health: A nursing advocacy approach*, ed., J. Griffith-Kennedy. Menlo Park, CA: Addison Wesley.

Solberg, L.I., Maxwell, P.L., Kottke, T.E., Gepner, G.J., and Brekke, L.M. 1990. A systematic primary care office-based smoking cessation program. *The Journal of Family Practice* 30:647–654.

Soman, L.A., Dunn-Malhota, E., and Halfon, N. 1991. Model of care for chemically dependent pregnant and postpartum women and their drug exposed children from birth to age three. *Technical Assistance Report from the California Policy Seminar, University of California.* Center for the Vulnerable Child, Oakland, CA.

Sorby, N.O.D., Reavley, W., and Huber, J.W. 1991. Self-help programme for anxiety in general practice: Controlled trial of an anxiety management booklet. *British Journal of General Practice* 41:471–420.

Stewart, D.E., Robinson, G.E., Goldbloom, D.S., and Wright, C. 1990. Infertility and eating disorders. *American Journal of Obstetrics and Gynecology* 163:1196–1199.

Still, J.M. 1993. Smoking-cessation therapy: Current medical management. *Ob/Gyn Nursing and Patient Counseling* 5:5–9.

Taha-Cisse, A. H. 1990. Issues for African-American women. In *Alcohol and drugs are women's issues*, ed.

P. Roth. Metuchen, NJ: Women's Action Alliance and Scarecrow Press.

Taylor, C.B., Houston-Miller, N., Killen, J.D., and DeBusk, R.F. 1990. Smoking cessation after acute myocardial infarction: Effects of a nurse-managed intervention. *Annals of Internal Medicine* 113:118–123.

Texas Department of Health, Bureau of Emergency Management, Sexual Assault Prevention and Crisis Services Program. 1992. *Texas Evidence Collection Protocol.* Austin, TX: the Author.

Timmreck, T.C., and Randolph, J.R. 1993. Smoking cessation: Clinical steps to improve compliance. *Geriatrics* 48(4):63–70.

United States Department of Health and Human Services. 1989. *Reducing health consequences of smoking: 25 years of progress. Report of the Surgeon General.* Washington, DC: the Author.

United States Department of Health and Human Services, Public Health Service. 1990. *Healthy people 2000* (Section 18: HIV infection). Rockville, MD: the Author.

Walker, L. 1984. *The battered woman syndrome.* New York: Springer.

Wallace, B.C. 1990. Crack cocaine smokers as adult children of alcoholics: The dysfunctional family link. *Journal of Substance Abuse Treatment* 7:89–100.

Wallace, J. 1990. The new disease model of addiction. *Western Journal of Medicine* 152(5):502–505.

Walsh, B.T., Gladis, M., Roose, S.P., Stewart, J.W., Stetner, F., and Glassman, A.H. 1988. Phenelzine v. placebo in 50 patients with bulimia. *Archives of General Psychiatry* 45:471–475.

Warshaw, C. 1989. Limitations of the medical model in the care of battered women. *Gender and Society* 3(4):506–517.

Weltzin, T.E., Hsu, L.K.G., Pollice, C., and Kaye, W. 1991. Feeding patterns in bulimia nervosa. *Biological Psychiatry* 30:1093–1110.

Wong, J.G. 1993. How to help your patients quit smoking: Strategies that work. *Postgraduate Medicine* 94:197–201.

Wurtele, S.K., Kaplan, G.M., and Keairnes, M. 1990. Child sexual abuse among chronic pain patients. *The Clinical Journal of Pain* 6:110–113.

Wynder, E.L., and Graham, E.A. 1950. Tobacco smoking as a possible etiologic factor in bronchiogenic carcinoma. *Journal of the American Medical Association* 143:329–336.

Yanovsky, S.Z. 1991. Bulimia nervosa: The role of the family physician. *Association of Family Physicians* 44(4):1231–1238.

Yates, A.J., and Sambrailo, F. 1984. Bulimia nervosa: A description and therapeutic study. *Behavioral Research Therapy* 22:503–577.

Zahnd, E.G., Coates, T.J., Richard, R.J., and Cummings, S.R. 1990. Counseling medical patients about cigarette smoking: A comparison of the impact of training on nurse practitioners and physicians. *Nurse Practitioner* 15:10–18.

Zierler, S., Feingold, L., Laufer, D., Velentgas, P., Kantrowitz-Gordon, I., and Mayer, K. 1991. Adult survivors of childhood sexual abuse and subsequent risk of HIV infection. *American Journal of Public Health* 81(5):572–575.

SECTION 15

Occupational Health

Barbara J. Burgel, R.N., M.S., A.N.P., C.O.H.N.

Occupational Health

The field of occupational health is focused on the recognition and prevention of work-related injury and illness. The primary care provider should include occupational etiology within the differential diagnosis when evaluating and treating symptoms, and when making return-to-work determinations.

Work-related conditions do not receive the recognition they deserve. This is because occupational illnesses mimic other chronic diseases with long latency periods, and because of the difficulty in obtaining and interpreting data on various types and levels of exposures. With accurate recognition of work-site exposures, primary prevention measures can be instituted at the work site to protect patient health and the health of other workers.

The following are criteria important in the management of work-related injury and illness:

→ Interpreting symptoms and diagnosing an occupational injury or illness, including appropriate reporting (e.g., occupational asthma from a cotton dust exposure).

→ Treating an occupational injury and illness, including making recommendations regarding return to work and correction of the workplace hazard (e.g., prescribing physical therapy and non-steroidal anti-inflammatory agents for an acute back strain, with three days of bed rest/ temporary disability. Work-site recommendations include dividing up the 50-pound loads, and raising the work table to keep the load within the lifting zone).

→ Determining if someone is temporarily or permanently disabled from a particular job—

based on a work-related injury/illness—including communicating with a workers' compensation insurance carrier (e.g., following a keypunch operator for recurrent wrist tendinitis. There have been several failed attempts to return to work, even though the number and force of key strokes have been decreased. Vocational rehabilitation may be indicated, if this benefit is provided in the state's particular workers' compensation benefit package).

→ Rendering a placement decision, in compliance with the Americans with Disabilities Act (ADA), regarding an individual's ability—physically and mentally—to do a particular job (e.g., whether an individual with past or current substance abuse qualifies for a driver's license to drive a bus).

→ Making recommendations to employers for reasonable accommodations to any necessary work restrictions based on an individual's health status (e.g., a woman on chemotherapy for breast cancer may be physically able to work only four hours/day during her treatment).

It is critical that the primary care provider is familiar with criteria specific to women at risk for work-related injury and illness. The number of women in the work force is continuing to increase, with many in the reproductive age group (16 years to 44 years). In addition, 80 percent of all women workers are concentrated in low-paying jobs in approximately 20 industries, many of which use suspected teratogenic agents (Rudolph and Forest 1990).

The primary care provider should:

→ Complete a preconception occupational health (OH) history for both women and men planning a pregnancy, including identifying OH risk factors and making recommendations to prevent adverse reproductive outcomes (e.g., the woman painter who may be exposed to lead-based paint during burning and scraping operations should have the exposure evaluated and may need to wear a half-face dust/mist/fume respirator).

→ Identify any work restrictions necessary during pregnancy, including making recommendations for reasonable accommodations (e.g., the pregnant utility repair person who is precluded from climbing ladders after 20 weeks gestation. The accommodation could be office work for the remaining 20 weeks of her pregnancy).

→ Evaluate adverse reproductive outcomes for all possible occupational risk factors (e.g., the dental hygienist, with a spontaneous abortion, who has had radiation and nitrous oxide exposure).

→ Counsel working women on the dual demands of career and child-rearing. This would include striving for more family-oriented workplace policies (e.g., counseling a new mother on breast-feeding techniques to use upon returning to work).

DATABASE

SUBJECTIVE

→ OH history is critical for accurate diagnosis (Occupational Health Committee 1983). See **Figure 15.1, Occupational/Environmental History Form,** for a suggested format.

→ For a screening OH history, obtain information regarding:
- type and duration of all past and present positions.
- description of job duties.
- history or presence of injuries or exposures with these positions.
- use of protective equipment (e.g., respirator, earplugs, gloves).
- environmental exposures (e.g., hobbies at home, passive smoking).

→ For a diagnostic OH history, obtain additional information regarding:

- any change(s) in work process that coincide(s) with symptom onset.
- decrease or absence of symptoms on weekends or vacations.
- similar complaints from co-workers.

OJBECTIVE

→ Do complete physical examination.

→ For exposure, document route of exposure (i.e., inhalation, skin, ingestion) and amount of dose.

→ Document whether the toxicology of the exposure matches the symptoms/target organ damage.

→ Document whether condition is on the list of ten leading work-related injuries/illnesses from the National Institute of Occupational Safety and Health (NIOSH) (see **Table 15.1, Suggested List of Ten Leading Work-Related Diseases and Injuries.** If so, consider an occupational etiology.

→ Document applicable Occupational Safety and Health Administration (OSHA) standards, including permissible exposure levels.

→ Document baseline/past medical surveillance data—environmental monitoring data (e.g., noise levels) and/or biological monitoring data (e.g., audiometry results).

→ Document applicable material safety data sheet (MSDS) information (describes toxicology and health hazards for specific hazardous substances).

→ Document job analysis data if making a placement or return to work decision. Provided by the employer, they detail the physical requirements of the job—e.g., the number of hours and weight requirement for lifting, grasping, or repetitive pinching, or if the job requires working in various temperatures or rotating shifts.

ASSESSMENT

→ Occupational exposure
- Assess exposure relative to OSHA standard. **NOTE:** Biological effects occur *below* legally established permissible exposure levels

→ R/O nonoccupational exposure

→ R/O contributing nonoccupational exposure (e.g., smoking)

→ Occupational injury or illness

→ R/O nonoccupational injury or illness

Figure 15.1. OCCUPATIONAL/ENVIRONMENTAL HISTORY FORM

I.   IDENTIFICATION

Name: _____   Soc. Sec. _____

Address: _____   Sex: M   F

_____   Birthday: _____

Telephone: home _____   work _____

II. OCCUPATIONAL PROFILE
Fill in the table below listing all jobs at which you have worked, including short-term, seasonal, and part-time employment. Start with your present job and go back to the first. Use additional paper if necessary.

Workplace (Employer's Name & Address or City)	Dates Worked From	To	Did You Work Full Time?	Type of Industry (Describe)	Describe Your Job Duties	Known Health Hazards in Workplace (Dusts, Solvents, etc.)	Protective Equipment Used	Were You Ever off Work for a Health Problem or Injury?

Continued

III. OCCUPATIONAL EXPOSURE INVENTORY

    1. Please describe any health problems or injuries you have experienced connected with your present or past jobs:

    2. Have any of your co-workers also experienced health problems or injuries connected with the same jobs?................... No   Yes
       If yes, please describe:

    3. Do you or have you ever smoked cigarettes, cigars, or pipes?.. No   Yes
       If so, which and how many per day:

    4. Do you smoke while on the job, as a general rule?.. No   Yes

    5. Do you have any allergies or allergic conditions?... No   Yes
       If so, please describe:

    6. Have you ever worked with any substance which caused you to break out in a rash?................................. No   Yes
       If so, please describe your reaction and name the substance:

    7. Have you ever been off work for more than a day because of an illness or injury related to work?........................ No   Yes
       If so, please describe:

    8. Have you ever worked at a job which caused you trouble breathing, such as cough, shortness of wind, wheezing?............. No   Yes
       If so, please describe:

    9. Have you ever changed jobs or work assignments because of any health problems or injuries?........................... No   Yes
       If so, please describe:

  10. Do you frequently experience pain or discomfort in your lower back or have you been under a doctor's care for back
       problems?.. No   Yes
       If so, please describe:

  11. Have you ever worked at a job or hobby in which you came into direct contact with any of the following substances by breathing, touching, or direct exposure? If so, please check the box beside the substance.

☐ Acids	☐ Beryllium	☐ Chromates	☐ Heat (severe)	☐ Nickel	☐ Radiation	☐ Trichloroethylene
☐ Alcohols	☐ Cadmium	☐ Coal dust	☐ Isocyanates	☐ Noise (loud)	☐ Rock dust	☐ Trinitrotoluene
(industrial)	☐ Carbon	☐ Cold (severe)	☐ Ketones	☐ PBBs	☐ Silica powders	☐ Vibration
☐ Alkalis	tetrachloride	☐ Dichlorobenzene	☐ Lead	☐ PCBs	☐ Solvents	☐ Vinyl chloride
☐ Ammonia	☐ Chlorinated	☐ Ethylene dibromide	☐ Manganese	☐ Perchloroethylene	☐ Styrene	☐ Welding fumes
☐ Arsenic	naphthalenes	☐ Ethylene dichloride	☐ Mercury	☐ Pesticides	☐ Talc	☐ X-rays
☐ Asbestos	☐ Chloroform	☐ Fiberglass	☐ Methylene	☐ Phenol	☐ Toluene	
☐ Benzene	☐ Chloroprane	☐ Halothane	chloride	☐ Phosgene	☐ TDI or MDI	

       If you have answered "yes" to any of the above, please describe your exposure on a separate sheet of paper.

IV. ENVIRONMENTAL HISTORY

    1. Have you ever changed your residence or home because of a health problem?.. No   Yes
       If so, please describe:

    2. Do you live next door to or very near an industrial plant?.. No   Yes
       If yes, please describe:

    3. Do you have a hobby or craft which you do at home?... No   Yes
       If so, please describe:

    4. Does your spouse or any other household member have contact with dusts or chemicals at work or during leisure
       activities?... No   Yes
       If so, please describe:

    5. Do you use pesticides around your home or garden?.. No   Yes
       If so, please describe:

    6. Which of the following do you have in your home? (Please check those that apply.)
       ☐ Air conditioner   ☐ Air purifier   ☐ Humidifier   ☐ Gas stove   ☐ Electric stove   ☐ Fireplace   ☐ Central heating

Source: Reprinted with permission of the Occupational Health Committee. 1983. Taking the occupational history. *Annals of Internal Medicine* 99:641-650.

Table 15.1. SUGGESTED LIST OF TEN LEADING WORK-RELATED DISEASES AND INJURIES*

1. Occupational lung diseases: asbestosis, byssinosis, silicosis, coal workers' pneumonconiosis, lung cancer, occupational asthma

2. Musculoskeletal injuries: disorders of the back, trunk, upper extremity, neck, lower extremity; traumatically induced Raynaud's phenomenon

3. Occupational cancers (other than lung): leukemia; mesothelioma; cancers of the bladder, nose, and liver

4. Severe occupational traumatic injuries: amputations, fractures, eye loss, lacerations, and traumatic deaths

5. Occupational cardiovascular diseases: hypertension, coronary artery disease, acute myocardial infarction

6. Disorders of reproduction: infertility, spontaneous abortion, teratogenesis

7. Neurotoxic disorders: peripheral neuropathy, toxic encephalitis, psychoses, extreme personality changes (exposure-related)

8. Noise-induced loss of hearing

9. Dermatologic conditions: dermatoses, burns (scaldings), chemical burns, contusions (abrasions)

10. Psychological disorders: neuroses, personality disorders, alcoholism, drug dependency

*The conditions listed under each category are to be viewed as *selected examples*, not comprehensive definitions of the category.

Source: Reprinted from the Association of Schools of Public Health. 1986. *Proposed national strategies for the prevention of leading work-related diseases and injuries, Part I.* Washington, DC: U.S. Department of Health and Human Services.

PLAN

DIAGNOSTIC TESTS

→ Commonly ordered tests in occupational health include:
- spirometry or full pulmonary function tests (PFTs) with histamine challenge testing to evaluate more fully reactive airway disease for respiratory complaints.
- liver function tests (LFTs) for hepatotoxins.
- kidney function tests for nephrotoxins.
- neurobehavioral testing for mentation/behavior changes for solvent exposure.
- nerve conduction tests for paresthesias/motor changes.
- skin patch testing with work-site allergens for dermatitis.
- audiometry for hearing loss.
- x-ray/magnetic resonance imaging (MRI) for musculoskeletal complaints.
- serum heavy metal testing for specific exposure (e.g., lead or cadmium).
- complete blood count (CBC) for any exposure affecting the hematopoietic system.
- urinalysis (spot or 24-hour collection) for specific exposures (e.g., arsenic or cadmium).

→ Work-site evaluations are a critical diagnostic tool. A firsthand look at the work process is highly educational, and helps determine if an exposure has occurred. A videotape of the work process is helpful for determination of return to work and job modification.
- A collaborative relationship with the employer facilitates implementation of control measures at the work site.

- Gaining access to the work site is often a challenge, and should be done with the support of the patient and, if available, a union representative.

→ An industrial hygienist may assist in environmental monitoring to evaluate the extent and scope of the exposure (e.g., collecting wipe samples for lead dust, air monitoring for a methylene chloride level and/or use of smoke tubes to check adequacy of ventilation).

TREATMENT/MANAGEMENT

→ Occupational health exposures are managed through a *hierarchy of controls*, which includes: *substitution, engineering controls, administrative controls*, and *personal protective equipment*.
- *Substitution:* substitute a less hazardous substance for the offending agent (e.g., fiberglass substituted for asbestos).
- *Engineering controls:* focus on work process by "engineering the problem out" (e.g., ventilation systems to remove lead fumes).
- *Administrative controls:* focus on reducing dose to any one person (e.g., job rotation of 4-hour shifts to a specific work task).
- *Personal protective equipment:* while customarily viewed as temporary until engineering controls can be implemented, may be only viable option to control an exposure (e.g., gloves, masks, earplugs).

→ Temporary modified duty: often used until there is full recovery and/or a change in the work process.
- This is a critical component of a treatment plan and maintains the injured employee within the social support of the work group.

- Also helps to maintain income level and prolongs benefits.

→ Work hardening approach: very valuable, especially with musculoskeletal work injuries; often includes physical/occupational therapy.

→ Delayed recovery is important to recognize because depression often accompanies injury/ illness where there is a loss of full function and fear of losing income. Often, timely referral to on-site employee assistance programs is beneficial (Burgel and Gliniecki 1986).

→ Reporting requirements:

- "Doctor's First Report of Injury" (or other state-required form). Often there are additional forms the injured employee/employer may have to complete before a workers' compensation claim is initiated.
- "Mandatory Reporting of Occupational Diseases by Clinicians" (CDC 1990). Each state has a listing of those infectious/occupational diseases which must be reported to the local health department.
- there may be additional state-specific requirements. For example, in California, if there is suspected or actual pesticide exposure, the provider must report it to the local health officer within 24 hours.

CONSULTATION

→ Consultation with occupational health medical/ nursing expert, if available.

- Referral to occupational medicine consultant for toxic exposures, when expected rate of recovery is delayed, and for medical/legal evaluations.
- Consultation with patient's employer. Depending on the size and type of industry, some of these resources (e.g., occupational health nurse, industrial hygienist) will be available at the specific industry. The primary care provider can call (with employee permission) to discuss work abilities/work restrictions and/or need for environmental testing.
- Consultation with workers' compensation insurance carriers, especially for case management nursing services for a disabled employee or to request environmental monitoring data.
- Consultation with federal OSHA program or state OSHA program. Anonymous complaints about hazardous working conditions can be made to OSHA. Free OSHA consultation for

employers may be a component of your OSHA program.

- Consultation with local health departments, which often have occupational health consultants, poison control centers, or toxicology information lines for health providers. For example, in California there is a teratogen hotline for patients and providers.
- On-line occupational health and safety databases are available through the National Library of Medicine or Dialog (LaDou 1990).

PATIENT EDUCATION

→ Explain relationship between exposure and symptoms, and ways to prevent future exposure.

→ Explain meaning of workers' compensation system, and how best to maximize benefits.

→ Clarify expected rates of recovery, and the need to continue modified duty, if prescribed.

→ Acknowledge loss, anger, and fear, and refer for counseling if indicated.

→ Educate patient regarding limits of confidentiality with the workers' compensation system, and assure her that she will receive copies of all written reports sent to her insurance carrier.

→ Educate patient about her legal rights to be informed regarding potential hazards at the work site, specifically as outlined in the OSHA Standards on Hazard Communication (29 CFR §20.1992) and Access to Employee Exposure and Medical Records (29 CFR §1200.1992).

→ Advocate self-care approach, and empower patients, teaching them to use resources available at their work site—e.g., the on-site occupational health nurse and/or the union health and safety committee.

FOLLOW-UP

→ Close follow-up for re-evaluation whenever time off work is prescribed.

→ Evaluate progression of modified duty assignments during recovery.

→ There is often a requirement for the treating provider for the work-related injury or illness to file monthly status reports with the workers' compensation insurance carrier.

→ Document in progress notes and problem list.

Bibliography

American College of Obstetrics and Gynecology and National Institute of Occupational Safety and Health, U.S. Department of Health, Education and Welfare (Pub. No. 78-118). *Guidelines on pregnancy and work.* Washington, DC: U.S. Government Printing Office.

American Medical Association Council on Scientific Affairs. 1984. Effects of physical forces on the reproductive cycle. *Journal of the American Medical Association* 251(2): 247–250.

———. 1984. Effects of pregnancy on work performance. *Journal of the American Medical Association* 251(15): 1995–1997.

———. 1985. Effects of toxic chemicals on the reproductive system. *Journal of the American Medical Association* 253(23): 3431–3437.

Association of Schools of Public Health. 1986. *Proposed national strategies for the prevention of leading work-related diseases and injuries, Part 1.* Washington, DC: U.S. Department of Health and Human Services.

Burgel, B.J. 1993. Pregnancy and work restrictions: Implications for the occupational health nurse. American Association of Occupational Health Nurses CE Update, Volume 5, Lesson 5. Skillman, New Jersey: Continuing Professional Education Center, Inc.

Burgel, B.J., and Gliniecki, C.M. 1986. Disability behavior: Delayed recovery in employees with work compensable injuries. *American Association of Occupational Health Nurses Journal* 34(1): 26–30.

Centers for Disease Control. 1990. Mandatory reporting of infectious diseases by clinicians, and mandatory reporting of occupational diseases by clinicians. *Morbidity and Morality Weekly Report* 39(No. RR-9): 1–28.

LaDou, J. 1990. Approach to the diagnosis of occupational illness. In *Occupational medicine*, ed. J. LaDou, pp. 5–16. Norwalk, CT: Appleton & Lange.

Occupational Health Committee. 1983. Taking the occupational history. *Annals of Internal Medicine* 99: 641–650.

Office of Technology Assessment, U.S. Congress. 1985. *Reproductive health hazards in the workplace: Summary* (OTA-BA-267). Washington, DC: U.S. Government Printing Office.

Rosenberg, M.J., Feldblum, P.J., and Marshall, E.G. 1987. Occupational influences on reproduction: A review of the recent literature. *Journal of Occupational Medicine* 29(7): 584–591.

Rudolph, L., and Forest, C.S. 1990. Female reproductive toxicology. In *Occupational medicine*, ed. J. LaDou, pp. 275–287. Norwalk, CT: Appleton & Lange.

SECTION 16

General Nutrition Guidelines

Rozane Moon Gee, R.D., M.S.

General Nutrition Guidelines

To lead healthier lives, Americans are changing their habits. The new emphasis is on wellness and preventive medicine. The best way to stay healthy includes a program of regular exercise, adequate rest, and proper nutrition.

Food is what is eaten, *nutrition* is how the food is utilized in the body. Food is the sustenance of life, an important part of health and well-being, giving energy for everyday living, affecting weight and height and, to a great extent, strength. The nutrients in food are needed to nourish the body with protein, carbohydrates, fats, vitamins, minerals, and water.

Knowledge of the nutritive content of foods, the best sources of the various nutrients, and how to combine them into a healthful, balanced diet, is important for the women's health care provider. This section provides basic information on the nutritive value of food and guidelines for establishing a healthy diet. The role of the clinician in health promotion and maintenance is discussed.

Variety of Foods

A person needs more than 40 different nutrients (including vitamins and minerals) for good health. These nutrients should come from a variety of foods, not from a few highly fortified foods or supplements. Any food that supplies calories and nutrients can be part of a nutritious diet but it is the content of the total daily or weekly diet that matters.

No single food can supply all necessary nutrients in the necessary amounts. For example, milk supplies calcium but little iron; meat supplies iron but little calcium. To have a nutritious diet, a person must eat a variety of foods, including foods from each of the five major food groups.

The **Food Guide Pyramid, Figure 16.1,** is a general guide from which to choose a healthful diet. It calls for eating a variety of foods to get needed nutrients and the right amount of calories to maintain normal, healthy weight. It starts with six to 11 servings of bread, cereal,

Figure 16.1. THE FOOD GUIDE PYRAMID, A GUIDE TO DAILY FOOD CHOICES

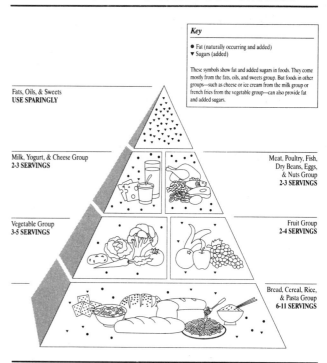

Source: Reprinted from U.S. Department of Agriculture Human Nutrition Information Service. 1992. *The food guide pyramid.* Hyattsville, MD: the Author.

rice, and pasta; three to five servings of vegetables; two to four servings of fruit; two to three servings from the milk group; and two to three servings from the meat/poultry group. Fats, oils, and sweets, the foods in the small tip of the pyramid, should be eaten in moderation.

Major Nutrients

Of the major categories of nutrients, only three—protein, carbohydrates, and fat—supply energy (measured in calories) to the body. A healthy diet usually consists of 12 percent to 15 percent from protein, 50 percent to 65 percent from carbohydrates, and 20 percent to 25 percent from fats.

PROTEIN

Every cell in the body contains protein. Protein helps build muscle tissue, which holds the bony skeleton together and provides the body with the strength to move and work. Protein is part of the hemoglobin molecule and the antibody system. Protein is also part of bone, cartilage, skin, blood, and lymph. After water and possibly fat, it is the most plentiful substance in the body. Enzymes, which control the processes that keep the body working, are made of protein.

Protein that is eaten is not directly assimilated. Instead, dietary protein must first be broken down into its component parts in the digestive tract and then absorbed into the bloodstream. The building blocks of protein are called *amino acids*. The particular amino acid arrangement determines the properties of the resulting protein.

The body is able to produce most amino acids, with the exception of eight or nine that must be provided by foods. Indispensable to humans, these are called the *essential amino acids*.

Because the body has no storage organ for protein, this nutrient needs to be consumed daily for proper nourishment. Even after one day without protein in the diet, the body will begin to break down non-essential tissue (e.g., muscle) and use it to reconstruct the proteins needed by organs vital for survival.

The body can use protein most efficiently when it is consumed frequently during the day. Four to six small meals containing some protein, rather than two to three larger ones, allow the body to make better use of the nutrient.

Most Americans get more than enough protein in their diets. Lean meats, poultry, fish, milk, cheese, and eggs provide ample quantities. Bread and cereal, soybeans, chickpeas, and dried beans are also good sources. It is not necessary to load up on meat, poultry, or eggs to get adequate protein. Combining cereal or vegetable foods can also provide adequate amounts. (See "Meatless Diet" section.)

The amount of protein each person requires is determined by physical size and age. Based on the *Recommended Dietary Allowance* (RDA) (National Academy of Sciences 1989), a 120-pound woman between 25 years to 50 years old could satisfy her recommended requirement of 50 grams of protein by eating 3 ounces of tuna, 2 slices of bread, 2 cups of skim milk, and ¾ cup of broccoli.

Table 16.1. PROTEIN IN "PROTEIN" FOODS

Food	Serving Size	Grams Protein
Beef, chuck roast	3 ounces cooked	24.0
Beef, lean ground	¼ pound cooked	23.4
Cheese, cheddar	1 ounce	7.1
Cheese, cottage	½ cup	15.0
Chicken	1 drumstick	12.2
Eggs	2 medium	11.4
Flounder	3 ounces	25.5
Ham, boiled	3 slices (3 ounces)	16.2
Liver, chicken	1 liver	6.6
Milk, skim	1 cup	8.8
Peanut butter	2 tablespoons	8.0
Scallops	3 ounces	16.0
Shrimp	3 ounces	11.6
Tuna, canned	3 ounces drained	24.4
Turkey	3 ounces	26.8
Yogurt	1 cup	8.3

Source: Adapted from Brody, J., 1981. *Jane Brody's Nutrition Book*, pp. 49-50. New York: W.W. Norton.

Table 16.2. PROTEIN IN OTHER FOODS

Food	Serving Size	Grams Protein
Banana	1 medium	1.3
Barley	¼ cup raw	4.1
Bean curd (tofu)	1 piece	9.4
Beans, kidney	½ cup cooked	7.2
Bran flakes (40%)	1 cup	3.6
Bread, whole wheat	1 slice	2.6
Broccoli	½ cup	2.4
Bulgur	1 cup cooked	8.4
Lentils	½ cup cooked	7.8
Macaroni	1 cup cooked	6.5
Noodles, egg	1 cup cooked	6.6
Oatmeal	1 cup cooked in water	4.8
Pancakes	3"-4" cakes	5.7
Potato	7 ounces baked	4.0
Potato, sweet	5 ounces baked	2.4
Rice, brown	1 cup cooked	4.9
Rice, white	1 cup cooked	4.1
Soup, tomato	1 cup with milk	6.5
Walnuts	10 large	7.3

Source: Adapted from Brody, J., 1981. *Jane Brody's Nutrition Book*, pp. 49-50. New York: W.W. Norton.

Tables 16.1, Protein in "Protein Food," and **16.2, Protein in Other Foods,** illustrate a variety of ways to fulfill the protein requirement, and demonstrate how little of the concentrated sources of protein must be eaten to meet the body's needs.

CARBOHYDRATES

Carbohydrates are the major source of energy in the diet. There are two basic types—the *sugars,* or *simple carbohydrates,* and the *starches,* called *complex carbohydrates.*

All carbohydrates are made up of one or more molecules of sugar. The sugars may be single molecules such as *glucose, fructose,* and *galactose,* or double molecules such as *sucrose* (combination of glucose and fructose), *maltose* (combination of two glucose molecules), and *lactose* (combination of glucose and galactose). The starches are branched chains of dozens of molecules of glucose.

All carbohydrates are readily broken down by digestive enzymes into their component sugars and absorbed into the bloodstream. The liver converts the fructose and galactose into glucose, which is the body's main energy source.

The chief sources of carbohydrates are grains, vegetables, fruits, and sugars. The majority of carbohydrates—both simple and complex—are present in foods like corn, wheat, rice, milk, fruits, and vegetables and in cookies, cakes, and pies.

Grains are the major carbohydrate source of food for people throughout the world. They can also supply a major portion of dietary protein. They are the cheapest, most easily obtainable, and most readily digested form of energy. Since many foods that are high in carbohydrates—bread, cereals, potatoes, and other root vegetables—are relatively inexpensive, the proportion of carbohydrates in the diet is greater than that of other nutrients, especially protein, for people at the lower economic levels.

Carbohydrate sources such as fruits and vegetables have a prominent place in a healthy diet. Despite recent concerns over pesticide residues, which demand strict regulation, the health benefits of eating fresh produce vastly outweigh any risk posed by pesticide. A diet rich in fruits and vegetables, especially the *cruciferous* vegetables like broccoli and cauliflower, has been shown to reduce the risk of certain cancers and is a good source of antioxidant vitamins (see "Vitamins and Minerals" section).

FATS

Fats provide energy and add flavor and variety to foods. Fats are plentiful in butter, salad oils, cream, most cheeses, mayonnaise, nuts, and bacon. Ounce for ounce, fats provide more than twice as many calories as protein or carbohydrate.

Fats carry Vitamins A, D, E, and K and are an essential part of the cell structure that makes up body tissue. Body fat protects vital organs by providing a cushioning effect.

There is evidence that high-fat diets may increase the risk of cancer of the colon, breast, and endometrium. Diets low in fat may reduce these risks while assisting in weight control and reduction of the incidence of heart disease.

In the typical American diet, about 40 percent of calories come from fat. The American Heart Association recommends that this figure be reduced to 30 percent; others recommend a fat intake as low as 20 percent. For example, a diet for an average woman usually contains about 1800 calories per day. If a woman chooses to reduce fat consumption to 30 percent of calories from fat, 540 calories would come from fat; the remaining calories would come from protein and carbohydrate sources (see **Figure 16.2, Formula to Determine Grams of Fat to Stay within 30 Percent Limit**).

Figure 16.2. FORMULA TO DETERMINE GRAMS OF FAT TO STAY WITHIN 30 PERCENT LIMIT

To determine grams of total fat allowed in the daily diet, first multiply the total number of calories by 30 percent, then divide by 9 (there are 9 calories per gram of fat).

Example: 1800 calories x .30 = 540 calories from fat

$$\frac{540 \text{ fat calories}}{9} = 60 \text{ grams fat} \quad \text{(goal of total fat per day)}$$

This chart lists grams of fat recommended per day at several different caloric levels:

Calories	Total Fat to Stay within 30%
1200	40 grams
1500	50 grams
2000	67 grams
2500	83 grams

FATS AND CHOLESTEROL

There are four main fats in foods: *saturated, polyunsaturated, monounsaturated,* and *cholesterol*. The first three are fatty acids; cholesterol is a fat-like substance. Of the fatty acids, only saturated fat raises blood cholesterol. Cholesterol obtained from food also can raise blood cholesterol (see **Table 16.3, Cholesterol and Fat Content of Selected Foods**).

→ SATURATED FATS

Saturated fatty acids are the main dietary culprits in raising blood cholesterol. They come from both animal and plant products. Saturated fats are usually solid at room temperature and are found largely in meat fat, whole milk products, butter, lard, cocoa butter, coconut oil, palm oil, and palm kernel oil.

During food processing, trans-fatty acid may be formed when manufacturers partially hydrogenate—i.e., partially saturate—liquid oils. The trans-fats that are formed do appear to raise blood cholesterol levels.

In the case of margarine, the process of hydrogenation allows an oil to be partially hardened and molded into tub or stick form. Hydrogenation increases the time it takes before oils become rancid, so they stay fresh longer. Hydrogenation of oils can be found mostly in fried fast foods, cookies, pies, doughnuts, and margarine.

Here are some ways to avoid trans-fat:
→ Eat less fat. Avoid deep-fried foods. Choose lower-fat crackers, cookies, and other processed foods.
→ Use canola or olive oils instead of butter, margarine, or shortening.
→ Look for foods that are labeled "saturated-fat-free." They're also low in trans-fat.

Saturated fat intake should not exceed one-third of the total fat intake (between seven percent to ten percent). The remainder of fat intake should come from polyunsaturated or monounsaturated fats.

→ POLYUNSATURATED FATS

There are two types of polyunsaturates. One type is *omega-6 fatty acids*. Vegetable oils such as safflower, sunflower seed, soybean, and corn contain these in large amounts. The other type, *omega-3 polyunsaturates*, is found mostly in fish oils. Polyunsaturated fatty acids should be limited to no more than 10 percent of total calories.

Some studies have shown this kind of fatty acid to be beneficial in reducing risks of heart disease, but these studies are as yet inconclusive. It is, however, beneficial to include fish in the diet regularly. Fish is very low in saturated fat and a better choice than red meat.

→ MONOUNSATURATED FATS

High amounts of monounsaturates are found in olive, canola, and peanut oils, high-monounsaturated forms of sunflower seed and safflower oils, avocados, and most nuts. Recent research suggests that these may be effective in lowering cholesterol levels when used in place of saturated fatty acids in the diet.

→ CHOLESTEROL

Cholesterol is a soft, fat-like substance found in all body cells. It is used to form certain hormones, cell membranes, and other important tissues. Because it cannot dissolve in the blood, cholesterol has to be transported to and from the cells by special carriers called *lipoproteins*. *Low-density lipoprotein (LDL)* is the major cholesterol carrier in the blood. Excess circulating LDL can form plaque on the inner walls of the coronary and cerebral arteries. The LDL-cholesterol level is used as a predictor of heart attack risk. (See **Hypercholesterolemia** Protocol.)

Approximately one-third to one-fourth of blood cholesterol is carried by another kind of lipoprotein—*high-density lipoprotein or HDL*, produced mostly in the liver. HDL tends to carry cholesterol away from the arteries and back to the liver, where it is metabolized. It is known as "good" cholesterol because a high level seems to guard against heart attack.

The average American consumes about 400 milligrams of cholesterol a day. Although some dietary cholesterol is eliminated through the liver, the American Heart Association recommends a daily intake of cholesterol of below 300 milligrams.

All dietary cholesterol comes from animal products. Egg yolks and organ meats contain the most cholesterol, but some is also found in all meats, fish, poultry, and animal fats. It is relatively easy to reduce blood cholesterol by eating more low-fat (particularly, low in saturated fats), low-cholesterol foods.

■ *Low-fat, low-cholesterol diet.*

• FATS AND OILS
  –Fats and oils used sparingly in cooking.
  –Small amounts of salad dressing and spreads, such as butter, margarine, and mayonnaise, fat-free or reduced-fat dressings and spreads.
  –Liquid vegetable oils (lower in saturated fat).
  –Cooking methods requiring little or no fat (boiling, broiling, baking, roasting, poaching, steaming, or microwaving).

• MEAT, POULTRY, FISH, DRY BEANS, AND EGGS
  –Lean cuts of beef (sirloin, round), poultry, fish; no more than 6 ounces (cooked) per day.
  –Fresh fish and shellfish, canned fish packed in water.
  –Meat and poultry without visible fat/skin.
  –Soups and stews without hardened fat.
  –Main dishes featuring pasta, rice, beans and/or vegetables. (These foods can be mixed with small amounts of lean meat, fish, or poultry to create a "low-meat meal.")
  –Egg yolks (maximum four per week) and organ meats in moderation.

• MILK AND MILK PRODUCTS
  –Skim or 1% extra-light milk and non-fat or low-fat yogurt and cheeses.

• SNACKS
  –Fresh or frozen fruits and vegetables.
  –Air-popped popcorn, low-salt pretzels.
  –Less pastry and deep-fried foods.

Table 16.3. CHOLESTEROL AND FAT CONTENT OF SELECTED FOODS

Food	Cholesterol (mg)	Saturated Fat (gms)
Milk, whole (1 cup)	33	5.1
Milk, non-fat (1 cup)	4	0.3
Cheese, cheddar (1 ounce)	30	6.0
Cheese, mozzarella, part-skim (1 ounce)	16	2.9
Egg, 1 whole	213	1.7
Egg, white	0	0.0
Butter (1 teaspoon)	11	2.5
Tub margarine -safflower oil (1 teaspoon)	0	0.4
Liver, beef (4 ounces)	545	3.0
Bacon, 4-5 slices	24	5.0
Flounder, sole, clams (4 ounces)	76	0.3
Shrimp (4 ounces)	220	0.3
McDonald's Egg McMuffin	226	4.0
Burger King Whopper w/cheese	113	17.0
Beans, fruit (exc. avocado), vegetables	0	0-1.0

Source: Adapted from Liebman, B., 1989. Cutting cholesterol. *Nutrition Action Health Letter* 16(7):5.

A MEATLESS DIET

Meats such as beef, pork, veal, and lamb provide protein and many vitamins and minerals the body needs to maintain good health. At the same time, some cuts of meat are high in total fat, saturated fatty acids, and cholesterol. The recommendation is to limit consumption to a total of 6 ounces of lean meat, seafood, or poultry daily. In addition, fish can be substituted for meat, and meatless (i.e., vegetarian) meals can be eaten at least twice a week.

A considerable body of scientific data suggests positive relationships between vegetarian diets and risk reduction for several chronic, degenerative diseases and conditions, including obesity, coronary artery disease, hypertension, diabetes mellitus, and several types of cancer.

The vegetarian diet consists mainly of plant foods—fruits, vegetables, legumes, grains, seeds, and nuts. Eggs and other dairy products can be included as well. Plant sources of protein alone can provide adequate amounts of the essential and non-essential amino acids.

Although most vegetarian diets meet or exceed the recommended dietary allowances for protein, they often provide less protein than non-vegetarian diets. This lower protein may be associated with better calcium retention and improved kidney function in individuals with a history of kidney damage. Further, lower protein intakes may result in a lower fat intake with its inherent advantages, because foods high in protein are also frequently high in fat.

A basic principle for preparing meatless meals is the mixing of grains with legumes or low-fat dairy products (see **Table 16.4, Daily Food Guide for Vegetarians**). This provides ample protein, which is naturally lower in fat and cholesterol. It is not necessary to add fat or sodium when preparing these grains, legumes, and dairy products. The use of cooking oils and spreads, creams and cheese-based sauces should be limited. Also, use a variety of fruits and vegetables, including a good food source of Vitamin C.

Grain products include brown or white rice, barley, pasta, kasha, whole grain bread, rolls, crackers, and cereals. Legumes include lentils, all beans, chickpeas, tofu, and other soy products. Low-fat dairy products include skim or 1% milk, low-fat or non-fat yogurt, and cheese with 5 grams of fat or less per ounce.

A meatless meal can be planned for any time of the day. Suggestions include:

■ *Breakfast.*

• Ready-to-eat or hot cereal and skim or 1% milk.
• Pancakes or waffles topped with low-fat or non-fat yogurt.
• Whole grain bread, rolls, bagels, or English muffin with low-fat cheese, 1% cottage cheese.

Table 16.4. DAILY FOOD GUIDE FOR VEGETARIANS

Food group	Suggested daily servings	Serving sizes
Breads, cereals, rice, and pasta	6 or more	1 slice bread ½ bagel or English muffin ½ cup rice or cooked cereal 1 oz. dry cereal
Vegetables	4 or more	½ cup cooked or 1 cup raw
Legumes and other meat substitutes	2 to 3	½ cup cooked beans 4 oz. tofu 8 oz. soy milk 2 tbsp. nuts or seeds (These tend to be high in fat, so use sparingly if you are following a low-fat diet.)
Fruits	3 or more	1 piece fresh fruit ¾ cup fruit juice ½ cup canned or cooked fruit
Dairy products	Optional—up to 3 servings daily	1 cup low-fat or skim milk 1 cup low-fat or nonfat yogurt 1½ oz. low-fat cheese
Eggs	Optional—limit to 3 to 4 yolks per week	1 egg or 2 egg whites
Fats, sweets, and alcohol	Go easy on these foods and beverages	Oil, margarine, and mayonnaise Cakes, cookies, pies, pastries, and candies Beer, wine, and distilled spirits

Source: Copyright the American Dietetic Association. Reprinted with permission from *Journal of the American Dietetic Association* 93(11):138.

■ *Lunch.*
- Whole grain crackers or roll with low-fat or non-fat yogurt.
- Meatless sandwiches—e.g., low-fat cheese and tomato, drained canned beans or tofu with lettuce and tomato.
- Lentil, bean, vegetable, or barley soup with whole grain crackers or bread.
- Salads of vegetables, beans, fruits, low-fat cheeses; dressings to be used sparingly or substituted with low-fat/fat-free brands.

■ *Dinner.*
- Whole grain pasta with tomato-based sauce, vegetables (mushrooms, onions, green peppers) and/or beans can be added.
- Bean-filled enchiladas and burritos.
- Rice and beans, vegetarian chili.
- Barley, kasha and/or brown rice mixed with beans and corn kernels, diced peppers; can be served with low-fat or non-fat yogurt.

FIBER

In the group of polysaccharides (ten or more glucose units), there is *fiber*, the portion of plant foods that human bodies cannot digest. There are two types of fiber: *insoluble* and *soluble*.

→ INSOLUBLE FIBER

Insoluble fiber, usually referred to as *roughage*, includes the woody or structural parts of plants, such as fruit and vegetable skins and the outer coating (bran) of wheat kernels. Insoluble fiber such as whole grain cereals, breads and crackers, and brown and wild rice may help accelerate intestinal transit, slow starch hydrolysis, delay glucose absorption, and guard against colon cancer and other diseases.

→ SOLUBLE FIBER

Soluble fiber is a substance that dissolves and thickens in water to form gels. Beans, oatmeal, barley, broccoli, raw carrots, and citrus fruits all contain soluble fiber. Oat bran is an especially rich source. There is evidence that soluble fiber may be helpful in improving glucose tolerance and in reducing blood cholesterol levels.

Normal gastrointestinal (GI) tract function is facilitated by both insoluble and soluble fiber. Fiber absorbs water and combats constipation by softening and enlarging the stool. Foods high in fiber also help with weight control as they tend to be lower in calories, are more filling, and take longer to chew. (see **Table 16.5, High-Fiber Favorites**, and **Table 16.6, Sample Menu with Fiber Content in Each Meal**).

■ *Increase fiber in the diet.*

- Increase fiber intake gradually. Too much, too quickly can cause gas, cramps, and/or diarrhea.
- Obtain fiber from a variety of sources—fruits, vegetables, and grains ensure a variety of nutrients.
- Include plenty of water. Fiber, especially soluble, absorbs large amounts of water. A high-fiber diet can actually cause constipation if not accompanied by liberal amounts of liquids (six to eight glasses a day).
- Include fiber foods in every meal. Breakfast offers an especially good opportunity for incorporating bran, whole grain cereals, and breads, along with fresh fruits.
- Substitute rather than add. Whole grain breads and flours should be used in place of the more refined varieties. Eat fruits and vegetables with skins intact and bran-containing cereals instead of low-fiber breakfast foods.
- Limit fats. Heavy sauces for high-fiber starch dishes (cheese sauce on broccoli, creamy dressing on salads) should be avoided. Advertisements for "high-fiber" cereals can be misleading because of the undesirable saturated fat content in some of these products.
- It is recommended that healthy adults eat 25 grams to 40 grams of dietary fiber a day. Most Americans eat far less.

WATER

Water is a very important nutrient and is necessary for all the digestive processes. Nutrients dissolve in water to

Table 16.5. HIGH-FIBER FAVORITES

Food	Portion size	Fiber (grams)
Apple	large	4.7
Banana	medium	1.8
Orange	medium	3.1
Strawberries	½ cup	2.0
Carrots	½ cup	2.3
Corn	½ cup	3.1
Sweet potato	medium	3.4
Beans, cooked		
pinto	¾ cup	14.2
navy	¾ cup	9.0
kidney	¾ cup	13.8
Bulgur (cracked wheat)	1 cup	8.1
Bran flakes	¾ cup	5.0
Oatmeal	⅔ cup	2.7
Air-popped popcorn	3 cups	3.9
Whole wheat bread	1 slice	2.0
Quaker rice cakes	2 cakes	0.6

Source: Adapted from Hurley, J., 1990. Rough it up. *Nutrition Action Health Letter* 17(2):8-9.

Table 16.6. SAMPLE MENU WITH FIBER CONTENT IN EACH MEAL

Meal	gm fiber
Breakfast:	
1 cup shredded wheat with milk	3.0
½ cup strawberries	2.0
1 slice whole wheat bread w/1 tsp. margarine	1.0
Snack:	
3 Triscuits crackers	2.0
Water	
Lunch:	
½ cup split pea soup	5.2
Tuna salad sandwich on whole grain bread w/lettuce	4.0
1 cup fruit salad (pear, cantaloupe, peach)	4.0
Snack:	
1 large apple, unpeeled	4.7
Dinner:	
½ grapefruit	0.7
Stir-fried chicken and broccoli	2.0
1 cup brown rice	3.3
½ cup vanilla yogurt	
Snack:	
3 cups popcorn, air-popped	3.9
Total	**36 grams fiber**

allow them to pass through the intestinal wall and into the bloodstream for use throughout the body. Water carries out waste and helps to regulate body temperature.

At least six to eight glasses of fluids daily are recommended. Coffee and tea, fruit juices and milk, soup, and fruits and vegetables are all sources.

VITAMINS AND MINERALS

One out of every four Americans takes a vitamin/mineral supplement daily. The American Medical Association (AMA), the National Academy of Sciences (NAS), and the American Dietetic Association (ADA) do not advocate supplements if a balanced diet is maintained. However, some studies suggest that certain vitamins or minerals may help prevent cancer, eye disorders, heart disease, neural-tube defects, and other serious chronic diseases.

The *recommended dietary allowances* (RDAs) (see **Table 16.7, Food and Nutrition Board, National Academy of Sciences Recommended Dietary Allowances**) are a set of guidelines that define the daily amounts of essential nutrients considered to be adequate to meet the known nutritional needs of most healthy persons. The levels are not strict recommendations; instead, they are calculated to be well over the requirements of most individuals so that nearly every person's needs will be met without adverse health effects.

A diet consisting of foods selected from among lean meats, low-fat dairy products, whole grains and ce-

Table 16.7. FOOD AND NUTRITION BOARD, NATIONAL ACADEMY OF SCIENCES—NATIONAL RESEARCH COUNCIL RECOMMENDED DIETARY ALLOWANCES,[a] Revised 1989

Designed for the maintenance of good nutrition of practically all healthy people in the United States

Category	Age (years) or Condition	Weight[b] (kg)	(lb)	Height[b] (cm)	(in)	Protein (g)	Vitamin A (µg RE)[c]	Vitamin D (µg)[d]	Vitamin E (mg α-TE)[e]	Vitamin K (µg)	Vitamin C (mg)	Thiamine (mg)	Riboflavin (mg)	Niacin (mg NE)[f]	Vitamin B6 (mg)	Folate (µg)	Vitamin B12 (µg)	Calcium (mg)	Phosphorus (mg)	Magnesium (mg)	Iron (mg)	Zinc (mg)	Iodine (µg)	Selenium (µg)
Infants	0.0–0.5	6	13	60	24	13	375	7.5	3	5	30	0.3	0.4	5	0.3	25	0.3	400	300	40	6	5	40	10
	0.5–1.0	9	20	71	28	14	375	10	4	10	35	0.4	0.5	6	0.6	35	0.5	600	500	60	10	5	50	15
Children	1–3	13	29	90	35	16	400	10	6	15	40	0.7	0.8	9	1.0	50	0.7	800	800	80	10	10	70	20
	4–6	20	44	112	44	24	500	10	7	20	45	0.9	1.1	12	1.1	75	1.0	800	800	120	10	10	90	20
	7–10	28	62	132	52	28	700	10	7	30	45	1.0	1.2	13	1.4	100	1.4	800	800	170	10	10	120	30
Males	11–14	45	99	157	62	45	1,000	10	10	45	50	1.3	1.5	17	1.7	150	2.0	1,200	1,200	270	12	15	150	40
	15–18	66	145	176	69	59	1,000	10	10	65	60	1.5	1.8	20	2.0	200	2.0	1,200	1,200	400	12	15	150	50
	19–24	72	160	177	70	58	1,000	10	10	70	60	1.5	1.7	19	2.0	200	2.0	1,200	1,200	350	10	15	150	70
	25–50	79	174	176	70	63	1,000	5	10	80	60	1.5	1.7	19	2.0	200	2.0	800	800	350	10	15	150	70
	51+	77	170	173	68	63	1,000	5	10	80	60	1.2	1.4	15	2.0	200	2.0	800	800	350	10	15	150	70
Females	11–14	46	101	157	62	46	800	10	8	45	50	1.1	1.3	15	1.4	150	2.0	1,200	1,200	280	15	12	150	45
	15–18	55	120	163	64	44	800	10	8	55	60	1.1	1.3	15	1.5	180	2.0	1,200	1,200	300	15	12	150	50
	19–24	58	128	164	65	46	800	10	8	60	60	1.1	1.3	15	1.6	180	2.0	1,200	1,200	280	15	12	150	55
	25–50	63	138	163	64	50	800	5	8	65	60	1.1	1.3	15	1.6	180	2.0	800	800	280	15	12	150	55
	51+	65	143	160	63	50	800	5	8	65	60	1.0	1.2	13	1.6	180	2.0	800	800	280	10	12	150	55
Pregnant						60	800	10	10	65	70	1.5	1.6	17	2.2	400	2.2	1,200	1,200	320	30	15	175	65
Lactating	1st 6 months					65	1,300	10	12	65	95	1.6	1.8	20	2.1	280	2.6	1,200	1,200	355	15	19	200	75
	2nd 6 months					62	1,200	10	11	65	90	1.6	1.7	20	2.1	260	2.6	1,200	1,200	340	15	16	200	75

[a]The allowances, expressed as average daily intakes over time, are intended to provide for individual variations among most normal persons as they live in the United States under usual environmental stresses. Diets should be based on a variety of common foods in order to provide other nutrients for which human requirements have been less well defined. See text for detailed discussion of allowances and of nutrients not tabulated.

[b]Weights and heights of Reference Adults are actual medians for the U.S. population of the designated age, as reported by NHANES II. The median weights and heights of those under 19 years of age were taken from Hamill et al. (1979) (see pages 16–17). The use of these figures does not imply that the height-to-weight ratios are ideal.

[c]Retinol equivalents. 1 retinol equivalent = 1 µg retinol or 6 µg β-carotene. See text for calculation of Vitamin A activity of diets as retinol equivalents.

[d]As cholecalciferol. 10 µg cholecalciferol = 400 IU of Vitamin D.

[e]α-Tocopherol equivalents. 1 mg d-α tocopherol = 1 α-TE. See text for variation in allowances and calculation of Vitamin E activity of the diet as α-tocopherol equivalents.

[f]1 NE (niacin equivalent) is equal to 1 mg of niacin or 60 mg of dietary tryptophan.

Source: Reprinted with permission from National Academy of Sciences. 1989. *Recommended dietary allowances*, 10th ed. Copyright 1989 by the National Academy of Sciences. Courtesy of National Academy Press, Washington, DC.

reals, legumes, and fresh fruits and vegetables will provide ample amounts of vitamins and minerals. A varied diet will provide safe and balanced levels of all essential nutrients. However, if a person's lifestyle prohibits eating wisely most of the time, or if less than 1200 calories per day are consumed, supplementing the diet with a vitamin/mineral pill that supplies no more than 100 percent of the RDAs for each nutrient may be a healthy recommendation.

Self-dosing with vitamins in amounts many times greater than the RDA is usually worthless and may be hazardous. Megadoses of certain vitamins can have drug-like effects quite apart from their usual role as vitamins, and can pose risks just as serious to health as deficiencies of those vitamins (e.g., fat-soluble vitamins are stored in the body and can build up toxic levels if too high a volume is consumed).

→ CALCIUM

Many women are not consuming enough calcium to maintain bone strength. Although the effects of insufficient dietary calcium are evident later in life, the most critical time to increase calcium consumption is during the years of bone formation and growth, from 11 years to 24 years of age. During this time, the RDA is 1200 mg/day, the amount of calcium found in four cups of milk. When the critical period of bone formation is over, the RDA drops to 800 mg/day.

Post-menopausal women who consume less than 1200 mg of calcium daily and find it difficult to eat enough calories to reach this calcium level, may be candidates for calcium supplementation. To attain maximum calcium absorption from the GI tract, some experts believe that calcium supplements should be taken with meals, since lactose and glucose enhance calcium absorption. Others believe calcium supplements should be taken alone, since the phytates and oxalates in food interfere with calcium absorption.

A recent study by Davis (1989) found that taking a calcium supplement (or milk) with a light meal increased calcium absorption by 10 percent to 30 percent above levels gained when the same amount of calcium was ingested between meals.

Table 16.8 lists some relatively easy to find lower-fat calcium sources that occur naturally in food.

→ IRON

Many women do not get enough iron-rich food to meet the RDA for iron. Women are likely to ingest fewer calories either because they are dieting or because they have smaller frames that require less food. Iron losses in blood during menstruation and pregnancy can also increase a woman's iron requirements.

Table 16.8. LOWER-FAT CALCIUM SOURCES

Food	Serving Size	Calcium (mg)
Milk, 1%, skim	1 cup	302
Swiss cheese	1 oz.	272
Provolone cheese	1 oz.	214
Part-skim mozzarella cheese	1 oz.	183
Low-fat yogurt (fruit)	1 cup	314
Low-fat yogurt (plain)	1 cup	415
Broccoli (cooked)	1 cup	178
Collard greens (cooked)	1 cup	304
Kale, cooked	1 cup	180
Salmon, canned w/bone	3 oz.	203
Sardines, canned w/ bone	3 oz.	372

Source: Adapted from Pennington, J. 1989. *Bowes & Church's food values of portions commonly used.* Philadelphia: J.B. Lippincott.

Iron-rich foods should be included regularly in the diet. Some excellent sources include lean, fat-trimmed cuts of meat (up to 6 oz. daily), enriched or fortified whole grain products (e.g., hot and cold cereal, bread, crackers, pasta), and dried apricots, prunes, lentils, and beans.

→ ANTIOXIDANT NUTRIENTS (VITAMINS C AND E AND BETA-CAROTENE)

Antioxidants are a group of compounds that help protect the body from damage by unstable molecules known as *free radicals*. Free radicals damage healthy cells and are thought to contribute to cancer, heart disease, immune diseases, cataracts, and aging. The body produces free radicals as byproducts of oxidation, the process by which the body burns fuel. Free radicals can also enter the body from outside—e.g., in cigarette smoke, exhaust fumes, and environmental toxins.

There are some built-in antioxidants to protect against free radical damage, levels of which are largely fixed. Additional antioxidant intake depends on the diet. Fruits and vegetables are particularly good sources. These and other sources are listed in **Table 16.9.**

Table 16.9. ANTIOXIDANT FOOD SOURCES

Fruits (2-4 servings daily)
Apricots, cantaloupe, grapefruit, oranges, strawberries, watermelon, peaches

Vegetables (3-5 servings)
Broccoli, carrots, kale, red cabbage, spinach, yams

Whole grains/cereals (6-11 servings)
Whole wheat, rye, pumpernickel, corn or oat bread, muffins or crackers; oatmeal, barley, grits, buckwheat, brown rice, whole-grain cereals

Fish and seafood (up to 6 oz./day)
Cod, halibut, salmon, lobster, scallops, shrimp, tuna, swordfish

Diet, Weight and Exercise

MAINTAIN A HEALTHY WEIGHT

Being underweight or overweight increases the chances of developing health problems. Whether or not the weight is healthy depends on how much of the weight is fat, the location of the body fat, and whether there are concomitant weight-related medical problems.

Extra pounds can increase the risk of heart disease, diabetes, and other illnesses. Being too thin is a less common problem in the United States. It occurs with anorexia nervosa and is linked with osteoporosis in women and greater risk of early death in both women and men.

The tables that follow can be used to help determine if a client's weight is healthy. The body frame size must be measured first. To do this, have the client extend one arm and bend the forearm upward at a 90-degree angle. Keep the fingers straight and turn the inside of the wrist toward the body. Feel the two prominent bones on either side of the bent elbow. Measure the elbow width between these bones. Compare the measurement with **Table 16.10, Elbow Measurements for Medium-Frame Women**. Measurements lower than those listed (for height) indicate a small frame. Higher measurements indicate a large frame. The **Ideal Weight for Height (and Frame Size) for Women Age 25 Years and Over** is listed in **Table 16.11.**

Another useful chart to determine whether weight for height is in a healthy range is the *body mass index* (BMI) chart (see **Figure 16.3**). The BMI is calculated as weight (in kg) divided by height (in square meters). It can be used to determine if a woman is a health risk because she is underweight (BMI <19.8), moderately overweight (BMI 26.1-29.0), or very overweight (BMI >29.0).

Draw a line from the client's weight (left column) to height (right column) to determine if the BMI is in the healthy range.

NOTE: There will be some discrepancy in the categorization of women as underweight or overweight depending on whether the weight-for-height chart or the BMI chart is used. Therefore, only *one method* should be used for assessing risk.

The client should consider losing weight if she falls above the recommended ranges for a healthy weight for height. Substantial weight loss is difficult, however, and may pose health risks of its own. Before a client attempts to lose weight, it should be determined how great a risk the weight poses, and how much weight needs to be lost to lower that risk. People with diabetes and

Table 16.10. ELBOW MEASUREMENTS FOR MEDIUM-FRAME WOMEN

Height of Woman	Elbow Breadth
4'10"–5'3"	2¼"–2½"
5'4"–5'11"	2⅜"–2⅝"
6'0"	2½"–2¾"

Source: Adapted from Shils, M., and Young, V. 1988. *Modern nutrition in health and disease,* 7th ed. Philadelphia: Lea and Febiger.

Table 16.11. IDEAL WEIGHT FOR HEIGHT (AND FRAME SIZE) FOR WOMEN AGE 25 YEARS AND OVER*

Height of Woman	Small Frame (lbs.)	Medium Frame (lbs.)	Large Frame (lbs.)
4'10"	102-111	109-121	118-131
4'11"	103-113	111-123	120-134
5'0"	104-115	113-126	122-137
5'1"	106-118	115-129	125-140
5'2"	108-121	118-132	128-143
5'3"	111-124	121-135	131-147
5'4"	114-127	124-138	134-151
5'5"	117-130	127-141	137-155
5'6"	120-133	130-144	140-159
5'7"	123-136	133-147	143-163
5'8"	126-139	136-150	146-167
5'9"	129-142	139-153	149-170
5'10"	132-145	142-156	152-173
5'11"	135-148	145-159	155-176
6'0"	138-151	148-162	158-179

*Women with indoor clothing that weighs 3 lbs; shoes with 1" heels.

Source: Reprinted courtesy of Metropolitan Life Insurance Company. 1983. *1983 Metropolitan weight/height tables.* New York: the Author.

high blood pressure are especially likely to improve their health when extra pounds are shed.

Heredity and metabolism play key roles in keeping some people overweight despite their best efforts to reduce. For such people, striving to attain a recommended weight may be futile and even damaging. Nonetheless, a client can do well to follow a high-carbohydrate, low-fat diet and exercise regularly.

EXERCISE

Proper diet and exercise improve the odds of losing weight and help maintain health at whatever weight is attained. Inactivity may play an even greater role in weight gain than a high-calorie diet. Exercise can help shed pounds and maintain a healthier weight, as well as improve overall fitness and quality of life.

Aerobic exercise is a good choice because it burns fat from all over the body. It works the larger muscles and uses plenty of oxygen to fuel them. Walking, running, bicycling, and swimming are all aerobic.

Figure 16.3. BODY MASS INDEX

Weight		Height, in. (and cm)																							
		55.9	56.7	57.5	58.3	59.1	59.8	60.6	61.4	62.2	63.0	63.8	64.6	65.4	66.1	66.9	67.7	68.5	69.3	70.1	70.9	71.7	72.4	73.2	74.0
lb	kg	(142)	(144)	(146)	(148)	(150)	(152)	(154)	(156)	(158)	(160)	(162)	(164)	(166)	(168)	(170)	(172)	(174)	(176)	(178)	(180)	(182)	(184)	(186)	(188)
220	100	49.6	48.2	46.9	45.7	44.4	43.3	42.2	41.1	40.1	39.1	38.1	37.2	36.3	35.4	34.6	33.8	33.0	32.3	31.6	30.9	30.2	29.5	28.9	28.3
218	99	49.1	47.7	46.4	45.2	44.0	42.8	41.7	40.7	39.7	38.7	37.7	36.8	35.9	35.1	34.3	33.5	32.7	32.0	31.2	30.6	29.9	29.2	28.6	28.0
216	98	48.6	47.3	46.0	44.7	43.6	42.4	41.3	40.3	39.3	38.3	37.3	36.4	35.6	34.7	33.9	33.1	32.4	31.6	30.9	30.2	29.6	28.9	28.3	27.7
213	97	48.1	46.8	45.5	44.3	43.1	42.0	40.9	39.9	38.9	37.9	37.0	36.1	35.2	34.4	33.6	32.8	32.0	31.3	30.6	29.9	29.3	28.7	28.0	27.4
211	96	47.6	46.3	45.0	43.8	42.7	41.6	40.5	39.4	38.5	37.5	36.6	35.7	34.8	34.0	33.2	32.4	31.7	31.0	30.3	29.6	29.0	28.4	27.7	27.2
209	95	47.1	45.8	44.6	43.4	42.2	41.1	40.1	39.0	38.1	37.1	36.2	35.3	34.5	33.7	32.9	32.1	31.4	30.7	30.0	29.3	28.7	28.1	27.5	26.9
207	94	46.6	45.3	44.1	42.9	41.8	40.7	39.6	38.6	37.7	36.7	35.8	34.9	34.1	33.3	32.5	31.8	31.0	30.3	29.7	29.0	28.4	27.8	27.2	26.6
205	93	46.1	44.8	43.6	42.5	41.3	40.3	39.2	38.2	37.3	36.3	35.4	34.6	33.7	33.0	32.2	31.4	30.7	30.0	29.4	28.7	28.1	27.5	26.9	26.3
202	92	45.6	44.4	43.2	42.0	40.9	39.8	38.8	37.8	36.9	35.9	35.1	34.2	33.4	32.6	31.8	31.1	30.4	29.7	29.0	28.4	27.8	27.2	26.6	26.0
200	91	45.1	43.9	42.7	41.5	40.4	39.4	38.4	37.4	36.5	35.5	34.7	33.8	33.0	32.2	31.5	30.8	30.1	29.4	28.7	28.1	27.5	26.9	26.3	25.7
198	90	44.6	43.4	42.2	41.1	40.0	39.0	37.9	37.0	36.1	35.2	34.3	33.5	32.7	31.9	31.1	30.4	29.7	29.1	28.4	27.8	27.2	26.6	26.0	25.5
196	89	44.1	42.9	41.8	40.6	39.6	38.5	37.5	36.6	35.7	34.8	33.9	33.1	32.3	31.5	30.8	30.1	29.4	28.7	28.1	27.5	26.9	26.3	25.7	25.2
194	88	43.6	42.4	41.3	40.2	39.1	38.1	37.1	36.2	35.3	34.4	33.5	32.7	31.9	31.2	30.4	29.7	29.1	28.4	27.8	27.2	26.6	26.0	25.4	24.9
191	87	43.1	42.0	40.8	39.7	38.7	37.7	36.7	35.7	34.9	34.0	33.2	32.3	31.6	30.8	30.1	29.4	28.7	28.1	27.5	26.9	26.3	25.7	25.1	24.6
189	86	42.7	41.5	40.3	39.3	38.2	37.2	36.3	35.3	34.4	33.6	32.8	32.0	31.2	30.5	29.8	29.1	28.4	27.8	27.1	26.5	26.0	25.4	24.9	24.3
187	85	42.2	41.0	39.9	38.8	37.8	36.8	35.8	34.9	34.0	33.2	32.4	31.6	30.8	30.1	29.4	28.7	28.1	27.4	26.8	26.2	25.7	25.1	24.6	24.0
185	84	41.7	40.5	39.4	38.3	37.3	36.4	35.4	34.5	33.6	32.8	32.0	31.2	30.5	29.8	29.1	28.4	27.7	27.1	26.5	25.9	25.4	24.8	24.3	23.8
183	83	41.2	40.0	38.9	37.9	36.9	35.9	35.0	34.1	33.2	32.4	31.6	30.9	30.1	29.4	28.7	28.1	27.4	26.8	26.2	25.6	25.1	24.5	24.0	23.5
180	82	40.7	39.5	38.5	37.4	36.4	35.5	34.6	33.7	32.8	32.0	31.2	30.5	29.8	29.1	28.4	27.7	27.1	26.5	25.9	25.3	24.8	24.2	23.7	23.2
178	81	40.2	39.1	38.0	37.0	36.0	35.1	34.2	33.3	32.4	31.6	30.9	30.1	29.4	28.7	28.0	27.4	26.8	26.1	25.6	25.0	24.5	23.9	23.4	22.9
176	80	39.7	38.6	37.5	36.5	35.6	34.6	33.7	32.9	32.0	31.3	30.5	29.7	29.0	28.3	27.7	27.0	26.4	25.8	25.2	24.7	24.2	23.6	23.1	22.6
174	79	39.2	38.1	37.1	36.1	35.1	34.2	33.3	32.5	31.6	30.9	30.1	29.4	28.7	28.0	27.3	26.7	26.1	25.5	24.9	24.4	23.8	23.3	22.8	22.4
172	78	38.7	37.6	36.6	35.6	34.7	33.8	32.9	32.1	31.2	30.5	29.7	29.0	28.3	27.6	27.0	26.4	25.8	25.2	24.6	24.1	23.5	23.0	22.5	22.1
169	77	38.2	37.1	36.1	35.2	34.2	33.3	32.5	31.6	30.8	30.1	29.3	28.6	27.9	27.3	26.6	26.0	25.4	24.9	24.3	23.8	23.2	22.7	22.3	21.8
167	76	37.7	36.7	35.7	34.7	33.8	32.9	32.0	31.2	30.4	29.7	29.0	28.3	27.6	26.9	26.3	25.7	25.1	24.5	24.0	23.5	22.9	22.4	22.0	21.5
165	75	37.2	36.2	35.2	34.2	33.3	32.5	31.6	30.8	30.0	29.3	28.6	27.9	27.2	26.6	26.0	25.4	24.8	24.2	23.7	23.1	22.6	22.2	21.7	21.2
163	74	36.7	35.7	34.7	33.8	32.9	32.0	31.2	30.4	29.6	28.9	28.2	27.5	26.9	26.2	25.6	25.0	24.4	23.9	23.4	22.8	22.3	21.9	21.4	20.9
161	73	36.2	35.2	34.2	33.3	32.4	31.6	30.8	30.0	29.2	28.5	27.8	27.1	26.5	25.9	25.3	24.7	24.1	23.6	23.0	22.5	22.0	21.6	21.1	20.7
158	72	35.7	34.7	33.8	32.9	32.0	31.2	30.4	29.6	28.8	28.1	27.4	26.8	26.1	25.5	24.9	24.3	23.8	23.2	22.7	22.2	21.7	21.3	20.8	20.4
156	71	35.2	34.2	33.3	32.4	31.6	30.7	29.9	29.2	28.4	27.7	27.1	26.4	25.8	25.2	24.6	24.0	23.5	22.9	22.4	21.9	21.4	21.0	20.5	20.1
154	70	34.7	33.8	32.8	32.0	31.1	30.3	29.5	28.8	28.0	27.3	26.7	26.0	25.4	24.8	24.2	23.7	23.1	22.6	22.1	21.6	21.1	20.7	20.2	19.8
152	69	34.2	33.3	32.4	31.5	30.7	29.9	29.1	28.4	27.6	27.0	26.3	25.7	25.0	24.4	23.9	23.3	22.8	22.3	21.8	21.3	20.8	20.4	19.9	19.5
150	68	33.7	32.8	31.9	31.0	30.2	29.4	28.7	27.9	27.2	26.6	25.9	25.3	24.7	24.1	23.5	23.0	22.5	22.0	21.5	21.0	20.5	20.1	19.7	19.2
147	67	33.2	32.3	31.4	30.6	29.8	29.0	28.3	27.5	26.8	26.2	25.5	24.9	24.3	23.7	23.2	22.6	22.1	21.6	21.1	20.7	20.2	19.8	19.4	19.0
145	66	32.7	31.8	31.0	30.1	29.3	28.6	27.8	27.1	26.4	25.8	25.1	24.5	24.0	23.4	22.8	22.3	21.8	21.3	20.8	20.4	19.9	19.5	19.1	18.7
143	65	32.2	31.3	30.5	29.7	28.9	28.1	27.4	26.7	26.0	25.4	24.8	24.2	23.6	23.0	22.5	22.0	21.5	21.0	20.5	20.1	19.6	19.2	18.8	18.4
141	64	31.7	30.9	30.0	29.2	28.4	27.7	27.0	26.3	25.6	25.0	24.4	23.8	23.2	22.7	22.1	21.6	21.1	20.7	20.2	19.8	19.3	18.9	18.5	18.1
139	63	31.2	30.4	29.6	28.8	28.0	27.3	26.6	25.9	25.2	24.6	24.0	23.4	22.9	22.3	21.8	21.3	20.8	20.3	19.9	19.4	19.0	18.6	18.2	17.8
136	62	30.7	29.9	29.1	28.3	27.6	26.8	26.1	25.5	24.8	24.2	23.6	23.1	22.5	22.0	21.5	21.0	20.5	20.0	19.6	19.1	18.7	18.3	17.9	17.5
134	61	30.3	29.4	28.6	27.8	27.1	26.4	25.7	25.1	24.4	23.8	23.2	22.7	22.1	21.6	21.1	20.6	20.1	19.7	19.3	18.8	18.4	18.0	17.6	17.3
132	60	29.8	28.9	28.1	27.4	26.7	26.0	25.3	24.7	24.0	23.4	22.9	22.3	21.8	21.3	20.8	20.3	19.8	19.4	18.9	18.5	18.1	17.7	17.3	17.0
130	59	29.3	28.5	27.7	26.9	26.2	25.5	24.9	24.2	23.6	23.0	22.5	21.9	21.4	20.9	20.4	19.9	19.5	19.0	18.6	18.2	17.8	17.4	17.1	16.7
128	58	28.8	28.0	27.2	26.5	25.8	25.1	24.5	23.8	23.2	22.7	22.1	21.6	21.0	20.5	20.1	19.6	19.2	18.7	18.3	17.9	17.5	17.1	16.8	16.4
125	57	28.3	27.5	26.7	26.0	25.3	24.7	24.0	23.4	22.8	22.3	21.7	21.2	20.7	20.2	19.7	19.3	18.8	18.4	18.0	17.6	17.2	16.8	16.5	16.1
123	56	27.8	27.0	26.3	25.6	24.9	24.2	23.6	23.0	22.4	21.9	21.3	20.8	20.83	19.8	19.4	18.9	18.5	18.1	17.7	17.3	16.9	16.5	16.2	15.8
121	55	27.3	26.5	25.8	25.1	24.4	23.8	23.2	22.6	22.0	21.5	21.0	20.4	20.0	19.5	19.0	18.6	18.2	17.8	17.4	17.0	16.6	16.2	15.9	15.6
119	54	26.8	26.0	25.3	24.7	24.0	23.4	22.8	22.2	21.6	21.1	20.6	20.1	19.6	19.1	18.7	18.3	17.8	17.4	17.0	16.7	16.3	15.9	15.6	15.3
117	53	26.3	25.6	24.9	24.2	23.6	22.9	22.3	21.8	21.2	20.7	20.2	19.7	19.2	18.8	18.3	17.9	17.5	17.1	16.7	16.4	16.0	15.7	15.3	15.0
114	52	25.8	25.1	24.4	23.7	23.1	22.5	21.9	21.4	20.8	20.3	19.8	19.3	18.9	18.4	18.0	17.6	17.2	16.8	16.4	16.0	15.7	15.4	15.0	14.7
112	51	25.3	24.6	23.9	23.3	22.7	22.1	21.5	21.0	20.4	19.9	19.4	19.0	18.5	18.1	17.6	17.2	16.8	16.5	16.1	15.7	15.4	15.1	14.7	14.4
110	50	24.8	24.1	23.5	22.8	22.2	21.6	21.1	20.5	20.0	19.5	19.1	18.6	18.1	17.7	17.3	16.9	16.5	16.1	15.8	15.4	15.1	14.8	14.5	14.1
108	49	24.3	23.6	23.0	22.4	21.8	21.2	20.7	20.1	19.6	19.1	18.7	18.2	17.8	17.4	17.0	16.6	16.2	15.8	15.5	15.1	14.8	14.5	14.2	13.9
106	48	23.8	23.1	22.5	21.9	21.3	20.8	20.2	19.7	19.2	18.8	18.3	17.8	17.4	17.0	16.6	16.2	15.9	15.5	15.1	14.8	14.5	14.2	13.9	13.6
103	47	23.3	22.7	22.0	21.5	20.9	20.3	19.8	19.3	18.8	18.4	17.9	17.5	17.1	16.7	16.3	15.9	15.5	15.2	14.8	14.5	14.2	13.9	13.6	13.3
101	46	22.8	22.2	21.6	21.0	20.4	19.9	19.4	18.9	18.4	18.0	17.5	17.1	16.7	16.3	15.9	15.5	15.2	14.9	14.5	14.2	13.9	13.6	13.3	13.0
99	45	22.3	21.7	21.1	20.5	20.0	19.5	19.0	18.5	18.0	17.6	17.1	16.7	16.3	15.9	15.6	15.2	14.9	14.5	14.2	13.9	13.6	13.3	13.0	12.7
97	44	21.8	21.2	20.6	20.1	19.6	19.0	18.6	18.1	17.6	17.2	16.8	16.4	16.0	15.6	15.2	14.9	14.5	14.2	13.9	13.6	13.3	13.0	12.7	12.4
95	43	21.3	20.7	20.2	19.6	19.1	18.6	18.1	17.7	17.2	16.8	16.4	16.0	15.6	15.2	14.9	14.5	14.2	13.9	13.6	13.3	13.0	12.7	12.4	12.2
92	42	20.8	20.3	19.7	19.2	18.7	18.2	17.7	17.3	16.8	16.4	16.0	15.6	15.2	14.9	14.5	14.2	13.9	13.6	13.3	13.0	12.7	12.4	12.1	11.9
90	41	20.3	19.8	19.2	18.7	18.2	17.7	17.3	16.8	16.4	16.0	15.6	15.2	14.9	14.5	14.2	13.9	13.5	13.2	12.9	12.7	12.4	12.1	11.9	11.6
88	40	19.8	19.3	18.8	18.3	17.8	17.3	16.9	16.4	16.0	15.6	15.2	14.9	14.5	14.2	13.8	13.5	13.2	12.9	12.6	12.3	12.1	11.8	11.6	11.3

Note: BMI (metric = (kg/m²) × 100; BMI (English) = (lb/in.²) × 100. BMI (metric) × 0.142 = BMI (English); BMI (English) × 7 = BMI (metric). BMIs < 19.8 = low; BMIs 26.1 - 29.0 = high; BMIs > 29.0 = obesity (see shaded area above heavy line).

Source: Reprinted with permission from Institute of Medicine. 1990. *Nutrition during pregnancy–Pt. 1, weight gain, Pt. 2, nutritional supplements.* Washington, DC: National Academy Press.

Thirty minutes or more a day of moderate-intensity activity, like walking, is a good recommendation. A 30-minute walk, or three ten-minute walks can get more or less comparable results. Vigorous or high-intensity aerobic exercise for a certain amount of time may strengthen the heart, but regular, moderate activity can also substantially reduce the risk of disease.

The key is to get up and move. The total energy spent in physical activity is the most important factor. See **Table 16.12**, for **Calories Used per Minute of Exercise**. One can spend 300 calories by running three miles in half an hour, or one can spend it in six ten-minute brisk walks throughout the day. The benefits may not be exactly the same, but they're comparable.

Exercise increases the level of HDL, the "good" cholesterol carrier. (See "Cholesterol" section.) It also lowers blood pressure (significantly lowering both systolic and diastolic blood pressure by an average of ten points), increases insulin sensitivity in the muscles, and lowers the risk of forming blood clots.

There is consistent, strong epidemiological evidence that exercise is associated with a lower rate of colon cancer in humans, perhaps increasing the speed with which food travels through the intestinal tract, thus lessening the time the colon is exposed to any potential carcinogens in food. In addition, exercise may stimulate the natural immunity along the mucosal lining of the intestines. For the skeletal system, a moderate, weight-bearing exercise like walking or dancing, rather than swimming, may improve bone mineral density.

TOTAL ENERGY REQUIREMENT

In the body's use of nutrients, the energy requirement of an individual takes precedence over all other needs: the body's minimum energy needs must be met first. The *basal metabolic rate* (*BMR*) is the minimum amount of energy needed by the body at rest in the fasting state. This includes cellular metabolism, circulation, and maintenance of body temperature.

Since it is technically difficult to measure an individual's BMR, it is calculated using one of many formulas. Frequently, the calculated BMR is referred to as the *basal energy expenditure* or *BEE*. To be most accurate, these formulas should take into account age, sex, and body surface area.

The following *Harris and Benedict formula* (Krause and Mahan 1984, 15) gives the standard BEE for women plus a physical activity factor:

$$655 + 9.56\,(W) + 1.85(H) - 4.68(A) = BMR$$

$$BMR \times physical\ activity = total\ calories\ required\ per\ day$$

W = weight in kg. H = height in cm. A = age in years.

Physical Activity—If:

sedentary — BMR × 1.3 (or 30% additional kcal above BMR)

moderate — BMR × 1.5 (or 50% additional kcal above BMR)

active — BMR × 2.0 (or 100% additional kcal above BMR)

Example: 35-yr.-old, 5'5", 140-pound moderately active woman

$655 + (9.56 \times 64kg) + (1.85 \times 165cm) - (4.68 \times 35) =$ BMR = 1408

$1408 \times 1.5 = 2112$ *kcalories required per day*

The energy or kcalories calculated is the amount required to maintain weight. To lose one pound of weight a week, the average person needs to reduce caloric intake by 3500 kcalories or increase energy expenditure (calories used) by that much.

Table 16.12. CALORIES USED PER MINUTE OF EXERCISE

Activity	Calories Burned Weight (115 lbs.-150 lbs.)	Weight (150 lbs.-195 lbs.)
Aerobic dancing	6-7	8-9
Basketball	9-11	11-15
Bicycling	5-6	7-8
Golf	3-4	4-5
Jogging (5 mph)	9-10	12-13
Jogging (7 mph)	10-11	13-14
Rowing machine	5-6	7-8
Skiing (downhill)	8-9	10-12
Skiing (cross-country)	11-12	13-16
Swimming	5-6	7-10
Tennis (doubles)	5-7	7-8
Walking (2 mph)	2-3	3-4
Walking (4 mph)	4-5	6-7

Source: Adapted from Morgan, B., 1987. *Nutrition prescription*, p. 403. New York: Ballantine Books.

The Best Nutrition Advice

By adhering to the nutritional guidelines that follow, clients can maintain better health and reduce their chances of developing certain diseases such as heart disease, as well as high blood pressure and certain cancers.

→ Eat a variety of foods.

→ Eat a diet low in fat, saturated fat, and cholesterol.

→ Include plenty of vegetables, fruits, grain products and fiber-rich foods.

→ Consume sugars, sodium, and alcoholic beverages in moderation.

→ Maintain a healthy weight.

→ Exercise regularly.

Tables 16.13, Healthy Substitutes, and **Table 16.14, Eating Chart,** may be helpful in planning a healthy diet/menu.

Role of the Clinician

Clinicians should include nutritional services in the periodic health care of women, counseling them to improve nutrition to prevent certain chronic diseases. Basic nutritional advice should consider the dietary intake of calories, fat (especially saturated fat), cholesterol, fiber, and supplemental vitamins and minerals if indicated.

When the clinician, through basic nutritional care, detects serious nutritional problems or complex medical conditions that complicate the care, referral to a registered dietitian or other nutrition professional is required. Special nutritional care usually includes detailed assessments, complex diet modifications, dietary counseling, and close follow-up. For successful nutritional interventions to occur and for the new patterns that are set up to be maintained, additional reinforcement and follow-up must be provided by the primary care practitioner (Abrams and Berman 1993).

BASIC NUTRITIONAL CARE FOR ALL WOMEN

(Abrams and Berman 1993)

→ Assess weight-for-height status, hemoglobin or hematocrit, dietary practices, and exercise habits.

→ Based on family history, risk factors, and age, consider screening for total cholesterol and, if necessary, a more extensive fasting lipoprotein panel. (See **Hypercholesterolemia** Protocol.)

Table 16.13. HEALTHY SUBSTITUTES

Instead of	Try
Dairy Products	
Whole milk	1% or skim milk
Regular cottage cheese	Low-fat or non-fat cottage cheese
Regular cream cheese	Light cream cheese
Regular cheese	Light/reduced-fat cheese (<5gm fat/oz.)
Regular ice cream	Light ice milk, fat-free frozen yogurt, sherbet, fruit ice
Cream	Evaporated non-fat milk (undiluted) Liquid non-dairy creamer w/ polyunsaturated oil
Sour cream	Non-fat sour cream, plain low-fat yogurt
Butter	Margarine (liquid oil first ingredient listed) Olive oil
Meat, Poultry	
Chuck steak, untrimmed	Round steak, trimmed
Lean ground beef	Ground turkey
Chicken drumstick with skin	Chicken drumstick without skin
Skinless chicken breast	Skinless turkey breast
Pork chop	Pork tenderloin
Regular bacon	Canadian bacon
Beef franks	Turkey franks
Tuna in oil	Tuna in water
Whole egg	egg white or egg substitute
Regular peanut butter	Old-fashioned peanut butter
Grain/Starch/Snacks	
Cereal, sweetened	Cereal, unsweetened
French fries	Baked potato
White rice	Brown rice
Crackers	Rice cake, melba toast, Ak-Mak
Regular potato chips	Light potato chips, popcorn, pretzels
Baked goods	Fat-free baked products
Chocolate chip cookies	Fig Newtons, ginger snaps
Hot chocolate	Hot cocoa
Condiments	
Regular mayonnaise	Light or fat-free mayonnaise
Soy sauce	Low-sodium soy sauce
White sauce	Red sauce (tomato-based)
Fast Foods	
McDonald's Quarter Pounder	McDonald's McLean Deluxe
McDonald's McChicken Sandwich	Burger King BK Broiler
Burger King Vanilla Shake	McDonald's Vanilla Shake
McDonald's Blue Cheese Dressing	McDonald's Lite Vinaigrette
McDonald's Apple Danish	McDonald's Apple Bran Muffin
Burger King Croissant	Burger King Bagel
Taco Bell Double Beef Supreme	Taco Bell Chicken Fajita, Burrito
Baskin-Robbins Waffle Cone	Baskin-Robbins Plain or Sugar Cone
Kentucky Fried Thighs & Wings	Kentucky Fried Chicken Breasts
Kentucky Fried Original Recipe	Kentucky Fried Skinless Recipe
Arby's Regular Roast Beef	Arby's French Dip Roast Beef

Source: Adapted from Liebman, B. 1990. Fat savings plan, *Nutrition Action Health Letter* 17:(7).

Table 16.14. EATING CHART

Cereals, Grains and Starchy Vegetables	Fruits and Vegetables	Milk and Milk-Type Products	Meat and Meat Alternatives	Fats, Oils, Beverages, and Condiments
CHOOSE FROM				
Breads *(all varieties, preferably whole grain)* Bagels (except egg) English muffins Tortillas (corn and fat-free flour) Sourdough/French **Crackers** *(1 g or less of fat per serving)* Flatbread Matzoh Melba toast Rice/popcorn cakes **Grains/Pasta** Barley Bulgur Cereals, hot or cold, unsweetened (2 g or less of fat per serving) Cereal, instant* Couscous Pasta (not egg) Rice (plain) Quinoa **Snacks**** Angel food cake Fat-free cookies Fat-free baked goods Popcorn (plain, unsalted) Unsalted pretzels **Starchy Vegetables** Corn Green peas Lima beans Potatoes Sweet potatoes	**Fruits** Applesauce (unsweetened) Canned in own juice Dried Fresh: Apples, Melons Apricots, Nectarines Bananas, Oranges Berries, Papaya Cherries, Peaches Grapefruit, Pears Grapes, Pineapple Kiwi, Plums Mangos, Tangerines Frozen (unsweetened) Fruit juice (unsweetened) **Vegetables** *(raw, baked, boiled, or steamed, without added fat or cheese sauce):* Fresh: Artichokes, Green pepper Asparagus, Lettuce Beets, Mushrooms Broccoli, Onions Brussel sprouts, Parsnips Cabbage, Radishes Carrots, Spinach Cauliflower, Sprouts Celery, Summer squashes Collard greens, Tomatoes Cucumbers, Water chestnuts Eggplant Green beans Frozen vegetables, plain	**Cheese** *(very low in fat, 2 g or less of fat per oz.)* Cottage cheese (non-fat or low-fat) Hoop Pot Sapsago ***Dessert*** Pudding made with skim milk Fat-free dairy desserts Non-fat frozen yogurt **Milk** *(non-fat/skim, 1%, 2 g or less of fat per oz.)* Buttermilk (from skim milk) Cocoa made with skim milk Evaporated skim milk Non-fat milk Powdered milk beverage made with skim milk (except eggnog) **Yogurt** *(non-fat)* All flavors except chocolate **Condiments** Fat-free sour cream	**Fish** *(baked, microwaved, broiled, poached)* Bass Canned (water-packed tuna)* Cod, Perch Flounder, Pike Haddock, Red snapper Halibut, Sole **Lunch meat*** Low-fat varieties: *(2 g or less of fat per oz.)* **Meat** *(trim visible fat, 10% or less fat or 3 g or less of fat per oz.)* Beef (look for ROUND or LOIN cuts) Lamb (look for LEG or LOIN cuts) Pork (Canadian bacon*, CENTER CUT, ham,* LOIN) Veal (choose all cuts *except* BREAST) Wild game **Poultry** *(light meat without skin)* Chicken, Turkey Cornish hen, Turkey ham* **Protein-Rich Foods** Canned beans (drained and rinsed) Dried beans and lentils Egg substitutes (without added fat) Egg whites Tofu **Shellfish** *(not fried)* Abalone Canned (water-packed clams, crab, oysters)* Clams, Scallops Crab, Surimi (imitation shellfish) Crayfish†, Shrimp† Lobster†, Squid† Oysters	**Beverages** Herbal tea Mineral water or club soda **Condiments** Catsup* Fat-free mayonnaise Herbs and spices Hot pepper sauce Jams, jellies, preserves Lemon juice Mustard* Salad dressing, fat-free (homemade low-fat, low-salt types) Salsa Vinegar **Fats and Oils‡** Canola oil Corn oil Diet margarine or margarine with liquid as the first ingredient Olive oil Peanut oil Safflower oil Soybean oil Sunflower oil Walnut oil **Miscellaneous** Bouillon* Chestnuts Chocolate syrup Cocoa powder Frozen fudge bars Gelatin Ices Juice bars Sorbet
CHOOSE LESS OFTEN				
Breads/Crackers *(low-fat varieties)* Animal crackers Bread sticks Oyster crackers Soda crackers Tortillas with added fat **Grains/Pasta** Egg noodles	**Fruits** "Fruit" drinks **Vegetables** Canned* Pickles* Relishes* Sauerkraut* Tomato juice* Vegetable juice* Vegetable soup*	**Cheese** *(part-skim, no more than 5g fat per oz.)* Farmer's (part-skim) Low-calorie natural or processed cheese/cheese slices Light cream cheese Mozzarella (part-skim) Parmesan/Romano (2 tbsp. grated) Ricotta (part-skim) String	**Fish** Canned (water-packed salmon)* Herring (pickled)* Mackerel Salmon Trout **Meat** *(trim visible fat)* Beef (FLANK and RUMP) Lamb (RIB) Veal (BREAST)	**Beverages** Diet soft drinks Tea and coffee (without cream) **Condiments** Chocolate syrup Low-fat mayonnaise Salad dressing (most non-creamy types)* Sauces or gravies made with appropriate ingredients Soy sauce (low-sodium)*

Choose From

Homemade Baked Goods
(made with appropriate ingredients and low in fat, 5 g or less of fat per serving)
Cookies Pancakes
Muffins Waffles
Snacks**
Fig bars
Ginger snaps
Graham crackers
Low-fat/light microwave popcorn*
Vanilla wafers
Starchy Vegetables
Sweet potatoes, candied

Desserts
Ice milk or "light" ice cream
Low-fat frozen yogurt
Milk (2%)
Buttermilk (from low-fat milk)
Chocolate low-fat milk
Low-fat milk
Yogurt (low-fat)
All flavors

Poultry
Dark meat turkey and chicken
Self-basting turkey
Protein-Rich Foods
Egg substitute with cheese
Peanut butter

Fats and Oils‡
Cottonseed oil
Nuts/Seeds (unsalted)
Almonds Pistachios
Hazelnuts Sesame seeds
Peanuts Sunflower seeds
Pecans Walnuts

CHOOSE LEAST OFTEN

Breads/Crackers*
Biscuits
Croissants, scones, or other buttery rolls
Croutons
Egg bagels or egg bread
Packaged stuffing
Commercial Baked Goods*
Cakes Muffins
Cookies Sweet rolls/Pastries
Doughnuts Waffles
Grains/Pasta*
Cereals (most granola and pre-sweetened varieties)
Commercial rice and noodle mixes (macaroni & cheese, etc.)
Snacks*
Cakes
Candy (especially chocolate, peanut butter, and carob)
Cheese snacks
Chips (corn, potato, or tortilla)
Cookies
Pies
Popcorn (buttered, salted, or microwaved)*
Starchy Vegetables*
French fries
Hash browns
Potato dishes with butter, cream, or cheese
Potato salad

Fruits
Avocado or guacamole
Coconut
Vegetables*
Cole slaw
Olives
Onion rings (fried)
Any vegetable prepared as follows:
buttered
creamed
fried
in cheese sauce

Cheese (whole milk)
Blue
Brie
Cheddar
Cream cheese
Jack
Muenster
Swiss
Condiments
Blue cheese dressing
Cream
Cream sauces
Evaporated milk
Half & half
Non-dairy coffee creamer or whipped topping
Sour cream
Sour half & half
Sweetened condensed milk
Whipped cream
Desserts
Cheese cake
Custards, puddings
Ice cream
Milk (whole)
Egg nog
Extra-rich milk
Hot chocolate (regular)
Whole milk products
Soups*
Creamed varieties

Fish*
Anchovies
Canned (sardines, tuna in oil)
Caviar
Herring (creamed)
Lunch meat*
Bologna Pastrami
Bratwurst Salami
Meat
Bacon or "light" bacon*
Corned beef brisket
Dried meat (jerky)*
Domesticated game
Hamburgers
Hot dogs*
Lamb chops
Organ meats (brain, heart, liver, kidney, gizards)
Pig's feet
Polish/Italian sausage*
Pork chops
Rabbit
Salt pork*
Sausage*
Spareribs
Untrimmed red meat
Meat Alternatives*
Custards Quiches
Egg Yolks Souffles
Omelettes
Poultry
Duck Goose Fried chicken
Soup*
Chunky or creamy varieties

Condiments
Fudge toppings
Guacamole
Regular mayonnaise
Regular gravies, sauces
Salad dressings (most creamy types)
Salt, seasoned salts*
Soy sauce (regular)*
Fats and Oils‡
Bacon drippings
Butter
Cocoa butter
Coconut oil
Lard, suet
Margarine (other than these listed above)
Palm kernel oil
Palm oil
Salt pork*
Vegetable shortening
Miscellaneous
Carob
Chocolate
Nuts/Seeds (higher in saturated fats)
Brazil nuts
Cashews
Macadamia nuts
Pine nuts
Pumpkin seeds
All salted nuts and seeds*

*May be high in sodium. Read product labels to determine sodium content.

**Always check labels. Some varieties may be low in fat and some acceptable products may have fat added.

†Shrimp, crayfish, and squid are higher in cholesterol than other types of fish, but lower in fat than most meats and poultry.

‡Limit all fats and oils. When using fats and oils, select from the "Choose From" category most often.

Source: Reprinted with permission from American Heart Association (San Francisco Chapter). 1993. *Eat heart smart.* San Francisco: the Author.

→ Assess for nutritional risk factors, making recommendations for dietary change or supplementation. Refer to dietitian, social services, or substance abuse cessation program if necessary. Nutritional risk factors include:
- obesity, eating disorders, food allergies, anemia, extreme underweight, unusual or restrictive dietary patterns.
- metabolic or chronic diseases.
- substance (cigarettes, alcohol, or drugs) abuse.
- adolescence.
- limited income, education, motivation, or knowledge about food and nutrition.
- homelessness.

→ Emphasize food rather than supplements as the main source of nutrients. Encourage women to eat a daily minimum of five servings of fruits and vegetables; six servings of grains; a minimum of two low-fat, calcium-rich dairy products; and moderate amounts of protein-rich foods such as legumes, fish, poultry, and lean meats. Individualize recommendations to reflect the woman's food preferences, lifestyle, and economic situation.

→ Encourage regular physical activity or exercise.

→ Recommend vitamin/mineral supplement(s) when it is difficult or impossible for a woman to get adequate dietary intake or when nutritional risk factors (e.g., eating disorders) exist.

→ Document nutritional assessments and interventions in the progress notes and problem list.

Bibliography

Abrams, B., and Berman, C. 1993. Women, nutrition and health. *Current Problems in Obstetrics, Gynecology and Fertility* 16(1):39–41.

American Dietetic Association. 1992. Eating well—the vegetarian way. Chicago: the Author.

———. Nov. 1993. Vegetarian diets. *Journal of the American Dietetic Association* 93(11):1317–1318.

———. Dec. 1993. Health implications of dietary fiber. *Journal of the American Dietetic Association*: 1446.

American Heart Association. 1993. *Cholesterol and your heart*. Dallas, TX: the Author.

American Heart Association, San Francisco Chapter. 1993. *Eat heart smart*. San Francisco: the Author.

Brody, J. 1981. *Jane Brody's nutrition book*, pp. 49–50. New York: W.W. Norton.

California Department of Health Services. 1990. *Nutrition during pregnancy and the post-partum period: A manual for health care professionals*. Sacramento, CA: Maternal and Child Health Branch, WIC Supplemental Food Branch.

Center for Science in the Public Interest. Nov. 1993. The great trans wreck. *Nutrition Action Health Letter.* 20(9):10.

———. Dec. 1993. These feet were made for walking. *Nutrition Action Health Letter.* 20(10):11.

Davis, R. 1989. Calcium absorption. *American Journal of Clinical Nutrition.* 49:372.

Hurley, J. 1990. Rough it up. *Nutrition Action Health Letter* 17(2):8–9.

Krause, M.V., and Mahan, L.K. 1984. Food, nutrition, and diet therapy, 7th ed., p. 15. Philadelphia: W.B. Saunders.

Liebman, B. 1989. Cutting cholesterol. *Nutrition Action Health Letter* 16(7):5.

———. 1990. CSPI's Fat Savings Plan. *Nutrition Action Health Letter* 17(7).

Metropolitan Life Insurance Company. 1983. *1983 Metropolitan height/weight tables*. New York: the Author.

Morgan, B. 1987. *Nutrition prescription*. New York: Ballantine Books.

National Academy of Sciences, National Research Council. 1989. *Recommended Dietary Allowances*, 10th ed. Washington, DC: National Academy Press.

Owen, A. 1989. *Fiber in your diet*. New York: Healthteam Interactive Communications.

Pennington, J. 1989. *Bowes & Church's food values of portions commonly used*, 15th ed. Philadelphia: J.B. Lippincott.

Shils, M., and Young, V. 1988. Modern nutrition in health and disease, 7th ed. Philadelphia: Lea and Fiebiger.

Spence, W.R. 1990. *Cholesterol—Keeping your heart healthy*. Waco, TX: Health Edco.

U.S. Department of Agriculture Human Nutrition Information Service. 1992. *The food guide pyramid*. Hyattsville, MD: the Author.